DC Dutta's

Textbook of Gynecology

including Contraception

ONLINE VIDEO CONTENT LIST

- Total Abdominal Hysterectomy with Bilateral Salpingo-oophorectomy
- Vaginal Hysterectomy
- Diagnostic Laparoscopy with Chromopertubation
- Laparoscopic Ovarian Cystectomy

OTHER BOOKS BY THE SAME AUTHOR

- Textbook of Obstetrics
- Bedside Clinics & Viva-Voce in Obstetrics and Gynecology
- Manual of Obstetrics and Gynecology for the Postgraduates
- A Guide to Clinical Obstetrics and Gynecology
- Emergencies in Manipulative and Operative Obstetrics

DC Dutta's

Textbook of Gynecology including Contraception

Eighth Edition

DC Dutta MBBS DGO MO (Cal)
Professor and Head, Department of Obstetrics and Gynecology
Nilratan Sircar Medical College and Hospital, Kolkata, India

Edited by

Hiralal Konar (Hons; Gold Medalist)
MBBS (Cal) MD (PGI) DNB (India)
MNAMS FACS (USA) FRCOG (London)
FOGSI Representative to Asia Oceania Federation of Obstetricians and Gynecologists (AOFOG)
Member, Oncology Committee of AOFOG
Professor and Head, Department of Obstetrics and Gynecology
Agartala Govt. Medical College and G B Pant Hospital, Tripura, India
Chairman, Indian College of Obstetricians and Gynecologists (2013)
Formerly Professor, Department of Obstetrics and Gynecology
Calcutta National Medical College and Hospital, Kolkata
One-time Professor and Head, Department of Obstetrics and Gynecology
Midnapore Medical College and Hospital, West Bengal University of Health Sciences, Kolkata, India
Rotation Registrar in Obstetrics, Gynecology and Oncology
Northern and Yorkshire Region, Newcastle-upon-Tyne, UK
Examiner-National: MBBS, DGO, MD and PhD of different Indian Universities
and National Board of Examination, New Delhi, India
International: Royal College of Obstetricians and Gynaecologists, (MRCOG), London,
Royal College of Physicians of Ireland (MRCPI)
Recipient, "Pride of FOGSI" award – 2019, for exemplary efforts toward upliftment of Women's Health in India

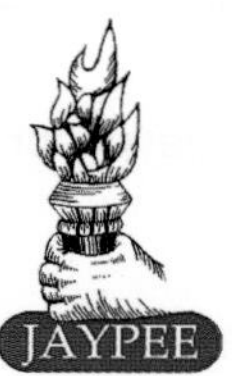

JAYPEE BROTHERS MEDICAL PUBLISHERS
The Health Sciences Publisher
New Delhi | London

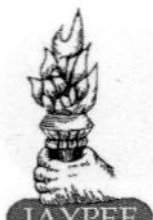

Jaypee Brothers Medical Publishers (P) Ltd

Headquarters

Jaypee Brothers Medical Publishers (P) Ltd
4838/24, Ansari Road, Daryaganj
New Delhi 110 002, India
Phone: +91-11-43574357
Fax: +91-11-43574314
Email: jaypee@jaypeebrothers.com

Overseas Office

J.P. Medical Ltd
83 Victoria Street, London
SW1H 0HW (UK)
Phone: +44 20 3170 8910
Fax: +44 (0)20 3008 6180
Email: info@jpmedpub.com

Website: www.jaypeebrothers.com
Website: www.jaypeedigital.com

Medical knowledge and practice change constantly. This book is designed to provide accurate, authoritative information about the subject matter in question. However, readers are advised to check the most current information available on procedures included and check information from the manufacturer of each product to be administered, to verify the recommended dose, formula, method and duration of administration, adverse effects and contraindications. It is the responsibility of the practitioner to take all appropriate safety precautions. Neither the publisher nor the author(s)/editor(s) assume any liability for any injury and/or damage to persons or property arising from or related to use of material in this book.

Inquiries for bulk sales may be solicited at: jaypee@jaypeebrothers.com

DC Dutta's Textbook of Gynecology
Seventh Edition: 2016
Eihth Edition: 2020
Reprint: ***2023***
ISBN: 978-93-89587-88-3
Printed at: Samrat Offset Pvt. Ltd.

Dedicated to

The students of gynecology—
past and present

Preface to the Eighth Edition

***Dutta's Textbook of Gynecology* has stepped in its 8th edition through its journey over the last 31 years.** Its first edition was in photo-type setting in 1989 with 450 pages. Concept was to provide students with the knowledge of "Medical Gynecology" as maternity care was the need of those days. The contribution of this great teacher to the medical fraternity was monumental. This provided a huge impetus to the successors to follow his footsteps. Significant development has been observed in each edition of this book concurrent to the progress of science, technology and imaging. This textbook has now been considered the classic in the field both nationally and internationally. The advances observed in all the areas of subspeciality like: reproductive endocrinology, infertility, urogynecology, oncology, endoscopy and general gynecology are adequately reflected in this edition. Consistency and uniformity with updated information in all the chapters are the special features of this book.

Dutta's Gynecology is comprehensive and user friendly with its easy-to-read format. The presentation of this book with its quality of graphics, design, profuse illustrations (366), high quality photographs (330) and imaging studies are the special attraction. Numerous tables, boxes, flowcharts, and algorithms are there, for ease of study and reproducibility. The key points are at the end of each chapter to provide an outline synopsis of the entire chapter. This is of value for quick and easy revision. **The state-of-the-art in the book lies in the presentation** which is simple, lucid, clear and concise. Above all, it provides a balanced distillation of evidence-based information upon which a student, trainee resident, a practitioner and a nurse can fully depend.

All the chapters have been exhaustively revised, updated and many of these thoroughly rewritten. **Practical gynecology (Chapter 38), contains a total of 107 high quality photographs and plates of imaging studies.** Few hundreds of viva questions along with answers and explanations are presented to enable the students to face the clinical and viva voce part of examination. **The total information given in Chapter 38 amounts to a "mini-textbook-cum color atlas" of gynecology.**

Considering the vast amount of scientific information and the research, it is practically impossible to limit the subject matter within the few pages of the book. Arrangements have been made through electronic media for the readers who wish to know more. Information regarding the examination situation (theory, viva voce, multiple choice questions and answers, operation video clips) have been provided through the electronic resources (www.dcdutta.com/www.hiralalkonar.com).

My aim in this book has always been to help the students, residents and clinicians to remain updated with the knowledge that has passed the test of clinical relevance. I do hope this comprehensive textbook will continue to be an immense educational source to readers as ever. The readers will enjoy this edition and learn as much as they can in this ever-evolving field, in order to provide a quality care to women.

According to the author's desire, the book is therefore dedicated once again ***"to the students of gynecology: past and present"***.

Hiralal Konar

h.kondr@gmail.com
P–13, New CIT Road
Kolkata–700014

Preface to the First Edition

Since my publication of Textbook of Obstetrics about 5 years back, I have been pressed hard by my esteemed colleagues and the students all over the country and abroad to write a Textbook on Gynecology of similar style to fill up the deficit. Initially, I was hesitant to proceed with the stupendous task but considering the fact that a compact, comprehensive and practical-oriented fundamental book in gynecology is not available to the undergraduates, I have decided to comply with their request.

The book has been written in a lucid language in author's own style. Extensive diagrams, photographs, and flowcharts (schemes) have been depicted throughout the text to give clarity of the subject. Due attention has been paid to project the fundamental principles and practice of gynecology. As such, more emphasis has been given on medical gynecology. But for that, indications, limitations, and principles of techniques of operations have received adequate consideration. The book is thus made invaluable not only to the medical students but also the practising physicians and students of nursing.

The author wishes to acknowledge gratitude to his esteemed colleague Dr N Chowdhury, MBBS, DGO, MO (Cal), for his contribution to the topic "Hormone Therapy in Gynecological practice". Dr Santosh Kr Paul, MBBS, DGO, MO(Cal), Prof, Dept of Obst and Gyne, NRS Medical College, Calcutta, deserves full appreciation for his contribution in a lucid way to the topic "Radiotherapy and Chemotherapy in Gynecology". The author has much pleasure in expressing grateful thanks to Dr BN Chakravorty, MBBS, DGO, MO (Cal), FRCOG (Eng), and Dr KM Gun, MBBS, DGO, MO (Cal), FRCOG (Eng), FRCS (Edin), FACS (USA), for their valued suggestions as and when required and their contribution of photographs to enrich the text. I gratefully record my thanks to Dr Subir Kumar Dutta, MBBS, DCP, MD (Path & Bact), Prof, Dept of Pathology and Bacteriology, University College of Medicine, Calcutta, for the microphotographs depicted throughout the text. The author records his thanks to Dr SM Dali Prof, Obst and Gyne; Dr Bhola Rijal, Associate Prof, Obst and Gyne of Teaching Hospital, and Dr (Mrs) Dibya S Malia, Director, Maternity Hospital, Kathmandu, Nepal, for their contribution of few outstanding photographs to enrich the text.

The author expresses much pleasure all the time to the House Surgeons, Internees and students of Nilratan Sircar Medical College, Calcutta, for the help they have rendered in preparation of the final drafts of the manuscripts, check up of the proofs and compiling the index. Their help is invaluable and unforgettable and without which the book could never have been published.

The author wishes to thank Mr Biren Das for his exhaustive number of drawings and flowcharts which enrich the lucidity of the book. The author also thanks Mr Ranjit Sen for preparation of photographs (black and white) depicted throughout the text. The author has much pleasure in expressing his appreciation to Mr Bimal Bhattacharya, MSc, LLB (Cal), DSW, DHE, Lecturer, Health Education and Family Welfare, Postpartum Unit, NRS Medical College, Calcutta for the patience shown in dealing with correction of manuscripts and proofs.

In preparing the textbook, the author has utilized the knowledge of number of stalwarts in his profession and consulted many books and publications. The author wishes to express his appreciation and gratitude to all of them including the related authors and publishers.

The author still confesses that as a teacher, he has learnt a lot from the students and more so while writing this book and as such he could not think to dedicate the book to anyone else than the ***students of gynecology—past and present***.

DC Dutta

Acknowledgments

A textbook of this standard could never be completed without the help and advice of many. The editor thanks many distinguished persons for their support in updating the book. I have consulted many outstanding teachers in the profession, multitude of eminent authors and many current evidence-based studies. The legacy is gratefully acknowledged. I express my sincere thanks to many of my esteemed colleagues throughout the country and abroad for their valued suggestions and criticisms. I sincerely acknowledge the support of all the students (undergraduates and postgraduates) of different medical institutions in the country for their opinions and criticisms that have helped to enrich this book. As before, I welcome the views of students and teachers who regularly write to me, offering their suggestions and ideas on email: *h.kondr@gmail.com*.

At the outset, I am indebted wholeheartedly for the support provided by the *Department of Health and Family Welfare, Government of Tripura: Prof Chinmoy Biswas, Director of Medical Education; Prof Kamal Krishna Kundu, Principal, and Dr Ranjit Kumar Das, Medical Superintendent-cum-Vice-Principal, AGMC, Tripura.*

I am specially grateful to Dr KM Gun, MD, FRCOG, FRCS, Prof (Late); Dr BN Chakravorty, MD, FRCOG, DSc, Prof (Rtd), Director, Institute of Reproductive Medicine, Kolkata for the contributions on the topics; Neuroendocrinology in Relation to Reproduction (Chapter 7); Infertility (Chapter 17); Disorders of Sexual Development (Chapter 28); Amenorrhea (Chapter 29) and Hormones in Gynecological Practice (Chapter 32). Thanks are due to Dr A Mazumder, MD, Prof for his support in revising the chapter—Basic Principles of Radiation Therapy, Chemotherapy, Immunotherapy and Gene Therapy in Gynecology (Chapter 31). The editor sincerely thanks Dr Subir K Dutta, MD, Prof (Pathology) for the microphotographs depicted in the text.

I sincerely acknowledge the following teachers across the country and abroad for their valuable feedback for Dutta's books. Their comments and suggestions have helped to shape this new edition. I hope I have listed all those who have contributed and apologize if any name has been accidentally omitted.

My sincere thanks are due to Sir Prof Sabaratnam Arulkumaran, Emeritus Prof, St George's University of London, President FIGO (Past); Prof Lesley Regan, President, RCOG; Mr Michael O'Connel, Royal College of Physicians, Dublin; Prof PS Chakraborty, IPGMER, Kolkata; Prof P Mukherjee, Calcutta MCH; Prof C Das, NRSMCH; Prof A Majhi, RG Kar MC, Kolkata; Prof S Pati, CNMC, Kolkata; Prof PK Biswas and Dr Aftabuddin Mondal, CNMCH; Prof Picklu Choudhury, Rampurhat Medical College, West Bengal; Dr Annie Regi, CMC, Vellore; Prof KK Ray and Dr Neerja Bhatla, AIIMS, New Delhi; Prof V Das, KGMC, Lucknow; Prof RL Singh, RIMS, Imphal; Prof Subroto Ponda, NEGRIMS, Shillong; Prof Kavita Singh, NSCBMC, Jabalpur; Prof V Das, PGIMER, Chandigarh; Prof NR Agarwal and Prof Uma Pandey, Banaras Hindu University, Banaras; Prof Abha Rani Sinha, Muzaffarpur, Bihar; Prof Hemali Sinha, AIIMS, Patna; Prof K Pandey, GSVM MCH, Kanpur; Prof Hemant Deshpande and Prof Himadri Bal, Dr DY Patil MCH, Pune; Prof Pranay Phukan, Dibrugarh; Prof R Talukdar and Prof Saswati Sanyal Choudhry, Guwahati; Prof S Dutta, NBMCH, Siliguri; Prof M Sarkar and Dr Santyandra Manna, MMCH, Malda; Prof N Jana and Dr Arindam Halder, CRSS, Kolkata; Prof J Mukherjee, Kishanganj MCH, Bihar; Prof Hafizur Rahman, Gangtok; Prof DK Bhowmik, TMCH, Tripura; Prof Anindya Kumar Das, Bankura; Prof Chandra Kiran, PMCH, Patna; Prof Farhana Dewan and Prof Kohinoor Begum, Dhaka; Prof Rokeya Begum, Chittagong; Prof Rowshan Ara Begum and Prof Sabera Khatun, Dhaka; Prof Jyoti Bindal, GRMC, Gwalior; Prof Seema Hakim, AMU, Aligarh; Prof Beena Bhatnagar, NIMS, Jaipur; Prof Manpreet Kaur, DMC, Ludhiana; Prof MB Bellad, Belagavi; Prof Ajith, Kannur; Prof Malik Goonewardene, University of Ruhuna, Sri Lanka; Prof HR Seneviratne, Colombo, Sri Lanka; Prof Pratap Kumar, KMC, Manipal; Prof Nilesh Dalal, MGMC, Indore; Prof Sudesh Agarwal, SPMC, Bikaner; Prof Pushpa Dahiya, Rohtak, PIMS; Prof Mary Daniel, PIMS, Puducherry; Prof Sasikala, SMVMCH, Puducherry; Prof Atiya Sayed, AIIMS, J&K; Prof N Chaudhury, HIMS, Dehradun; Prof S Nanda, PGI, Rohtak; Prof N Chutani and Prof SS Gulati, SMC, Greater Noida; Prof Raksha Arora, SMC, Ghaziabad; Prof Jaya Chaturvedi, AIIMS, Rishikesh; Prof Abha Singh, JNMCH, Raipur; Prof Rehana Nazam, TMU, Moradabad; Prof Bharati Misra, MKCG, Berhampur; Prof Neelam Pradhan and Prof Meeta Singh, Tribhuvan University Teaching Hospital (TU & TH), Kathmandu; Prof Sujatha Sharma, GMC, Amritsar; Prof Promila Jindal; PIMS, Jalandhar; Prof R Shahnaz Taing, Government MCH, Srinagar; Prof Surinder Kumar, Government MCH, Jammu; Prof Alka Sehgal, Government MCH, Chandigarh; Prof Arun H Nayak, LTMG MCH, Mumbai; Prof Ashok Anand, Grant MCH, Mumbai; Prof B Sarala, Osmania MCH, Hyderabad; Prof D Rajyalakshmi, Rangaraya MCH, Hyderabad; Prof J Fidvi, GMC, Nagpur; Prof Chellamma, KMCT MCH, Kozhikode; Prof Nirmala, Govt MCH Thiruvananthapuram, Prof Chandrika, Govt MCH, Palakkad; Prof Abha Singh, LHMC, Delhi; Prof Asmita Rathore, Maulana Azad MCH, Delhi; Prof Vinita Das, KGMC, Lucknow; Prof Nisha Rani Agrawal, BHU, Banaras; Prof Geeta, GMC, Haldwani; Prof N Palaniappan, SRMC, Chennai; Prof Sujatha, JSS MCH, Mysuru; Prof Ravi Gowda, JJM MCH, Davangere; Prof Girija MK, BR Ambedkar MCH, Bengaluru; Prof Dharma Vijay, MVJ MCH, Bengaluru; Prof Rajini Uday, MS Ramaiah MCH, Bengaluru; Prof Dhanjaya, Sri Siddartha MCH, Tumakuru; Prof Savitha C, Bangalore MCH & Research Institute, Bengaluru; Prof Shridhar Venkatesh, Vydehi Institute of Medical Sciences, Bengaluru;

Prof Kamal P Patil, JN MCH, Belagavi; Prof MM Umadi, BIMS, Belagavi; Prof Asha Neravi, SDM Institute of Medical Sciences, Dharwad; Prof Vidya A Thobbi, Al-Ameen MCH, Vijayapura; Prof Muralidhar Pai, Kasturba MCH, Manipal; Prof PA Uikey, IGGMC, Nagpur; Prof Sarita Agrawal, AIIMS, Raipur; Prof K Pushpalatha, AIIMS, Bhopal; Prof Rekha Sapkal, Peoples MCH, Bhopal; Prof Aruna Kumar, GMC, Bhopal; Prof Nilufar Sultana, Dhaka MCH, Dhaka; Prof Fatema Ashraf, Shaheed Suhrawardy MCH, Nepal; Prof Bekha Mana, Institute of Medicine, Nepal; Prof Kavita, Government MCH, Ludhiana; Prof Alauddin and Prof S Choudhury, Midnapore MCH; Prof Soubhagya Kr Jena, AIIMS, Bhubaneswar; Prof Meenakshi Chauhan, IPGMER, Rhotak; Prof B Sil and Dr Chatterjee, Murshidabad MCH, WB; Prof Sunesh Kumar, AIIMS, Delhi; Prof Tusar Kar, SCB MCH, Cuttack; Prof Apurva Bhattacharya, JORHAT MCH, Assam; Prof Manidip Pal, Kalyani MCH, WB; Prof P Sengupta, BMCH, Bardhaman, and Prof N Arora, ESI MCH, Joka, Kolkata; Prof Panchanan Das, Tezpur MCH and Dr Monidipa Roy, Barpeta, MCH, Assam.

I am specially indebted to my esteemed colleagues, the beloved residents of the Dept. of Obst & Gyne and the faculties of the Dept of Radiology, AGMC, Agartala, Tripura, India for their all round support to enrich this edition.

I would like to extend my thanks to the readers, including the residents and students, who have contacted me with suggestions and seeking clarifications through e-mails. Their inputs have been invaluable and much appreciated. I wish I could mention their names individually.

I am grateful to many colleagues, who have generously provided few of the illustrations and photographs. They are duly acknowledged.

I sincerely thank Dr A Ray, Professor (Rtd) for his professional guidance and suggestions. I am extremely grateful to Mrs Madhusri Konar, MA, BEd for all her insightful secretarial accomplishments in support of the book through eight edition.

I gratefully acknowledge the help of especially Shri Jitendar P Vij (Group Chairman), Mr Ankit Vij (Managing Director), Mr MS Mani (Group President), Dr Madhu Choudhary (Publishing Head–Education), Ms Pooja Bhandari (Production Head), Ms Sunita Katla (Executive Assistant to Group Chairman and Publishing Manager), Mr Rajesh Sharma (Production Coordinator) of Jaypee Brothers Medical Publishers (P) Ltd, New Delhi for their all-round support as and when needed.

I wish to thank Ms Seema Dogra (Cover Visualizer), Mr Ajeet Rathore (Typesetter), Ms Geeta Rani and Mr Laxmidhar Padhiary (Proofreaders) and Mr Ankush Sharma (Graphic Designer), who worked in this project.

Dr Madhu Choudhary (Publishing Head–Education) needs special appreciation for her endless support and expertise in shaping and collation to bring out this enlarged and eighth edition.

I acknowledge the support of MD Jakir Hossain, who diligently and expertly worked with me to accomplish the final phase of the eighth edition of this book.

Lastly, I am grateful to all who have taught me, most of all the patients and my beloved students.

I do hope this comprehensive Dutta's Textbook of Gynecology will continue to be an essential educational resource to the readers as ever.

Hiralal Konar

Contents

Abbreviations

ACOG	American College of Obstetricians and Gynecologists
ACTH	Adrenocorticotropic Hormone
ADD	Androstenedione
AFS	American Fertility Society
AGC	Atypical Glandular Cells
AH	Assisted Hatching
AI	Anal Incontinence
AID	Artificial Insemination Donor
AIDS	Acquired Immunodeficiency Syndrome
AIS	Adenocarcinoma In Situ
AMH	Anti-Müllerian Hormone
ART	Assisted Reproductive Technology
ASC-US	Atypical Squamous Cells of Undetermined Significance
ASRM	American Society of Reproductive Medicine
AUB	Abnormal Uterine Bleeding
BMD	Bone Mineral Density
BMI	Body Mass Index
BOC	Breast Ovarian Cancer
BSE	Breast Self-examination
BUN	Blood Urea Nitrogen
BV	Bacterial Vaginosis
CAD	Coronary Artery Disease
CAM	Complementary and Alternative Medicine
CBE	Clinical Breast Examination
CC	Clomiphene Citrate
CCNS	Cell Cycle Nonspecific Agents
CDC	Center for Disease Control and Prevention
CEA	Carcinoma Embryonic Antigen
CECT	Contrast Enhanced Computed Tomography
CEE	Conjugated Equine Estrogen
CGIN	Cervical Glandular Intraepithelial Neoplasia
CIN	Cervical Intraepithelial Neoplasia
CIS	Carcinoma In Situ
CNB	Core Needle Biopsy
COCS	Combined Oral Contraceptives
COS	Controlled Ovarian Stimulation
COX	Cyclooxygenase
CPT	Complete Perineal Tear
CRH	Corticotropin Releasing Hormone
CTU	Computed Tomography Urogram
CUSA	Cavitational Ultrascan and Surgical Aspiration
D&C	Dilatation and Curettage
DES	Diethylstilbestrol
DEXA	Dual-energy X-ray Absorptiometry
DMPA	Depot Medroxyprogesterone Acetate
DO	Detrusor Overactivity
DSD	Disorders of Sexual Development
DUB	Dysfunctional Uterine Bleeding
EAS	External Anal Sphincter
EB	Endometrial Biopsy
EBRT	External Beam Radiation Therapy
ECC	Endocervical Curettage
EIN	Endometrial Intraepithelial Neoplasia
EMI	Endometrial-myometrial Interface
FDG	18F-fluoro-2 deoxyglucose
FIGO	International Federation of Gynecology and Obstetrics
FNAC	Fine-needle Aspiration Cytology
FRAX	Fracture Risk Assessment Tool
FSH	Follicle-stimulating Hormone
GABA	γ-aminobutyric Acid
GHRH	Growth Hormone-releasing Hormone
GIFT	Gamete Intrafallopian Transfer
GnRH	Gonadotropin Releasing Hormone
GSI	Genuine Stress Incontinence
GTD	Gestational Trophoblastic Disease
GTN	Gestational Trophoblastic Neoplasia
GTT	Glucose Tolerance Test
HAART	Highly Active Antiretroviral Therapy
HAIR-AN	Hyperandrogenism Insulin Resistance-Acanthosis Nigricans
HGSOC	High Grade Serous Ovarian Carcinoma
HIV	Human Immunodeficiency Virus
HMB	Heavy Menstrual Bleeding
HMG	Human Menopausal Gonadotropins
HNPCC	Hereditary Nonpolyposis Colorectal Cancer
HPO	Hypothalamic-pituitary-ovarian
HPV	Human Papilloma Virus
HR HPV	High-risk Human Papilloma Virus
HSDD	Hypoactive Sexual Desire Disorder
HSG	Hysterosalpingography
HSIL	High-grade Squamous Intraepithelial Lesion
HSV	Herpes Simplex Virus
HT	Hormone Therapy
IAS	Internal Anal Sphincter
ICSI	Intracytoplasmic Sperm Injection
ICS	International Continence Society
IGF-BP	Insulin-like Growth Factor-binding Protein
IGF	Insulin-like Growth Factor
IMRT	Intensity Modulated Radiation Therapy
IR	Insulin Resistance
ISSVD	International Society for the Study of Vulvovaginal Diseases
IUCD	Intrauterine Contraceptive Device
IUD	Intrauterine Device
IUI	Intrauterine Insemination

IVD	Intravenous Drug Abuser
IVF-ET	In Vitro Fertilization and Embryo Transfer
IVM	In Vitro Maturation
IVP	Intravenous Pyelogram
IVU	Intravenous Urography
JZ	Junctional Zone
LAM	Lactional Amenorrhea Method
LAM	Lymphangioleiomyomatosis
LARC	Long Acting Reversible Contraceptive
LAVH	Laparoscopically Assisted Vaginal Hysterectomy
LBC	Liquid-based Cytology
LH	Luteinizing Hormone
LHRH	Luteinizing Hormone Releasing Hormone
LMS	Leiomyosarcoma
LNG-IUS	Levonorgestrel Intrauterine System
LOD	Laparoscopic Ovarian Drilling
LPD	Luteal Phase Defect
LRHPV	Low-risk Human Papillomavirus
LSIL	Low-grade Squamous Intraepithelial Lesion
LUF	Luteinized Unruptured Follicle
LUNA	Laparoscopic Uterine Nerve Ablation
MAS	Minimally Access Surgery
MCP-1	Monocyte Chemotactic Protein-1
MDCT	Multidetector Computed Tomography
MESA	Microsurgical Epididymal Sperm Aspiration
MGY	Mammography
MI	Maturation Index
MIS	Minimally Invasive Surgery
MMMT	Malignant Mixed Müllerian Tumors
MRgFUS	Magnetic Resonance Guided Focused Ultrasound
MRI	Magnetic Resonance Imaging
MRKH	Mayer-Rokitansky-Küster-Hauser
MRSA	Methicillin-Resistant *Staphylococcus Aureus*
MSH	Melanocyte Stimulating Hormone
NAAT	Nucleic Acid Amplication Testing
NACT	Neoadjuvant Chemotherapy
NNRTI	Non-nucleoside Reverse Transcriptase Inhibitors
NRTI	Nucleoside Reverse Transcriptase Inhibitors
NSAIDS	Nonsteroidal Anti-inflammatory Drugs
NSV	No Scalpel Vasectomy
OAB	Overactive Bladder
OER	Oxygen Enhancement Ratio
OGN	Oestrogen
OHSS	Ovarian Hyperstimulation Syndrome
OMI	Oocyte Maturation Inhibition
PAF	Platelet Activating Factor
PALM-COEIN	Polyps, Adenomyosis, Leiomyoma, Malignancy-Coagulopathy, Ovulatory Disorders, Endometrial Causes, Iatrogenic, Not Classified
PBS	Painful Bladder Syndrome
PCOS	Polycystic Ovarian Syndrome
PCT	Postcoital Test
PDGF	Platelet Derived Growth Factor
PDT	Photodynamic Therapy
PESA	Percutaneous Epididymal Sperm Aspiration
PET	Positron Emission Tomography
PGD	Preimplantation Genetic Diagnosis
PGN	Progesterone
PID	Pelvic Inflammatory Disease
PMDD	Premenstrual Dysphoric Disorder
PMS	Premenstrual Syndrome
POD	Pouch of Douglas
POP-Q	Pelvic Organ Prolapse-Quantification
POP	Pelvic Organ Prolapse
POST	Peritoneal Oocyte and Sperm Transfer
PSI	Prostaglandin Synthetase Inhibitors
PTH	Parathyroid Hormone
RAIR	Rectoanal Inhibitory Reflex
RANZCOG	Royal Australian and New Zealand College of Obstetricians and Gynecologists
RNTCP	Revised National Tuberculosis Control Program
RU 486	Mifepristone
RVF	Rectovaginal Fistula
RVS	Rectovaginal Septum
SCCA	Squamous Cell Carcinoma Antigen
SCJ	Squamocolumnar Junction
SCMCT	Sperm Cervical Mucus Contact Test
SDs	Standard Deviations
SERMs	Selective Estrogen Receptor Modulators
SHBG	Sex Hormone Binding Globulin
SIS	Saline Infusion Sonography
SLN	Sentinel Lymph Node
SSI	Surgical Site Infections
SSRI	Selective Serotonin Reuptake Inhibitors
STD	Sexually Transmitted Disease
STIC	Serous Tubal Intraepithelial Carcinoma
SUI	Stress Urinary Incontinence
SUZI	Subzonal Insemination
TAS	Transabdominal Sonography
TDF	Testicular Determining Factor
TENS	Transcutaneous Electrical Nerve Stimulation
TESE	Testicular Sperm Extraction
TO Mass	Tubo-ovarian Mass
TOT	Trans Obturator Tape
TPHA	Treponema Pallidum Hemagglutination
TPI	Treponema Pallidum Immobilization
TPJ	Tubal Peritoneal Junction
TV-CDS	Transvaginal Color Doppler Sonography
TVS	Transvaginal Sonography
TVT	Tension-free Vaginal Tape
TZ	Transformation Zone
UAE	Uterine Artery Embolization
UTI	Urinary Tract Infections
VAIN	Vaginal Intraepithelial Neoplasia
VCU	Videocystourethrography
VIN	Vulvar Intraepithelial Neoplasia
VVF	Vesicovaginal Fistula
WHO	World Health Organization
ZIFT	Zygote Intrafallopian Transfer

CHAPTER

1 Anatomy of the Female Pelvic Organs

CHAPTER OUTLINE

- External Genital Organs
- Internal Genital Organs
  - Vagina
  - Uterus
  - Fallopian Tube
  - Ovary
  - Female Urethra
- Other Internal Organs
  - Urinary Bladder
  - Pelvic Ureter
  - Rectum
  - Anal Canal
- Pelvic Muscles
- Perineum
- Pelvic Fascia and Cellular Tissue
- Ligaments

EXTERNAL GENITAL ORGANS (SYN: VULVA, PUDENDUM)

The vulva includes mons veneris, labia majora, labia minora, clitoris, vestibule and conventionally the perineum. These are all visible on external examination. It is, therefore, bounded anteriorly by the mons veneris, laterally by the labia majora and posteriorly by the perineum (Fig. 1.1).

MONS VENERIS (MONS PUBIS)

It is the pad of subcutaneous adipose connective tissue lying in front of the pubis and, in the adult female, is covered by hair.

LABIA MAJORA

The vulva is bounded on each side by the elevation of skin and subcutaneous tissue, which form the labia majora. They are continuous where they join medially to form the posterior commissure in front of the anus. The inner surface of the labia majora are hairless. The labia majora are covered with squamous epithelium and contain sebaceous glands, sweat glands and hair follicles. Beneath the skin, there are dense connective tissue and adipose tissue. The adipose tissue is richly supplied by venous plexus, which may produce hematoma, if injured during childbirth. **The labia majora are homologous with the scrotum in the male**. The round ligaments terminate at its anterior third.

LABIA MINORA

Labia minora are two thick folds of skin, devoid of fat, on either side just within the labia majora. Except in the parous women, they are only exposed when the labia majora are separated. Anteriorly, they are divided to enclose the clitoris and unite with each other in front and behind the clitoris to form the prepuce and frenulum, respectively. The lower portion of the labia minora fuses across the midline to form a fold of skin known as fourchette. It is usually injured during childbirth. **Between the fourchette and the vaginal orifice is the fossa navicularis. The labia minora do not contain hair follicle**. The folds contain connective tissues, numerous sebaceous glands, erectile muscle fibers and numerous vessels and nerve endings. **It is homologous to the ventral aspect of the penis**.

CLITORIS

Clitoris is a small cylindrical erectile body, measuring about 2.5 cm situated in the most anterior part of the vulva. It consists of glans, a body and two crura. The glans is covered by squamous epithelium and is richly supplied with nerves. The vessels of the clitoris are connected with the vestibular bulb and are liable to be injured during childbirth. **Clitoris is an analog to the penis in the male**, but it differs basically in being entirely separate from the urethra. It is attached to the undersurface of the symphysis pubis by the suspensory ligament.

VESTIBULE

Vestibule is a triangular space bounded anteriorly by the clitoris, posteriorly by the fourchette and on either side by labium minus. **There are four openings into the vestibule (Fig. 1.1)**.

Urethral Opening

The opening is situated in the midline, just in front of the vaginal orifice about 1–1.5 cm below the pubic arch. The paraurethral ducts open either on the posterior wall of the urethral orifice or directly into the vestibule.

Vaginal Orifice and Hymen

The vaginal orifice lies in the posterior end of the vestibule and is of varying size and shape. In virgins and nulliparae, the opening is closed by the labia minora but in parous, it may be exposed. It is incompletely closed by a septum of mucous membrane, called hymen. The membrane varies in shape but is usually circular or crescentic in virgins. The hymen is usually ruptured at the consummation of marriage. During childbirth, the hymen is extremely lacerated and is later represented by cicatrized nodules

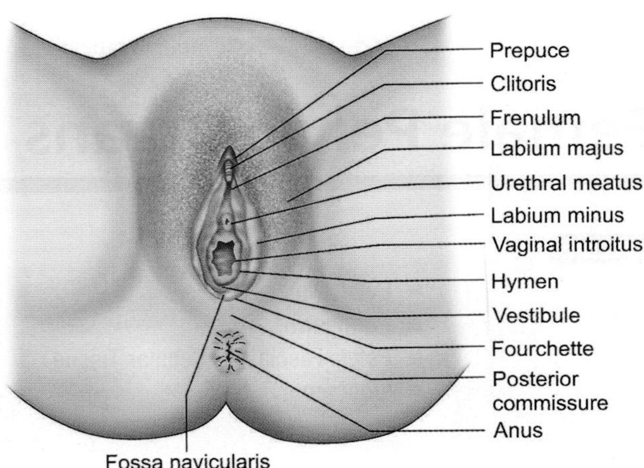

Fig. 1.1: The virginal vulva (external genitalia).

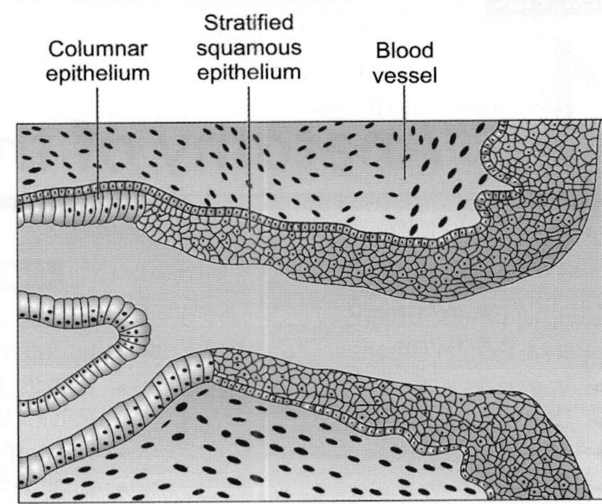

Fig. 1.2: Mucous lining of Bartholin's duct.

of varying sizes, called the **caruncülae myrtiformes.** On both sides, it is lined by stratified squamous epithelium.

BARTHOLIN'S GLAND

The Bartholin's glands are situated in the superficial perineal pouch, close to the posterior end of the vestibular bulb. They are pea-sized, of about 0.5 cm and yellowish-white in color. During sexual excitement, it secretes abundant alkaline mucus which helps in lubrication. Contraction of bulbocavernosus helps squeeze the secretion. The glands are compound racemose variety and are lined by columnar epithelium. **Each gland has got a duct which measures about 2 cm** and opens into the vestibule, outside the hymen at the junction of the anterior two-thirds and posterior one-third in the groove between the hymen and the labium minus. **The duct is lined by columnar epithelium but near its opening by stratified squamous epithelium** (Fig. 1.2). **The Bartholin's gland corresponds to the bulbourethral gland of male.**

Vestibular Bulbs

These are bilateral elongated masses of erectile tissues situated beneath the mucous membrane of the vestibule. Each bulb lies on either side of the vaginal orifice in front of the Bartholin's gland and is incorporated within the bulbocavernosus muscles. **They are homologous to the single bulb of the penis and corpus spongiosum in the male.** They are likely to be injured during childbirth with brisk hemorrhage (Fig. 1.3).

PERINEUM

The details of the anatomy of perineum are described later in this Chapter (p. 15).

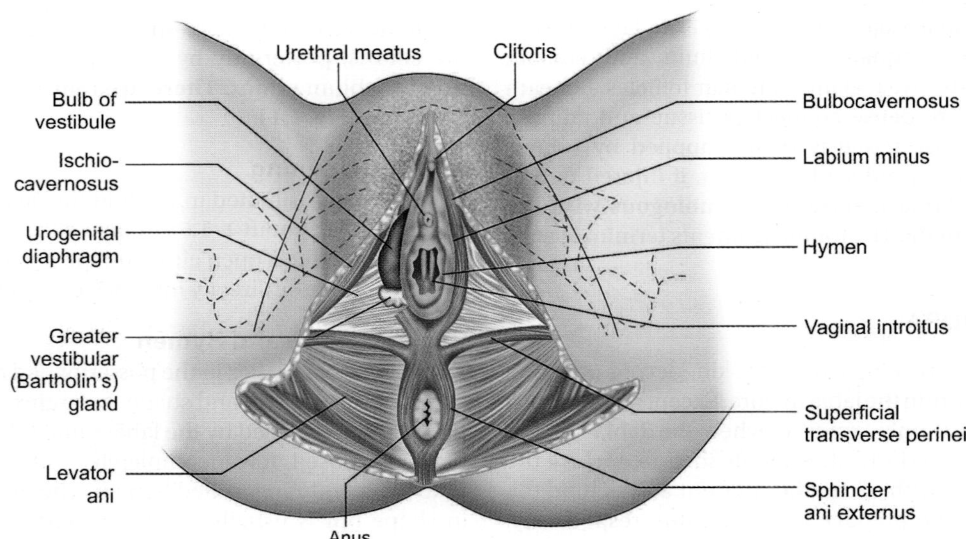

Fig. 1.3: Exposition of superficial perineal pouch with vestibular bulb and Bartholin's gland.

BLOOD SUPPLY OF THE VULVA

Arteries: (a) Branches of internal pudendal artery—the chief being labial, transverse perineal, artery to the vestibular bulb and deep and dorsal arteries to the clitoris and (b) branches of femoral artery—superficial and deep pudendal.
Veins: The veins form plexuses and drain into—(a) Internal pudendal vein; (b) Vesical or vaginal venous plexus; (c) Long saphenous vein. Varicosities during pregnancy are not uncommon and may rupture spontaneously causing visible bleeding or hematoma formation.

NERVE SUPPLY OF THE VULVA

The supply is through bilateral spinal somatic nerves. Anterosuperior part is supplied by the cutaneous branches from the ilioinguinal and genital branch of genitofemoral nerve (L_1 and L_2) and the posteroinferior part by the pudendal branches from the posterior cutaneous nerve of thigh ($S_{2,3,4}$). Between these two groups, the vulva is supplied by the labial and perineal branches of the pudendal nerve ($S_{2,3,4}$).

INTERNAL GENITAL ORGANS

The internal genital organs in female include vagina, uterus, fallopian tubes, and the ovaries. These organs are placed internally and require special instruments for inspection.

VAGINA

The vagina is a fibromusculomembranous sheath communicating the uterine cavity with the exterior at the vulva. It constitutes the excretory channel for the uterine secretion and menstrual blood. It is the organ of copulation and forms the birth canal of parturition. The canal is directed upwards and backwards forming an angle of 45° with the horizontal in erect posture. The long axis of the vagina almost lies parallel to the plane of the pelvic inlet and at right angle to that of the uterus. The diameter of the canal is about 2.5 cm, being the widest in the upper part and the narrowest at its introitus. It has got enough power of distensibility as evident during childbirth.

Walls

Vagina has got an anterior, a posterior, and two lateral walls. The anterior and posterior walls are apposed together but the lateral walls are comparatively stiffer especially at its middle, as such it looks 'H' shaped on transverse section. **The length of the anterior wall is about 7 cm and that of the posterior wall is about 9 cm (Figs. 1.4A and B)**. The upper end of vagina is above the pelvic floor.

Fornices

The fornices are the clefts formed at the top of vagina (vault) due to the projection of the uterine cervix through the anterior vaginal wall, where it is blended inseparably with its wall. There are four fornices—one anterior, one posterior, and two lateral; the posterior one being deeper and the anterior, most shallow one.

Relations

Anterior: The upper one-third is related with base of the bladder and the lower two-thirds are with the urethra, the lower half of which is firmly embedded with its wall (Figs. 1.4A and B).
Posterior: The upper one-third is related with the pouch of Douglas, the middle-third with the anterior rectal wall separated by rectovaginal septum, and the lower-third is separated from the anal canal by the perineal body (Fig. 1.5).
Lateral walls: The upper one-third is related with the pelvic cellular tissue at the base of broad ligament in which the ureter and the uterine artery lie approximately 2 cm from the lateral fornices. The middle-third is blended with the levator ani and the lower-third is related with the bulbocavernosus muscles, vestibular bulbs, and Bartholin's glands (Fig. 1.6).

Structures

Layers from within outwards are: (a) Mucous coat which is lined by stratified squamous epithelium without any secreting glands; (b) Submucous layer of loose areolar vascular tissues; (c) Muscular layer consisting of indistinct inner circular and outer longitudinal and; (d) Fibrous coat derived from the endopelvic fascia which is tough and highly vascular (Fig. 1.7).

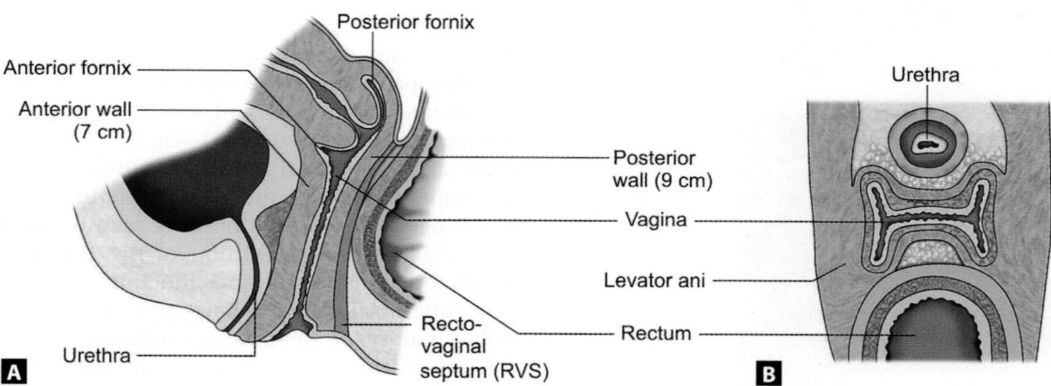

Figs. 1.4A and B: (A) Relation of the anterior and posterior vaginal wall; (B) 'H' shaped on cross-section.

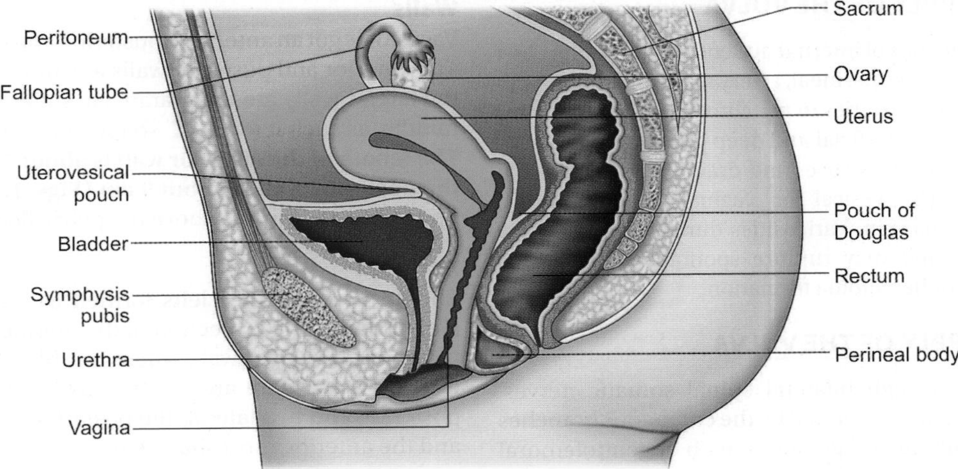

Fig. 1.5: Mid-sagittal section of the female pelvis showing relative positions of the pelvic organs.

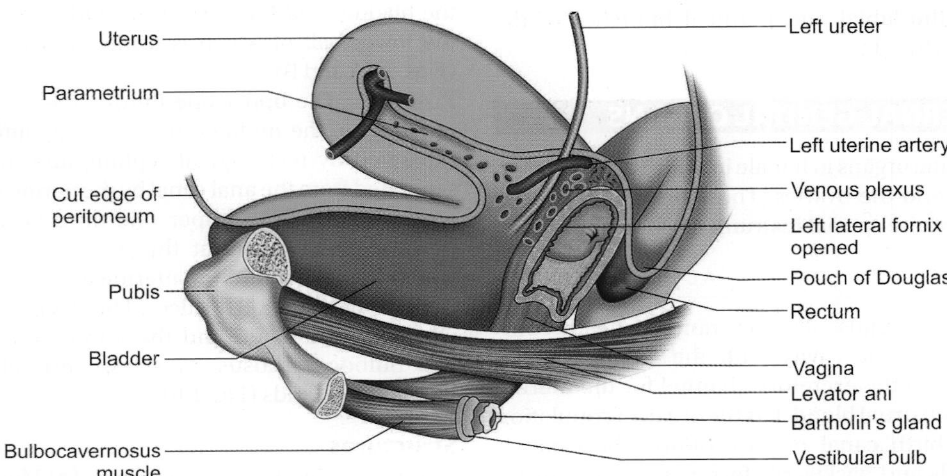

Fig. 1.6: Lateral relations of vagina.

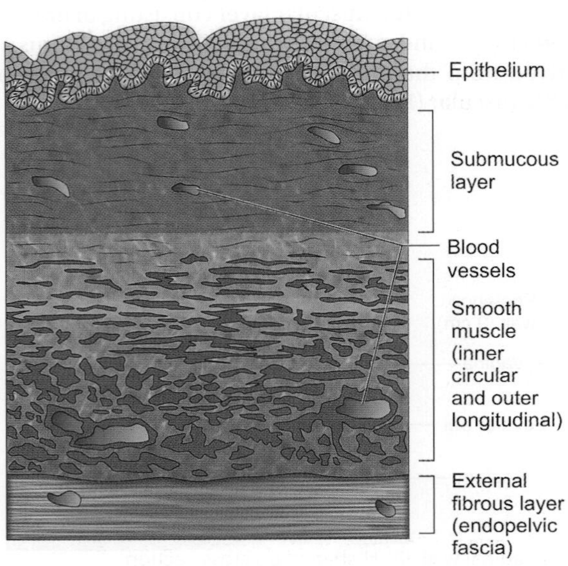

Fig. 1.7: Structure of vaginal wall.

Epithelium

The vaginal epithelium is under the action of sex hormones (Fig. 1.8). **At birth and up to 10–14 days**, the epithelium is stratified squamous under the influence of maternal estrogen circulating in the newborn. Thereafter, up to prepuberty and in postmenopause, the epithelium becomes thin, consisting of few layers only.

From puberty till menopause, the vaginal epithelium is stratified squamous and devoid of any gland. Three distinct layers are defined—basal cells, intermediate cells, and superficial cornified cells. The intermediate and superficial cells contain glycogen under the influence of estrogen. These cells become continuous with those covering the vaginal portion of the cervix and extend up to the squamocolumnar junction at the external os. The superficial cells exfoliate constantly and more so in inflammatory or neoplastic condition. Replacement of the superficial cells occurs from the basal cells. When the epithelium is exposed to the dry external atmosphere, keratinization occurs. **Unlike skin, it does not contain hair follicle, sweat, and sebaceous gland**.

	ESTROGEN	EPITHELIUM	GLYCOGEN	pH	FLORA
BIRTH TO 2 WEEKS	+	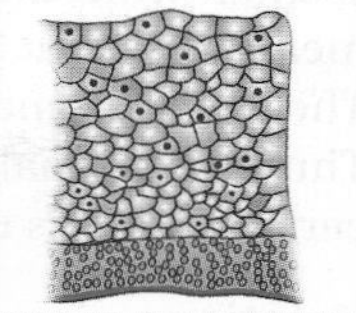	+	ACIDIC 4–5	STERILE ↓ DODERLEIN'S BACILLI SECRETION ABUNDANT
2 WEEKS TO PREPUBERTY	–	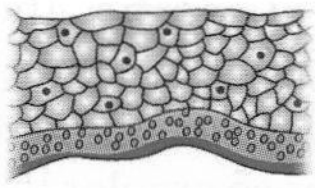	–	ALKALINE >7	DODERLEIN'S BACILLI ABSENT SECRETION SCANT
PREPUBERTY	APPEARS	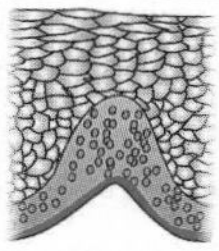	– ⟶ +	ALKALINE ↓ ACIDIC	SPARSE, COCCAL ↓ RICH BACILLARY
REPRODUCTIVE PERIOD	++	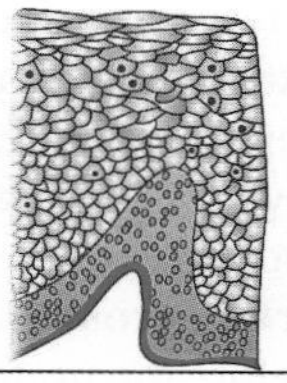	+	ACIDIC 4–5	DODERLEIN'S BACILLI APPEAR SECRETION ABUNDANT
POSTMENOPAUSE	+ ⟶ –	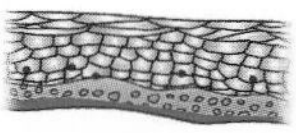	–	NEUTRAL OR ALKALINE 6 –>7	DODERLEIN'S BACILLI ABSENT SECRETION SCANT

Fig. 1.8: Estrogenic effect on vaginal epithelium and flora at different ages.

Secretion

The vaginal secretion is very small in amount, sufficient to make the surface moist. Normally, it may be little excess in mid-menstrual or just prior to menstruation, during pregnancy, and during sexual excitement. **The secretion is mainly derived from** the glands of the cervix, uterus, transudation of the vaginal epithelium, and Bartholin's glands (during sexual excitement).

The pH is acidic and varies during different phases of life and menstrual cycle. Conversion of glycogen in the exfoliated squamous cells to lactic acid by the **Doderlein's bacilli** is dependent on estrogen. As such, the pH is more towards acidic during childbearing period and ranges **between 4 and 5.5 with average of 4.5.** The pH is highest in upper vagina because of contaminated cervical secretion (alkaline). The **vaginal secretion consists** of tissue fluid, epithelial debris, some leukocytes (never contains more than an occasional pus cell), electrolytes, proteins, and lactic acid (in a concentration of 0.75%). Apart from Doderlein's bacilli, it contains many pathogenic organism including *Clostridium welchii.* **The glycogen content is highest** in the vaginal fornix to the extent of 2.5–3 mg% and is lowest in the lower-third being 0.6–0.9 mg%.

Doderlein's bacillus: It is a rod-shaped gram-positive bacillus which grows anaerobically on acid media. It appears in the vagina 3–4 days after birth and disappears after 10–14 days. It appears again at puberty and disappears after menopause. It probably comes from the intestine. Its presence is dependent on estrogen, and its function is to convert the glycogen present in the vaginal mucosa into lactic acid so that the vaginal pH is maintained towards acidic side. This acidic pH prevents growth of the other pathogenic organisms (Fig. 1.8).

Blood Supply

The arteries involved are: (a) Cervicovaginal branch of the uterine artery; (b) Vaginal artery—a branch of anterior division of internal iliac or in common origin with the uterine; (c) Middle rectal; (d) Internal pudendal. These anastomose with one another and form two azygos arteries—anterior and posterior.

Veins drain into internal iliac and internal pudendal veins.

Nerve Supply

The vagina is supplied by sympathetic and parasympathetic nerves from the pelvic plexus. The lower part is supplied by the pudendal nerve.

UTERUS

The uterus is a hollow pyriform muscular organ situated in the pelvis between the bladder in front and the rectum behind (Fig. 1.5).

Position

Its normal position is one of the **anteversion** and **anteflexion**. The uterus usually inclines to the right (dextrorotation) so that the **cervix is directed to the left (levorotation)** and comes in close relation with the left ureter.

Measurements and Parts

The uterus measures about 8 cm long, 5 cm wide at the fundus and its walls are about 1.25 cm thick. Its weight varies from 50–80 g. It has got the following parts (Fig. 1.9).

- **Body or corpus**
- **Isthmus**
- **Cervix**

Body or corpus: The body is further divided into **fundus**—the part which lies above the openings of the uterine tubes. The **body** properly is triangular and lies between the openings of the tubes and the isthmus. The superolateral angles of the body of the uterus project outwards from the junction of the fundus and body and are called the cornua of the uterus. The uterine tube, round ligament, and ligament of the ovary are attached to each cornu.

Isthmus: The isthmus is a constricted part measuring about 0.5 cm situated between the body and the cervix. It is limited above by the anatomical internal os and below by the histological internal os (Aschoff). Some consider isthmus as a part of the lower portion of the body of the uterus.

Cervix: The cervix is the lowermost part of the uterus. It extends from the histological internal os and ends at external os which opens into the vagina after perforating the anterior vaginal wall. It is almost cylindrical in shape and measures about 2.5 cm in length and diameter. It is divided into a supravaginal part—the part lying above the vagina and a vaginal part which lies within the vagina, each measuring 1.25 cm. In **nulliparous**, the vaginal part of the cervix is conical with the external os looking circular, whereas **in parous**, it is cylindrical with the external os having bilateral slits. The slit is due to invariable tear of the circular muscles surrounding the external os and gives rise to anterior and posterior lips of the cervix.

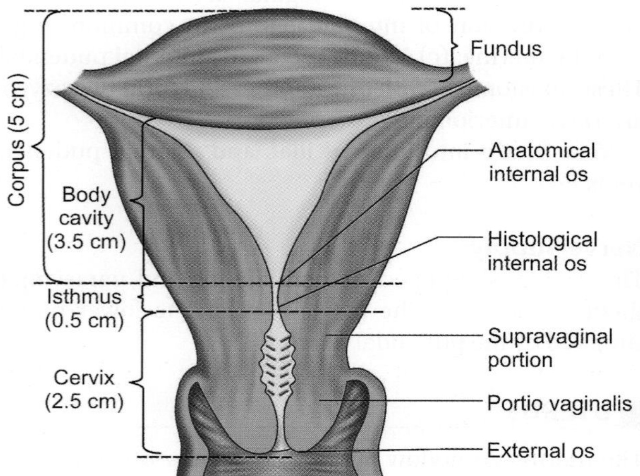

Fig. 1.9: Coronal section showing different parts of uterus.

Cavity

The cavity of the uterine body is triangular on coronal section with the base above and the apex below. It measures about 3.5 cm. There is no cavity in the fundus. The cervical canal is fusiform and measures about 2.5 cm. Thus, the normal length of the uterine cavity including the cervical canal is usually 6–7 cm (Fig. 1.9).

Relations

Anteriorly: Above the internal os, the body forms the posterior wall of the uterovesical pouch. Below the internal os, it is separated from the base of the bladder by loose areolar tissue (Fig. 1.10).

Posteriorly: It is covered by peritoneum and forms the anterior wall of the pouch of Douglas containing coils of intestine (Fig. 1.10).

Laterally: The double folds of peritoneum of the broad ligament are attached laterally between which the uterine artery ascends up. Attachment of the Mackenrodt's ligament extends from the internal os down to the supravaginal cervix and lateral vaginal wall. About 1.5 cm away at the level of internal os, a little nearer on the left side is the crossing of the uterine artery and the ureter. **The uterine artery crosses from above and in front of the ureter**, soon before the ureter enters the ureteric tunnel (Fig. 1.11).

Structures

Body

The wall consists of three layers from outside inwards:

1. *Perimetrium:* It is the serous coat which invests the entire organ except on the lateral borders. The peritoneum is intimately adherent to the underlying muscles.
2. *Myometrium:* It consists of thick bundles of smooth muscle fibers held by connective tissues and are arranged in various directions. During pregnancy, however, three distinct layers can be identified—outer longitudinal, middle interlacing, and inner circular.
3. *Endometrium:* The mucous lining of the cavity is called endometrium. As there is no submucous layer, the endometrium is directly apposed to the muscle coat. It

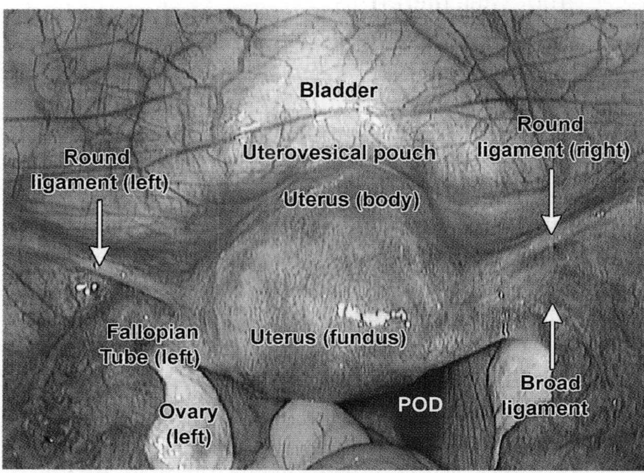

Fig. 1.10: Laproscopic view of the anterior surface of the uterus. (POD: pouch of Douglas)

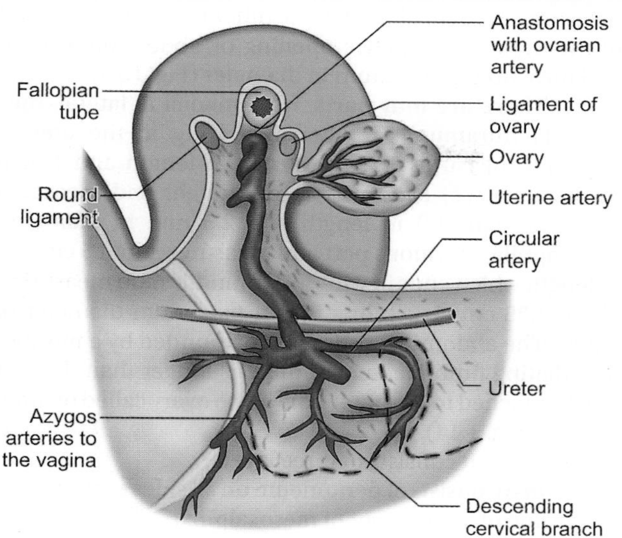

Fig. 1.11: The relation of the ureter to the uterine artery.

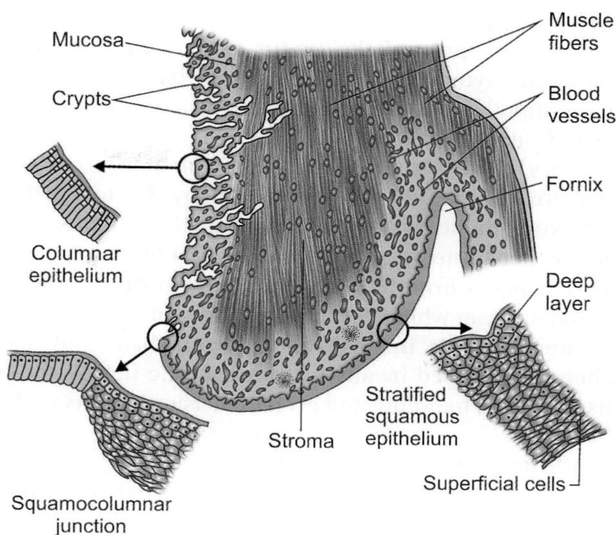

Fig. 1.12: Character of the lining epithelium of the cervix.

consists of lamina propria and surface epithelium. The surface epithelium is a single layer of ciliated columnar epithelium. The lamina propria contains stromal cells, endometrial glands, vessels and nerves. The glands are simple tubular and lined by mucus secreting non-ciliated columnar epithelium which penetrate the stroma and sometimes even enter the muscle coat. All the components are changed during menstrual cycles (Ch. 8). The endometrium is changed to decidua during pregnancy.

Cervix

The cervix is composed mainly of fibrous connective tissues. The smooth muscle fibers average 10–15%. Only the posterior surface has got peritoneal coat (Fig. 1.5).

Epithelial lining of the cervix

Endocervical canal and glands: There is a median ridge on both the anterior and posterior surface of the canal from which transverse folds radiate. This arrangement is called arbor vitae uteri. The canal is lined by single layer of tall columnar epithelium with basal nuclei. Those placed over the top of the folds are ciliated. There are patches of cubical basal or reserve cells underneath the columnar epithelium. These cells may undergo squamous metaplasia or may replace the superficial cells.

The glands which dip into the stroma are of complex racemose type and are lined by secretory columnar epithelium. There is no stroma unlike the corpus and the lining epithelium rests on a thin basement membrane. The change in the epithelium and the glands during menstrual cycle and pregnancy are not so much as those in the endometrium.

Portio vaginalis: It is covered by stratified squamous epithelium and extends right up to the external os where there is abrupt change to columnar type.

The transitional zone (transformation zone) may be of 1–10 mm width with variable histological features. The zone consists of endocervical stroma and glands covered by squamous epithelium. **The zone is not static but changes with hormone level of estrogen.** The site is constantly irritated not only by hormones but also by infection and trauma. Thus, **there is more chance of severe dysplasia, carcinoma in situ or even invasive carcinoma at this zone (Fig. 1.12) (p. 269).**

Secretion: The endometrial secretion is scanty and watery. The physical and chemical properties of the cervical secretion change with menstrual cycle and with pregnancy. The cervical glands secrete an alkaline mucus with **pH 7.8**. The mucus is rich in fructose, glycoprotein, and mucopolysaccharides. It also contains sodium chloride. The fructose has got nutritive function to the spermatozoa. Under estrogenic stimulation, glycoprotein network is arranged parallel to each other thus facilitating sperm ascent. Progesterone produces interlacing bridges thereby preventing sperm penetration. Cervical mucus contributes significantly to the normal vaginal discharge. A part forms the mucus plug which functionally closes the cervical canal and has got bacteriolytic property.

Pelvic Peritoneum in Relation to the Uterus

This is described later in the chapter.

Blood Supply

Arterial supply: The arterial supply is from the uterine artery—one on each side. The artery arises directly from the anterior division of the internal iliac or in common with superior vesical artery. The other sources are ovarian and vaginal arteries to which the uterine arteries anastomose. **The uterine artery crosses the ureter anteriorly about 1.5 cm away at the level of internal os** before it ascends up along the lateral border of the uterus in between the leaves of broad ligament. The internal blood supply of the uterus is shown in Figure 2.1.

Veins: The venous channels correspond to the arterial course and drain into internal iliac veins.

Nerve Supply

The nerve supply of the uterus is derived principally from the sympathetic system and partly from the parasympathetic system. Sympathetic components are from T_5 and T_6 (motor) and T_{10} to L_1 spinal segments (sensory). The somatic distribution of uterine pain is that area of the abdomen supplied by T_{10} to L_1. The parasympathetic system is represented on either side by the pelvic nerve which consists of both motor and sensory fibers from S_2, S_3, S_4 and ends in the ganglia of Frankenhauser which lies on either sides of the cervix.

The cervix is insensitive to touch, heat and also when it is grasped by any instrument. The uterus, too is insensitive to handling and even to incision over its wall.

Changes of Uterus with Age

At birth, the uterus lies in the false pelvis; the cervix is much longer than the body. **In childhood**, the proportion is maintained but reduced to 2:1. **At puberty**, the body is growing faster under the action of ovarian steroids (estrogens) and the proportion is reversed to 1:2 and following childbirth, it becomes even 1:3. **After menopause** the uterus atrophies; the overall length is reduced; the walls become thinner, less muscular but more fibrous (Figs. 5.1A to E).

Position of the Uterus

The normal position of the uterus is anteversion and anteflexion. **Anteversion relates** the long axis of the cervix to the long axis of vagina which is about 90°. **Anteflexion relates** the long axis of the body to the long axis of the cervix and is about 120°. In about 15–20%, normally the uterus remains in retroverted position. In erect posture, the internal os lies on the upper border of the symphysis pubis and the external os lies at the level of ischial spines.

FALLOPIAN TUBE (SYN: UTERINE TUBE)

The uterine tubes are paired structures, measuring about 10 cm (4") and are situated in the medial three-fourth of the upper free margin of the broad ligaments. Each tube has got two openings, one communicating with the lateral angle of the uterine cavity, called uterine opening and measures 1 mm in diameter, the other is on the lateral end of the tube, called pelvic opening or abdominal ostium and measures about 2 mm in diameter (Fig. 1.13).

Parts: There are four parts, from medial to lateral, they are—(1) Intramural or interstitial lying in the uterine wall and measures 1.25 cm (1/2") in length and 1 mm in diameter; (2) Isthmus almost straight and measures about 2.5 cm (1") in length and 2.5 mm in diameter; (3) Ampulla—tortuous part and measures about 5 cm (2") in length which ends in wide; (4) Infundibulum measuring about 1.25 cm (1/2") long with a maximum diameter of 6 mm. The abdominal ostium is surrounded by a number of radiating fimbriae, one of these is longer than the rest and is attached to the outer pole of the ovary called ovarian fimbria (Fig. 1.14).

Structures—it consists of three layers:

1. ***Serous:*** Consists of peritoneum on all sides except along the line of attachment of mesosalpinx.
2. ***Muscular:*** Arranged in two layers—outer longitudinal and inner circular.
3. ***Mucous membrane*** is thrown into longitudinal folds. It is lined by columnar epithelium, partly ciliated, others secretory nonciliated and 'Peg cells'. The epithelium rests on delicate vascular reticulum of connective tissue. There is no submucous layer nor any glands. Changes occur in the tubal epithelium during menstrual cycle but are less pronounced and there is no shedding (Fig. 1.14).

Functions: The important functions of the tubes are—(1) Transport of gametes; (2) To facilitate fertilization; (3) Survival of zygote through its secretion.

Blood supply: Arterial supply is from the uterine and ovarian. Venous drainage is through the pampiniform plexus into the ovarian veins.

Nerve supply: The nerve supply is derived from the uterine and ovarian nerves. The tube is very much sensitive to handling.

OVARY

The ovaries are paired sex glands or gonads in female which **are concerned with:**

1. Germ cell maturation, storage and its release
2. Steroidogenesis.

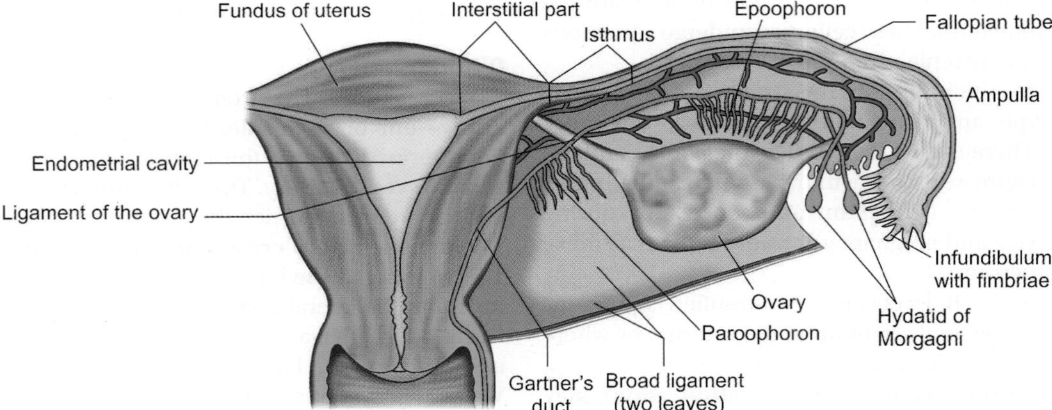

Fig. 1.13: Half of uterine cavity and fallopian tube of one side are cut open to show different parts of the tube. The vestigial structures in the broad ligament are shown.

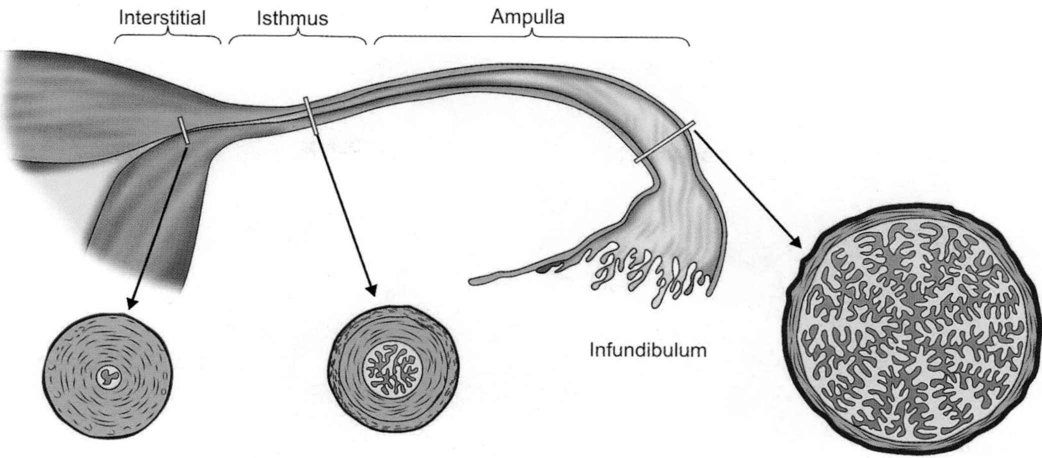

Fig. 1.14: Cut section of the tube showing complex mucosal pattern.

Each gland is oval in shape and pinkish-gray in color and the surface is scarred during reproductive period. It measures about 3 cm in length, 2 cm in breadth and 1 cm in thickness. Each ovary presents two ends—tubal and uterine, two borders—mesovarium and free posterior and two surfaces—medial and lateral.

The ovaries are intraperitoneal structures. In nulliparae, the ovary lies in the ovarian fossa on the lateral pelvic wall. **The ovary is attached** to the posterior layer of the broad ligament by the mesovarium, to the lateral pelvic wall by infundibulopelvic ligament and to the uterus by the ovarian ligament.

Relations: Mesovarium or anterior border—a fold of peritoneum from the posterior leaf of the broad ligament is attached to the anterior border through which the ovarian vessels and nerves enter the hilum of the gland. **Posterior border** is free and is related with tubal ampulla. It is separated by the peritoneum from the ureter and the internal iliac artery. **Medial surface** is related to fimbrial part of the tube. **Lateral surface** is in contact with the **ovarian fossa** on the lateral pelvic wall.

The ovarian fossa is related superiorly to the external iliac vein, posteriorly to ureter and internal iliac vessels and laterally to the peritoneum separating the obturator vessels and nerves (Fig. 1.15).

Structures

The ovary is covered by a single layer of cubical cell known as germinal epithelium. It is a misnomer as germ cells are

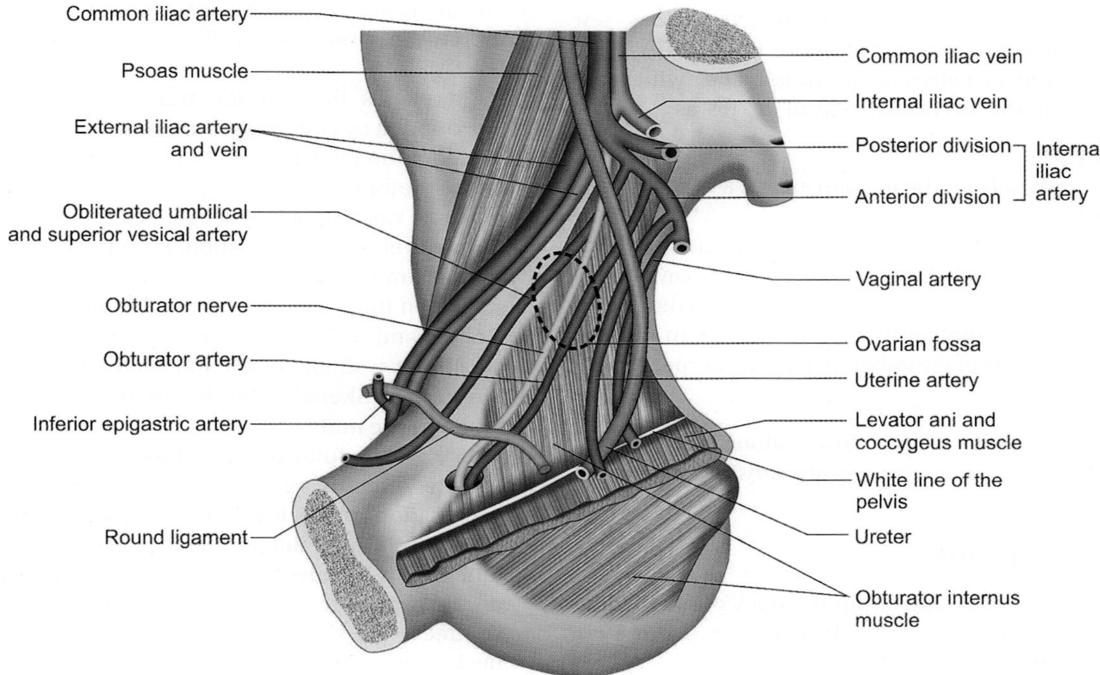

Fig. 1.15: The structures in the lateral pelvic wall of ovarian fossa.

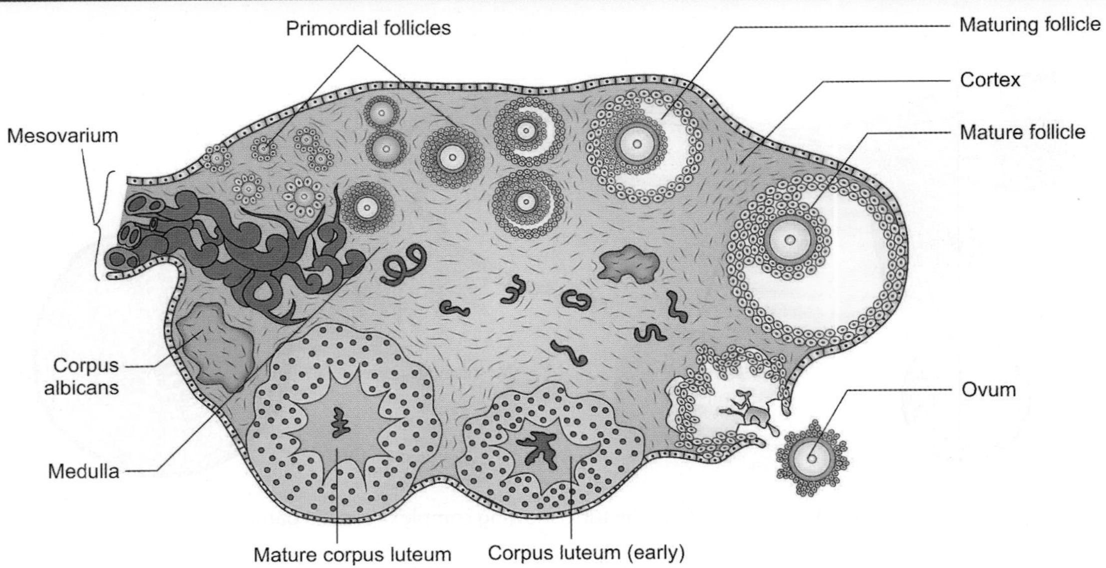

Fig. 1.16: Histological structures of the ovary.

not derived from this layer. The substance of the gland consists of outer cortex and inner medulla (Fig. 1.16).

Cortex: It consists of stromal cells which are thickened beneath the germinal epithelium to form tunica albuginea. During reproductive period (i.e. from puberty to menopause), the cortex is studded with numerous follicular structures, called the functional units of the ovary in various phases of their development. These are related to sex hormone production and ovulation. **The structures include** primordial follicles, maturing follicles, Graafian follicles and corpus luteum. Atresia of the structures results in formation of atretic follicles or corpus albicans (Fig. 1.16). The structural changes during ovular cycle are described in Chapter 8 (p. 69).

Medulla: It consists of loose connective tissues, few unstriped muscles, blood vessels, and nerves. There are small collection of cells called "hilus cells" which are homologous to the interstitial cells of the testes.

Blood Supply

Arterial supply is from the ovarian artery, a branch of the abdominal aorta.

Venous drainage is through pampiniform plexus, that forms the ovarian veins which drain into inferior vena cava on the right side and left renal vein on the left side. Part of the venous blood from the placental site drains into the ovarian and thus may become the site of thrombophlebitis in puerperium.

Nerve Supply

Sympathetic supply comes down along the ovarian artery from T_{10} segment. Ovaries are sensitive to manual squeezing.

FEMALE URETHRA

The female urethra extends from the neck of the bladder to the external urethral meatus. **It measures about 4 cm and has a diameter of about 6 mm.**

The bladder base forms an angle with the posterior wall of the urethra called posterior urethrovesical angle (PUV) which normally measures 100°. The urethra runs downwards and forwards in close proximity of the anterior vaginal wall. About 1 cm from the lower end, it pierces the triangular ligament. It ultimately opens into the vestibule about 2.5 cm below the clitoris.

Relations

Posteriorly: It is related to the anterior vaginal wall to which it is loosely separated in the upper two-third but firmly adherent in the lower-third.

Anteriorly: It is related to the posterior aspect of symphysis pubis. The upper two-third is separated by loose areolar tissue; the lower one-third is attached on each side of the pubic rami by fibrous tissue called—pubourethral ligament.

Laterally:

- As it passes through the triangular ligament, it is surrounded by compressor urethra.
- Whether the medial fibers of puborectalis get attached to the urethra while passing by its sides to get attached to lateral vaginal walls is debatable.
- Bulbocavernosus and vestibular bulb.

Glands: Numerous tubular glands called paraurethral glands open into the lumen through ducts. Of these, two are longer and called Skene's ducts which open either on the posterior wall just inside the external meatus or into the vestibule. **Skene's glands are homologous to the prostate in the male.**

Sphincters—the following are the sphincters:

- At the urethrovesical junction, there is intricate decussation of the involuntary muscles. This has the effect of forming anterior and posterior slings which function as an involuntary internal sphincter. This is the lissosphincter. When the detrusor muscle actively contracts, the slings relax → funneling of the bladder neck → urine flows into the urethra (Fig. 1.17).

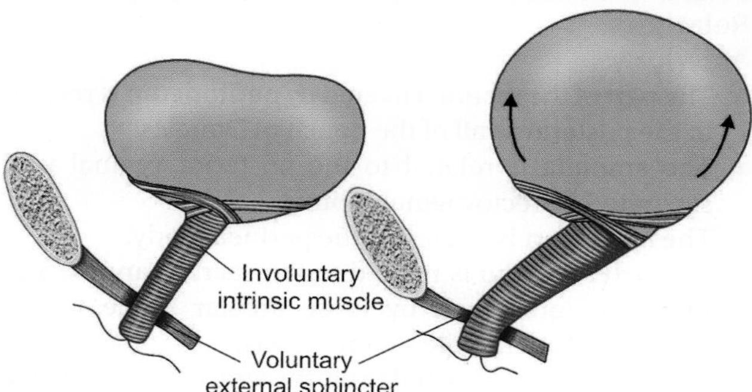

Fig. 1.17: Urethral sphincters.

- The wall of the urethra is composed of involuntary muscles and the fibers are arranged in the form of crossed spirals. The fibers are continuous with those of the bladder detrusor. The tone and elasticity of these muscles keep it close except during micturition.
- Sphincter urethra in the urogenital diaphragm. This sphincter allows the voluntary arrest of urine flow.
- Although debatable, puborectalis part of levator ani which surrounds the lower-third of the urethra acts as an external sphincter.
- Superficial perineal muscles, bulbocavernosus and ischiocavernosus form an accessory external sphincter.

Structures: Mucous membrane is lined by transitional epithelium except at the external urethral meatus where it becomes stratified squamous. Submucous coat is vascular. Muscle coat is composed of involuntary muscles and the fibers are arranged in the form of crossed spirals.

Blood Supply

Arterial supply: Proximal part is supplied by the inferior vesical branch and the distal part by a branch of internal pudendal artery.

The veins drain into vesical plexus and into internal pudendal veins.

Lymphatics

P. 24.

Nerves

The urethra is supplied by the pudendal nerve.

Development

The urethra is developed from the vesicourethral portion of the cloaca.

APPLIED ANATOMY

- Because of shortness and its close proximity to the vagina and anus, the infection is likely and that commonly spreads upwards to involve the bladder.
- Because of close proximity of the anterior vaginal wall, the urethra may be injured during the process of childbirth.
- The paraurethral glands are the sites of infection and occasional development of benign adenoma or malignant changes.

OTHER INTERNAL ORGANS

URINARY BLADDER

The bladder is a hollow muscular organ with considerable power of distension. Its capacity is about 450 mL (15 oz) but can retain as much as 3–4 liters of urine. When distended, it is ovoid in shape. It has got: (a) An apex; (b) Superior surface; (c) Base; (d) Two inferolateral surfaces; (e) Neck, which is continuous with the urethra. **The base and the neck remain fixed even when the bladder is distended.**

Relations: The superior surface is related with the peritoneum of the uterovesical pouch (Fig. 1.5). The base is related with the supravaginal cervix and the anterior fornix. The ureters, after crossing the pelvic floor at the sides of the cervix, enter the bladder on its lateral angles. In the interior of bladder, the triangular area marked by three openings—two ureteric and one urethral, is called the trigone. The **inferolateral surfaces are related with the space of Retzius**. The neck rests on the superior layer of the urogenital diaphragm.

Structures—from outside inwards:

- Outer visceral layer of the pelvic fascia.
- Muscle layer composed of muscles running in various directions. Near the internal urethral opening, the circular muscle fibers provide involuntary sphincter.
- Mucous coat is lined by transitional epithelium with no gland. **There is no submucous coat.**

Blood supply: The arterial supply is through superior and inferior vesical arteries. **The veins** drain into vesical and vaginal plexus and thence to internal iliac veins.

Lymphatics: Lymphatics drain into external and internal iliac lymph nodes.

Nerve supply: The sympathetic supply is from the pelvic plexus and the parasympathetic via the pelvic plexus from the nervi erigentes ($S_{2,3,4}$). **The parasympathetic** produces contraction of the detrusor muscles and relaxation of the internal sphincter (nerve of evacuation). Sympathetic conveys afferent painful stimuli of overdistension.

Development: The urinary bladder is developed from the upper part of the urogenital sinus.

PELVIC URETER

The pelvic ureter extends from its crossing over the pelvic brim up to its opening into the bladder. **It measures about 13 cm in length and has a diameter of 5 mm.**

Course and relations: The ureter enters the pelvis in front of the bifurcation of the common iliac artery over the sacroiliac joint behind the root of the mesentery on the right side and the apex of the mesosigmoid on the left side. As it courses downwards in contact with the peritoneum, it lies anterior to the internal iliac artery and behind the ovary and forms the posterior boundary of ovarian fossa (Fig. 1.15). On reaching the ischial spine, it lies over the pelvic floor and as it courses forwards and medially on the base of the broad ligament, **it is crossed by the uterine artery anteriorly (Fig. 1.11)**. Soon, it enters into the ureteric tunnel and lies close to the supravaginal part of the cervix, about 1.5 cm lateral to it. After traversing a short distance on the anterior fornix of the vagina, it courses into the wall of the bladder obliquely for about 2 cm by piercing the lateral angle before it opens into the base of the trigone. **In the pelvic portion, the ureter is comparatively constricted**:

- Where it crosses the pelvic brim.
- Where crossed by the uterine artery.
- In the intravesical part.

Structures: From outside inwards—(a) Fibers derived from the visceral layer of the pelvic fascia; (b) Muscle coat consisting of three layers—outer and inner longitudinal and intermediate circular; (c) Mucous layer lined by transitional epithelium.

Blood supply: The ureter has got segmental supply from nearly all the visceral branches of the anterior division of the internal iliac artery. The venous drainage corresponds to the arteries (uterine, vaginal, vesical, middle rectal, and superior gluteal).

Lymphatics: The lymphatics from the lower part drain into the external and internal iliac lymph nodes and the upper part into the lumbar lymph nodes.

Nerve supply: Sympathetic supply is from the hypogastric and pelvic plexus; parasympathetic from the sacral plexus.

Development: The ureter is developed as an ureteric bud from the caudal end of the mesonephric duct.

APPLIED ANATOMY

The ureter is recognized by the following features:
- Pale glistening appearance.
- Longitudinal vessels on the surface.
- Peristalsis.

The ureter is likely to be damaged during pelvic surgery.

Abdominal hysterectomy: The common sites of ureteric injury are—(a) infundibulopelvic ligament; (b) by the side of the cervix (clamping the cardinal ligament along with descending cervical artery); (c) vaginal angle as the ureter traverses along the anterior fornix; (d) during pelvic peritonization (ureter lies in the posterior leaf of the peritoneum).

The chances of injury are more in cases of endometriosis, pelvic inflammation or broad ligament tumor. Injury is more common during reclamping than primary clamping.

Radical hysterectomy: Direct injury is not common. Sloughing necrosis may occur due to stripping the ureter off the peritoneum → devitalization → sloughing.

RECTUM

The rectum commences at the level of the third piece of the sacrum in continuation of pelvic colon and ends in anal canal. It measures 12–15 cm. The rectum follows the curve of the sacrum. It curves twice to the left and once to the right before it passes down to continue as anal canal.

Peritoneal coverings: Rectum is covered anteriorly and laterally in its upper-third, only anteriorly in the middle-third. Whole of the posterior surface and the entire lower-third remain uncovered.

Relations

Anteriorly
- The part of the rectum covered by peritoneum is related to the posterior wall of the pouch of Douglas.
- The ampulla is related to the posterior vaginal wall separated by rectovaginal septum.
- The lower part is related to the perineal body.

Posteriorly: Rectum is related to the sacrum and coccyx from which intervened by loose areolar tissue, sacral nerve trunks, and middle sacral vessels.

Laterally: Rectum is related to uterosacral ligament, pelvic plexus of nerves, and ureter. Near the anorectal junction, it is related to puborectalis part of levator ani. Below the muscle, it is related to ischiorectal fossa.

Structures

Rectum is surrounded by rectal fascia. Muscle coat consists of outer longitudinal and inner circular fibers. Submucous layer is loose and contains venous plexuses. Mucous membrane is lined by columnar epithelium.

ANAL CANAL

The anal canal measures about 2.5 cm. It is directed backwards almost at right angles to the ampulla and at the site of insertion of puborectalis part of levator ani. It ends at the anal orifice. At the junction of the upper two-third and lower one-third is the white line (Hilton's line).

Relations

Anteriorly: It is related to perineal body and posteriorly to the anococcygeal body.

Anal Sphincters

The anal canal has got two sphincters:
- Involuntary internal sphincter is formed by thickening of circular layer of the upper two-third of the anal canal.
- Voluntary sphincter ani externus which surrounds the entire length of the canal, **consists of three parts:**
  1. *Subcutaneous part*—it is attached to the skin.
  2. *Superficial part*—it starts from the perineal body and is inserted posteriorly to the tip of the coccyx.
  3. *Deep part*—it is separated from the sphincter ani internus by levator ani (Fig. 1.18).

Lining Epithelium

The upper two-third is lined by columnar epithelium but the lower-third with stratified squamous epithelium.

Blood Supply of Rectum and Anal Canal

Arterial supply is from:
- *Superior rectal*—branch of inferior mesenteric artery.
- *Middle rectal*—branch of internal iliac artery.
- *Inferior rectal*—branch of the internal iliac artery.

Venous drainage: The rectum and upper-third of the anal canal drain via superior rectal veins to portal circulation. The lower-third of the anal canal drains on both sides into inferior rectal veins (systemic system).

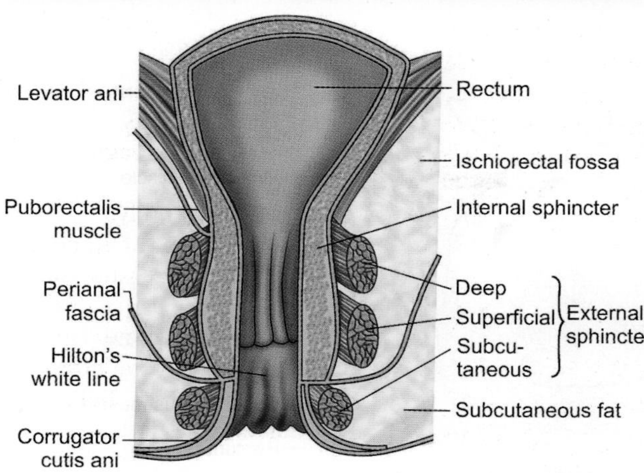

Fig. 1.18: Rectum and anal canal with anal structures.

Lymphatics of Rectum and Anal Canal

The lymphatics from the rectum and upper-third of the anal canal drain into internal iliac and preaortic nodes, while the lower-third of the anal canal drains into the superficial inguinal nodes.

Nerve Supply of Rectum and Anal Canal

The rectum and the upper two-third of the anal canal are supplied by autonomic through pelvic plexuses. The lower-third of the anal canal is supplied by inferior hemorrhoidal nerve.

Development of Rectum and Anal Canal

The rectum and the upper two-third of the anal canal are developed from the dorsal part of cloaca (endoderm). The lower one-third of the anal canal is developed from the anal pit (ectoderm).

PELVIC MUSCLES

The most important muscle supporting the pelvic organs is the levator ani which forms the pelvic floor. The small muscles of the perineum also have got some contribution in the support.

PELVIC FLOOR (SYN: PELVIC DIAPHRAGM)

Pelvic floor is a muscular partition which separates the pelvic cavity from the anatomical perineum. It consists of three sets of muscles on either side—**pubococcygeus, iliococcygeus, and ischiococcygeus. These are collectively called levator ani.** Its upper surface is concave and slopes downwards, backwards, and medially and is covered by parietal layer of pelvic fascia. The inferior surface is convex and is covered by anal fascia. The muscle with the covering fascia is called the **pelvic diaphragm. Levator ani** is a strong and fatigue resistant striated muscle. It is slug like a hammock around the midline pelvic effluents—urethra, vagina and anal canal (Figs. 1.19 and 1.20).

Origin

Each levator ani arises from the back of the pubic rami, from the condensed fascia covering the obturator internus **(white line)** and from the inner surface of the ischial spine (Fig. 1.20).

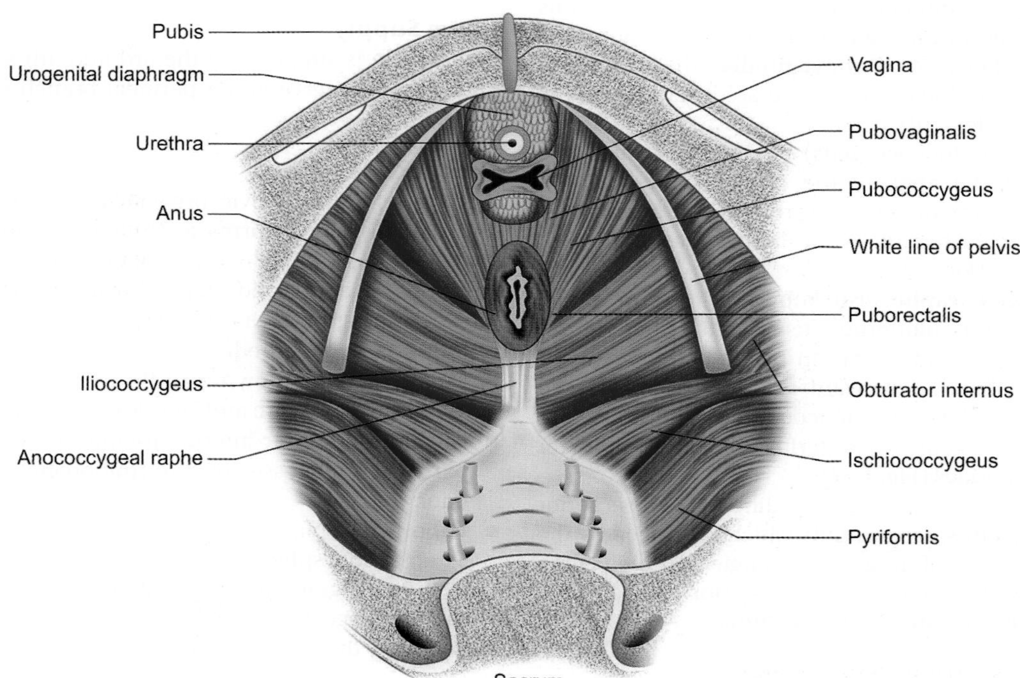

Fig. 1.19: Levator ani muscles viewed from above.

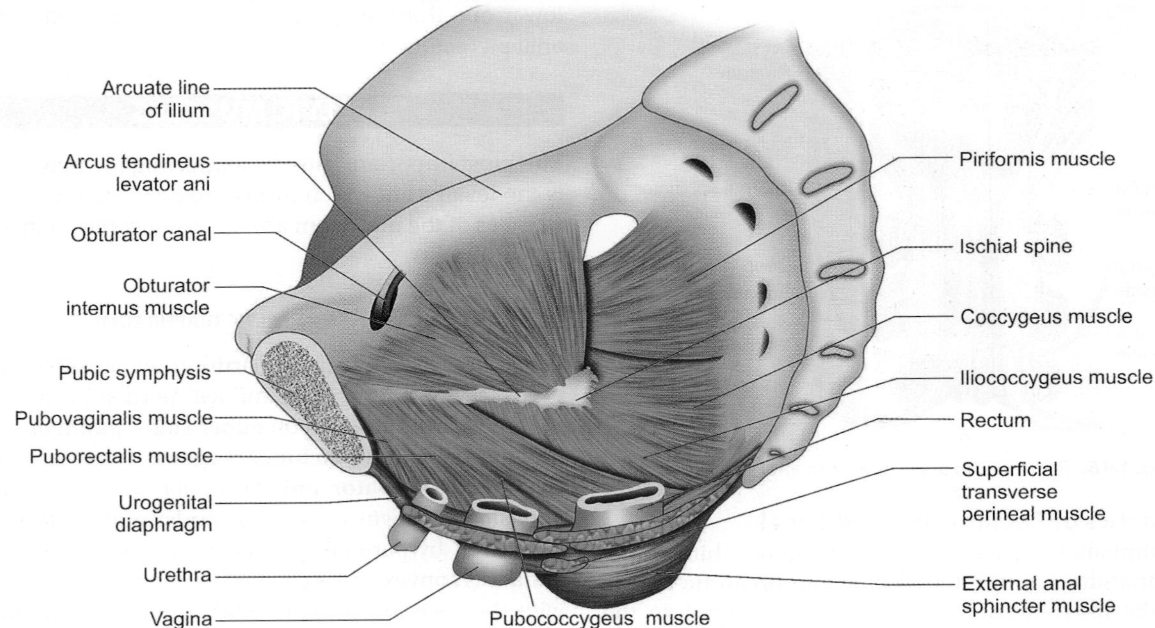

Fig. 1.20: Lateral (sagittal) view of the pelvis showing the muscles of the pelvic diaphragm.

Insertion

The pubococcygeus—the fibers pass backwards and medially and are inserted as follows: (a) The posterior fibers are inserted into the anococcygeal raphe and tip of the coccyx; (b) **Puborectalis**—these fibers wind round the anorectal junction and are continuous with the similar fibers of the opposite side forming a 'U' shaped loop known as puborectal sling; (c) **Puboanalis**—these fibers run between the sphincter and externus and internus and are inserted in the wall of the anal canal along the longitudinal fibers; (d) **Pubovaginalis**—these anterior fibers pass by the side of vagina and are inserted into the perineal body (Fig. 1.19).

Coccygeus (ischiococcygeus) is triangular in shape. It arises from the apex of the ischial spine and the sacrospinous ligament and is inserted by its base into the sides of the upper two pieces of the coccyx and the last piece of sacrum (Fig. 1.19).

Anococcygeal raphe also known as **levator plate**, is a layered musculofibrous tissue. It extends from the anorectal junction to the tip of the coccyx. It comprises from above downwards: (a) Presacral fascia; (b) Tendinous plate of pubococcygeus; (c) Muscular raphe of iliococcygeus; (d) Superficial fibers of sphincter ani externus muscles (Fig. 1.19).

Gaps: There are two gaps in the midline—(1) The anterior one is called **hiatus urogenitalis** which is bridged by the muscles and fascia of urogenital triangle and pierced by the urethra and vagina; (2) The posterior one is called **hiatus rectalis**, transmitting the rectum.

Structure in Relation to Pelvic Floor

The superior surface is related with the following:

- Pelvic organs from anterior to posterior are bladder, vagina and rectum.
- Pelvic cellular tissues between the pelvic peritoneum and upper surface of the levator ani which fill all the available spaces.
- Ureter lies on the floor in relation to the lateral vaginal fornix. **The uterine artery lies above and the vaginal artery lies below it.**
- Pelvic nerves.

The inferior surface is related to the anatomical perineum.

Nerve Supply

The muscle is supplied by the 3rd and 4th sacral nerve, inferior rectal nerve and a perineal branch of pudendal nerve ($S_{2,3,4}$).

Functions

- To support the pelvic organs (Table 1.1)—the pubovaginalis which forms a 'U' shaped sling, supports the vagina which in turn supports the other pelvic organs—bladder and uterus. Weakness or tear of this sling during parturition is responsible for prolapse of the organs concerned.
- Counteracts the downward thrust of increased intra-abdominal pressure and guards the hiatus urogenitalis.
- Facilitates anterior internal rotation of the presenting part when it presses on the (puborectal sling) pelvic floor.
- Puborectalis plays an ancillary role to the action of the external anal sphincter.
- Ischiococcygeus helps to stabilize the sacroiliac and sacrococcygeal joints.
- To steady the perineal body.

Pelvic Floor During Pregnancy and Parturition

During pregnancy, levator muscles hypertrophy, become less rigid and more distensible. Due to water retention,

TABLE 1.1: Biomechanical basis of uterovaginal support (Delancy, 1992).

Level	Site of vagina	Structures involved	Type of defects
I *Or* ***Suspension axis***	**Upper**	▪ Ligaments • Uterosacral • Mackenrodt	▪ Prolapse • Uterovaginal • Enterocele • Vaginal vault
II *Or* ***Attachment axis***	**Middle**	▪ Fascia • Arcus tendineus • Pubocervical	▪ Defects • Paravaginal • Pararectal ▪ Urinary incontinence
III *Or* ***Fusion axis (strongest)***	**Lower**	▪ Urogenital diaphragm ▪ Perineal muscles ▪ Perineal body ▪ Levator plate	▪ Cystocele ▪ Rectocele ▪ Urinary incontinence ▪ Anal incontinence

it swells up and sags down. In the second stage, the pubovaginalis and puborectalis relax and the levator ani is drawn up over the advancing presenting part in the second stage. Failure of the levator ani to relax at the crucial moment may lead to extensive damage of the pelvic structures. The effect of such a displacement is to elongate the birth canal, which is composed solely of soft parts below the bony outlet. The soft canal has got deep lateral and posterior walls and its axis is in continuation with the axis of the bony pelvis.

PERINEUM

ANATOMICAL PERINEUM

Anatomically, the perineum is bounded above by the inferior surface of the pelvic floor, below by the skin between the buttocks and thighs. Laterally, it is bounded by the ischiopubic rami, ischial tuberosities and sacrotuberous ligaments and posteriorly, by the coccyx. The diamond-shaped space of the bony pelvic outlet is divided into two triangular spaces with the common base formed by the free border of the urogenital diaphragm. The anterior triangle is called the urogenital triangle which fills up the gap of the hiatus urogenitalis and is important from the obstetric point of view. The posterior one is called the anal triangle.

Urogenital Triangle

It is pierced by the terminal part of the vagina and the urethra. The small perineal muscles are situated in two compartments formed by the ill-defined fascia. The compartments are superficial and deep perineal pouch. **The superficial pouch** is formed by the deep layer of the superficial perineal fascia (Colles fascia) and inferior layer of the urogenital diaphragm (perineal membrane). **The contents are** (Figs. 1.3 and 1.21) superficial transverse perinei (paired), bulbocavernosus covering the bulb of the vestibule, ischiocavernosus (paired) covering the crura of the clitoris and the Bartholin's gland (paired). The **deep perineal pouch** is formed by the inferior and superior layer of the urogenital diaphragm—together called urogenital diaphragm or triangular ligament. Between the layers, there is a potential space of about 1.25 cm. **The contents are** the following muscles—deep transverse perinei (paired) and sphincter urethrae membranacea. Both the pouches contain vessels and nerves (Fig. 1.21).

Anal Triangle

The triangle has got no obstetric importance. It contains the terminal part of the anal canal with sphincter ani externus, anococcygeal body, ischiorectal fossa, blood vessels, nerves, and lymphatics.

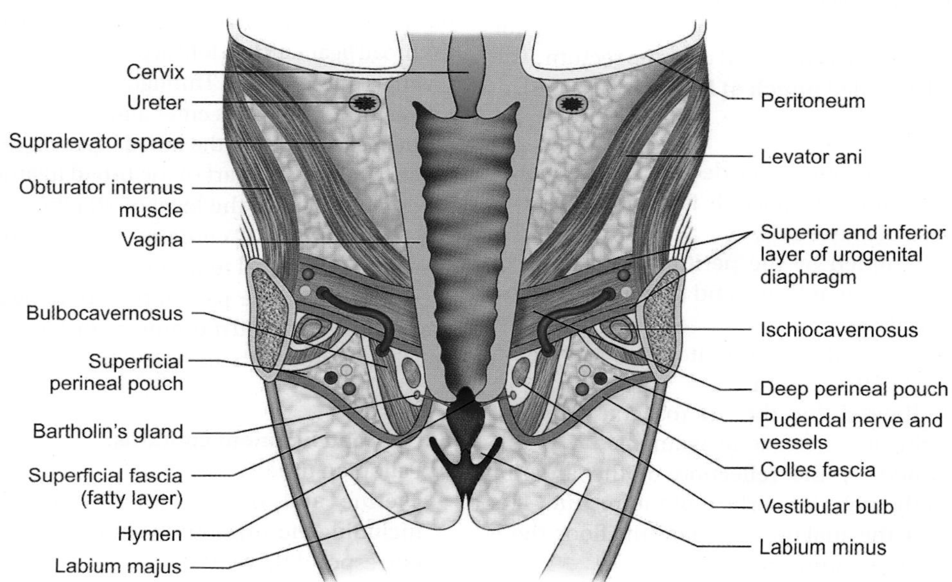

Fig. 1.21: Schematic diagram showing pelvic muscles, fascia and cellular tissue as seen from the front.

OBSTETRICAL PERINEUM

(SYN: PERINEAL BODY, CENTRAL POINT OF PERINEUM)

The pyramidal-shaped tissue where the pelvic floor and the perineal muscles and fascia meet in between the vaginal and the anal canal is called the obstetrical perineum. It measures about 4 cm × 4 cm (1½") with the base covered by the perineal skin and the apex is pointed and is continuous with the rectovaginal septum.

The Musculofascial Structures Involved

- *Fascia:* (a) Two layers of superficial perineal fascia—superficial fatty layer and deeper layer called Colles fascia; (b) Inferior and superior layers of urogenital diaphragm, together called triangular ligament.
- *Muscles:* (a) Superficial and deep transverse perinei (paired); (b) Bulbospongiosus; (c) Levator ani—pubococcygeus part (paired) situated at the junction of the upper two-third and lower one-third of the vagina; (d) Sphincter ani externus (few fibers).

Importance

- It helps to support the levator ani which is placed above it.
- By supporting the posterior vaginal wall, it indirectly supports the anterior vaginal wall, bladder and the uterus.
- It is vulnerable to injury during childbirth.
- Deliberate cutting of the structures during delivery is called episiotomy.

PELVIC PERITONEUM

Traced anteriorly, the peritoneum covering the superior surface of the bladder reflects over the anterior surface of the uterus at the level of the internal os. The pouch, so formed, is called **uterovesical pouch**. The peritoneum, thereafter, is firmly attached to the anterior and posterior walls of the uterus and upper one-third of the posterior vaginal wall where from it is reflected over the rectum. The pouch, so formed, is called **pouch of Douglas** (Fig. 1.6).

Pouch of Douglas

This is a narrow peritoneal cul-de-sac in the pelvis situated in the rectouterine space. It is continuous with the pararectal fossa of either side.

Anteriorly, it is bounded by the peritoneal covering of the cervix, posterior vaginal fornix and upper-third of the posterior vaginal wall.

Posteriorly, it is bounded by the peritoneal covering on the anterior surface of the rectum.

Laterally, it is limited by the uterosacral folds of peritoneum covering the uterosacral ligaments.

The floor is formed by the reflection of the anterior peritoneum onto the anterior surface of the rectum. It is about 6–7 cm above the anal orifice. Below the floor, there is a thin fibrous tissue septum (rectovaginal).

Contents: It may remain empty but may contain coils of intestine or omentum.

Surgical Importance

- As it is the most dependent part of the peritoneal cavity, intraperitoneal blood or pus usually settles down to the pouch to produce either pelvic hematocele or pelvic abscess.
- Herniation of the pouch through the posterior fornix may occur producing the clinical entity of enterocele.
- Vaginal ligation is done through opening the pouch.
- Culdoscopy, culdocentesis or at time pneumoperitoneum may be done through the pouch.
- Nodules deposited in the pouch can help in the clinical diagnosis of pelvic malignancy, endometriosis or genital tuberculosis.

BROAD LIGAMENT

The double fold of peritoneum which extends from the lateral border of the uterus to the lateral pelvic wall of pelvis is called broad ligament. These are two, one on each side. These, truly are not ligaments (Fig. 1.13).

Each broad ligament consists of two layers, anterior and posterior. The layers are continuous at its upper free border embracing the fallopian tube. The lower part of the broad ligament is wider from before backwards and the layers are reflected above the pelvic diaphragm. The anterior leaf is reflected forwards at the level of the internal os as uterovesical pouch. The posterior leaf descends a little down to cover the upper-third of the posterior vaginal wall to form the posterior layer of the pouch of Douglas.

Parts of Broad Ligament

Infundibulopelvic ligament (Syn: Suspensory ligament of the ovary): It includes the portion of the broad ligament which extends from the infundibulum of the fallopian tube to the lateral pelvic wall. It contains ovarian vessels and nerves and lymphatics from the ovary, fallopian tube, and body of the uterus.

Mesovarium: The ovary is attached to the posterior layer of the broad ligament by a fold of peritoneum called mesovarium (ovarian mesentery). Through this fold, ovarian vessels, nerves, and lymphatics enter and leave the hilum. The ovary is not enclosed within the broad ligament (Fig. 1.13).

Mesosalpinx: The part of the broad ligament between the fallopian tube and the level of attachment of the ovary is the mesosalpinx. It contains utero-ovarian anastomotic vessels and vestigial remnants (Fig. 1.13).

Mesometrium: The part of the broad ligament below the mesosalpinx is called mesometrium. It is the longest portion which is related with the lateral border of the uterus.

Contents

Each broad ligament contains:

- Fallopian tube.
- Uterine and ovarian arteries with their branches, including the anastomotic branches between them and corresponding veins.
- Nerves and lymphatics from the uterus, fallopian tube, and ovary.

- Proximal part of the round ligament which raises a peritoneal fold on the anterior leaf.
- Ovarian ligament which raises a peritoneal fold on the posterior leaf.
- Parametrium containing loose areolar tissue and fat. The terminal part of the ureter, uterine artery, paracervical nerve, and lymphatic plexus are lying at the base of the broad ligament.
- Vestigial structures, such as duct of Gartner, epoophoron, and paroophoron.

Development

The broad transverse fold which is established as the two Müllerian ducts approach each other is developed into broad ligament.

Function

Along with the loose areolar tissue (packing material), it has got steadying effect to maintain the uterus in position.

PELVIC FASCIA AND CELLULAR TISSUE

PELVIC FASCIA

For descriptive purpose, the pelvic fascia is grouped under the heading that covers the pelvic wall, the pelvic floor, and the pelvic viscera.

Fascia on the Pelvic Wall

The fascia is very tough and membranous. It covers the obturator internus and pyriformis and gets attached to the margins of the bone. The pelvic nerves lie external to the fascia but the vessels lie internal to it.

Fascia on the Pelvic Floor

The fascia is not tough but loose. The superior and the inferior surfaces are covered by the parietal layer of the pelvic fascia which runs down from the white line to merge with the visceral layer of the pelvic fascia covering the anal canal (Fig. 1.21).

Fascia Covering the Pelvic Viscera

The fascia is not condensed and often contains loose areolar tissue to allow distension of the organs.

PELVIC CELLULAR TISSUE

The cellular tissue lies between the pelvic peritoneum and the pelvic floor, and fills up all the available empty spaces. It contains fatty and connective tissues and unstriped muscle fibers. **Collectively, it is known as endopelvic fascia.** Its distribution round the vaginal vault, supravaginal part of the cervix and into the layers of the broad ligament is called **parametrium**. Condensation occurs especially near the cervicovaginal junction to form ligaments, which extend from the viscera to the pelvic walls on either side. **The deep endopelvic connective tissue condenses to form:** (a) Uterosacral ligaments; (b) Cardinal ligaments; (c) Pubocervical ligament; (d) Rectovaginal septum; (e) Pubovesical fascia.

MACKENRODT'S LIGAMENTS (SYN: CARDINAL LIGAMENT, TRANSVERSE CERVICAL)

Origin: Condensation of parietal fascia covering the obturator internus.

Insertion: Lateral supravaginal cervix and upper part of lateral vaginal wall in a fan-shaped manner. This insertion is continuous with the endopelvic and pericervical fascial ring.

Content: Uterosacral plexus of autonomic nerves, uterine artery, and vein, smooth muscle fiber. **Distal part of ureter passes under the uterine artery within the upper part of the cardinal ligament.** It is situated inferior to the uterosacral ligament with which it is blended (Fig. 1.22).

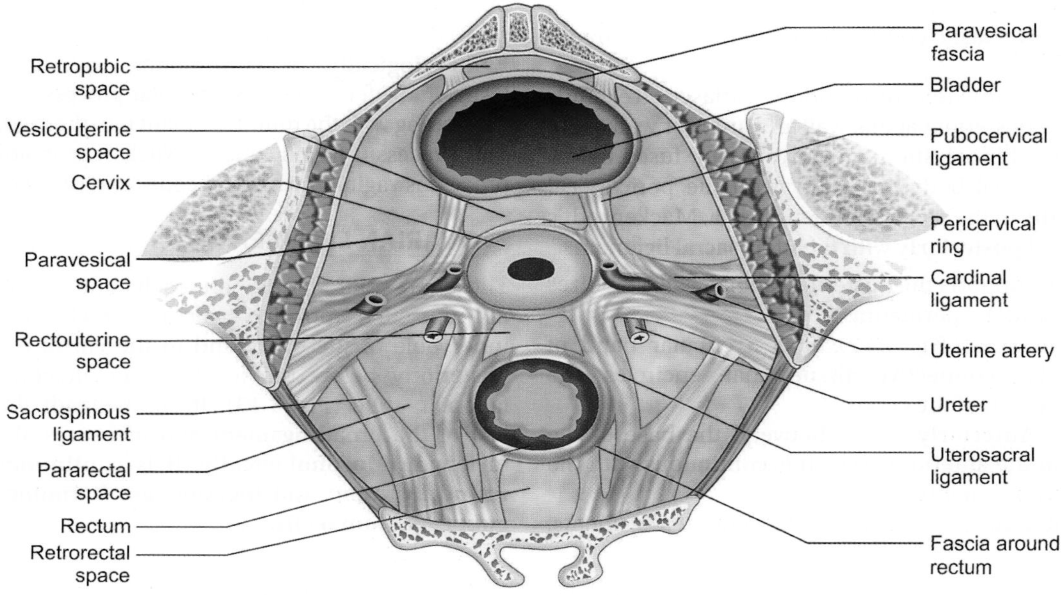

Fig. 1.22: The main supporting ligaments of the uterus viewed from above.

Function: (a) Lateral stabilization to the cervix at the level of ischial spine; (b) Primary vascular conduits of the uterus and vagina.

UTEROSACRAL LIGAMENTS

Origin: Periosteum of sacral vertebra 2, 3, and 4.
Insertion: Posterolateral surface of the cervix at the level of internal os. Here it blends with the endopelvic fascial ring. These are formed by condensation of peritoneum.
Content: Uterosacral plexus of autonomic nerves. Smooth muscle and minimal vessels.
Function: These are the primary proximal suspensory ligaments of the uterovaginal complex. They hold the cervix posteriorly at the level of the ischial spines. Uterus is thus maintained anteflexed and the vagina is suspended over the levator plate.

PUBOCERVICAL FASCIA (BLADDER PILLAR)

Origin: Back of the pubic bone and the arcus tendineus fascia laterally.
Insertion: Anterolateral supravaginal cervix and blends with the pericervical ring of endopelvic fascia and the cardinal ligaments.
Content: Artery and veins of the bladder pillar.
Function: These ligaments are poorly developed. They serve mainly as vascular conduit and provide less cervical stabilization force.
Vesicovaginal septum: It is a fibroelastic connective tissue with some smooth muscle fibers.
Extension: Laterally, it extends from pubic tubercles, pubic arch. Arcus tendineus fascia (white line) and centrally to the pubocervical ring, blending with the pubocervical and cardinal ligaments, and pelvic visceral fascia.
Function: It supports the bladder and the anterior vaginal wall.
Rectovaginal septum (RVS) (Fascia of Denonvilliers'): It is also a fibroelastic connective tissue with few smooth muscle fibers.
Extension: It is an extension of endopelvic fascia. It extends between the posterior vaginal wall and anterior wall of the rectum. This fibroelastic connective tissue fuses **below** with the perineal body, **centrally** with the pericervical ring, **laterally** to the arcus tendineus fascia, Mackenrodt's ligament and **posteriorly** with the uterosacral ligaments.

Function: It supports the posterior vaginal wall, stabilizes the rectum and the perineum.
Pericervical ring (Fig. 1.22): It is a circular band of fibromuscular connective tissue that encircles the supravaginal part of the cervix.
Extension: **Anteriorly**, it lies between the base of the bladder and the anterior cervix. It is continuous with the pubocervical ligaments.
Laterally: It is continuous with the Mackenrodt's ligaments.
Posteriorly: It is located between the posterior surface of the cervix and the rectum behind. It extends posteriorly as the uterosacral ligaments.
Function: It stabilizes the cervix at the level of ischial spines.

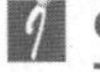

CLINICAL SIGNIFICANCE OF THE PELVIC CELLULAR TISSUE AND THEIR CONDENSATION

- To support the pelvic organs.
- To form protective sheath for the blood vessels and the terminal part of the ureter.
- Infection spreads along the track, so from outside the pelvis to the perinephric region along the ureter, to the buttock along the gluteal vessels, to the thigh along the external iliac vessels and to the groin along the round ligament.
- Marked hypertrophy occurs during pregnancy to widen up the spaces.

ROUND LIGAMENTS

These are paired, one on each side. Each measures about 10–12 cm. It is attached at the cornu of the uterus below and in front of the fallopian tube. It courses beneath the anterior leaf of the broad ligament to reach the internal abdominal ring (Figs 1.11 and 1.15). After traversing through the inguinal canal, it fuses with the subcutaneous tissue of the anterior third of the labium majus. During its course, it runs anterior to obturator artery and lateral to the inferior epigastric artery (Fig. 1.15). It contains plain muscles and connective tissue. It is hypertrophied during pregnancy and in association with fibroid. Near the uterus, it is flat but more distally, it becomes round. It corresponds developmentally to the gubernaculum testis and is morphologically continuous with the ovarian ligament. The blood supply is from the utero-ovarian anastomotic vessels. The lymphatics from the body of the uterus pass along it to reach the inguinal group of nodes. While it is not related to maintain the uterus in anteverted position, but its shortening by operation is utilized to make the uterus anteverted.
Embryologically, it corresponds with gubernaculum testis. In the fetus, there is a tubular process of peritoneum continuing with the round ligament into the inguinal region. This process is called canal of Nuck. It is analogous to the processus vaginalis which precedes to descent of the testis.

OVARIAN LIGAMENTS

These are paired, one on each side. Each one is a fibromuscular cord-like structure which attaches to the inner pole of the ovary and to the cornu of the uterus posteriorly below the level of the attachment of the fallopian tube (Fig. 1.13). It lies beneath the posterior leaf of the broad ligament and measures about 2.5 cm in length. **Morphologically, it is continuous with the round ligament and together are homologous to the gubernaculum testis.**

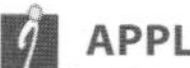

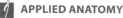

APPLIED ANATOMY

Supports of the uterus and pelvic organ prolapse (p. 166)

Paravaginal defect (p. 177)

Normally, the pubocervical fascia is attached laterally to the arcus tendineus fascia (white line) of the pelvis. Paravaginal defect may be due to:

- Complete detachment of pubocervical fascia from the arcus tendineus fascia.
- Detachment of arcus tendineus fascia from the pelvic side wall. However, pubocervical fascia remains attached to it.
- The arcus tendineus fascia may spit. One part remains attachment to the pelvic side wall while the other part sags down with the attached pubocervical fascia.

Defect in the posterior compartment

Posterior compartment defect (Fig. 1.4A) may be due to any one or a combination of the following five defects as mentioned below:

1. Detachment of the rectovaginal septum (RVS) from the pericervical ring and from the uterosacral ligaments (Figs. 1.4 and 1.22)
2. Break or tear of the RVS in its central or lateral part at the level of midvagina (Fig. 1.4A)
3. Detachment of the RVS from the perineal body (Figs. 1.4A and 1.5)
4. Disruption of the perineal body (Fig. 1.5)
5. Disruption or attenuation of the sphincter anus externus (Fig. 1.18).

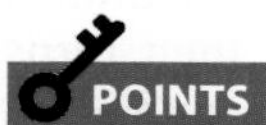

KEY POINTS

- **The labia majora** contain sebaceous, sweat glands, and hair follicles. The labia minora are devoid of fat and do not contain hair follicle.
- **There are four openings in the vestibule**—vaginal orifice, urethral opening, and opening of paired Bartholin's ducts. Rarely, paraurethral ducts open into the vestibule.
- **Bartholin's gland** is situated in the superficial perineal pouch and measures about 0.5 cm. The duct measures 2 cm. The gland is compound racemose and lined by columnar epithelium. The duct is lined by columnar epithelium except near the opening, where it is lined by stratified squamous epithelium.
- The length of the anterior vaginal wall is 7 cm and that of posterior wall is 9 cm. Ureter lies about 2 cm from the lateral fornix. Vagina is lined by stratified squamous epithelium. It has no glands. The pH ranges between 4 and 5.5. Doderlein's bacillus is gram-positive anaerobic organism. The glycogen content is **highest in** the vaginal fornix being 2.5–3 mg%.
- **Uterus measures** 8 cm and weighs 50–80 g. Isthmus is bounded above by the anatomical internal os and below by the histological internal os. Isthmus measures 0.5 cm. Normal length of uterine cavity is 6–7 cm. Uterine artery crosses the ureter anteriorly from above. The epithelium, called endometrium is ciliated columnar type. The glands are simple tubular. There is no submucous layer. Cervical canal is lined by tall columnar epithelium. The cervical glands are compound racemose type.
- **Fallopian tube** has got four parts—interstitial (1 mm diameter), isthmus, ampullary (fertilization takes place), and infundibulum (6 mm diameter). It is lined by ciliated columnar epithelium, secretory nonciliated epithelium, and 'peg' cells. The tube measures 10 cm.
- **Ovary** is attached to the posterior leaf of the broad ligament by the mesovarium. The **ovarian fossa** is related posteriorly to ureter. The cortex is studded with follicular structures and the medulla contains hilus cells which are homologous to the interstitial cells of the testes.
- **Female urethra** measures 4 cm with a diameter of 6 mm. Posterior urethrovesical angle measures 100°. Mucous coat in the upper two-thirds is lined by stratified transitional epithelium and in the distal one-third by stratified squamous epithelium. There is no submucous coat.
- **Pelvic part of the female ureter** measures 13 cm with a diameter of 5 mm. It lies close to the supravaginal part of the cervix (1.5 cm). It is comparatively constricted (i) where it crosses the brim, (ii) where crossed by the uterine artery, and (iii) in the intravesical part. The ureter is likely to be damaged during hysterectomy at the infundibulopelvic ligament, by the side of the cervix, at the vaginal angle and during posterior peritonization. The ureter in the pelvis could be identified by (a) seeing peristalsis after simulation with a surgical instrument and (b) by the plexus of longitudinal blood vessels.
- **Superficial perineal pouch** is formed by the deep layer of the superficial perineal fascia and inferior layer of the urogenital diaphragm. The deep perineal pouch is formed by the inferior and superior layer of the urogenital diaphragm. Obstetrical perineum is the fibromuscular structure, pyramidal-shaped with the base covered by the perineal skin and situated in between the vaginal and anal canal. It measures 4 cm × 4 cm.
- **Pelvic cellular tissues** (endopelvic fascia), ligaments, perineal body, pelvic floor muscles (levator ani), support the pelvic organs and counteracts the downward thrust of increased intra-abdominal pressure. This prevent pelvic organ prolapse (Table 16.1). Functions of levator ani muscle are many (p. 14).
- **Broad ligament** has got four parts—infundibulopelvic ligament, mesovarium, mesosalpinx and mesometrium. Broad ligament contains Fallopian tube, round ligament, ovarian ligament, parametrium, utero-ovarian anastomotic vessels, nerves, lymphatics of the uterus, tubes and ovaries and vestigial structures—duct of Gartner, epoophoron, and paroophoron.
- **Round ligament** measures 10–12 cm. One end is attached to cornu of the uterus and the other end terminates in the anterior third of the labium majus.
- The pelvic diaphragm is the major support to all the pelvic and abdominal viscera. The levator ani muscle is the main part of the pelvic diaphragm.

CHAPTER

2 Blood Vessels, Lymphatic Drainage and Innervation of Pelvic Organs

CHAPTER OUTLINE

PELVIC BLOOD VESSELS

- **Arterial supply**
- **Venous drainage**

ARTERIAL SUPPLY

Sources

- Anterior division of internal iliac artery
- Ovarian artery
- Superior rectal artery.

Internal Iliac Artery

Internal iliac artery is one of the bifurcations of the common iliac artery. **The bifurcation occurs over the sacroiliac articulation.** It measures about 2 cm. Ureter lies anteriorly and the internal iliac vein, posteriorly. It soon divides into anterior and posterior divisions. Only the anterior division supplies the pelvic viscera. The branches are schematically mentioned overleaf (Flowchart 2.1).

Uterine Artery

Origin

The uterine artery arises either directly from the internal iliac artery or in common with the obliterated umbilical artery.

Course (Figs. 1.11 and 1.15)

It runs downwards and forwards along the lateral pelvic wall almost in the same direction as the ureter until it reaches the base of the broad ligament. It then turns medially and crosses the ureter anteriorly from above and at right angle to it; about 1.5–2 cm lateral to, at the level of internal os. On reaching the side of the uterus, it runs upwards and takes a spiral course along the lateral uterine wall between the layers of broad ligament. It ultimately anastomoses end on with the tubal branch of the ovarian artery in the mesosalpinx.

Branches

The following branches are given off:

- Ureteric—as it crosses it
- Descending cervical
- **Circular artery to the cervix:** This is formed by anterior and posterior branches of the artery to the cervix of both sides
- **Segmental arcuate arteries:** These are the branches from the ascending part. These pierce about one-third of the myometrium and then divide into anterior and posterior branches. These anastomose with the corresponding branches of the opposite side in the midline. Thus, the middle of the uterus is comparatively avascular. From the arcuate arteries, a series of radial

Flowchart 2.1: Branches of internal iliac artery.

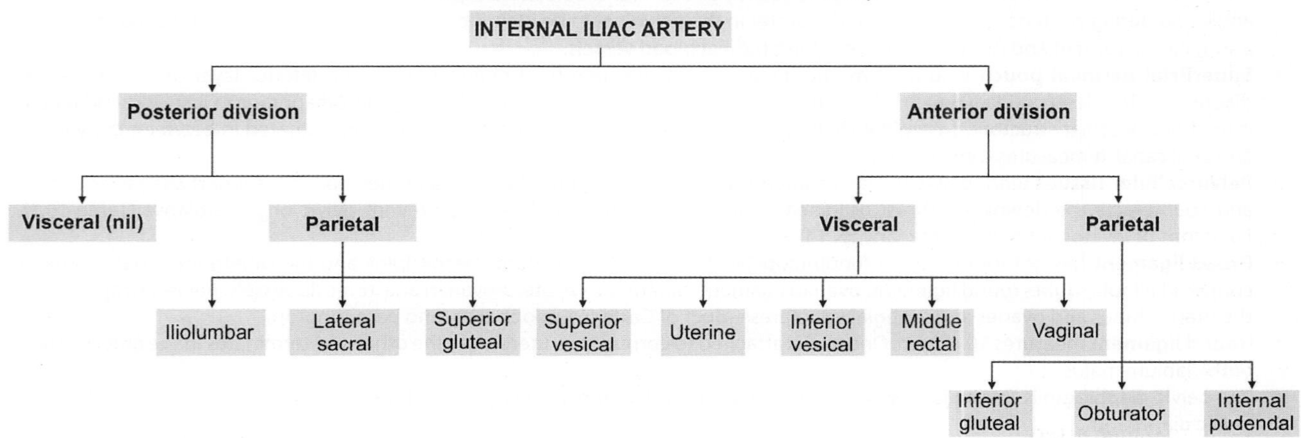

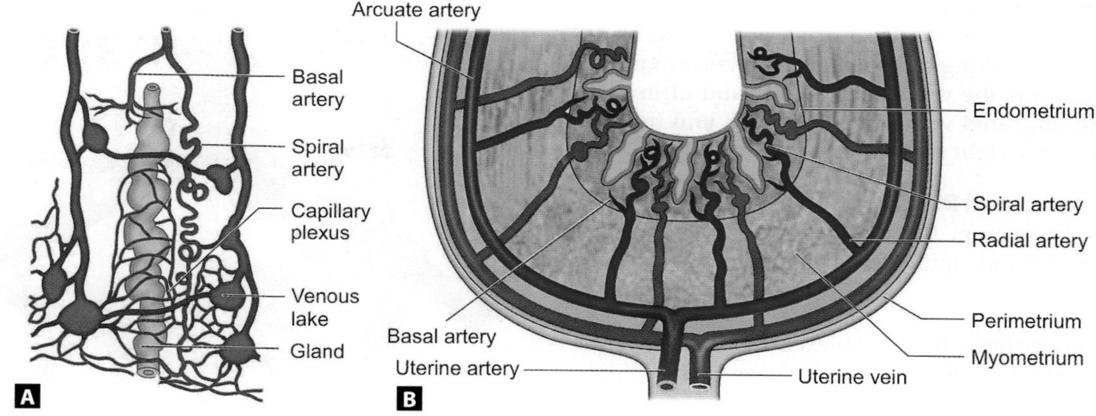

Figs. 2.1A and B: (A) Showing pattern of basal and spiral arteries in the endometrium; (B) Internal blood supply of the uterus.

arteries arise almost at right angles, which stretch through the entire length of the myometrium. Near the myoendometrial junction, the radial arteries are divided into:

- Short basal artery—supplies the basal endometrium.
- Spiral artery which proceeds as far as superficial portion of the endometrium and ends finally in extensive capillary plexuses (Figs. 2.1A and B).

- Fundal branch
- Twigs to round ligament
- Tubal branch
- Ovarian anastomotic branch.

Vaginal Artery

Origin

The vaginal artery arises either from the uterine artery or directly from the anterior division of the internal iliac artery. It is in relation to the lateral fornix and then runs down along the lateral wall of the vagina. Numerous transverse branches are sent off anteriorly and posteriorly, which anastomose with the similar branches of the other side to form azygos arteries of the vagina—one anterior and one posterior.

Other arteries contributing to azygos arteries are:
(a) Descending cervical; (b) Circular artery to the cervix; (c) Inferior vesical; (d) Internal pudendal.

Vesical Arteries

These are variable in number. They supply the bladder and the terminal part of the ureter. Inferior vesical artery supplies the middle-third of vagina and urethra.

Middle Rectal

It arises either directly from the **anterior division of the internal iliac** or in common with inferior vesical artery. It supplies the lower-third of the vagina.

Internal Pudendal Artery

It is one of the parietal branches of the anterior division of the internal iliac artery. It leaves the pelvic cavity along with its vein and pudendal nerve through the greater sciatic foramen and re-enters the ischiorectal fossa to lie in the **pudendal canal (Alcock's canal)** after winding round the ischial spine. Here, it gives off inferior rectal artery. Thereafter, it sends numerous branches to supply the perineal and vulvar structures, including the vestibular bulb and clitoris. The terminal branches of the artery anastomose with superficial and deep pudendal arteries—branches of the femoral artery. This will help in maintaining the blood supply of the bladder when the vesical branch of the internal iliac artery is ligated.

Ovarian Artery

Each ovarian artery arises from the **front of the aorta**, a little below the renal artery. It enters the pelvic cavity after crossing the external iliac vessels. It then runs medially along the **infundibulopelvic ligament to enter the mesovarium**. As it enters the hilum of the ovary, it breaks up into numerous branches to supply the organ.

Branches given to structures other than the ovary are:

- Ureter
- Uterine tube
- Round ligament
- Uterine anastomotic.

Superior Rectal Artery

This artery is a continuation of the **inferior mesenteric artery** and descends down to the base of pelvic mesocolon. It then divides into two and each courses down on either side of the rectum to supply it by numerous branches.

PELVIC VEINS

The peculiarities of the pelvic veins are:

- There is a tendency to form plexuses
- The plexuses anastomose freely with each other
- The veins may not follow the course of the artery
- They have no valves.

Ovarian Veins

The ovarian veins on each side begin from the pampiniform plexus, which lies in between the layers of broad ligament near the mesovarium. Beyond the infundibulopelvic ligament, there are two ovarian veins on each side, which ascend up along the course of the corresponding artery. Higher up, the veins become one and **ultimately drains into left renal vein on the left side and inferior vena cava on the right side.**

Uterus, Vagina and Bladder

Venous drainage from the uterine, vaginal, and vesical plexuses chiefly drain into internal iliac vein.

Rectum

Venous drainage from the rectal plexus drains via superior rectal vein into the inferior mesenteric vein. The middle and inferior rectal veins drain into the internal pudendal vein and thence to the internal iliac vein.

APPLIED ANATOMY

- The free anastomosis between the superior rectal veins of the portal with the middle and inferior rectal veins of the systemic circulation, explains the liver metastases from the genital organ.
- The uterine veins communicate with the vaginal plexus; thus, accounting for vaginal metastases in endometrial carcinoma or choriocarcinoma.
- A free communication between pelvic plexuses with the sacral and lumbar channels of the vertebral venous plexus explains not only the development of vertebral metastases but also explains the intracranial malignant metastases bypassing the lungs through jugular vein. This collateral pathway is also related with supine hypotension syndrome in late pregnancy.

PELVIC LYMPHATICS

The knowledge of the lymphatic channels and the draining lymph nodes from the genital organs is of paramount importance either in inflammatory or especially in malignant diseases. The following groups of nodes are involved:

INGUINAL NODES (FIG. 2.2)

Superficial

There are two groups. One lying horizontally and parallel to the inguinal ligament and the other is placed vertically along the long saphenous vein.

- **Superficial group** receive afferents from gluteal region, anterior abdominal wall below the umbilicus, vulva, perineum, vagina below the hymen, anal canal below the Hilton's line and cornu of the uterus (along the round ligament). The efferents from the superficial inguinal lymph nodes drain into the deep inguinal nodes and external iliac lymph nodes passing through the inguinal canal.
- **Deep inguinal lymph nodes:** These nodes receive afferents from deep femoral vessels, glans clitoris and few from superficial inguinal nodes. They are 5–6 in number and lie on the medial side of the femoral vein. The uppermost gland of this group is called the **gland of Cloquet or the gland of Rosenmüller,** which lies beneath the inguinal ligament in the femoral canal. Efferents from the deep nodes pass through the femoral canal and drain to the **external iliac nodes.**

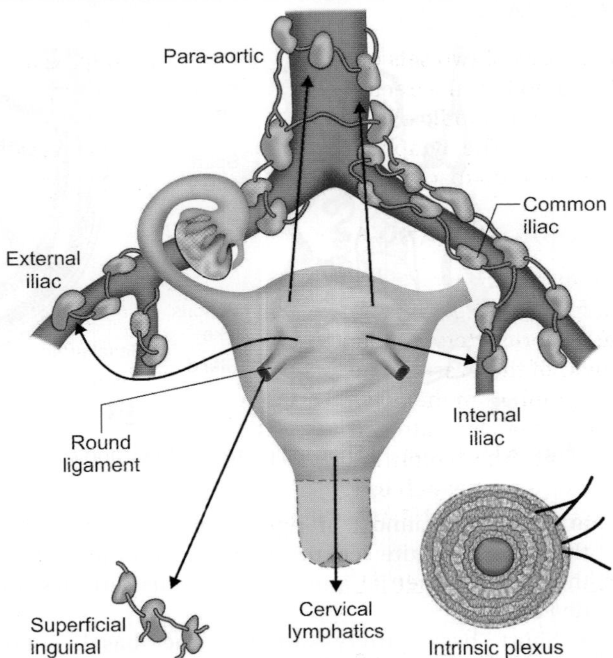

Fig. 2.2: Schematic representation of the lymphatic drainage of the body of uterus.

PARAMETRIAL NODE

It is of small size, inconsistently present in the parametrium near the crossing of the ureter with the uterine artery.

Internal iliac nodes receive afferents from all the pelvic viscera, deeper perineum, and muscles of the thigh and buttock. These glands receive the afferents from the obturator (obturator canal) and the sacral nodes (along the median and lateral sacral vessels).

EXTERNAL ILIAC NODES

There are three groups: (1) Lateral—lateral to external iliac artery; (2) Middle (anterior)—in between the artery and vein; (3) Medial—medial to the vein. These glands receive drainage from the cervix, upper vagina, bladder, lower abdominal wall and from the inguinal nodes. Afferents are from internal iliac, inferior epigastric, circumflex iliac, obturator nodes and parauterine nodes. The efferents ultimately drain into the **common iliac group. In carcinoma cervix, the medial and middle groups are involved.**

Common iliac lymph nodes are arranged in three groups: (1) Lateral; (2) Intermediate; (3) Medial. They receive **afferents** from external and internal iliac nodes and send **efferents** to the lateral aortic nodes.

SACRAL GROUP

It consists of two sets of glands; one lateral group, which lies lateral to the rectum and a medial group lying in front of the middle of the sacrum and medial to the sacral foramina. The lymphatics from these groups pass on either to the subaortic group or to the common iliac group.

SUBAORTIC AND AORTIC NODES

It consists of two sets of glands: (1) Inferior group lies in front of the aorta below the origin of the inferior mesenteric artery; (2) Superior group, which lies near the origin of the ovarian artery. These two groups receive all the lymph from the pelvic organs. Thereafter, it passes up to cisterna chyli situated over the body of 12th thoracic vertebra. The lymph is finally carried upwards via the **thoracic duct which opens into the left subclavian vein at its junction with left internal jugular vein.**

LYMPHATICS OF THE CORPUS (FIG. 2.2)

Intrinsic Plexus

Two plexuses are demonstrated: (1) Basal layer of the endometrium and (2) Subserosal layer. The lymphatics from the basal layer run through the myometrium in close relation to the blood vessels to reach the subserosal plexus.

Extrinsic Drainage

- From the fundus and the adjoining part of the body → along ovarian lymphatics → superior lumbar (para-aortic) group of nodes.
- From the cornu → along the round ligament → superficial inguinal (horizontal group).
- Rest of the body of uterus → external iliac group.
- Adjacent to cervix → into cervical lymphatics.

LYMPHATICS OF THE CERVIX (FIG. 2.3)

The lymphatics from the cervix drain into the following lymph nodes coursing along the uterine veins.

Primary Groups

- Parametrial group—inconsistent
- Internal iliac group
- Obturator group
- External iliac—anterior and medial group
- Sacral group.

Secondary Group

The lymphatics from all the primary groups drain into common iliac and superior lumbar group.

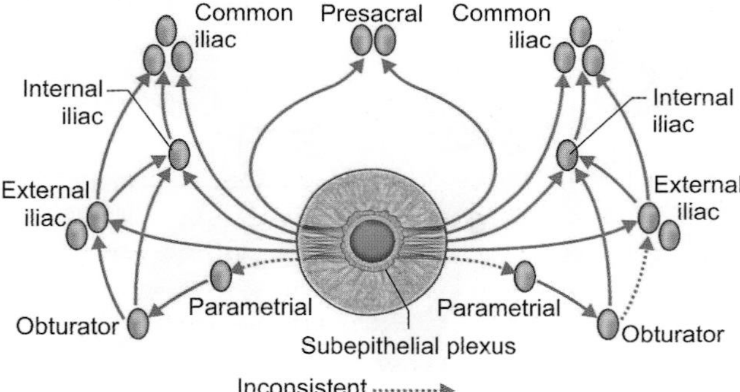

Fig. 2.3: Schematic representation of the lymphatic drainage of the cervix.

LYMPHATICS FROM THE FALLOPIAN TUBE AND OVARY

The intrinsic plexuses of the fallopian tube are situated in the mucosal and subperitoneal layers. The afferents from these plexuses pass up along with ovarian lymphatics to superior lumbar group. There is free anastomosis between the ovarian lymphatics of each side across the uterosacral ligament or via the subperitoneal lymphatic plexus of the fundus of the uterus.

LYMPHATICS OF THE VAGINA

The intrinsic plexuses are situated in the mucosal and muscle layers: (a) Upper two-thirds drain into the nodes like those of the cervix (external iliac, common iliac, internal iliac and obturator nodes); (b) Lower one-third drains into superficial inguinal and at times external iliac nodes; (c) The posterior wall lymphatics anastomose with the rectal lymphatics and drain to the rectal nodes, inferior gluteal and sacral nodes.

LYMPHATICS OF THE VULVA (FIG. 2.4)

There are dense lymphatic plexuses in the dermis of the vulva, which intercommunicate with those of subcutaneous tissue (p. 510).

- The lymphatics of each side freely communicate with each of them.
- The lymphatics hardly cross beyond the labiocrural fold.

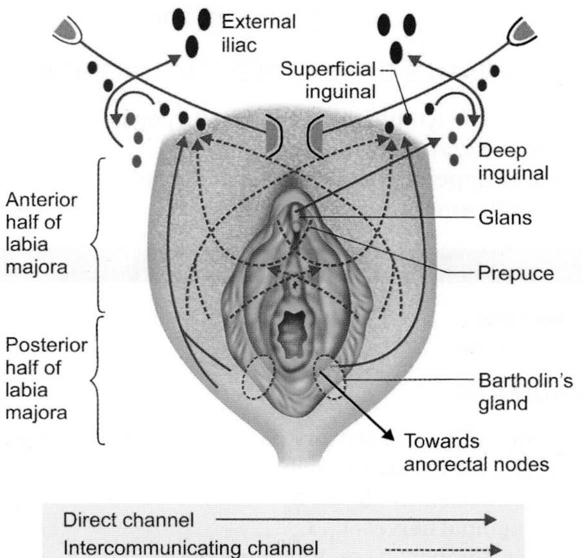

Fig. 2.4: Schematic representation of the vulvar lymphatics.

- The vulvar lymphatics also anastomose with the lymphatics of the lower-third of the vagina and drain into external iliac nodes.
- Lymphatics from the deep tissues of the vulva accompany the internal pudendal vessels to the internal iliac nodes.
- Superficial inguinal lymph nodes are the primary lymph nodes that act as the sentinel nodes of the vulva. Deep inguinal lymph nodes are secondarily involved. It is unusual to find positive pelvic glands without metastatic disease in the inguinal nodes.
- Gland of Cloquet or Rosenmüller, which is the upper most deep femoral nodes is absent in about 50% of cases.

Labia Majora (Anterior Half)

Lymphatics intercommunicate with the opposite side in the region of mons veneris → superficial inguinal nodes. Thus, there is bilateral and contralateral spread of metastasis in malignancy affecting the areas.

Labia Majora (Posterior Half)

Drains into → superficial inguinal → deep inguinal → external iliac.

Labia Minora and Prepuce of Clitoris

Intercommunicating with the lymphatics of the opposite side in the vestibule and drains into superficial inguinal nodes.

Glans of clitoris: Drains directly into the deep inguinal and external iliac nodes.

Bartholin's glands: The lymphatics drain into superficial inguinal and anorectal nodes.

Node of Cloquet: It was previously thought to be the main relay node through which the efferents from the superficial inguinal nodes pass to the external iliac nodes. Recent study shows its insignificant involvement in vulvar malignancy, and thus, it is not considered to be the relay node. The efferents from the superficial inguinal may reach the external iliac group bypassing the node of Cloquet.

LYMPHATICS OF BLADDER AND URETHRA

Bladder: The lymphatics drain into hypogastric group of glands → external iliac.

Urethra: Upper half drains like that of bladder; lower half drains into superficial inguinal node.

PELVIC NERVES

- **Somatic**
- **Autonomic**

SOMATIC

Both the motor and sensory part of the somatic supply to the pelvic organs are through:

- Pudendal nerve—S_2, S_3, S_4
- Ilioinguinal nerve—L_1, L_2
- Genital branch of genitofemoral nerve—L_1, L_2
- Posterior cutaneous nerve of thigh.

Pudendal Nerve

The sensory component supplies the skin of the vulva, external urethral meatus, clitoris, perineum, and lower vagina. The motor fibers supply all the voluntary muscles of the perineal body, levator ani and sphincter ani externus. Levator ani, in addition, receives direct supply from S_3 and S_4 roots.

While the anterior half of vulvar skin is supplied by the ilioinguinal and genital branch of genitofemoral nerves, the posterior part of the vulva, including the perineum is supplied by the posterior cutaneous nerve of thigh.

AUTONOMIC

The autonomic supply is principally from the sympathetic and partly from the parasympathetic systems.

Sympathetic

The sympathetic system carries both the sensory and motor fibers. The motor fibers arise from the segments T_5 and T_6 and the sensory fibers from the segments T_{10} to L_1. The fibers from the preaortic plexus of the sympathetic system are continuous with those of the superior hypogastric plexus. This plexus lies in front of 5th lumbar vertebra and more often wrongly called presacral nerve. While passing over the bifurcation of aorta, it divides into right and left hypogastric nerves. The hypogastric nerve joins the pelvic parasympathetic nerve of the corresponding side and forms the pelvic plexus (right and left) or inferior hypogastric plexus or Frankenhauser plexus (Fig. 2.5).

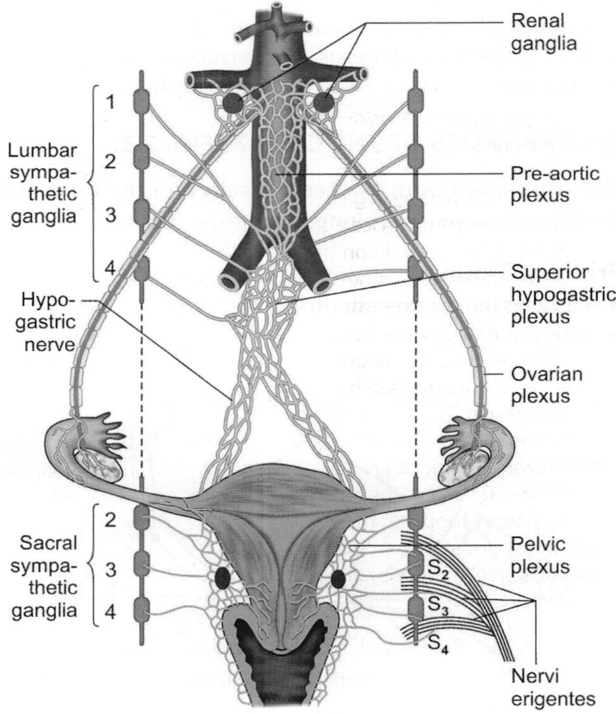

Fig. 2.5: Diagram showing nerve supply of the internal genital organs.

This plexus lies in the loose cellular tissue, posterolateral to the cervix below the uterosacral folds of peritoneum. The pelvic plexus then continues along the course of the uterine artery as paracervical plexus.

- Pelvic parasympathetics: S_2–S_4
- Pelvic sympathetics via hypogastric plexus: T_{11}–T_{12}, L_1
- Via aortic and superior mesenteric plexus: T_9–T_{10} via renal and aortic plexus: T_9–T_{10}

APPLIED ANATOMY

- Epidural analgesia or paracervical block during labor is effective due to blocking of the sensory impulses carried via sympathetic or parasympathetic fibers.
- Presacral neurectomy, although rarely done, either for intractable dysmenorrhea or endometriosis is to divide the sensory impulses carried from the uterus.
- While simple hysterectomy rarely disturbs the paracervical plexus, but the radical hysterectomy does and, in such cases, there may be marked atonicity of the bladder because of the division of the sacral connection of the uterovaginal plexus.
- Myometrium contains both alpha and beta adrenergic and cholinergic receptors. Strong stimulation of the receptors with beta mimetic drugs, such as isoxsuprine will inhibit myometrial activity.

Parasympathetic

The parasympathetic fibers (nervi erigentes) are derived from the S_2, S_3, and S_4 nerves and join the hypogastric nerve of the corresponding side to form pelvic plexus. The fibers are mainly sensory to the cervix. Thus, from the vaginal plexus, the nerve fibers pass on to the uterus, upper-third of vagina, urinary bladder, ureter, and rectum.

OVARIAN PLEXUS

Ovarian plexus is derived from the celiac and renal ganglia. The fibers accompany the ovarian vessels to supply to ovary, fallopian tube and the fundus of the uterus. The sensory supply of the tube and ovary is from T_{10}–T_{12}.

APPLIED ANATOMY

LIGATION OF INTERNAL ILIAC ARTERY AND DEVELOPMENT OF COLLATERAL CIRCULATION IN THE PELVIS

Systemic artery		Internal iliac artery
1. Lumbar (A) →	with	← Iliolumbar
2. Middle sacral (A) →	with	← Lateral sacral
3. Superior rectal (inferior mesenteric artery) (A) →	with	← Middle rectal and inferior rectal artery
4. Ovarian (A) →	with	← Uterine
5. Inferior epigastric (E) →	with	← Obturator
6. Lateral circumflex femoral (F) →	with	← Superior gluteal
7. Medial circumflex femoral (F) →	with	← Inferior gluteal
8. Deep circumflex iliac (E) →	with	← Superior gluteal
9. Vertebral (A)	with	← Iliolumbar
10. Lumbar (A)	with	← Iliolumbar

(A: aorta; E: external iliac; F: femoral)

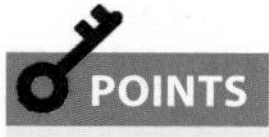

POINTS

- Only the anterior division of the internal iliac artery supplies the pelvic viscera.
- The uterine artery arises either directly from the internal iliac artery or in common with obliterated umbilical artery.
- Vaginal artery arises either from the uterine artery or directly from the anterior division of internal iliac artery. The azygos arteries (two) are formed by vaginal, descending cervical, inferior vesical, and internal pudendal arteries.
- The ovarian artery arises from the aorta below the renal artery. The ovarian veins drain into inferior vena cava on the right side and into the left renal vein on the left side.
- The free anastomosis between the superior rectal veins of the portal, the middle and inferior rectal veins of the systemic system explains the liver metastases from the genital organs.
- The gland of Cloquet lies beneath the inguinal ligament in the femoral canal.
- From the cornu of the uterus, the lymphatics course along the round ligament to superficial inguinal group of glands.
- Levator ani is supplied by pudendal nerve and receives direct supply from S_3 and S_4 nerve roots. Levator ani muscle supports the pelvic viscera and prevents pelvic organ prolapse (p. 166).
- The motor fibers of the sympathetic arise from the segments D_5 and D_6 and the sensory fibers from the segments D_{10}–L_1. The parasympathetic fibers are derived from the S_2, S_3 and S_4 nerves. The sensory supply of the tube and ovary is from D_{10}–D_{12}.
- Myometrium contains both alpha and beta adrenergic and cholinergic receptors.
- The arterial supply of the pelvis has multiple collaterals and numerous anastomosis.
- The development of collateral circulation after ligation of internal iliac artery depends on the site of ligation. The vessels that develop collateral circulation are: (a) Branches from the aorta; (b) Branches from external iliac; and (c) Branches from the femoral arteries (p. 20).

CHAPTER

3 Development of Genital Organs and Gonads

CHAPTER OUTLINE

DEVELOPMENT OF EXTERNAL GENITAL ORGANS

The external genital organs start developing almost simultaneously with the development of the internal genital organs. The site of origin is from the **urogenital sinus** (Fig. 3.1). The endodermal cloaca is divided by a coronally oriented vertical partition, known as **urorectal septum**. The urorectal septum contains a pair of **paramesonephric ducts** close to the midline and a pair of **mesonephric ducts** laterally. The dorsal part of the endodermal cloaca, thus formed, differentiates to form the **rectum and anal canal**. The ventral portion, known as **urogenital sinus**, differentiates into three parts (Fig. 3.3).

1. **Upper vesicourethral part** forms the **mucous membrane of the bladder except the trigonal area**. It also contributes to the major part of **female urethra**.
2. **Middle pelvic part of urogenital sinus:** It receives the united caudal end of the two paramesonephric ducts in the midline. Derivatives of this part differentiates into the epithelium of the vagina, Bartholin's gland, and the hymen.
3. **The lower phallic part of the urogenital sinus:** It is lined by the bilaminar urogenital membrane (see below). It contributes to **vestibule of vagina**.

The site of fusion between the urorectal septum and the cloacal membrane is the **primitive perineal body**.

The part of the cloacal membrane in front of the primitive perineal body is called **urogenital membrane** and the part behind is called **anal membrane**. When the urogenital membrane ruptures, the genital folds do not reunite in female (e.f. male). They persist as **labia minora**. The perineal cleft persists as **vestibule**, into which the urethra and the vagina open. The ectodermal swelling, one on either side and lateral to the genital fold is called **labioscrotal swelling**. Eventually they form the **labia majora**.

The genital folds meet at the cephalic end of the cloacal membrane to form an elevation. This elevation is known as **genital tubercle**, which ultimately differentiates into the **clitoris**.

Development up to this stage is the same in the male and the female [50 mm crown-rump (CR) length, 10 weeks].

If the gonads become ovaries, the external genitalia will attain the female characteristics (Table 3.1).

- **Clitoris** is developed from the genital tubercle.
- **Labia minora** are developed from the genital folds (urogenital membrane).
- **Labia majora** are developed from the genital swellings (labioscrotal swelling).

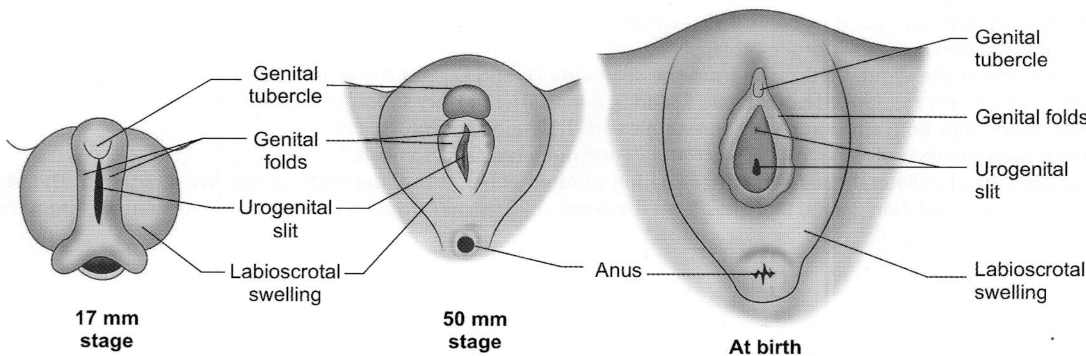

Fig. 3.1: Diagrammatic representation showing differentiation of the female external genitalia.

TABLE 3.1: Male and female derivatives of embryonic urogenital structures.

	Derivatives	
Embryonic structure	***Male***	***Female (Fig. 3.2)***
Labioscrotal swelling	Scrotum	Labia majora
Urogenital folds	Ventral aspect of penis	Labia minora
Genital tubercle	Penis	Clitoris
Urogenital sinus	▪ Urinary bladder ▪ Urethra except navicular fossa ▪ Prostate gland ▪ Prostatic utricle ▪ Bulbourethral glands	▪ Urinary bladder, urethra ▪ Urethral and paraurethral glands ▪ Vagina ▪ Bartholin's glands ▪ Vestibule
Paramesonephric duct (Müllerian duct)	▪ Appendix of testes ▪ Prostatic utricle	Uterus, cervix, fallopian tubes, vagina (muscular wall), hydatid of Morgagni
Mesonephric duct (Wolffian duct)	▪ Duct of epididymis ▪ Vas deferens and seminal vesicles, part of bladder, prostatic urethra	▪ Duct of epoophoron ▪ Gartner's duct, part of bladder and urethra
Mesonephric tubules	▪ Ductuli efferentes ▪ Paradidymis	▪ Epoophoron ▪ Paroophoron
Undifferentiated gonad	Testis	Ovary
Cortex	Seminiferous tubules	Ovarian follicles
Medulla	Rete testis	Rete ovarii
Gubernaculum	Gubernaculum testis	▪ Ovarian ligament ▪ Round ligament
Müllerian tubercle	Seminal colliculus	Hymen

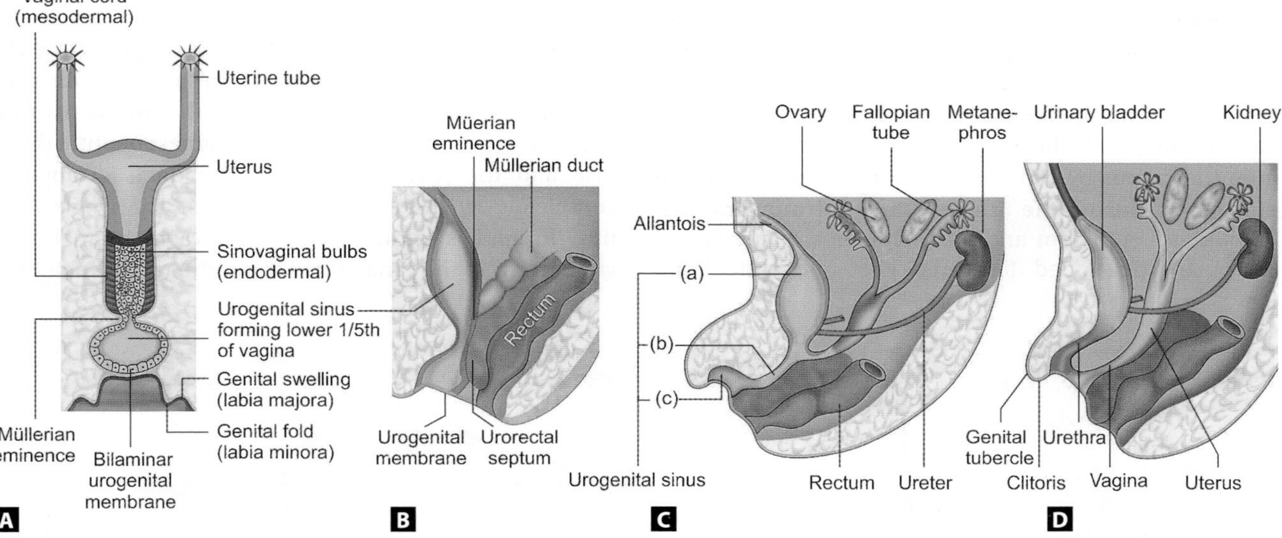

Figs. 3.2A to D: Schematic representation (coronal and sagittal view) of the development of genitourinary system (internal genital organs): (A) Coronal view of paramesonephric ducts, uterovaginal canal, with urogenital sinus, formation of Müllerian eminence; (B) Earliest development of vaginal plate and paramesonephric duct; (C and D) Further development of the paramesonephric ducts and urorectal septum, permanent (metanephric) kidney and urogenital sinus: (a) vesicle, (b) pelvic, and (c) phallic parts and development of urinary bladder and anorectal canal.

- **The Bartholin's glands** are developed as outgrowths from the caudal part of the urogenital sinus and correspond to the bulbourethral glands of male.
- **The vestibule:** The inferior portion of the pelvic part (Fig. 3.2D) and whole of the phallic part of the urogenital sinus expand to form the **vestibule** of the vagina (at about 5th month). It receives the openings of urethra, the vagina and Bartholin's ducts (Fig. 3.1).

DEVELOPMENT OF INTERNAL GENITAL ORGANS

- **Fallopian tubes**
- **Uterus**
- **Broad ligaments**
- **Vagina**

The major part of the female genital tract develops from the **Müllerian ducts.** The duct forms one on each side as an ingrowth of **coelomic epithelium** in the lateral aspect of mesonephros at about 5–6 weeks (10 mm CR length). The ingrowth forms a groove and then a tube, which goes beneath the surface. While it grows downwards, it has developed three parts—(1) cranial vertical; (2) middle horizontal; and (3) caudal vertical after crossing the Wolffian duct anteriorly. In the absence of **androgen** (testosterone) and **anti-Müllerian hormone (AMH)**, as in a normal female, there is further growth and development of the Müllerian duct system with regression of the Wolffian ducts (Figs. 3.4 and 3.5).

FALLOPIAN TUBES

Fallopian tube is developed from **upper vertical part and the adjoining horizontal part of the Müllerian duct.** The coelomic opening of the duct becomes the **abdominal ostium** (Figs. 3.3 and 3.4).

UTERUS

Uterus is developed by the fusion of the **intermediate horizontal and the adjoining vertical part of the Müllerian ducts**, which begins at 7–8 weeks (22 mm CR length) and completes by 12th week. Cervix is developed from the fused lower vertical parts of the two paramesonephric ducts. The cervix is differentiated from the corpus by 10th week. **The intervening septum disappears during the 5th month of intrauterine life.** The lining epithelium and the glands of the uterus and cervix are developed from the coelomic epithelium. Myometrium and endometrial stroma are developed from the **mesoderm of the paramesonephric ducts** (Figs. 3.2 and 3.3).

BROAD LIGAMENTS

When the Müllerian ducts approach each other in the midline, a broad transverse fold is established. It extends from the lateral side of the fused Müllerian ducts up to the lateral pelvic walls, which is named as broad ligament. All the vestigial remnants of mesonephric tubules, i.e. **epoophoron** (situated above the ovary), **paroophoron** (between ovary and uterus) and the duct, remnant as **Gartner's duct** are found in the broad ligament in the mesosalpinx (Fig. 3.3). **Kobelt's tubules** on the outer set are said to be of pronephric origin.

VAGINA

Development of vagina is composite, partly from the Müllerian (paramesonephric) ducts and partly from the urogenital sinus (Figs. 3.3 and 3.4).

The **paramesonephric ducts** develop at about **sixth week**, as an invagination of coelomic epithelium lateral to each mesonephric (Wolffian) duct. Each paramesonephric duct passes ventral to the corresponding mesonephric duct and then meets its counterpart from the opposite side in the midline (Fig. 3.3). The lower vertical parts of the two paramesonephric (Müllerian) ducts pass caudal wards in the urorectal septum and meet each other. **The cephalic vertical and most of horizontal parts of each paramesonephric duct form the respective fallopian tube. The distal open end forms the abdominal ostium.** The caudal vertical parts of both paramesonephric ducts fuse and the partition between the ducts disappears completely by the end of 12th weeks. The single duct thus formed is known as the uterovaginal canal. The cranial part of the canal forms the entire uterus including

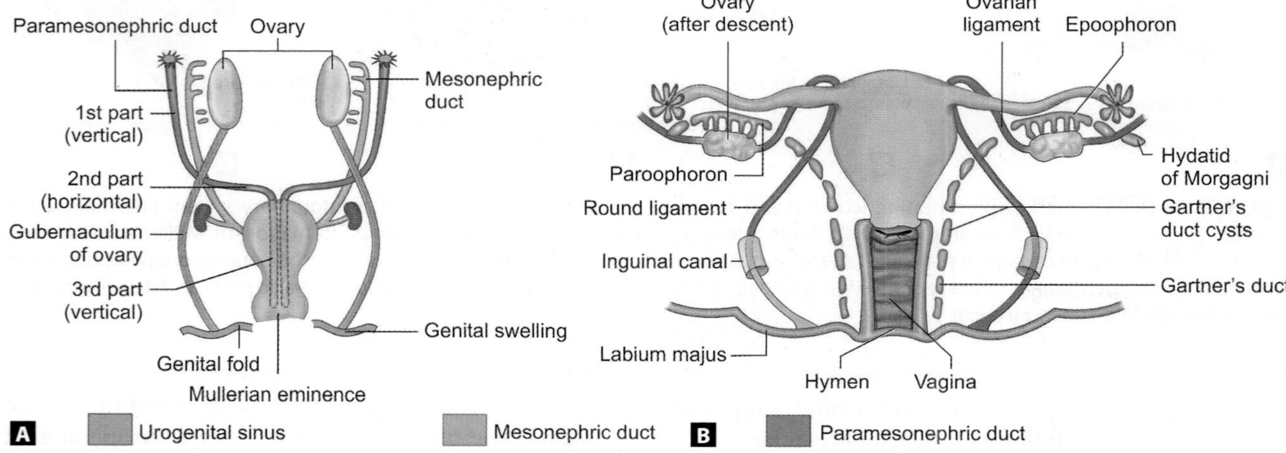

Figs. 3.3A and B: (A) Coronal view of the female gonads, mesonephric and paramesonephric ducts; (B) Differentiation of the different parts of the paramesonephric ducts and regression of the mesonephric ducts in a female, are seen before the descent of the ovary.

the fundus. The endometrium is developed from the paramesonephric ducts. The myometrium and the endometrial stroma are derived from the mesenchyme of the genital cord. Therefore, uterus is entirey mesodermal in origin. Around 9th week, the solid caudal tip of the fused vertical parts of the Müllerian ducts project blindly into the dorsal wall of the urogenital sinus as **Müllerian tubercles (Fig. 3.2A)**.

The united lower vertical parts of the two paramesonephric ducts form the **uterovaginal canal** and the fused Müllerian tubercles form the **Müllerian eminence**.

The endodermal cells from the dorsal wall of the urogenital sinus proliferate and form the **sinovaginal bulb** (Fig. 3.2B). These endodermal cells further proliferate and extend cranially into the central axis to form a solid plate, called **vaginal plate**. This vaginal plate elongates thereby increasing the distance between the urogenital sinus (below) at the cervix (above).

At about 20 weeks the vaginal plate undergoes canalization with the disintegration of the central cells. The upper end of the canal forms the vaginal fornices and communicates with the cervical canal and uterine cavity.

Central cells of the **Müllerian eminence** disintegrate, so that the vaginal canal now opens into the urogenital sinus (Fig. 3.2C). The tissue at the periphery persists as **hymen**. It is lined by sinus epithelium (endodermal origin) on either side with a thin mesoderm in between. Thus, whole of the vagina is lined by endoderm of the urogenital sinus and the muscle in the wall is derived from the mesoderm of the Müllerian ducts.

Finally, the urogenital membrane ruptures and the genital folds persist as the labia minora.

Eventually, the vaginal segment grows and is extended between the paramesonephric derived cervix at the top and the sinus derived vestibule at the bottom.

SUMMARY

Development of female reproductive organs

Fallopian tubes are developed from the cephalic vertical and most of the intermediate horizontal parts of the respective paramesonephric duct.

Uterus is developed from the cephalic part of the uterovaginal canal which is formed by the fusion of the vertical parts of both the paramesonephric ducts. Segments of horizontal parts of the paramesonephric ducts also contribute to the fundus of the uterus.

Vagina

Vagina is developed mainly from the Mullerian ducts and partly from the urogenital sinus.

- **Upper four-fifths:**
  - Mucous membrane is developed from the endoderm of the canalized sinovaginal bulb.
  - Musculature is developed from the mesoderm of the united lower vertical parts of the two paramesonephric ducts.
- **Lower one-fifth (below the hymen)** is developed from the endoderm of the urogenital sinus
- **External vaginal orifice (vaginal introitus)** is developed from the ectoderm of the genital folds after rupture of the bilaminar urogenital membrane.

DEVELOPMENT OF THE OVARY

- Site
- Sources
- Indifferent or primitive gonad
- Definitive gonad
- Descent of the ovary

SITE

The ovary is developed on either side from the genital or gonadal ridge. This ridge is formed in a four-week embryo between the dorsal mesentery (medially) and the mesonephric ridge (laterally) by the multiplication of the coelomic epithelium along with condensation of the underlying mesenchyme (Fig. 3.4).

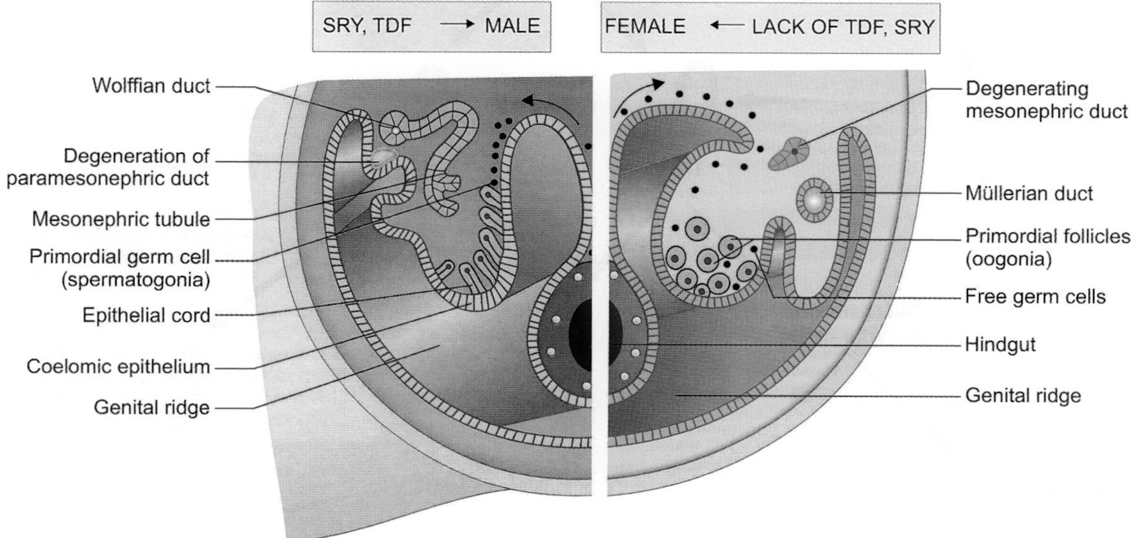

Fig. 3.4: Differentiation of the indifferent gonads into ovary and testis with migration of the germ cells into the genital ridge. (TDF: testicular determining factor, SRY: sex determining region on Y).

SOURCES

The cortex and the covering epithelium are developed from the coelomic epithelium and the medulla from the mesenchyme. **The germ cells are of endodermal origin.** They migrate from the **yolk sac** to the genital ridge along the dorsal mesentery by ameboid movement between 20 and 30 days. The germ cells undergo a number of rapid mitotic divisions and differentiate into oogonia. **The number of oogonia reaches its maximum at 20th week numbering about 7 million.** The mitotic division gradually ceases and the majority enter into the prophase of the first meiotic division and are called **primary oocytes**. These are surrounded by flat cells (granulosa cells) and are called **primordial follicles**. At birth, there is no more mitotic division and all the oogonia are replaced by primary oocytes. **The estimated number at birth is about 2 million (details p. 67).**

INDIFFERENT OR PRIMITIVE GONAD

Initially, the gonads do not acquire male or female morphological characteristics until the **seventh week of development.** Around the time of arrival of germ cells, the coelomic epithelium of the genital ridge proliferates. The irregular cords of cells (primitive sex cords) invaginate the underlying mesenchyme. These cords of cells surround the primordial germ cells and still have connection with the surface epithelium. It is difficult at this stage to differentiate between an ovary and testis.

DEFINITIVE GONAD

In a XX individual, without the active influence of Y chromosome, **the bipotential gonad develops into an ovary about two weeks later than testicular development. SRY gene located on the short arm of Y chromosome directly controls the differentiation of testis from the bipotential gonad.** Apart from SRY, autosomal genes are also essential for differentiation of the gonads. Absence of SRY gene leads to female sex differentiation (Fig. 3.5).

- **Genetic control** is of prime importance for differentiation of bipotential gonad. Genes that regulate the process are: Wilms' tumor gene (WTI), FTZI and SRY.
- **Second gene** involved in development of testis is SOX9 and anti-Müllerian hormone (produced by Sertoli cells). DAXI gene expression is involved in ovarian differentiation. DAXI antagonizes the action of SRY gene.

The surface becomes thicker and continues to proliferate extensively. It sends down secondary cords of cells into the mesenchyme (cortical cords), but unlike testis, maintains connection with the surface epithelium. In the fourth month, these cords split into clusters of cells, which surround the germ cells.

The germ cells will be the future oogonia and the epithelial cells will be the future **granulosa cells**. From 20th week, the oocytes that are not surrounded by the granulosa cell envelope, are destroyed. The stromal mesenchymal cells also surround the follicular structure to form the future theca cells. Thus, a basic unit of a follicle is completed.

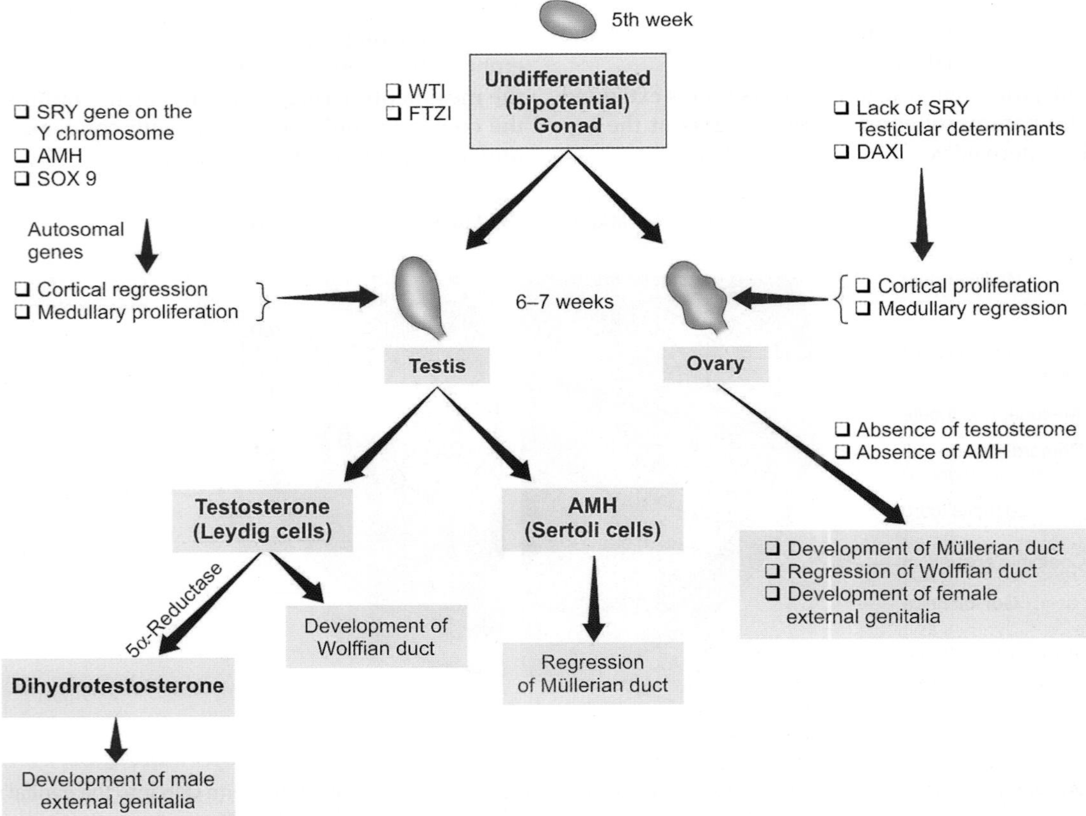

Fig. 3.5: Schematic representation of the development of the reproductive system in the male and female.

By 28th week, number of these follicles are exposed to maternal gonadotropin and undergo various degrees of maturation (little short of antrum formation) and atresia. Anti-Müllerian hormone (AMH) is produced by the Sertoli cells. In the absence of AMH paramesonephric ducts develop and mesonephric duct systems are suppressed.

DESCENT OF THE OVARY

The cranial part of the genital ridge becomes the infundibulopelvic ligament (Fig. 3.3). From the lower pole of the ovary, genital ligament (gubernaculum) is formed, which is attached to the genital swelling (labial). Gubernaculum is a fibromuscular band. The genital ligament gets an intermediate attachment as it comes close to Müllerian ducts (angle of the developing uterus). The part between **the ovary and the Müllerian attachment is the ovarian ligament and the part between the cornu of the uterus to the end is the round ligament. The ovaries descend during the seventh to ninth months, and at birth, they are situated at the pelvic brim**.

DEVELOPMENTAL ANOMALIES OF FEMALE REPRODUCTIVE ORGANS

Imperforate hymen: This is due to failure of disintegration of the central cells of Müllerian eminence.

Congenital agenesis of vagina: This is due to failure of canalization of the sinovaginal bulbs.

Congenital vesicovaginal or rectovaginal fistula: Rarely, the Müllerian eminence ruptures in the vesico-urethral part of the cloaca, instead of the urogenital sinus. This results in congenital vesicovaginal fistula.

Similarly, the Müllerian eminence at times projects into the rectal segment of the cloaca due to incomplete development of the urorectal septum. This result in recto-vaginal fistula.

Septate vagina: This is due to the failure of resorption of the median partition in the caudal part of the uterovaginal canal.

Transverse vaginal septa: Failure of the complete disintegration of the central cells of the sinovaginal bulb.

Uterus didelphys: This is due to the complete failure of fusion of the paramesonephric ducts. This is clinically manifested by double uterus, double cervix and double vaginal canals.

Uterus bicornis bicollis: It clinically presents with double uterus, double cervix and single vagina. There is due to failure of resorption of the partition from the upper part of the uterovaginal canal.

Septate uterus: A septum divides the uterine cavity into the two parts. This is due failure resorption of the partition in the upper part of uterovaginal canal.

Subseptate uterus: This is similar to septate uterus but the partition extents from the fundus partly and is incomplete.

Arcuate uterus: The fundus is concave otherwise the uterus is normal.

Unicornuate uterus: This is due to unilateral suppression of a paramesonephric duct.

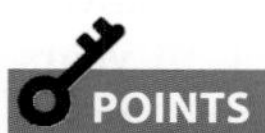

POINTS

- The external genital organs start developing almost simultaneously with the development of the internal genital organs.
- Clitoris is developed from the genital tubercle, labia minora from the genital folds and labia majora from the genital swellings.
- Bartholin's glands are developed from the caudal part of the urogenital sinus.
- Major part of the vagina is developed from urogenital sinus.
- SRY (sex-determining region of the Y chromosome) gene directly controls the testicular differentiation from the bipotential gonad. SRY gene encodes the testicular determining factor (TDF), which induces the differentiation. Testicular development is an active event whereas ovarian development is a default pathway due to absent SRY gene.
- An individual with absent SRY gene, though the chromosomal complement is 46, XY, the gonadoductal development is towards female (XY gonadal dysgenesis).
- The ovary is developed from the gonadal ridge. The cortex and the covering epithelium are developed from the coelomic epithelium and the medulla from the mesenchyme. The germ cells are endodermal in origin and migrate from the yolk sac to the genital ridge. The number of oogonia reaches its maximum at 20th week numbering about 7 million. The estimated number at birth is about 2 million.
- Two functional X chromosomes are necessary for optimal development of the ovary.
- **The bipotential gonad** develops into an ovary about two weeks later than the testicular development.
- The cranial end of the genital ridge becomes the infundibulopelvic ligament.
- The ovary is developed from the middle part of the genital ridge.
- The part of the gubernaculum (genital ligament) between the lower pole of the ovary and the Müllerian attachment is the ovarian ligament. The part between the cornu of the uterus (Müllerian attachment) to the end (external genitalia) is the round ligament.
- The ovaries descend during seventh to ninth months, and at birth, they are situated at the pelvic brim.
- **The paramesonephric duct** in female differentiates into fallopian tube, uterus, and cervix. The **mesonephric duct** in male gives rise to epididymis, vas deferens and seminal vesicles. The sinovaginal bulbs, which grow out from the posterior aspect of the urogenital sinus, differentiates into vagina. The genital tubercle differentiates into clitoris (female) or penis (male). The urinary bladder develops from the urogenital sinus.
- Urinary bladder develops from the upper vesicourethral part of the urogenital sinus except the trigone.
- A cyst of the vagina, especially on the anterolateral vaginal wall, is usually Gartner's duct cyst (embryonic cyst).
- Adult kidney develops from the metanephros, and its collecting system (ureter and calyceal system) from the ureteric bud of the mesonephric duct.

CHAPTER

4 Congenital Malformation of Female Genital Organs

CHAPTER OUTLINE

- Developmental Anomalies of the External Genitalia
- Vaginal Abnormalities
- Uterine Anomalies
- Other Abnormalities

INTRODUCTION

From the embryological considerations, the following facts can be deduced:

- Developmental anomalies of the external genitalia along with ambiguity of sex are **usually genetic in origin**.
- Major anatomic defect of the genital tract is usually associated with **urinary tract abnormality (40%), skeletal malformation (12%)**, and **normal gonadal function**.
- While minor abnormality escapes attention, it is the moderate or severe form, which will produce gynecologic and obstetric problem.

DEVELOPMENTAL ANOMALIES OF THE EXTERNAL GENITALIA

PERINEAL OR VESTIBULAR ANUS

The entity is detected at birth. The usual anal opening site is evidenced by anal pit. The anal opening is situated either close to the posterior end of the vestibule or in the vestibule. Rarely, it is situated in the vagina (congenital rectovaginal fistula). The opening is usually sufficiently big and continence is present. There is no problem in future reproduction. The delivery should be by cesarean section (p. 37).

If there are features of obstruction or the opening is situated high in the vagina, pull-through operation is to be done, bringing the anal end to the anal pit with prior colostomy.

ECTOPIC URETER

The additional ureteric opening is usually in the vestibule close to the urethra or in the vagina. The main symptom is uncontrollable wetness. Partial nephrectomy and ureterectomy may be indicated or implantation of the ectopic ureter into the bladder may be done.

VAGINAL ABNORMALITIES

The significant abnormalities include:

- **Narrow introitus**
- **Hymen abnormality**
- **Septum**
- **Agenesis**
- **Associated abnormalities.**

NARROW INTROITUS

The existence is revealed after marriage. Dyspareunia may be the first complaint, or it may be detected during investigation of infertility. Treatment is effective by manual stretching under general anesthesia or by surgical enlargement (Perineoplasty/Fenton's operation, p. 497).

HYMEN ABNORMALITY

Gross hymenal abnormality of significance is **imperforate hymen.** It is due to failure of disintegration of the central cells of the **Müllerian eminence** that projects into the **urogenital sinus** (p. 34). The existence is almost always unnoticed until the girl attains the age of 14–16 years. Overall incidence is 1 in 1,000 live born females. As the uterus is functioning normally, the menstrual blood is pent up inside the vagina behind the hymen (cryptomenorrhea). Depending upon the amount of blood so accumulated, it first distends the vagina (hematocolpos). The uterus is next involved and the cavity is dilated (hematometra). In the late and neglected cases, the tubes may also be distended after the fimbrial ends are closed by adhesions **(hematosalpinx)** (Fig. 4.1).

Clinical features: The girl is aged about 14–16 years. The chief complaints are periodic lower abdominal pain, which may be continuous, primary amenorrhea and urinary symptoms, such as frequency, dysuria or even retention of urine. In fact, in significant cases the presenting feature may be the retention of urine. **The cause of retention is due to elongation of the urethra** (Fig. 4.1).

Abdominal examination reveals a suprapubic swelling, which may be uterine or full bladder. Prior catheterization reveals the true state.

Vulvar inspection reveals a tense bulging membrane of bluish coloration (Fig. 4.3). In majority, however, it is not the true hymen but the obstructing membrane is a transverse vaginal septum close to the inner aspect of the hymen. Rectal examination reveals the bulged vagina. **Ultrasonography** can make the diagnosis of **hematometra and hematocolpos** (Fig. 4.2).

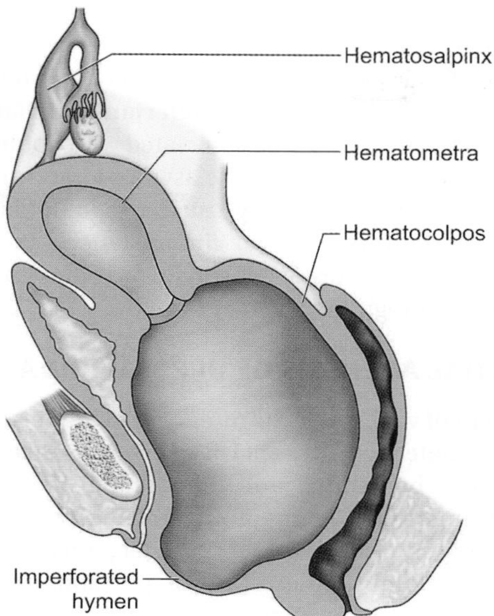

Fig. 4.1: Hematocolpos and hematometra due to imperforate hymen. Note the elongation of the urethra due to distension of the vagina by blood.

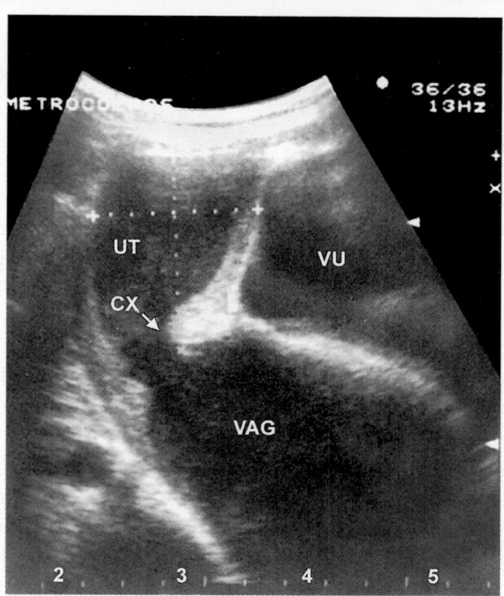

Fig. 4.2: Ultrasonographic view of hematometra and hematocolpos in a girl with imperforate hymen.

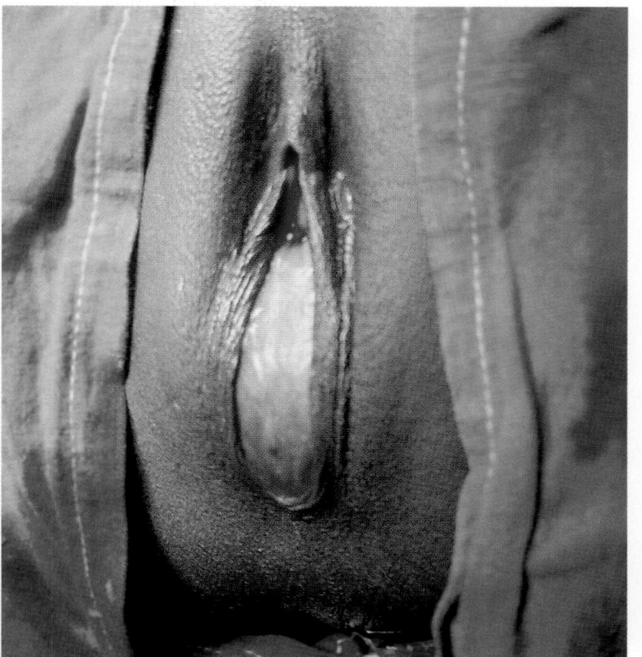

Fig. 4.3: Tense bulging of the hymen in hematocolpos.

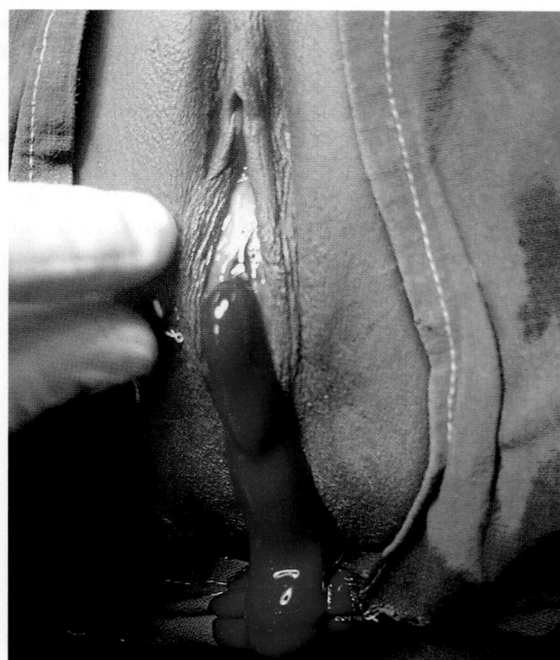

Fig. 4.4: Spontaneous escape of dark tarry blood following incision.

In newborn (usually within one week of birth), accumulated mucus behind the imperforate membrane gives the clinical entity of mucocolpos. The secretion is either from the desquamated vaginal epithelial cells or from the cervical glands.

Treatment: Cruciate incision is made in the hymen. The quadrants of the hymen are partially excised not too close to the vaginal mucosa. Spontaneous escape of dark tarry colored blood is allowed (Fig. 4.4).

Pressure from above should not be given. Internal examination should not be done. The patient is put to bed with the head end raised. Antibiotic should be given. The residual pathology, if any, may be detected by internal examination after the next period is over.

Partial hymenal perforation: This may be microperforation, cribiform, septate or incomplete perforation. Women face the difficulty of inserting a tampoon or sexual activity. Surgical correction is needed to restore the normal hymenal anatomy.

VAGINAL MALDEVELOPMENTS

Common Variations of Vaginal Maldevelopments

- Agenesis of vagina
- Hypoplasia
- Failure of vertical fusion
- Failure of lateral fusion.

Etiological factors for Müllerian malformations are not clearly understood. The probable causes are polygenic, multifactorial, teratogens or environmental.

Pathology of Müllerian Malformation

It may be due to failure of formation of the vaginal plate or due to its failure of canalization or cavitation.

- **Vertical fusion defects** result in failure of fusion of the Müllerian system with urogenital sinus. It may also be due to incomplete or segmental canalization of the vagina.
- **Disorders of lateral fusion** are also due to failure of the two Müllerian ducts to unite. This results in double uterovaginal canals. Such malformation may be obstructive or nonobstructive.
- **Transverse vaginal septa** (Fig. 4.5) are due to faulty fusion or canalization of the urogenital sinus and the Müllerian ducts. **About 45% occur in the upper vagina, 40% in midvagina and 15% in the lower vagina.** Septum located in the lower vagina is often complete and the signs and symptoms are similar to that of imperforate hymen. **Ultrasonography** is a useful investigation to detect hematometra, hematocolpos, and also urinary tract malformations. **The principles of surgical treatment** are the same. Septum in the upper vagina is often perforated. Incision of a complete (imperforate) septum becomes easy when the upper vagina is distended. This reduces the risk of injury to adjacent organs. Otherwise abdominovaginal approach is made.
- **Longitudinal septum** of the vagina may be present when the distal parts of the **Müllerian ducts fail to fuse** (fusion failure). It may be associated with double uterus and double cervix. It may be asymptomatic and needs no treatment. But it may cause dyspareunia or may obstruct delivery. In such circumstances, the septum is to be excised. Results of surgery are good in terms of achieving pregnancy.

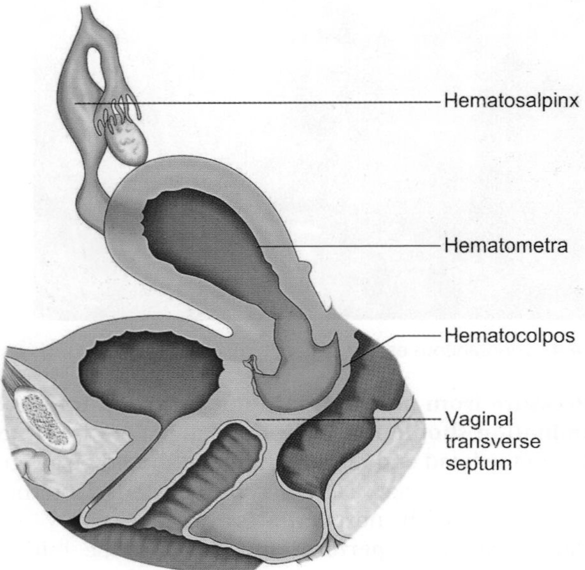

Fig. 4.5 Hematocolpos, hematometra and hematosalpinx are seen due to transverse vaginal septum. Hematometra develops after puberty. Cyclic lower abdominal pain is a common presentation.

PARTIAL AGENESIS OF UPPER VAGINA

A segment of vagina may be atretic in the upper-third. It is often associated with hypoplasia or even absence of cervix. Uterus may be normal and functioning or malformed. Primary amenorrhoea (cryptomenorrhea), hematometra, hematocolpos, cyclic lower abdominal pain and presence of lower abdominal mass (as felt per abdomen or per rectum) point to the diagnosis. Conventional treatment is hysterectomy. Currently, abdominovaginal approach is made to establish communication between the uterovaginal canal above and the newly created vagina below. Prosthesis is used to prevent restenosis. The result is, however, not always satisfactory though successful pregnancy and live birth have been reported. When hysterectomy is considered, ovaries should be conserved. This gives the benefit of endogenous estrogen. Assisted reproductive technology would be the option, when desired, using a surrogate uterus.

Complete Agenesis

Complete agenesis of the vagina is almost always associated with absence of uterus. Some women may have rudimentary uterine horns. Some rudimentary horns are functional as they contain endometrial lining. There is menstruation, and the gonads are the healthy ovaries. The tubes are usually normal. The patient is phenotypically female, with normal female karyotype pattern. **The entity is often associated with urinary tract (40%) and skeletal (12%) malformation. This is called Mayer-Rokitansky-Küster-Hauser syndrome.** The patient usually seeks advice for primary amenorrhea and dyspareunia.

Treatment of such patients need psychological counseling. Often they are depressed concerning their sexual and reproductive life. **Treatment options are:** (1) **Nonsurgical** and (2) **Surgical**.

Objective of treatment is to create a neovagina:

- **Nonsurgical method:** Repeated use of graduated vaginal dilators for a period of 6–12 months. Presence of a vaginal dimple (1 cm) is often seen. This method (Frank, 1938) is a simple and effective one.
- **Surgical methods:** The goal of operation is to create a potential space between the bladder and rectum. Various procedures of vaginal reconstruction (vaginoplasty) are done.
  - **McIndoe-Reed procedure (1938):** A space is created digitally between the bladder and the

rectum. Split thickness skin graft is used over a mold. This mold is kept in this neovaginal space.

- **Williams vulvovaginoplasty (1976):** A vaginal pouch is created from skin flaps of labia majora in the midline. This is not done these days.
- **Vaginoplasty with amnion graft** (Chakraborty, Konar, 2004).

Complications of vaginoplasty: During surgery vesicovaginal fistula (VVF), rectovaginal fistula (RVF), infection, and bleeding are the important ones. Dyspareunia, restenosis are the common late complications.

ASSOCIATED ABNORMALITIES

Associated abnormalities with:

- **Vesicovaginal fistula** is formed when the Müllerian eminence ruptures into the vesicourethral part of the cloaca instead of the pelvic part of the urogenital sinus (Fig. 3.2D).
- **Rectovaginal fistula** when the Müllerian eminence opens in the dorsal segment of the endodermal cloaca.
- **Persistent urogenital sinus** with various irregularities of urethral and vaginal orifices in the sinus.

UTERINE ANOMALIES

Uterine anomalies are often associated with vaginal maldevelopment.

American Society of Reproductive Medicine (ASRM) Classification of Müllerian anomalies (1988) are shown in Figures 4.6A to G:

ASRM Classification

- **Type I:** Segmental hypoplasia or agenesis, involving vagina, cervix, uterus or tubes.
- **Type II:** Unilateral hypoplasia or agenesis.
- **Type III and IV:** Failure of fusion of Müllerian ducts.
- **Type V:** Nonresorption of midline septum.
- **Type VI:** Arcuate uterus (Fig. 4.7F).
- **Type VII:** Anomalies related to in utero diethylstilbestrol (DES) exposure.

Incidence of Müllerian abnormalities: It varies between 3 and 4%. The incidence is found to be high in women suffering from recurrent miscarriage or preterm deliveries (5–20%).

Abnormalities of the Uterus (AFS Classification, 1988)

Category I and II (Figs. 4.6A and B): These abnormalities are due to failure of development (complete or partial) of one or both the Müllerian ducts.

Category III and IV (Figs. 4.6C and D): These anomalies are due to failure of midline fusion (varying degree) of both the ducts.

Category V and VI (Figs. 4.6E and F): These anomalies are due to failure of resorption of the midline septum to a varying degree.

With this classification, associated anomalies of the vagina, cervix, fallopian tubes and urinary system must be documented separately. There are many anomalies that are beyond the common theory of Müllerian development.

Types of fusion anomalies (Figs. 4.6A to G)

- **Arcuate (18%):** The cornual parts of the uterus remains separated. The uterine fundus looks concave with heart-shaped cavity outline—Category-VI (Fig. 4.6F)].
- **Uterus didelphys (8%):** There is complete lack of fusion of the Müllerian ducts with a double uterus,

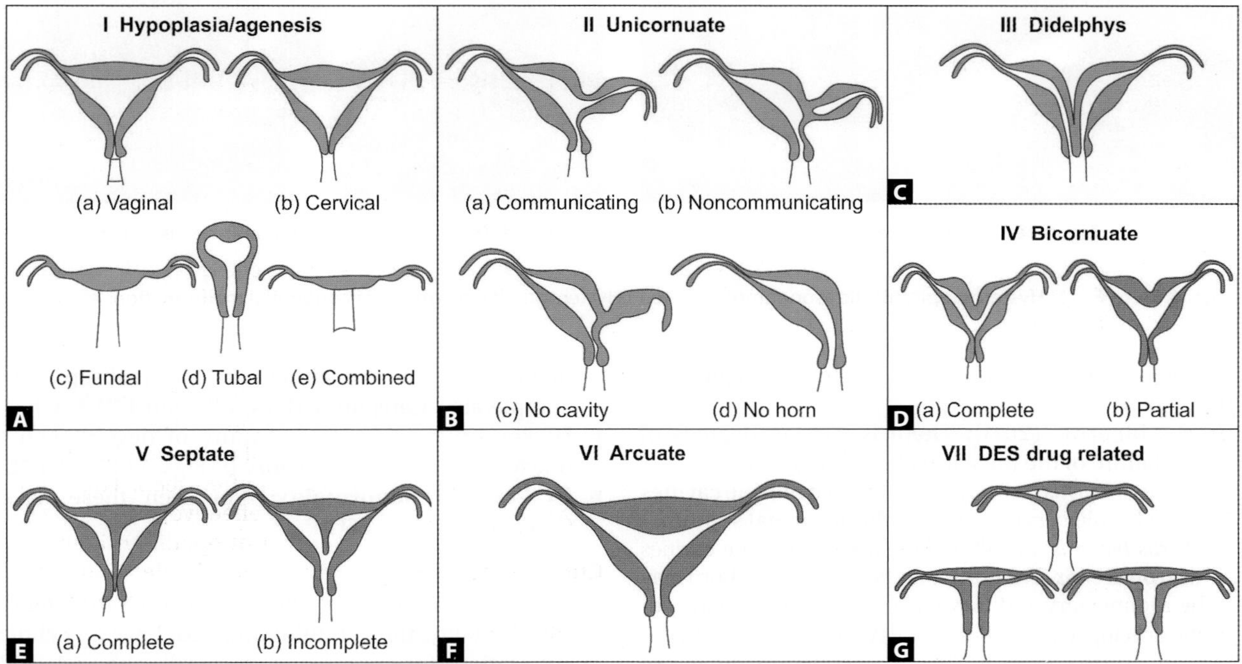

Figs. 4.6A to G: Classification of Müllerian anomalies (Based on classification of American Fertility Society – 1988).

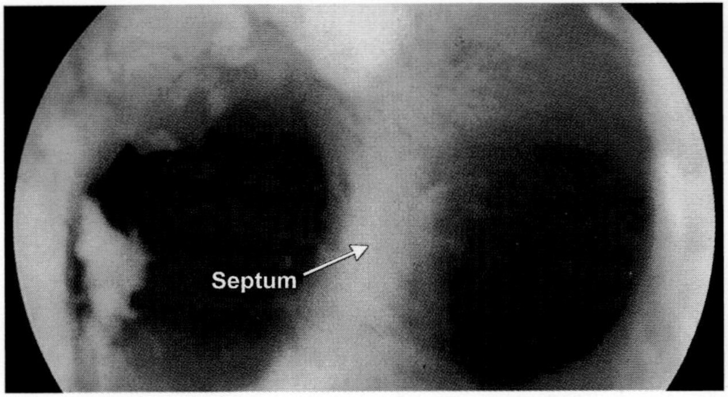

Fig. 4.7A: Hysteroscopic view of a septate uterus.

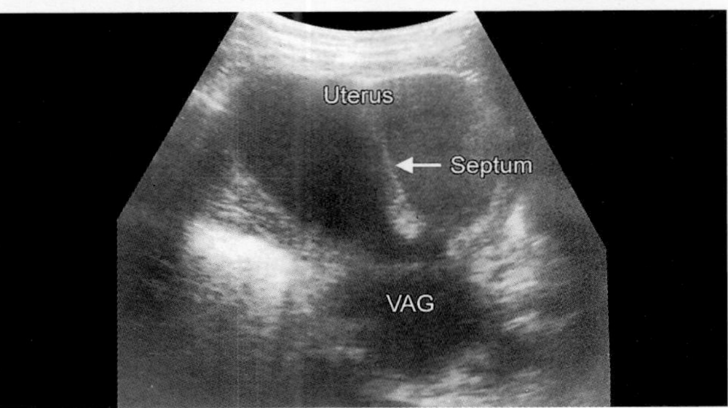

Fig. 4.7B: Ultrasonographic view of a septate uterus.

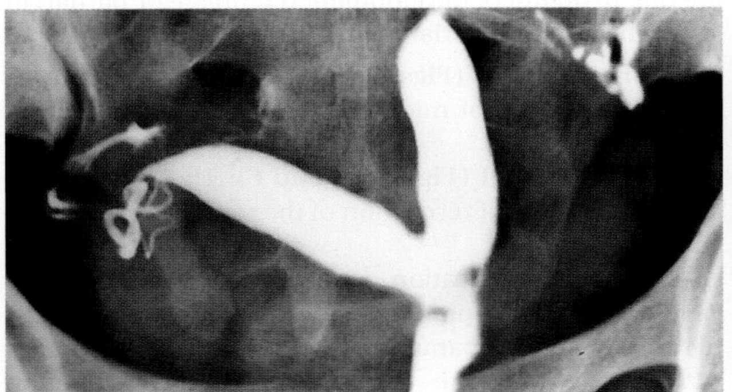

Fig. 4.7C: Hysterographic view of a septate uterus (*Courtesy*: Dr SS Murmu, RMO-clinical tutor, BSMCH).

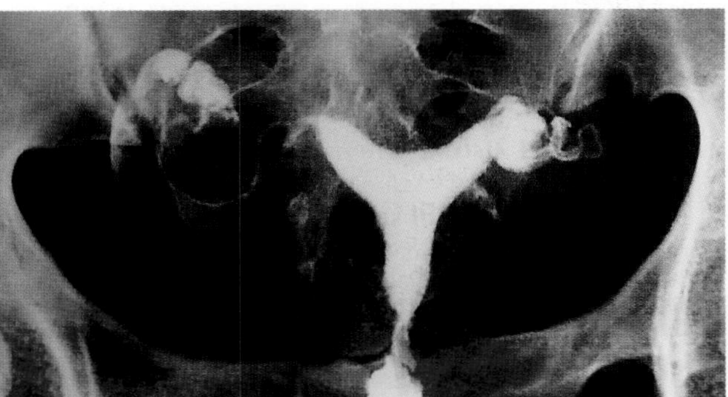

Fig. 4.7D: Hysterographic view of an arcuate uterus confirmed by laparoscopy.

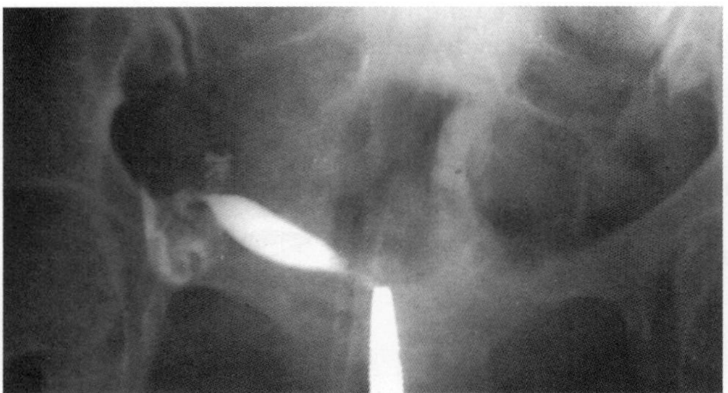

Fig. 4.7E: Unicornuate uterus.

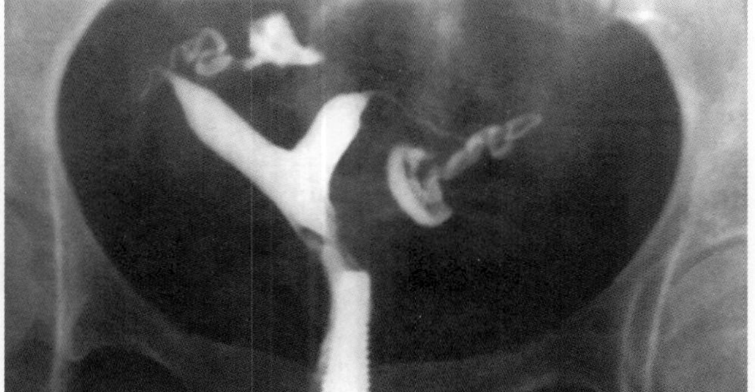

Fig. 4.7F: Bicornuate uterus confirmed by laparoscopy.

Figs. 4.6A to F: (A) Hysteroscopic; (B) Ultrasonographic; (C to F) Hysterographic diagnosis of congenital malformations of uterus.

double cervix and a double vagina—Category III (Fig. 4.6C).

- **Uterus bicornis (26%):** There is varying degrees of fusion failure of the muscle walls of the two ducts.
  - *Uterus bicornis bicollis:* There are two uterine cavities with double cervix with or without vaginal septum.
  - *Uterus bicornis unicollis:* There are two uterine cavities with one cervix. The horns may be equal or one horn may be rudimentary and may have no communication with the developed horn—Category IV (Figs. 4.6D and 4.7F).
- **Septate uterus (35%):** The two Müllerian ducts are fused together but there is persistence of septum in between the two either partially (subseptate) or completely—Category V (Figs. 4.6E and 4.7A to C).
- **Uterus unicornis (10%):** Failure of development of one Müllerian duct—Category II (Figs. 4.6B and 4.7E).
- **DES-related abnormality:** Not seen these days—Category VII (Fig. 4.6G).

Clinical Features

As previously mentioned, depending on the extent of the abnormality, the condition may not have any clinical manifestation (asymptomatic patient). Otherwise she may have many symptoms.

The symptoms are: Amenorrhea due to uterine hypoplasia/aplasia or obstructive anomaly.

Gynecological

- **Infertility and dyspareunia** are often related in association with vaginal septum.
- **Dysmenorrhea**, cyclic or noncyclic pain in bicornuate uterus or due to cryptomenorrhea (pent up menstrual blood in rudimentary horn).
- **Menstrual disorders: Hematometra** retrograde menstruation, cryptomenorrhea and endometriosis or menorrhagia) are seen. Menorrhagia is due to increased surface area in bicornuate uterus and abnormal uterine bleeding (AUB) may be present.

Obstetrical

- **Midtrimester miscarriage** which may be recurrent.
- **Rudimentary horn pregnancy** may occur due to transperitoneal migration of sperm or ovum from the opposite side. Cornual pregnancy (ectopic) inevitably ends in rupture around 16th week.
- **Cervical incompetence**.
- **Increased incidence of malpresentation**—transverse lie in arcuate or subseptate, breech in bicornuate, unicornuate or complete septate uterus.
- **Preterm labor, fetal growth restriction, IUD.**
- **Prolonged labor**—due to incoordinate uterine action.
- **Obstructed labor**—obstruction by the nongravid horn of the bicornuate uterus or rudimentary horn.
- Increased cesarean delivery
- Uterine horn pregnancy may end up with rupture uterus causing an emergency
- **Retained placenta** and **postpartum hemorrhage** where the placenta is implanted over the uterine septum.

Diagnosis

Internal examination reveals septate vagina and two cervices. Passage of a sound can diagnose two separate cavities. In fact, in significant number of cases, the clinical diagnosis is made during uterine curettage, manual removal of placenta or cesarean section. For exact diagnosis of the malformation, internal as well as external architecture of the uterus must be visualized. For this reason several investigations in different combinations are done. Three-dimensional (3D) ultrasonography are helpful in most cases. Other investigations are: **Hysterography, hysteroscopy, laparoscopy, ultrasonography (vaginal probe) (Figs. 4.7A to F). Magnetic resonance imaging (MRI) is the gold standard for the diagnosis of such anomalies (p. 101).** 3D ultrasonography and MRI are noninvasive procedures. Urological tract is also evaluated at the same time. **The renal tract abnormality in association with Müllerian abnormality is about 40%. Skeletal system anomaly (12%) is also associated**.

Treatment

Mere presence of any uterine malformation per se is not an indication of surgical intervention. Women with obstructive anomilies need surgery.

Reproductive outcome: Better obstetric outcome in **septate uterus (86%), bicornuate uterus (50%)** has been mentioned following surgical correction. **Unicornuate uterus has very poor (40%) pregnancy outcome**. No treatment is generally effective. **Uterus didelphys** has best possibility of successful pregnancy (64%). Unification operation is generally not needed. **Other causes of infertility or recurrent fetal loss must be excluded.**

- **Rudimentary horn** should be excised to reduce the risk of ectopic pregnancy (8%).
- **Unification operation (in bicornuate uterus)** is, indicated in otherwise unexplained cases with uterine malformation. Abdominal metroplasty is done by an unification operation (Strassman, Jones, and Jones). Success rate of abdominal metroplasty in terms of live birth is high (85%).

Hysteroscopic metroplasty is more commonly done in cases with septate uterus. Resection of the septum can be done either by a resectoscope by scissors or by laser.

Advantages are: (a) High success rate (80–89%); (b) Short hospital stay; (c) Reduced postoperative morbidity (infection or adhesions); and (d) Subsequent chance of vaginal delivery is high compared to abdominal metroplasty where cesarean section is mandatory.

ABNORMALITIES OF THE FALLOPIAN TUBES

The tubes may be unduly elongated; may have accessory ostia or diverticula. Rarely, the tube may be absent on one side either complete or segmental. These conditions may lower the fertility or favor ectopic pregnancy.

ANOMALIES OF THE OVARIES

There may be **streak gonads** or gonadal dysgenesis, which are usually associated with errors of sex chromosomal pattern. No treatment is of any help. **Accessory ovary** (division of the original ovary into two) may be rarely (1 in 93,000) present. Rarely, **supernumerary ovaries** may be found (1 in 29,000) in the broad ligament, omentum or elsewhere. This can explain a rare event where menstruation continues even after removal of two ovaries.

WOLFFIAN REMNANT ABNORMALITIES

The outer end of the Wolffian (Gartner) duct may be cystic, size of pea, often pedunculated (hydatid of Morgagni) and attached near the outer end of the tube. The tubules of the Gartner's duct may be cystic, the outer ones are Kobelt's tubules, the middle set, the epoophoron and the proximal set, the paroophoron. Small cyst may arise from any of the tubules. **A cystic swelling from the Gartner's duct** may appear in the anterolateral wall of the vagina, which may be confused with cystocele.

PAROVARIAN CYST

It arises from the vestigial remnants of Wolffian tissue situated in the mesosalpinx between the tube and the ovary. This can attain a big size. The cyst is unilocular; the wall is thin and contains clear translucent fluid. The ovarian fimbria with the ovary is stretched over the cyst

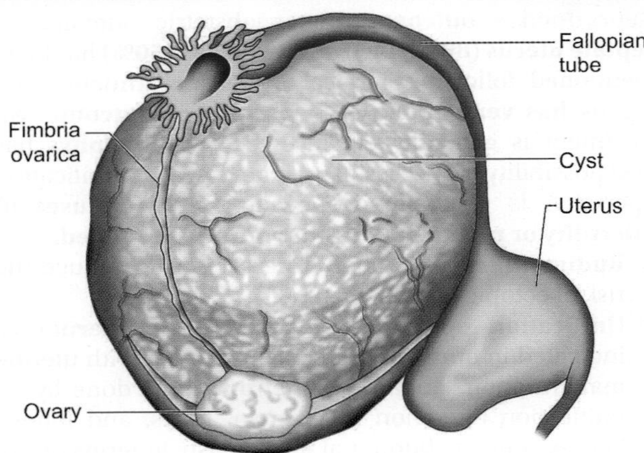

Fig. 4.8: Parovarian cyst.

(Fig. 4.8). The wall consists of connective tissue lined by single layer of low columnar epithelium.

OTHER ABNORMALITIES

- **Labia minora:** Labial fusion—(a) True due to developmental defect; (b) Inflammatory.
- **Labia majora:** (a) Hyperplastic or hypoplastic labia; (b) Abnormal fusion in adrenogenital syndrome (p. 373).
- **Clitoral abnormalities:** Clitoris normally measures 1-1.5 cm. Clitoral anomalies are uncommon. It may be clitoral duplication, bifid clitoris (bladder exstrophy) clitoromegaly, or a phalic utethra. Clitoromegaly (clitoral index >10 mm^2) may be due to intrauterine exposure of excess androgens and often associated with various disorders of sexual development [congenital adrenal hyperplasia (CAH) and androgen insensitivity syndrome (AIS)].
- **Perineum:** Perineum differentiates from the area of contact between the urorectal septum (mesoderm) and the dorsal wall of cloaca (endoderm) at about 7th week. This site of contact between the two is the perineal body. Malformations of the perineum are rare. Imperforate anus, anal stenosis or fistula are the result of abnormal development of the urorectal septum (p. 32). This is due to the posterior deviation of the septum as it approaches the cloacal membrane. Anal agenesis and fistula are rare. **The anal fistula may open into the posterior aspect of the vestibule of the vagina** (anovestibular fistula p. 32).

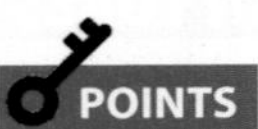
POINTS

- Developmental anomalies of the external genitalia along with ambiguity of sex are usually genetic in origin.
- The clinical features with imperforate hymen usually appear at 14–16 years. Retention of urine may be the first symptom. Cruciate incision of the hymen is the treatment. Major anatomic defect of the genital tract is usually associated with normal gonadal function and urinary tract abnormalities.
- While minor abnormality escapes attention, it is the moderate or severe form which will produce gynecologic and obstetric problems (p. 37). For exact diagnosis of malformation both the internal and external architecture of the uterus must be viewed. Failure of fusion of Müllerian ducts may lead to arcuate, bicornuate, septate or didelphys uterus.
- Gynecological symptoms are pelvic pain, hematometra, dysmenorrhea, endometriosis, abnormal bleeding, but at times, they may produce infertility or obstetric problems, such as recurrent miscarriage, cornual pregnancy, preterm labor, malpresentation, IUGR, or even obstructed labor.
- Presence of uterine malformation per se is not an indication of surgical correction. Unification operation is indicated in otherwise unexplained cases of infertility or repeated pregnancy wastage. Hysteroscopic metroplasty has got many advantages.
- Vaginal agenesis is most commonly due to Mayer-Rokitansky-Küster-Hauser syndrome. In such a case urologic (40%) and skeletal (12%) anomalies are associated. Treatment may be nonsurgical or surgical (p. 34).
- Nearly 15–20% of women with recurrent miscarriage are associated with malformation of the uterus.
- Turner's syndrome is the most common cause of primary amenorrhea and MRKH syndrome is the next common cause.
- Women with septate uterus can be easily treated with hysteroscopic resection. Alternatively the septum can be incised with a scissor or any cutting device. It improves reproductive outcome significantly (86%).

CHAPTER

5 Puberty—Normal and Abnormal

CHAPTER OUTLINE

PUBERTY

DEFINITION

Puberty in girls is the period, which links childhood to adulthood. It is the **period of gradual development of secondary sexual characters.** There are profound biological, morphological, and psychological changes that lead to full sexual maturity and eventually fertility.

MORPHOLOGICAL CHANGES

As described by Tanner and Marshall, **five** important physical changes are evident during puberty. **These are breast, pubic and axillary hair growth, growth in height, and menstruation.** Most of the changes occur gradually but only the menarche can be dated. Moreover, there is a lot of variations in the timing of the events. **The most common order is beginning of the growth spurt → breast budding (thelarche) → pubic and axillary hair growth (adrenarche) → peak growth in height → menstruation (menarche).** All these changes are usually completed between the age of 10 years and 16 years.

Important controlling factors for onset of puberty are genetic, nutrition, body weight, psychologic state, social and cultural background, and exposure to light and others. A girl, living in urban areas with good nutrition, adequate body weight and whose mother and sisters have early menarche, starts puberty early. Blind girls start menarche early.

ENDOCRINOLOGY IN PUBERTY

The levels of gonadal steroids and gonadotropins (FSH, LH) are low until the age of 6–8 years. This is mainly due to the negative feedback effect of estrogen to the hypothalamic pituitary system (gonadostat). The gonadostat remains very sensitive (6–15 times) to the negative feedback effect, even though the level of estradiol is very low (10 pg/mL) during that time. As puberty approaches this negative feedback effect of estrogen is gradually lost. This results in some significant changes in the endocrine function of the girl.

- **Hypothalamopituitary gonadal axis:** The gonadotropin-releasing hormone (GnRH) pulses from hypothalamus results in pulsatile gonadotropin secretion (first during the night then by the day time).

  GnRH → FSH, LH → Estradiol

  The tonic and episodic secretion of gonadotropins in prepubertal period is gradually changed to one of cyclic release in postpubertal period (details in p. 59).
- **Thyroid gland** plays an active role in the hypothalamo-pituitary gonadal axis.
- **Adrenal glands** (adrenarche) increase their activity of sex steroid synthesis [androstenedione, dehydroepiandrosterone (DHA), dehydroepiandrosterone sulfate (DHAS) from about 7 years of age. Increased sebum formation, pubic and axillary hair, and change in voice are primarily due to adrenal androgen production.
- **Gonadarche:** Increased amplitude and frequency of GnRH → ↑ secretion of FSH and LH → ovarian follicular development → ↑ estrogen. Gonadal estrogen is responsible for the development of uterus, vagina, vulva, and also the breasts.
- **Leptin**, a peptide, secreted in the adipose tissue is also involved in pubertal changes and menarche. Leptin is important for feedback involving GnRH and LH pulsatility. Leptin plays a major link between body composition (body fat proportion), H-P-O axis and thus the menstrual cyclicity.
- **Kisspeptin:** It is a hypothalamic hormone. It stimulates the release of GnRH. Kisspeptin is thought to initiate puberty. During puberty, there is accelerated growth, skeletal maturation and epiphyseal closure (p. 42).

Menarche

The onset of first menstruation in life is called menarche. It may occur anywhere between 10 and 16 years, the **peak time being 13 years**. There is endometrial proliferation due to ovarian estrogen but when the level drops temporarily, the endometrium sheds and bleeding is visible. It denotes an intact hypothalamic pituitary-ovarian axis, functioning ovaries, presence of responsive endometrium to the endogenous ovarian steroids and the presence of a patent uterovaginal canal. The **first period is usually anovular**. The ovulation may be irregular for a

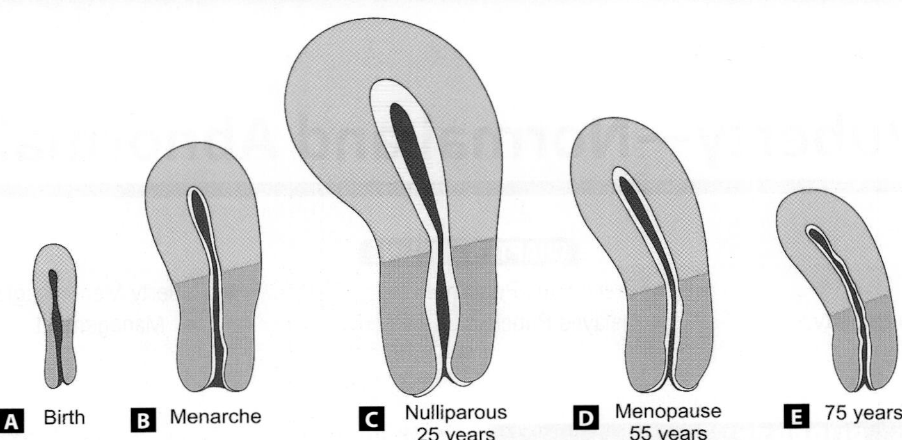

Figs. 5.1A to E: Changes in the size of the uterus from birth to 75 years of age. Note the change in relation of the cervix to the body.

variable period following menarche and may take about 2 years for regular ovulation to occur. The menses may be irregular to start with.

Growth

Growth of height in an adolescent girl is mainly due to hormones. The important hormones are growth hormone, estrogen, and insulin-like growth factor-1 (IGF-1). The bone or skeletal age is determined by X-ray of hand or knee.

Changes in Genital Organs

Ovaries change their shape, the elongated shape becomes bulky and oval. The ovarian bulk is due to follicular enlargement at various stages of development and proliferation of stromal cells.

The uterine body and the cervix ratio at birth is about 1:2, the ratio becomes 1:1 when menarche occurs. Thereafter, the enlargement of the body occurs rapidly, so that the ratio soon becomes 2:1 (Figs. 5.1A to E).

The vaginal changes are more pronounced. A few layers of thin epithelium in a child become stratified epithelium of many layers. The cells are rich in glycogen due to estrogen. Doderlein's bacilli appear which convert glycogen into lactic acid; the vaginal pH becomes acidic, ranging between 4 and 5.

The vulva is more reactive to steroid hormones. **The mons pubis and the labia minora** increase in size.

Breast changes are pronounced. Under the influence of estrogen, there is marked proliferation of duct systems and deposition of fat. The breast becomes prominent and round. Under the influence of progesterone, the development of acini increases considerably.

Tanner Staging

According to Tanner, breast and pubic hair development at puberty are divided into five stages (Table 5.1).

COMMON DISORDERS OF PUBERTY

- Precocious puberty
- Delayed puberty
- Menstrual abnormalities (amenorrhea, menorrhagia, dysmenorrhea)
- Others (infection, neoplasm, hirsutism, etc.), Ch. 33.

PRECOCIOUS PUBERTY

Definition

The term precocious puberty is reserved for girls who exhibit any secondary sex characteristics before the age of 8 (before age 7 in whites) or menstruate before the age of 10.

Precocious puberty may be isosexual where the features are due to excess production of estrogen. It may be heterosexual where features are due to excess production of androgen (from ovarian and adrenal neoplasm).

Precocious puberty is more common in girls (20 times) than boys.

TABLE 5.1: Tanner stages of pubertal development in girls.

Stage	Breast	Pubic hair
Stage I	Prepubertal state, elevation of papilla only	No pubic hair present
Stage II	Breast buds and papilla slightly elevated, areola begins to enlarge (Median age: 9.8 years)	Sparse, long pigmented hair on either side of labia-majora (Median age: 10.5 years)
Stage III	Further enlargement of entire breast tissue	Darker, coarser, and curly hair over the mons pubis
Stage IV	Secondary mound of areola and papilla projecting above the breast tissue (Median age: 12.1 years)	Adult type hair covering the mons only (Median age: 12 years)
Stage V	Areola recessed to general contour of breast (Median age: 14.6 years)	Adult hair with an inverse triangle distribution (female escutcheon) covering the medial thighs (Median age: 13.7 years)

Types or Causes

The causes are tabulated in the Table 5.2.

Etiopathology

Constitutional

It is due to premature activation of hypothalamo-pituitary-ovarian axis. There is secretion of gonadotropins and gonadal steroids due to premature release of GnRH. Bone maturation is accelerated, leading to premature closure of the epiphysis and curtailed stature. If menstruation occurs, they may be ovulatory. The changes in puberty progress in an orderly sequence.

Intracranial Lesions

Meningitis, encephalitis, craniopharyngioma, neurofibroma or any tumor—hypothalamic or pineal gland.

McCune-Albright syndrome is characterized by the features of sexual precocity, multiple cystic bone lesions (polyostotic fibrous dysplasia), endocrinopathies and café-au-lait spots on the skin. Sexual precocity is due to early and excessive estrogen production from the ovaries. McCune–Albright syndrome is due to mutation in G3 protein leading to activation of adenylyl cyclase. There is stimulation of LH, FSH, TSH and GH. First sign is vaginal bleeding. There is life time increased risk of malignancy. There may be associated hyperthyroidism, hyperparathyroidism, and acromegaly. Girls with McCune-Albright syndrome is treated with aromatase inhibitors (anastrozole). Pure estrogen receptor antagonist, fulvestrant, monthly injections have been found helpful.

Premature thelarche

It is the isolated development of breast tissue before the age of 8 and commonly between 2 and 4 years of age. Either one or both the breasts may be enlarged (Fig. 5.2). There is no other feature of precocious puberty. Life-threatening neoplasms of ovary, adrenal gland or central nervous system (CNS) are excluded on priority.

TABLE 5.2: Causes of precocious puberty.

GnRH dependent—80% (complete, central, isosexual or true)	
▪ Constitutional—most common ▪ Primary hypothyroidism ▪ CNS lesions (30%)—trauma, infection (tuberculosis, encephalitis), and some degenerative, neoplastic or congenital defects ▪ **Incomplete** • Premature thelarche • Premature puberche • Premature menarche	
GnRH independent (precocious puberty of peripheral origin) (excess estrogen or androgen)	
Ovary	**Adrenal**
▪ Granulosa cell tumor ▪ Theca cell tumor ▪ Leydig cell tumor ▪ Chorionic epithelioma ▪ Androblastoma ▪ McCune-Albright syndrome	▪ Hyperplasia ▪ Tumor
Liver	
Hepatoblastoma	
Iatrogenic (factitious)	
Estrogen or androgen, combined oral contraceptives (COCs)	

Premature pubarche

Premature pubarche is isolated development of axillary and/or pubic hair prior to the age of 8 without other signs of precocious puberty. The premature hair growth may be due to unusual sensitivity of end organs to the usual low level of hormones in the blood during childhood. Rarely, there may be signs of excess androgen production due to adrenal hyperplasia or tumor or androgenic ovarian tumor (Leydig cell tumor, androblastoma, etc.).

Premature menarche

Premature menarche is an isolated event of cyclic vaginal bleeding without any other signs of secondary sexual development. The cause remains unclear but may be related to unusual endocrine sensitivity of the endometrium to the low level of estrogens.

Chorionic epithelioma, hepatoblastoma are the ectopic sources of human chorionic gonadotropin and may cause sexual precocity.

Diagnosis

Meticulous history taking and physical examination are essential.

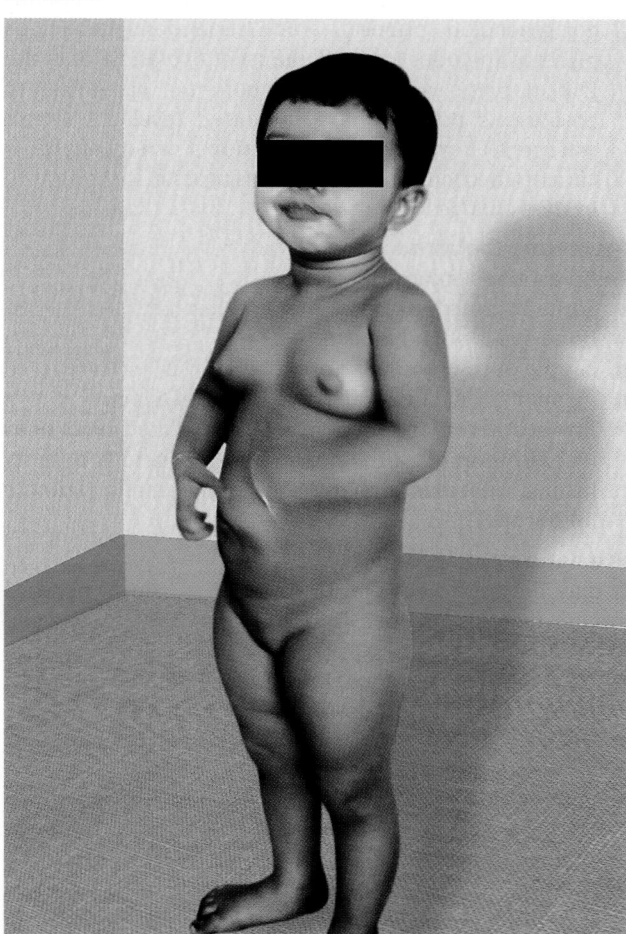

Fig. 5.2: Precocious puberty in a girl aged 2 years and 3 months.

True Precocious

Constitutional type is the most common one but the rare one is to be kept in mind. The diagnosis is made by:

- During puberty there is accelerated growth, skeletal maturation, and epiphyseal closure.
- The pubertal changes occur in orderly sequence.
- Tanner stages.
- No cause could be detected in majority (90%).

Basic investigations for evaluation of a girl with precocious puberty:

- Serum hCG, FSH, LH and prolactin (PRL).
- Thyroid profile (TSH, T_4).
- Serum estradiol, testosterone, 17-OH progesterone, DHEA.
- USG, CT or MRI of the abdomen and pelvis to rule out pathology of ovaries, adrenals or uterus.
- Skull X-ray, CT scan, or MRI brain—to exclude intracranial lesion (hypothalamic hamartoma).
- Electroencephalogram (EEG): Abnormal EEG is often associated with CNS disease.
- X-ray hand and wrist (nondominant) for bone age. Acceleration of growth is one of the earliest clinical features of precocious puberty.
- **GnRH stimulation test**: 100 μg of GnRH is administered (SC) and serum level of LH is measured. Value of LH >15 mIU/mL suggests gonadotropin dependent precocious puberty. GnRH dependent precocious puberty includes normal menses, ovulation and the risk of pregnancy. However, both the categories of precocious puberty have increased levels of serum estrogen. The causes of constitutional variety of precocious puberty are unknown. Kisspeptine is thought to initiate changes in puberty.

Premature thelarche

- Breast buds enlarge to 2–4 cm.
- Somatic growth pattern is not accelerated.
- Bone age is not advanced.
- Nipple development is absent.
- Vaginal smear shows negative estrogen effect.
- Breast buds enlargement may be an isolated event or as a continuum of GnRH dependent precocious puberty having follicular activity. This child needs periodic follow up.

Premature pubarche

It may be due to adrenal or ovarian or central nervous system disease. As such, the investigations are directed accordingly.

- An ovarian enlargement may not be palpable clinically. Examination under anesthesia or sonography is helpful.
- USG, CT or MRI scan is required to detect ovarian or adrenal tumor.
- Estimations of serum 17-α-hydroxyprogesterone, DHEA-S and serum testosterone are to be done in suspected cases of adrenal pathology—hyperplasia or tumor.

If nothing abnormal is detected, then the diagnosis of idiopathic pubarche is made.

Premature menarche

The other causes of vaginal bleeding, such as foreign body or injury has to be excluded. If the bleeding is cyclic, the diagnosis is confirmed.

Remarks

Investigations must be carried out to rule out any pathology in the CNS, ovary, and adrenal. It should be borne in mind that even in cases when no cause can be detected in any of the types mentioned, the periodic evaluation at 6 monthly intervals is to be made to detect any life-threatening pathology at the earliest.

Treatment

The treatment depends upon the cause and the speed of progress of the disease. The exogenous estrogen therapy or its inadvertent intake should be stopped. Cortisone therapy for adrenal hyperplasia and surgery to remove the adrenal or ovarian tumor eliminate the excess source of either androgen or estrogen. The intracranial tumor requires neurosurgery or radiotherapy. Primary hypothyroidism needs thyroid replacement therapy.

Constitutional or Idiopathic Type

Goals are

- To reduce gonadotropin secretions.
- To suppress gonadal steroidogenesis or counteract the peripheral action of sex steroids.
- To decrease the growth rate to normal and slowing the skeletal maturation.
- To protect the girl from sex abuse.
- Assessment of the speed of maturation process.

Drugs used are

GnRH agonist therapy arrests the pubertal precocity and growth velocity significantly. The agonists suppress the premature activation of hypothalamopituitary axis due to down regulation and thereby diminished estrogen secretion. **GnRH agonist therapy is the drug of choice in cases with GnRH dependent precocious puberty**. Therapy should be started as soon as the diagnosis is established. GnRH agonist therapy suppresses FSH, LH secretion, reverses the ovarian cycle, establishes amenorrhea, causes regression of breast, pubic hair changes, and other secondary sexual characteristics. This drug is safe and effective. It should be continued till the median age of puberty (p. 39) to allow development of maximum adult height.

Dose

Depot forms (goserelin or leuprolide) once a month can be used (p. 441). Dose is adjusted to maintain the serum estradiol below 10 pg/mL. Leuprolide acetate can be given (7.5 mg) 4 weekly although 3 months regimen are available.

Other durgs used:

- **Medroxyprogesterone acetate**—30 mg daily orally or 100–200 mg. IM weekly to suppress gonadal steroids. It can suppress menstruation and breast development but cannot change the skeletal growth rate.
- **Precocious puberty** of peripheral origin (ovarian tumors) needs specific management (p. 41, Table 5.2).

Duration of therapy

The drugs should be used up to the age of 11 years. However, individualization is to be done.

Prognosis

Counseling to the parents is essential. The girl needs to be protected from sexual abuse. Prognosis varies considerably depending on the etiology. Overall prognosis is good with primary hypothyroidism, adrenal or ovarian tumors following treatment. For the CNS group, prognosis depends on neurological involvement. Apart from the short stature due to accelerated bone maturation, **the idiopathic group** have got a normal menstrual pattern in future. The fertility rate is also expected to be normal.

DELAYED PUBERTY

Puberty is said to be delayed when the breast tissue and/or pubic hair have not appeared by 13–14 years or menarche appears as late as 16 years (Table 5.3). The normal upper age limit of menarche is 15 years. It is more common in boys than in girls.

Delayed Menarche

Before the onset of menarche, pubertal (Tanner stage 1 through 5) changes are breast budding followed within few months by the appearance of pubic hair. Breast budding is the earliest sign and menarche is the latest sign of puberty.

Onset of menarche is related to body composition (ratio of body fat to total body weight) rather than total body weight. Moderately obese girls between 20% and 30% above the ideal body weight have earlier onset of menarche. Malnutrition is known to delay the onset of puberty.

Diagnosis

Details of history taking and physical examination are done.

Examination of secondary sexual characters:

- **Mature:** To evaluate for Müllerian agenesis/dysgenesis.
- **Asynchronous** development of breasts, pubic hair → androgen insensitivity syndrome.

TABLE 5.3: Causes of delayed puberty.

■ **Hypergonadotropic hypogonadism** • Gonadal dysgenesis, 45 XO • Pure gonadal dysgenesis 46 XX, 46 XY • Ovarian failure 46 XX
■ **Hypogonadotropic hypogonadism** • Constitutional delay • Chronic illness, malnutrition • Primary hypothyroidism • Isolated gonadotropin deficiency (Kallmann's syndrome) • Intracranial lesions—tumors: Craniopharyngioma, pituitary adenomas
■ **Eugonadism** • Anatomical causes (Ch. 4) – Müllerian agenesis – Imperforate hymen – Transverse vaginal septum • Androgen insensitivity syndrome

- **Immature** secondary sexual characters: Serum FSH, PRL, TSH, T_4.
  - ↑FSH: Karyotype for gonadal dysgenesis/premature gonadal failure.
  - Low/normal FSH → **sellar CT/MRI** → **normal** → constitutional/chronic illness/malnutrition.
- **Abnormal sellar CT/MRI** → hypopituitarism/CNS tumor
- **TSH:** ↑ TSH → hypothyroidism.

Treatment

Treatment is directed according to the etiology. Assurance, improvement of general health and treatment of any illness may be of help in nonendocrinal causes. Cases with hypogonadism may be treated with cyclic estrogen. Unopposed estrogen 0.3 mg (conjugated estrogen) daily is given for first 6 months. Then combined estrogen and progestin, sequential regimen is started (Ch. 6). Cases of hypergonadotropic hypogonadism should have chromosomal study to exclude intersexuality.

PUBERTY MENORRHAGIA

Menstrual abnormality in adolescents are common. The periods may be heavy, irregular or scanty initially. Eventually, the majority of these teenaged girls establish a normal cycle and are fertile.

Important Causes of Menorrhagia

- **Dysfunctional uterine bleeding** (95%): Anovulatory cycles → unopposed estrogen → endometrial hyperplasia → prolonged and heavy periods (p. 156).
- **Endocrine dysfunction**
  - Polycystic ovary syndrome [(PCOS), p. 384)]
  - Hypothyroidism or hyperthyroidism.
- **Hematological**
  - Idiopathic thrombocytopenic purpura (p. 156)
  - Von-Willebrand's disease (p. 156)
  - Leukemia.
- **Pelvic tumors**
  - Fibroid uterus (p. 224).
  - Sarcoma botryoides (p. 329).
  - Estrogen producing ovarian tumor (p. 309).
- **Pregnancy complications** (abortion).

Diagnosis

Diagnosis is made by careful history taking and through clinical examination.

Evaluation is especially indicated if the menstrual interval is <22 days or >44 days, lasts longer than one week or the bleeding is too heavy that anemia develops.

Investigations

Investigations are planned according to the clinical diagnosis. Investigations include, routine hematological examination, including bleeding time, clotting time, platelet count. Thyroid profile (TSH, T_3, T_4), coagulation parameters [PT, PTT, factor VIII and von Willebrand factor (VWF)], and imaging study of the pelvis by ultrasonography or MRI to exclude pelvic pathology may be needed. Examination under anesthesia (EUA) and uterine curettage may be needed to exclude any pelvic pathology (pregnancy complications). The curetted material is sent for histopathological study.

Management

The girl needs adequate explanation, reassurance and psychological support. Rest and correction of anemia are helpful in majority of the cases.

Therapy with hematinics or even blood transfusion may be needed. In refractory cases, progestogens, such as medroxyprogesterone acetate or norethisterone 5 mg thrice daily is given till bleeding stops. Usually, the bleeding is controlled within 3–7 days. Medication is continued for 21 days. The condition usually becomes normal following 2–3 courses and then normal cycles resume. In emergency, conjugated equine estrogen 20–40 mg IV is given every 6–8 hours. Once the bleeding is controlled, combined oral pills are started (Flowchart 5.1). GnRH analogs can be used for short-term.

Regular menstrual cycle will be established once the hypothalamic-pituitary-ovarian axis is matured.

Flowchart 5.1: Management protocol of puberty menorrhagia.

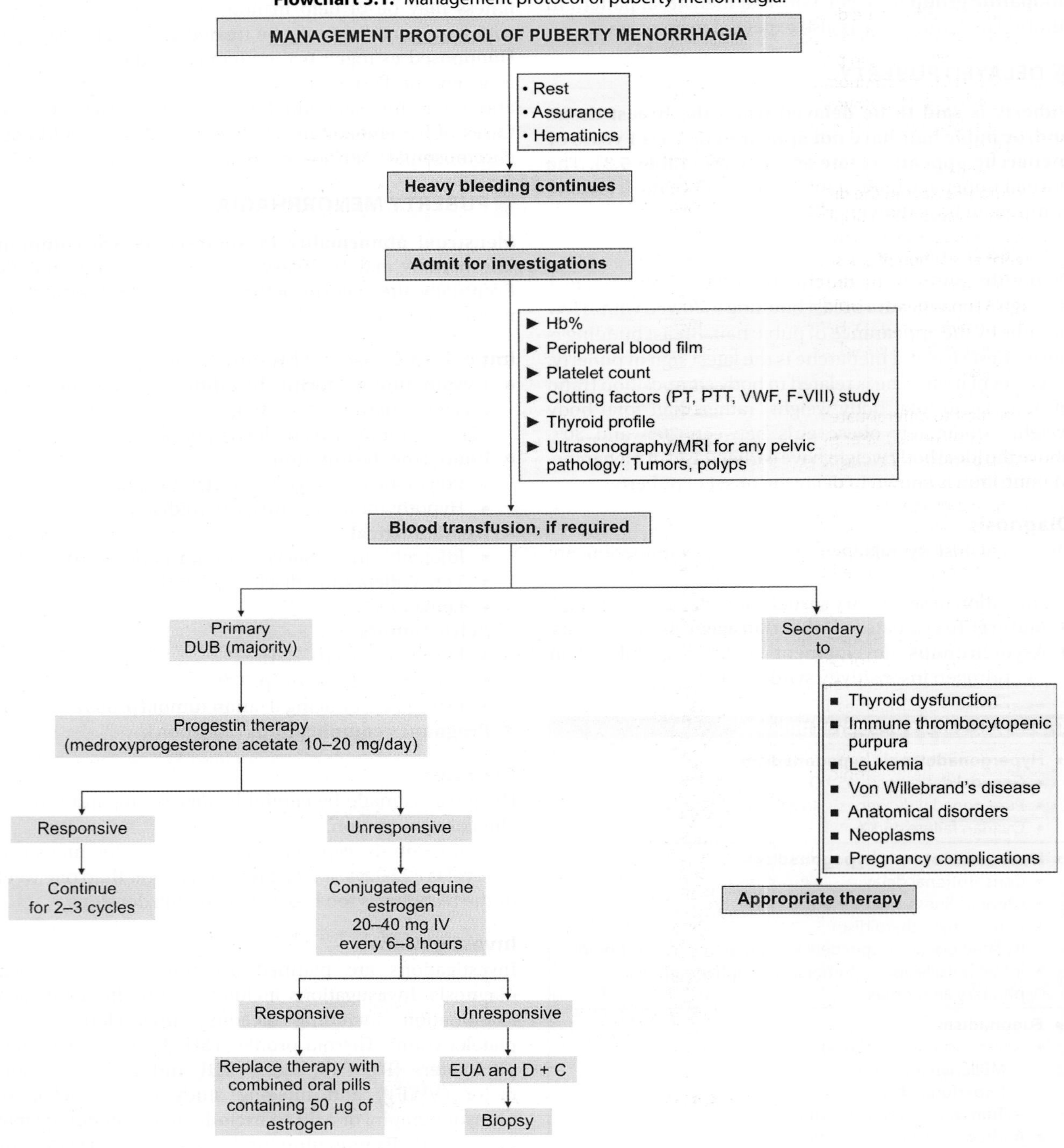

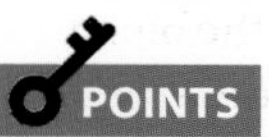

- **Puberty in girls** is the period that binds childhood to adulthood.
  The most common order of changes is beginning of growth spurt → enlargement of the breast buds → appearance of pubic hair → axillary hair → peak growth in height → menstruation (menarche).
- Uterine body and cervix ratio becomes 1:1 at menarche from 1:2 at birth. The ratio is 2:1 in adult.
- **The term precocious puberty** is reserved to those who exhibit any secondary sex characteristic before the age of 8 or menstruate before the age of 10. The common cause being constitutional.
- **The exact etiology** of GnRH dependent (true) precocious puberty is not known. Central nervous system disease may be present in nearly 30% of cases. GnRH independent (pseudo) precocious puberty is mostly related to an ovarian or adrenal pathology.
- **Life-threatening neoplasms** (ovary, adrenal or CNS) must be ruled out when a girl with precocious puberty is seen.
- **The basic investigations include:** Serum level of hCG, FSH, CH, prolactin, thyroid profila, serum estradiol, testosterone, 17-OH progesterone and dehydroepiandrosterone (DHEA).
- **Imaging studies** to be done are: Pelvic sonography, skull X-ray, CT or MRI abdomen, brain and electroencephalogram.
  Interpretation of hormone results for a girl with isosexual development:
  - LH ↑: Gonadotropin producing neoplasm
  - hCG ↑: Choriocarcinoma, hepatoblastoma
  - TSH ↑, T_4 ↓: Hypothyroidism
  - LH, FSH: Low or equivocal → serum E_2 → high → estrogen-producing neoplasm (isosexual development).
  - **Heterosexual development:** Serum levels of T, DHEAS, 17-OHP; High ↑ T → androgen producing neoplasm; ↑17-OHP/↑DHEAS → adrenal hyperplasia.
- Hormone assays in the differentiation of precocious puberty.
- Serum levels of: LH, FSH, TSH, T_4, Estradiol, hCG.
- **The primary aim of management** for a girl with precocious puberty is to: (a) Reduce the secretion of gonadotropins; (b) Block the peripheral action of sex steroids; and (c) Slow down the growth rate, including skeletal maturation.
- **GnRH agonist** is the drug of choice. It suppresses FSH, LH secretion, reverses ovarian cycle, establishes amenorrhea, causes regression of breast, pubic hair changes, and other secondary sexual characteristics. CNS diseases present with headaches, seizures, encephalitis or trauma. Hamartomas secrete GnRH.
- **Delayed puberty** is said to occur when the breast tissues and/or pubic hair have not appeared by 13–14 years or menarche as late as 17 years.
- **Ovarian failure and chromosomal anomalies** are the common causes of delayed puberty. Estimation of serum gonadotropins is important to differentiate hypogonadotropic from hypergonadotropic causes (Table 5.3).
- **Menstruation** just after puberty and just before menopause are mostly anovulatory and often irregular in frequency.
- **Initial periods** following menarche may be excessive due to anovulation.
- **The important causes of puberty menorrhagia are:** DUB, PCOS, thyroid disorders, hematological, pelvic tumors or pregnancy complications (p. 43).
- **Pubertal menorrhagia** should be treated with rest, assurance, hematinics and blood transfusions. Hypothyroidism and thrombocytopenic purpura are to be excluded. Pelvic ultrasonography is needed to exclude any organic lesion. In refractory cases, progestins or conjugated estrogen are effective failing which, EUA and uterine curettage are to be done. The materials should be histologically examined.
- The major concerns for the girl with precocious puberty are the psychosocial maturation of the girl, risk of sexual abuse and the ultimate reduced height due to premature closure of epiphyseal centers.
- Most common cause of GnRH independent precocious puberty is a functioning ovarian tumor (granulosa cell tumor: 60%).
- **Adrenal:** Levels of dehydroepiandrosterone sulfate (DHEAS) decline.
- Menstrual abnormalities in adolescent girls are common. Abnormal uterine bleeding (AUB) is common. This is mostly due to anovulation and unopposed estrogen effects.
- Girls need to be investigated to exclude the other causes when the bleeding is alarming. The other pathologies are: Endocrine dysfunction, hematological causes, pelvic tumors or even pregnancy related complications (p. 154).

CHAPTER

6 Menopause

CHAPTER OUTLINE

DEFINITION

Menopause means *permanent cessation of menstruation at the end of reproductive life due to loss of ovarian follicular activity. It is the point of time when last and final menstruation occurs.*

The clinical diagnosis is confirmed following stoppage of menstruation (amenorrhea) for twelve consecutive months without any other pathology. **As such, a woman is declared to have attained menopause only retrospectively**. Serum follicle-stimulating hormone (FSH) level is found elevated around the period of menopause (45–55 years).

Menopause transition is the period of time during which a woman passes from the reproductive to the non-reproductive stage. This phase covers 4–7 years on either side of menopause.

Menopause transition is associated with elevated serum FSH levels and variable length of menstrual cycle and/or missed menses.

Perimenopause is the time starting few years before continuing after the period of onset of menopause.

Climacteric refers to the time after the cessation of reproductive function.

Postmenopause is the phase of life that comes after the menopause.

AGE OF MENOPAUSE

Age at which menopause occurs is genetically predetermined. The age of menopause is not related to age of menarche or age at last pregnancy. It is variably related to lactation, use of oral pill, socioeconomic condition, race, height. Thinner women have early menopause. However, cigarette smoking and severe malnutrition living in high altitude may cause early menopause. The age of menopause ranges between 45–55 years, average being 47 years. **Late menopause** is seen in women with high parity or higher BMI, **Earlier menopause** is seen in cases following chemotherapy, ovarian resection.

CLINICAL IMPORTANCE

Due to increased life expectancy, especially in affluent society, about one-third of life span will be spent during the period of **estrogen deficiency stage** with long-term symptomatic and metabolic complications.

ENDOCRINOLOGY OF MENOPAUSAL TRANSITION AND MENOPAUSE

HYPOTHALAMO-PITUITARY GONADAL AXIS

Few years prior to menopause, along with depletion of the ovarian follicles, the follicles become resistant to pituitary gonadotropins. As a result, effective folliculogenesis is impaired with diminished estradiol production. There is a significant fall in the serum level of estradiol from 50–300 pg/mL before menopause to 10–20 pg/mL after menopause. **This decreases the negative feedback effect on hypothalamo-pituitary axis resulting in increase in FSH. The increase in FSH is also due to diminished inhibin.** Inhibin, a peptide, is secreted by the granulosa cells of the ovarian follicle. The increase of luteinizing hormone (LH) occurs subsequently. Anti-Müllerian hormone (AMH), a glycoprotein is secreted by the granulosa cells. Levels of AMH decrease progressively during the menopause transition (p. 62).

Disturbed folliculogenesis during this period may result in anovulation, oligoovulation, premature corpus luteum or corpus luteal insufficiency. The sustained level of estrogens may even cause endometrial hyperplasia and clinical manifestation of menstrual abnormalities prior to menopause.

The mean cycle length is significantly shorter. This is due to shortening of the follicular phase of the cycle. Luteal phase length remains constant. In late menopausal transition, there is accelerated rate of follicular depletion. Ultimately, no more follicles are available and even some exist, they are resistant to gonadotropins. Estradiol production drops down to the optimal level of 20 pg/mL → no endometrial growth → absence of menstruation.

ESTROGENS

Following menopause, the predominant estrogen is estrone and to a lesser extent estradiol. Serum level of estrone (30–70 pg/mL) is higher than that of estradiol (10–20 pg/mL). The major source of estrone is peripheral conversion (aromatization) of androgens from adrenals (mainly) and ovaries. The aromatization occurs at the level of muscle and adipose tissue. The trace amount of estradiol is derived from peripheral conversion of estrone and androgens. Compared to estradiol, estrone is biologically less (about one-tenth) potent.

With times, the sources fail to supply the precursors of estrogen and about 5–10 years after menopause, there is a sharp fall in estrogen and also the trophic hormones. The woman is said to be in a state of true menopause.

ANDROGENS

After menopause, the stromal cells of the ovary continue to produce androgens because of increase in LH. The main androgens are androstenedione and testosterone. Though the secretion of androgens from postmenopausal ovary are more, their peripheral levels are reduced due to conversion of androgens to estrone in adipose tissue. However, the cumulative effect is decrease in—estrogen: androgen ratio. This results in increased facial hair growth and change in voice.

As the obese patient converts more androgens into estrone, they are less likely to develop symptoms of estrogen deficiency and osteoporosis. But, they are vulnerable to endometrial hyperplasia and endometrial carcinoma.

PROGESTERONE

A trace amount of progesterone detected is probably adrenal in origin. AMH levels are decreased markedly (p. 62) due to loss of ovarian reserve.

GONADOTROPINS

The secretions of both FSH and LH are increased due to **absent negative feedback effect of estradiol and inhibin** or due to enhanced responsiveness of pituitary to gonadotropin-releasing hormone (GnRH). Rise in FSH is about 10–20 fold whereas that of LH is about 3-fold. GnRH pulse section is increased both in frequency and amplitude. During menopause, there is fall in the level of prolactin and inhibin. Fall in the level of inhibin (Ch. 7), lead to increase in the level of FSH from the pituitary. Ultimately, due to physiologic aging GnRH and both FSH, LH decline along with decline of estrogens.

ORGAN CHANGES SYMPTOMS

- **Ovaries** shrink in size, become wrinkled and white. There is thinning of the cortex with increase in medullary components. There is abundance of stromal cells which have got secretory activity.
- **Fallopian tubes** show feature of atrophy. The muscle coat becomes thinner, the cilia disappear and the plicae become less prominent.
- **The uterus** becomes smaller and the ratio between the body and the cervix reverts to the 1:1 ratio. The endometrium becomes thin and atrophic. In some women, however, with high endogenous estrogens, the endometrium may be proliferative or even hyperplastic. The cervical secretion becomes scanty.
  Menstrual changes: Abnormal uterine bleeding (AUB) is common. This is mostly due to anovulation and unopposed estrogen effects.
- **The vagina** becomes narrower due to gradual loss of elasticity. The vaginal epithelium becomes thin. The rugae progressively flatten. There is no glycogen. Doderlein's bacillus is absent. The vaginal pH becomes alkaline. Maturation index (parabasal, intermediate and superficial cells) is 10/85/5.
- **The vulva** shows features of atrophy. The labia becomes flattened and the pubic hair becomes scantier. The end result is a narrow introitus.
- **Breast fat** is reabsorbed and the glands atrophy. The nipples decrease in size. Ultimately, the breasts become flat and pendulous.
- **Bladder and urethra** undergo similar changes to those of the vagina. The epithelium becomes thin and is more prone to damage and infection. There may be dysuria, frequency, urge or even stress incontinence.
- **Loss of muscle tone** leads to pelvic relaxation, uterine descent and anatomic changes in the urethra and neck of the bladder. The pelvic cellular tissues become scanty and the ligaments supporting the uterus and vagina lose their tone. As such pre-existing weakness gets aggravated.
- **Adrenal:** Levels of dehydroepiandrosterone sulfate (DHEAS) decline.

BONE METABOLISM

Normally, bone formation (osteoblastic activity) and bone resorption (osteoclastic activity) are in balance depending on many factors (age, endocrine, nutrition and genetic). Following menopause, there is a loss of bone mass by about 3–5% per year. This is due to deficiency of estrogen. **Osteoporosis** is a condition where there is reduction in bone mass but bone mineral to matrix ratio is normal.

Bone mineral density (BMD) is reported as T-Scores (WHO, 2014). **Normal BMD** has the T score between +2.5 and –1.0 (below). This means that the patient's BMD lies between 2.5 standard deviations (SDs) above and 1 SD below the young adult mean.

Bone Disease Based on Bone Mineral Density (WHO – 2014)

- Normal BMD: T-score between + 2.5 and –1.0
- Osteopenia: T-score between –1.0 and –2.5
- Osteoporosis: T-score at or below –2.5
- Severe osteoporosis: T-score ≤–2.5 with one or more fracture.

Postmenopausal woman runs a high risk for fracture of bones due to osteoporosis. Parathyroid hormone (PTH) and interleukin-I (IL-I) are involved in osteoporosis. Estrogen prevents osteoporosis by several mechanisms.

It inhibits osteoclastic activity and inhibits release of IL-I by monocytes. Estrogen increases absorption of calcium from the gut, stimulates calcitonin secretion from the C cells of the thyroid and increases 1, 25-dihydroxyvitamin D. All these lead to increased bone mineralization.

CARDIOVASCULAR SYSTEM

Risk of cardiovascular disease is high in postmenopausal women **due to deficiency of estrogen. Estrogen prevents cardiovascular disease by several ways.** It increases high-density lipoprotein (particularly HDL2) and decreases low-density lipoprotein (LDL) and total cholesterol. It inhibits platelet and macrophage (foam cell) aggregation at the vascular intima. It stimulates the release of nitric oxide (NO) and prostacyclin from vascular endothelium to dilate the blood vessels. It prevents atherosclerosis by its **antioxidant property**.

MENSTRUATION PATTERN PRIOR TO MENOPAUSE

Any of the following patterns are observed:
- Abrupt cessation of menstruation (rare).
- Gradual decrease in both amount and duration. It may be spotting or delayed and ultimately lead to cessation.
- Irregular with or without excessive bleeding. One should exclude genital malignancy prior to declare it as the usual premenopausal pattern.

MENOPAUSAL SYMPTOMS

In majority, apart from cessation of menstruation, no more symptoms are evident. In some women, symptoms appear. **The important symptoms and the health concerns of menopause:**
- Vasomotor symptoms
- Urogenital atrophy
- Osteoporosis and fracture
- Cardiovascular disease
- Cerebrovascular diseases
- Psychological changes
- Skin and hair
- Sexual dysfunction
- Dementia and cognitive decline.

RISK FACTORS FOR VASOMOTOR SYMPTOMS

▪ Early menopause ▪ Surgical menopause ▪ Smoking	▪ Use of SERMs ▪ Sedentary lifestyle ▪ White women

Vasomotor symptoms: The characteristic symptom of menopause is 'hot flash'. **Hot flash is characterized by sudden feeling of heat followed by profuse sweating.** There may also be the symptoms of palpitation, fatigue and weakness. The physiologic changes with hot flashes are **perspiration** and **cutaneous vasodilation**. Both these two functions are under central thermoregulatory

SYMPTOMS OF MENOPAUSAL TRANSITION

A. Menstrual changes	D. Sexual dysfunction
▪ Shorter cycles (common) ▪ Irregular bleeding	▪ Vaginal dryness ▪ Dyspareunia ▪ Decreased libido
B. Vasomotor symptoms	**E. Urinary**
▪ Hot flashes ▪ Upper body sweating ▪ Anxiety, lack of sleep	▪ Incontinence ▪ Urgency ▪ Dysuria
C. Psychological	**F. Others**
▪ Irritability ▪ Mood swings ▪ Poor memory ▪ Depression	▪ Back aches ▪ Joint aches ▪ Weight gain ▪ Palpitations

control. Low estrogen level is a prerequisite for hot flash. Hot flash coincides with GnRH pulse secretion with increase in serum LH level. It may last for 1–10 minutes and may be at times unbearable. Sleep may be disturbed due to night sweats. The **thermoregulatory center in association with GnRH center in the hypothalamus is involved in the etiology of hot flash.** Gonadotropins (LH) are thought to be involved.

Neurotransmitters (norepinephrine, serotonin) are involved to lower the threshold of thermoregulatory zone.

Genital and urinary system: Steroid receptors have been identified in the mucous membrane of urethra, bladder, vagina and the pelvic floor muscles. Estrogen plays an important role to maintain the epithelium of vagina, urinary bladder and the urethra. Estrogen deficiency produces atrophic epithelial changes in these organs. This may cause dyspareunia and dysuria.

Dyspareunia: Estradiol deficiency leads to vaginal dryness or atrophy. Estrogen replacement reverses atropic changes. It can be given orally or vaginally. 17 β-estradiol tablet or conjugated equine estrogen (CEE) cream is effective in relieving symptoms. Risks of endometrial hyperplasia is less with vaginal tablets than that of cream. Vaginal lubricants (water soluble) and moisturizers (K-Y jelly) are commonly used.

Vagina: Minimal trauma may cause vaginal bleeding. Dyspareunia, vaginal infections, dryness, pruritus and leukorrhea are also common. **The urinary symptoms are** urgency, dysuria and recurrent urinary tract infection and stress incontinence.

Sexual dysfunction: Estrogen deficiency is often associated with decreased sexual desire. This may be due to psychological changes (depression anxiety) as well as atrophic changes of the genitourinary system.

Skin and hair: There is thinning, loss of elasticity and wrinkling of the skin. Skin collagen content and thickness decrease by 1–2% per year. *'Purse string'* wrinkling around the month and *'crow feet'* around the eyes are the characteristics. Estrogen receptors are present in the skin and maximum are present in the facial skin. Estrogen replacement can prevent this skin loss during menopause. After menopause, there is some loss of pubic and axillary hair and slight balding. This may be due to low level of estrogen with normal level of testosterone.

Psychological changes: There is increased frequency of anxiety, headache, insomnia, irritability, dysphasia and depression. They also suffer from dementia, mood swing and inability to concentrate. Estrogen increases opioid (neurotransmitter) activity in the brain and is known to be important for memory.

Dementia: Estrogen improves cerebral perfusion and cognition. However, it is not clear whether estrogen therapy prevents vascular dementia and Alzheimer disease.

Bone structure and metabolism: Bone types are—(a) Cortical bone: Peripheral bones (arms, legs) and (b) Trabecular bone: Bone of axial skeleton—vertebrae, pelvic, proximal femur. During menopause, there is loss of bone mass by 2–5% per year for the first 5 to 10 years. Then it slows down by 1% per year. Bone remodeling is maintained by bone forming cells (osteoblasts) and the bone resorption by the osteoclast cells. Increased osteoporosis by the osteoclasts in postmenopausal women is mediated by the receptor activator of Nuclear Factor-κB (RANK) ligand pathway. RANK, RANK ligand and osteoprotegerin (OPG) are the major components in this pathway.

Osteoporosis and fracture: Osteoporosis is a state of reduced bone mass (in trabecular bones) and ultimately ends in fracture (Table 6.1). Osteopenia is the precursor to osteoporosis. Common fracture sites are: Vertebra, femoral neck and the wrist bones. Fractures are the cause of significant morbidity and mortality. **Osteoporosis** may be **primary (Type 1)** due to estrogen loss, age, deficient nutrition (calcium, vitamin D) or hereditary. It may be **secondary (Type 2)** to endocrine abnormalities (parathyroid, diabetes) or medication (Table 6.1). **Fracture may be due to fall of the woman** (fall risk factors). This occurs due to reduced muscle mass or due to comorbid conditions like visual or **cognitive impairment**. Osteoporosis may lead to back pain, loss of height and kyphosis. Fracture of bones is a major health problem. Fracture may involve the vertebral body, femoral neck or distal forearm (Colles' fracture). Morbidity and mortality in elderly women following fracture is high.

Detection of osteoporosis: Computed tomography (CT) and especially the dual-energy X-ray absorptiometry (DEXA) are reliable methods to assess the bone mineral density. Total radiation exposure is high with CT than DEXA.

Fracture risk assessment tool (FRAX) WHO - 2004 (*www.shef.ac.uk/FRAX*) is used to calculate the 10 year fracture risk probability of an individual. Eleven risk factors are considered and femoral neck raw BMD value (g/cm^2) are calculated. FRAX is useful to identify a person with BMD in osteopenic category when pharmacotherapy may be beneficial.

TABLE 6.1: Risk factors for osteoporosis in a women.

▪ **Family history** ▪ **Age**— >65 years ▪ **Race**—Asian, white race ▪ **Lack of estrogen** ▪ **Body weight**—low BMI ▪ **Fragility fracture** ▪ **Osteopenia** ▪ **Osteoporosis** ▪ **Hypogonadism** ▪ **Fall risk factors**	▪ **Early menopause**—surgical, radiation ▪ **Dietary**—↓ calcium and ↓ vitamin D, ↑ caffeine, ↑ smoking, ↑ alcohol ▪ **Sedentary habit** ▪ **Medications**—heparin, corticosteroids, GnRH analog and anticonvulsants ▪ **Diseases**—rheumatoid arthritis, hyperparathyroidism, malabsorption, multiple myeloma, thyroid disorders

TABLE 6.2: Risk factors for cardiovascular disease.

▪ Hypertension	▪ Smoking habit
▪ Familial hyperlipidemia	▪ Impaired glucose tolerance

FALL RISK FACTORS

Fall risk (fragility) fracture
Comorbid conditions ▪ Impaired vision ▪ Reduced balance ▪ Reduced muscle mass ▪ Poor lighting ▪ Medications (sedatives)

Biochemical parameters to detect bone loss are measurement of urinary calcium/creatinine and hydroxyproline/creatinine ratios.

Cardiovascular and cerebrovascular effects: Due to estrogen deficiency oxidation of LDL and foam cell formation cause vascular endothelial injury, cell death and smooth muscle proliferation. These women develop insulin resistance and central (android) obesity. All these lead to vascular atherosclerotic changes, vasoconstriction and thrombus formation (p. 48).

Risks of ischemic heart disease, coronary artery disease and strokes [cardiovascular disease (CVD)] are increased due to estrogen deficiency when compared to premenopausal women.

Clotting factor: CVD risks are further increased due to increase in clotting factors (fibrinogen, plasminogen activator inhibitor, factor VII). This creates a hypercoagulable state.

DIAGNOSIS OF MENOPAUSE

- Cessation of menstruation for consecutive 12 months during climacteric.
- Average age of menopause: 50 years.
- Appearance of menopausal symptoms 'hot flash' and 'night sweats'.
- Vaginal cytology—showing maturation index of at least 10/85/5 (features of low estrogen).

- Serum estradiol: <20 pg/mL.
- Serum FSH and LH: >40 mlU/mL (three values at weeks interval required).

MANAGEMENT

PREVENTION

Spontaneous menopause is unavoidable. However, **artificial menopause** induced by surgery (bilateral oophorectomy) or radiation (gonadal) or chemotherapy during reproductive period can to some extent be prevented or delayed.

Counseling: Every woman with postmenopausal symptoms should be adequately explained about the physiologic events. This will remove her fears and minimize or dispel the symptoms of anxiety, depression and insomnia. Reassurance is essential.

TREATMENT

Nonhormonal Treatment

- **Lifestyle modification:** This includes physical activity (weight-bearing), reducing high coffee intake, smoking and excessive alcohol. There should be adequate calcium intake (300 mL of milk), reducing medications that causes bone loss (corticosteroids).
- **Nutritious diet:** Balanced with calcium and protein is helpful.
- **Supplementary calcium:** Daily intake of 1–1.5 g can reduce osteoporosis and fracture.
- **Exercise:** Weight-bearing exercises, walking and jogging.
- **Vitamin D:** Supplementation of vitamin D_3 (1500–2000 IU/day) along with calcium can reduce osteoporosis and fractures. Exposure to sunlight enhances synthesis of cholecalciferol (vitamin D_3) in the skin.
- **Cessation of smoking and alcohol.**
- **Bisphosphonates** prevent osteoclastic bone resorption. It improves bone density and prevents fracture. It is preferred for older women. Women should be monitored with bone density measurement. Drug should be stopped when there is severe pain at any site. Commonly used drugs are ibandronate, risedronate and alendronate. Residronate is also effective and have less side effects. Bisphosphonates when used alone cannot prevent hot flashes, atrophic changes and cardiovascular disease. It is taken in empty stomach. Nothing should be taken by mouth for at least 30 minutes after oral dosing. Patient should remain upright for 30 minutes. **Side effects include** gastric and esophageal ulceration and bleeding, osteomyelitis and osteonecrosis of the jaw.
- **Denosumab:** It is a human monoclonal antibody to RANK ligand. It inhibits osteoclast development and bone resorption. It reduces the risk of fracture.
- **Calcitonin** inhibits bone resorption by inhibiting osteoclasts. It is a polypeptide hormone. Simultaneous therapy with calcium and vitamin D should be given. It has an analgesic effect. It is given either by nasal spray (200 IU daily) or by injection (SC) (50–100 IU daily). It is used when estrogen therapy is contraindicated.
- **Selective estrogen receptor modulators (SERMs)** are tissue specific in action. Of the many SERMs, **raloxifene** has shown to increase bone mineral density, reduce serum LDL and to raise HDL2 level. Raloxifene inhibits the estrogen receptors at the breast and endometrial tissues. **Risks of breast cancer and endometrial cancer are therefore reduced. Raloxifene does not improve hot flashes or urogenital atrophy.** Evaluation of bone density (hip) should be done periodically. Risks of venous thromboembolism is increased.
- **Bazedoxifene:** It is a nonhormonal agents to control the vasomotor symptoms. Bazedoxifene is a SERM and is combined with conjugated equine estrogen. It is used for management of vasomotor symptoms in women with intact uterus. It is well-tolerated and effective.
- **Clonidine**, an α_2 adrenergic agonist may be used to reduce the severity and duration of hot flashes. It is helpful where estrogen is contraindicated (hypertension). **Side effects are** hypotension, dry mouth and constipation.
- **Paroxetine,** venlafaxine, sertraline and fluoxetine are under the group of selective serotonin reuptake inhibitors. These are effective antidepressants.
  Side effects of selective serotonin reuptake inhibitors (SSRIs) are: Nausea, headache, diarrhea, insomnia, fatigue and sexual dysfunction.
- **Gabapentin** is an analog of gamma-aminobutyric acid (GABA). It is a neurotransmitter and effective to control hot flashes.
- **Parathyroid hormone:** Teriparatide is a recombinant parathyroid hormone. It increases osteoblast number and activity and reduces apoptosis of osteoblasts. It is given by daily subcutaneous injection for women who are at high-risk of fracture. It is safe and well-tolerated.
  Side effects are: Nausea, headache, leg cramps. Risk of osteosarcoma in rats has been observed.
- **Phytoestrogens** containing isoflavones are found to lower the incidence of vasomotor symptoms, osteoporosis and cardiovascular disease.
- **Soy protein** is also found effective to reduce vasomotor symptoms. Soy protein acts as SERM.
- **Vitamin E** reduces hot flash (25%).

Hormone Therapy

The hormone therapy (HT) is indicated in menopausal women to overcome the short-term and long-term consequences of estrogen deficiency.

Indications of Hormone Therapy

- Relief of menopausal symptoms (p. 48)
- Relief of vasomotor symptoms
- Prevention of osteoporosis (p. 49)
- To maintain the quality of life in menopausal years.

Special group of women to whom HT should be prescribed:

- Premature ovarian failure
- Gonadal dysgenesis
- Surgical or radiation menopause.

BENEFITS OF HORMONE THERAPY

- Improvement of vasomotor symptoms (70–80%)
- Improvement urogenital atrophy
- Increase in bone mineral density (2–5%)
- Decreased risk in vertebral and hip fractures (25–50%)
- Reduction in colorectal cancer (20%)
- Possibly cardioprotection

HT and Osteoporosis

HT prevents bone loss and stimulate new bone formation. HT increases BMD by 2–5% and reduces the risk of vertebral and hip fracture (25–50%). Estrogen is to play a direct role, on the osteoblast receptors of the bones. Women receiving HT should supplement their diet with an extra 500 mg of calcium daily. Total daily requirement of calcium in postmenopausal women is 1.5 g.

HT is thought to be cardiovascular protective. LDL on oxidation produces vascular endothelial injury and foam cell (macrophage) formation. These endothelial changes ultimately lead to intimal smooth muscle proliferation and atherosclerosis. Estrogen prevents oxidation of LDL, as it has got **antioxidant properties.**

In postmenopausal women, there is some amount of insulin resistance and hyperinsulinemia. Hyperinsulinemia induces atherogenesis. Estrogen improve glucose metabolism.

Risks of Hormone Therapy

- **Endometrial cancer:** When estrogen is given alone to a woman with intact uterus, it causes endometrial proliferation, hyperplasia and carcinoma. It is therefore advised that a progestin should be added to estrogen replacement therapy (ERT) to counterbalance such risks.
- **Breast cancer:** Combined estrogen and progestin replacement therapy for a long-term, increases the risk of breast cancer slightly (RR 1.26). Adverse effects of hormone therapy are related to the dose and duration of therapy.
- **Venous thromboembolic (VTE) disease** has been found to be increased with the use of combined oral estrogen and progestin (Table 6.3). Transdermal estrogen use does not have the same risk compared to oral estrogen.
- **Coronary heart disease (CHD):** Combined HT therapy shows a relative hazard (RR 1.29) of CHD. Hypertension has not been observed to be a risk of HT.

TABLE 6.3: Contraindications to hormone therapy.

- Known, suspected or history of breast cancer
- Undiagnosed genital tract bleeding
- Estrogen-dependent neoplasm in the body
- History of venous thromboembolism or active deep vein thrombosis (DVT)
- Active liver disease
- Prior chotestatic jaundice (caution)
- Gallbladder disease
- Prior endometriosis (caution)

- **Lipid metabolism:** An increased incidence of gallbladder disease has been observed following ERT due to rise in cholesterol (in bile).
- **Dementia, Alzheimer** disease not benefited.

Available Preparations for Hormone Therapy

The principal hormone used in HT is estrogen. This is ideal for a woman who had her uterus removed (hysterectomy) already. But in a woman with an intact uterus, only estrogen therapy leads to endometrial hyperplasia and even endometrial carcinoma. Addition of progestins for last 12–14 days each month can prevent this problem. **Commonly used estrogens** are conjugated estrogen (0.625–1.25 mg/day) or micronized estradiol (1–2 mg/day). **Progestins** used are medroxyprogesterone acetate (MPA) (1.5–5 mg/day), micronized progesterone (100–300 mg/day) or dydrogesterone (5–10 mg/day).

Considering the risks, hormone therapy should be used with the lowest effective dose and for a shortest period of time. Low dose oral conjugated estrogen 0.3 mg daily is effective and has got minimal side effects. Dose interval may be modified as daily for initial 2–3 months then it may be changed to every other day for another 2–3 months and then every third day for the next 2–3 months. It may be stopped thereafter if symptoms are controlled.

- **Oral estrogen regime:** CEE, 0.3 mg or 0.625 mg is given daily for woman who had hysterectomy.
- **Estrogen and cyclic progestin:** For a woman with intact uterus, estrogen is given continuously for 25 days and progestin is added for last 10 days.
- **Continuous estrogen and progestin therapy:** Continued combined therapy can prevent endometrial hyperplasia. There may be irregular bleeding with this regimen.

  Transdermal administration: This route avoids the 'first pass hepatic metabolism'. Effects of oral estrogens on lipids, clotting factors may be beneficial. Risks of venous thromboembolism or gallbladder disease are not increased compared to oral route.
  - **Subdermal implants:** Implants are inserted subcutaneously over the anterior abdominal wall using local anesthesia. 17 β-estradiol implants 25 mg, 50 mg or 100 mg are available and can be kept for 6 months. This method is suitable in patients after hysterectomy. Implants maintain physiological E2 to E1 ratio.
  - **Percutaneous estrogen gel:** 1 g applicator of gel, delivering 1 mg of estradiol daily, is to be applied onto the skin over the anterior abdominal wall or thighs. Effective blood level of estradiol (90–120 pg/mL) can be maintained.
  - **Transdermal patch:** It contains 3.2 mg of 17 β-estradiol, releasing about 50 μg of estradiol in 24 hours. Physiological level of E_2 to E_1 is maintained. It should be applied below the waist line and changed twice a week. Skin reaction, irritation and itching have been noted with their use.

Vaginal cream: Conjugated equine vaginal estrogen cream 1.25 mg daily is very effective especially when associated with atrophic vaginitis. It also reduces urinary frequency, urgency and recurrent infection. Women with symptoms of urogenital atrophy and urinary symptoms and who do not like to have systemic HT, are suitable for such treatment.

- **Progestins:** In patients with history of breast carcinoma or endometrial carcinoma, progestins may be used. It may be effective in suppressing hot flashes and it prevents osteoporosis. MPA, 2.5–5 mg/day can be used.
- **Levonorgestrel intrauterine system (LNG-IUS)** (p. 399) with daily release of 10 mg (*see* below) of levonorgestrel per 24 hours, it protects the endometrium from hyperplasia and cancer. At the same time it has got no systemic progestin side effects. Estrogen can be given by any route. It can serve as contraception and HT when given in a perimenopausal women.
- **Tibolone:** Tibolone is a steroid (19-nortestosterone derivative) having weak estrogenic, progestogenic and androgenic properties. It prevents osteoporosis, atrophic changes of vagina and hot flashes. It increases libido. Endometrium is atrophic. A dose of 2.5 mg per day is given.
- **Testosterone:** Androgen replacement in women with hypoactive sexual desire disorder (HSDD) is found beneficial. It improves mood, bone, muscle mass and quality of life. Short-term use is suggested.
- **Parathyroid hormone (PTH):** Recombinant PTH (teriparatide) is given by injection (SC) to prevent osteoporosis and fracture. It increases the number of osteoblast cells and their activity and reduces apoptosis of osteoblast cells. PTH is safe and well-tolerated. At low daily doses (20 μg/day, SC) teriparatide, its anabolic effects predominate. Side effects are leg cramps, nausea and headache. Use for more than 2 years is not recommended.
- **Complementary and alternative medicine (CAM):** Acupuncture decreases hot flash frequency and intensity significantly.

Duration of HT Use

Generally, use of HT for a shortest period as long as the benefits outweigh the risks. Individual woman need counseling with annual or semiannual review. Reduction of dosage should be done as soon as possible. Menopausal women should maintain optimum nutrition, ideal body weight and perform regular exercises.

Individual woman should be informed with updated knowledge as regard the relative merits and possible risks of continuing HT (Table 6.4).

Progress in Hormone Therapy

Low dose HT: Women with intact uterus with 0.3 mg CEE and MPA 1.5 mg is found effective to control the vasomotor symptoms. Similarly 1 mg of estradiol and norethisterone acetate 0.5 mg orally, are also effective and have significant bone sparing effect. Progestogen is added in the HT to minimize the adverse effects of estrogen.

TABLE 6.4: Monitoring prior to and during hormone therapy.

A base level parameter of the following and their subsequent check up (at least annually) are mandatory.

- Physical examination including pelvic examination.
- Blood pressure recording.
- Breast examination (p. 82) and mammography (p. 475).
- Cervical cytology (p. 89).
- Pelvic ultrasonography (TVS) to measure endometrial thickness (normal < 5 mm).
- Any irregular bleeding should be investigated thoroughly (endometrial biopsy, hysteroscopy).
- Ideal serum level of estradiol should be 100 pg/mL during HT therapy. Serum level of estradiol is useful to monitor the HT therapy rather than that of serum FSH.

Hormone therapy should be used with lowest effective dose and for the shortest period of time as possible (ACOG, 2008). Dose interval may be modified (*see* above) before stopping the therapy. To minimize the systemic adverse effects of progestogen, LNG-IUS is being used. It is primarily used as a contraceptive. Estrogen component is delivered by oral or by transdermal route or as an implant. A small size LNG-IUS has been developed that releases 10 μg LNG per day. This reduced size LNG-IUS is suitable for the postmenopausal women as the size of the uterus is also small.

ABNORMAL MENOPAUSE

- **Premature menopause:** If the menopause occurs at or below the age of 40, it is said to be premature (details in p. 390). Often, there is familial diathesis. Treatment by replacement therapy is of value (details in p. 446).
- **Delayed menopause:** If the menopause fails to occur even beyond 55 years, it is called delayed menopause.

  The common causes are constitutional, uterine fibroids, diabetes mellitus and estrogenic tumor of the ovary. The cases should not be neglected. In the absence of palpable pelvic pathology, diagnostic curettage should be done and an early decision of hysterectomy should be taken in the face of increased incidence of endometrial carcinoma.
- **Artificial menopause:** Permanent cessation of ovarian function done by artificial means, e.g. surgical removal of ovaries by radiation or chemotherapy is called artificial menopause.
- **Surgical menopause:** Menstruating women who have bilateral oophorectomy, experience menopausal symptoms (p. 50). It is sometimes more troublesome than natural menopause.
- **Radiation menopause:** The ovarian function may be suppressed by external gamma radiation in women below the age of 40. The castration is not permanent. The menstruation may resume after 2 years and even conception is possible. Intracavity introduction of radium can cause castration effect by destroying the endometrium and also by depressing the ovarian function. The menopausal symptoms are not so intense as found in surgical menopause or menopause following external radiation.

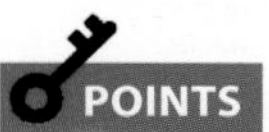

- **Menopause** means permanent cessation of menstruation at the end of reproductive life due to ovarian follicular inactivity. The average age being 50 years. Menopause is genetically predetermined. It is not related to the number of pregnancies, race, socioeconomic conditions, education, height, weight, age at menarche or age of last childbirth.
- **The initial endocrine change** with the onset of menopause is decreased ovarian inhibin production and increase in pituitary FSH release. The amount of estrogen replacement in menopause is not dependent upon the level of FSH.
- There is gradual elevated levels of first the FSH and then LH. Simultaneously, estradiol levels fall to optimal 20 pg/mL when menopause sets in. There is increased androgen secretion from the ovarian stroma and from the adrenal. A trace amount of progesterone is adrenal in origin.
- **Diagnosis** is from the classic symptom of 'hot flash' (50%) and confirmed by elevated FSH levels to >100 mIU/mL and serum estradiol <20 pg/mL.
- **In menopause**, there is depletion of ovarian follicles with degeneration of granulosa and theca cells. Stromal cells produce androgens, which are converted to estrogens in peripheral body fat. Obese postmenopausal women, have higher levels of estrone, less hot flashes and osteoporosis. But risk of developing endometrial cancer is high for them.
- **Benefits of HT are** improvement in vasomotor symptoms, urogenital atrophy, increase in BMD, reduced risk of vertebral and hip fractures, reduction colorectal cancer and possibly cardioprotection (p. 51). Estrogen reduces the risk of late onset Alzheimer's disease. It is beneficial in symptomatic women.
- **Risks of HT are** endometrial cancer, breast cancer, VTE and coronary heart disease (p. 51).
- **For a woman with intact uterus**, progestin (for last 12–14 days) must be combined with estrogen. Otherwise unopposed estrogen therapy will increase the risk of endometrial hyperplasia and adenocarcinoma. Estrogen without a progestin is recommended for a postmenopausal women who had hysterectomy.
- **Contraindications to HT** include undiagnosed genital tract bleeding, estrogen dependent neoplasm in the body, history of venous thromboembolism, active liver disease and gallbladder disease (p. 51).
- **Estrogen may be administered** orally, subdermal implants, vaginal cream, percutaneous gel or by transdermal patch. Provided the women is monitored during the period of therapy (Table 6.4). HT can be continued as long as the benefits are desired. However, low dose and short period of therapy (3–5 years) is currently recommended.
- **Dual energy X-ray absorptiometry (DEXA)** is the most accurate method to measure bone density. At least 25% of bone needs to be lost before osteoporosis can be diagnosed by routine radiographic examination.
- **Indications of estrogen therapy in menopause are** presence of vasomotor symptoms, prevention of atrophic vaginitis, urethritis and osteoporosis. Estrogen increases calcium absorption and reduces bone reabsorption.
- LDL cholesterol increases the risk of coronary artery disease (CAD) while HDL protects CAD. Estrogen therapy decreases LDL cholesterol and increases HDL.
- **Premature menopause** is one when the menstruation stops at or below the age of 40. **Delayed menopause** is one when menopause fails to occur even beyond 55 years.
- **Counseling should be done** as regard life style measures, HT and the alternatives.
- **Androgen therapy** may be needed for women with hypoactive sexual desire disorder (HSDD).
- **Fall risk factors** are increased in situation due to physiological changes (diminished vision, reduced muscle mass), comorbid conditions (arthritis, cognitive impairment), use of medications (sedatives) or environmental (poor lighting).
- Female reproductive aging criteria can guide health management in menopause, rather than using the chronological age of the woman. Stages of Reproductive Aging Workshop (STRAW, 2012) guides are followed.
- The Stages of Reproductive Aging Workshop (STRAW): STRAW considers final menstrual period (FMP) as the anchor age (O). FMP is preceded by 5 stages (as: –5, –4, –3, –2 and –1). FMP is again followed by two stages (+2 and +1). Stage –5 to –3 considers early reproductive period (–5), reproductive period (–4) and the late reproductive period (–3) respectively. Stage –2 is the early Menopausal Transition (MT), and –1 is the late MT. Stage +1 indicates 1 year after menopause and +2 indicates 2 years after menopause. Duration of the stages are often variable. Menstrual cycles vary from normal to variable (skipped cycles >2 or phases of amenorrhea), to permanent amenorrhea. Important endocrine changes ranges from normal levels of FSH (during the phases of –5, –4 and –3) to mild to moderate rise (during the phases of –2 and –1) and gradually to the levels of significant FSH rise (+1, +2).

CHAPTER

7 Neuroendocrinology in Relation to Reproduction

CHAPTER OUTLINE

The neuroendocrine mechanisms are the basic factors in the reproductive cycle. A transducer concept has been evolved in which the specialized neural cells of the hypothalamus function as the final common pathway to guide the appropriate anterior pituitary hormonal response.

HYPOTHALAMUS

Hypothalamus plays an important role in the neuroendocrine regulation. Three well-defined areas are demarked—(a) supraoptic area; (b) tuberal region; and (c) mamillary region. Each region is further subdivided into areas, or nuclei (Fig. 7.1). Both a tonic and a cyclic center are located within the hypothalamus resulting in changes in gonadotropin releasing hormone (GnRH) production.

CONNECTIONS

- **Cortical**
- **Pituitary**

Cortical

During recent years, the neural connection between the higher cortical centers and the hypothalamus has been well established. Apart from this, there are numerous output connections to pituitary gland as well other areas of the central nervous system (CNS), e.g. amygdala, hippocampus (limbic system), the thalamus and the pons (Fig. 7.8). Through this system, the ovarian and consequently the menstrual cycle are affected by various emotional and environmental factors.

Pituitary

The hypothalamus is connected with the anterior lobe of the pituitary (**adenohypophysis**) through a special hypothalamo-pituitary portal system of vessels. However, it is directly connected with the posterior lobe of the pituitary (**neurohypophysis**) by the supraoptic and paraventricular nuclei (Fig. 7.1).

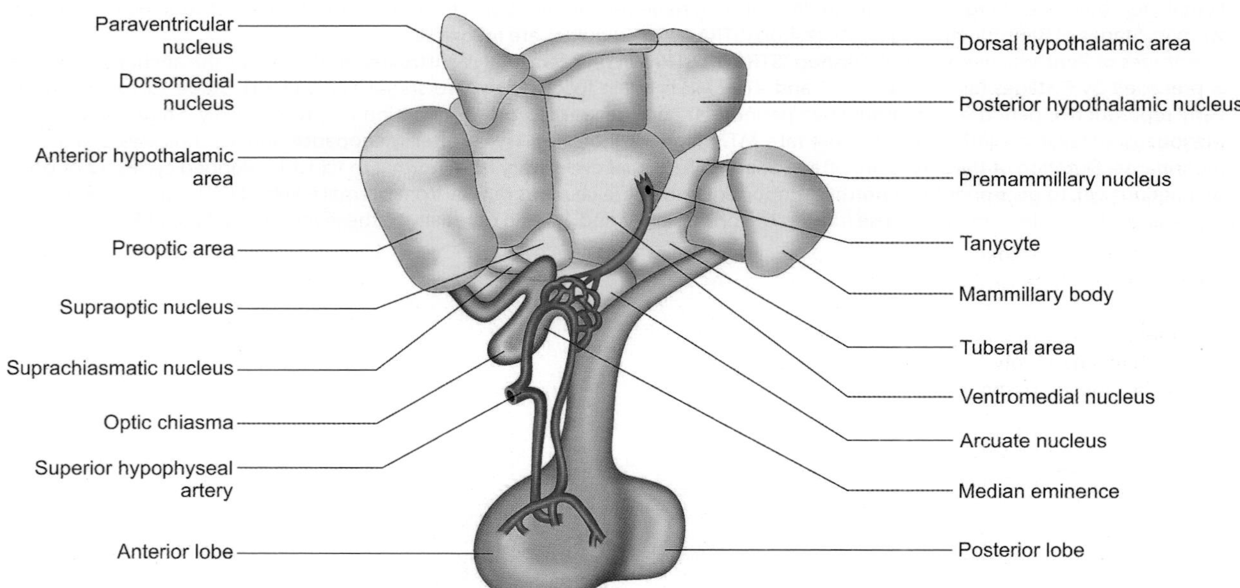

Fig. 7.1: Anatomy of the hypothalamus and pituitary. The hypothalamus, anterior pituitary and the portal system of blood supply is shown.

SECRETIONS

The hypothalamus produces a series of specific releasing and inhibiting hormones which have got effect on the production of the specific pituitary hormones. These hormones are synthesized by the hypothalamic neurons and are released at the nerve endings around the tuber cinereum. Thereafter, these are drained to the pituitary through the hypothalamo-pituitary portal system of vessels.

Gonadotropin-releasing Hormone (GnRH) (Ch. 32)

The GnRH is also named as *luteinizing hormone-releasing hormone* (LHRH). **GnRH is a decapeptide** and is concerned with the release, synthesis and storage of both the gonadotropins [follicle-stimulating hormone (FSH) and luteinizing hormone (LH)] from the anterior pituitary. The divergent patterns of FSH and LH in response to a single GnRH are due to modulating influence of the endocrine environment especially the feedback effects of steroids on anterior pituitary gland. **GnRH is secreted by the arcuate nucleus of the hypothalamus (Fig. 7.1) in a pulsatile fashion.** Developmentally, these neurons originated from the olfactory area. The half-life of GnRH is very short (2–4 minutes). This is due to the cleavage of amino acid bonds between 5–6, 6–7 and 9–10 in circulation (Fig. 7.2). GnRH is secreted into the portal circulation in **pulsatile fashion.** This pulse secretion varies in **frequency and amplitude** at different phases of menstrual cycle (*see* below). **GnRH stimulates anterior pituitary** for synthesis, storage and secretion of gonadotropins. There is decrease in receptor sensitivity when gonadotroph cells (adenohypophysis) are exposed to GnRH stimulation continually. This is called **'downregulation'**. On the contrary, intermittent exposure of GnRH to gonadotrophs, increase the receptor sensitivity. This is called **'upregulation'**. This variable response of anterior pituitary gonadotrophs to GnRH have been utilized in different clinical situation to get therapeutic benefits.

GnRH gene is located on the short arm of chromosome 8. Several forms of GnRH decapeptides have been identified. The principal GnRH is GnRH-2 and thus differs from GnRH by 3 amino acids.

The GnRH axons terminate within the capillary plexus in the median eminence where GnRH is released. Hypophyseal portal vessels descend along the pituitary stalk to terminate in another capillary plexus within the anterior lobe of pituitary.

The mechanisms involved in pulsatile release of GnRH is thought to be due to kisspeptin (Kiss 1). In general estradiol decreases GnRH pulse amplitude and progesterone decreases GnRH pulse frequency.

Prolactin Inhibitory Factor (PIF)

Prolactin secretion from the anterior pituitary seems to be under chronic inhibition by PIF. **Dopamine is the physiological inhibitor.**

Thyrotropin-releasing Hormone (TRH)

The hormone TRH, a tripeptide stimulates the release of not only the thyrotropin but also prolactin from the pituitary.

Corticotropin-releasing Hormone (CRH)

It is a tetradecapeptide.

Other secretions are—growth hormone-releasing hormone (GHRH) and melanocytic releasing factor.

CONTROL OF GnRH SECRETION

The neurohormonal control of GnRH secretion is modulated by five ways:
1. Neurotransmitters and neuromodulators
2. Peptides
3. Ultrashort feedback loop
4. Short feedback loop
5. Long feedback loop.

Neurotransmitters and Neuromodulators

The control of GnRH secretion is highly complex and dependent on a number of inhibitory or excitatory pathways involving neurotransmitters and neuromodulators with interaction of ovarian steroids (Flowchart 7.1). The neurotransmitters and neuromodulators within the brain act through a neural input.

The important neurotransmitters are catecholamines—dopamine, norepinephrine (noradrenaline) and serotonin.

Norepinephrine exerts a stimulatory effect on the release of GnRH, while **dopamine** exerts its inhibitory effect. **Serotonin** plays an inhibitory role in GnRH release.

Catecholamines are capable of changing the frequency of GnRH pulse. Thus, pharmacological agents, psychological factors which affect the brain catecholamines, are likely to affect the pulsatile release of GnRH.

The principal neuromodulators are endogenous opioids, peptides and prostaglandins.

Endogenous opioids: The important endogenous opioids are endorphins, encephalins and dynorphins. They inhibit GnRH release and thereby inhibit gonadotropin secretion.

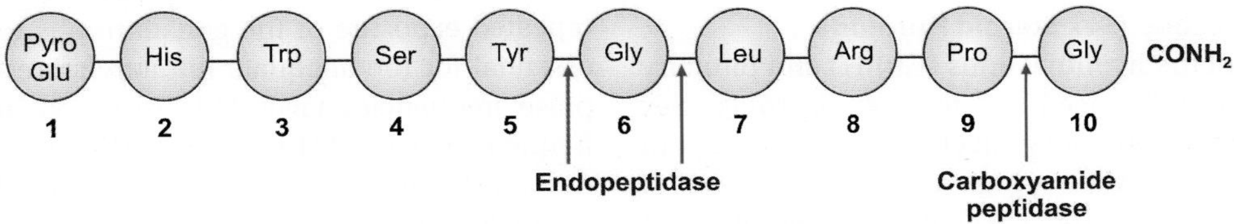

Fig. 7.2: Gonadotropin-releasing hormone (GnRH).

Flowchart 7.1: Neurohormonal control of GnRH secretion.

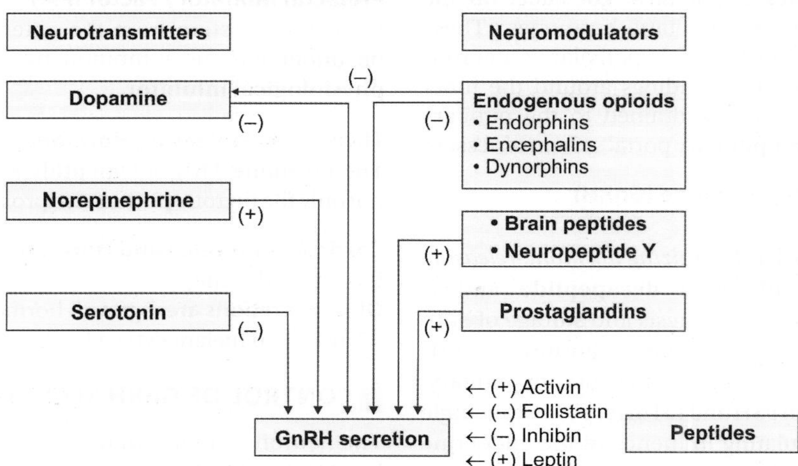

The endorphins may suppress both the dopamine and GnRH pathway leading to increase in prolactin secretions. Increased endogenous opioids has been actively implicated in hypothalamic amenorrhea and elevated prolactin levels observed in association with stress and exercise. **Prostaglandin E** produced locally, increases the release of GnRH.

Role of Peptides

A number of peptides like activin, inhibin and follistatin are produced by GnRH from pituitary cells as well as from the granulosa cells of the ovary. Activin stimulates but follistatin inhibits GnRH secretion. Inhibin blocks GnRH receptors. LH secretion is regulated by GnRH. Inhibin, activin or follistatin has no effect on it.

Ultrashort Feedback Loop

It refers to autoregulation of the releasing hormone of the hypothalamus on its own synthesis. If the GnRH production is more, it will suppress and if it is less, it will stimulate its own production.

GnRH can regulate the concentration of its own pituitary receptors.

Short Feedback Loop (Gonadotropins)

It relates to the secretion of the GnRH by the interplay between the neurotransmitters and the pituitary gonadotropins. FSH and LH are believed to exert negative feedback effect on hypothalamic production of GnRH.

Long Feedback Loop (Sex Steroid Hormones)

The secretion of the hypothalamus (GnRH) and pituitary (FSH, LH) are influenced by the sex steroids. Sex steroids exert their inhibitory effect throughout except in preovulatory period, when a high and sustained level of estradiol exerts a stimulatory effect in the release of GnRH through catechol estrogen.

Nature of Secretion

The secretion and release of GnRH are tonic, cyclic and pulsatile.

The tonic center is controlled primarily by the negative feedback of sex steroids, probably via dopaminergic activity.

The cyclic center is stimulated by the positive feedback effect of preovulatory sustained and high rise of estradiol resulting in increased GnRH secretion.

The pulsatile release (i.e. secretion of GnRH into portal circulation) is presumably regulated by the neurotransmitters and neuromodulators. The pulse secretion of GnRH has an amplitude and frequency. **Amplitude signifies** the amount of GnRH delivered into portal circulation. **Frequency means** at what interval the GnRH is delivered into portal circulation. The frequency is rapid in the follicular phase, about one pulse per hour and lower in the luteal phase about one pulse every 2–3 hours. In the follicular phase the amplitude is low but it is high in luteal phase.

GnRH Action on Anterior Pituitary (Self-priming of Gonadotrophs)

GnRH, on reaching the anterior lobe of the pituitary, stimulates the synthesis and release of both LH and FSH from the same cell (gonadotrophs) in the pituitary gland.

GnRH is involved not only in release of stored LH and FSH but it is of importance in maintaining the synthesis of gonadotropins. It has been demonstrated that repeated exposure of the gonadotrophs to GnRH seems essential for the adequate pituitary stores. Lower GnRH pulse frequencies favor FSH secretion and the higher frequencies favor LH secretion. This response has been termed 'self-priming'. It has got a cyclic relationship and is greatest with the higher levels of estrogen. Estrogen preferentially induces more LH than FSH release.

Physiological Control Mechanism of Gonadotropin Release

There are two pools of gonadotropins. One is readily releasable by the initial exposure to GnRH (primary pool) and a second one—called reserve pool (secondary pool). GnRH makes this larger reserve pool to be more readily released by a subsequent repeated exposure. Thus, this is suggestive of a transfer of gonadotropins from one pool to the other.

Mechanism of Action of GnRH on Pituitary Cell (Fig. 7.3)

GnRH binds to the specific receptors on the cell membrane of the gonadotrophs. Within a second, there is activation of the enzyme, adenyl cyclase which catalyzes the conversion of adenosine triphosphate (ATP) to cyclic adenosine monophosphate (cAMP). cAMP-receptor protein complex then activates protein kinase C. Intracellular free Ca^{++} concentration increases. Protein kinase C causes phosphorylation and activation of specific enzymes. Ca^{++}, protein kinase C and cAMP then interact to stimulate the release of stored FSH and LH and their subsequent biosynthesis.

However, if GnRH continues to be infused, gonadotropin secretion is inhibited, probably because the receptors are saturated and are unable to stimulate the release of second messenger. This is known as **desensitization or downregulation**.

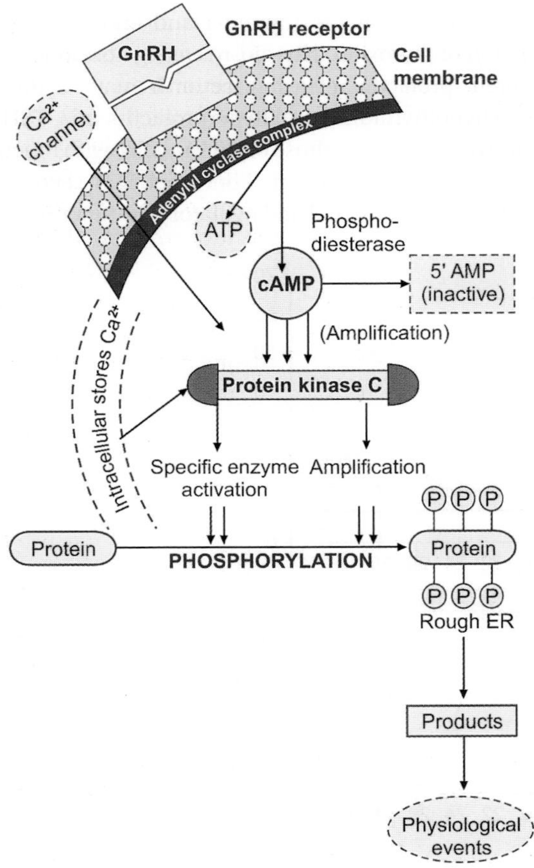

Fig. 7.3: Schematic representation of hormone GnRH receptor signal activation.

PITUITARY GLAND

The pituitary gland lies in a bony cavity called sella turcica. The gland, principally consists of two parts—the anterior pituitary (adenohypophysis) and the posterior pituitary (neurohypophysis).

ANTERIOR PITUITARY

The anterior pituitary is a large, compact and highly vascular gland. It consists of cells arranged in nests or columns. The cells are of two types:

1. **Chromophobes** or parent cells—these are small cells without affinity for any dye.
2. **Chromophils**—these are larger cells which stain easily.
   - Acidophils or eosinophils or alpha cells which stain red with eosin. These cells produce growth hormone and lactogenic hormone (prolactin).
   - Basophils or beta cells which stain blue with hematoxylin.

These beta cells are of three types. **The oval ones produce gonadotropins**; the angular ones produce thyrotropin and the lightly granulated ones produce corticotropin.

Secretions from Anterior Pituitary

Gonadotropins

There are two gonadotropic hormones secreted from the anterior pituitary—(a) Follicle-stimulating hormone (FSH) and (b) Luteinizing hormone (LH).

Site of secretion and chemical nature

The mechanisms of hormone synthesis, storage and release of the anterior pituitary hormones are poorly understood. While pulsatile stimulation of hypothalamic GnRH is required by the pituitary for the synthesis and release of gonadotropins, ovarian hormones determine the cyclic pattern of FSH and LH as they occur in normal cycle. FSH and LH are secreted from the beta cells in a pulsatile fashion in response to pulsatile GnRH. **These are water-soluble glycoproteins** of high molecular weight. They have got two subunits. The amino acid composition of the α subunits of FSH, LH and human chorionic gonadotropins (hCG) are similar. The hormone specificity being determined by the difference between the β subunits.

Functions of FSH

The function of FSH is predominantly morphogenic, related to the growth and maturation of the Graafian follicle. It acts primarily on the granulosa cells. In conjunction with LH, it is also involved in maturation of oocyte, ovulation and steroidogenesis.

- **Morphological effects**
- **Biochemical effects**

Morphological effects of FSH

- FSH rescues follicles from apoptosis
- Stimulates formation of follicular vesicles (antral follicle)

- Stimulates proliferation of granulosa cells
- Helps full maturation of the Graafian follicle (dominant follicle) as it converts the follicular microenvironment from androgen dominated to estrogen dominated (p. 69).

Biochemical effects of FSH

- **Synthesizes its own receptors** in the granulosa cells.
- **Synthesizes LH receptors** in the theca cells.
- **Synthesizes LH receptors** in the granulosa cells.
- **Induces aromatization** to convert androgens to estrogens in granulosa cells (p. 75).
- **Enhances autocrine and paracrine function** (IGF-II, IGF-I) in the follicle.
- **Stimulates granulosa cells** to produce activin and inhibin.
- **Stimulates plasminogen activator** necessary for ovulation.

The FSH level tends to rise soon following the onset of menstruation and attains its peak at the twelfth day of the cycle (preovulatory) and gradually declines to attain the base level at about the eighteenth day (Figs. 7.4A and B).

Functions of LH

The main function of LH is steroidogenic as it acts primarilly on theca cells. Along with FSH, it is responsible for full maturation of the Graafian follicle and oocyte and ovulation.

- **Biochemical effects**
- **Morphological effects**

Biochemical effects (steroidogenic) of LH

- **Activation of LH receptors** in the theca cells which stimulates the enzymes necessary for androgen production → diffuse into the granulosa cells → estrogens.
- **Luteinization of the granulosa cells** → to secrete progesterone.
- Synthesizes prostaglandins.

Morphological effects of LH

- **Stimulates resumption** of meiosis with extrusion of first polar body (p. 76).
- **Helps in the physical act of ovulation.**
- **Formation and maintenance of corpus luteum.**

Therefore FSH receptors are present primarily on the granulosa cells. Receptors for LH are present on the theca cells at all stages of the cycle. They are also present on the granulosa cells after the follicle matures.

LH levels remain almost static throughout the cycle except at least 12 hours prior to ovulation, when it attains its peak, called LH surge (Figs. 7.4A and B).

Prolactin

Prolactin is secreted from the alpha cells and **is a polypeptide.**

Its role in the human reproductive physiology is not clearly understood. Its role in the maintenance of corpus luteum in human is not well-documented, but the fact remains that there is high incidence of anovulation in women with elevated plasma prolactin levels (p. 486). The mechanism of amenorrhea with hyperprolactinemia is due to the alterations of GnRH pulsatility.

Thyrotropic Hormone

Thyroid-stimulating hormone (TSH) is produced by the beta cells. It acts on the thyroid gland and regulate the production of thyroxine. Thyroid-releasing hormone (TRH) is a potent prolactin releasing factor. It may be the link between hypothyroidism and hyperprolactinemia. TSH has got α and β subunits like those of FSH and LH, with functions of β subunits being different. Abnormal TSH secretion is associated with menstrual and ovulatory dysfunction.

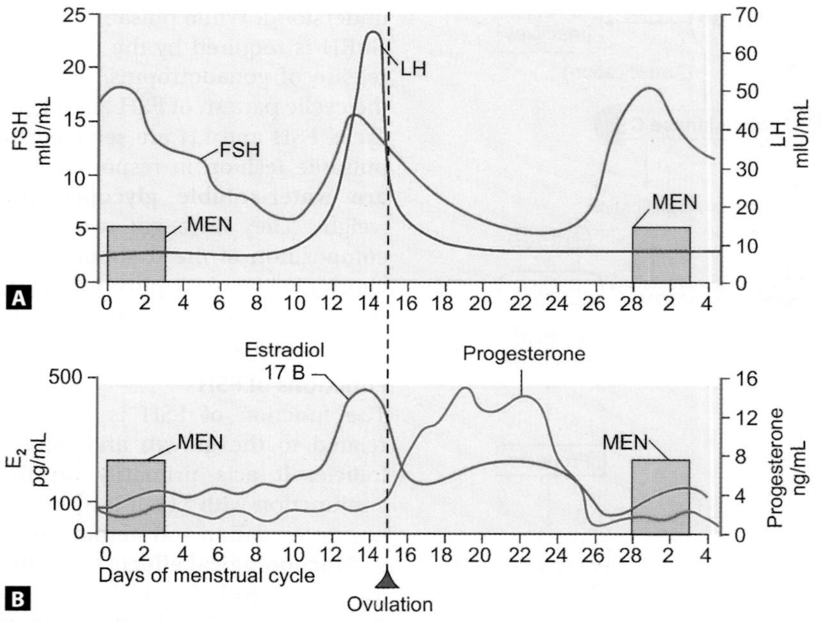

Figs. 7.4A and B: Fluctuations of levels of different gonadotropins (A) and the steroid hormones (B) during a normal menstrual cycle (ovulatory).

Corticotropin Releasing Hormone (CRH)

CRH consists of 41 amino acids. CRH stimulates adrenocorticotropic hormone (ACTH) biosynthesis and secretion. CRH is under negative feedback regulation of circulating cortisol. Increased levels of CRH inhibit GnRH secretion. This may be the reason for hypercortisolism and menstrual abnormalities.

Adrenocorticotropic Hormone (ACTH)

ACTH is also secreted by the beta cells. It stimulates the production of corticosteroids in the adrenal cortex.

Growth Hormone-releasing Hormone (GHRH)

Growth hormone (GH) is regulated by GHRH and inhibited by somatostatin.

Similar to GnRH, GHRH secretion is in a pulsatile fashion. Exercise, stress, sleep and hypoglycemia stimulate GH release.

Somatotropin or Growth Producing Hormone

It is secreted from the alpha cells of the pituitary and acts directly on the skeletal system.

GH stimulates skeletal and muscle growth. GH induces insulin resistance and may precipitate diabetes mellitus.

Melanocyte-stimulating Hormone (MSH)

It is clearly linked with ACTH. The hormone is increased during puberty and in pregnancy. It is probably responsible for the pigmentary changes during those periods.

POSTERIOR PITUITARY

The hormones oxytocin and vasopressin are formed in the hypothalamus and transported within the neurons in the hypothalamohypophyseal tract. Both the hormones are bound to polypeptides called neurophysins.

Oxytocin is a nonapeptide. It is produced by the paraventricular nucleus of the hypothalamus. Oxytocin acts on the myometrial contractile system, especially during labor and also causes contraction of the myoepithelial cells in the breast ductules during lactation.

Arginine-vasopressin is also a nonapeptide, with two amino acid composition different from that of oxytocin. It is produced by the supraoptic nucleus. It regulates plasma osmolality and circulating blood volume.

OVARY

The gross anatomy (Ch. 1) and the structure of the functional unit of the ovary (Ch. 8) are described in the appropriate chapters. **The functions of the ovary** are ovulation and production of hormones (steroidogenesis). The ovulation is dealt in the Ch. 8.

OVARIAN STEROIDOGENESIS

The principal hormones secreted from the ovaries are—(a) Estrogens; (b) Progesterone; (c) Androgens; and (d) Inhibin.

Estrogens

Site of Production

The estrogen is predominantly estradiol (E_2) and to a lesser extent estrone.

The sites of production in the ovary are:

- Predominant sites are granulosa cells of the follicles and from the same cells after luteinization to form corpus luteum.
- Small quantity is also produced from the theca cells and ovarian stroma.

Mechanism of Steroid Hormone Production (Figs. 7.5A and B)

Two cell, two gonadotropin, concept of ovarian steroidogenesis establishes the fact that two cells **(theca cells and granulosa cells)** produce different hormones under the influence of **two gonadotropins (LH and FSH)**. During the **follicular phase**, under the influence of LH, androgens (androstenedione and testosterone) are produced in the theca cells. These androgens diffuse into the granulosa cells where they are aromatized under the influence of FSH to estrogens—estradiol predominantly and to lesser extent estrone (Figs. 7.5 to 7.7).

After ovulation, progesterone is synthesized in the luteinized granulosa cells under the influence of LH. The precursor- low density lipoproteins (LDL) is available to the site after vascularization of the granulosa cells following ovulation. During luteal phase, androstenedione produced by the theca luteal cells diffuses into the granulosa luteal cells (Fig. 7.7) to be converted into estradiol by LH. During follicular phase, it is the FSH that enhances aromatase activity in the granulosa cells. Whereas during the luteal phase it is the LH that enhances the aromatase activity in the luteinized granulosa cells for the conversion of androstenedione to estradiol. Therefore, during luteal phase, a two cell (theca luteal and granulosa luteal)—one gonadotropin (LH) system works for estradiol biosynthesis.

Metabolism

The estrogens are bound to albumin (30%) and sex hormone binding globulin (SHBG) in 69% and the remaining free 1% is biologically active. Unlike trophic hormones, steroid hormones enter the cell and mediate action via receptors within the nucleus as shown diagrammatically in Figures 7.6 and 7.7 to produce specific response.

Following this, the estrogens are quickly inactivated by converting to estriol. Of the three classic estrogens, **estradiol is the most potent**, being ten times as potent as estrone which is ten times as potent as estriol.

The estriol is conjugated in the liver with glucuronic acid. The conjugated estrogen is excreted partly in the bile and partly in the urine. The bile fractions on reaching the intestine are broken down by microorganisms and then reabsorbed as active hormones (enterohepatic circulation). The disturbances of liver function or of the intestinal flora can thus alter this mechanism with consequent disturbances of menstrual cycles.

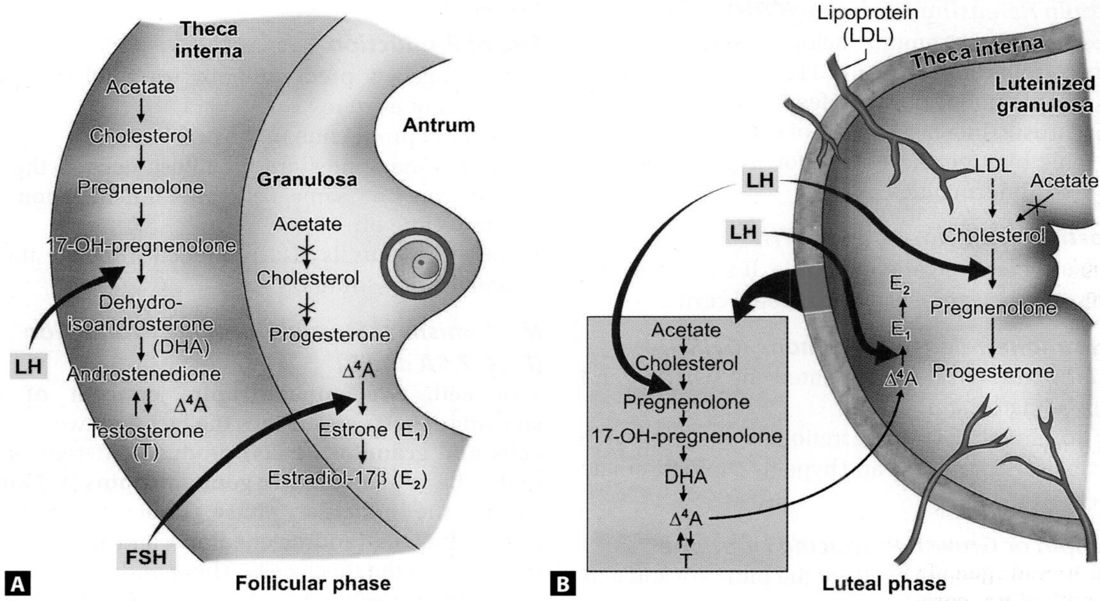

Figs. 7.5A and B: Schematic representation of the ovarian steroidogenesis (Two cell, two gonadotropin 7.4A and two cell, one gonadotropin 7.4B concept).

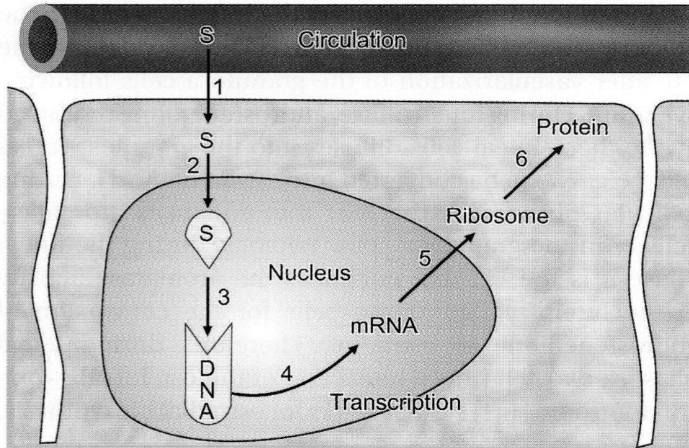

Fig. 7.6: Mechanism of action of steroid hormone: The precise mechanism of action of steroid hormones includes: (1) Diffusion of steroid hormone through the cell membrane; (2) Steroid hormone receptor complex within the nucleus; (3) Interaction of this complex with nuclear DNA; (4) Synthesis of messenger RNA (mRNA); (5) mRNA combines with ribosome in the cytoplasm; (6) Synthesis of protein and desired activity.

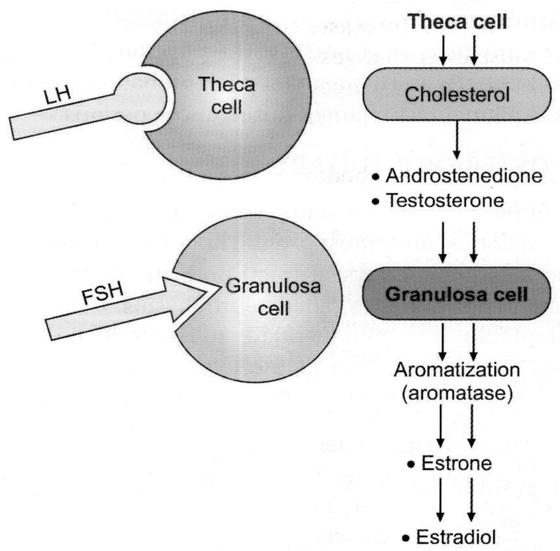

Fig. 7.7: Two cell and two gonadotropin theory of ovarian steroidogenesis.

Amount of Estrogen Production and Blood Level (Table 7.1)

Total daily production of estradiol is estimated to be about 50 μg during the early follicular phase reaching 150–300 μg at ovulation.

The blood level rises to about 300–600 pg/mL at ovulation. After a sharp fall, it rises again to about 150–200 pg/mL in the luteal phase (Fig. 7.4).

Total quantity of estradiol production during a cycle from ovulatory ovary is estimated to be 10 mg.

Physiological Action

Two isoforms of estrogen receptors (ERα; ERβ) have been observed to be encoded by two separate genes. They are variably expressed in tissues. Both the receptors are required for normal ovarian function.

Secondary sex characters: Estrogen tends to induce feminine characteristics. The hormone is responsible for feminine body configuration and feminine mental make up including shyness. There is secretion in apocrine glands, change in voice and deposition of fat on the breasts, thighs and hips. The growth of axillary and pubic hair is dependent predominantly on androgens of adrenal origin.

Action on the genital organs: Under the action of estrogen, the genital organs not only develop into maturity but induce cyclic changes for reproduction. After menopause, with the fall in the estrogen level, atrophic changes of the organs occur.

TABLE 7.1: Daily production, serum values and urinary excretion of hormones.

Hormones	Follicular phase	At ovulation	Luteal phase
Daily production			
Estradiol (μg)	50	150–300	100
Progesterone (mg)	2–3		20–30
Serum values			
Estradiol (pg/mL)	50	300–600	150–200
Progesterone (ng/mL)	<1		>5
FSH (mIU/mL)	10	15–20	10
LH (mIU/mL)	5	60	5
Daily excretion			
Total estrogen (μg)	10–25	35–100	25–75
Pregnanediol (mg)	<1		3–6

Vulva and vagina: All the structures are influenced by the estrogens. The vaginal vascularity and epithelial activity are related to estrogen. Estrogen induces thickening of the lining epithelium, cornification of the superficial cells and deposition of glycogen which is converted into lactic acid by the Doderlein's bacilli. As such, the vaginal flora is maintained by estrogen.

Uterus: There is increased vascularity with hyperplasia of the muscles. It changes the uterus from the infantile to adult form. Cyclic changes in the endometrium includes regeneration and proliferation of the endometrium. **It produces receptors for progesterone**. Withdrawal of estrogen causes shedding of the endometrium and menstruation.

Cervix: Estrogen causes hypertrophy of the cervix and increases the cervical gland secretion. The secretion is more watery, alkaline with less protein and more electrolytes. These favor penetration of the sperm.

Fallopian tubes: There is increased vascularity with increased motility of the tubes.

Breasts: There is increased proliferation of the ducts and stromal tissues. There is also increased vascularity and pigmentation of the areola. Accumulation of fat also occurs. Breast secretion, however, cannot occur.

Blood: Estrogen increases the coagulability of blood by increasing many procoagulants, chiefly fibrinogen. The platelets become more adhesive.

Locomotor system: Estrogen conserves calcium and phosphorus and encourages bone formation.

General: Estrogen increases sodium, nitrogen and fluid retention of the body. It lowers the blood cholesterol and lowers the incidence of coronary heart disease in women prior to menopause. It has got widespread capillary vasodilatation effect.

Endocrine System

- *Hypothalamopituitary axis.*

Negative Feedback

Estrogen exerts a negative feedback effect on the release of FSH. This is by:

- Direct action on pituitary, decreasing the sensitivity of the gonadotroph to GnRH.
- Direct action on the hypothalamus with a decrease in GnRH secretion, possibly via increased inhibitory dopaminergic activity.

Positive Feedback

High levels of estrogen (>200 pg/mL) exert a positive feedback effect on LH (mid cycle LH surge). Sustained (24–48 hours) elevated levels of estrogen lead to sustained and elevated LH secretion. It may be due to:

- Increasing pituitary responsiveness to GnRH
- Stimulating the hypothalamus in secreting GnRH.

The positive feedback effect cannot occur in the postovulatory phase because of the presence of progesterone.

- ***Ovary*:** The presence of E_2 and FSH in the antral fluid is essential for sustained proliferation of granulosa cells and continued follicular growth.
- It increases the binding globulin in circulation and raises the blood levels of protein bound iodine and protein bound cortisol.

Progesterone

Site of Secretion

The progesterone is secreted from the luteinized theca granulosa cells of the corpus luteum. A trace amount is however, secreted from the theca granulosa cells of the follicle and also from the ovarian stroma.

Metabolism

Progesterone is bound mainly to albumin (79%) and corticosteroid binding globulin (17.7%).

It is metabolized in the liver and excreted as sodium pregnanediol glucuronide (pregnanediol) in the urine. This metabolite has no progestational activity. Only 20% of secreted progesterone is conjugated and appears in the urine as pregnanediol. The fate of the remainder is not clear.

17-α-hydroxyprogesterone is an important product of the ovary. It is metabolized in the liver and reduced to pregnanetriol.

Amount of Production and Blood Level (Table 7.1)

Daily production of progesterone is 2–3 mg in follicular phase and 20–30 mg in luteal phase.

Daily excretion of pregnanediol in the urine is less than 1 mg in follicular phase and 3–6 mg in luteal phase.

Serum value of progesterone is less than 1 ng/mL in follicular phase and 5–15 ng/mL in midluteal phase (Fig. 7.4).

Physiological Action

PGN mediates its receptor action though multiple isoforms eneoded by a single gene. The PRA; PRB are al most identical. Progesterone acts on all the organs of the genital tract and on the breasts provided they are sensitized by estrogen.

- **Uterus:** Progesterone produces myohyperplasia and diminishes the contractility of the myometrium. It however, increases the tone of the circular muscle fibers at the isthmus. It produces secretory activity in the endometrium; enhances secretion of the glands rich in glycogen. The character of the cervical mucus is changed and become more thick and viscid preventing sperm penetration.

- **Vagina:** The maturation of the vaginal epithelium is hindered. There is more shedding of the intermediate cells with folded edges and a tendency to clump.
- **Fallopian tubes:** The epithelial cells are stimulated to secrete clear mucus which helps in migration of the ovum. Tubal motility is however, decreased which may predispose to tubal pregnancy.
- **Breasts:** Along with estrogen, it produces hypertrophy and growth of the acinar structures.
- **General:** Progesterone is thermogenic, raises the basal body temperature by 0.2–0.5°C. There may be enhanced deposition of fat in the tissues. It relaxes smooth muscles and ligaments—especially during pregnancy. It promotes the secretion of sebum by the skin. Like other steroids, it causes fluid retention.

Endocrine System

- **Hypothalamo-pituitary axis:** The principal negative feedback action of progesterone is upon the midcycle gonadotropin surge and it may be responsible for its short duration.

  Progesterone by itself does not appear to exert a positive feedback effect. However, its rise during preovulatory period is related with the FSH surge by its positive feedback action. The positive feedback effect of estradiol in the secretory phase is inhibited by progesterone.
- **GnRH secretion:** Progesterone first (low level) stimulates, then (high level) inhibits the production of GnRH.
- **Ovary:** Progesterone acts through both intraovarian and central negative feedback mechanisms to suppress new follicular growth. It is postulated that increased intraovarian progesterone concentration prevents follicular maturation in that ovary in the subsequent cycle.

Androgens

The androgens are produced in the ovary by all three types of cells—stroma, theca and granulosa, but mainly by the theca interna of the follicles. The production of androgens is primarily under the control of LH. **The principal androgens secreted are**—dehydroepiandrosterone, androstenedione and testosterone.

The principal site of metabolism is liver. The androgens are reduced to androsterone and etiocholanolone. These can be measured in the urine as 11 deoxy-17 ketosteroids.

Total daily production of androstenedione is 3 mg and of testosterone 0.2–0.3 mg.

Plasma level of androstenedione is 1.3–1.5 ng/mL, that of testosterone 0.3–0.6 ng/mL and of SHBG 38–103 nmol/L.

Peptides and their Role

- **Inhibin, activin and follistatin** are the polypeptides, secreted by the granulosa cells in response to FSH. Inhibin and activin are glycoproteins. Inhibin, inhibits FSH secretion. Activin is produced by the pituitary and granulosa cells. **Activin** stimulates FSH release from the pituitary. It also enhance FSH action in the ovary. Follistatin, suppresses FSH activity by inhibiting activin.
- **Inhibin:** It is secreted by the granulosa cells of the ovarian follicle in response to FSH. It has got a preferential negative feedback effect on FSH release. FSH and inhibin bear a reciprocal relationship. Inhibin A and inhibin B block the synthesis and secretion of FSH.
- **Leptin** is a peptide and is produced by adipose cells. It enhances the release of GnRH. Leptin level is elevated in obesity. It has a possible role in implantation.

ANTI-MÜLLERIAN HORMONE

- Anti-Müllerian hormone (AMH) is a peptide produced by the granulosa cells of primordial follicles (<6 mm) and by the Sertoli cells of fetal testes.
- AMH belongs to transforming growth factor-β super family.
- It causes Müllerian duct regression during male sexual differentiation.
- AMH levels reflect the number of growing follicles in the ovary.
- It helps oocyte maturation and follicular development and recruitment of dominant follicle. It favours monofollicular development.
- Low levels of AMH is observed with rise of FSH and E_2 levels and also with increasing age of the women (as the follicle number declines).
- AMH levels correlates with ovarian primordial follicle number more strongly than FSH or inhibin levels.
- Estimation of serum AMH is independent of menstral cycle. It is used as a predictor of ovarian reserve (p. 443).
- AMH is used for assessing ovarian reserve. It suppresses FSH stimulation. Serum levels decreases with age.
- Levels around 0.05 ng/mL indicates menopause within 4–5 years.
- Levels >2 ng/mL suggest good reserve, levels <0.5 ng/mL suggest decreased ovarian reserve.
- High levels of AMH suggest polycystic ovarian syndrome.
- Role of AMH in follicular development: AMH inhibits initial recruitment of primordial follicles into the pool of growing follicles. It also decreases responsiveness of follicles to FSH. It prevents premature depletion of the follicular pool.
- **Interleukin-1 (IL-1)** is a polypeptide cytokine. It is produced by macrophages and also by the theca and granulosa cells following follicular rupture. It has antigonadotropic activity and it suppresses luteinization of granulosa cells.

Relaxin

Relaxin is secreted from the preovulatory follicle and corpus luteum. It probably facilitates follicular rupture during ovulation.

Growth factors are polypeptides and they act locally through paracrine and autocrine way. Important growth factors are: Insulin-like growth factors (IGF), epidermal growth factor, tumor necrosis factor (TNF) α and interleukin-1 system.

Insulin-like growth factors (IGF)—are most abundant. IGF-II is produced in theca cells, granulosa cells and luteinized granulosa cells. IGF-II enhances gonadotropin (FSH and LH) actions to stimulate granulosa cell proliferation, aromatase activity, and progesterone synthesis.

THYROID GLANDS

The thyroid gland consists of numerous acini and follicles. Between the follicles, there are parafollicular or 'C' cells. The follicular cells synthesize iodine containing thyroxine (T_4) and triiodothyronine (T_3) under the influence of TSH of the anterior pituitary (Table 7.2). These hormones are related to body growth and metabolic needs. Ovarian function is markedly related to the thyroid activity. Normal enlargement of the gland occurs during puberty, pregnancy and menopause. Menstrual function may be significantly disturbed in thyroid dysfunction. Calcitonin is secreted from the parafollicular cells in response to elevated blood calcium.

ADRENAL GLANDS

Adrenal gland consists of two zones—outer cortex and inner medulla. The medulla secretes adrenaline and noradrenaline.

CONTROL OF CORTICAL SECRETIONS

Zona glomerulosa: Aldosterone is secreted from this zone. The secretion is principally controlled by the renin-angiotensin mechanism and is not markedly affected by ACTH. It produces retention of sodium and increased excretion of potassium through the renal tubules.

Zona reticularis and fasciculata: They act as a single unit. The principal hormones that are secreted are cortisol, corticosterone (glucocorticoids); androstenedione, androsterone and dehydroepiandrosterone (collectively called androgens) and to some extent estrogen and progesterone (Table 7.1). These constitute the extraovarian sources of steroids.

The control of cortisol synthesis through ACTH is regulated by the negative feedback, diurnal rhythm and stress. Stress can override the negative feedback mechanism and diurnal rhythm. A rise of plasma cortisol causes a rapid suppression of ACTH. A fall in cortisol level leads to increased production of ACTH probably through release of CRH from the hypothalamus.

The biosynthetic pathway in the secretion of cortisol through series of enzymatic action (predominantly 21-hydroxylase) is as follows (Flowchart 7.2):

- **Action of glucocorticoids**
  The main action of cortisol is anabolic.
  - Antagonistic to insulin and tends to raise the blood sugar.
  - Suppression of inflammatory reaction.
  - Lipogenic effect.

TABLE 7.2: Normal serum values of thyroid profile.

TSH	0.4–5 mmol/L	(3 μU/mL)
T_3	1.1–2.3 nmol/L	(70–190 ng/100 mL)
T_4	10–25 pmol/L	(5–12 μg/100 mL)

- **The action of androgens and adrenal steroids** are anabolic to antagonize the catabolic effects of the glucocorticoids.

HYPOTHALAMO-PITUITARY-OVARIAN AXIS

The hormones liberated from the hypothalamus, pituitary and ovary are dependent to one another. A well-coordinated axis is formed called hypothalamo-pituitary-ovarian axis (Fig. 7.8). The secretion of hormones from these glands is modified through feedback mechanism operating through this axis. The axis may also be modified by hormones liberated from the thyroid or adrenal glands. The enzymes required for steroidogenesis are shown in Flowchart 7.2.

FEEDBACK LOOP

- The long feedback loop refers to the feedback effects of the ovarian steroids on both the hypothalamus and pituitary. It is usually inhibitory (negative) but may be stimulatory (positive-preovulatory).
- The short feedback loop relates the secretion of GnRH by gonadotropins by interplay between the neurotransmitters and the pituitary gonadotropins. FSH and LH exert negative feedback effect on the hypothalamic production of GnRH.

Flowchart 7.2: Ovarian and adrenal steroidogenic pathways. The enzymes required for steroidogenesis are shown.

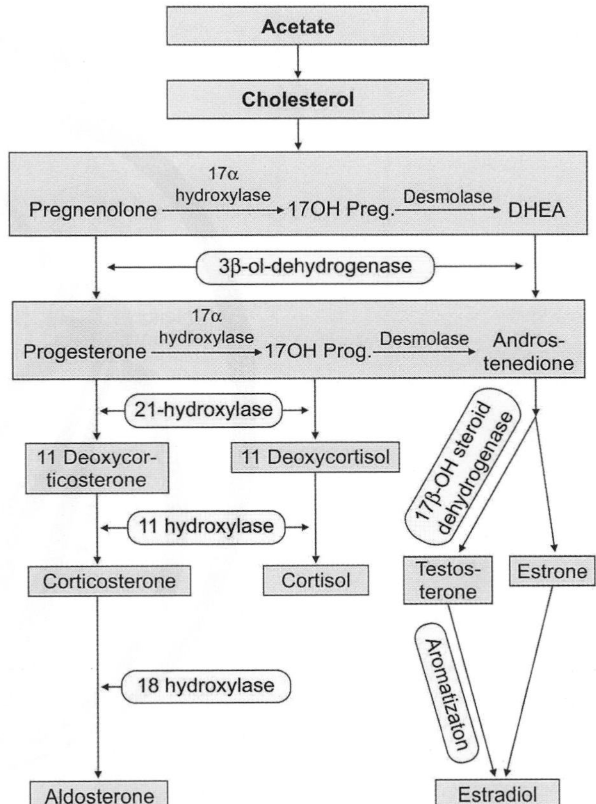

(17OH Preg.: 17OH pregnenolone; DHEA: dehydroepiandrosterone; 17OH Prog.: 17OH progesterone)

- Ultrashort feedback loop refers to autoregulation of the releasing hormones of the hypothalamus on its own synthesis (Fig. 7.8).

FETAL LIFE

In terms of hormone production, the hypothalamo-pituitary-ovarian axis is active and functional from approximately 20 weeks of fetal life. In fact, the circulatory gonadotropin levels remain at a higher level in fetal life than during neonatal period. The development of ovarian follicles in the fetus depends upon the gonadotropins released from the fetal pituitary.

INFANCY AND CHILDHOOD

The high level of FSH and to a lesser degree of LH at birth gradually decline and the minimum levels are achieved by two years of age. The FSH levels are highly sensitive to exogenous estrogen.

PREPUBERTY AND PUBERTY

The hypothalamo-pituitary-gonadal feedback system is in operation for many years prior to puberty. Prior to puberty, the hypothalamus is very much sensitive to the negative feedback by even a small amount of extragonadal steroids (estrogens produced by peripheral conversion of androgens from adrenals). As a result, the release of gonadotropin releasing hormone (GnRH) from the hypothalamus and that of FSH and LH from the anterior pituitary are kept in abeyance. As puberty approaches, the hypothalamic centers involved in the release of GnRH becomes more and more sensitive to the positive feedback of ovarian steroids. This may be related to increasing androgens from adrenals. There is augmented GnRH pulse release. This results in gradually increasing gonadotropin secretion (LH > FSH) → increasing ovarian stimulation → increasing estrogen levels → tonic and pulsatile discharge of gonadotropins.

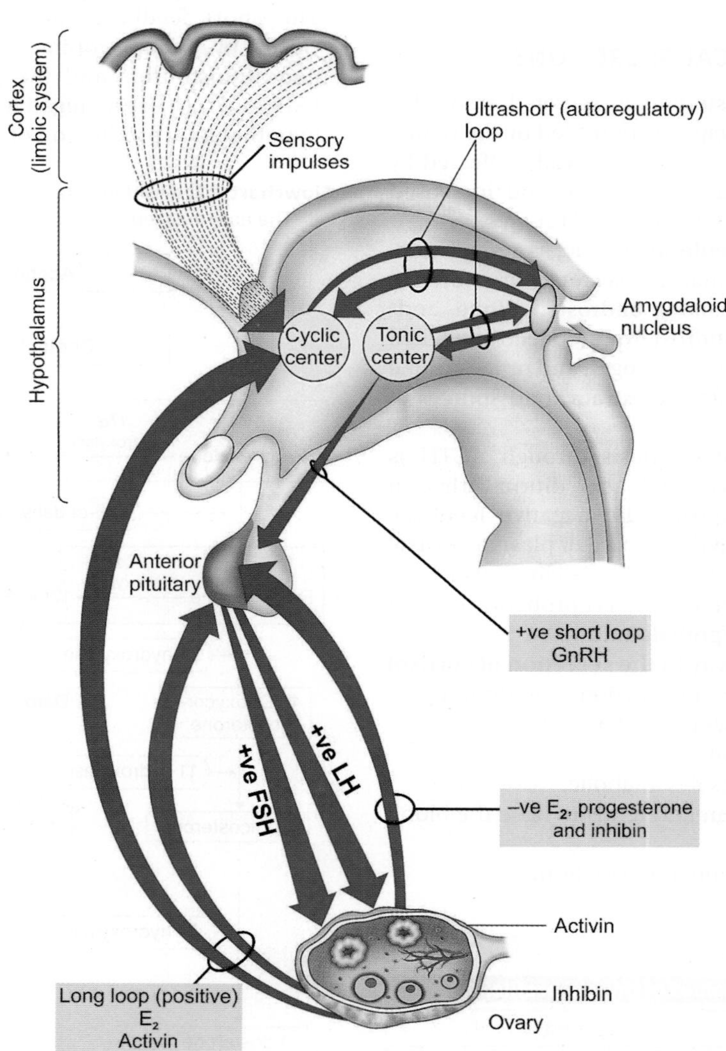

Fig. 7.8: Interplay of hormones along the hypothalamo-pituitary-ovarian axis through feedback mechanism.

This increasing level of estrogen is responsible for the growth and initiation of thelarche and finally menarche. The development of the positive feedback response to estrogen resulting in cyclic release of gonadotropins occurs after a variable period following menarche. As such, the first few cycles are expected to be anovulatory. The growth of pubic and axillary hair is related to increase in the secretion of adrenal androgens. The onset of this increase is called adrenarche which occurs at age 8–10 years.

OVARIAN AND MENSTRUAL CYCLE

Pregnancy and during 'Pill' intake: As the estrogen level is high in both the conditions, the pituitary gonadotropins remain static at low levels by the negative feedback mechanism.

FOLLOWING DELIVERY

During pregnancy, there is hypofunction of the axis induced by high level of estrogen. The hypothalamic hypofunction results in low levels of GnRH. In the immediate postpartum period, there is pituitary refractoriness to GnRH resulting in low FSH and LH levels. High prolactin levels render the ovary less sensitive to the already low gonadotropin stimulation resulting in ovarian inactivity, low estrogen status and anovulation. Even when ovarian activity resumes, raised levels of prolactin give rise to short luteal phase and reduced fertility. Lactating mother, usually ovulate 10 weeks after delivery as opposed to non lactating mother where ovulation occurs as early as 4 weeks (LAM) (Ch. 30, p. 422).

Thus, the picture of the first three weeks postpartum is one of hypothalamo-pituitary-ovarian inactivity which is prolonged by lactation under the influence of prolactin secretion.

MENOPAUSAL TRANSITION PERIOD

Few years prior to menopause, the ovarian follicles become gradually resistant to the pituitary gonadotropins. As a result of impaired folliculogenesis, less estrogen is secreted. There is decrease in the negative feedback effect of estrogen on the hypothalamic-pituitary-axis, resulting in increase of FSH. The increase of FSH may also be due to diminished follicular inhibin (p. 46).

When menopause sets in, the estradiol level comes down to basal 20 pg/mL and cannot have any negative feedback effect on hypothalamo-pituitary-axis (p. 46). As a result, GnRH release is enhanced resulting in increased synthesis and release of gonadotropins. The pulsatile pattern is maintained and while the frequency remains unaltered, the amplitude is markedly increased.

Gradually with senescence, the GnRH secretion is diminished and so also the gonadotropins and estrogens, when the true menopause sets in.

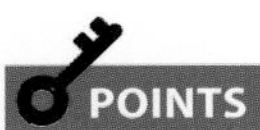

POINTS

- **Hypothalamus** has got neural connection with the cortex and through hypothalamo-portal system of vessels, connected with the anterior pituitary.
- Among the specific **releasing hormones**, the important releasing hormones are: GnRH, TRH, CRH and the prolactin secretion is inhibited by PIF. Dopamine is a physiological inhibitor.
- **GnRH** is a decapeptide with a very short half-life.
- **GnRH** is secreted in a pulsatile manner. The amplitude and frequency vary in the menstrual cycle. The frequency is rapid (one pulse/hour) in the follicular phase but slower (1 pulse/2–3 hours) in the luteal phase.
- **GnRH stimulates** the release and synthesis of both LH and FSH from the same cells of the anterior pituitary in pulsatile manner.
- **GnRH binds** to the specific receptor on the surface membrane of the gonadotrophs. A second messenger is activated combining Ca^{++}, protein kinase C and cAMP together to stimulate the release of stored LH and FSH and their subsequent synthesis (Fig. 7.3).
- **The neurohormonal control of GnRH** secretion is very complex. A number of neurotransmitters and neuromodulators are involved to play their inhibitory (endogenous opioids, dopamine, inhibin) and stimulatory (norepinephrine, prostaglandin, activin) roles (p. 55).
- **Gonadotropins** are secreted from the beta cells of anterior pituitary. These are glycoproteins. The hormone specificity is ascertained by β subunits.
- **Downregulation** is the decrease in sensitivity of the gonadotroph (adenohypophysis) receptors, due to continued stimulation of GnRH. Upregulation is the increase in receptor sensitivity due to intermittent exposure to GnRH.
- **GnRH analog** are produced by substitution of amino acids in the parent molecule at the 6 and 10 positions. The agonists have greater potencies and longer half-lives than the parent GnRH.
- Ovarian hormones determine the cyclic pattern of FSH and LH release (Fig. 7.8).
- The half-life of LH is 30 minutes and that of FSH is 3.9 hours. LH acts primarily on the theca cells to produce androgens. Granulosa cells convert androgens to estrogen by the enzyme aromatase.
- **FSH is predominantly** morphogenic but in conjunction with LH, it is involved in maturation of oocyte, ovulation and steroidogenesis. LH is predominantly steroidogenic. It also stimulates resumption of meiosis, helps in ovulation and formation and maintenance of corpus luteum.
- **LH acts primarily** on theca cells to produce androgens, whereas FSH acts primarily on the granulosa cells to produce estrogens by aromatization of androgens. LH also acts on the granulosa cells after the follicle matures under the influence of FSH and estradiols. The ovary secretes three principal steroid hormones: estradiol from the follicle, progesterone from the corpus luteum and androstenedione from the stroma.

Contd...

Contd...

- **Prolactin** is secreted from the alpha cells and is a polypeptide. Thyrotrophic hormone is produced by the beta cells.
- **The α subunits** of LH, FSH, TSH and hCG are similar. It is due to the different β subunits which provide specific biologic activity for each hormone.
- LH, FSH have the same α subunit of TSH and hCG. The β subunits of all these hormones have different amino acids and carbohydrates. These provide specific biologic activity of each hormone.
- **A number of peptides** like activin, inhibin and follistatin are produced by GnRH from pituitary cells as well as from the granulosa cells of the ovary. Inhibin inhibits FSH. Follistatin inhibits GnRH secretion. Activin stimulates FSH release.
- **Two cell, two gonadotropin concept** of ovarian steroidogenesis states that LH stimulates the theca cells to produce androgens, which are subsequently aromatized in the granulosa cells by FSH to produce estrogens (Figs. 7.5 and 7.7).
- **LH acts** upon the luteinized granulosa cells to produce progesterone. Estrogen is also produced in luteal phase under the influence of FSH and LH.
- ***The midcycle LH surge*** *initiates the resumption of meiosis-I. The primary oocyte under goes first meiotic division giving rise to secondary oocyte and first polar body (p. 76).*
- **The second meiotic division** is completed only after fertilization by a sperm. The ovum and second polar body is then developed (p. 68).
- **The sites** of production of estrogens, predominantly the estradiol, are granulosa cells, luteinized granulosa cells, theca cells and stroma of the ovary. The estrogens are produced by two-cell two gonadotropin concept (Figs. 7.5A and 7.7).
- **Androstenedione** is converted to estrone in the adipose tissue. Estradiol and estrone are interconvertible. Estrone sulfate is the major circulating estrogen and has a long half-life.
- **Estradiol** exerts a negative feedback effect on the hypothalamo-pituitary-axis. However, when the level is raised to more than 200 pg/mL and sustained for 24–48 hours, it has got positive feedback effects. The positive feedback effect cannot occur in the luteal phase because of progesterone.
- *Progesterone and corticosteroids have 21 carbon atoms, androgens have 19 carbon atoms and estrogens have 18 carbon atoms. All have the cyclopentanoperhydrophenanthrene nucleus. Cholesterol is the common biosynthetic precursor of steroid hormones.*
- The progesterone is secreted from the luteinized theca granulosa cells of the corpus luteum, theca granulosa cells of the follicle and from the stroma. Trace amount of 17-α-hydroxyprogesterone in the preovulatory period is essential for final maturation of the oocyte and involved in LH surge.
- *Kisspeptin (Kiss 1) plays a key role in the regulation of GnRH release.*
- **Serum progesterone** levels are <1 ng/mL before ovulation and reach 10–20 ng/mL at the mid luteal phase.
- **Progesterone** has got negative feedback on the hypothalamo-pituitary-axis; principally upon the midcycle gonadotropin surge and is responsible for its short duration.
- **Estrogen** stimulates the synthesis of both estrogen and progesterone receptors in target tissues. Progestins inhibit the synthesis of both the receptors. Progesterone has antimitotic and antiproliferative action.
- **Anti-Müllerian hormone (AMH)** is a peptide secreted by the granulosa cells of primordial follicles (<6 mm). AMH levels reflect the number of growing follicles in the ovary. Low levels of AMH is observed with rise of FSH. AMH levels are used as a predictor of ovarian reserve and response to ovarian stimulation protocol (p. 443).
- Normal enlargement of **thyroid gland** occurs during puberty, pregnancy and menopause.
- Menstrual function is significantly disturbed in thyroid dysfunction.
- The biosynthetic pathway in the secretion of cortisol is through series of enzymatic action from cholesterol via 17-α-hydroxy progesterone. Ovarian and adrenal steroidogenic pathways lead to biosynthesis of androgens, estrogens and corticosteroids. These involve a series of enzymatic action (p. 76).
- *Due to absence of 21-hydroxylase, 11-β hydroxylase and 18-hydroxylase reductase activity, ovaries cannot synthesize mineralocorticoids and glucocorticoids.*
- The **hypothalamo-pituitary**-axis is active and functional from 20 weeks of fetal life.
- **At puberty**, increasing estrogen levels result in pulsatile release of gonadotropins. The development of positive feedback effect occurs 2–3 years following menarche.
- **During pregnancy** and 'pill' taking period, gonadotropins remain static at low levels.
- **During first three weeks** postpartum, there is hypothalamo-pituitary-ovarian inactivity due to high level of prolactin. As menopause approaches, there is less production of estrogens and the remaining ovarian follicles become resistant to gonadotropins. There is decrease in follicular inhibin. The combined effects result in increase in FSH and later on LH also. When the estradiol level falls below 20 pg/mL, menopause sets in.
- **GnRH release** is also enhanced because of decrease in negative feedback effect of estrogen. This results also in increased release and synthesis of gonadotropins.
- **Dominant follicle** is selected by days 5 and 7 of the cycle. The dominant follicle on ultrasonography has a maximum diameter of about 20 mm and a volume of 3.8 mL. It secretes more estradiol which in turn induces more FSH receptors (p. 69, Figs. 8.2 and 8.4).
- **FSH induces** LH receptors on granulosa cells.
- **The actions of FSH and LH** on the follicles are modulated by a group of peptides and growth factory by autocrine and paracrine nodes. Inhibin, secreted in the granulosa cells by FSH, directly suppresses FSH. Activin augments FSH secretion and action.
- **Successful development of a follicle** depends on the FSH induced aromatase activity in the granulosa cells to convert the follicular microenvironment from androgen dominated to an estrogen dominated one.

CHAPTER

8 Menstruation

CHAPTER OUTLINE

DEFINITION

Menstruation is the visible manifestation of cyclic physiologic uterine bleeding due to shedding of the endometrium following invisible interplay of hormones mainly through hypothalamo-pituitary-ovarian axis. **For the menstruation to occur**, the axis must be actively coordinated, endometrium must be responsive to the ovarian hormones (estrogen and progesterone) and the outflow tract must be patent.

ANATOMICAL ASPECT

The period extending from the beginning of a period (mens) to the beginning of the next one is called menstrual cycle. The first menstruation (menarche) occurs between 11 and 15 years **with a mean of 13 years**. It is more closely related to bone age than to chronological age. For the past couple of decades, the age of menarche is gradually declining with improvement of nutrition and environmental condition. Once the menstruation starts, it continues cyclically at intervals of 21–35 days with a mean of 28 days. Physiologically, it is kept in abeyance due to pregnancy and lactation. Ultimately, it ceases between the ages 45–50 when menopause sets in. **The duration of menstruation (mens) is about 4–5 days and the amount of blood loss is estimated to be 20–80 mL with an average of 35 mL. Nearly 70% of total menstrual blood loss occurs in the first 2 days. The menstrual discharge consists** mainly of dark altered blood, mucus, vaginal epithelial cells, fragments of endometrium, prostaglandins, enzymes and bacteria.

FOLLICULAR GROWTH AND ATRESIA

- Germ cells
- Primordial follicle
- Cyclic maturation of the follicle (ovarian cycle)
  - Ovulation
  - Corpus luteum
- Follicular atresia.

GERM CELLS

Origin

The germ cells migrate from the endoderm of the yolk sac in the region of hindgut. From there, they migrate into the genital ridge (between 5 and 6 weeks of gestation), passing through the dorsal mesentery of the hindgut. A peptide, called, telopheron directs this anatomic migration. The migration is probably through amoeboid activity or by chemotactic mechanism between 4 and 6 weeks gestation. In the gonadal ridge, the oogonia are surrounded by clumps of epithelial cells (Fig. 3.4).

Multiplication

The germ cells undergo rapid mitotic division and **by 20 weeks, the number reaches about 7 million**. While majority of the oogonia continue to divide until 7th month of gestation, some enter into the prophase of first meiotic division and **are called primary oocytes**. These are surrounded by flat cells from the stroma (pregranulosa cells) and are called **primordial follicles**. The primary oocytes continue to grow through various stages of prophase (leptotene, zygotene, pachytene and diplotene) and ultimately reach to the stage of diplotene or else become atretic. Primary oocytes are then arrested in the diplotene stage of prophase of first meiotic division, until ovulation.

Total number of oocytes at 20 weeks' of intrauterine life is about 6–7 million. At birth, the total number of primordial follicles is estimated to be about 2 million. The primary oocytes do not finish the first meiotic division until puberty is reached. **At puberty, some 4,00,000 primary oocytes are left behind, the rest become atretic. During the entire reproductive period, some 400 are likely to ovulate**. Thus, the important feature is the tendency of the sex cells to undergo degeneration. **The degeneration starts in the intrauterine life** and continues throughout childhood and the childbearing period. As a result, no more follicles with ova can be detected in menopausal women.

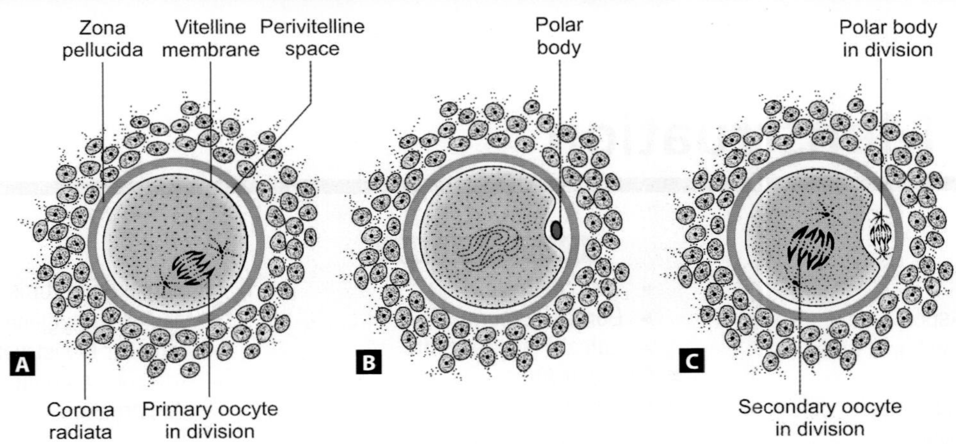

Figs. 8.1A to C: Morphology of the oocyte.

Maturation

The essence of maturation is reduction of the number of chromosomes to half. The primary oocyte remains in diplotene phase until shortly before ovulation unless it undergoes atresia. **It is the midcycle LH surge that initiates the resumption of meiosis-1**. The primary oocyte undergoes **first meiotic division** giving rise to secondary oocyte and **one polar body**. The two are of unequal size, the secondary oocyte contains haploid number of chromosomes (23, X) but nearly all the cytoplasm. The small polar body also contains haploid number of chromosome (23, X) but with scanty cytoplasm. **The formation of secondary oocyte occurs** with full maturation of Graafian follicle just prior to ovulation.

The secondary oocyte immediately begins the **second meiotic division** but stops at metaphase. **The secondary oocyte completes the second meiotic division (homotypical) only after fertilization by a sperm in the fallopian tube**. The division results in the formation of the two unequal daughter cells each possessing 23 chromosomes (23, X). The larger one is called the ovum (female pronucleus) and the smaller one is the **second polar body. In the absence of fertilization, the secondary oocyte, does not complete the second meiotic division and degenerates as such**. Thus, the first stage of maturation of the oocyte occurs within the follicle but the final stage is achieved only after fertilization in the fallopian tube.

The arrested meiotic division of the oocyte prior to ovulation is probably due to oocyte maturation inhibition (OMI) factor present in the follicular fluid. OMI is secreted by the granulosa cells. The resumption of meiosis occurs due to the midcycle LH surge.

PRIMORDIAL FOLLICLE

The primordial follicle consists of an oocyte, which is surrounded by a **single layer of flattened granulosa cells.** The follicle measures about 0.03–0.05 mm. The oocyte (primitive ovum) measures about 18–24 μ in diameter, nucleus 12 μ and nucleolus 6 μ. Throughout childhood, the primordial follicles grow very slowly. **Thin growth is not dependent on gonadotropin.**

Morphology of the Oocyte

With the maturation of the follicle, there is simultaneous enlargement of the oocyte although at a slower pace. While the follicle continues to enlarge until just prior to ovulation, the oocyte ceases to enlarge around the time of antrum formation. **The morphological features of the primary oocyte just prior to ovulation (often erroneously called mature ovum) are as follows.**

It measures about 130 microns and the nucleus measures 20–25 microns. This is in contrast with 20 microns and 10 microns, respectively in the primordial follicle. The radially arranged granulosa cells surrounding the oocyte are called **corona radiata.** The oocyte is surrounded by an outer envelope called **zona pellucida**, a glycoprotein layer, secreted by the growing oocyte (Figs. 8.1A to C). The cytoplasm, also called vitellus contains nutritive yolk granules and is limited by a definite membrane called **vitelline membrane**. The space between the vitelline membrane and the zona pellucida is called **perivitelline space**. The spherical nucleus is located near the center of the cytoplasm. The nucleolus is large with sparsely distributed chromatin. **Shortly before ovulation, meiosis is reinitiated.** At the completion of the first and second meiotic division, the number of chromosomes in the oocyte is halved (23, X) and the two polar bodies which are formed are pushed to the perivitelline space. **The first polar body is formed just prior to ovulation and the second one just after fertilization (Figs. 8.1 and 8.2).**

MENSTRUAL CYCLE

Ovarian Cycle

Definition

The development and maturation of a follicle, ovulation and formation of corpus luteum and its degeneration constitute an ovarian cycle. All these events occur within 4 weeks.

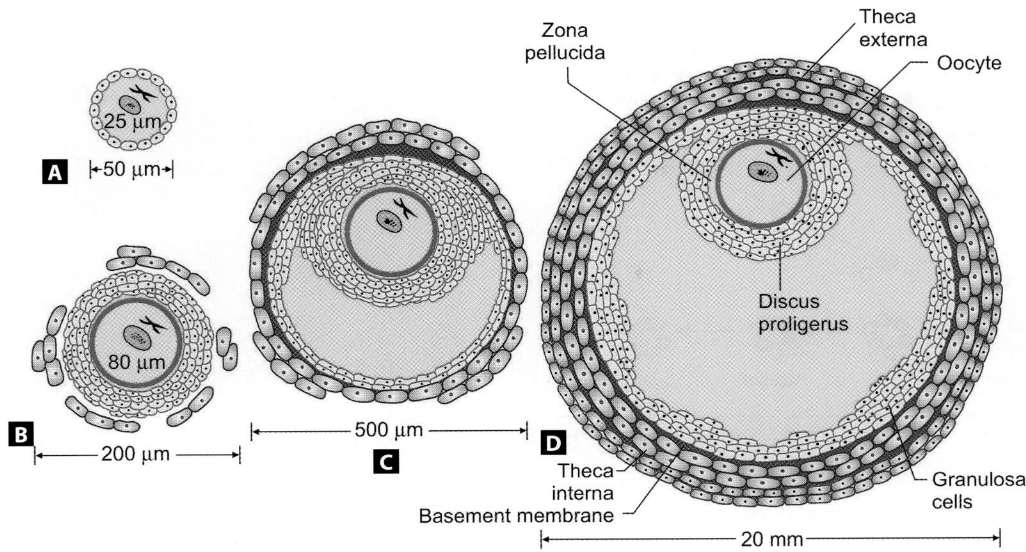

Figs. 8.2A to D: Development of Graafian follicle.

Thus, the ovarian cycle consists of:

- Recruitment of cohort of follicles
- Selection of dominant follicle and its maturation
- Ovulation
- Corpus luteum formation
- Demise of the corpus luteum.

Recruitment of Groups of Follicles (Preantral Phase)

The cohort of the growing follicles undergoes a process of development and differentiation which takes about **85 days and spreads over 3 ovarian cycles**.

It is not clear as to how many and which of the primordial follicles amidst several thousands are recruited for a particular cycle. **It is presumed that about 20 antral follicles (about 5–10 per ovary) proceed to develop in each cycle**.

The initial recruitment and growth of primordial follicles are not under the control of any hormone. After a certain stage (2–5 mm in size) the growth and differentiation of primordial follicles are under the control of follicle-stimulating hormone (FSH). **Unless the follicles are rescued by FSH at this stage, they undergo atresia**.

The predominant change is in the oocyte which is enlarged out of proportion to the size of the follicle. The oocyte is now surrounded by an acellular barrier of glycoprotein produced by the follicular cells and is called **zona pellucida. The flattened outer single layer pregranulosa cells become cuboidal and multilayered—now called granulosa cells**. There is appearance of channels (gap junctions) between the granulosa cells and the oocyte. Through these gap junctions nutrition to the oocyte is maintained. There is noticeable beginning of differentiation of the theca interna layer of ovarian stroma surrounding the follicle. The granulosa cells now acquire FSH receptors.

Selection of a Dominant Follicle and its Maturation

The Graafian follicle is named after the **Dutch physician and anatomist Regnier de Graaf (1641–1673).** The development of antrum containing secondary or vesicular follicle from the solid primary follicle depends on FSH.

There is accelerated growth of all the components of the follicles of the preantral phase. The granulosa cells grow faster than the theca cells. There is production of follicular fluid which is primarily an ultrafiltrate of blood from the vessels within theca interna. The fluid-filled space is formed amidst the granulosa cells. The spaces coalesce to form an antrum.

Dominant Follicle

As early as day 5–7, one of the follicles out of so many becomes dominant and undergoes further maturation. It seems probable that the **one with highest antral concentration of estrogen and lowest androgen—estrogen ratio (estrogenic microenvironment) and whose granulosa cells contain the maximum receptors for FSH, becomes the dominant follicle**. The rest of the follicles become atretic by day 8 (Fig. 8.3).

There is marked enlargement of the granulosa cells with lipid inclusion. The granulosa cells surround the ovum to form cumulus oophorus or discus proligerus which infact anchors the ovum to the wall of the follicle (Fig. 8.3). The cells adjacent to the ovum are arranged radially and is called corona radiata. At this stage, **FSH induces LH receptors on the granulosa cells of the dominant follicle.** LH receptor induction is essential for the midcycle LH surge to induce ovulation, luteinization of the granulosa cells to form corpus luteum and secretion of progesterone (two cell, two gonadotropin therapy—p. 59).

Theca cells becomes vacuolated and more vascular than those of other antral follicles. The theca cells are

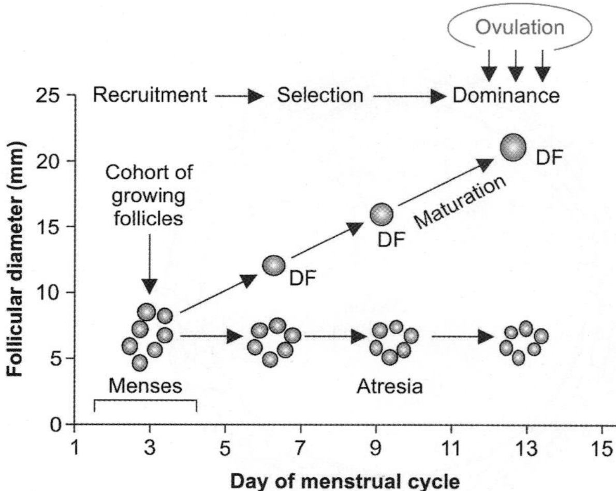

Fig. 8.3: Selection and maturation of the dominant follicle (DF) during a natural cycle.

separated from the granulosa cells by a polymerized membrane called membrana granulosa. Just prior to ovulation, LH may act to depolymerize this membrane to facilitate vascularization of the granulosa cells.

The follicular fluid is increased in amount. **The fluid contains** estrogens, FSH, trace amount of androgen, prolactin, OMI, luteinization inhibitor (LI), inhibin—which acts centrally to inhibit FSH, proteolytic enzymes, plasmin, etc.

The fully mature Graafian follicle just prior to ovulation measures about 20 mm, and is composed of the following structures from outside inward (Figs. 8.4 and 8.5).

- Theca externa
- Theca interna
- Membrana granulosa (limitans)
- Granulosa cell layer
- Discus proligerus in which the ovum is incorporated with cells arranged radially (corona radiata)
- Antrum containing vesicular fluid.

As previously mentioned, it takes 3 months for the follicle to grow and mature to ovulation—2 months to reach an antral stage measuring 1 mm; 2 weeks to reach 5 mm and another 2 weeks to reach 20 mm before ovulation.

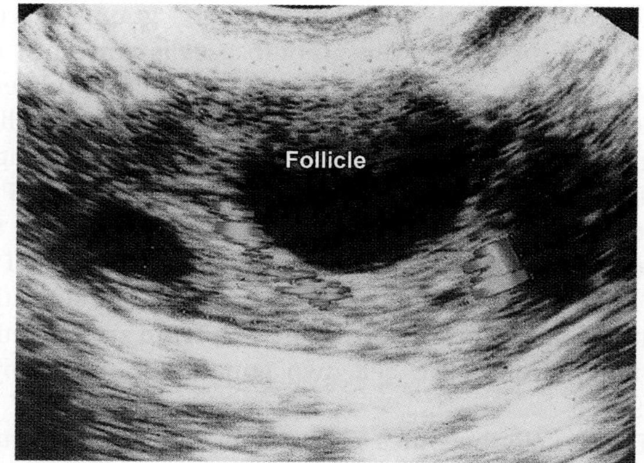

Fig. 8.4: Color Doppler (TV) sonogram showing a mature Graafian follicle prior to ovulation.

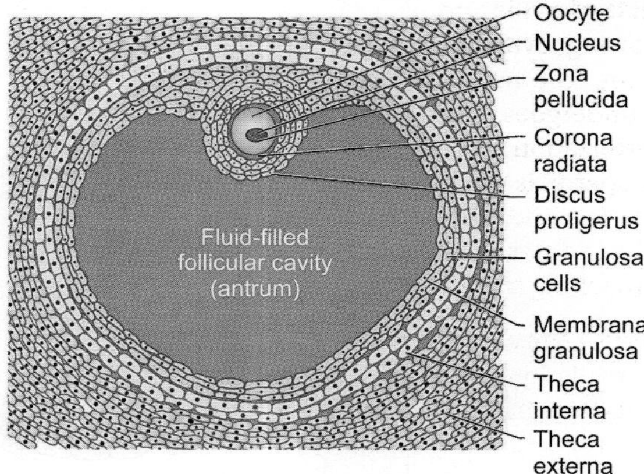

Fig. 8.5: A mature Graafian follicle.

Ovulation

The dominant follicle, shortly before ovulation reaches the surface of the ovary. The cumulus becomes detached from the wall, so that the ovum with the surrounding cells (corona radiata) floats freely in the liquor folliculi. **The oocyte completes the first meiotic division with extrusion of the first polar body** which is pushed to the perivitelline space. The follicular wall near the ovarian surface becomes thinner. The stigma develops as a conical projection which penetrates the outer surface layer of the ovary and persists for a while (30–120 seconds) as a thin membrane. The cumulus escapes out of the follicle by a slow oozing process, taking about 60–120 seconds along with varying amount of follicular fluid. The stigma is soon closed by a plug of plasma.

Causes

The following are the possible explanations which may operate singly or in combination.

Endocrinal

- **LH surge:** Sustained peak level of estrogen for 24–48 hours in the late follicular phase results in LH surge from the anterior pituitary (positive feedback effect). Effective LH surge persists for about 24 hours. The **LH surge stimulates completion of reduction division of the oocyte and initiates luteinization of the granulosa cells, synthesis of progesterone and prostaglandins.**
- **FSH rise:** Preovulatory rise of 17-α-hydroxyprogesterone facilitates the positive feedback action of estrogen to induce FSH surge → increase in plasminogen activator → plasminogen → plasmin → helps lysis of the wall of the follicle.

Thus, the combined LH/FSH midcycle surge is responsible for the final stage of maturation, rupture of the follicle and expulsion of the oocyte.

Stretching factor

It is more a passive stretching causing necrobiosis of the overlying tissue rather than rise in intrafollicular pressure which remains static at about 10–15 mm Hg.

Contraction of the micromuscles

It occurs in the theca externa and ovular stroma due to increased local prostaglandin secretion.

Effects of ovulation

Following ovulation, the follicle is changed to corpus luteum. The ovum is picked up into the fallopian tube and undergoes either degeneration or further maturation, if fertilization occurs. Life span of ovum is 24 hours and sperm is 72 hours. **Menstruation is unrelated to ovulation and anovular menstruation is quite common during adolescence**, following childbirth and in women approaching menopause.

Corpus Luteum

After ovulation, the ruptured Graafian follicle develops into corpus luteum. The life cycle is divided into four stages:

1. **Proliferation**
2. **Vascularization**
3. **Maturation**
4. **Regression**.

Stage of proliferation

The collapsed walls of the empty follicle form convolutions. The opening through which the ovum escapes soon becomes plugged with fibrin. The granulosa cells undergo hypertrophy without multiplication. The cells become larger, polyhedral with pale vesicular nuclei and frothy cytoplasm. The cells are called granulosa lutein cells. The color of the corpus luteum at this stage is grayish yellow due to presence of lipids (Fig. 8.6).

Stage of vascularization

Within 24 hours of rupture of the follicle, small capillaries grow into granulosa layer towards the lumen accompanied by lymphatics and fibroblasts. The sprouting vessels may rupture and bleed in the cavity.

Stage of maturation

By fourth day, the luteal cells have attained the maximum size. Approximately about 7–8 days following ovulation, the corpus luteum attains a size of about 1–2 cm and reaches its secretory peak. There is hypertrophy of the theca interna cells. The cells persist in the periphery and in the septa and are called paralutein cells. Some theca lutein cells called 'K' cells invade the granulosa layer. The lutein cells become greatly enlarged and develop lipid inclusion, giving the cells a distinctive yellowish color. **The color is due to the pigment carotene.** The cavity may be small containing scanty fluid.

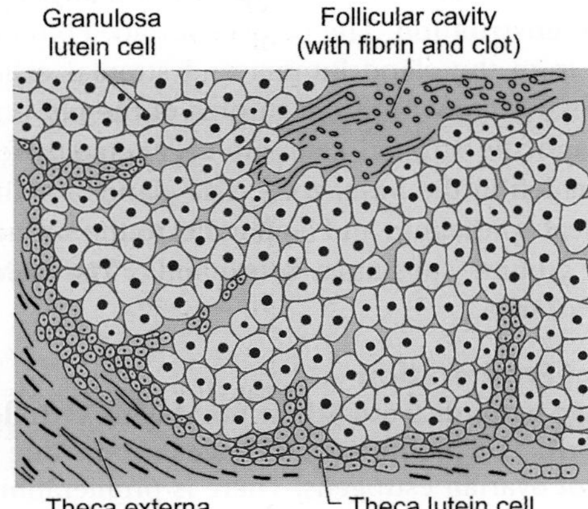

Fig. 8.6: Histological appearance of a section of corpus luteum.

Stage of regression

On the day 22–23 of cycle, retrogression starts. The first evidence of degeneration is appearance of vacuolation in the cells. There is deposition of fat in the lutein cells and appearance of hyaline tissue between them. The lutein cells atrophy and the corpus luteum becomes corpus albicans. Regression of corpus luteum is due to withdrawal of tonic LH support.

If, however, fertilization occurs in the particular cycle, regression fails to occur, instead it is converted into corpus luteum of pregnancy.

Hormones in relation to formation and maintenance of corpus luteum

- FSH in presence of high level of estrogen induces LH receptors in the granulosa cells of the dominant follicle. Thereafter midcycle LH surge causes luteinization of the granulosa cells and progesterone secretion. LH secretion must be continued for the function of corpus luteum, failing which the corpus luteum will regress.
- Adequate folliculogenesis in the preovulatory phase with increased secretion of estradiol and of 17-α-hydroxyprogesterone is a prerequisite for adequate corpus luteum formation.
- Low level of prolactin: **Corpus luteum has a lifespan of about 12–14 days.** The cause of degeneration of corpus luteum in an infertile cycle is not clear. It has been suggested that prostaglandin-F2-α liberated from the ovary is luteolytic. Estradiol is also considered to have luteolytic effect. The role of prolactin is not clear.

Corpus luteum of pregnancy

There is a surge of hyperplasia of all the layers between 23rd to 28th day due to chorionic gonadotropin. hCG, like LH will stimulate the corpus luteum to secrete progesterone. The 'K' cells are also increased in number. The growth reaches its peak at about 8th week when it measures about 2–3 cm. It looks bright orange, later on becomes yellow and finally pale. Regression occurs following low levels of chorionic gonadotropin and the degenerative changes take place most frequently at about 6 months of gestation.

Hormone secretion

Hormones—predominantly progesterone is secreted by the corpus luteum to support the endometrium of the luteal phase. There is also secretion of estrogen, inhibin and relaxin. Progesterone along with estrogen from corpus luteum maintain the growth of the fertilized ovum. This is essential till the luteal function is taken over by the placenta.

This turn over of function from corpus luteum of pregnancy to placenta is called luteal-placental shift. This transition period continues from 7–10 weeks. In the absence of pregnancy, there is fall in the levels of **serum estradiol, progesterone and inhibin**. This removes the inhibitory control of GnRH and FSH. Gradual increase in FSH is responsible for fresh recruitment of follicles for the next cycle.

Implantation Window

The timing and endometrial receptivity for implantation of a human blastocyst is defined as the implantation window. It extends from day 20 to day 24 of a normal menstrual cycle. Trophectoderm attaches to endometrial epithelial cells and invades subsequently into endometrial stroma. Endometrial maturation involves development of cellular protrusions, called **pinopods formation.** Pinopod formation is dependent on progesterone secretion. Different adhesion molecules are also involved in implantation. These molecules in the endometrium are: Integrins, selectins, cadherins and mucins.

Important Events and Ovulation

- Occurs 34–36 hours after onset of LH surge
- 10–12 hour after LH peak
- 83 hours after E2 rise
- Ovulation is preceded by completion of 1st meiotic division.
- Extrusion of 1st polar body in perivitelline space
- Leutinization of granulosa cells
- Formation of corpus luteum
- Synthesis of progesterone
- Beginning of secretory phase
- Ovulation occurs around D14 of a regular 28 days cycle.

FOLLICULAR ATRESIA

Atresia is a continued process which actually starts at 20th week of intrauterine life and **ends at menopause.** It may affect a follicle at any stage of development. However, the following descriptions are related to atretic changes of a maturing follicle which is ultimately left out in the race of a dominant follicle.

Changes in the ovum occur first. The ovum swells and undergoes hyaline and fatty degeneration. Granulosa cells then regress at a faster rate than the cells of theca interna. Hyaline tissue is deposited beneath the membrana granulosa to form the glass membrane which is the classic feature of follicular degeneration. Liquor folliculi is gradually absorbed with increasing formation of hyaline tissue in the glass membrane. Eventually, the follicle collapses; its cavity is obliterated when the opposing surfaces of the glass membranes come in contact. In the periphery, deep staining theca interna cells persist and are called interstitial cells of the ovary. These cells atrophy after menopause.

Causes of Germ Cell Loss and Follicular Atresia

Exact factors are unknown. The following are the possible explanations for follicular degeneration and atresia:

- Oogonia having no granulosa cell layer envelope
- Follicles that do not enter the germ cell meiotic division
- Follicles not rescued by FSH
- Follicles not having estrogen induced FSH receptors
- Follicles loosing FSH receptors due to negative feedback effect of estrogen secreted by the dominant follicle
- Follicles loosing FSH receptors due to high androgen: Estrogen ratio (androgenic follicular microenvironment)
- Genetic influence—as in 45, X individual
- Apoptosis—programed cell death.

Under the action of LH, more **androgens** are formed from these thecal cells which perhaps have got two functions: (1) **to enhance the process of atresia** of the small follicles; and (2) **to stimulate libido** especially noticed in midmenstrual period.

ENDOMETRIAL CYCLE

The endometrium is the lining epithelium of the uterine cavity above the level of internal os. It consists of **surface epithelium, glands, stroma and blood vessels.** Two distinct divisions are established—**basal zone (stratum basalis) and the superficial functional zone.**

BASAL ZONE

It is about one-third of the total depth of the endometrium and lies in contact with the myometrium. It consists of stromal cells which stain deeply and are compactly placed. The base of the endometrial glands extends into the layer. **The zone is supplied by the basal arteries. The zone is uninfluenced by hormone and as such, no cyclic changes are observed.** After shedding of the superficial part during menstruation, the regeneration of all the components occurs from this zone. **It measures about 1 mm.**

FUNCTIONAL ZONE

This zone is under the influence of fluctuating cyclic ovarian hormones, estrogen and progesterone. The changes in different components during an ovulatory cycle has been traditionally divided into four stages (Figs. 8.7 to 8.9).

1. Regenerative phase
2. Proliferative phase
3. Secretory phase
4. Menstruation.

Phase of Regeneration

Regeneration of the endometrium starts even before the menstruation ceases and is **completed 2–3 days after the end of menstruation**. The cubical surface epithelium is derived from the gland lumina and stromal cells. New blood vessels grow from the stumps of the old one. The glands and the stromal cells are regenerated from the remnants left in the basal zone. The glands are lined by the cubical epithelium and lie parallel to the surface. The stromal ground substance re-expands. **The thickness averages 2 mm.**

Phase of Proliferation

This stage extends from 5th or 6th day to 14th day (till ovulation). The proliferative changes occurs due to rise in level of ovarian estrogens. There is proliferation of all the elements—at first slowly but later on at a rapid pace. **The glands** become tubular and lie perpendicular to the

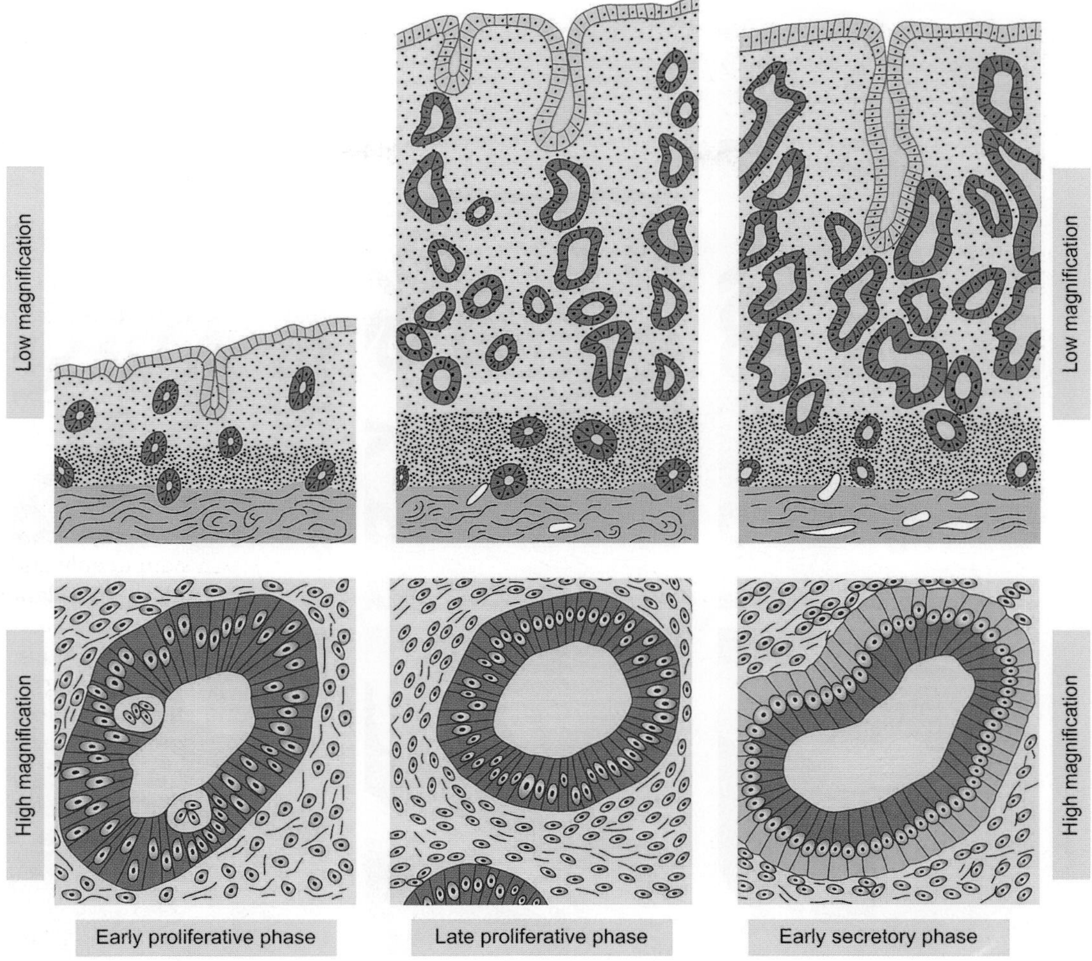

Fig. 8.7: Endometrium in proliferative and early secretory phase. Note the tendency of tortuosity of the glands and the characteristic subnuclear vacuolation in early secretory phase (cf compare with those of proliferative phase).

surface. **The epithelium** becomes columnar with the nuclei placed at the base. The epithelium of one gland becomes continuous with the neighboring gland. Abundant mitosis is evident in the epithelial cells. Before ovulation the cells lining the glandular lumen undergo pseudostratification. **The stromal cells** become spindle-shaped with evidences of mitosis and are compact. **The spiral vessels** extend unbranched to a region below the epithelium where they form loose capillary network. There may be evidences of subepithelial congestion. **The thickness measures about 10–12 mm** at the time of ovulation.

Secretory Phase

The changes of the components are due to the combined effects of estrogen and progesterone liberated from the corpus luteum after ovulation. The endometrium contains receptors for progesterone which are induced by estrogen. **Thus, the progesterone can only act on the endometrium previously primed by estrogen.**

All the components display their growth. **It begins on day 15 and ceases 5–6 days prior to menstruation. The surface epithelium** becomes more columnar and ciliated at places. The glands show predominant changes. **The glands** increase in size. The lining epithelium become taller. There is appearance of vacuoles due to secretion of glycogen between the nuclei and the basement membrane. This is called **subnuclear vacuolation**, which is the **earliest (36–48 hours) evidence of progesterone effect (ovulation). The subnuclear vacuolation persists until about 21st day of cycle.** The intracellular secretion then enters the gland lumina on the way to the uterine cavity pushing the nuclei back towards the basement membrane. The effect is a **saw-toothed** glandular epithelium. The fluid has got nutritive value for any fertilized ovum reaching the uterus during that time. **The glands become corkscrew-shaped. The blood vessels undergo marked spiraling.**

The stromal cells become swollen, large and polyhedral and after the 21st day tend to collect more superficially around the neck of the glands. The deeper spongy layer is composed of convoluted glands, coiled arterioles and comparatively few stromal cells in edematous stroma. Histochemical studies show increase in glycogen and acid phosphatase. Histological staining is eosinophilic.

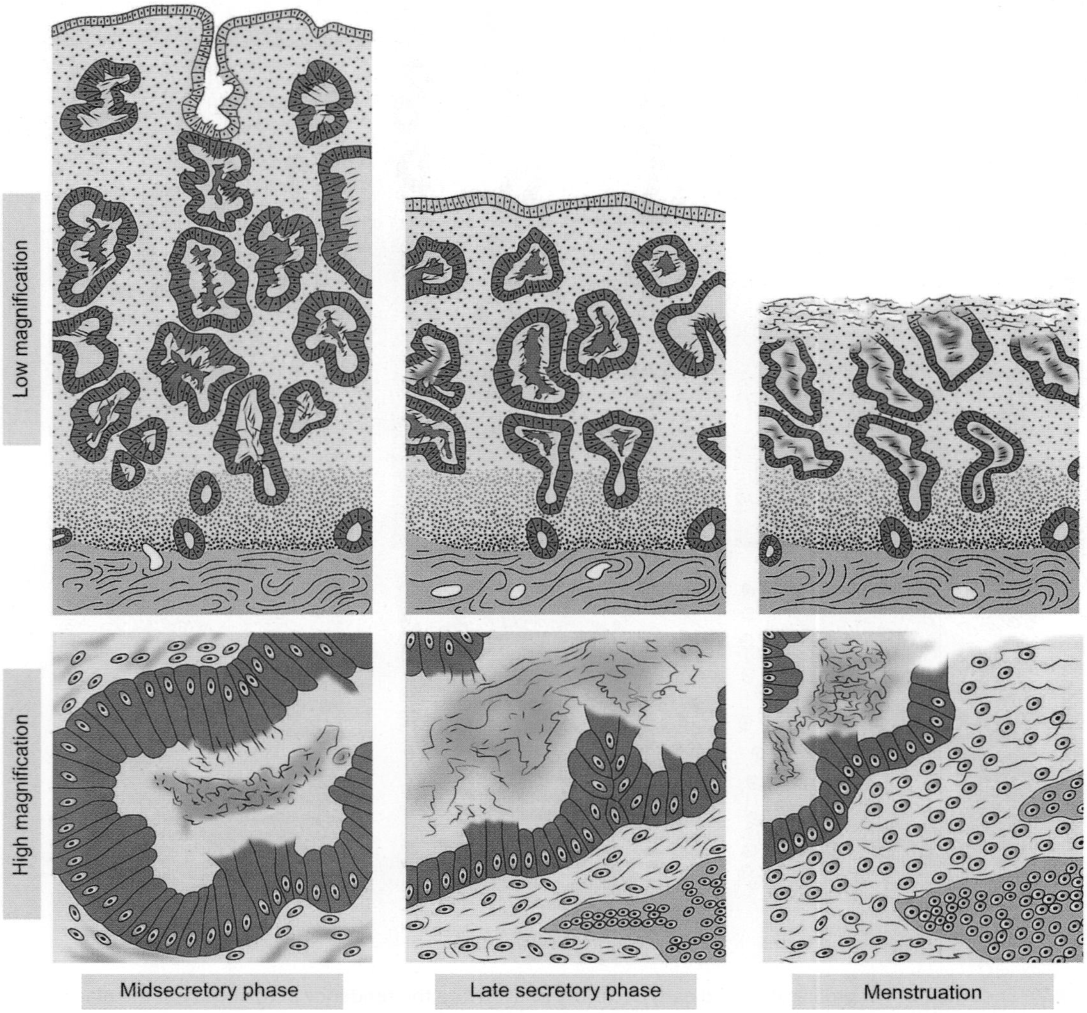

Fig. 8.8: Endometrium in secretory and menstrual phase. Note the marked tortuosity of the glands with secretion in the lumen in the midsecretory phase. The nucleus is pushed to the base.

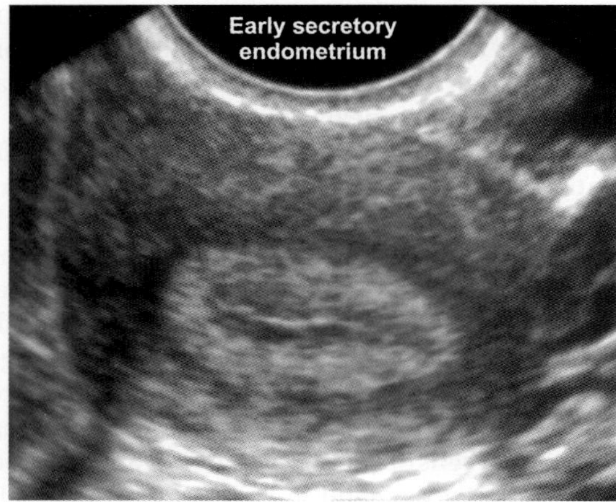

Fig. 8.9: Transvaginal scan demonstrating thickened, triple line endometrium (preovulatory phase).

The thickness of the endometrium remains its highest (12 mm) (Fig. 8.8).

Several glycoproteins including glycodelin, insulin-like growth factor binding protein-1 (IGFBP-1), leukemia inhibitory factor, are produced by the secretory endometrium. These play an integral part for blastocyst implantation and continuation of pregnancy.

The endometrial growth ceases 5-6 days prior to menstruation (22nd or 23rd day of cycle) in an infertile cycle. This is due to dehydration of the glands. The subepithelial capillaries and the spiral vessels are engorged. **The regressive changes in the endometrium are pronounced 24–48 hours prior to menstruation.** There is marked spiraling of the arteries and the withdrawal of hormones estrogen and progesterone causes intense spasm of the spiral arterioles at the basal part. These two lead to stasis and tissue anoxemia. There are evidences of infiltration of leukocytes and monocytes in the stroma.

Menstrual Phase

It is essentially degeneration and casting off an endometrium prepared for a pregnancy. **Regression of corpus**

luteum with fall in the level of estrogen and progesterone is an invariable preceding feature. As a result of withdrawal of hormone support, there is retrogressive changes in the endometrium as mentioned earlier.

MECHANISM OF MENSTRUAL BLEEDING

Stasis of blood and **spasm** of the arterioles lead to damage of the arteriolar walls. Phase of relaxation leads to escape of blood out of the vessels through the damaged walls. There is breakdown of endometrial tissues by proteolytic enzymes belonging to the members of matrix metalloproteinase family (MMPs). These enzymes are stimulated by the process of inflammation. **So there is enzymatic autodigestion of the functional zone. The bleeding occurs** from the broken arteries, veins and capillaries and also from the stromal hematoma. The blood along with the superficial functional layer is shed into the uterine cavity. The blood **coagulates** in the uterine cavity but soon liquefies by **plasmin** unless the bleeding is very brisk and rapid. **The menstrual flow** stops as a result of combined effect of prolonged vasoconstriction, myometrial contraction and local aggregation of platelets with deposition of fibrin around them. Endothelin and platelet activating factor present in the endometrium are potent vasoconstrictors. Resumption of estrogen secretion leads to clot formation over the decapitated stumps of endometrial vessels. There is simultaneous repair of endometrium. This is under control of estrogen and different growth factors.

ROLE OF PROSTAGLANDINS

It is likely that the arteriolar constriction and endometrial necrosis are caused by prostaglandins. The endometrium and partly the myometrium, synthesize the prostaglandins from arachidonic acid by the enzyme cyclooxygenase. Different prostaglandins have got different action. *$PGF_2\alpha$ causes* myometrial contraction and vasoconstriction. It seems to play a dominant role in normal cycle. PGE_2 produces myometrial contraction but causes vasodilatation. PGI_2 (prostacyclin) causes myometrial relaxation and vasodilatation. It also inhibits platelet activity. Thus, the menstrual pain and blood flow are probably related to the relative proportion of different prostaglandins present in the endometrium.

HORMONES IN RELATION TO OVARIAN AND MENSTRUAL CYCLE

The outcome in relation to hormonal interplay in normally menstruating women includes:

- Growth and development of the Graafian follicle
- Ovulation
- Maintenance and demise of corpus luteum
- Endometrial growth and shedding.

Growth and Development of the Follicle (Fig. 8.10)

At the **beginning of a menstrual** cycle, a low level of estrogen and inhibin secreted from the previous weaning corpus luteum maintains a high FSH level through release of negative feedback of estrogen. The FSH increases not only its own receptors in the granulosa cells but also LH receptors in theca cells. Initial sustained low level of LH stimulates the production of estrogen. Under the synergistic effect of FSH and estrogen, multiplication of the granulosa cells, formation of the follicular fluid and synthesis of more LH receptors in the theca cells occur.

With increased secretion of estrogen, the FSH level is lowered through a negative feedback mechanism. Thus, the initial high level of FSH comes down to a static base level by day 5. Paradoxically, the increasing LH level with the rising estrogen level stimulates androgen production in the theca cells. Granulosa cells now utilize the increased

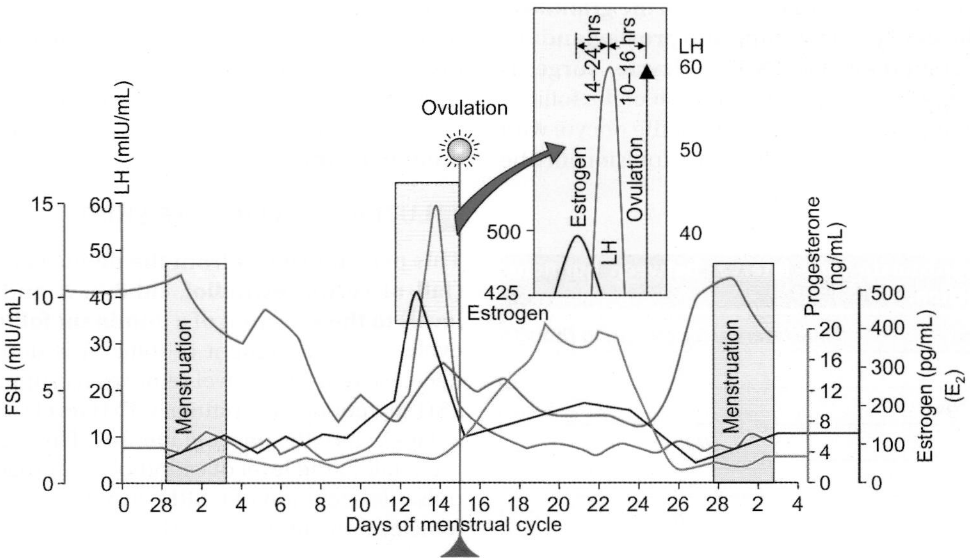

Fig. 8.10: Fluctuation of serum levels of ovarian steroids and gonadotropins in a normal ovulatory cycle.

androgen produced from the theca cells for the synthesis of estrogen.

The falling FSH level with peak rise of estrogen in the late follicular phase increases the LH receptors in the granulosa cells. Final maturation of the follicle is thus achieved by the combined effect of FSH and LH.

Role of Peptides and Growth Factors (p. 62)

- **Peptides:** FSH stimulates the granulosa cells to produce a number of peptides like inhibin, activin and follistatin. Activin is also secreted by the pituitary gland. Inhibin directly inhibits FSH, whereas activin stimulates FSH.
- **Growth factors:** Insulin like growth factors (IGF), epidermal growth factors and others, modulate the action of FSH, LH and the peptides. IGF-II, is produced in the theca cells. It stimulates aromatase activity and progesterone synthesis in the granulosa cells.

Ovulation

LH surge initiates luteinization acting through its receptors about 24–48 hours. Prior to ovulation. A trace amount of 17-α-hydroxyprogesterone is formed which is probably responsible for completion of the first meiotic division of the oocyte and compounds the effect of estrogen for LH surge. Progesterone also facilitates the positive feedback action to induce FSH surge → increase in plasminogen activator → plasminogen → plasmin → helps lysis of the follicular wall.

After the estradiol reaches beyond the critical level of 200 pg/mL and is sustained for about 48 hours, it exerts a positive feedback action to LH from the anterior pituitary (LH surge). Ovulation occurs approximately 12–16 hours after the LH peak or 32–36 hours after the onset of LH surge. A threshold of LH surge generally persists for 24 hours. Ovulation coincides approximately 24–36 hours after the peak estradiol level (Table 8.1). LH surge stimulates completion of the reduction division of the oocyte and initiates luteinization of the granulosa cells and synthesis of progesterone and prostaglandins.

Thus, the **combined LH/FSH midcycle surge** is responsible for the final stage of maturation of the follicle, completion of the first meiotic division of the oocyte with extrusion of the first polar body and expulsion of the oocyte (ovulation).

TABLE 8.1: Approximate time interval between hormone levels and ovulation.

Events	*Time interval for ovulation (hour)*
Estradiol rise	83
Onset of LH surge	34–36
Estradiol peak	24–36
LH peak	12–16
Progesterone rise	8

The drop in LH level following its peak may be due to desensitization of LH receptors or due to negative feedback effect of progesterone. This down regulation results in a refractory state during which there is diminished steroidogenesis.

Maintenance and Demise of Corpus Luteum

Soon following the LH surge, the level of estrogen drops down within an hour and the LH peak after 24 hours. LH initiates and maintains the corpus luteum from which both progesterone and estrogen are secreted. The estrogen attains a lower level and maintains a plateau curve as against a peak rise in follicular phase. 17-α-hydroxyprogesterone parallels with the estradiol level in the luteal phase. **Progesterone attains its highest peak about 8 days after the LH peak**. Through intraovarian and central negative feedback mechanisms, **progesterone acts to suppress new follicular growth**. As the estrogen and progesterone attain their highest peak, they exert a negative feedback effect on LH and FSH in an infertile cycle and the level of LH and FSH drops down to a minimum. The lysis of the corpus luteum occurs and so the secretion of progesterone and estrogen falls. **The lifespan of corpus luteum is about 12–14 days**. With the fall of estrogen and progesterone, FSH level again rises under the influence of GnRH to exert its effect on follicular growth and maturation for the next cycle (Figs. 8.10 and 8.11).

Endometrial Growth and Shedding

Estrogen secreted in the follicular phase produces proliferative changes in the endometrium and induces receptors for progesterone. In the luteal phase, progesterone acts on the estrogen primed endometrium having sufficient number of receptors and produces secretory changes. In the infertile cycle, with the fall of estrogen and progesterone, the endometrium becomes unsupported to the hormones and degeneration occurs → menstruation (Fig. 8.10).

Endometrial sample biopsy and histology can precisely determine the date of menstrual cycle. Any discrepancy of **more than 2 days** when examined in the postovulatory phase is called **luteal phase defect**. This method of endometrial examination is called **dating of endometrium**.

LUTEAL–FOLLICULAR SHIFT

This period extends from the demise of corpus luteum (fall of serum estradiol, inhibin-A and progesterone level) to the selection of a dominant follicle for the next cycle. The recruitment of follicles is done by FSH. The decrease in inhibin level removes its suppressive effect of FSH secretion in the pituitary. FSH level starts rising about 2 days before the onset of menses. The increase FSH : LH ratio, fall in the level of estradiol and progesterone allows pulsatile secretion of GnRH. Rising FSH level rescues the follicles from atresia and selects the dominant follicle.

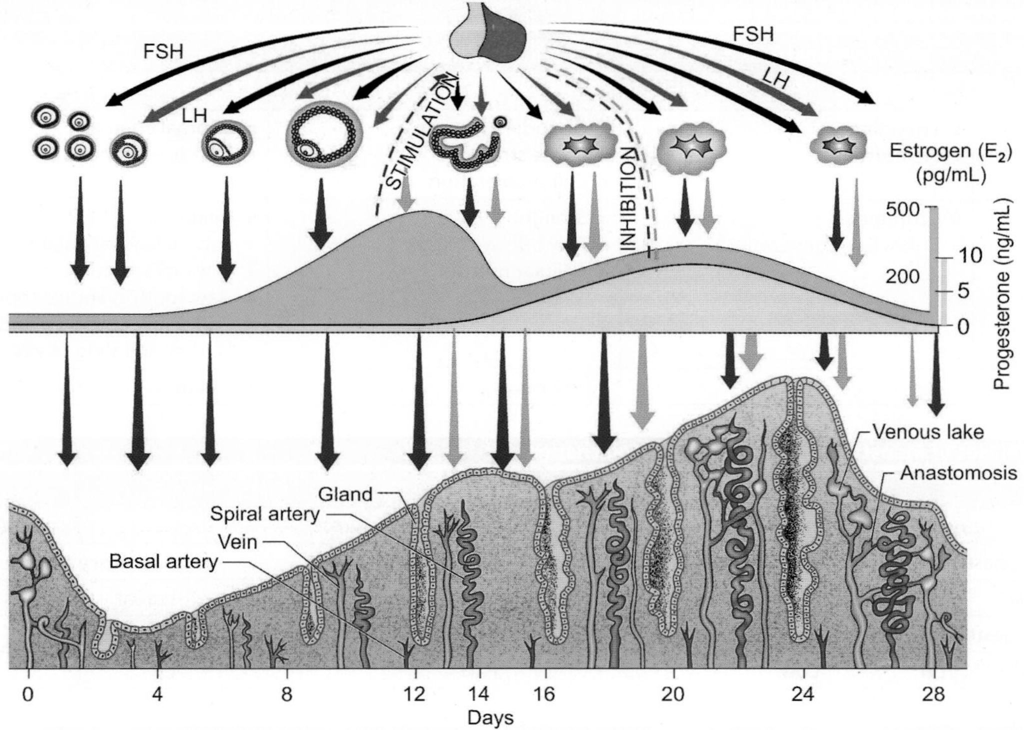

Fig. 8.11: Hormones controlling the ovarian and endometrial cycles.
(FSH: follicle-stimulating hormone; LH: luteinizing hormone)

MENSTRUAL SYMPTOMS

In majority, apart from bleeding per vaginam there is no symptom. Initially, it begins as pink discharge but on day 2 and 3 it becomes dark red. In teenagers or nulliparous, there may be associated tolerable colicky pain at the beginning due to uterine contraction. If the pain is of sufficient magnitude so as to incapacitate the day-to-day activities, it is called dysmenorrhea (Ch. 14). There may be premonitory symptoms such as pelvic discomfort, backache, fullness of the breasts or mastalgia just prior to menstruation. Headache or depression may be present. If these premonitory symptoms are predominant, these are grouped into a syndrome called "premenstrual syndrome" and is dealt separately in Ch. 14.

MENSTRUAL HYGIENE

Sympathetic and careful handling of the young girls experiencing first menstruation is of paramount importance. This should be done by the mother explaining the physiological and other associated changes during period. The girls should continue with their normal activities. The daily bath should not be suspended. During initial few periods, the girl may use sanitary pads comfortably but with experience may be changed to tampon, if so desired.

ANOVULAR MENSTRUATION

In an anovulatory cycle, the follicles grow without any selection of dominant follicle. The estrogen is secreted in increasing amount. There may be imbalance between estrogen and FSH or because of temporary unresponsiveness of the hypothalamus to the rising estrogen, GnRH is suppressed → no ovulation. The net effect is unopposed secretion of estrogen till the follicles exist. The endometrium remains in either proliferative or at times hyperplastic state. There is inadequate structural stromal support and the endometrium remains fragile. When the estrogen level falls, there is asynchronous shedding of the endometrium and menstruation. The bleeding may be heavy or prolonged and irregular.

This type of bleeding is mostly found during adolescence, following childbirth and abortion and in premenopausal period.

ARTIFICIAL POSTPONEMENT OF MENSTRUATION

Artificial alteration of the date of menstrual flow should be judiciously comply with. It should not be taken lightly. **It is preferable to defer than to advance the date** as the artificial withdrawal bleeding may be continued for a variable period which may spoil the purpose.

The hormones used for deferment of the period are—combined oral pill, 2 tablets daily or progestogen such as

TABLE 8.2: Important changes in the endometrium.

	Menstrual	Proliferative	Secretory
Day	*1–5*	*6–14*	*15–28*
Stroma	▪ Shedding ▪ Hemorrhage	▪ Abundant mitosis ▪ Loose stroma ▪ Cell proliferation	▪ Stromal edema ▪ Decidual changes
Glands	▪ Crumbing ▪ Epithelial regeneration	▪ Straight ▪ Few tightly coiled ▪ Cellular mitosis	▪ Dilatation ▪ Subnuclear vacuolation ▪ Luminal secretion ▪ 'Saw tooth' glandular epithelium ▪ Corkscrew-shaped glands ▪ Marked spiraling of vessels
Layer thickness	1–2 mm	10–12 mm	12–14 mm

TABLE 8.3: Phases of menstrual cycle and the related changes.

Menstrual cycle			
Cycle days	*1–5*	*6–14*	*15–28*
Endometrial phase	**Menstrual (bleeding) phase**	**Proliferative phase**	**Secretory phase**
Ovarian phase	Early follicular	Late follicular	Luteal
Estrogen/Progesterone	Low	Estrogen↑	Progesterone↑
Gonadotropins FSH/LH	Low	FSH↑	LH↑

TABLE 8.4: Cervical cycle in follicular and luteal phase.

Cervical characters	*Follicular phase*	*Luteal phase*
Internal os	Funnel-shaped	Tightly closed
Cervical mucus	Thin and watery	Thick and viscid
Stretchability (spinberkeit)	Increased to beyond 10 cm	Lost
Fern tree pattern	Present	Lost
Glycoprotein network	Parallel, thus facilitating sperm penetration	Interlacing bridges, preventing sperm penetration
Glandular epithelium	Taller	More branched

TABLE 8.5: Vaginal cycle in follicular and luteal phase (Fig. 8.12).

Cellular characters	*Follicular phase*	*Luteal phase*
Cytology	Showing preponderance of superficial large cornified cells with pyknotic nuclei	Preponderance of intermediate cells with folded edges (navicular cells)
Background of the smear	Clear	Dirty due to presence of leukocytes and bacilli

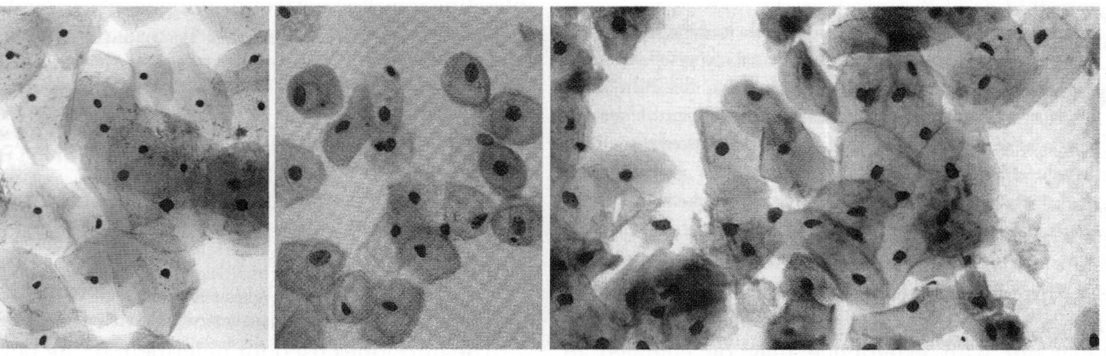

Fig. 8.12: Vaginal cytology—in the late proliferative phase, there are preponderance of superficial large cornified cells with pyknotic nuclei. The background is clear. In the premenstrual phase, there is preponderance of navicular cells. The background is dirty.

TABLE 8.6: General changes in follicular and luteal phase.

Preovulatory	Ovulatory	Premenstrual
No symptom	■ Pain abdomen on either iliac fossa ■ Slight vaginal bleeding ■ Mucoid vaginal discharge	■ Irritability, lethargy, constipation ■ Acne ■ Pelvic discomfort ■ Abnormal gain in weight ■ Mastalgia

norethisterone 5 mg twice daily. The drug should be taken at least 3–6 days before the expected date of the period and continued until the crisis is over. The period is expected 2–3 days after the drug is suspended.

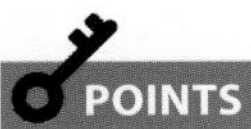

POINTS

- **Menstruation** is the visible manifestation of cyclical physiologic uterine bleeding due to shedding of the endometrium as a result of invisible interplay of hormones mainly through hypothalamo-pituitary-ovarian axis.
- **Average age of menarche** is 13 years. The average menstrual blood loss is 35 mL (may be up to 80 mL). Average loss of iron in each menses is 13 mg and about 70% of total menstrual blood loss (MBL) occurs in the first 2 days (p. 154). Alkali hematin method is most precise to measure the MBL.
- **The primordial follicle measures** 0.03–0.05 mm. Primitive ovum measures 18–24 microns in diameter.
- **The primary oocyte** undergoes first meiotic division giving rise to secondary oocyte and one polar body just prior to ovulation. The measurement of a primary oocyte just prior to ovulation (mature ovum) is 130 microns.
- **The secondary oocyte** completes the second meiotic division only after fertilization by a sperm in the fallopian tube.
- It is presumed that those follicles which are less exposed to progesterone environment are likely to run in the race for dominance in the next cycle.
- **One follicle with highest antral concentration of estrogen and lowest androgen:** Estrogen ratio and the granulosa cells containing the maximum receptors for FSH becomes the dominant follicle. The fully mature Graafian follicle measures about 20 mm with a volume of 3.5 mL.
- **With ultrasound** the dominant follicle mean diameter is about 19.5 mm.
- **LH surge stimulates** the completion of first meiotic division, luteinization of granulosa cells, synthesis of progesterone and prostaglandins. Subnuclear vacuole is the first histologic evidence of progesterone effect.
- **Preovulatory FSH surge** (which is progesterone dependent) enhances conversion of plasminogen to plasmin for the lysis of follicular wall.
- **Estradiol (E_2)** exerts negative feedback effect to FSH but bears a positive feedback effect to LH.
- **Both FSH and LH regulates follicular** development through a number of growth factors and peptides by autocrine and paracrine mechanism (p. 57).
- **Insulin growth factor-II** (IGF-II) is produced by theca and granulosa cells. IGF-II stimulates granulosa cell proliferation and aromatase activity (p. 58).
- **Inhibin is a peptide**, secreted by the granulosa cells in response to FSH. Inhibin is a potent inhibitor of FSH. Activin, another peptide secreted by the granulosa cells and by the pituitary, stimulates FSH.
- **Sustained peak level of estradiol** for about 24 hours beyond 200 pg/mL in late follicular phase results in LH surge (positive feedback effect). Ovulation occurs about 32–36 hours after the onset of LH surge and about 10–12 hours of the LH peak levels. The mean duration of LH surge is about 24 hours. The peak LH levels plateau for about 14 hours. The cause of LH decline is probably due to acute down regulation or due to negative feedback effect of progesterone (Table 8.1).
- **After ovulation**, the ruptured Graafian follicle becomes corpus luteum.
- The yellowish color is due to lipid and pigment carotene. Regression starts on day 22–23 of infertile cycle.
- **LH hormone**, with adequate number of LH receptors in the granulosa cells, as induced during folliculogenesis with increased secretion of estradiol, is the key factor of adequate corpus luteum formation (p. 76).
- **The hormones**—estrogen and progesterone are secreted from the corpus luteum.
- **The follicles containing high Androgen: Estrogen ratio** are destined to undergo atresia. Under the action of LH, more androgens are produced from the active thecal compartments (p. 72).
- **The functional zone of the endometrium** is under the influence of fluctuating cyclic ovarian hormones, estrogen and progesterone. Progesterone can only act on the endometrium previously primed by estrogen. Subnuclear vacuolation is the earliest evidence of ovulation and appears on 18th day and persists up to 21st day (Table 8.2). The mechanism of menstrual bleeding is due to degenerative changes predominantly of vascular origin. The menstrual flow stops as a result of combined effect of prolonged vasoconstriction, myometrial contraction and local aggregation of platelets.
- **$PGF_2\alpha$ causes myometrial contraction** and vasoconstriction, PGE_2 produces myometrial contraction but causes vasodilatation, **PGI_2 (prostacyclin) causes myometrial** relaxation and vasodilatation.
- **Under the synergistic effect of FSH and estrogen**, multiplication of the granulosa cells, formation of the follicular fluid and synthesis of more LH receptors in the theca cells occur. The falling FSH level with peak rise of estrogen in the late follicular phase increases the LH receptors in the granulosa cells. Final maturation of the follicle is achieved by the combined effect of FSH and LH.

Contd...

Contd...

- **Preovulatory FSH surge** increases the plasmin which helps lysis of the follicular wall. LH surge stimulates completion of reduction division of the oocyte and initiates luteinization of the granulosa cells and synthesis of progesterone and prostaglandins.
- **Progesterone attains its highest peak about 8 days** after the LH peak. Through intraovarian and central negative feedback mechanisms, progesterone acts to suppress new follicular growth.
- **When the endometrium** becomes unsupported by the fall of estrogen and progesterone, degeneration occurs resulting in menstruation. The regressive changes in the endometrium are pronounced 24–48 hours prior to menstruation (p. 74).
- **There is intense breakdown of the endometrium**, by proteolytic enzymes belonging to the members of matrix metalloproteinases family (MMPs). These enzymes are stimulated by the process of inflammation.
- **LH stimulates granulosa cell proliferation** and **luteinization** and production of progesterone.
- **The theca cells** and the stroma of atretic follicles produce more androgens in the midcycle. This raised androgen level enhances further atresia of the small follicles. This also increases libido.
- **Demise of corpus luteum** is due to the luteolytic action of estrogen, prostaglandin $F\alpha_2$, nitric oxide, endothelin, TNFα and the proteolytic enzymes. hCG rescues the corpus luteum, if pregnancy occurs.
- **Luteal-placental shift** is the turnover of function from corpus luteum of pregnancy to placenta. This transition period continues from 7–10 weeks. This is essential for the growth of the fertilized ovum (p. 71).
- **Luteal-follicular shift** is the period that extends from the demise of corpus luteum to the selection of a new dominant follicle for the next cycle. It is due to fall in the levels of estradiol, progesterone and inhibin. There is simultaneous rise in the levels of GnRH and FSH (p. 76).
- **Rising in FSH level** rescues follicles from apoptosis and selects the dominant follicle.
- **Phases of menstrual cycle** is associated with other changes like cervical, vaginal and general (Table 8.3). The cervical cycle includes changes in the ovary, endometrium, hormones, cervix and cervical mucus (Table 8.4). Vaginal cytology varies with the phases of menstruation (Table 8.5). General changes includes the different systemic symptoms (Table 8.6).
- Kisseptin (Kiss 1) plays an important role in the regulation of GnRH release. Transvaginal sonography (TVS), can detect steady and progressive increase in the follicular diameter and the volume. With this, there is parallel rise in the levels of estradiol. The dominant follicle has the maximum mean diameter of 19.5 mm (range of 18–25 mm) before ovulation. The maximum follicular volume is 3.8 mL.
- Approximate interval of time between rise in hormones and ovulation is as mentioned below. Ovulation occurs: ♦ 24 hours after the serum estradiol peak ♦ 32 hours after the onset of rise in serum LH ♦ 12–16 hours after the serum LH surge.

CHAPTER

9 Examination of a Gynecological Patient and the Diagnostic Procedures

CHAPTER OUTLINE

INTRODUCTION

The clinical examination should be thorough and meticulous. These include **in-depth history taking and examinations**—general, abdominal and internal. It should be emphasized that a meticulous history taking alone can give a positive diagnosis in majority of cases without any physical examination. The examination should in fact proceed with the provisional diagnosis in mind. On occasion, ancillary aids are required to confirm the diagnosis. For a careful history taking, the following outlines are of help:

Name .... Age ....
Address ....
Marital status .... Parity ....
Socialstatus ....
Chiefcomplaint ....

A patient hearing should be given about the complaints made by the patient in her own words. In order to substantiate the guess made out of her complaints, some pertinent questions (open-ended or specific) may be asked tactfully and judiciously. Looking at the patient with eye to eye contact (direct observation) before speaking may give many clues (nonverbal) to the diagnosis, e.g. fear, sadness, apathy or anger.

HISTORY

This should be taken in details. If multiple symptoms are present, their chronologic appearances are to be noted. Integration of the symptomatology to one pathology is to be tried first before embarking on the diagnosis of multiple pathology. Enquiry should be made about the bowel habits and urinary trouble, if any.

Menstrual History

Enquiries should be made about:
- Age of onset of the first period (menarche)
- Regularity of the cycle
- Duration of period
- Length of the cycle
- Amount of bleeding—excess is indicated by the passage of clots or number of pads used
- First day of the last menstrual period (LMP).

The menstrual history can be reproduced as 13/4/28, representing that the onset of period was at the age of 13, bleeding lasts for 4 days and occurs every 28 days.

Past Medical History

Relevant medical disorders—systemic, metabolic or endocrinal (diabetes, hypertension, hepatitis) should be enquired. Their presence requires care during operative procedure. Next pertinent point is the interrogation about sexually transmitted diseases.

Family History

It is of occasional value. Malignancy of the breast, colon, ovary or endometrium is often related.

Obstetric History

If the patient had been previously pregnant, details are to be enquired as per tabulation below. Many a times, the complaints may be related to the pregnancy complications or lactation.

Sl. No. / Date	*Year and events*	*Pregnancy events*	*Labor delivery*	*Method of delivery*	*Puerperium*	*Baby weight and sex. Birth asphyxia. Duration of breastfeeding, contraception*
1.						
2.						

The obstetric history is to be summed up as:

No. of living children .... Boys .... Girls ....
Health status of the baby ....
Immunization .... Last child birth ....

Past Surgical History

This includes general, obstetrical or gynecological surgery. The nature of the operation, anesthetic procedures, bleeding or clotting complication if any, postoperative convalescence are to be enquired. Any histopathological report or relevant investigation related to the previous surgery is most often helpful.

Personal History

Occupation, marital status—married, widow, divorced or separated should be enquired. If married—details of sexual history should be taken, including Pap smear screening and human papillomavirus (HPV) vaccination. **Sexual history** includes any sexual dysfunction or dyspareunia. **Contraceptive** practice, if any should be enquired—especially relevant in pill users or cases having intrauterine contraceptive devices (IUCD), as these methods often produce some adverse symptoms. History of taking medications for a long time or allergy to certain drugs is to be noted.

EXAMINATION

The examination includes:

- General and systemic examination
- Gynecological examination
  - Breast examination
  - Abdominal examination
  - Pelvic examination.

GENERAL AND SYSTEMIC EXAMINATION

The general and systemic examination should be thorough and meticulous.

- *Built*—too obese or too thin—may be the result of endocrinopathy and related to menstrual abnormalities
- *Nutrition*—average/poor
- *Stature*—including development of secondary sex characters
- Body mass index (BMI)
- Pallor
- Jaundice
- Lymph nodes
- Edema of legs
- *Teeth, gums and tonsils*—for any septic foci
- *Neck*—palpation of thyroid gland and lymph nodes, especially the left supraclavicular glands
- Cardiovascular and respiratory systems—any abnormality may modify the surgical procedure, if it seems necessary
- Pulse
- Blood pressure.

GYNECOLOGICAL EXAMINATION

Breast Examination (Figs. 9.1A to F)

This should be a routine especially in women above the age of 30 to detect any breast pathology, the important being carcinoma. In India, **breast carcinoma is the second most common** malignancy in female, next to carcinoma cervix.

A. **Self-breast examination (SBE)** is done by the patient herself (p. 475). If they feel or see any concerning symptoms or abnormality such as redness, pain, skin changes or a mass.
B. **Clinical breast examination (CBE)** is done by a skilled professional. CBE includes visual inspection combined with palpation of the breasts and axilla (ACOG - 2014). Clinical breast examination is recommended every 1 to 3 years for women aged 20 to 39 years and yearly thereafter (ACOG, ACS and NCCN - 2014) is done. Palpation of the entire breast tissue from mid sternum to posterior axillary line and from inframammary crease to the clavicle (Table 9.1).

Abdominal Examination

Prerequisites

- **Bladder should be empty.** The only exception to the procedure is the presence of history suggestive of stress incontinence. If history is suggestive of chronic retention of urine, catheterization should be done taking aseptic precautions, using sterile simple rubber catheter.
- The patient is to lie flat on the table with the thighs slightly flexed and abducted to make the abdominal muscles relaxed.
- The physician usually prefers to stand on the right side.
- Presence of a chaperone (a female) for the support of the patient and the physician.

Actual Steps

- **Inspection**
- **Palpation**
- **Percussion**
- **Auscultation**

Inspection

The skin condition of the abdomen—presence of old scar, striae, prominent veins or eversion of the umbilicus is to be noted. By asking the patient to strain, one can elicit either incisional hernia or divarication of the rectus abdominis muscles. In pelvic peritonitis, the lower abdomen is only distended with diminished inspiratory movements. In ascites, one can find fullness only in the flanks with the center remaining flat. A huge pelvic tumor is more

TABLE: 9.1 Observations with inspection and palpation of the breasts

Skin	*Nipple*	*Breast tissue*
▪ Dimpling, flattening ▪ Erythema ▪ Edema	▪ Retraction ▪ Eczema ▪ Discharge (p. 475)	▪ Fixation ▪ Thickening ▪ Masses ▪ Tenderness

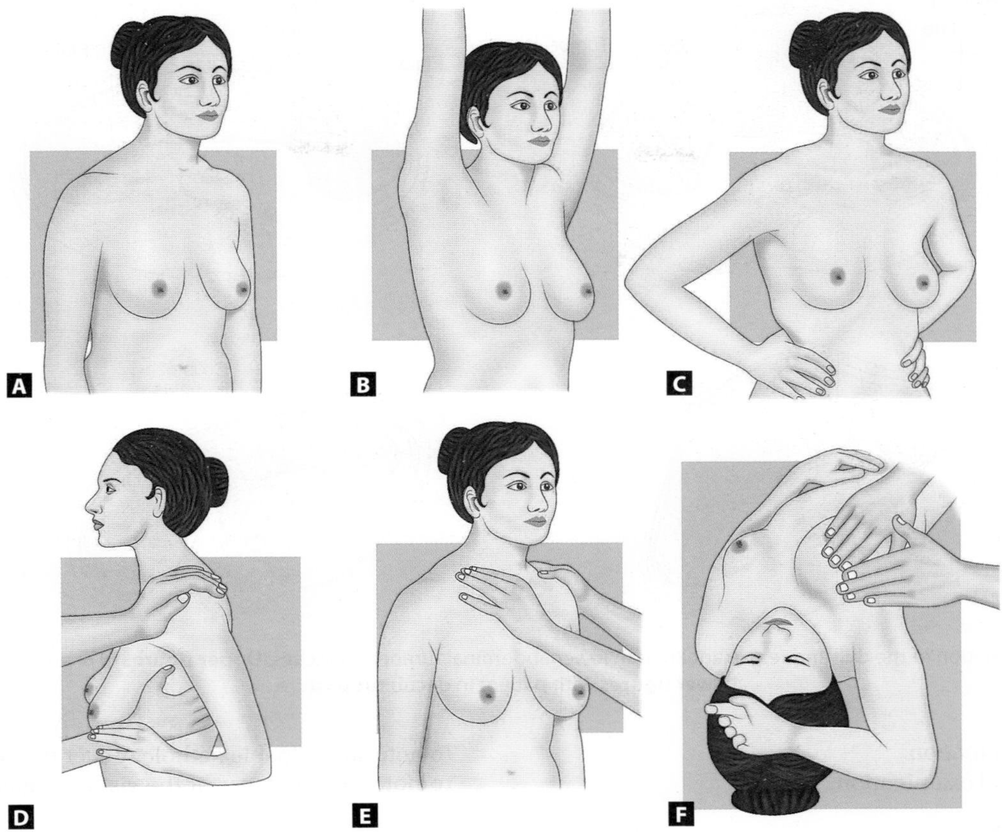

Figs. 9.1A to F: Clinical examination of the breast. (A, B and C) Visualization is for symmetry of the breast and nipples: (A) Inspection with the arms at her sides; (B) Inspection with the arms raised above the head; (C) Inspection with hands at the waist (with contracted pectoral muscle); (D) Palpation of the axillary nodes; (E) Palpation of the supraclavicular nodes; (F) Palpation in supine position with her arms above her head to examine the outer half of the breast (a pillow is placed under the patient's shoulder).

prominent in the hypogastrium situated either centrally or to one side. Female escutcheon over the mons pubis is noted.

Palpation

The palpation should be done with the flat of the hand gently rather than the tips of the fingers. If **rigidity** of the abdominal muscles is encountered, it may be due to high tension or due to **muscle guard**. If **a mass is felt** in the lower abdomen, its location, size above the symphysis pubis, consistency, feel, surface, mobility from side to side and from above to down, and margins are to be noted. Whether the lower border of the mass can be reached or not should be elicited. In general, lower border cannot be reached in pelvic tumor, but in ovarian tumor with a long pedicle one can go below the lower pole. If the tumor is cystic and huge, one can exhibit a fluid thrill felt with a flat hand placed on one side of the tumor when the cyst is tapped on the other side of the tumor with the other hand. Whether a mass is felt or not, routine palpation of the viscera (for any organomegaly) includes—liver, spleen, cecum and appendix, pelvic colon, gallbladder and kidneys.

Percussion

A pelvic tumor is usually dull on percussion with resonance on the flanks. However, if there are intestinal adhesions or the tumor is retroperitoneal, it will be resonant. In presence of ascites, the flanks will be dull on percussion and the shifting dullness, if elicited, confirms the diagnosis of free fluid in the peritoneal cavity. It is, however, mandatory to elicit presence of free fluid in the peritoneal cavity in every case of pelvic tumor (Fig. 9.2).

Auscultation

Ordinarily, auscultation reveals only the intestinal sounds. Hypoactive bowel sounds are found in paralytic ileus, hyperactive bowel sounds may be due to intestinal obstruction. The uterine souffle may be heard over a pregnant uterus or vascular fibroid, which is synchronous with the patient's pulse. If the tumor is of pregnant uterine origin, fetal heart sound can be heard after 24 weeks.

Pelvic Examination

Pelvic examination includes:

- Inspection of the external genitalia
- Vaginal examination
  - Inspection (using a speculum) of the cervix and vaginal walls.
  - Palpation of the vagina and vaginal cervix by digital examination.
  - Bimanual examination of the pelvic organs (uterus adnexa).

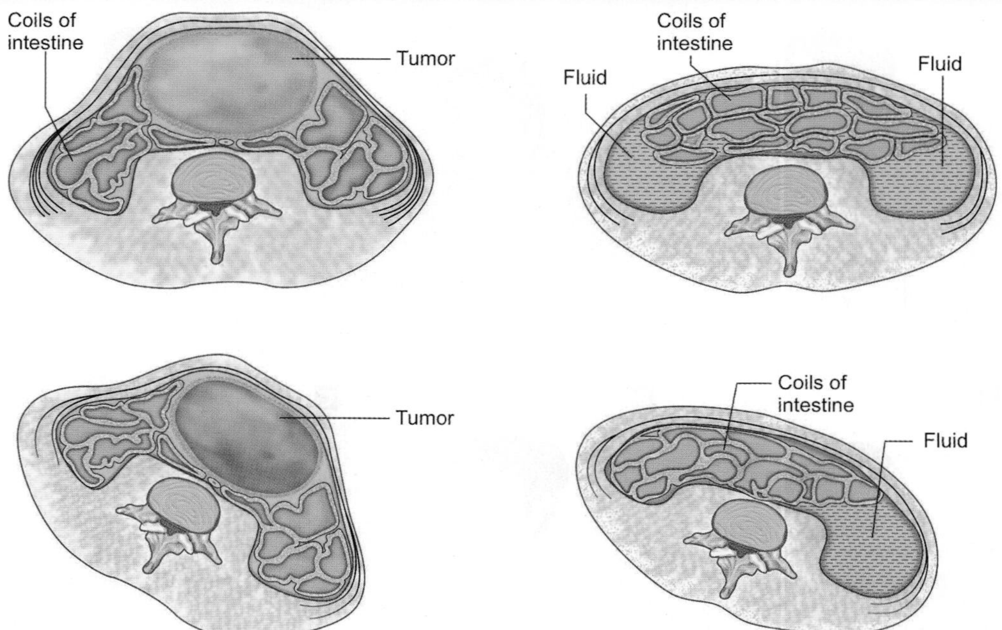

Fig. 9.2: Relation of the dull and reasonant areas in lower abdominal tumor and ascites; **Upper figures** in recumbent posture. **Lower figures** with patient in decubitus posture.

- Rectal examination
- Rectovaginal examination.

Prerequisites

- The patient's bladder must be empty—the exception being a case of stress incontinence.
- A female attendant (nurse or relative of the patient) should be present by her side.
- To examine a minor or unmarried, a consent from the parent or guardian is required.
- Lower bowel (rectum and pelvic colon) should preferably be empty.
- A light source should be available.
- Sterile gloves, sterile lubricant (preferably colorless without any antiseptics), speculum, sponge holding forceps and swabs are required.

Position of the Patient (Figs. 9.3A to D)

The patient is commonly examined in **dorsal position** with the knees flexed and thighs abducted. The physician usually stands on the right side. This position gives better view of the external genitalia and the bimanual pelvic examination can be effectively performed.

However, the patient can be examined, in any position of the physician's choice. **Lateral or Sims' position** seems ideal for inspecting any lesion in anterior vaginal wall as the vagina balloons with air as soon as the introitus is opened by a speculum. **Lithotomy position** (patient lying supine with her legs on stirups) is ideal for examination under anesthesia.

Inspection of the Vulva (Fig. 9.4)

- To note any anatomical abnormality starting from the pubic hair, clitoris, labia and perineum.
- To note any palpable pathology over the areas.
- To note the character of the visible vaginal discharge, if any.
- To separate the labia using fingers of the left hand to note external urethral meatus, visible openings of the Bartholin's ducts (normally not visible unless inflamed) and character of the hymen.
- To ask the patient to strain to elicit:
  - Stress incontinence—urine comes out through urethral meatus (p. 335).
  - Genital prolapse and the structures involved—cystocele, uterus alone or rectocele or all the three (p. 166).
- Lastly, to look for hemorrhoids, anal fissure, anal fistula or perineal tear.

Vaginal Examination

Inspection of the vagina and cervix

Which one is to be done first—speculum examination or palpation?

Speculum examination should preferably be done prior to bimanual examination. **The advantages are:**

- Cervical scrape cytology and endocervical sampling can be taken as 'screening' in the same sitting.
- Cervical or vaginal discharge can be taken for bacteriological examination.
- The cervical lesion may bleed during bimanual examination, which makes the lesion difficult to visualize.

Two types of speculum are commonly used—Sims' or Cusco's bivalve. **While in dorsal position, Cusco's is widely used** but in lateral position, Sims' variety has got advantages (Figs. 9.5A and B).

The cervix is best visualized with the Cusco's or Pederson's variety. While the vaginal fornices are only

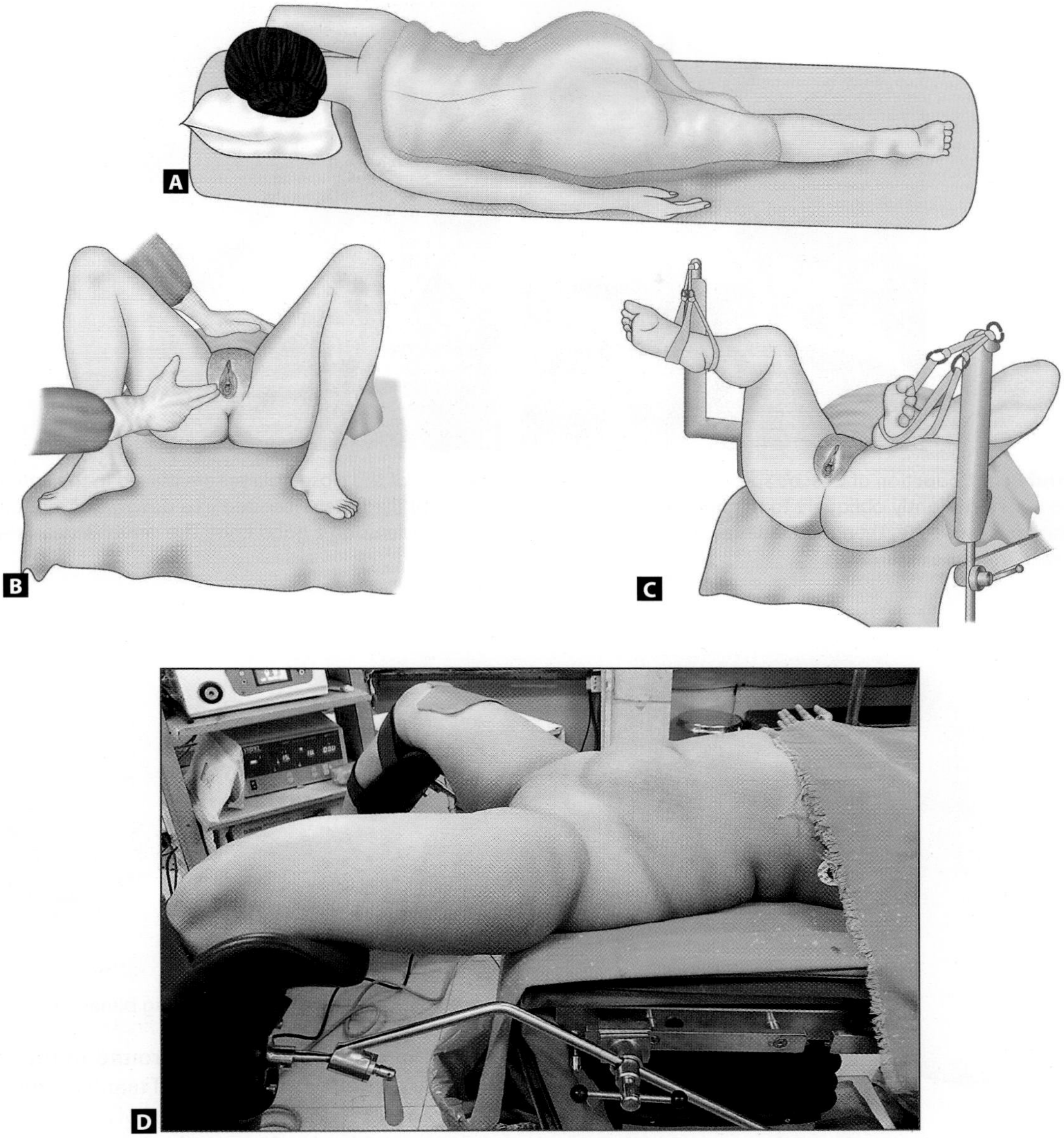

Figs. 9.3A to D: Positions of the patient for gynecological examination: (A) Sims' position—the patient lies on her left side with right knee and thigh drawn up towards the chest, the left arm along the back; (B) Dorsal position; (C) Lithotomy position; (D) Dorsal low lithotomy position for laparoscopic and hysteroscopic surgeries.

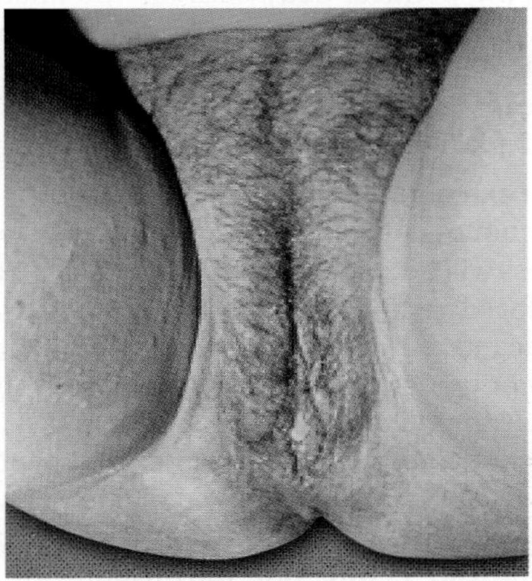

Fig. 9.4: Inspection of vulva in dorsal position.

visualized by Cusco's, and **the anterior vaginal wall is to be visualized by Sims' variety**. Sims' speculum is advantageous in cases of genital prolapse.

Apart from inspection, collection of the discharge (chlamydia) from the cervix or from the vaginal fornices or from the external urethral meatus is taken for bacteriological examination (NAAT).

It is a routine practice to take **cervical scrape cytology and endocervical sampling for cytological examination in all patients** as a screening procedure, if not done recently.

Digital examination

Digital examination is done using a gloved index finger lubricated with sterile lubricant. In virgins with intact hymen, this examination is withheld but can be employed under anesthesia.

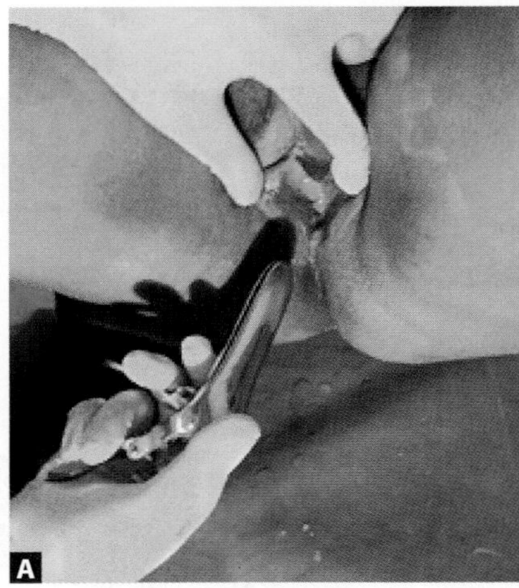

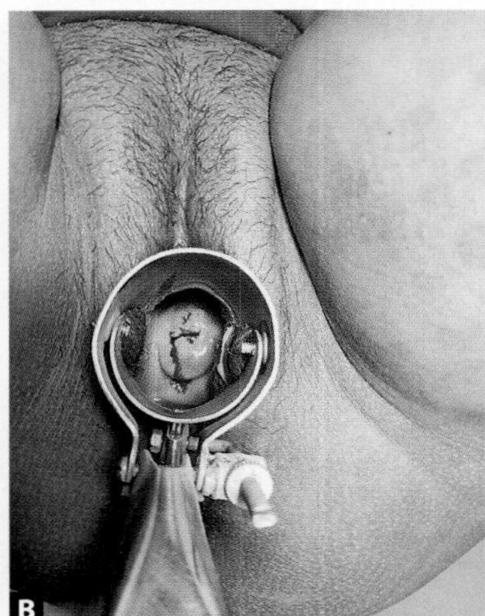

Figs. 9.5A and B: Introduction of Cusco's speculum: (A) The transverse diameter of the closed blades are placed in the anteroposterior position and inserted slightly obliquely to minimize pressure on the urethra; (B) Blades are inserted in a downward motion and then rotated. Rotation is made 90°, then the blades are opened. Inspection is then made using a good light. The cervix is clearly seen. Some bleeding is seen from the external os.

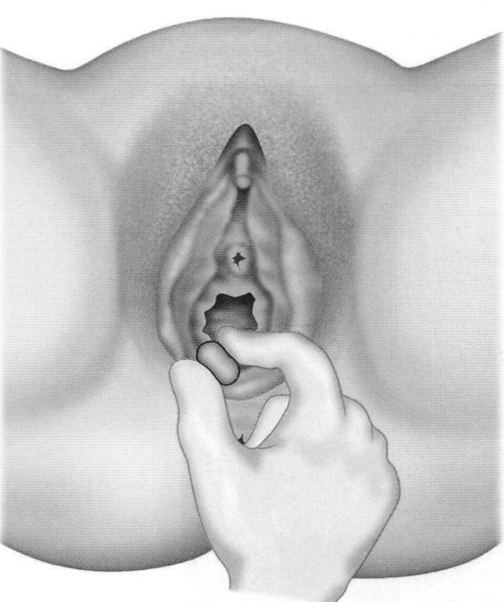

Fig. 9.6: Palpation of a labial swelling (Bartholin's gland).

Palpation of any labial swelling (commonly Bartholin's cyst or abscess) is made with the finger placed internally and thumb placed externally (Fig. 9.6). The **urethra** is now pressed from above down for any discharge escaping out through the meatus.

Palpation of the vaginal walls is to be done from below upwards to detect any abnormality either in the wall or in the adjacent structures.

The vaginal portion of cervix is next palpated to note:

- **Direction:** In anteverted uterus, the anterior lip is felt first and in retroverted position either the external os or the posterior lip is felt first.
- **Station:** Normally, the external os is at the level of ischial spines.
- **Texture:** In nonpregnant state, it feels firm like tip of the nose.
- **Shape:** It is conical with smooth surface in nulliparae but cylindrical in parous women.

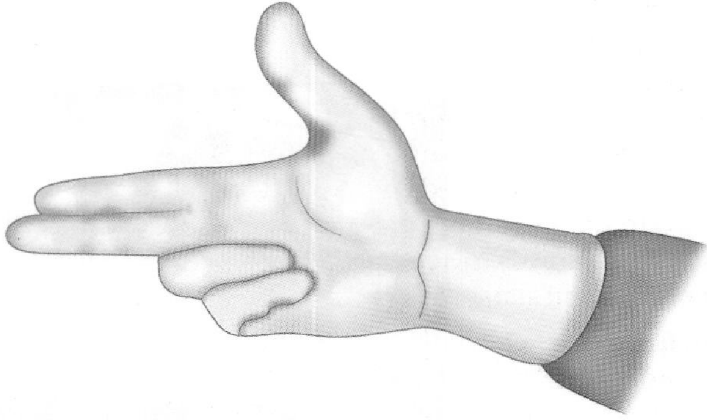

Fig. 9.7: Position of the fingers during bimanual examination.

- **External os:** It is smooth and round in nulliparae but may be dilated with evidence of tear in parous women.
- **Movement:** Painful or not.
- Whether it bleeds when touched.

Integrity and tone of the perineal body are to be elicited by flexing the internal finger posteriorly and palpating the perineal body between the internal finger and the thumb placed externally. The finger is now turned laterally above the level of levator ani muscles. The muscles can be palpated between the vaginal finger and the thumb placed externally over the labium majus.

Bimanual examination

The techniques are difficult to describe in words but perfectness will be achieved only through experience.

The gloved right index and middle fingers smeared with lubricants are inserted into the vagina. If the introitus is narrow or tender, one finger may be used. The relative position of the fingers during introduction is shown in Figure 9.7. The left hand is placed on the hypogastrium well above the symphysis pubis so that the pelvic organs can be palpated between them. **The examination should be methodical, gentle but purposeful.** To be more informative, abdominal hand is to be used more than the vaginal fingers and the patient is asked to breathe through the mouth for better relaxation of the abdominal muscles.

The information obtained by bimanual examination includes:

- Palpation of the uterus
- Palpation of the uterine appendages
- Pouch of Douglas.

Palpation of the uterus

The two internal fingers, which are placed in the anterior fornix exert a pushing force at the uterocervical junction in an upward direction towards the lumbar vertebrae and not towards the symphysis pubis. The pressure exerted by the left hand should not be only downwards but from behind forward (Fig. 9.8). The uterine outline between the two hands can thus be palpated clearly as anteverted. If the uterus is retroverted, it will not be so felt apparently can be felt if the internal fingers push up the uterus through the posterior fornix. After the uterine outline is defined, one should note its position, size, shape, consistency and mobility. **Normally**, the uterus is anteverted, pear shaped, firm and freely mobile in all directions.

Palpation of the uterine appendages

For palpation of the adnexa, the vaginal fingers are placed in the lateral fornix and are pushed backwards and upwards. The counter pressure is applied by the abdominal hand placed to one side of the uterus in a backward direction. **The normal uterine tube cannot be palpated.** A normal ovary may not be felt. If it is palpable; it is mobile and sensitive to manual pressure.

Pouch of Douglas

The pouch of Douglas can be examined effectively through the posterior fornix. Normally, the fecal mass in the rectosigmoid or else the body of a retroverted uterus is only felt. Some pathology detected in the pouch of Douglas should be supplemented by rectal examination.

Rectal or Rectoabdominal Examination

Rectal examination can be done in isolation or as an adjunct to vaginal examination.

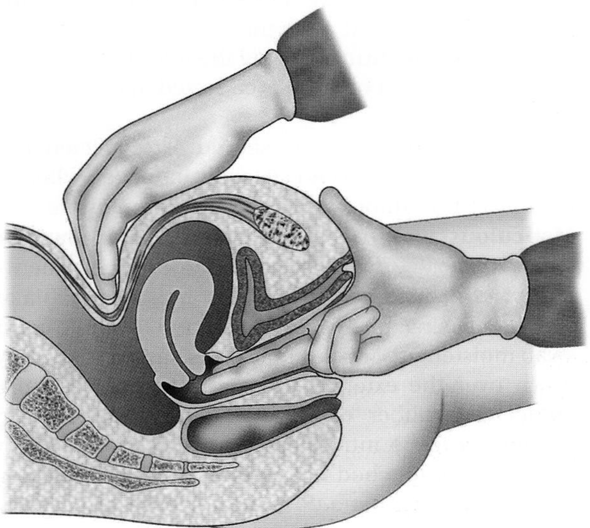

Fig. 9.8: Bimanual examination of the uterus.

Indications of rectal examination

- Children or in adult virgins
- Painful vaginal examination
- Carcinoma cervix—to note the parametrial involvement (base of the broad ligament and the uterosacral ligament can only be felt rectally) or involvement of the rectum
- To corroborate the findings felt in the pouch of Douglas by bimanual vaginal examination
- Atresia (agenesis) of vagina
- Patients having rectal symptoms
- To diagnose rectocele and differentiate it from enterocele.

The lower bowel should preferably be empty. The rectoabdominal procedure is almost the same as that of vaginal examination except that only the gloved index finger smeared with vaseline is to be introduced into the rectum (Fig. 9.9A). The rectum is palpated in all around. Anal sphincter, anal fissures, hemorrhoids and masses if present can also be felt.

Rectovaginal Examination

The procedure consists of introducing the index finger in the vagina and the middle finger in the rectum. This examination may help to determine whether the lesion is in the bowel or between the rectum and vagina. Any thickening or beaded appearance of uterosacral ligaments or presence of endometriotic nodules are noted. This is of special help to differentiate a growth arising from the ovary or rectum (Fig. 9.9B).

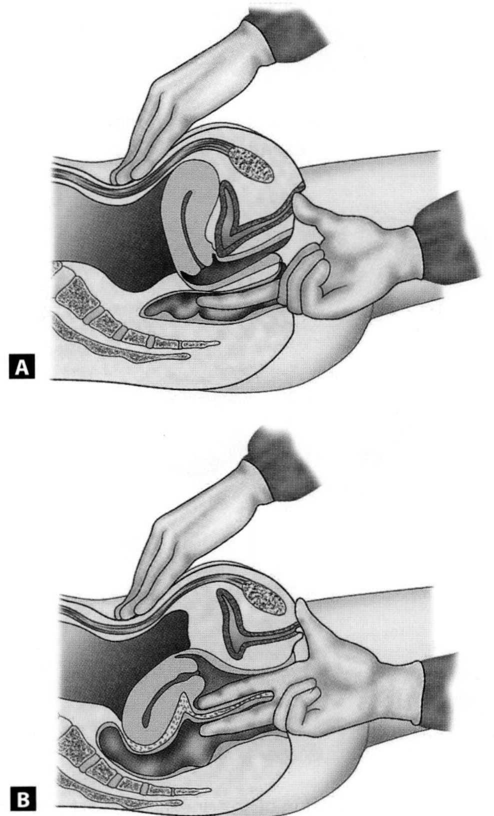

Figs. 9.9A and B: (A) Rectoabdominal; (B) Rectovaginal examination.

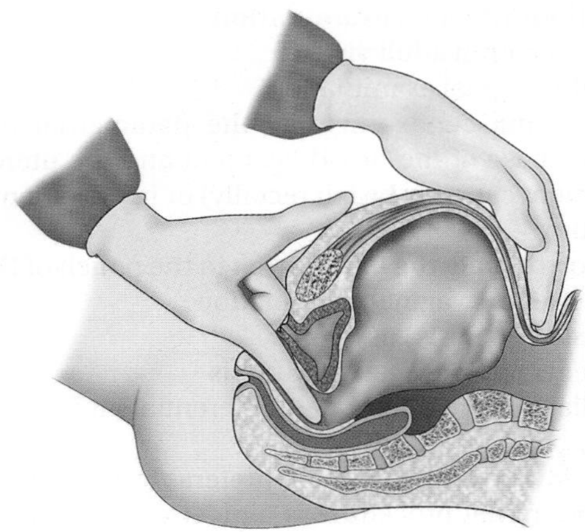

Fig. 9.10: Identification of an uterine tumor in bimanual examination.

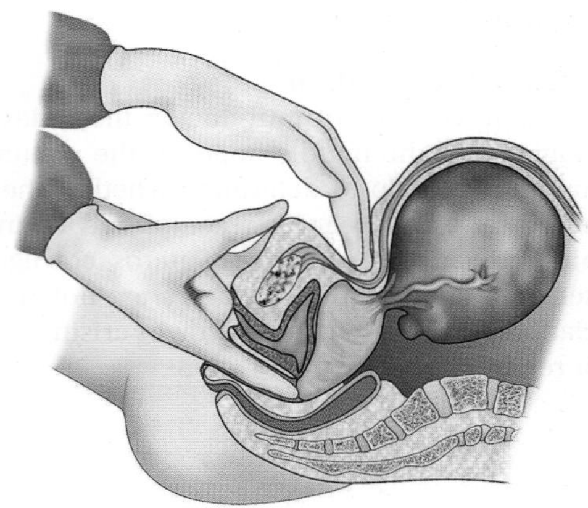

Fig. 9.11: Identification of ovarian tumor in bimanual examination.

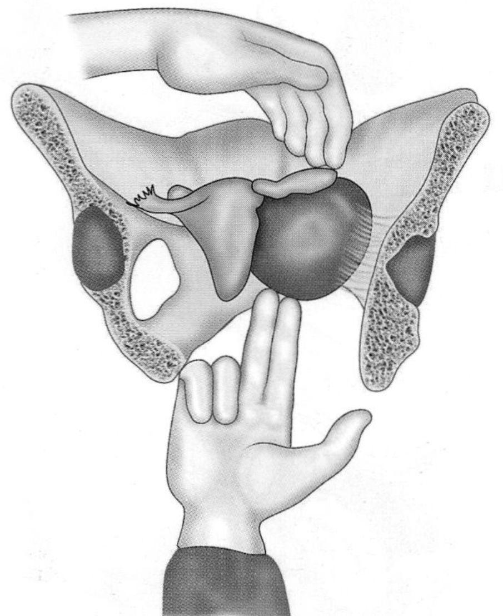

Fig. 9.12: Identification of an adnexal mass in bimanual examination.

Identification of a mass felt on bimanual examination

Uterine tumor (Fig. 9.10)

- Uterus is not separated from the mass.
- Movements of the mass felt on abdomen are transmitted to the cervix and vice versa, the exception being one of subserosal pedunculated fibroid.

Adnexal mass

- The uterus is separated from the mass (Figs. 9.11 and 9.12).
- Movement of the mass (tumor) is not transmitted to the cervix, the exception being one, if the mass is fixed with uterus.

DIAGNOSTIC PROCEDURES

For confirmation of diagnosis or rarely in cases with diagnostic difficulty, ancillary aids are required.

BLOOD VALUES

Hemoglobin estimation should be done in all cases of excessive bleeding. Total and differential count of white blood cells and erythrocyte sedimentation rate (ESR) are helpful in diagnosis of pelvic inflammation. Serological investigation includes blood for venereal disease research laboratory (VDRL) to be done in selected cases of HIV. Platelet count, bleeding and coagulation time are helpful in pubertal menorrhagia.

URINE

Routine and microscopic examination for the presence of protein, sugar, pus cells and casts are done. In the presence of excessive vaginal discharge, it is preferable to collect the midstream urine (vide infra).

Culture and drug sensitivity test is done in suspected cases of urinary tract infection. Any of the following methods are used to collect the urine for the purpose.

- **Midstream collection:** The patient herself should separate the labia with the fingers of left hand. A sterile cotton swab moistened with sterile water is passed over the external urethral meatus from above down and is then discarded. With the vulva still separated the patient is to pass urine. During the middle of the act of micturition, a part of urine is collected in a sterile wide mouth container.
- **Catheter collection:** This should be collected by a doctor or a nurse. This is especially indicated when the patient is not ambulant or having chronic retention. **Meticulous washing of the hands with soap and wearing sterile gloves are mandatory.** The patient is in dorsal position with the thighs apart. The labia are separated using the fingers of left hand. A sterile cotton swab moistened with sterile water is passed from above down over the external urethral meatus. The sterile autoclaved rubber catheter or a disposable plastic catheter is to be introduced with the proximal 4 cm remaining untouched by the fingers. With meticulous asepsis, the technique does not increase urinary tract infection (Figs. 9.13A and B).

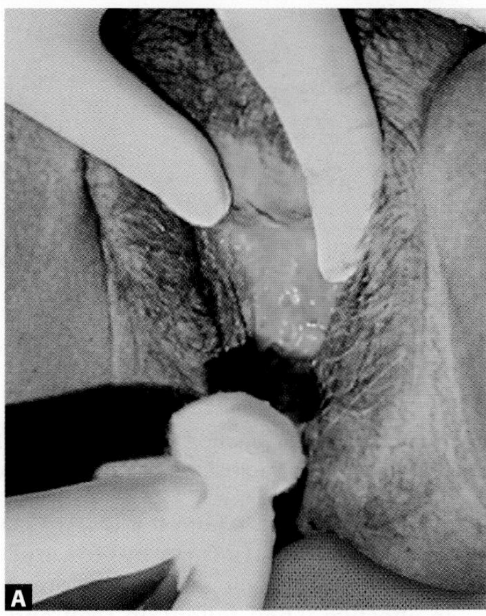

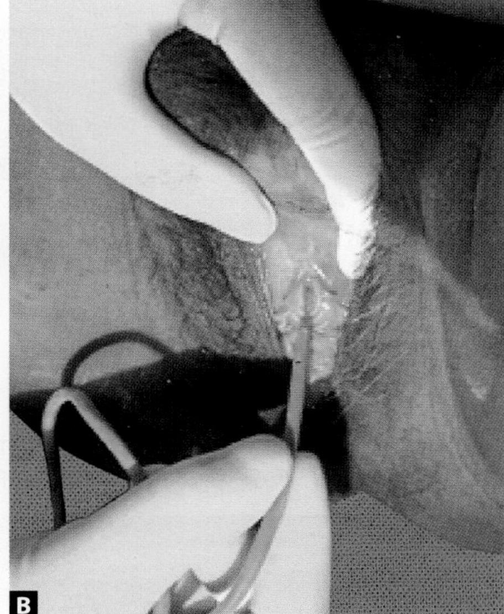

Figs. 9.13A and B: Methods of catheterization by rubber catheter: (A) Cleansing of the vestibule from above down by a moist swab; (B) Note the use of left fingers for disposition of the external urethral meatus and holding the catheter well away from the tip by the right hand.

- **Suprapubic bladder puncture:** The result is more reliable and bladder infection is minimum. The patient is asked not to void urine to make the bladder full. A fine needle fitted with a syringe is passed through the abdominal wall just above the symphysis pubis into the bladder. About 5–10 mL of urine is collected. **The patient is asked to void urination immediately**.

  Whatever method employed in the collection of urine, **the sample should be sent immediately to the laboratory**. There may be multiplication of the organisms with time.
  - **Urethral discharge:** With a sterile gloved finger, the urethra is squeezed against the symphysis pubis from behind forwards. The discharge through the external urethral meatus is collected with sterile swabs. One swab may be sent for culture and the other to be spread on to a slide, stained and examined under microscope.
  - **Vaginal or cervical discharge**: The patient is advised not to have vaginal douche at least in previous 24 hours. **Cusco's bivalve speculum is introduced without lubricant and prior to internal examination.** The material collected in the posterior blade or from the cervical canal as the case may be, is taken either by a platinum loop or swab stick.

For culture: The cotton swab stick is put in a sterile container with a stopper and to be sent immediately to the laboratory. The culture is usually unnecessary in vaginal infection. For trichomoniasis, Kupferberg's media or Feinberg Whittington media; for *Candida albicans*—Nickerson's or Sabouraud's media is used.

Identification of Organisms in a Slide

- ***Trichomonas vaginalis:*** The material is dropped over a slide and then mixed with one drop of normal saline. It is then covered with a coverslip. Actively motile trichomonas can be seen under microscope easily (Fig. 13.2). It can be effectively visualized after staining with 1% brilliant cresyl violet; leukocytes and other bacteria will not take up the dye.
- ***Monilia:*** One drop of the discharge is mixed with one drop of 10% potassium hydroxide and is covered with a coverslip. The mycelia of the fungus can be seen under microscope. Alternatively, the discharge is spread over a slide, dried and stained with methylene blue to demonstrate the mycelia (Fig. 13.4).

CERVICAL AND VAGINAL SMEAR FOR EXFOLIATIVE CYTOLOGY

The indications are:
- **As a screening procedure**
- **For cytohormonal study**
- **Others**

Screening Procedure

Collection of material: The cervix is exposed with a Cusco's vaginal speculum without lubricant and prior to bimanual examination. Lubricants tend to distort cell's morphology.

Cervical scraping: The material from the cervix is best collected using Ayre's spatula made of plastic. Whole of the squamocolumnar junction has to be scrapped to obtain good material (Figs. 9.14A to C and 9.15).

Pap Testing Procedure

Transformation zone is the squamocolumnar junction, which is the area of meeting point for the squamous epithelium of the ectocervix with the columnar epithelium of the endocervix. Smear is collected by a plastic spatula from the ectocervix. The endocervical cells are collected using an endocervical brush or using the broom (Fig. 9.15).

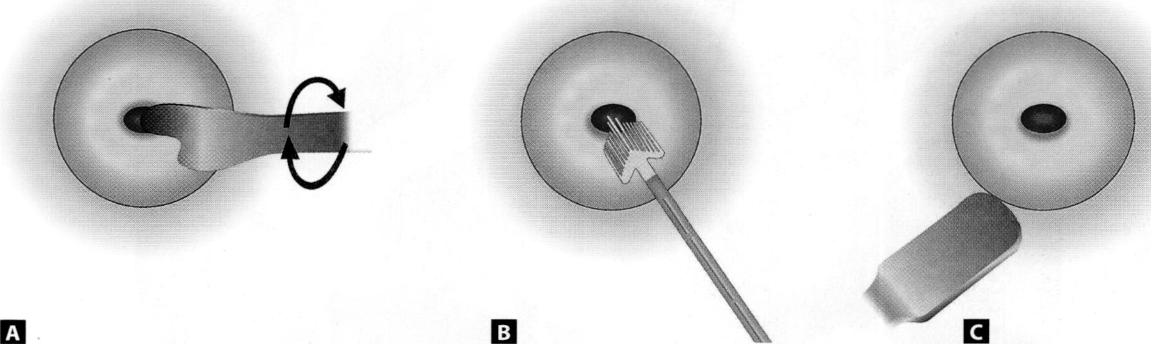

Figs. 9.14A to C: Collection of smear: (A) Using Ayre's spatula from the squamocolumnar junction for screening; (B) By cervical broom taking endocervical sampling for screening; (C) By plastic spatula from the lateral vaginal fornix for cytohormonal study.

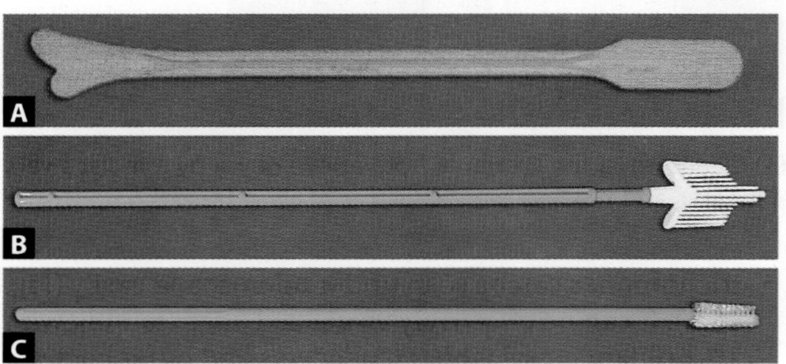

Fig. 9.15: (A) Ayre spatula; (B) Rocket endocervical broom—it's for both ecto and endocervical smear. It has conical shape with plastic bristles; (C) Endocervical brush.

The sample is placed on a glass slide and fixed with ethyl alcohol. For LBC, this sample is placed in a liquid medium for transport to the laboratory where the slide is prepared. This liquid medium is also used for HPV DNA testing. Cervical cytology reporting: The Bethesda system (TBS) is followed.

Unsatisfactory sample is defined as:

- Absence of a label
- Loss of transport medium
- Scant cellularity
- Presence of contamination
- Absence of endocervical cells.

Fixation and Staining

The material so collected should be immediately spread over a microscopic slide and at once fixed with ethyl alcohol (95%) before drying. After fixing of the slide sent to the laboratory. The slide so sent is stained either with Papanicolaou's or Sorr's method and examined by a trained cytologist. Indeed, **trained cytopathologist and cytotechnologist are vital for the success of any screening program.**

- **Benefits:** The objective of screening is to reduce the incidence and mortality from cervical cancer. Even a single smear in a lifetime, if appropriately timed, will produce some benefits. The lifetime risk of developing cervical cancer by the age of 74 is 0.9% in developed countries compared to 1.6% in low and middle income countries (LMICs). Lifetime risk of death from cervical cancer is 0.3% in developed countries compared to 0.9% in LMICs. **Pap smear test has been effective reducing the incidence of cervical cancer by 80% and the mortality by 70%.** Opportunistic screening done by a trained staff is effective when follow-up (call and recall) is maintained. Pap testing after total hysterectomy, done for benign lesion is not recommended.
- **Intervals:** The high risk group should be screened with cytology and HPV cotesting **(p. 272). The negative predictive value of one negative HPV DNA test and two negative cytology tests are almost 100%.** High risk HPV (HPV 16, 18) testing alone without cytology screening for women aged ≥30 years is recommended. When both the test results are negative, test is performed every 5 years. Colposcopy is recommended when HPV test results are persistently positive.

Cervical Cytology Screening Program (ACOG, FOGSI – 2011, ACS, USPSTF – 2012)

1. Initial screening—to begin at 25 years (*30 years by GOI*) of age regardless of sexual activity to continue upto the age of 65 years.
   Women's age (years): Screening interval
2. Age: 25–29—every 3 years
3. Age: 30 and 65
   a. Pap testing (alone): Every 3 years
   b. **Cotesting:** Pap plus high risk HPV: Every 5 years
4. Women of age > 65 years: No screening provided normal testing over past 10 years. No high grade dysplasia (CIN 2/3) in past 20 years.
   Exceptions: Women with HIV seropositivity, immunosuppression, exposure to DES in utero: All these women need annual screening.
5. Women following total hysterectomy. No follow up Pap screening is needed when hysterectomy was done for benign conditions.
6. Women with subtotal hysterectomy: Usual screening as in 1, 2, 3, 4 (mentioned above).

Morphological Abnormalities of the Nucleus (Dyskaryosis)

- Disproportionate nuclear enlargement
- Irregularity of the nuclear outline
- Abnormalities of the nucleus—in number, size and shape
- Hyperchromasia

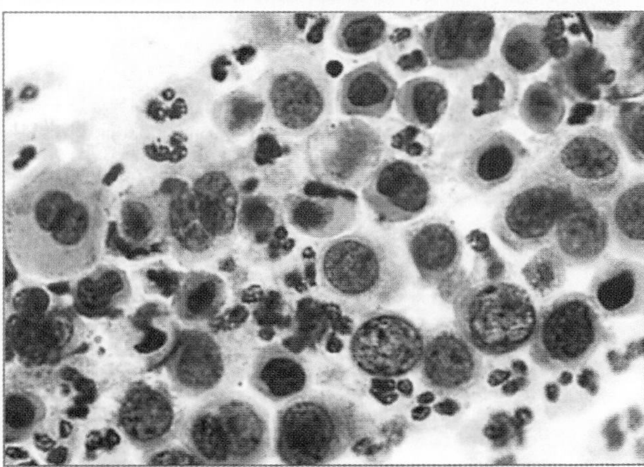

Fig. 9.16: Severe dyskaryosis.

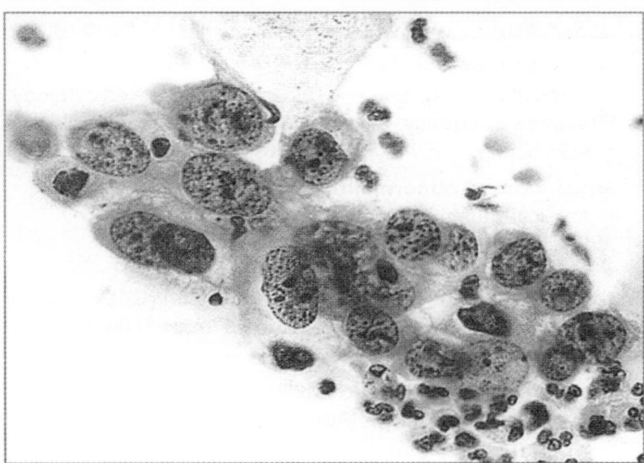

Fig. 9.17: Carcinoma in situ.

- Condensation of chromatin material
- Multinucleation.

Abnormal cells are:

- **Mild dyskaryosis:** Cells are of superficial or intermediate type squamous cells. Cells have angular borders with translucent cytoplasm. The nucleus occupies less than half of the total area of cytoplasm. Binucleation is common. Mild dyskaryosis correlates with cells from surface of cervical intraepithelial neoplasia (CIN 1) (p. 268).
- **Moderate dyskaryosis:** The cells are of intermediate, parabasal or superficial type squamous cells. Cells have more disproportionate nuclear enlargement and hyperchromasia compared to mildly dyskaryotic cells. The nucleus occupies one half to two-thirds of the total area of the cytoplasm.
- **Severe dyskaryosis** (Fig. 9.16): Cells are of basal type, looking round, oval, polygonal or elongated in shape. The abnormal cells may occur in clumps or singly. The abnormal nucleus either practically fills the cell or there may be a thick, dense and narrow rim of cytoplasm around it. The nucleus is irregular with coarse chromatin pattern. The cells may be different in size and shape. Severely dyskaryotic cells when elongated, are sometimes called **fiber cells.** A severely dyskaryotic cell with an elongated tail of cytoplasm is described as a **tadpole cell.** Severely dyskaryotic cells **correlate with CIN 3.**
- **Koilocytosis** is the nuclear abnormalities associated with human papilloma virus infection. Cells show typical central clearing (perinuclear halo) with peripheral condensation of cytoplasm. The nucleus is irregularly enlarged and shows hyperchromasia with multinucleation. Patients with koilocytosis on repeated smear, need colposcopic evaluation.
- **Carcinoma in situ** (Fig. 9.17): Cells are parabasal type with increased nuclear cytoplasmic ratio. The nucleus may be irregular sometimes multiple. The chromatin pattern is granular; cytoplasm is scanty.
- **Invasive carcinoma:** Cells are single or grouped in clusters. The cells show irregular nuclei and clumping of nuclear chromatin, which is also coarse. **Large tadpole cells are seen.**

Reporting System

Reporting system on the grade basis (Papanicolaou's) is made with two remarks only—normal or abnormal. **Currently the Bethesda system (TBS) is followed (p. 268).**

Accuracy

A single Pap smear has a diagnostic sensitivity of about 60%. False negative results may be up to 25%. False negative rate of Pap smear after three consecutive negative tests is less than 1%. There are several reasons for false-negative smear. This may be due to technical error where smear is too scanty, too thick, too bloody, poorly stained or due to misinterpretation by the cytologist. Error in cytology could be reduced further by liquid-based thin layer slide preparation and automated (computer) screening methods. Abnormal cytology is an indication of colposcopic evaluation and directed biopsy. If colposcopy is not available, biopsy is to be taken from the unstained areas following application of acetic acid (VIA) or Schiller's or Lugol's iodine (Ch. 23). In the presence of infection, repeat cytology has to be done after the infection is controlled (Table 9.2). A doubtful or inconclusive smear dictates repeat smear.

Liquid-based cytology (LBC) (Fig. 9.18): Cervical smear is taken using a plastic spatula and the broom. The spatula and the broom are rinsed or broken off in the liquid media. Cells are separated by centrifugation. Thin layer smears are made.

LBC has the following advantages: (a) Improved cell collection and preparation quality; (b) Even distribution of abnormal cells that makes easy detection. Whereas with conventional Pap smear cells are clustered and obscured. LBC avoids the risk of false-positive, false-negative or unsatisfactory smears.

Cytohormonal Study

The vaginal epithelium is highly sensitive to the hormones estrogen and progesterone. The noninvasive study of the

TABLE 9.2: The Bethesda System cytology (2014).

▪ **Specimen type:** • Conventional Pap test • Thin layer liquid-based cytology ▪ **Specimen adequacy:** • Satisfactory • Unsatisfactory
▪ **Squamous cell abnormalities** • Atypical squamous cells (ASC) – ASC of undetermined significance (ASC-US) – ASC, cannot exclude high grade lesion (ASC-H) ▪ **Low-grade squamous intraepithelial lesion (LSIL)** ▪ **High-grade squamous intraepithelial lesion (HSIL)** ▪ **Squamous cell carcinoma (SCC)**
▪ **Glandular cell abnormalities** • Atypical glandular cells (AGC): Endocervical, endometrial or not specified • AGC favor neoplastic endocervical or not otherwise specified • Adenocarcinoma (endocervical) in situ (AIS) • Adenocarcinoma
▪ **Other cancers** (e.g. lymphoma, metastasis, sarcoma)
Significance of epithelial cell abnormalities
▪ **ACS-US** is the most common cytologic abnormality. Risk of CIN 2 or 3 is about 3–7%; risks of invasive carcinoma is about 0.2%. These patients should undergo repeat cytology at 12 months or reflex HPV testing. When HPV test is positive, colposcopy is done, if negative, routine screening at 5 years. ▪ **Low-grade squamous intraepithelial lesion (LSIL)**: LSIL is mainly due to HPV infection (CIN 1). Risks of CIN 2 and 3 and is up to 19% to 5%. HPV DNA testing is not useful in women with age <30 years. LSIL may resolve spontaneously or may progress to more severe dysplasia (ASCCP – 2013). If both cytology and HPV testing are negative, repeat testing should be done in 5 years. If cytology is positive and HPV is negative, cytology is repeated at 1 year. If both are positive, colposcopy and biopsy are to be done. ▪ **Atypical squamous cells, cannot exclude HSIL (ASC-H):** ACS-H is seen in about 5–10% of cytologic abnormalities. These women need colposcopy to exclude CIN 2/ 3 lesions. ▪ **High-grade squamous intraepithelial lesion (HSIL):** Risks of underlying CIN2 or 3 is 69–47% respectively. Risks of cervical cancer is 7%, if left untreated. All women with HSIL should be evaluated with colposcopy (ASCCP – 2013). Majority of the women are treated with excision or ablation depending on age, colposcopy and biopsy reports (p. 271, Ch. 23). ▪ **Glandular cell abnormalities**: Risks of endometrial cancer is high. The risks of neoplasia in this group is increased. ▪ **Atypical glandular cells (AGS):** Risks of underlying invasive cancer is 3–17% (ACOG, 2013). All such women should have colposcopy with endocervical and endometrial sampling.

epithelium for hormonal status is steadily increasing owing to the speed, cheapness and accuracy.

Instructions to the Patient

- To avoid intercourse for about 48 hours
- Not to use vaginal douche for 24 hours
- To withhold use of hormonal drugs.

Procedures: **The lateral wall of the upper-third of the vagina (most sensitive to hormonal influence)** is lightly scraped

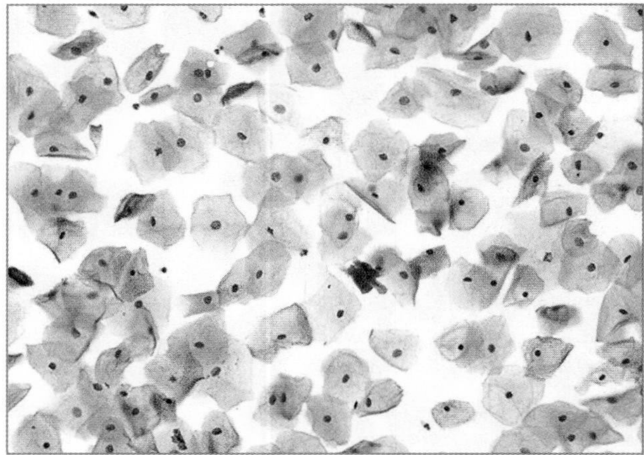

Fig. 9.18: Liquid-based cytology—normal squamous cells and endocervical cells.

with a plastic spatula after taking due precautions mentioned earlier. The material so collected is to be fixed and stained as mentioned earlier. **The physician should mention the following information**, such as age, first day of the last period, menstrual pattern and any hormone therapy.

Inferences: The exfoliated vaginal epithelial cells normally include parabasal, intermediate and superficial cells. The **parabasal** cells are small, round and basophilic; the **intermediate cells** are transparent and basophilic while the **superficial cells** are large, thin acidophilic with pyknotic nuclei. The estrogen produces superficial cell maturation; progesterone, androgen, corticosteroids, 'pill' and pregnancy produce intermediate cell maturation, whereas lack of any hormonal activity produces parabasal cell dominance (Table 9.3).

The estrogenic smear is suggested by preponderance of large eosinophilic cells with pyknotic nuclei (cornified cells). The background remains clear (Fig. 8.12).

The progesterone smear is of predominantly basophilic cells with vesicular nuclei. The background looks dirty (Fig. 8.12).

Interpretations: The number of cornified cells per 100 cells counted is expressed as **cornification or karyopyknotic index**. It is mostly replaced by a more appropriate expressive method—called **maturation index (MI)**. The maturation index relates to the relative percentage of parabasal, intermediate and superficial cells per 100 cells counted. It is expressed in three numbers; the left one parabasal percentage, the intermediate in the centre and on the right, the percentage of the superficial cells (Table 9.3).

Other Indications of Cytology Study

- **The exfoliative cell cytology is used** in follow-up cases of carcinoma cervix treated either by surgery or radiotherapy.
- **Sex chromatin study:** The materials are from scraping of buccal mucosa and to be stained with Papanicolaou stain. The presence of Barr body in more than 25% cells is diagnostic of female sex.
- **Aspirated fluids:** Ascitic fluid from the cysts or pleural space, are subjected to Papanicolaou stain for evidences of malignant cells.

TABLE 9.3: Vaginal cells maturation index from birth to menopause.

Age	MI	Smear features	Inference
At birth	0/95/5	—	Combined effect of circulating maternal hormones: Estrogen, progesterone and corticoids
Childhood	80/20/0	—	MI shifting to left due to diminished steroid hormones
Reproductive period ▪ Preovulatory	0/40/60	Smear clear, cells are discrete	Estrogen ++
▪ Mild secretory	0/70/30	Smear dirty, cells in clusters	Estrogen +; Progesterone ++
▪ During pregnancy	0/95/5	Marked folding of the intermediate cells—'navicular cells'	Estrogen ++; Progesterone ++; Corticosteroids +
▪ Postpartum	100/0/0	—	Parabasal maturation
Postmenopausal	0/100/0 or 100/0/0	—	Lack of estrogen

EXAMINATION OF CERVICAL MUCUS

- **Bacteriological study**
- **Hormonal status**
- **Infertility investigation**

Bacteriological Study

Cusco's bivalve speculum is introduced without lubricant. With the help of a sterile cotton swab, the cervical canal is swabbed. The material is either sent for culture or spread over a microscopic slide for Gram staining.

Hormonal Status

The physical, chemical and cellular components of the cervical secretion are dependent on hormones—estrogen and progesterone. Estrogen increases the water and electrolyte content with decrease in protein. As such, the mucus becomes copious, clear and thin. Progesterone, on the other hand, decreases the water and electrolytes but increases the protein. As a result, the mucus becomes scanty, thick and tenacious. The influence of the hormones on the cervical mucus is utilized in detection of ovulation in clinical practice.

- pH around the time of ovulation is about 6.8–7.4.
- **Spinnbarkeit** (stretchability or elasticity)—during the midcycle, the cervical secretion is collected with a pipette and placed over a glass slide. Another glass slide is placed over it. Because of increased elasticity due to high estrogen level during this period, the mucus placed between the slides **can withstand stretching up to a distance of over 10 cm.** After ovulation when corpus luteum forms, progesterone is secreted. Under its action, the cervical mucus looses its property of elasticity and while attempting the above procedure, the mucus fractures when put under tension much earlier. **This loss of elasticity after its presence in the midcycle is the indirect evidence of ovulation.**
- **Fern test**—during the midcycle, the cervical mucus is obtained by a platinum loop or pipette and spread on a clean glass slide and dried. When seen under low power microscope, it shows characteristic pattern of fern formation. **It is due to high sodium chloride,** low protein content in the mucus, high estrogen in the midmenstrual phase prior to ovulation. After ovulation with increasing progesterone, the ferning disappears completely after 21st day. **Thus, the presence of ferning even after 21st day suggests anovulation and its disappearance is presumptive evidence of ovulation** (Fig. 9.19).

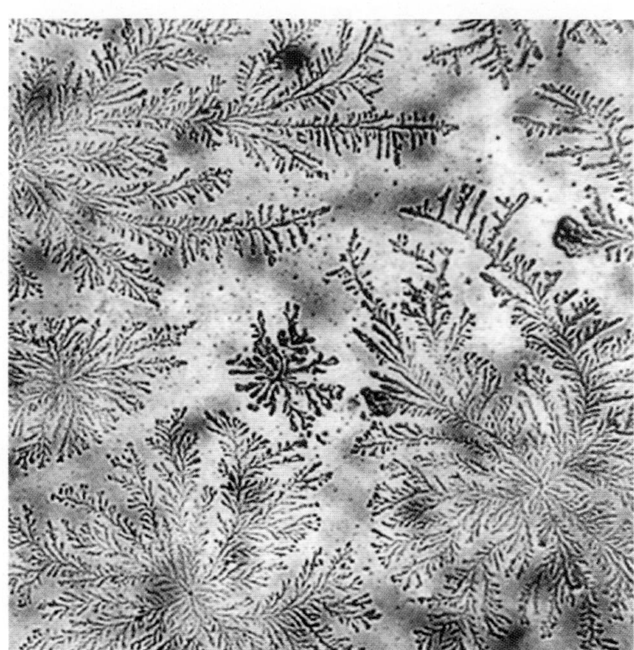

Fig. 9.19: Typical fern pattern appearance of cervical mucus.

Infertility Investigations

Postcoital test (PCT)—Marion Sims (1866) and Max Huhner (1913). Not commonly done these days.

COLPOSCOPY

The instrument was devised by Hinselmann in 1925. **Colposcope and colpomicroscope are the low-power binocular microscope, mounted on a stand.** It is designed to magnify the surface epithelium of the vaginal part of the cervix including entire transformation zone. The magnification is to the extent of 15–40 times in

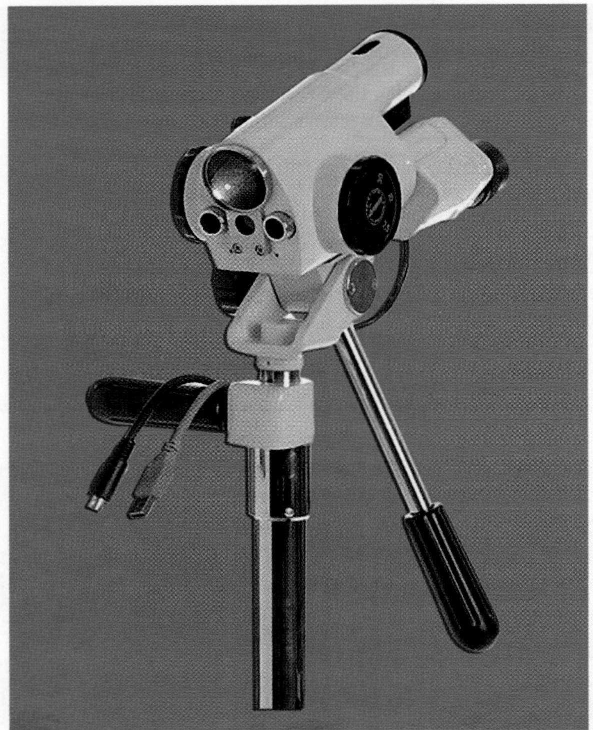

Fig. 9.20: Technique of colposcopy needs ease of maneuver (frontal distance of 225–250 mm), magnification (6–16 times), adequate light source (30,000 lux), the stand to permit mobility and the examination table for patient's comfort.

colposcopy and about 100–300 times in colpomicroscopy (Fig. 9.20). Some of the terms used in colposcopy are listed in Table 9.4.

TABLE 9.4: Colposcopic terminology.

I	**Normal colposcopic findings** A—Normal squamous epithelium B—Columnar epithelium C—Transformation zone
II	**Abnormal colposcopic findings (p. 273)** **A—A typical transformation zone** a. Mosaic b. Punctuation c. Acetowhite epithelium d. Keratosis e. Atypical vessels f. Iodine negativity **B—Suspected frank invasive cancer:** The cancer is evident only colposcopically
III	**Satisfactory colposcopy:** Entire transformation zone is seen. **Unsatisfactory colposcopy:** Entire transformation zone not seen as it extends to the endocervical canal, or the examiner is unable to determine the presence or extent of abnormal tissue. In such a situation, endocervical curettage (ECC) is recommended. Cervical biopsy is done if any acetowhite lesions are noted. Any bleeding following biopsy is controlled by Monsel's solution containing ferric subsulfate. Biopsy specimens are very small. The biopsy sites heal spontaneously.
IV	**Other findings** Condyloma, ectopy and papilloma are of importance

Procedure

The patient is placed in lithotomy position. The cervix is visualized using a Cusco's speculum (Fig. 9.5). Cervical infections are to be treated before hand. Colposcopic examination of the cervix and vagina is done using low power magnification (6–16 fold). Cervix is then cleared of any mucus discharge using a swab soaked with normal saline. Green filter and high magnification can be used now. Next, the cervix is wiped gently with 3–5% acetic acid and examination repeated after 30–60 seconds. Acetic acid is a mucolytic agent. It causes coagulation of nuclear protein which is high in CIN. This prevents transmission of light through the epithelium, which is visible as white (acetowhite) areas (Fig. 23.7A).

Lugol solution: Stains mature squamous epithelial cells to dark brown color due to the presence of abundant glycogen content. Dysplastic cells appear yellowish due to lack of glycogen.

Important parameters of colposcopic examinations are: (a) Margin of the lesion; (b) Color; (c) Vascular patterns; and (d) Lugol solution staining (Reid index). Following application of acetic acid to cervical epithelium, the epithelial color, degree and rapidity of whiteness, sharpness of the lesion borders and vascular pattern (Table 9.4) are observed.

Reid colposcopic index: Assessment is based on four features of the lesion: (a) Margin; (b) Color; (c) Vascular pattern and (d) Lugol solution staining effect. Each category is scored from 0, 1 and 2, maximum 8. There is a numeric index that correlates the histology.

ENDOMETRIAL SAMPLING

Endometrial sampling is one of the diagnostic tests, most frequently performed as an outdoor procedure. This rapid, safe and inexpensive test is employed in the clinical work up of women with infertility or abnormal uterine bleeding or for periodic screening during hormone replacement therapy (HRT). The instrument commonly used is either a Vabra aspirator or a Sharman curette. **Currently, endometrial sampler (Pipelle) is used as an outpatient procedure** (Fig. 9.21). A thin plastic cannula (2–4 mm diameter), with a plunger within is negotiated within the uterus. **It is done as an outpatient procedure.** When the plunger is withdrawn, adequate endometrium is obtained due to suction action. This procedure is reliable and is accepted by the patient.

Indications of endometrial sampling are:

- Dysfunctional uterine bleeding
- Abnormal bleeding following the use of hormone replacement therapy and
- Abnormal perimenopausal or menopausal bleeding. Pipelle is the instrument of first choice for endometrial sampling. The failure rate of the procedure is less than 8%. To study the hormonal effect, material from

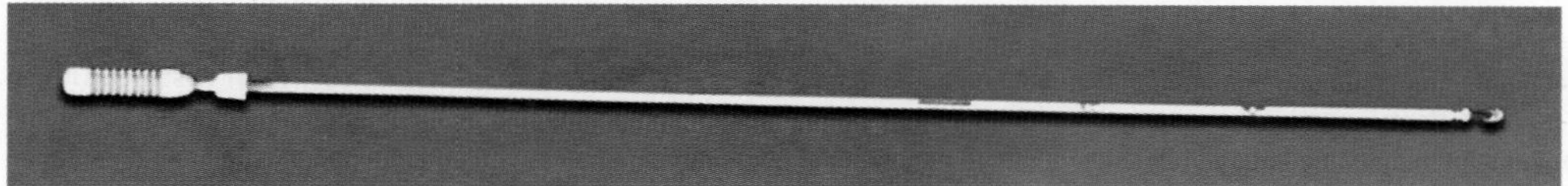

Fig. 9.21: Endometrial sampler.

the fundus and upper part of the body is to be taken. However, additional diagnostic procedures, such as hysteroscopy should be done when needed. When a large tissue mass is needed for histological studies, a thorough endometrial curettage is to be done under anesthesia as in endometrial tuberculosis or postmenopausal bleeding.

Endometrial Biopsy

The most reliable method to study the endometrium is by obtaining the material by curettage after dilatation of the cervix usually under general anesthesia. Its clinical application is described in appropriate chapters (p. 159, 534).

Tests for Tubal Patency

These are described in the Ch. 17 (p. 196).

Cervical Biopsy

To confirm the clinical diagnosis of the cervical pathology, biopsy is mandatory. It can be done in the outpatient department or indoor. Biopsy can be taken safely at the outpatient department, if the pathology is detectable—for wider tissue excision as in cone biopsy, it should be done as an inpatient procedure. The details are described in page 541.

CULDOCENTESIS

Definition

Culdocentesis is the transvaginal aspiration of peritoneal fluid from the cul-de-sac or pouch of Douglas.

Indications

- In suspected disturbed ectopic pregnancy or other causes producing hemoperitoneum.
- In suspected cases of pelvic abscess.

Steps

- The procedure is done under sedation.
- The patient is put in lithotomy position.
- Vagina is cleaned with Betadine.
- A posterior vaginal speculum is inserted.
- An 18 gauge spinal needle fitted with a syringe is inserted at a point 1 cm below the cervicovaginal junction in the posterior fornix (Figs. 9.22A and B).
- After inserting the needle to a depth of about 2 cm, suction is applied as the needle is withdrawn.
- **If unclotted blood is obtained, the diagnosis of intraperitoneal bleeding is established.** If no blood or fluid is obtained, the needle is withdrawn slowly while intermittent suction should be maintained. If the tap is found dry, another attempt is to be made.

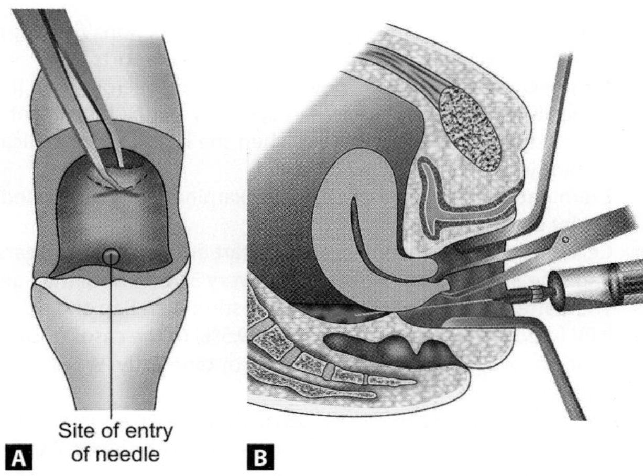

Figs. 9.22A and B: Culdocentesis: (A) Front view; (B) Lateral view.

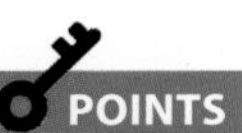

POINTS

- **The clinical examination** should be thorough and meticulous. The examination should in fact proceed with the provisional diagnosis in mind. A patient hearing should be given about the complaints made by the patient in her own words.
- **Menstrual history includes age** of menarche, cycle length, regularity, duration of period, amount of flow and the first day of the last menstrual period.
- **Integration of the symptomatology** to a single pathology is to be tried first before embarking on the diagnosis of multiple pathology.
- **The general and systemic examination** should be thorough and meticulous.
- **Clinical breast examination (CBE)** should be a routine part of the gynecologic examination (Fig. 9.1). Annual CBE of women with age more than 40 years is recommended (ACOG).
- **CBE** begins with inspection and then a thorough palpation (p. 474). The examiner should check for nipple discharge (p. 474) as well as the axillary lymph nodes (p. 474).
- **Bladder** should be empty prior to examination.
- **Abdominal palpation** should be done with the flat of the hand rather than the tips of the fingers. Whether a mass is felt or not, routine palpation of the viscera includes liver, spleen, cecum, pelvic colon, gallbladder and kidneys.
- **It is mandatory** to elicit presence of free fluid in the peritoneal cavity in all cases of pelvic tumors.

Contd...

Contd…

- **Pelvic examination** includes inspection of external genitalia, vaginal examination (inspection with a speculum, palpation and bimanual examination), rectal examination and rectovaginal examination.
- **Rectovaginal examination** is of special help to differentiate a growth arising from the ovary or rectum.
- **Dyskaryosis** is the morphological abnormality of the nucleus. It may be mild, moderate or severe. Koilocytosis is associated with human papilloma virus infection.
- **As a screening procedure,** the material from the cervix is best collected using Ayre's spatula. About 5 cases of cervical intraepithelial neoplasia are diagnosed per 1000 patients and invasive carcinoma of the cervix in order of 1 in 1000. A complete gynecological evaluation should include menstrual history, sexual history, contraceptive history, history of Pap smear, HPV vaccination and medications.
- **Diagnostic accuracy of Pap smear** after three consecutive negative tests is about 99%.
- **For cytohormonal study,** the smear is taken from the lateral wall of the upper-third of the vagina. The estrogenic smear is suggested by preponderance of large eosinophilic cells with pyknotic nuclei. The progesterone smear is predominantly basophilic with vesicular nuclei. The background is dirty.
- **Maturation index (MI),** is expressed by three numbers as the percentage of parabasal, intermediate and superficial cells written from left to the right. There is significant shift in maturation index from birth to menopause.
- **Examination of cervical mucus** is done for bacteriological study, to know the hormonal status and in infertility investigation.
- Nucleic acid amplification testing (NAAT) of vaginal and cervical discharge for detection of infections (chlamydia, gonorrhea).
- **Estrogenic mucus** is clear, abundant and has got the power of elasticity and shows pattern of fern tree formation. Progesterone smear is thick and viscid, loses its property of elasticity and ferning disappears.
- **Menstrual cycles** after puberty and before menopause are frequently anovulatory and irregular.
- **Endometrial sampling** is useful in the clinical **work-up** of women with infertility or abnormal perimenopausal bleeding. It can be performed in the OPD using a narrow plastic cannula (pipelle).
- **Culdocentesis** is indicated in suspected cases of hemoperitoneum (ectopic pregnancy) or pelvic abscess.
- **Pap test (cervical smear test)** is the most effective cancer screening procedure. It reduces the incidence of cancer cervix by 80% when used regularly.
- **Cervical cancer** is caused by HPV (p. 270) infection. Virtually most HPV infections regress spontaneously. An HPV-DNA test can be used to triage women with ASC-US cytology reports.
- **Colposcope** is a lower power binocular microscope. It is employed in cases with abnormal cervical smear and with clinically suspicious cervices, especially with history of contact bleeding even if the smear is negative. Colposcopy directed biopsy is the best one when the lesion is not clinically detected. Colposcope is used to evaluate women with abnormal cytology (p. 93, 272).
- Examination of the breasts or pelvic examination will be based on patient's age and presenting symptoms, risk factors and following a joint discussion.
- Cervical cytology screening should start at the age of 25 years or 30 years regardless of the onset of sexual activity.
- Pap smear should be performed at every 3 years until the age of 29 years.
- Thereafter, from 30 to 65 years: Co-testing with Pap and HPV, every 5 years or Pap testing alone every 3 years.
- HPV infection is the cause of most (99.5%) of the cases of cancer cervix.
- Majority of HPV infections regress spontaneously. Women with persistent and high risk HPV infection develop cervical dysplasia and cancer.
- Pap smear testing can reduce cervical cancer by approximately 70 to 80%.
- Colposcopy is used to evaluate women with abnormal Pap tests.

CHAPTER

10 Imaging Techniques, Other Diagnostic Procedures and Laser in Gynecology

CHAPTER OUTLINE

IMAGING TECHNIQUES IN GYNECOLOGY

- **X-ray**
- **Ultrasonography**
- **Uterine artery embolization**
- **CT scan**
- **MRI**
- **PET**

X-RAY

A chest X-ray and intravenous urogram are essential for investigation in urogynecology and pelvic malignancy, cervical cancer in particular, prior to staging. Plain X-ray of the pelvis is helpful to locate an intrauterine contraceptive device (IUCD) (Fig. 30.6) or to look for shadows of teeth or bone in benign cystic teratoma (Fig. 21.14). Special X-ray using contrast media are:

- Hysterosalpingography (HSG) (details in p. 494).
- Lymphangiography—to locate the lymph nodes involved in pelvic malignancy.
- Intravenous urography.

CASE SUMMARY

A 47-year-old lady underwent laparotomy due to advanced pelvis endometriosis and multiple fibroid uterus. She had previous three laparotomies due to left-sided ovarian cystectomy (once) and cesarean delivery (twice). Total abdominal hysterectomy and bilateral salpingooophorectomy was done. Initial recovery was uneventful, but later on she developed intermittent leakage of urine through the vagina. She also passed urine normally. Intravenous urogram was done (Fig. 10.1).

Intravenous Urography (IVU)

Excretion radiography is an important investigation in urogynecology. Initially, a scout film is taken to identify any radiopaque urinary calculi. An intravenous contrast media is used that contains iodine atom to absorb X-rays. The chemical (urografin) when injected intravenously, is filtered by the glomeruli and is not absorbed by the tubules. It rapidly passes through the renal parenchyma into the urine. Films are taken early within 1–3 minutes of injection of the medium to show the renal parenchyma (nephrogram phase). Later films show the ureters, bladder and urethra (pyelogram phase). IVU is useful to detect any tumor, calculi,

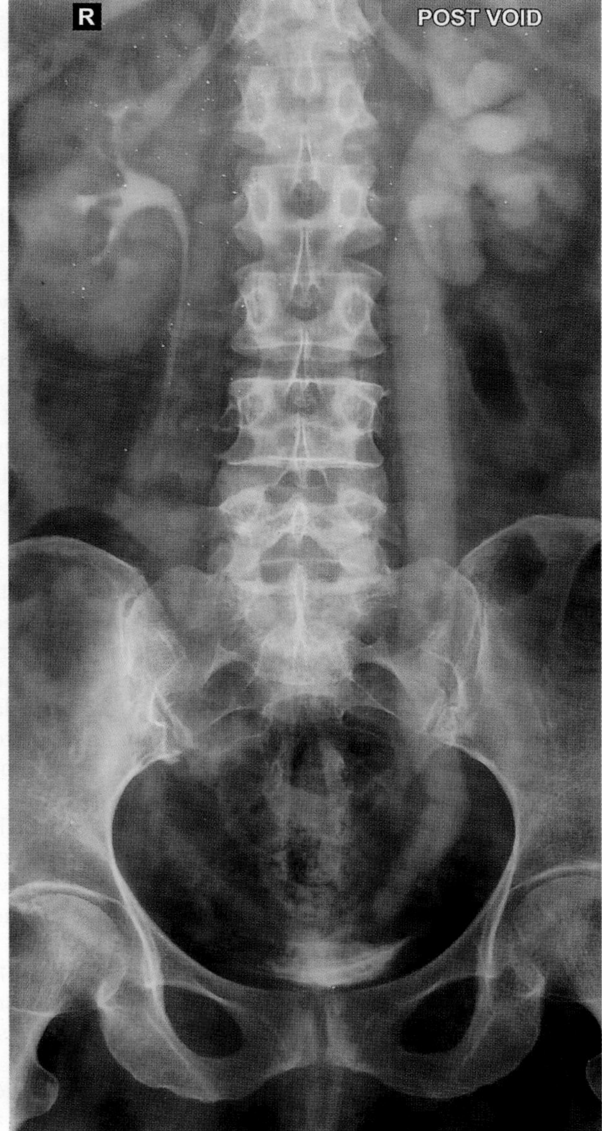

Fig. 10.1: Intravenous urogram showing marked changes in the left ureter. Greatly enlarged renal pelvis, dilated 'clubbed' calyces and hydronephrosis, hydroureter are seen. Right ureter is normal.

obstruction, stricture or fistula communication within the urinary tract. Normal peristaltic waves of the ureters could be seen during the procedure. Changes in the kidney, pelvis, calyces, ureter, bladder, urethra and urinary tract anomalies could be seen. Presently, computed tomography (CT) based urography imaging is done as a part of cervical cancer staging. CT allows imaging of the cervix, parametrial lymph nodes, uterus, adnexa, retroperitoneal lymph nodes, kidney, ureters and bladder simultaneously.

Disadvantages: Hypersensitivity reaction may occur (rarely). Ultrasonography or CT can provide more information compared to IVU.

ULTRASONOGRAPHY

Ultrasound is a noninvasive imaging procedure that utilizes high frequency sound waves. It was first introduced by Ian Donald (Glasgow—1950) in the field of medicine. Sonography is used widely in gynecology either with the transabdominal (TAS) or with the transvaginal (TVS) probe. Because of safety, high patient acceptance and relatively low cost, ultrasonography has become a common diagnostic modality in gynecology, these days.

- **Transabdominal sonography (TAS):** It is done with a linear or curvilinear array transducer operating at 3–5 MHz. TAS requires full bladder to displace the bowel out of pelvis. Full bladder serves as an **acoustic window** for the high-frequency sound waves. Ultrasound is very accurate (>90%) in recognizing a pelvic mass but cannot stabilize a tissue diagnosis. Tissue resolution of <0.2 mm can be obtained with sonography. **TAS is best used** for large masses like fibroid or ovarian tumor. Higher is the frequency of ultrasound wave, better is the image resolution but lesser is the depth of tissue penetration.
- **Transvaginal sonography (TVS):** It is done with a probe, which is placed close to the target organ. There is no need of a full bladder. It also avoids the difficulties due to obesity, faced in TAS. TVS operates at a high frequency (5–10 MHz). **Therefore, detailed evaluation of the pelvic organs (within 10 cm of the field) is possible with TVS.** But the drawbacks of TVS are mainly due to narrow vagina as in virgins, postmenopausal women or post-radiation vaginal stenosis.
- **Transvaginal color Doppler sonography (TV–CDS):** It provides additional information of blood flow to, from or within an organ (uterus or adnexae). This flow can be measured by analysis of the waveform using the pulsatility index.
- **Three-dimensional sonography (3D sonography):** It is more accurate. It can provide details of information as regard to the ovarian volumes, follicular dimensions, complex ovarian masses and uterine malformations.
- **Harmonic imaging:** Improves tissue visualization and quality by using several frequencies instead of just a single frequency. Visual artifacts are reduced. Post processing features improve image resolution.

Compression sonography is combined with color Doppler sonography. It is used to detect deep vein thrombosis (DVT).

Normal Sonographic Findings

- Uterine stroma: Low level uniform echoes
- Endometrium: Linear echogenic stripe (Fig. 8.9)
- Ovary: Solid and ellipsoid structures
- Small amount of fluid is normal finding in POD following ovulation
- Normal tubes are not visible (c.f. hydrosalpinx)
- Blood is echogenic.

Use of Ultrasound in Gynecology

- **TVS** is commonly used in asesment of ovarian reserve by counting AF. Count <10 predict poor reserve.
- **Infertility workup**
  - TVS is commonly used in the assessment of ovarian vesserve
  - Serial measurement of ovarian follicular diameter (folliculometry) and endometrial thickness are done using TVS. **Mature follicle** should measure between 18 and 20 mm in diameter. The favorable periovulatory endometrium should be between 7 and 11 mm thick (Ch. 17).
  - Ultrasound can provide presumptive evidence of ovulation. **Following ovulation**, internal echoes appear within ruptured follicle and free fluid is observed in pouch of Douglas.
  - To detect **correct timing of ovulation** by folliculometry in conjunction with plasma estradiol. This helps in induction of ovulation, artificial insemination and ovum retrieval in vitro fertilization (IVF).
  - Sonographic guided **oocyte retrieval** in IVF and gamete intrafallopian transfer (GIFT) programs, is now accepted as the best method.
- **Ectopic pregnancy** can be detected on TVS as a "**tubal ring**", separate from the ovary in a patient with empty uterine cavity. **TV–CDS** is of more help to detect the vascularity of "tubal ring" when it is unruptured.
- **Pelvic mass** can be evaluated as regard to its location and consistency. Uterine fibroid, ovarian mass, endometrioma, tubo-ovarian mass, etc. can be delineated when there is confusion in clinical diagnosis. However, major limitation is due to its lack of specificity.
- **Oncology:** TV-CDS can assess the vascularity, neovascularization of the mass. Low flow impedance with high flow velocity raises the suspicion of a malignant tumor.

  Presence of papillary excrescences, mural nodules, septations, cystic lesion with solid components, snow storm appearance (hydatidiform mole) and ascites are the other sonographic features of malignancy.
- **Endometrial disease:** Women with unexplained uterine bleeding, or postmenopausal bleeding are better studied with TVS. An endometrial thickness of less than 5 mm is considered atrophic. Endometrial biopsy is needed for postmenopausal women with thicker endometrium.
- **To locate missing IUD (p. 403).**
- **Transrectal sonography** can be used where TVS cannot be used due to vaginal narrowing.
- **Endoanal USG:** Used for asessment of anal sphincter injury following CPT (Ch. 27).
- **Endorectal USG** can detect pelvic pathology like endometriosis.

TABLE 10.1: Saline infusion sonography (SIS)

Benefits in diagnosis	Indications	Contraindications	Complications
▪ Evaluation of • Uterine cavity anatomy • Detection of – Polyp – Submucous fibroids ▪ Tubes evaluation—tubal patency	▪ Evaluation of • Postmenopausal bleeding • Abnormal uterine bleeding (endometrial polyps) • Recurrent miscarriage • Release of intrauterine adhesions • Infertility	▪ Pelvic infection ▪ Hematometra ▪ Presence of uterine bleeding ▪ Pregnancy	▪ Infection (<1%) ▪ Pain

- **Interventional sonography**
- **Sonographically guided procedures:** A needle guide is attached to the shaft of the vaginal probe. With the use of real time, TVS can guide the needle course in a safe path. This technique can be utilized for many diagnostic and therapeutic purposes:
  - Aspiration of cystic masses, e.g. chocolate cyst (p. 261).
  - Follicular aspiration, e.g. ovum retrieval in IVF.
  - Aspiration of tubo-ovarian abscess.
  - Biopsies.
- **Focused ultrasound therapy:** Ultrasound beam carries a high level of energy. When the beam is focused, then energy is converted to heat. Cells die due to coagulative necrosis when the target spot temperature rises >55°C. MR/US guided high-intensity focused ultrasound (HIFU) is based on this principle.
- **Saline infusion sonography (SIS):** Infusion of normal saline into the uterine cavity and performing transvaginal (high resolution) sonography is helpful for the diagnosis of many focal intracavity pathology. SIS catheter (17F) is inserted through the cervical os. Normal saline is infused slowly (10–20 mL) when the uterus is imaged with vaginal ultrasound. It is done within the first 10 days of the cycle (Table 10.1 and Fig. 10.2).

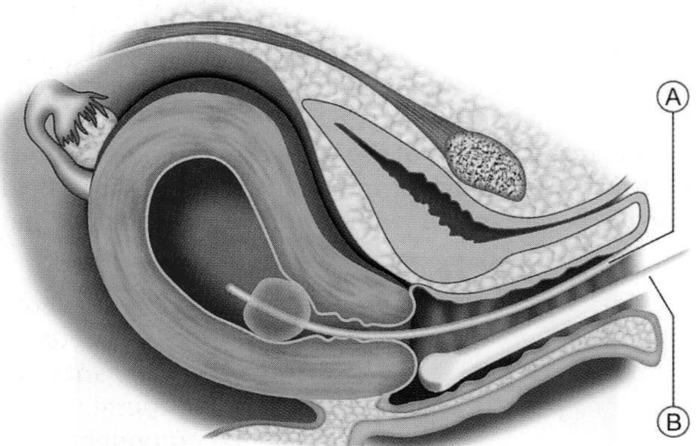

Fig. 10.2: Saline infusion sonography (SIS) or sonohysterography: (A) SIS catheter; (B) TVS probe.

Selective Salpingography (SS)

It is the procedure of transcervical tubal catheterization under fluoroscopic guidance. It is done in the follicular phase of the cycle. The catheter is advanced by tactile sensation to the tubal ostium. Contrast dye (water or oil based) is injected thereafter to outline the tubal lumen. A guide wire may be threaded through the catheter to overcome any resistance. This procedure is useful in cases with proximal tubal blockage when seen by hysterosalpingogram (HSG). The contrast media is injected after the guidewire is withdrawn. This fluoroscopic tool is effective in diagnosing and treating proximal tubal blockage.

Usually proximal tubal cannulation is done under hysteroscopic guidance.

UTERINE ARTERY EMBOLIZATION

Uterine artery embolization (UAE) is an angiographic interventional procedure. It is the treatment procedure of uterine myomas (p. 234). Pelvic angiography is done for visualization and occlusion of both the uterine arteries by embolization. It stops the blood flow through uterine arteries. This results in ischemic necrosis of fibroids. Polyvinyl alcohol (PVA) microspheres are commonly used. The catheter is placed in the femoral artery and is advanced to uterine artery under fluoroscopic guidance. Women with significant symptoms despite medical management, are considered for UAE. Conservation of uterus is the benefit (Figs. 10.3A and B). It is also obstetrics to control PPH.

Indications: Treatment of leiomyoma of uterus after failed medical treatment.

The benefits, contraindications and complications are mentioned in Table 10.2.

TABLE 10.2: Uterine artery embolization.

Benefits	Contraindications	Complications
▪ Reduction in size of fibroid ▪ Reduced bleeding and pain. ▪ Reduced need of hysterectomy or myomectomy ▪ Less hospital stay ▪ Early return to daily activities ▪ Relief of pressure symptoms	▪ Pregnancy ▪ Pelvic infection ▪ Suspected genital tract malignancy ▪ Desire for future pregnancy ▪ Coagulopathy ▪ Renal impairment ▪ Large uterus (>20 weeks) ▪ Prior use of GnRH agonist	▪ Pain ▪ Pelvic infection (<1%) ▪ Fever ▪ Nausea ▪ Vomiting ▪ Amenorrhea ▪ Necrosis of the pelvic tissues ▪ Ovarian failure, Post embolization syndrome

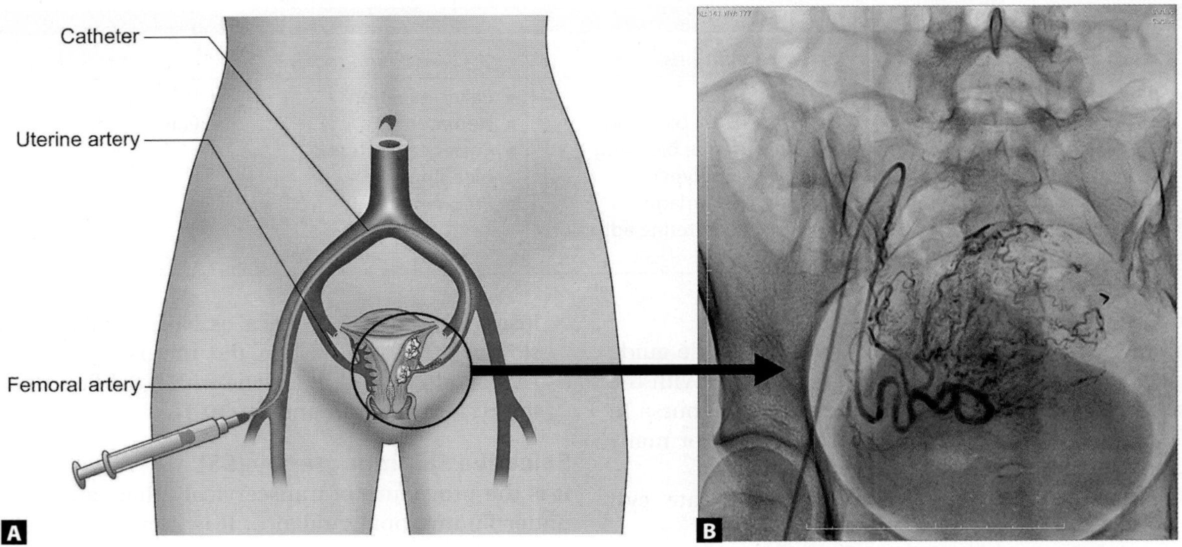

Figs. 10.3A and B: Uterine artery embolization: (A) Pelvic angiography is done through femoral artery catheterization; (B) Uterine artery embolization is done through the catheter.

(*Courtesy:* Dr M Saha, Consultant Radio-interventionist, Apollo Glen eagles Hospital, Kolkata)

COMPUTED TOMOGRAPHY (CT SCAN)

The CT scan provides high resolution two-dimensional images. Cross-sectional images of the body are taken at very close intervals (few millimeters thick) in the form of multiple slices. CT can differentiate tissue densities and this gray-scale pictures can be read on an X-ray film or a television monitor. **Pelvic organs** could be differentiated from gastrointestinal and urinary systems using contrast media. Contrast media can be given orally, intravenously (IV) or rectally. CT is most useful in the **diagnosis of lymph node metastases**, depth of **myometrial invasion** in endometrial cancer, ovarian mass and uterine myomas. Unlike USG or MRI, endometrium is poorly delineated by CT. CT can detect enlarged lymph nodes but cannot differentiate between benign hyperplasia and metastatic carcinoma. **However, lymph nodes must be enlarged at least by 2 cm to be detected by CT. Cerebral metastases of choriocarcinoma or microadenoma of the pituitary** can best be detected by CT procedure. CT scan also facilitates the percutaneous **needle biopsy** of suspicious lymph nodes. In obese or in cases of distended stomach or gut, it is an ideal alternative to sonar. CT is useful in assessing tumor extent and detecting metastases (Fig. 10.4). CT enhances the lateral margins of the cervix and the parametria. It is useful in assessing gynecologic malignancy. Visualization and delineation of pelvic ligaments and ureters in a case with cancer cervix are done well. CT has its role in staging of ovarian cancer as it can detect peritoneal, omental and serosal deposits in addition to liver and nodal (retroperitoneal and intraperitoneal) metastasis. It is superior to ultrasound. Lower limit of detectable **intraperitoneal implants** between 1 and 5 mm. CT scans are useful in evaluating **pituitary tumors**. The best images from CT are obtained when there are significant differences in tissue densities. Helical CT is a current modification and has many advantages. Helical CT has replaced pulmonary angiography and ventilation-perfusion scans for the diagnosis of **pulmonary embolism**.

However, it is more costly and there is chance of surface radiation. Surface radiation dose of CT scan of the abdomen and pelvis is between 2 and 10 cGY. However, value of CT in the assessment of pelvic organ malignancy is limited. MRI is preferred where available. Use of CT should be avoided in pregnancy.

MAGNETIC RESONANCE IMAGING (MRI)

The phenomenon of nuclear magnetic resonance was first described by Felix Bloch and Edward Purcell in 1946. MR as a basis for an imaging technique was employed in practice about 30 years later by Lauterbur.

MRI creates images of the body using a combination of radiowaves (nonionizing radiation) and magnetic fields. Biologic tissue nuclei with protons or neutrons have

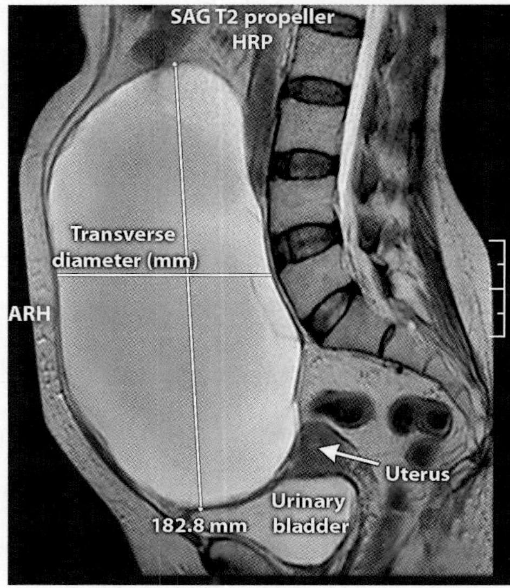

Fig. 10.4: MRI of the pelvis showing a huge ovarian mass.

got magnetic properties. When a pulse of radiowaves is imposed on the nuclei a strong resonance will occur and the energy is absorbed by the nuclei. A signal is detected in a receiver coil, situated close to the tissue, when the energy is emitted by the nuclei. The strength of the emitted signal varies directly with the proton density. With the technology of MRI, images are constructed based on the radiofrequency signal emitted by hydrogen nuclei. These hydrogen nuclei have been excited by the radiofrequency pulses in the presence of a strong magnetic field. On T_1-weighted images, urine in the bladder appears dark (low signal intensity). On T_2-weighted images, the same urine will appear bright (high signal intensity). In gynecology, resolution is 0.5–1 mm. The strength of the magnetic field within the bore of the magnets is measured in tesla (T) (1 tesla = 10,000 gauss). The standard technique of T_1 and T_2-weighted sequences are obtained in two planes—axial and sagittal. The radiowaves penetrate bone and air without attenuation. Respiratory movements have got little effect on the pelvic organs. Sagittal and coronal views can be obtained without moving the patient. Gadolinium is used as IV contrast for better visualization of organs and their abnormalities. MR imaging is able to achieve superior soft tissue contrast. Ovaries are seen on T_2-weighted images. Used safely in pregnancy regardless of trimester.

Uses of MRI

- MRI can differentiate the different zones (endometrium, inner and outer myometrium) of the uterus and the cervix clearly. It can measure the depth of myometrial penetration of endometrial cancer preoperatively.
- MRI can detect accurately the parametrial invasion of cervical cancer but cannot identify lymph node metastases reliably. It is more reliable in distinguishing post-treatment fibrosis and recurrence.
- MRI is superior to CT or ultrasound in diagnosing adenomyosis, myomas and endometrial cancer (including myometrial invasion).
- MR-HIFU therapy is safe, feasible and minimally invasive for leiomyoma treatment (p. 233).
- Endovaginal or endorectal coils produce high resolution images of the cervix and parametrium. Tumor volume can be measured with 3D imaging system. Coronal and axial planes are used to determine the invasion of the bladder, rectum, parametrium and uterine body.
- **Urogynecology:** MRI provides detailed soft tissue imaging of female urethra, levator ani muscles, in women with pelvic organ prolapse (POP). MR defecography is useful for women with POP, incontinence and defecatory dysfunction.
- **Ovarian cancer:** MRI is useful due to its superior contrast resolution for detection of peritoneal, lymph node metastasis and tumor extension to omentum, bowel, bone and vessels.
- MRI is found to be safe in pregnancy and is not mutagenic.
- Leiomyomas are better diagnosed with MRI (Fig. 38.87). MRI is superior in diagnosing adnexal pathology with superior contrast resolution.
- Thickness of the low signal intensity junctional zone >12 mm is diagnostic of adenomyosis on T_2-weighted images. A normal junctional zone is up to 8 mm. For endometrial polyps, hyperplasia, MRI is useful.
- MRI is a noninvasive tool in the diagnosis of endometriosis. MRI is superior in diagnosis for deep infiltrating endometriosis (DIE).
- MRI is superior to CT in the evaluation of metastatic lymph nodes or recurrent pelvic tumor. However, neither CT nor MRI can detect microscopic malignant disease. MRI is twice more expensive than CT.
- **Detection of Müllerian duct abnormalities:** Diagnosis of septate, unicornuate or bicornuate uterus.

Safety

There are no harmful or any teratogenic effects observed till date with MRI when used clinically with field strength less than 3 tesla. Use of MRI in pregnancy is safe regardless of the trimester. Imaging in pregnancy is limited to 1.5 T. Gadolinium contrast is not used routinely in pregnancy.

Contraindications

Presence of mechanically, electrically or magnetically activated implant devices such as cardiac pacemakers, cochlear implants. Cardiac defibrillators, and electronic infusion pumps are contraindicated. Some of the implanted devices are safe: IUCDs (Mirena), others are Essure, Filshie clips, Implants (Implanon), silicone breast.

Hazards are electroconvulsions and atrial fibrillation. This is due to rapidly changing magnetic field. Hence, caution should be exercised with epileptic patients and who had recent myocardial infarction. Other limitation of MRI is patient acceptance. Many patient feel 'trapped' in the machine (psychological distress).

POSITRON EMISSION TOMOGRAPHY (PET)

The PET is based on the tissue uptake of 18F-fluoro-2 deoxyglucose (FDG). FDG-PET can measure the difference between the normal tissue and cancerous tissue. Cancer tissues process this glucose analogue differently compared to that of normal tissues. This glucose analogue is given intravenously. FDG-PET scan is then done and the images are interpreted.

FDG-PET scan is more sensitive for detection of metastatic disease and recurrence of ovarian or cervical malignancy. It is also useful to assess the response following tumor therapy. FDG-PET scan is found to be more sensitive and specific compared to CT or MRI.

FDG-PET scan can also be used for postsurgical monitoring of patients with endometrial or ovarian cancer.

Sensitivity of PET in detecting pelvic node metastasis is 80% compared to MRI (70%) and CT (48%).

PET is poor modality for detecting the detailed anatomy. For this, CT scans are done and the combination allows correlation of metabolic and the anatomic data. Currently PET/CT has become a vital tool for diagnosis and management of cancers.

FDG-PET/CT is used for:

- Staging of cervical cancer
- Assessment of nodal status in cervical cancer
- Treatment planning: Prior to lymph node radiation
- To guide IMRT with anatomic data obtained with PET/CT.
- It reduces the amount of radiation to the normal tissues.

INTERVENTIONAL PROCEDURES UNDER RADIOLOGIC GUIDANCE

- USG or CT-guided procedures
  - Fine-needle aspiration cytology (FNAC) from pelvic/abdominal mass
  - FNAC of lymph nodes
  - Aspiration of peritoneal fluid for cytology evaluation
  - Drainage of pus, ascetic fluid.
- **MRI-guided focused ultrasound surgery (p. 100).**

CONCLUSION

All the imaging systems have got their role in gynecological practice.

- **X-ray**, either plain or using contrast media, has got its place. It is cheaper and quite informative with minimal risks of irradiation.
- **Ultrasound** establishes a definite place in diagnostic evaluation. Ultrasound guided procedures are used for both the diagnostic and therapeutic purposes.
- **CT** is useful in the diagnosis of lymph node metastasis and depth of myometrial invasion in endometrial cancer. It may be employed in selected cases to detect microadenoma of pituitary or metastatic lesions in the brain or liver.
- **MRI**: Superior to CT or ultrasound. It is especially helpful to differentiate post-treatment fibrosis and tumor. It is safe in pregnancy.
- **PET** is helpful to differentiate normal tissues from cancerous one.

OTHER DIAGNOSTIC PROCEDURES IN GYNECOLOGY

ENDOSCOPY IN GYNECOLOGY (CH. 36)

Gynecological endoscopy includes the procedures as mentioned in Table 10.3.

LAPAROSCOPY

Laparoscopy is a technique of visualization of peritoneal cavity by means of a fiberoptic endoscope introduced through the abdominal wall (Fig. 10.5). Prior pneumoperitoneum is achieved by introduction of carbon dioxide or air. For diagnostic purposes, either local or general anesthesia may be used. Its use is gradually widening both in diagnostic and therapeutic field in gynecology. The details are in Ch. 36.

Indications

- **Diagnostic**
- **Operative (Ch. 36)**

Diagnostic

- Infertility work up (Ch. 17)
  - Peritubal adhesions
  - Chromopertubation

TABLE 10.3: Different methods of gynecological endoscopy.

Laparoscopy	Hysteroscopy	Salpingoscopy
Falloposcopy	Cystoscopy	Culdoscopy
Sigmoidoscopy and proctoscopy		Vaginoscopy

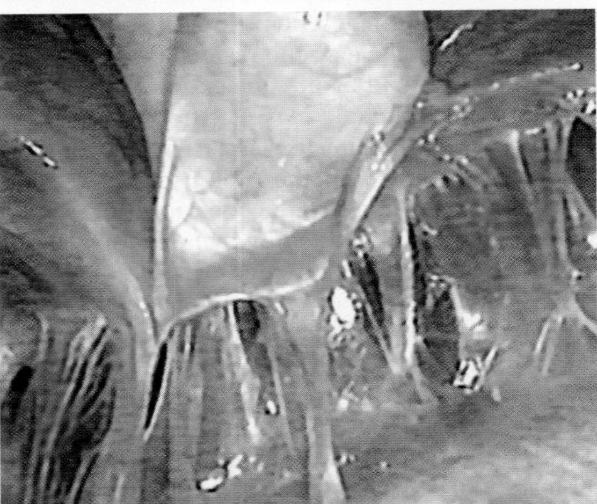

Fig. 10.5: Chlamydial infection causing perihepatic adhesions (Fitz-Hugh-Curtis syndrome) diagnosed by laparoscopy.

  - Minimal endometriosis
  - Ovulation stigma of the ovary
  - Before reversal of sterilization operation.
- Chronic pelvic pain (p. 467)
- Nature of a pelvic mass: Fibroid, ovarian cyst
- To diagnose an acute pelvic lesion
  - Ectopic pregnancy (p. 466)
  - Acute appendicitis
  - Acute salpingitis—diagnosis and collection of pus for culture
- Follow-up of pelvic surgery (second look)
  - Tuboplasty
  - Ovarian malignancy
  - Evaluation of therapy in endometriosis
- Investigation protocol of amenorrhea
- Diagnosis of suspected Müllerian abnormalities (p. 34).
- Uterine perforation.

Operative

Indications are almost similar to laparotomy (For detail Ch. 36).

Complications (p. 519)

Timing of Laparoscopy

In infertility work up, it may be done in the preovulatory period to facilitate chromopertubation and also diagnosis of ovulation. However, in endometriosis, it is preferably done in the premenstrual period when the ectopic endometrial implants increase in size.

HYSTEROSCOPY (P. 520)

Hysteroscopy is an operative procedure whereby the endometrial cavity can be visualized with the aid of fiberoptic telescope. **The uterine distension is achieved by** carbon dioxide, normal saline or glycine. The instrument is to pass transcervically, usually without dilatation of the cervix or local anesthesia. However, for operative hysteroscopy, either paracervical block or general anesthesia is required. **Diagnostic hysteroscopy should be performed in the postmenstrual period** for

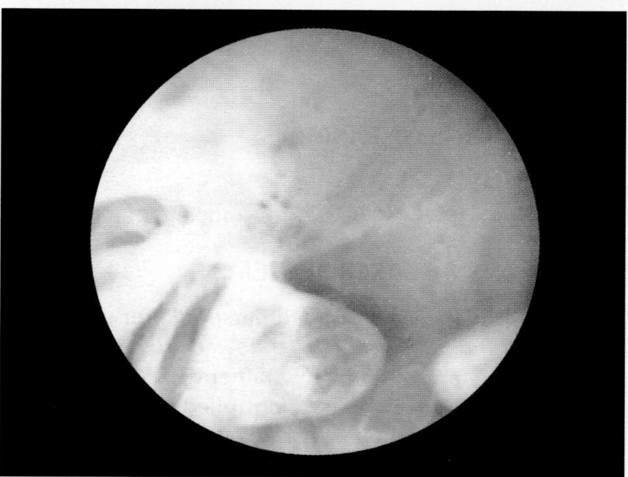

Fig. 10.6: Hysteroscopic view of a submucous fibroid polyp.

better view without bleeding. The chance of conception disturbance is absent.

Recently, contact hysteroscopy has become more popular since a distending medium is not needed. The interpretation of endometrial pathology is similar to colposcopy in that it depends on color, contour and vascular pattern.

Indications

- **Diagnostic**
- **Operative**

The technical details and operative hysteroscopy are dealt in Ch. 36.

Diagnostic

- Unresponsive irregular uterine bleeding to exclude uterine polyp, submucous fibroid or products of conception.
- Congenital uterine septum in recurrent abortion.
- Missing threads of IUD.
- Intrauterine adhesions (uterine synechiae).
- To visualize transformation zone with microcolpo-hysteroscopy when colposcopic finding (Fig. 10.6) is unsatisfactory.

Operative (p. 522)

Outpatient hystroscope: Ch. 36.

Complications (p. 523)

SALPINGOSCOPY

In salpingoscopy, a firm telescope is inserted through the abdominal ostium of the uterine tube so that the tubal mucosa can be visualized by distending the lumen with saline infusion. The telescope is to be introduced through laparoscope.

Salpingoscopy allows study of the physiology and anatomy of the tubal epithelium and **permits more accurate selection of patients for IVF rather than the tubal surgery**.

Falloposcopy: For detail p. 197.

Cystoscopy: The main use of cystoscopy in gynecology is to evaluate cervical cancer prior to staging and, to investigate the urinary symptoms including hematuria, incontinence and fistulae.

Culdoscopy: Culdoscopy is an optical instrument designed to visualize the pelvic structures through an incision in the pouch of Douglas. Its use has almost been replaced by laparoscopy.

Proctoscopy and sigmoidoscopy: For rectal involvement of genital malignancy, a digital examination or at best proctoscopy is usually adequate.

EXAMINATION UNDER ANESTHESIA (EUA)

It is indicated where bimanual examination cannot be conducted properly either because of extreme tenderness or inadequate relaxation of abdominopelvic muscles or non-cooperative patient. It should be done routinely in all cases of uterine malignancy for clinical staging. It is extended freely to examine virgins or in cases with pediatric gynecological problems.

URODYANAMIC STUDY

Urodyanamic studies are recommended in women when objective asessment is essential. This is specially so when initial management is unsuccesful and surgical management is planned. Common indications are: (a) Presence of mixed (GSI + OAB); (b) Associated nocturia, frequency; (c) Neuropathy; (d) Previous failed surgery.

LASER IN GYNECOLOGY

The word 'Laser' is an acronym for *light amplification by stimulated emission of radiation.*

PHYSICS OF LASER

The important physical properties of laser are:

- **Monochromacity**—light beams of a particular laser have got the same wavelength.
- **Coherent**—the light waves are all perfectly aligned and unidirectional.
- **Collimated**—the light beams run parallel and do not diverge.
- The laser beam can be converged by a convex lens to a sharp focus, called **spot size.**
- Power density is the measure of laser effects upon tissue. It is expressed as watts/cm^2.
- Smaller the spot size, greater is the power density.
- **Laser-tissue interaction**—the water in the cells (80% by volume) boils instantly at the temperature of 100°C. The cell explodes and vaporizes. The cell protein and minerals are incinerated and look charred.
- The depth of tissue destruction is very precise and there is very little lateral effect.
- Laser effect depends on power (watts), spot size, power density, and laser-tissue contact time.

TABLE 10.4: Common laser systems used in gynecology.

Laser type	*Wavelength*	*Tissue penetration*
Carbon dioxide	10.6 μm	0.1 mm
Neodymium-doped: Yttrium-aluminum garnet (Nd : YAG)	1.06 μm	0.6–4.2 mm
Potassium titanyl-phosphate (KTP 532)	0.532 μm	0.4–0.8 mm
Argon	0.5 μm	0.2 mm

- Beams of CO_2 and Nd:YAG laser are invisible. There is preferential absorption of laser by one tissue from another.

Common laser systems used in gynecology are carbon dioxide, Nd:YAG, KTP and Argon (Table 10.4).

Fiberoptic laser laparoscopy (KTP 532 and Argon) has the following advantages accurate targeting, higher precision, minimum effect on surrounding tissues, better hemostasis, contact modes of cutting, vaporization, coagulation and less laser plume production.

USES OF LASER IN GYNECOLOGY

Principal use of laser in gynecology is for the purpose of tissue cutting, coagulation or vaporization. It is used widely in genital tract surgery and with endoscopic surgery. It is commonly used in the management of:

- Cervical intraepithelial neoplasia (CIN) (p. 268).
- Conization of the cervix (p. 495).
- Vulvar intraepithelial neoplasia (VIN) (p. 266).
- Vaginal intraepithelial neoplasia (VAIN) (p. 267).
- Vaporization of pelvic endometriosis (p. 261).
- Laser laparoscopy for ovarian cystectomy, adhesiolysis, removal of ectopic pregnancy and presacral neurectomy.
- Laser laparoscopy assisted hysteroscopy, for dividing large pedicles that have been coagulated or suture ligated.
- Hysteroscopic surgery—laser ablation of endometrium, resection of uterine septum (metroplasty) and submucous fibroids.

LIMITATIONS OF LASER

- The equipment is expensive.
- Technical complexity—requires sufficient training.

HAZARDS OF LASER SYSTEMS

Laser must be used by a trained person. Laser protection guidelines must be strictly followed to protect the operator, assistant, the theater staff and the patient from the accidental hazards. A laser controlled area (LCA) must have warning signs when laser is in use. Special spectacles are used to protect the eyes. Common hazards are:
A—(a) Eyes—visual loss due to corneal or retinal damage; (b) Skin damage; and (c) Damage from laser smoke.
B—General: (a) Burn injury (use of spirit and paper drapes must be avoided in theater); (b) Inflammable anesthetic gases are to be used with great care; (c) Reflections of laser beam is dangerous. Shining instruments are not to be used; (d) Fire extinguisher should always be available, and (e) Plume of smoke should be extracted.

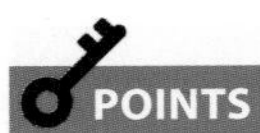

KEY POINTS

- **Use of X-ray** in gynecology is commonly done for urogynecology and pelvic malignancy. It is specifically done using contrast media for HSG, IVU and lymphangiography.
- **Ultrasonography** (TAS, TVS or TV-CDS) has become a common diagnostic modality in gynecology. It is widely used in infertility work up (sonohysterosalpingography, folliculometry, detection of ovulation and oocyte retrieval in IVF program), evaluation of pelvic mass, ectopic pregnancy and endometrial disease. Sonographically guided procedures provide added information. Compression sonography is combined with color Doppler sonography. It is used to detect DVT.
- **CT** is useful in detection of enlarged pelvic lymph nodes and microadenoma of pituitary. Helical CT is a modification that uses movement of the patient combined with rotation of several radiographic registers in a spiraling fashion. Vascular images are so high quality that it has replaced pulmonary angiography and ventilation-perfusion scans. Surface radiation dose from CT is between 2 and 10 rads.
- **Currently FDG-PET/CT** has become a vital tool for diagnosis and management of cancers. Combination of FDG-PET/CT allows correlation of metabolic and the anatomic data in the managements of cancers.
- **MRI** uses radiowaves (nonionizing) and magnetic fields. It accurately shows parametrial invasion of cervical cancer and identify the enlarged lymph nodes. It can measure the depth of myometrial penetration in endometrial carcinoma preoperatively. High resolution images in multiple planes are obtained. It can differentiate septate from bicornuate uterus. MR-guided HIFU is safe and a minimally invasive procedure. Tumor volume can be measured with 3D imaging system.
- **MRI** should not be used in patients with cochlear implants or pacemakers, it is safe in women with pregnancy or IUDs.
- **The use of laparoscopy** is wide indication are similar to laparotomy. The major diagnostic uses are infertility, chronic pelvic pain and to exclude pelvic lesion (Ch. 36). More complicated surgery like hysterectomy, pelvic and retroperitoneal lymphadenectomy are done.
- **Hysteroscopy** is gaining popularity as a diagnostic aid in unresponsive uterine bleeding, uterine synechiae, congenital uterine septum or missing threads of IUD (Ch. 36).
- **Salpingoscopy** is the evaluation of tubal mucosa with a telescope, introduced through the abdominal ostium of the tube.
- **Principal use of laser** in gynecology is for tissue cutting, coagulation or vaporization. Laser effects depend on power (watts), spot size, power density and laser-tissue contact time. Commonly used laser systems in gynecology are CO_2, Nd:YAG, KTP 532 and Argon (Table 10.4).
- **Power density** is the most important determinant of the laser effects. Greater the power density, the less the thermal effect and less is the hemostatic property.
- UAE is an angiographic interventional procedures. It is effective in cases with AUB due to fibroid. It has few contraindications also (p. ???).
- **Saline Infusion Sonography (SIS)** uses transvaginal (high resolution) sonography for the diagnosis of many focal intracavity pathology. Normal saline is infused slowly (10–20 mL) when the uterus is imaged with vaginal ultrasound. It is done within the first 10 days of the cycle (Table 10.1 and Fig. 10.2). It has many advantages (p. 99).

CHAPTER

11 Pelvic Infection

CHAPTER OUTLINE

DEFENSE OF THE GENITAL TRACT

As there is free anastomosis between the lymphatics and blood vessels, the infection of one pelvic organ usually spreads to the other more frequently. There is direct communication of the peritoneal cavity to the exterior through the vagina. In spite of these, the frequency and intensity of pelvic infection is kept lowered by the defense mechanism.

Vulvar Defense

Anatomic: (a) Apposition of the cleft by labia; (b) Compound racemose type of Bartholin's glands.

Physiologic: (a) Fungicidal action of the secretion (undecylenic acid) of the apocrine glands; (b) Natural high resistance to infection of the vulvar and perineal skin.

Vaginal Defense

Anatomic: (a) Apposition of the anterior and posterior walls with its transverse rugae; (b) Stratified epithelium devoid of glands.

Physiologic: This is maintained by the hormone estrogen (Table 11.1).

At Birth, under the influence of maternal estrogen circulating into the newborn, the vaginal epithelium becomes multilayered. The desquamated epithelium containing glycogen is converted into lactic acid by enzymatic action of vaginal ecosystem flora (Gram +ve Lactobacillus acidophilus). Subsequently, the Doderlein's bacilli appear probably from the gut and convert the glycogen into lactic acid. As a result, **for about 10–12 days following birth, the vaginal defense is good and infection is unlikely**.

Thereafter and up to puberty, there is no circulatory estrogen. The vaginal epithelium is reduced to few layers; glycogen is absent and so also the Doderlein's bacillus. The vaginal pH becomes neutral or alkaline. **During the reproductive period** with high estrogen, the vaginal defense is fully restored. After the onset of menopause with estrogen deficiency and lack of glycogen in vaginal epithelial cells, vaginal defense is lost. Vaginal pH rises (6.0–7.5) and lactic acid production is less.

It should be emphasized that only the **Doderlein's bacilli can grow in the acidic media with pH 4–4.5.** But when the pH increases, the other organisms normally present in the vagina will grow.

Phases of life when defense is lost:

- Following 10 days of birth till puberty is reached
- During reproductive period—in the following situation:
  - **During menstruation:** The vaginal pH becomes increased due to contaminated blood and fall of estrogen. The protective cervical mucus disappears and the endometrium sheds.
  - **Following abortion and childbirth:** The contaminated lochia increases the pH. The raw placental site, inevitable tear of the cervix, bruising of the vagina and presence of blood clots or remnants of decidua, favor nidation of the bacterial growth.
- During menopause.

Cervical Defense

Anatomic—(a) Racemose type of glands; (b) Mucus plug; and (c) *Physiologic*—bactericidal effect of the mucus.

Uterine Defense

(a) Cyclic shedding of the endometrium and (b) Closure of the uterine ostium of the fallopian tube with slightest inflammatory reaction in the endometrium.

TABLE 11.1: Defense of the vagina in relation to age.

	Newborn (0–10 days)	*Up to puberty*	*Childbearing period*	*Postmenopause*
Epithelium	Multilayered	Thin	Multilayered	Thin
Glycogen	++	(–)	++	(–)
Doderlein's bacillus	+	(–)	++	(–)
pH	Acidic (4–5)	Neutral or alkaline (6–8)	Acidic (4–5)	Neutral (6–7)

Tubal Defense

Anatomic—integrated mucus plicae and epithelial cilia.

Physiologic—peristalsis of the tube and also the movement of the cilia are towards the uterus.

Causative Organisms

The bacterial pathogens involved in upper genital tract infections are principally derived from the normal flora of the vagina and endocervix. Exogenous sources are sexually transmitted or following induced or unsafe abortion or during delivery in unhygienic surroundings.

Organisms

- **Pyogenic (50%):** This is the most common type—the organisms responsible are:
  Aerobes: **The gram-positive organisms are** *Staphylococcus,* Lactobacillus, Diphtheroids. **The gram-negatives are** *E. coli, Pseudomonas, Klebsiella, N. gonorrhoeae,* etc.
  Anaerobes: **The gram-positives** are anaerobic *Streptococcus, Clostridium welchii, C. tetani, Peptostreptococcus,* etc. **The gram-negatives** are mainly bacteroides (Fusobacterium, Viellonella) group of which *Bacteroides fragilis* is the commonest.
- **Sexually transmitted disease (STD):** The organisms are *N. gonorrhoeae, Chlamydia trachomatis, Treponema pallidum, Herpes simplex virus type II, Human papilloma virus, Gardnerella vaginalis (Haemophilus vaginalis), Haemophilus ducreyi, Donovan bodies, HIV I or II, Mycoplasma,* etc.
- **Parasitic:** *Trichomonas vaginalis*
- **Fungal:** *Candida albicans*
- **Viral:** Herpes simplex virus type II, human papillomavirus, HIV, Condylomata accuminata, etc.
- **Tubercular:** *Mycobacterium tuberculosis.*

Modes of spread of infections

The route of infection is most commonly ascending in nature. However, the classic modes of infection of some specific organisms are:

- **Through continuity and contiguity**—gonococcal infection (Fig. 11.1)
- **Through lymphatics and pelvic veins**—postabortal and puerperal infection—by pyogenic organisms other than gonococcus (p. 110)

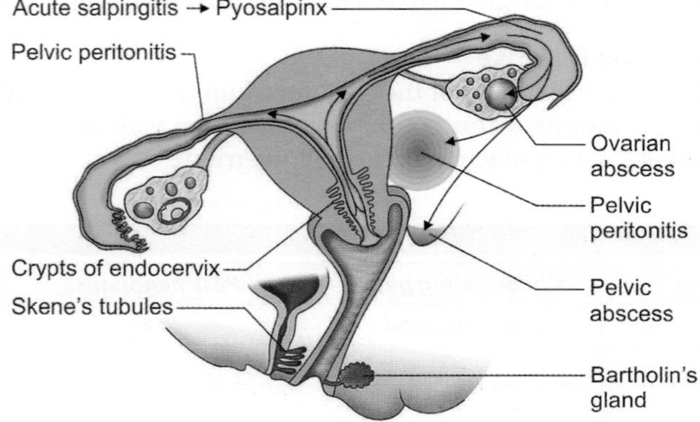

Fig. 11.1: Mode of spread in gonococcal infection.

- **Through bloodstream**—tubercular
- **From adjacent infected extragenital organs** like intestine.

ACUTE PELVIC INFECTION

- Pelvic inflammatory disease (PID)
- Following delivery and abortion
- Following gynecological procedures
- Following intrauterine devices (IUD)
- Secondary to other infections—appendicitis.

PELVIC INFLAMMATORY DISEASE

Definition

Pelvic inflammatory disease (PID) of the upper genital tract, **is a spectrum of infection and inflammation of the upper genital tract organs typically involving the uterus (endometrium), fallopian tubes, ovaries, pelvic peritoneum and surrounding structures (parametrium).** It is attributed to the ascending spread of microorganisms from the cervicovaginal canal to the contiguous pelvic structures. **The clinical syndrome is not related to pregnancy and surgery.**

The terminology is currently used to express the specific organ pathology. Thus infection may include any or all of the following anatomic sites and it is described as **endometritis, salpingitis, pelvic peritonitis, tubo-ovarian abscess or parametritis. Cervicitis is not included in the list.**

Many prefer the term salpingitis as it ultimately bears the brunt of acute infection.

Epidemiology

Despite better understanding of the etiology, pathogenesis, improved diagnostic tools such as ultrasound or laparoscopy and advent of wide range of antimicrobials, it still constitutes a health hazard both in the developed and more so in the developing countries. The incidence of pelvic infection is on the rise due to the rise in sexually transmitted diseases.

The ready availability of contraception together with increased permissive sexual attitude has resulted in increased incidence of sexually transmitted diseases and correspondingly, acute PID (more on p. 121).

The incidence varies from 1–2% per year among sexually active women. About 85% are spontaneous infection in sexually active females of reproductive age. The remaining 15% follow procedures, which favors the organisms to ascend up. Such iatrogenic procedures include endometrial biopsy, uterine curettage, insertion of IUD and hysterosalpingography. Two-thirds are restricted to young women of less than 25 years and the remaining **one-third limited among 30 years** or older.

Pelvic inflammatory disease is a major problem to the reproductive health of young women. PID may be asymptomatic or subclinical. Currently, there are **certain changes in the epidemiology of PID.** (A) Shift from *inpatient PID to outpatient PID.* (B) Change in clinical presentation. Less severe disease is commonly seen. (C) Shift in the microbial etiology of more *Chlamydia trachomatis* than gonococcus and others.

Teenagers have got low hormonal defense in response to genital tract infection. Wider area of cervical epithelium allows colonization of *Chlamydia trachomatis* and *N. gonorrhoeae*.

RISK FACTORS FOR PID

- Sexually active teenagers
- Younger age (<19 years)
- Multiple sexual partners
- Absence of contraceptive pill use
- Previous history of acute PID
- IUD users (not with LNG-IUS)
- Lower socioeconomic status
- Husband/sexual partner with urethritis or STI
- Genetic predisposition

Protective Factors

- **Contraceptive practice**
  - Barrier methods, especially condom, diaphragm with spermicides (p. 420).
  - Oral steroidal contraceptives have got two preventive aspects.
    - Produce thick mucus plug preventing ascent of sperm and bacterial penetration.
    - Decrease in duration of menstruation, creates a shorter interval of bacterial colonization of the upper tract.
  - Monogamy or having a partner who had vasectomy.
- **Others**
  - Pregnancy
  - Menopause
  - Vaccines: Hepatitis B, HPV (p. 274)
  - Postcoital washing (urethra, genital skin)

Microbiology

Acute PID is usually a **polymicrobial** infection caused by organisms ascending upstairs from downstairs.

The primary organisms are sexually transmitted and limited approximately to *N. gonorrhoeae* in 30%, *Chlamydia trachomatis* in 30% and *Mycoplasma hominis* in 10%.

The secondary organisms normally found in the vagina are almost always associated sooner or later. These are:

- **Aerobic organisms**—nonhemolytic *Streptococcus, E. coli*, group B *Streptococcus* and *Staphylococcus*.
- **Anaerobic organisms**—*Bacteroides* species—*fragilis* and *bivius, Peptostreptococcus* and *Peptococcus*.

Mode of Affection

- The classic concept is that the gonococcus ascends up to affect the tubes through mucosal **continuity and contiguity**. This ascent is facilitated by the sexually transmitted vectors such as sperm and trichomonas.
- **Reflux of** menstrual blood along with gonococci into the fallopian tubes is the other possibility.
- *Mycoplasma hominis* probably spreads across the **parametrium** to affect the tube.
- The secondary organisms probably affect the tube through **lymphatics**.
- Rarely, organisms from the gut may affect the tube **directly**.

Pathology

The involvement of the tube is almost always bilateral and usually following menses due to loss of genital defense.

The pathological process is initiated primarily in the endosalpinx. There is gross destruction of the epithelial cells, cilia and microvilli. In severe infection, it invades all the layers of the tube and produces acute inflammatory reaction; becomes edematous and hyperemic. The exfoliated cells along with the exudate pour into the lumen of the tube and agglutinate the mucosal folds. **The abdominal ostium is closed** by the indrawing of the edematous fimbriae and by inflammatory adhesions. The uterine end is closed by congestion. The closure of both the ostia results in pent up of the exudate inside the tube. **Depending upon the virulence, the exudate may be watery producing hydrosalpinx or purulent producing pyosalpinx**. The purulent exudate then changes the microenvironment of the tube which favors growth of other pyogenic and anaerobic organisms resulting in deeper penetration and more tissue destruction. The organisms spontaneously die within 2–3 weeks. As the serous coat is not much affected, **the resulting adhesions of the tube with the surrounding structures are not so dense**, in fact flimsy, unlike pyogenic or tubercular infection.

On occasions, the exudate pours through the abdominal ostium to produce pelvic peritonitis and pelvic abscess or may affect the ovary (the organisms gain access through the ovulation rent) producing ovarian abscess. A tubo-ovarian abscess is thus formed (Fig. 11.1).

Clinical Features

Symptoms

Patients with acute PID present with a wide range of non-specific clinical symptoms. Symptoms usually appear at the time and immediately after the menstruation.

- Bilateral lower abdominal and pelvic pain which is dull in nature. The onset of pain is more rapid and acute in gonococcal infection (3 days) than in chlamydial infection (5–7 days)
- There is fever, lassitude and headache
- Irregular and excessive vaginal bleeding is usually due to associated endometritis
- Abnormal vaginal discharge which becomes purulent and or copious
- Nausea and vomiting
- Dyspareunia
- Pain and discomfort in the right hypochondrium due to concomitant perihepatitis **(Fitz-Hugh-Curtis syndrome)** may occur in 5–10% of cases of acute salpingitis. **The liver is involved** due to transperitoneal or vascular dissemination of either gonococcal or chlamydial infection.

Laparoscopic examination reveals inflamed liver capsule with classic violin string adhesions to the parietal peritoneum and beneath the diaphragm.

Signs

- The temperature is elevated to beyond 38.3°C.
- Abdominal palpation reveals tenderness on both the quadrants of lower abdomen. The liver may be enlarged and tender (perihepatitis).
- Vaginal examination reveals: (a) Abnormal vaginal discharge which may be of purulent; (b) Congested external urethral meatus or openings of Bartholin's ducts through which pus may be seen escaping out on pressure; (c) Speculum examination shows congested cervix with purulent discharge from the canal and (d) Bimanual examination reveals bilateral tenderness on fornix palpation, which increases more with movement of the cervix (cervical motion tenderness). There may be thickening or a definite mass felt through the fornices.

Clinical Diagnostic Criteria of Acute PID (CDC - 2015)

- **Minimum criteria**
  - Lower abdominal tenderness or
  - Adnexal tenderness or
  - Cervical motion tenderness
- **Additional criteria for diagnosing PID**
  - Oral temperature >38°C
  - Mucopurulent cervical or vaginal discharge
  - Abundant WBCs on saline microscopy of cervical secretions
  - Raised C-reactive protein
  - Elevated ESR
  - Laboratory documentation of positive cervical infection with *Gonorrhea* or *C. trachomatis*
- **Definitive criteria**
  - Histopathologic evidence of endometritis on biopsy
  - Imaging study (TVS/MRI) showing evidence of thickened fluid filled tubes, ± free pelvic fluid or tubo-ovarian complex.
  - Laparoscopic evidence of PID (*see* below).
  - Although initial treatment can be made before bacteriologic diagnosis of *C. trachomatis* or *N. gonorrhoeae* infection, such a diagnosis emphasizes the need to treat sex partners.

Investigations

- **Identification of organisms:** The materials are collected from the following available sources:
  - Discharge from the urethra or Bartholin's gland
  - Cervical canal
  - Collected pus from the fallopian tubes during laparoscopy or laparotomy.

  The material so collected is subjected to Gram stain and culture (aerobic and anaerobic). The findings of gram-negative diplococci is very much suggestive of gonococcal infection. Except in highly sophisticated centers, the detection of *C. trachomatis* is difficult (for diagnosis p. 123). As the process of investigation is not specific and is time consuming, treatment for *C. trachomatis* should be started from the clinical diagnosis. A positive Gram stain smear from endocervical mucus is nonspecific and a negative smear does not rule out upper genital tract infection.
- **Blood:** Leukocyte count shows leukocytosis to more than 10,000 per cu mm and an elevated ESR value of more than 15 mm per hour. The results correlate with the severity of the inflammatory reactions of the fallopian tubes as seen on laparoscopy. **Serological test for syphilis should be carried out for both the partners in all cases.**
- **Laparoscopy:** Laparoscopy is considered the **"gold standard"**. While it is the **most reliable aid** to support the clinical diagnosis but it may not be feasible to do in all cases. It is reserved only in those cases in which differential diagnosis includes salpingitis, appendicitis or ectopic pregnancy. Nonresponding pelvic mass needs laparoscopic clarification.

Laparascopic Findings and Grading of PID

- **Mild:** Tubes—edema, erythema, no spontaneous purulent exudates and tubes are freely mobile
- **Moderate:** Gross purulent material present, erythema and edema, marked; tubes may not be freely movable, and fimbria stroma may not be patent
- **Severe:** Pyosalpinx or inflammatory complex, abscess
- **'Violin string'** like adhesions in the pelvis and around the liver suggests chlamydial infection (Fig. 10.5).

Laparoscopy helps to aspirate fluid or pus for microbiological study from the fallopian tube, ovary or pouch of Douglas.

- **Sonography:** It is of limited value. Dilated and fluid-filled tubes, fluid in the pouch of Douglas or adnexal mass are suggestive of PID. It may be employed where clinical examination is difficult or is not informative because of acute tenderness or obesity. MRI is also useful.
- **Culdocentesis:** Aspiration of peritoneal fluid and its white cell count, if exceeds 30,000/mL is significant in acute PID. Bacterial culture from the fluid is not informative because of vaginal contamination.

Investigations are also to be extended to male partner and smear and culture are made from urethral secretion.

Diagnosis

The anatomic diagnosis of infection to the upper genital tract is made from the following clinical features (Table 11.2).

Microbial diagnosis is difficult. But as already emphasized, one should not wait for the report, instead treatment should be started empirically. **The materials for identification of organisms are** from the cervical and urethral discharge and secretion from the Bartholin's gland, and laparoscopic or laparotomy collection of pus from the fallopian tubes. The materials are to be subjected to Gram stain and culture (aerobic and anaerobic).

Gram stain of the discharge may be positive for gram-negative intracellular diplococci of *N. gonorrhoeae*.

TABLE 11.2: Clinical features of acute PID.

- Fever >38°C
- Bilateral lower abdominal tenderness with radiation to the legs
- Abnormal vaginal discharge
- Abnormal uterine bleeding
- Deep dyspareunia
- Cervical motion tenderness } On bimanual examination
- Adnexal tenderness/mass } On bimanual examination
- Raised ESR

Bacteriologic diagnosis of *Chlamydia trachomatis* is difficult. However, the status of the sexual partner is the single most important clue to the diagnosis of chlamydial infection. **If the woman has a stable sexual relationship with an asymptomatic man, the clinical manifestations are unlikely to be due to chlamydial infection**.

Differential Diagnosis (Table 11.3)

The clinical condition may be confused with:

- Appendicitis
- Disturbed ectopic pregnancy
- Torsion of ovarian pedicle, hemorrhage or rupture of ovarian cyst
- Endometriosis
- Diverticulitis
- Urinary tract infection.

The two conditions—**acute appendicitis and disturbed ectopic pregnancy must be ruled out**, because both the conditions require urgent laparotomy whereas acute salpingitis is to be treated conservatively.

Complications of PID

Immediate

- Pelvic peritonitis or even generalized peritonitis
- Septicemia—producing arthritis or myocarditis.

Late

- Dyspareunia
- Infertility rate is 12%, after two episodes increases to 25% and after three raises to 50%. It is due to tubal damage or tubo-ovarian mass
- Chronic pelvic inflammation is due to recurrent or associated pyogenic infection
- Formation of adhesions or hydrosalpinx or pyosalpinx and tubo-ovarian abscess
- Chronic pelvic pain and ill health
- Increased risk of ectopic pregnancy (6-10 fold).

Treatment

***Essential steps in the prevention are*:**

- Community-based approach to increase public health awareness.
- Prevention of sexually transmitted infections with the knowledge of healthy and safer sex.
- Liberal use of contraceptives.
- Routine screening of high-risk population.

***The principles of therapy are*:**

- To control the infection
- To prevent infertility and late sequelae
- To prevent reinfection.
- Follow up examination of women within 48 to 72 hours for evaluation of response.

Outpatient Therapy

Apart from adequate rest and analgesic, antibiotics are to be prescribed even before the microbiological report is available. As because the infection is polymicrobial in nature, instead of single, combination of antibiotics should be prescribed. Antimicrobial coverage includes: *N. gonorrhoeae, C. trachomatis*, streptococci, *E. coli* and anaerobes. Outpatients antibiotic therapy for acute PID is given in the Table 11.4.

All patients treated in the outpatients are **evaluated after 48 hours and if no response, are to be hospitalized**.

Inpatient Therapy

The patients are to be hospitalized for antibiotic therapy in the conditions as mentioned in Table 11.5.

The patient is urged to take bed rest. Oral feeding is restricted. Dehydration and acidosis are to be corrected by intravenous fluid.

Intravenous antibiotic therapy is recommended for at least 48 hours but may be extended to 4 days, if necessary (Table 11.6).

TABLE 11.3: Clinical features of acute salpingitis, acute appendicitis and disturbed ectopic.

Clinical features	*Acute salpingitis (Table 13.3)*	*Acute appendicitis*	*Disturbed ectopic*
Pain	Acute lower abdominal on both sides	Starts near umbilicus but settles to right iliac fossa	Acute lower abdomen on one side
Amenorrhea and bleeding PV	Unrelated	Unrelated	Usually present
GI symptoms: Nausea, vomiting	Inconsistently present	Usual	Absent
General look	Face-flushed	Toxic	Pale
Tongue	No significant change	Furred	Pale
Pulse	Rapid but proportionate with temperature	Rapid, out of proportion to temperature	Persistent rise even with normal temperature
Temperature	More raised	Slightly raised	Not raised
Tenderness	Lower abdomen on both sides	On McBurney's point may have muscle guard	Lower abdomen more on one side
Per vaginam	Tenderness on both fornices. A mass may be felt	Tenderness on right fornix and high up	Mass may be felt through one fornix extending up to pouch of Douglas
Sonography (TVS)	Oedamatous tube	Oedamatous appendix may be seen	Empty uterine cavity, refer in POD see authors Textbook of Obstetrics
Additional features for diagnosis of disturbed ectopic pregnancy are: (a) VPT +ve; (b) USG findings; (c) Cervical motion tenderness and (d) Rarely evidence of hemodynamic instability.			

TABLE 11.4: Outpatient treatment of PID (CDC – 2015).

1. Ceftriaxone 250 mg IM single dose
   Or
   Cefoxitin, 2g IM single dose and probenecid, 1 g PO single dose
   Or
   Injection Cefotaxime IV
   Plus
2. Doxycycline 100 mg PO, bid for 14 days with or without Metronidazole 500 mg PO bid for 14 days
3. Minimum criteria: Empirical treatment of PID should be initiated.

TABLE 11.5: Indications for hospitalization (CDC – 2015).

- Suspected tubo-ovarian abscess
- Severe illness, vomiting, temperature >38°C
- Uncertain diagnosis—where surgical emergencies, (e.g. appendicitis) cannot be excluded
- Unresponsive to outpatient therapy for 48 hours
- Intolerance to outpatient oral antibiotics
- Coexisting pregnancy
- Patient is known to have HIV infection

However, no regimen is uniformly effective for all patients. Moreover superiority of one regimen over the other in respect to initial response or subsequent fertility is not yet established.

Improvement of the patient is evidenced by remission of temperature, improvement of pelvic tenderness, normal white blood cell count and negative report on bacteriological study.

Women need to be admitted if the resolution of clinical symptoms are not optimal.

Indications of Surgery

The indications of surgery are comparatively less. The unequivocal indications are:

- Generalized peritonitis
- Pelvic abscess
- Tubo-ovarian abscess which does not respond (48–72 hours) to antimicrobial therapy/or there is rupture
- Life-threatening infections.

To prevent reinfection: The following formalities are to be rigidly followed to prevent reinfection:

TABLE 11.6: Inpatient antibiotic therapy (CDC – 2015).

- **Parenteral regimen A**
  - Cefoxitin 2 g IV every 6 hours for 7 days
    Plus
  - Doxycycline 100 mg PO BID for 14 days
- **Parenteral regimen B**
  - Clindamycin 900 mg IV every 8 hours
    Plus
  - Gentamicin 2 mg/kg IV (loading dose), followed by 1.5 mg/kg IV (maintenance dose) every 8 hours
  - Aztreonam (2 g IV slowly) is similar to aminoglycoside and can be used. It has no renal toxicity and but is more expensive.
- **Alternative parenteral regimen**
  - Ampicillin-salbactum 3 g IV every 6 hours 3–5 days
    Plus
  - Doxycycline 100 mg orally BID for 14 days

- Educating the patient to avoid reinfection and the potential hazards of it
- The patient should be warned against multiple sexual partners
- To use condom
- The sexual partner or partners are to be traced and properly investigated to find out the organism(s) and treated effectively.

Follow up

Repeat smears and cultures from the discharge are to be done after 7 days following the full course of treatment. The tests are to be repeated following each menstrual period until it becomes **negative for three consecutive reports when the patient is declared cured.** Until she is cured and her sexual partner(s) have been treated and cured, the patient must be prohibited from intercourse.

PELVIC INFECTION FOLLOWING DELIVERY AND ABORTION

The common organisms producing acute infection following delivery are anaerobic *Streptococcus, Staphylococcus pyogenes,* nonhemolytic *streptococcus, E. coli* and *Bacteroides group.* Too often, multiple organisms are present and it is difficult to pinpoint a particular organism responsible for a particular type of infection.

Pathology

The infection is either localized to the cervix, producing acute cervicitis or may affect the placental site producing endometritis. The infection may spread to the myometrium producing endomyometritis which is limited by a leukocytic barrier. On occasion, the infection spreads to the parametrium, usually to one or both the sides, through lymphatics or directly through the tear of the cervix; thereby to cause parametritis. The infection may also spread upwards through the tubal openings into the tubal lumen producing **endosalpingitis. Therefore, the fallopian tube is affected either from outside following parametritis, through lymphatics producing perisalpingitis or through endosalpingitis**. The ovary may be affected through involvement of the tube or following pelvic peritonitis. Thus, an acute tubo-ovarian mass is formed (Fig. 11.2).

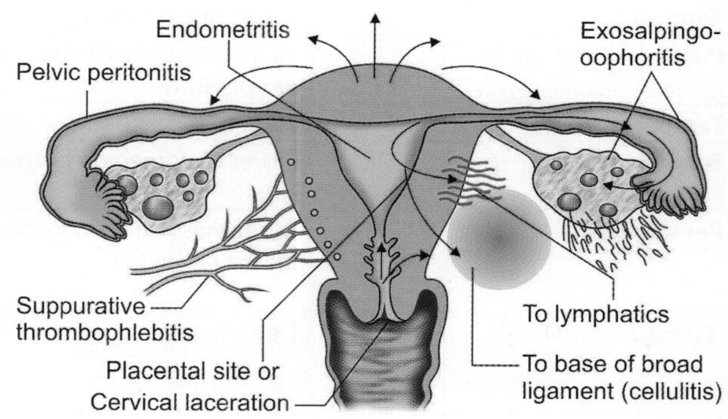

Fig. 11.2: Mode of spread in postabortal or puerperal infection.

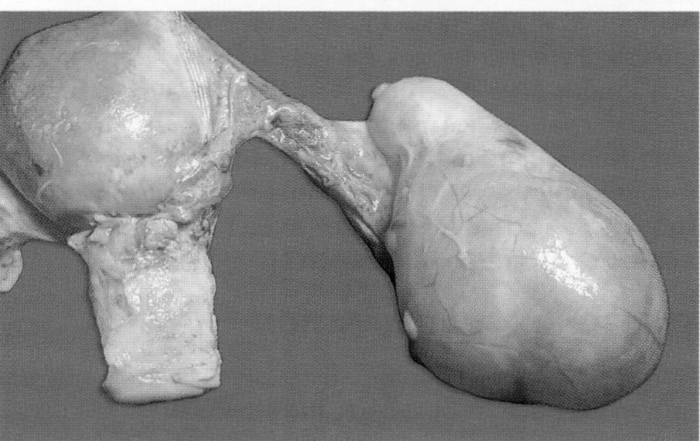

Fig. 11.3: Huge hydrosalpinx change of one tube.

Spread of Infection

Depending upon the virulence of the organisms and resistance of the host, the following events may occur.

The infection is localized principally to the cervix and subsequently develops into chronic cervicitis. **The parametrial exudate** may resolute completely leaving behind scarring or fibrosis or may undergo suppuration. The abscess so formed usually points above the inguinal ligament. **The tubal affection results in cornual block**, hydrosalpinx (Fig. 11.3) or pyosalpinx following blockage of the fimbrial end. **There may be peritonitis** either localized or at times generalized. In others, the tube may be adherent with the ovary, intestine and omentum producing tubo-ovarian mass, the abdominal ostium usually remaining patent. **The pelvic veins may be involved producing thrombophlebitis**, which is either confined to the pelvis or spreads upward along the ovarian veins or downwards along the iliofemoral veins.

Clinical Features

The **chief complaints** of varying magnitude are fever, lower abdominal and pelvic pain and offensive vaginal discharge following delivery or abortion.

On examination, **the patient looks ill and may be restless.** She likes to lie on her back with the legs flexed. Pulse rate is rapid and is out of proportion to the temperature. Abdominal examination reveals tenderness or even rigidity on lower abdomen.

Vaginal examination is painful. The discharge is offensive. The uterus is tender, more with movement of the cervix. The fornices are tender. Depending upon the spread, there may be unilateral or bilateral mass (tubo-ovarian), an unilateral tender indurated mass pushing the uterus to the contralateral side (parametritis) or a bulging fluctuating mass felt through the posterior fornix (pelvic abscess). Rectal examination is useful to corroborate the pelvic findings.

Complications of Acute PID Following Delivery/Abortion

- Endotoxic shock
- Oliguria or anuria
- DIC, gram-negative septicemia
- Tubo-ovarian abscess
- Peritonitis
- Parametritis
- Thrombophlebitis (after 7–10 days)
- Pulmonary embolism

(DIC: Disseminated intravascular coagulation)

Treatment

Prevention

(a) To maintain asepsis and antiseptic measures during labor; (b) To avoid traumatic and difficult vaginal deliveries; (c) To use prophylactic antibiotic when labor is delayed following rupture of the membranes or when there are intrauterine manipulations like forceps or manual removal of placenta; and (d) To encourage family planning acceptance to prevent the unwanted pregnancies.

Curative

- **Hospitalization**: The patient may be admitted if clinically indicated (Table 11.5).
- **Triple swabs** are to be taken—one from high vagina, one from the endocervix and the third from the urethra. These are to be sent for aerobic and anaerobic culture, drug sensitivity test and Gram stain. **The swabs are to be taken prior to bimanual examination.**
- Vaginal and rectal examinations are then made to note the extent of pelvic infection.

Investigations

Routine: (a) **Blood** is sent for hemoglobin estimation, total and differential count of white cells, depending on severity of infection blood culture and serum electrolytes are done; (b) **Urine** analysis including culture.

Special investigations are to be done as required: Ultrasonography of abdomen and pelvis to detect physometra or presence of any foreign body left behind in the uterus or in the abdominal cavity used for criminal interference.

Definitive Treatment

Antibiotics: Pending sensitivity report, potent bactericidal drugs such as gentamicin 2 mg/kg body weight and clindamycin IV 600 mg daily with IV metronidazole 500 mg are to be administered at every 6–8 hours interval. If the temperature does not subside by 48 hours, the antibiotic should be changed according to microbiology and sensitivity report.

Supportive Therapy

- Blood transfusion for anemia.
- Treatment for endotoxic shock, renal failure or disseminated intravascular coagulopathy need intensive care management.

Indications of Surgery in Septic Abortion

- Injury to the uterus
- Suspected injury to the bowels
- Presence of foreign body in the abdomen as evidenced by the USG or felt through the fornix on bimanual examination
- Unresponsive peritonitis suggestive of collection of pus
- Patient is not responding to the treatment

Types of Active Surgery

- Evacuation of uterus
- Posterior colpotomy
- Laparotomy—in a suspected case of acute appendicitis or ruptured tubo-ovarian abscess
- Laparoscopy: Drainage of abscess
- Removal of symptomatic mass

Late Sequelae of PID

- Infertility either due to cornual block, or damage to the wall of the tube
- Chronic infection
- Chronic pelvic pain, dysmenorrhea
- Pelvic adhesive disease
- Ectopic pregnancy
- Residual infection with periodic acute exacerbation
- Intestinal obstruction
- Chronic ill health
- Dyspareunia and marital disharmony
- Endometriosis
- May end in hysterectomy

PELVIC INFECTION FOLLOWING GYNECOLOGICAL PROCEDURES

Infection of the residual pelvic organs or cellular tissues is not uncommon following hysterectomy, more in vaginal than abdominal one.

Organisms: *Escherichia coli* and *Bacteroides fragilis* are the predominant organisms.

Pathology: The vaginal cuff may be indurated due to infected hematoma → cellulitis → abscess.

Clinical features: Fever and lower abdominal or pelvic pain of varying degrees appear few days (3–4) following surgery.

Per vaginam: Discharge is offensive and the vaginal vault is indurated and tender. Speculum examination may reveal exposed vaginal cuff with purulent discharge coming through the gaping vault. Rectal examination reveals induration on the vault or its extension to one side (parametritis). Rarely, a fluctuant mass may be felt (pelvic abscess).

Treatment prophylactic: Preoperative cleaning of the vagina with antiseptic lotion, perfect hemostasis during surgery and leaving behind the vault open in infected cases could reduce the postoperative infection. **Chemoprophylaxis** in potentially or actually infected cases using **intravenous metronidazole 500 mg 8 hourly for 3 such and intravenous ceftriaxone 1 g, given during the operation and 1–2 doses after the operation is quite effective to lower the risk of infection.**

Definitive treatment: Appropriate antibiotic (based on the culture and sensitivity report of the discharge), and drainage of pus through the vault are enough to arrest the infection.

IUCD AND PELVIC INFECTION

IUCD is one of the iatrogenic causes of pelvic infection in gynecology (Ch. 30). All types of IUCDs except the hormone containing ones are responsible. The incidence ranges from 2–10%. **The risk is, however, more in nulliparae.** It may flare up pre-existing pelvic infection. IUCD tail may be implicated in ascent of the organisms from the vagina in infections long after insertion. The bacteria may be carried from the cervix into the endometrium during insertion. Actinomycosis has been found rarely in association with the use of copper devices. Risk of PID is highest following first month after insertion. Again risk of PID is highest when the patient has multiple sexual partners.

Prevention: **It is better not to insert in cases with recent history of pelvic inflammatory disease.** Insertion should be carried out under strict aseptic condition. Actinomycosis responds well with penicillin.

CHRONIC PELVIC INFECTION

Chronic pelvic infection is a distressing clinical entity not only to the patients but also to the physicians. It results:

- Following acute pelvic infection—the initial treatment was delayed or inadequate
- Following low grade recurrent infection
- Tubercular infection.

The first two types are predominantly due to pyogenic organisms. There is often history of previous acute pelvic infection. Tubercular infection is chronic from the beginning and is described as a separate entity.

Pyogenic

Pathology

The pathology in the uterus is most often spared because of periodic shedding of the endometrium. The tubal changes are secondary to the changes induced by previous acute salpingitis. The tubal epithelium is usually lost, especially in gonococcal infection; the wall gets thickened with plasma cell infiltration and the openings are blocked. These result in hydrosalpinx, with loss of the lining mucosa with its plicae. The peritoneal surface is involved in recurrent infection producing **either flimsy (gonococcal) or dense (nongonococcal pyogenic) adhesions**. The tubes are thus kinked and may get adherent to the ovaries, uterus, intestine, omentum and pelvic peritoneum. A tubo-ovarian mass or a frozen pelvis results. The serum and lymphatic exudate in the parametrium of acute infection coagulates, which later either completely resolutes or becomes fibrotic. The fibrosis pulls the uterus, the cervix in particular to the same side.

Clinical Features

- The entity may remain asymptomatic.
- There may be previous history of acute pelvic infection following childbirth or abortion. Recurrent episodes of reinfection is often present. The use of IUCD is highly corroborative.

Symptoms

- Chronic pelvic pain of varying magnitude and the pain aggravates prior to menstruation due to congestion.
- Dyspareunia, which is deep and may be located unilaterally or bilaterally.
- Congestive dysmenorrhea.
- Lower abdominal pain.
- Menorrhagia or polymenorrhagia are due to congestion.

- Vaginal discharge is almost a constant manifestation and may be mucoid or mucopurulent.
- Infertility, which may be primary or more commonly secondary.

Important factors for infertility are—cornual block (Fig. 38.72), loss of cilia, loss of peristalsis due to thickening of the tubal wall, closure of the abdominal ostium and distortion of the tube due to peritubal adhesions.

On Examination

Per abdomen: There may be tenderness on one or both iliac fossa. An irregular tender pelvic mass may be felt.

Per vaginam: The findings are as mentioned in page 122.

Rectal examination corroborates the findings of vaginal examination and should not be omitted. The involvement of the parametrium and uterosacral ligaments are better assessed rectally.

Investigations

- Blood examination for evidences of leukocytosis, Hb estimation and ESR. Urine examination—routine and if necessary, culture sensitivity.
- **Laparoscopy:** This is helpful to confirm the diagnosis and to know the extent of the lesion especially in cases of infertility. However, in cases where too much adhesions are anticipated, diagnostic laparotomy is a safer substitute.

Management

- **General**
  - Improvement of general health and anemia.
  - Analgesics as required may be prescribed. Pelvic heat application by short wave diathermy is comforting to the patient.
- **Specific**
  - The IUCD is to be removed, if it is still inside.
  - Antibiotic therapy has got little benefit unless there is recent acute exacerbation. The long-term broad spectrum antibiotics to be administered include doxycycline or tetracycline or cephalosporin for three weeks. In proved cases of gonococcal infection, specific therapy is directed as outlined in acute infection (p. 123).
- **Surgery:** Surgery may be needed either by laparoscopy or by laparotomy in a few selected cases.

  Indications:
  - **Persistence** of symptoms in spite of adequate conservative treatment.
  - **Recurrence** of acute attacks.
  - **Increase in size** of the pelvic mass despite treatment.
  - **Infertility** for restorative tubal surgery or for adhesiolysis.

  Nature of surgery: Due consideration should be given to age, parity and extent of the lesion.

  Laparoscopic adhesiolysis, tubal restorative and reconstructive surgery are commonly done. Few cases may need salpingectomy or salpingo-oophorectomy.

  In general, the ideal surgery should be total hysterectomy with bilateral salpingo-oophorectomy for women that they have completed their family.

GENITAL TUBERCULOSIS

INCIDENCE

The incidence of female genital tuberculosis (FGTB) varies widely with the social status of the patient and her environment. The incidence is about 1% amongst the gynecological patients attending the outpatient department in the developing countries. Incidence is high (5–16%) amongst the patients with infertility. In US, the incidence of FGTB is 1% based on infertility clinic data. With the prevalence of HIV infection incidence of genital tuberculosis is rising (40–50%). About 10% of women with pelvic tuberculosis, have urinary tract tuberculosis.

PATHOGENESIS

The causative organism is *Mycobacterium tuberculosis* of human type. Very rarely the bovine type may affect the vulva. **Genital tuberculosis is almost always secondary to primary infection** elsewhere in the extragenital sites such as lungs (50%), lymph nodes, urinary tract, bones and joints. **The fallopian tubes are invariably the primary sites** of pelvic tuberculosis from where secondary spread occurs to other genital organs.

MODE OF SPREAD

Mode of spread

- Hematogenous (90%)
- Lymphatic
- Direct to other organ
- Ascending (rare)

Affection Rates of Genital Organs with Tuberculosis (%)	
Fallopian tubes	100%
Endometrium	50–60%
Cervix	5–15%
Ovaries	30%
Pelvic peritoneum	40–50%
Vulva, vagina	1%

Hematogenous: From any of the primary sites, the pelvic organs are involved by **hematogenous spread in about 90%** cases. If the post-primary hematogenous spread coincides with the growth spurt of the pelvic vessels, the genital organs, the tubes in particular, are likely to be affected. Thus, the pelvic organs are infected during puberty. If the spread precedes the growth phase, the genital organs are spared. The infection remains dormant for a variable period of time (4–6 years) until clinical manifestations appear (Fig. 11.4).

Lymphatic or direct: The pelvic organs are involved directly or by lymphatics from the infected organs such as peritoneum, bowel or mesenteric nodes.

Ascending: Although difficult to prove but **sexual transmission** from a male with urogenital tuberculosis is possible in vulvar, vaginal or cervical lesion.

PATHOLOGY OF PELVIC ORGANS

Fallopian tube: The most common site of affection is the fallopian tubes (100%). Both the tubes are affected simultaneously. The initial site of infection is in the submucosal layer (interstitial salpingitis) of the ampullary part of the tube.

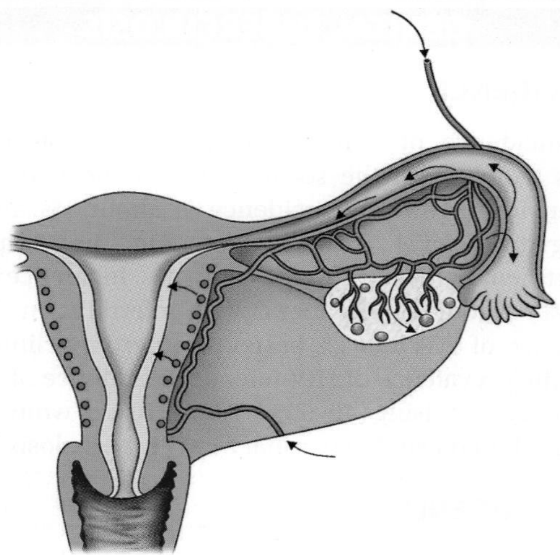

Fig. 11.4: Mode of spread in tubercular infection through bloodstream.

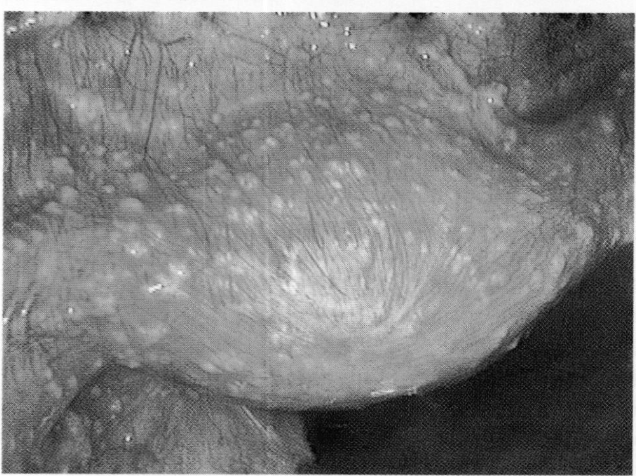

Fig. 11.5: Laparoscopic view miliary tuberculosis. Tubercles are seen over the uterus and the tube. Note also the peritoneum and intestines which are all studded with miliary tubercules. (*Courtesy:* Dr H Roy, Patna)

The infection may spread medially along the wall causing destruction of the muscles which are replaced by fibrous tissue. The walls get thickened, become calcified or even ossified. The thickening may at time become segmented. The infection may spread inwards; the mucosa gets swollen and destroyed. The fimbria are everted and **the abdominal ostium usually remains patent**. The elongated and distended distal tube with the patent abdominal ostium gives the appearance of "**tobacco-pouch**". Occlusion of the ostium may however occur due to adhesions. The tubercles burst pouring the caseous material inside the lumen producing tubercular pyosalpinx, which may adhere to the ovaries and the surrounding structures. Often the infection spreads outwards producing **perisalpingitis** with exudation, causing dense adhesions with the surrounding structures—tubercular **tubo-ovarian mass**. Rarely, **miliary tubercles** may be found on the serosal surface of the tubes, uterus, peritoneum or intestines. These are often associated with **tubercular peritonitis (Fig. 11.5)**.

However, not infrequently the tubes may look absolutely normal or nodular at places. If the nodules happen to be present in the isthmus near the uterine cornu, it constitutes salpingitis isthmica nodosa. **Salpingitis isthmica nodosa** is the nodular thickening of the tube due to proliferation of tubal epithelium within the hypertrophied myosalpinx (muscle layer). Exact etiology is unknown. It is diagnosed radiologically as a small diverticulum. It is however not specific to tubercular infection only (p. 141). It is also observed in pelvic endometriosis.

Uterus: The endometrium is involved in 60% of cases. The infection is from the tubes either by lymphatics or by direct spread through continuity. Cornual ends are commonly affected due to their dual blood supply, as well as their anatomical proximity to tubes. The tubercle is situated in the basal layer of the endometrium only to come to the surface premenstrually. After the endometrium is shed at each menstruation, reinfection occurs from the lesions in the basal layer or from the tubes. Endometrial ulceration may lead to **adhesion or synechiae formation (Asherman's syndrome)**. This may cause infertility, secondary amenorrhea or recurrent abortion (p. 384). Rarely, the infection spreads to the myometrium (2.5%) and if caseation occurs, a pyometra results, especially in postmenopausal women.

Cervix: The cervical affection is not so uncommon (5–15%). Primary infection of the cervix by sexual intercourse though rare, has been recorded. It may be ulcerative or may be bright nodular in type. Both may bleed to touch, thereby causing confusion with carcinoma. Histologically genital tuberculosis is associated with marked epithelial hyperplasia with some degree of atypia. This may lead to erroneous diagnosis of carcinoma.

Vulva and vagina: The affection of these sites is **very rare (1%)**. The lesion may be ulcerative with undermined edges. Rarely, the lesions may be of hypertrophic variety. The diagnosis is made only by histology.

Ovary: The ovaries are involved in **about 30% of tubercular salpingitis**. The manifestation may be surface tubercles, adhesions, thickening of the capsule or even caseating abscess in the substance of the ovary.

Urinary tract: About 10% of women with pelvic tuberculosis have urinary tract tuberculosis.

Pelvic Peritoneum

Pelvic peritonitis is present in about 40–50% of cases. Tuberculous peritonitis may be 'wet' (exudative type) or 'dry' (adhesive type).

In the **'wet' variety** there is ascites with straw colored fluid in the peritoneal cavity. The parietal and visceral peritoneum are covered with numerous small tubercles.

In the **'dry' (plastic) variety** there is dense adhesion with bowel loops, tubo-ovarian mass formation. The adhesion is due to fibrosis when the 'wet' variety heals.

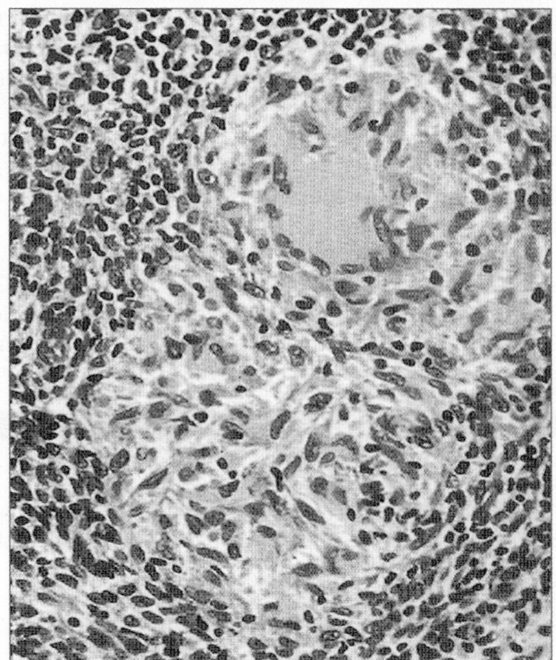

Fig. 11.6: A typical tubercular granuloma formed by lymphocytes, epithelioid cells and Langhans giant cells. Central area of caseation necrosis is seen.

Microscopic Appearance of the Lesion

Microscopic picture of the lesion is very characteristic irrespective of the organ involved. **Typical granuloma consists of infiltration of multinucleated giant cells (Langhans), chronic inflammatory cells and epithelioid cells, surrounding a central area of caseation necrosis (Fig. 11.6)**. Caseation may not be a constant feature.

CLINICAL FEATURES

Patient profile: The infection is restricted mostly (80%) to childbearing period (20–40 years). There may be past history of tubercular affection of the lungs or lymph glands. **Genital tuberculosis occurs in 10–20% of patients who have pulmonary tuberculosis in adolescence**. A family history of contact may be available. Onset is mostly insidious. A flare up of the infection may occur acutely either spontaneously or following diagnostic endometrial curettage or hysterosalpingography.

Symptoms

Symptoms vary considerably with the severity and stage of the disease. At one extreme, there is neither any symptom nor any palpable pelvic pathology. **Sometimes symptoms like** weakness, low-grade fever, anorexia, anemia or night sweats may be present. The lesion is accidentally diagnosed during investigation for infertility or dysfunctional uterine bleeding. These cases are often designated as "**silent tuberculosis**". **In others, the clinical manifestations appear**. Some of these manifestations are:

- *Infertility*: It may be primary or secondary and is present in about 70–80% cases of pelvic tuberculosis. In India, about 10% infertile women have got genital tuberculosis.

Common Causes of Infertility and Poor Pregnancy Outcome

- Tube: Block due to damage, adhesions.
- Endometrium: Destruction, synechae formation, implantation failure, miscarriage and preterm delivery.
- Ovary: Less commonly involved. Ovaries are resistant to gonadotropin stimulation, failure of IVF-ET (options for gestational surrogacy) (p. 206).

- *Menstrual abnormality*: In about 50%, the menstrual function is normal.

The menstrual abnormalities (20–30%) include:

- **Menorrhagia** or irregular bleeding is probably due to ovarian involvement, pelvic congestion or endometrial proliferative lesion. It is the early manifestation. These patients fail to respond with hormone therapy. Endometrial tuberculosis is a rare cause of puberty menorrhagia and postmenopausal bleeding.
- **Amenorrhea or oligomenorrhea**: Secondary amenorrhea is more common and may be the only presenting symptom that makes the patient seek medical advice. It may be due to **suppression of the ovarian function probably by tubercular toxin** (oophoritis). Else it may be result of endometrial destruction and uterine **synechiae formation**. It may be due to general debility also. As such, it is a late manifestation.

Others: **Chronic pelvic pain** is present in about 20–30% cases. It is often associated with **tubo-ovarian mass** and may be precipitated by tubal patency test. Secondary infection may aggravate the chronic pain to an acute one. **Vaginal discharge**—cervical or vaginal tuberculosis may be associated with postcoital bleeding or blood stained discharge. **Constitutional symptoms** such as loss of weight, malaise, anorexia, pyrexia and anemia are present in the acute phase of the disease.

Signs

- *Health status*: The general health usually remains unaffected. There may be constitutional symptoms like weakness, low-grade fever, anorexia, anemia and night sweats. There may be evidences of active or healed extragenital tubercular lesion.
- *Per abdomen*: Abdominal findings may be negative or rarely one may find an irregular tender mass in lower abdomen arising out of the pelvis. Abdomen may **feel doughy due to matted intestines**. Evidences of free peritoneal fluid are rare. **Tubercular ascites when encysted mimics an ovarian cyst.**
- *Per vaginam*: The pelvic findings may be negative in 50% cases. **Vulvar or vaginal ulcer** presents with undermined edges. There may be **thickening of the tubes** which are felt through the lateral fornices or nodules, felt through posterior fornix. At times, there is **bilateral pelvic mass** of varying sizes quite indistinguishable from that due to pyogenic infection. Per rectum, one may confirm the vaginal findings.

INVESTIGATIONS

The aims of investigations are:
- To identify the primary lesion
- To confirm the genital lesion.

Blood: The leukocyte count and ESR values may be raised. Periodic examination is of value to evaluate the progress of the lesion. **Interferon gamma release assay** from whole blood is more specific and it takes less time.

Mantoux test: It is less specific. Positive test with high dilution is suggestive that the patient is sensitized to tuberculoprotein. A negative test excludes tuberculosis.

Chest X-ray: It is taken for evidence of healed or active pulmonary lesion.

Diagnostic uterine curettage: This is to be done during the week preceding menstruation. The tubercles are likely to come to the surface during this period. **The material should be sent to the laboratory in two portions.**
- **One part in normal-saline for histopathological** examination to detect the giant cell system. Histology could detect tuberculosis in about 10% of cases only. False-positive histology may be due to the presence of chronic lesions (like talc or catgut granuloma) or sarcoidosis. False-negative result is due to improper timing of uterine curettage or due to less incidence of uterine infection.
- **One part in normal saline for:**
  - Culture in Löwenstein-Jensen media
  - Identification of the acid-fast bacilli by Ziehl-Neelsen's stain (AFB-microscopy)
  - Nucleic acid amplification
  - Guinea pig inoculation.

A positive culture is suggestive while a positive guinea pig inoculation test is diagnostic. Bacteriological test, if positive, should be able to type the bacilli and report on their drug sensitivity.

Liquid culture using automated bactec (460) is more sensitive. It takes less time (9–10 days) compared to LJ media (4–8 weeks). However, it needs more bacilus (>100) for test positivity.

Nucleic acid amplification (16S ribosomal DNA) techniques with polymerase chain reaction (PCR), **can identify *M. tuberculosis* from endometrium or menstrual blood (clinical specimens)**. PCR is more sensitive (85–95%) than microscopy and bacteriological culture. **This method can detect fewer than 10 organisms in clinical specimens compared to 10,000 necessary for smear positivity. Genital TB is usually paucibacillary.**

Gene expert (automated CBNATT) can detect *M. tuberculosis* and rifampicin resistance within two hours. It is a reliable test to start treatment. It uses PCR for detecting genetic material specific to the bacilli. A negative CBNAAT does not rule out TB.

First day menstrual discharge: This is to be collected by a pipette and the material subjected to **mycobacterial** nucleic acid amplification, culture and guinea pig inoculation. **It should be emphasized that while a positive report on AFB-microscopy, PCR, culture and histology gives the diagnosis, a negative report does not rule out tuberculosis.**

Serum ADA level is raised when pelvic peritonitis is present

Sputum and urine are to be cultured for tubercle bacillus.

Lymph node biopsy is to be done, especially from the neck in lymphadenitis.

Biopsy from the lesion in cervix, vagina or vulva.

Hysterosalpingography (HSG): In a proved case, HSG is contraindicated for the risk of reactivation of the lesion. HSG is done as a routine work up in the investigation of infertility. Few features may suggest the following diagnosis.

Suggestive Features for Pelvic Tuberculosis on HSG
- Vascular or lymphatic extravasation of dye (Fig. 11.7)
- Rigid (lead-pipe) tubes with nodulations at places
- 'Tobacco pouch' appearance with blocked fimbrial end beaded appearance of the tube with variable filling density (Fig. 11.8)
- Distal tube obstruction
- Coiling of the tubes or calcified shadow at places
- Bilateral cornual block (Fig. 38.72)
- Tubal diverticula and/or fluffiness of tubal outline
- Uterine cavity—irregular outline, honeycomb appearance or presence of uterine synechiae

Imaging: Abdominal and pelvic **ultrasound, IVU, CT or MRI** is helpful where a mass and/or ascites is present. However, it cannot confirm the diagnosis. For calcification of the tube or ovary (Fig. 11.9).

Laparoscopy: In the absence of endometrial evidence, one may take the advantage of laparoscopy for identification of

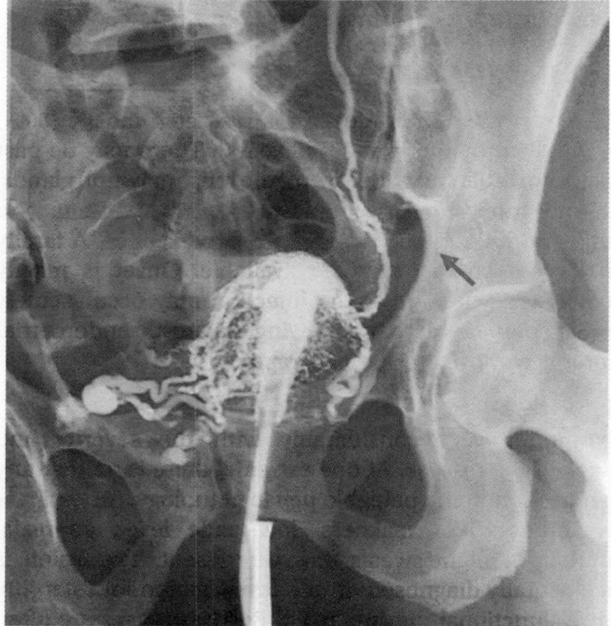

Fig. 11.7: Hysterosalpingogram showing marked extravasation of dye in venous and lymphatic channels (arrow). It was proved to be a case of tubercular endometritis.
(*Courtesy:* Dr H Roy, Patna)

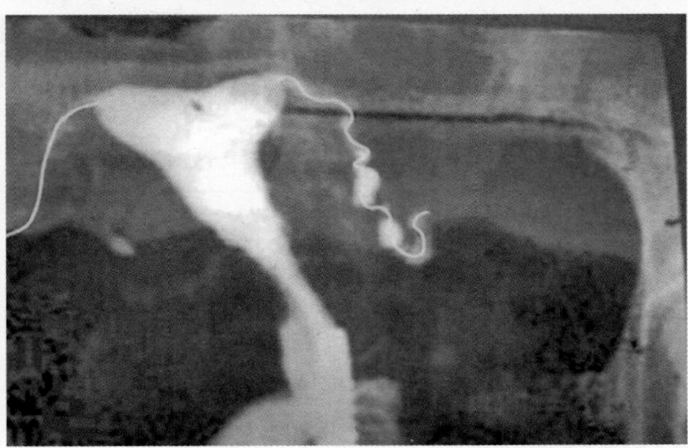

Fig. 11.8: Hysterosalpingogram showing beaded appearance of the tube with variable filling density. Pelvic tuberculosis was later confirmed.

(*Courtesy:* Dr P Panigrahi, Consultant Gynecologist, JLN Hospital, Bhilai)

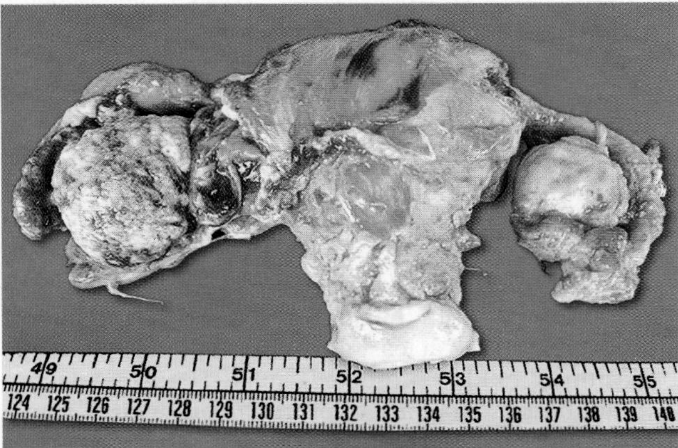

Fig. 11.9: Bilateral tubo-ovarian mass (calcification on the right) due to genital tuberculosis. TAH with BSO done following antitubercular drug therapy.

tubercles in the pelvic organs or characteristic segmented nodular appearance of the tubes. Other findings are: adhesions, ascites, hydrosalpinx change and peritoneal tubercles (Fig. 11.5). **Biopsy** may be taken from peritoneal tubercles for histology. **Aspiration of fluid** is done for culture. This may be accidentally discovered during diagnostic laparoscopy for infertility work up or for chronic pelvic pain.

Hysteroscopy: Early cases—the cavity and the tubal ostia appear normal. In advanced cases—cavity is reduced with intrauterine adhesion formation, ostia are closed. Complications of hysteroscopy are—flaring up of infection and uterine perforation or rupture.

DIAGNOSIS

Considering the high prevalence of extragenital tuberculosis, pulmonary in particular, the physicians of the low and middle income (LMIC) countries should look out for the presence of genital tuberculosis. For this, **the following guidelines may be prescribed**:

Differential diagnosis: The pelvic mass is often confused with: (a) Pyogenic tubo-ovarian mass; (b) Pelvic endometriosis; (c) Adherent ovarian cyst; and (d) Chronic disturbed ectopic pregnancy.

Clinical Diagnosis of Genital Tuberculosis

- The physician should be conscious of the entity.
- One should suspect and exclude genital tuberculosis in the following conditions:
  - Unexplained infertility or amenorrhea.
  - Recurrent episodes of pelvic infections, not responding with usual course of antibiotics.
- Presence of pelvic mass with nodules in the pouch of Douglas.

TREATMENT

- **General** ▪ **Chemotherapy** ▪ **Surgery**

- **General:** In the presence of active pulmonary tuberculosis, hospital admission is preferred. Otherwise, pelvic tuberculosis *per se* need not require hospitalization or bed rest except in acute exacerbation. To improve the body resistance, due attention is to be paid as regards diet and to correct anemia. Until the infection is controlled, the husband should use condom during intercourse to prevent possibility of contracting urogenital tuberculosis.
- **Chemotherapy:** Antitubercular chemotherapy is the treatment of first choice (Table 11.7).

RNTCP, Government of India,WHO National Strategic Plan (2019):

- **New cases:** (a) Initial phase: Four drugs are (WHO, RNTCP) used (2HRZE) daily for 2 months; (b) Continuation phase: Three drugs daily for 4 months (4 HRE)
- **Previously treated cases:** Relapse, treatment failure, and lost in follow up—initial phase 4 drugs daily for 2 months (2HRZE) and three drugs daily for 4 months (4 HRE).
  - **Initial phase:** Four drugs are used daily for 2 months to reduce the bacterial population and to prevent emergence of drug-resistance. The drugs used are (2HRZE) isoniazid, rifampicin, pyrazinamide and ethambutol. Ethambutol is essential to those who have been treated previously or are immunocompromised (HIV positive individual).
  - **Continuation phase:** Treatment is continued daily for a period of further 4 months with 3 drugs (4HRE) daily for 4 months—isoniazid, rifampicin and ethambutol.

This standard regimen may be used **during pregnancy and lactation.**

After about a year of treatment, diagnostic endometrial curettage is to be done. If the histological and/or bacteriological examination becomes positive, the treatment must be continued further. If these are negative, the endometrium is examined at interval of 6 months. **A patient may be considered cure**, if at least two reports including histological and bacteriological examination

TABLE 11.7: Antitubercular chemotherapy for initial treatment.

Drug	Daily oral dosage (adult)	Nature	Toxicity	Comments
Isoniazid	Max. 300 mg	Bactericidal	Hepatitis, peripheral neuropathy	▪ Check liver function ▪ Combine pyridoxine 50 mg daily
Rifampicin	Max. 600 mg	Bactericidal	Hepatic dysfunction, orange discoloration of urine. Febrile reaction	▪ Drug interaction (p. 400) ▪ Oral contraceptives to be avoided (p. 400) ▪ Monitor liver enzymes aspartate aminotransferase (AST)
Pyrazinamide	1.5 g/day	Bactericidal	Hepatitis, hyperuricemia, GI upset and arthralgia	▪ Active against intracellular dividing forms of *Mycobacterium* ▪ Monitor (AST)
Ethambutol	1200 mg/day	Bacteriostatic	Visual disturbances, optic neuritis, loss of visual acuity	▪ Ophthalmoscopic examination prior to therapy
Directly Observed Treatment, Short Course (DOTS)				
Revised National TB Control Program (RNTCP: 2018–2019): Government of India				
▪ **MDR cases:** are treated with 6 drug regimens. Drugs are used in different form combinations binding. Initial phase: for a period of 6–9 months and 18 months in the continuation phase. Drugs used are: Kanamycin (IM), Ofloxacin (PO), Ethionamide (PO), Pyrazinamide (PO), Ethanbutol (PO) and Cycloserine (PO). ▪ **XDR (extremely drug resistant) cases:** Capreomycin, Moxyfloxacilin, Ethionamide, Cycloserine, Linezolid or clofazimine are used for 24–30 months, in different combinations.				**RNTCP classifies TB patients into two treatment categories.** **(I): New and (II): Previously treated.** ▪ **New cases:** Initial phase—2HRZE + Continuation phase—4HRE. ▪ **Previously treated cases:** Initial phase—2HRZE + Continuation phase—4HRE

become negative. Majority of the patients (90–95%) respond well to chemotherapy.

Treatment should be started without waiting for the culture results, if clinical features and histology results are consistent with tuberculosis. Treatment should be continued even if initial culture results are negative.

Multidrug resistant (MDR) tuberculosis is defined as infection with ***M. tuberculosis*** that is resistant to two or more agents including isoniazid. HIV negative patients who are MDR have high mortality rate (80%). Such patients are treated with six drug regimens Center for Drug Control (CDC).

Treatment of woman with GTB along with positive HIV

Women with GTB and positive HIV have got high morbidity and mortality. Management options (RNTCP and NACO) are: (a) To complete TB treatment then to start ARV—therapy; (b) To treat TB (with rifampicin containing regimen) + efavirenz + 2 NRTIs (p. 129); (c) To treat TB [as above (b)] + 2 NRTIs; then to start HAART (maximally suppressive) regimen (p. 129).

- **Surgery**
  - **Indications:**
    - Unresponsiveness of the disease in spite of adequate antitubercular chemotherapy.
    - Tubercular pyosalpinx, ovarian abscess (Fig. 11.8) or pyometra.
    - Persistent menorrhagia and/or chronic pelvic pain causing deteriorating health status.
  - **Contraindications:** (a) Presence of active tuberculosis in extragenital site; (b) Favorable response to antimicrobial therapy with diminishing size of the pelvic mass and (c) Accidental discovery of tubercular tubo-ovarian mass on laparotomy in young patient. The abdomen is to be closed after taking tissue for biopsy.
- **Precautions:** Antitubercular drug therapy in full dosage should be instituted at least 6 weeks prior to surgery and similar treatment should be continued following surgery.
- **Type of surgery:** The ideal surgery should be total hysterectomy with bilateral salpingo-oophorectomy. In young women at least one ovary, if found apparently healthy, should be preserved. Isolated excision of tubo-ovarian mass, drainage of pyometra or repair of fistula may be done in selected cases.

RESULTS OF TREATMENT

In terms of future reproduction, the prognosis is most unfavorable. Pregnancy is rare (5–10%), and if occurs, chance of ectopic pregnancy is more (40%). While the pregnancy is intrauterine, the risks of miscarriage is high and a pregnancy going up to term is a rare event.

With the help of assisted reproductive technology (IVF-ET) better pregnancy rate is observed following successful chemotherapy. Ovulation is impaired due to gonadotropin resistance. Implantation failure, miscarriage. Preterm births are common. Gestational surrogacy is an option.

Contraception: As rifampicin is an enzyme inducer, (enzyme—P-450 cytochrome), COCs should be avoided.

Preconceptional Counseling: It is needed in view of adverse pregnancy outcome. ART may be an option. Pregnancy to be attempted once disease is free.

VULVAR TUBERCULOSIS

The patient complains of a painful and tender ulcer in the vulva. Confirmation is done by biopsy. The medical treatment is the same as that outlined in pelvic tuberculosis. In unresponsive cases, local vulvectomy is to be done.

CERVICAL TUBERCULOSIS

The presenting complaints are mucopurulent discharge and postcoital bleeding. Cervical tuberculosis on speculum examination (Fig. 11.10) appears as an ulcerated or hypertrophic growth which bleeds on touch.

Cervical cytology: May reveal multinucleated giant cells, epithelioid cells and dyskaryotic cells. Diagnosis is often confused with cervical cancer. **Biopsy** confirms the diagnosis. Antitubercular drug therapy as outlined in pelvic tuberculosis is prescribed (Table 11.7). In unresponsive cases, hysterectomy is justified.

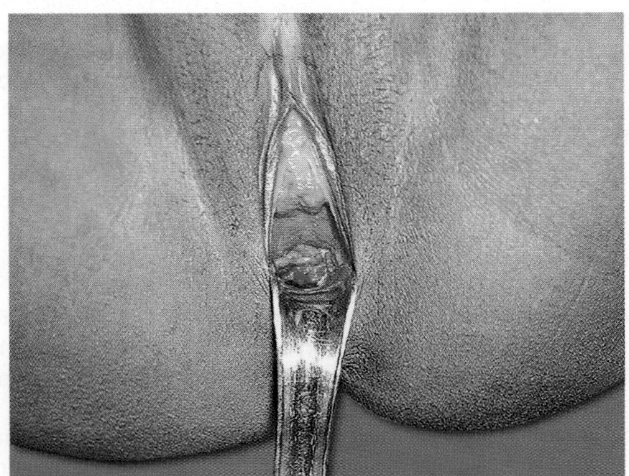

Fig. 11.10: Tubercular cervix proved by biopsy. The clinical diagnosis was confused with malignancy.
(*Courtesy:* Dr H Roy, Patna)

Chronic PID: The term chronic pelvic inflammatory disease has largely been abandoned. The long-term sequelae of acute PID such as adhesions or hydrosalpinx are bacteriologically sterile.

True chronic PID such as **genital tuberculosis and actinomycosis** is less although the former is not infrequent in the developing countries.

ACTINOMYCES INFECTION

It is a rare cause of upper genital tract infection. Infection is caused by *Actinomyces israelii*, a gram-positive anaerobe. It may be associated in IUCD users more with noncopper devices. Actinomyces causes chronic endometritis. There may be foul smelling vaginal discharge. **The diagnosis is usually made from tubo-ovarian abscess when the classic 'Sulfur granules' are observed histologically along with gram-positive filaments.** Presence of symptoms like fever, abdominal pain, abnormal uterine bleeding may necessitate the removal of IUCD. It is sensitive to penicillin, doxycycline or fluoroquinolones. **The treatment** should be continued for 12 weeks. Following the course of antibiotic treatment, Pap smear is repeated after 3 months.

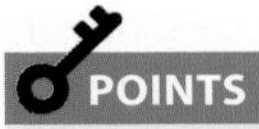

POINTS

- **The vaginal defense** is lost following 10 days of birth till puberty, in reproductive period-during menstruation, following abortion and childbirth and following menopause.
- **Pelvic inflammatory disease** according to anatomic location may be in the endometrium (endometritis), the oviducts (salpingitis), the ovary (oophoritis), the myometrium (myometritis), uterine serosa and broad ligaments (parametritis) and the peritoneum (pelvic peritonitis).
- **Infections of lower genital tract** involve the vulva, vaginal and the cervix. Patient presents with vaginal discharge and/or itching or with ulcers.
- **PID** is the infections of the upper genital organs; it is usually polymicrobial. It is due to the ascending infection from the vagina and cervix to the endometrium, tubal mucosa and the pelvic peritoneum.
- **The primary organisms of PID** are predominantly sexually transmitted. Acute PID is polymicrobial in nature. As the symptoms of PID are nonspecific, over treatment is preferred to missed diagnosis.
- **Clinical diagnostic criteria** for acute PID includes: Minimum and additional (routine and definitive) criteria (p. 108). PID should be diagnosed with a clinical approach and suspicion. It is always better to treat the woman rather than to leave her untreated for complication to develop.
- **Laparoscopy** is the optimum method for accurately diagnosing acute PID.
- **Gonococcal** affection of the tubes is by direct spread from downstairs to upstairs across the mucosal surface of the endometrium, reflux of the menstrual flow with gonococci into the tubes and carried along the spermatozoa or the trichomonas. The pathological process is initiated primarily in the endosalpinx.
- **For detection of *Gonococcus*,** the materials are collected from the urethra or Bartholin's duct, cervical smear and laparoscopic collection of pus from the uterine tube. Acute gonorrhea is treated by drugs (Table 12.2) to both the partners.
- **In acute condition,** the diagnosis is confused with acute appendicitis and disturbed ectopic pregnancy.
- **Immediate complications** include pelvic peritonitis and septicemia and late complications include infertility, chronic pelvic pain and chronic ill-health.
- **Repeat smears** and cultures from the discharge are to be done following each menstrual period until it becomes negative for 3 consecutive reports when the patient is declared cured.
- ***Chlamydia trachomatis,*** a gram-negative obligatory intracellular bacteria, is the most common organism proved to be sexually transmitted from the non-gonococcal urethritis in male consort. The clinical picture is almost the same to that of gonococcal infection but is milder in nature. Perihepatic inflammation (Fitz-Hugh-Curtis syndrome) is observed in 5–10% women with acute PID.

Contd...

Contd...

- **The late sequelae** include tubal obstruction, infertility, early abortion and ectopic pregnancy.
- **Detection** can be done by tissue culture. The specific antibody can be detected by immunofluorescent test or complement fixation test. Chlamydial nucleic acid amplification and detection by PCR is a very sensitive and specific test. The organism is sensitive to azithromycin, erythromycin or ofloxacin. The same treatment is to be given to the sexual partner.
- **The most common organisms** producing acute infection following delivery and abortion are anaerobic *Streptococcus, Staphylococcus pyogenes*, *Escherichia* and *Bacteroides* groups.
- **The fallopian tube** is affected either following parametritis through the lymphatics producing perisalpingitis or through endosalpingitis. Tubal affection to cause infertility depends on the severity and number of episodes of the disease.
- **Triple swabs** are to be taken prior to bimanual examination; one from the high vagina, one from the endocervix and the third from the urethra. These are to be sent for aerobic and anaerobic culture, Gram stain and drug sensitivity.
- **Clinical diagnostic criteria of PID** (CDC – 2015) include minimum and additional ones (p. 108). Diagnostic laparoscopy is considered the gold standard (p. 108). Women may be given antibiotic therapy either as an outpatient (Table 11.4) or as an inpatient (Table 11.6) depending on her evaluation (Table 11.5).
- **Surgical management** is needed for few patients (pelvic abscess, tubo-ovarian abscess) with laparotomy, posterior colpotomy or laparoscopy.
- **IUD** may produce pelvic infection (2–10%). The chance is more in nullipara. The highest risk is in the first month after insertion. Bacteria ascends along the nylon threads. Actinomycosis is often implicated.
- **Combined oral contraceptive use** offers some protection against PID causing thick cervical mucus and decrease in duration of menstrual flow. Contact tracing and treatment of sexual partner should be a routine for effective treatment of PID.
- **The incidence of genital tuberculosis** is about 1% amongst the gynecological patient. The pelvic organs are affected secondarily, the primary site is predominantly in lung. The spread is by hematogenous route. Fallopian tube is almost always (100%) affected by interstitial salpingitis, endometrium in 60% and cervix in 15% cases. Infertility is present in 70%. About 10% of the infertile couple have got genital tuberculosis.
- **Common causes of infertility are:** (a) Tubal—damage and block or adhesions; (b) Endometrium—destruction, synechiae formation, implantation failure, miscarriage and preterm delivery; (c) Ovary—anovulation, resistant to gonadotropin stimulation and failure of IVF-ET. Gestational surrogacy may be an option.
- Although menorrhagia may be the early symptom but more commonly, the patient presents with oligomenorrhea or amenorrhea. The diagnosis is confirmed by histological examination, culture in Löwenstein-Jensen media and guinea pig inoculation and identification of the bacteria by Ziehl-Neelsen's stain from the uterine curettage materials. PCR is more sensitive.
- **Contraception in a woman with ATD:** COCs should be avoided as rifampicin is an enzyme inducer.
- **The suggestive features of HSG** are extravasation of dye, rigid tubes with nodulation at places and tobacco-pouch appearance (p. 154). The result in terms of fertility following treatment (Table 11.7) is unsatisfactory. Pregnancy is rare and if occurs, risk of ectopic pregnancy is more. In uterine pregnancy, abortion is likely and a pregnancy up to term is a rarity.
- **Complications of PID are:** (a) immediate (pelvic peritonitis) or (b) Late (infertility, pelvic pain, dyspareunia, AUB, ectopic pregnancy) (p. 109). Amongst all the women with acute PID, one in four, suffer further sequelae including recurrent attacks of acute PID, ectopic pregnancy, chronic pelvic pain and chronic ill health.

CHAPTER

12 Sexually Transmitted Infections

CHAPTER OUTLINE

- Gonorrhea
- Syphilis
- Chlamydial Infections
- Chancroid (Soft Sore)
- Lymphogranuloma Venereum
- Granuloma Inguinale (Donovanosis)
- Bacterial Vaginosis
- Herpes Genitalis
- HIV and AIDS
- Genital warts (Condyloma Acuminata)
- Molluscum Contagiosum
- Pediculosis Pubis
- Scabies

INTRODUCTION

Sexually transmitted infections (STIs) include those infections, which are predominantly transmitted through sexual contact from an infected partner. Although the transmission of the infections is mostly due to sexual contact, other modes of transmission include placental human immunodeficiency virus (HIV) syphilis, by blood transfusion or infected needles (HIV, hepatitis B or syphilis), or by inoculation into the infant's mucosa when it passes through the birth canal (gonococcal, chlamydial, or herpes). Gynecological morbidities associated with sexually transmitted diseases (STIs) are high. Chronic pelvic infection, pain, infertility, ectopic pregnancy, vulvar, and cervical neoplasia are the long-term sequelae.

Transplacental infection (during pregnancy) to the fetus results in high perinatal morbidity and mortality. **There is rising trend of STIs throughout the globe.** With the improvement of diagnostic methods and increased interest on STIs, more and more diseases are included mostly of viral origin (HIV, hepatitis B and C, human papilloma virus).

Important sexually transmitted diseases are grouped in Table 12.1.

Reasons for Rising Incidence of STIs

- Rising prevalence of viral infections like HIV, hepatitis B and C.
- Increased use of 'pill' and intrauterine contraceptive device (IUCD) which cannot prevent STI and there is an increased promiscuity and permissiveness.
- Lack of sex education and inadequate practice of safer sex.
- Increased rate of overseas travel.
- Increased detection due to heightened awareness.

GONORRHEA

Gonorrhea still remains an important health problem. The causative organism is *Neisseria gonorrhoeae*—a gram-negative diplococcus. The incubation period is 3–7 days.

The principal site of invasion is the columnar and transitional epithelium of the genitourinary tract. As such, **the primary sites of infection are** endocervix, urethra, Skene's gland, and Bartholin's gland. It is an intracellular organism. The organism may be localized in the lower genital tract to produce urethritis, bartholinitis, or cervicitis. Other sites of infection are oropharynx, anorectal region, and conjunctiva. As squamous epithelium is resistant to gonococcal invasion, vaginitis in adult is not possible, but vulvovaginitis is possible in childhood. In about 15% of untreated cervicitis, gonococcal infection may ascend up to produce acute pelvic inflammatory disease (PID). Rarely, it may produce septicemia with distant involvement to cause tenosynovitis and septic arthritis. Upper genital organs are involved as the infection spreads along the spermatozoa. Gonococci attach to the spermatozoa and are being carried up. Endometritis and salpingitis are common. **It should be remembered that *N. gonorrhoeae* is often present with other sexually transmitted diseases and women with gonorrhea are considered to be at risk for incubating syphilis. One-third of such cases are associated with chlamydial infection.**

Clinical Features in Adult

About 50% of patients with gonorrhea are asymptomatic and even when the symptoms are present, they are nonspecific. The clinical features of acute gonococcal infection are described as follows:

- Local
- Distant or metastatic
- PID (Ch. 11).

Local

Symptoms

- Urinary symptoms such as dysuria (25%).
- Profuse, non-irritating, white to yellowish vaginal discharge (50%).
- Acute unilateral pain and swelling over the labia due to involvement of Bartholin's gland.

TABLE 12.1: Sexually transmitted infections (STIs).

Disease	*Agent*	*Prevention of STIs and RTIs*
■ **Bacterial** • **Gonorrhea** • **Non-gonococcal urethritis** • **Syphilis** • **Lymphogranuloma venereum** • **Chancroid** • **Granuloma inguinale** • **Nonspecific vaginitis** • **Mycoplasma infection**	 *Neisseria gonorrhoeae* *Chlamydia trachomatis* (D-K serotypes) *Treponema pallidum* *Chlamydia trachomatis* (L serotypes) *Haemophilus ducreyi* *Donovania granulomatis* *Haemophilus vaginalis* *Mycoplasma hominis*	■ **Safe sex as STIs are entirely preventable** ■ **Use of barrier contraception:** Condom, diaphragm, spermicides
■ **Viral** • **AIDS** • Genital herpes • Condyloma acuminata • CIN • Molluscum contagiosum • Viral hepatitis	 Human immunodeficiency virus (HIV 1 or HIV 2) Herpes simplex virus (HSV 2) Human papilloma virus (HPV) HPV – 16, 18 or 31 Pox virus Hepatitis B and C virus	■ **Reducing** the number of sexual partners—monogamous relationship reduces the risk of STIs and RTIs ■ **Contact tracing** and effective treatment
■ **Protozoal** • Bacterial vaginosis (BV) • Trichomonas vaginitis	 *Gardnerella vaginalis* *Trichomonas vaginalis*	■ **Screening** in asymptomatic or symptomatic cases for STIs and RTIs
■ **Fungal** • Monilial vaginitis	 *Candida albicans*	
■ **Ectoparasites** • Scabies • Pediculosis pubis	 *Sarcoptes scabiei* Crab louse (*Pthirus pubis*)	■ **Aseptic procedures** in delivery, MTP procedures and IUCD insertion

(AIDS: acquired immune deficiency syndrome; CIN: cervical intraepithelial neoplasia; STI: sexually transmitted infections; RTI: reproductive tract infection; MTP: medical termination of pregnancy; IUCD: intrauterine contraceptive device)

- There may be rectal discomfort due to associated proctitis from genital contamination.
- **Others**: Pharyngeal infection, intermenstrual bleeding.

Signs

- Labia may be swollen and look inflamed.
- The vaginal discharge is mucopurulent.
- The external urethral meatus and the openings of the Bartholin's ducts look congested. On squeezing the urethra and giving pressure on the Bartholin's glands, purulent exudate escapes out through the openings. **Bartholin's gland** may be palpably enlarged, tender with fluctuation, suggestive of formation of abscess.
- Speculum examination reveals congested ectocervix with occassional mucopurulent cervical secretions escaping out through the external os.

Distant or Metastatic

There may be features of **perihepatitis and septicemia**. Perihepatitis results from spread of infection to the liver capsule. There is formation of adhesions with the abdominal wall. This is not infrequently (5–10%) associated with acute PID.

Septicemia is characterized by low-grade fever, polyarthralgia, tenosynovitis, septic arthritis, perihepatitis, meningitis, endocarditis, and skin rash.

Complications

Acute pelvic inflammation leads to chronic pelvic inflammatory disease, unless adequately treated. Infertility, ectopic pregnancy (due to tubal damage), dyspareunia, chronic pelvic pain, tubo-ovarian mass, and Bartholin's gland abscess are commonly seen.

Diagnosis

Nucleic acid amplication testing (NAAT) of urine or endocervical discharge is done. First void morning urine sample (preferred) or at least one hour since the last void sample should be tested. **NAAT is very sensitive and specific (95%).**

In the acute phase, secretions from the urethra, Bartholin's gland, and endocervix are collected for Gram stain and culture.

A presumptive diagnosis is made following detection of gram-negative intracellular diplococci on staining. Culture of the discharge in Thayer-Martin medium further confirms the diagnosis. Drug sensitivity test is also to be performed.

Treatment

Preventive

- Adequate therapy for gonococcal infection and meticulous follow up are to be done till the patient is declared cured.

TABLE 12.2: Recommended drugs in acute gonorrhea (CDC – 2015).

▪ Ceftriaxone Plus	— 250 mg IM single dose
▪ Azithromycin	— 1 g PO once
▪ Doxycycline	— 100 mg PO BID × 7 days
Alternative regimen	
▪ Cefixime Plus	— 400 mg single dose
▪ Doxycycline	— 100 mg PO B1D x 7 days
Conjunctivitis of the newborn should be treated with a single dose of ceftriaxone (20–30 mg/kg) IM and gentamicin eye ointment (1%).	

- To treat adequately the **male sexual partner** simultaneously.
- To avoid multiple sex partners.
- To use condom till both the sexual partners are free from disease.

Curative

The specific treatment for gonorrhea is single dose regimen of any one of the following drugs (Table 12.2).

It should be borne in mind that the patient with gonorrhea must be suspected of having syphilis or chlamydial infection. As such, treatment should cover all the three.

Follow up

Cultures should be made 7 days after the therapy. Repeat cultures are made at monthly intervals following menses for three months. **If the reports are persistently negative, the patient is declared cured.**

SYPHILIS

Syphilis is caused by the anaerobic spirochete *Treponema pallidum*. Syphilitic lesion of the genital tract is acquired by direct contact with another person who has open primary or secondary syphilitic lesion. Transmission occurs through the abraded skin or mucosal surface.

Clinical Features

The incubation period ranges between 9 and 90 days.

The primary lesion (chancre) may be single or multiple and is usually located in the labia. Fourchette, anus, cervix, and nipples are the other sites of lesion. A small papule is formed, which is quickly eroded to form an ulcer. The margins are raised with smooth shiny floor. The ulcer is painless without any surrounding inflammatory reaction. The inguinal glands are enlarged, discrete, and painless. The **primary chancre** heals spontaneously in 1–8 weeks leaving behind a scar.

The tubes are not affected and infertility does not occur unless associated with gonococcal infection.

Secondary Syphilis

Within 6 weeks to 6 months from the onset of primary chancre, the secondary syphilis may be evidenced in the vulva in the form of **condyloma lata**. These are coarse, flat-topped, moist, necrotic lesions and teeming with treponemes. Patient may present with systemic symptoms like fever, headache, and sore throat. Maculopapular skin rashes are seen on the palms and soles. Other features include generalized lymphadenopathy, mucosal ulcers, and alopecia.

The primary and secondary stage can last up to two years and during this period, the woman is a source of infection.

Latent Syphilis

It is the quiescence phase after the stage of secondary syphilis has resolved. It varies in duration from 2 to 20 years. In this stage serology is positive without any symptoms or signs of the disease.

Tertiary Syphilis

About one-third of untreated patients progress from late latent stage to tertiary syphilis. It damages the central nervous, cardiovascular, and musculoskeletal systems. Patient may present with cranial nerve palsies (III, VI, VII, and VIII), hemiplegia, tabes dorsalis, aortic aneurysm, and gummas of skin and bones. The important pathology is endarteritis and periarteritis of small and medium sized vessels. **Tertiary syphilis is characterized by gumma.** A gummatous ulcer is a deep punched ulcer with rolled out margins. It is painless with a moist leather base. Serpiginous outline may also be produced.

The systemic manifestations of the secondary and tertiary syphilis are better dealt with in Textbook of Medicine.

Congenital Syphilis

See author's Textbook of Obstetrics (Ch. 20).

Diagnosis of Syphilis

1. **History** of exposure to an infected person.
2. **Identification** of the organism—*Treponema pallidum*, an anaerobe.
   A smear is taken from the exudate which is obtained after teasing the primary chancre (base and edge) with a swab dipped in normal saline. It is examined under dark ground illumination through a microscope. The treponemata appear as motile bluish white cork-screw shaped organisms.
3. **Serological tests:**
   a. VDRL: This is the common flocculation test performed and is **positive after 6 weeks of initial infection**. Biological False Positive (BFP) are seen in; (a) Pregnancy; (b) SLE. Serofast women may have persistant low titre.
   b. **The specific tests include** *Treponema pallidum* hemagglutination (TPHA) test, *Treponema pallidum* enzyme immunoassay (EIA), fluorescent treponemal antibody absorption (FTA-Abs) test and *Treponema pallidum immobilization (TPI)* test.
      - **Fluorescent treponemal antibody absorption test** (FTA-Abs). FTA-Abs is expensive but a confirmatory test. FTA-IgM is produced only in active treponemal infection and it declines after adequate treatment.
      - EIA test for treponemal specific IgG or IgM is now routinely used.
      - VDRL and TPHA tests are used for screening and FTA-Abs test is used for confirmation.
      - Serological tests are invariably positive in secondary syphilis.
   c. Currently immunoblotting and PCR tests are evaluated as more sensitive and confirmatory tests.
      After successful treatment, nonspecific tests become negative, whereas specific tests remain positive.

Treatment (CDC Recommendation – 2014)

Early syphilis (primary, secondary, and early latent syphilis of less than 1 year duration)

Benzathine penicillin G 2.4 million units is given intramuscularly in a single dose, half to each buttock.

In penicillin allergic cases, tetracycline 500 mg, PO, 4 times a day or doxycycline 100 mg BID PO for 14 days is effective.

Late syphilis (>1 year duration): Benzathine penicillin G 2.4 million units is given IM weekly for 3 weeks (7.2 million units total). This should be in consultation with the STI clinic.

Alternative regimen: Doxycycline 100 mg orally twice daily or tetracycline 500 mg orally 4 times a day for 4 weeks.

All women with syphilis should be tested for HIV infection and treated when found positive.

Sexual partners of women with syphilis should be evaluated clinically and serologically. The sexual partners should be treated presumptively.

Follow up: Serological test is to be performed 1, 3, 6, and 12 months after treatment of early syphilis. In late symptomatic cases, surveillance is for life; the serological test is to be done annually. All women with simultaneous syphilis and HIV infection may have high rate of treatment failure.

CHLAMYDIAL INFECTIONS

The causative organism is *Chlamydia trachomatis* (of D-K serotypes), an obligatory intracellular gram-negative bacteria. Its prevalence is more than *N. gonorrhoeae* as a causative agent for STI in developed countries. Chlamydia has longer incubation period (6–14 days) compared to gonorrhea (3–7 days).

The organisms affect the columnar and transitional epithelium of the genitourinary tract. It is an obligatory intracellular organisms. The lesion is limited superficially. As there is no deeper penetration, the pathological changes to produce symptoms may not be apparent. **The infection is mostly localized** in the urethra, Bartholin's gland, and cervix. It can ascend upwards like gonococcal infection to produce acute PID. Too often (20–40%), it is associated with gonococcal infection.

Clinical Features

These are nonspecific and asymptomatic in most cases (75%). Dysuria, dyspareunia, postcoital bleeding, and intermenstrual bleeding are the presenting symptoms.

Findings include mucopurulent cervical discharge, cervical edema, cervical ectopy, and cervical friability.

The clinical features of acute PID—has been mentioned in Chapter 11 (p. 107).

Complications

Urethritis and bartholinitis are manifested by dysuria and purulent vaginal discharge. Chlamydial cervicitis spreads upwards to produce endometritis and salpingitis. Chlamydial salpingitis is asymptomatic in majority of the cases. It causes tubal scarring resulting in infertility and ectopic pregnancy. It is the more common cause of perihepatitis **(Fitz-Hugh-Curtis syndrome)** than gonococcus. The spread to the liver from the pelvic organs is via lymphatics and the peritoneal cavity.

Diagnosis

In uncomplicated cases, the materials are to be collected from the urethra (Fig. 9.15):

Cytobrush is used for maximum endocervical/epithelial cell yield for appropriate sampling and culture as well.

Nucleic acid amplification testing (NAAT) of the endocervical cells is the most sensitive and specific test for identifying chlamydial infection.

Chlamydia can be demonstrated in **tissue culture**. (McCoy cell monolayers). It is 100% specific. It is expensive, technically difficult and takes 3–7 days to obtain result.

The sexual partner should also be treated with the same drug regimen to reduce drug resistance or recurrence.

Treatment failure with the above strict guidelines suggests either lack of patient compliance or reinfection.

Treatment (Table 12.3)

TABLE 12.3: Recommended drugs for chlamydial infections (CDC-2015).

▪ Azithromycin Or	— 1 g orally single dose
▪ Doxycycline Or	— 100 mg orally BID × 7 days
▪ Ofloxacin Or	— 300 mg orally BID × 7 days
▪ Erythromycin base	— 500 mg orally QID × 7 days

CHANCROID (SOFT SORE)

The causative organism is a gram-negative streptobacillus—*Haemophilus ducreyi*. The incubation period is very short 3–5 days or less.

The lesion starts as multiple vesicopustules over the vulva, vagina or cervix. It then sloughs to form shallow ulcers circumscribed by inflammatory zone. The lesion is very tender with foul purulent and hemorrhagic discharge. There may be cluster of ulcers. Unilateral inguinal lymphadenitis may occur which may suppurate to form abscess (buboes). The clinical significance is that chancroid genital ulcers facilitate the transmission of HIV infection.

Diagnosis

Syphilis must be ruled out first. Demonstration of *Ducreyi bacillus* in specialized culture media is confirmatory. Discharge from the ulcers or pus from the lymph glands is taken for culture. In the stained film (Gram-stain) the organisms appear classically as 'Shoal of fish'. It is difficult to grow this organism in culture method. Mostly the diagnosis is made clinically and by exclusion of other vulvar ulcers to cause STIs.

Treatment (CDC – 2015)

- Ceftriaxone 250 mg IM single dose is effective. Sexual partner should also be treated.
- Azithromycin 1 g PO single dose.
- Erythromycin 500 mg PO every 8 hours for 7 days can also be given.

Longer course of treatment is needed for patients who are positive with HIV.

LYMPHOGRANULOMA VENEREUM

Lymphogranuloma venereum (LGV) is caused by one of the aggressive L serotypes of *Chlamydia trachomatis* usually acquired sexually. It is an obligatory intracellular and gram-intermediate organism. The incubation period is 3–30 days. It is more commonly found in the sea ports of the far East, Malaysia, Africa, and South America.

Initial lesion is a painless papule, pustule or ulcer in the vulva (common site), urethra, rectum or the cervix. The inguinal nodes are involved and feel rubbery. There is acute lymphangitis and lymphadenitis. **The glands become necrosed and abscess (bubo) forms.** Within 7–15 days, the bubo ruptures and results in multiple draining sinuses and fistulas. The healing occurs with intense fibrosis with lymphatic obstruction. **The secondary phase** is noted by painful adenopathy. **The classical clinical sign of LGV is the "groove sign", a depression between the groups of inflamed nodes.** The lymphatic obstruction leads to vulvar swelling whereas lymphatic extension to the vulva, vagina, or rectum leads to ulceration, fibrosis, and stricture of the vagina or rectum.

Complications

- Vulvar elephantiasis
- Perineal scarring and dyspareunia
- Rectal stricture
- Sinus and fistula formation.

Diagnosis

- Culture and isolation (lymph node aspiration) of LGV (*Chlamydia* serotypes L1,2,3) is confirmatory.
- Detection of LGV antigen in pus obtained from a bubo with specific monoclonal antibodies using immunofluorescence method.
- Detection of LGV antigen by ELISA method.
- LGV complement fixation test—when positive with rising titer (>1 : 64).
- Intradermal Frei test is nonspecific and unreliable.

Treatment

Prevention: Use of condom or to avoid intercourse with a suspected infected partner.

Definitive treatment: Centers for disease control and prevention (CDC) recommends (2015) doxycycline 100 mg BID for at least 21 days. Alternatively, azithromycin 1 g PO weekly for 3 weeks or erythromycin 500 mg orally every 6 hours for 21 days is given (indicated for pregnant women). Sexual partner should also be treated.

Surgical: (a) Abscess should be aspirated but not be excised; (b) Manual dilatation of the stricture weekly. It is essential to use antibiotics during the perioperative period. Patient may need reconstructive surgery.

GRANULOMA INGUINALE (DONOVANOSIS)

This is a chronic progressive granulomatous diseases of the vulva, vagina, or cervix. It is commonly found in some tropics and subtropics like South China, South India, Papua New Guinea, and South America. **The causative organism is** a gram-negative intracellular bacillus—*Calymmatobacterium granulomatis* (*Donovania granulomatis*).

Clinical Features

The disease usually manifests itself 10–80 days after coitus with an infected partner. The lesion starts as pustules, which breakdown to ulcers and erode the adjacent tissues through continuity and contiguity. The ulcer looks hypertrophic (beefy red) due to indurated granulation tissue. The margins are rolled and elevated. Biopsy may be needed to exclude neoplasia. The lymph nodes do not undergo suppuration and abscess formation (cf. Lymphogranuloma venereum). If untreated, there is lymphatic obstruction due to scarring. This causes marked enlargement of the vulva.

Diagnosis

It is confirmed by demonstrating the *Donovan bodies* within the mononuclear cells, in the scraped material obtained from the ulcer. It is stained by the Giemsa method. **Donovan bodies are clusters of dark-staining bacteria with a bipolar (safety pin) appearance found within the cytoplasm of large mononuclear cells.**

Treatment (CDC – 2015)

- Doxycycline 100 mg BID for at least 3 weeks

  Or
- Azithromycin 1 g once a week for 3 weeks

  Or
- Erythromycin base 500 mg 6 hourly daily for 3 weeks.

Therapy to be continued till the lesions have healed completely. The residual destructive lesion in the vulva may need plastic surgery or vulvectomy.

BACTERIAL VAGINOSIS

The causative organism was previously thought to be *Gardnerella vaginalis* (*Haemophilus vaginalis*). The present concept is that along with *G. vaginalis*, anaerobic organisms such as *Bacteroides* species, *Peptococcus* species, mobiluncus, *Prevotella* and *Mycoplasma hominis* act synergistically to cause vaginal infection. There is marked decrease in lactobacilli. It is the most common cause of symptomatic vaginitis (15–50%).

Clinically, it is characterized by creamy vaginal discharge with fishy smell in the absence of any inflammation on biopsy of the vagina.

There is marked decrease in lactobacilli. Risk factors for bacterial vaginosis are: Multiple or new sexual partners, early age of SI, cigeratte smoking, IUCD, Immunosupression.

Clinical Features

Bacterial vaginosis (BV) is characterized by malodorous vaginal discharge. The term vaginosis is preferred as there is no vaginal inflammation. The discharge is homogeneous, grayish-white and adherent to the vaginal wall.

Complications

- Recurrent infections leading to PID.
- Development of PID following abortion.
- Vaginal cuff cellulitis following hysterectomy.
- Pregnancy complications—second trimester miscarriage, PROM, preterm birth, endometritis.
- **Pregnancy-related complications** are:
  - PPROM
  - Preterm labor
  - Endometritis
  - Pregnancy loss before 20 weeks
  - Decreased success rate with IVF treatment

Diagnosis

Diagnosis

- **Amsel's four diagnostic criteria are:**
  1. Homogeneous vaginal discharge
  2. Vaginal pH >4.5 (litmus paper test)
  3. Positive **whiff tests** (*see* below)
  4. Presence of **clue cells** (>20% of cells)

  Three of these four criteria are sufficient for the presumptive diagnosis. Bacterial vaginal culture has no role in the diagnosis.
- **Gram stained vaginal smear (Hay/Ison):** Presence of more *Gardnerella* or mobiluncus morphotypes with few or absent lactobacilli.

Whiff test: Fishy (amine) odor when a drop of discharge is mixed with 10% potassium hydroxide solution.

Clue cells: A smear of vaginal discharge is prepared with drops of normal saline on a glass slide and is seen under a microscope. Vaginal epithelial cells are seen covered with these coccobacilli and the cells appear as stippled or granular. At times, the cells are so heavily stippled that the cell borders are obscured. **These stippled epithelial cells are called "clue cells" (Fig. 12.1).** Presence of clue cells (>20% of cells) are diagnostic of BV.

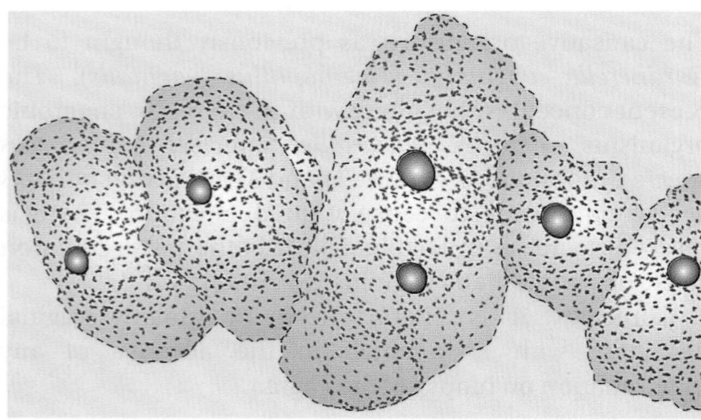

Fig. 12.1: Clue cells.

Treatment (CDC – 2015)

- Metronidazole 500 mg PO BID × 7 days
- Tinidazole 2 g orally for 3 days

Or

- Clindamycin 300 mg orally BID for 7 days and
- Clindamycin ovules 100 mg intravaginally, once at bed time for 3 days.

Sexual partner should be treated simultaneously. Cure rate is 80%.

HERPES GENITALIS

The causative organism is herpes simplex virus (HSV) type 1 and 2. It is usually transmitted sexually by an infected partner but may possibly be transmitted by orogenital contact. The incubation period is 2–14 days.

Clinical Features

Symptoms of the first attack usually appear less than 7 days after sexual contact. Initially, red painful inflammatory area appears commonly on the clitoris, labia, vestibule, vagina, perineum, and cervix. Multiple vesicles appear which progress into multiple shallow ulcers and ultimately heal up spontaneously by crusting. It takes about 3 weeks to complete the process. Inguinal lymphadenopathy occurs. Constitutional symptoms include fever, malaise, and headache. There may be vulvar burning, pruritus, dysuria, or retention of urine. Rarely, CNS infection causes encephalitis. The herpes virus resides in a latent phase in the dorsal root ganglia of S_2, S_3 and S_4.

First episodes are severe compared to the recurrent disease. Frequency of recurrent infection is high with HSV2.

Diagnosis

- Virus tissue culture and isolation—confirmatory.
- Detection of virus antigen by ELISA or immunofluorescent method.
- PCR test to identify the HSV DNA is the rapid, specific, and most accurate test.
- Western blot assay for antibodies to herpes is the most specific for diagnosing recurrent herpes.

Risks

- Physical and psychological trauma may precipitate recurrence.
- Adverse effects in primary infection during pregnancy.
  - Increased risks of miscarriage and preterm labor.
  - Transfer of infection from mother to neonates during vaginal delivery, if primary (50%) or recurrent (5%).
  - Baby may suffer from damage to central nervous system. Primary genital herpes is not an indication for MTP (TOP). Anomaly scan should be done at 20 weeks of gestation.
  - **Delivery by cesarean section is indicated with primary genital herpes infection at the time of delivery.**

Cautions

- **Recurrent episodes** are self-limiting and cause minor symptoms. Antiviral treatment is rarely needed.

- Daily suppressive therapy is given with valacyclovir 500 mg daily, at least for an year, when recurrences are >6 episodes per year.

Treatment (CDC – 2015)

Treatment of HSV 1 and HSV 2 is done as: **(a) Primary episode; (b) Recurrent episode; (c) Daily suppression.**

Rest and analgesics are helpful. **Acyclovir which inhibits the intracellular synthesis of DNA by the virus, has been found to be effective in acute attacks.**

Initial therapy	*Recurrent disease*	*Daily suppressive therapy*
▪ Acyclovir 200 mg five times daily × 7–10 days Or ▪ Valacyclovir 1 g twice daily × 7–10 days	▪ Acyclovir 400 mg thrice daily × 5 days Or ▪ Valacyclovir 1 g once daily × 5 days	▪ Acyclovir 400 mg twice daily Or ▪ Valacyclovir 1 g once daily

Acyclovir is effective in reducing the symptoms, duration of viral shedding, and helps in rapid healing. It has minimal toxicity. Its prophylactic use can reduce the episodes of recurrence.

HUMAN IMMUNODEFICIENCY VIRUS INFECTION AND ACQUIRED IMMUNODEFICIENCY SYNDROME

The Virus

The causative agents are human immunodeficiency viruses (HIV) of strains HIV1 and HIV2. HIV belongs to retrovirus (double-stranded RNA) family. Retroviruses possess the enzyme **reverse transcriptase** which allows viral RNA to be transcribed into DNA. The viral DNA when gets incorporated into the host cell genome, **chronic infection begins**. The basic structure of this icosahedral HIV (RNA-retrovirus) consists of a core protein (P-24) with glycoprotein (GP 120; GP 41) envelope. Of the various core antigens, **P-24 is most widely used for investigation study**. Antibodies to envelope proteins (GP 120) have got some protective role. The virus is destroyed by heating at 56°C for 30 minutes or by disinfectants with glutaraldehyde.

Incidence: The incidence is difficult to work out but the fact remains that the disease is spreading alarmingly fast both in the developed and developing countries and now has become a global problem (Table 12.4).

In South and South East Asia, an estimated 4 million people (more than 50% of them are women and children) were with HIV. In most Asian countries, infection rates are less than 0.5%.

TABLE 12.4: Risk factors for AIDS.

- Multiple sex partners
- Prostitution
- Homosexual males
- Intravenous drug abuser (IVDA)
- Multiple transfusions of blood or blood products
- Sexually transmitted disease
- Mother to infant

Predominent route of infection worldwide is heterosexual contact and vertical transmission.

Modes of Transmission of HIV

- **Sexual intercourse:** Women are affected more than the men because in female, larger mucosal surface is exposed and semen contains high viral load. Transmission of virus from male to female is high. Transmission is both by **heterosexual** and **homosexual contact**.
- **Intravenous drug abusers.**
- **Transfusion of infected** blood or blood products.
- **Use of contaminated needles**, needlestick injuries.
- **Breastfeeding:** Infected mothers may infect their children during breastfeeding through breast milk (10–20%). More so in presence of ulcers (cracked nipples).

  However, many health promoting benefits of breastfeeding may outweigh the risk of HIV transmission particularly in the developing world. For the other high-risk factors for AIDS (Table 12.4).
- **Perinatal transmission:** The vertical transmission to the neonates of the infected mothers is about 25–35%. The baby may be affected in utero (30%) through transplacental transfer, during delivery (70–75%) by contaminated secretions and blood of the birth canal.

Immunopathogenesis

The target for HIV is the CD4 receptor molecule. Cells within the immune system that have this molecule are: **CD4+ T lymphocytes** (predominantly affected), monocytes, macrophages and other antigen presenting cells like fibroblasts, neurons, renal, hepatic, and intestinal cells.

Following infection, there is profound cellular immunodeficiency as the CD4+ are progressively depleted by cytopathic effects of HIV.

Primary infection —3–6 weeks→ Acute syndrome —1 weeks to 3 months→
Immune response to HIV —1–2 weeks→ Clinical latency (7–10 years)

Immunological markers that are used to determine the **progression of the disease are:**

- CD4 T lymphocyte count—patients with count from 200–500 cells/mm^3 are more likely to have HIV-related symptoms and count <200 cells/mm^3 is taken into AIDS defining criteria.
- Measurement of HIV RNA levels by RT-PCR and the bDNA assays. Effectiveness of therapy is evaluated by monitoring of HIV RNA every 3–4 months.
- Raised P-24 (core) antigen titer—reflects the viral load.
- Raised serum β_2 microglobulin—reflects the immune response.

Clinical Presentation

Following exposure to HIV infection, a patient develops antibodies against HIV in about 8–12 weeks. The development of antibodies marks the stage of seroconversion and in some cases manifest clinically as a **'flu' like syndrome**.

Acute infection syndrome is characterized by fever, skin rash, arthralgia, lymphadenopathy, and diarrhea. This is called seroconversion illness. It lasts less than 2–3 weeks and resolves spontaneously.

After the initial exposure, the person remains asymptomatic for many years. The median time to develop AIDS is approximately 7–10 years. During this period, the patient shows progressive immune depletion. With increasing immunodeficiency, the person becomes susceptible to secondary infection by opportunistic organisms. Some individuals may just have persistent generalized lymphadenopathy during this period.

AIDS-related complex (ARC) refers to subjects having nonspecific clinical features of weight loss, fever, diarrhea, skin rash, lymphadenopathy, herpes simplex, oral or recurrent genital candidiasis, oral or genital ulcers, PID, tubo-ovarian abscess, and thrombocytopenia without full blown pictures of AIDS.

Any HIV infected individual with a CD4+ T cell count of <200/μL, has AIDS by definition regardless of the presence of symptoms or opportunistic diseases.

HIV-related Other Diseases

- Common secondary infections are: Atypical tuberculosis, pneumonia (*Pneumocystis carinii* pneumonia), systemic candidiasis, and meningitis.
- Encephalitis, myelopathy, and polyneuropathy are neurological manifestations.
- There is an increased incidence of high-grade lymphoid neoplasms, Kaposi sarcoma and non-Hodgkin's lymphoma.
- Viral infections with herpes simplex, human papilloma virus (HPV), and cytomegalovirus (CMV) are common.

Due to progressive immunosupression the woman is at risk of many opportunistic infections and tumors. Diagnostic criteria for AIDS are:

AIDS-defining Conditions

- Candidiasis of bronchi, trachea or lungs
- Cervical carcinoma (invasive)
- Cryptosporidiosis, chronic intestinal (1-month duration), encephalopathy HIV-related
- Kaposi's sarcoma
- Lymphoma (Burkitt's)
- Mycobacterium tuberculosis, any site
- Salmonella septicaemia (recurrent)
- Toxoplasmosis of brain
- Wasting syndrome, due to HIV

Gynecological Symptomatology

- **Infection of the genital tract** is high due to progressive immunodeficient state.
  - **Vaginitis** due to recurrent candidiasis. There may be oral, esophageal candidiasis also.
  - **Pelvic inflammatory diseases**—with other STIs (gonorrhea, syphilis, chlamydia) are more likely (p. 121, 123, 124).
- **Neoplasms of the genital tract are increased**
  - Increased incidence of CIN and carcinoma of the cervix. Colposcopy and cervical cytology screening should be routinely done.
  - Increased incidence of vulvar intraepithelial neoplasia (VIN).
- **Increased morbidity following gynecological surgery**
  - Increased risk of wound infection and chest infection, an intensive antibiotic therapy is needed.
- **Menstrual abnormality:** Menorrhagia, amenorrhea, or abnormal uterine bleeding may be due to associated weight loss, thrombocytopenia or opportunistic infections or neoplasms.
- **Fertility** is not generally affected.
- **Pregnancy does not worsen the disease** neither the disease affect pregnancy adversely.

Diagnosis

The effect on cellular immunity is manifested by decrease in CD4 cells. **An absolute CD4 cell count below 200/mm^3 is considered as cut off point when there is risk of opportunistic infections.**

The organism can be isolated from the blood, semen, vaginal secretions, breast milk, or saliva (body fluids) of the infected persons.

Diagnostic Tests for HIV

- Detection of IgG antibody to Gp 120 (envelope glycoprotein component) is **most commonly used.** Antibody production may take up to 3 months (window period) since the time of infection. These antibodies are not protective.
- Viral P-24 antigen can be detected very soon after the infection and it usually disappears by 8–10 weeks time.
- **ELISA (enzyme-linked immunosorbent assay)** is extremely sensitive (99.5%) but less specific. It is easy, cheap, and less time consuming (2–5 hours). As such, it can be employed as a screening procedure extended to 'at risk' persons.
- **Western blot or immunoblot:** It is highly specific but complicated and time consuming (1–2 days). It is expensive too.
- **HIV RNA by PCR** is **the gold standard for diagnosis of HIV**. Viral DNA is amplified following isolation of the virus from peripheral mononuclear cells. PCR amplification of cDNA generated from viral RNA is reliable up to 40 copies/mL of HIV RNA.

Causes of Death

- **Widespread infection** as it cannot be controlled effectively.
- **Profound immunodeficiency** leads to opportunistic infections and poor response to therapy.
- **Development** of unusual malignant lesions (lymphoma and Kaposi's sarcoma).

Treatment

- **Preventive**
- **Definitive**

Preventive Measures Include

- **'Safer sex'** practice with health education. Barrier methods (condoms and spermicides) are effective to reduce transmission (80%).

- **LNG-IUS with condoms** give excellent benefit.
- **Male circumcision** reduces transmission by 50%.
- **Use of blunt tipped needles** to avoid needle stick injury during surgery.
- **HIV negative blood** transfusion (screening of donors).
- **HIV negative** frozen semen to use for artificial donor insemination.
- **Postexposure prophylaxis** with zidovudine and lamivudine is advisable (described later).
- **Termination of pregnancy** in HIV positive women when requested.
- **Avoiding breastfeeding**—in the developing world, avoidance of breastfeeding may not be possible. Mother needs to be counseled as regard the risks and benefits of breastfeeding. **She is helped to make an informed choice**.
- **Infertility**—serodiscordant couples (female HIV negative) may have assisted conception with insemination following sperm washing.
- **Cervical cytology screening at yearly interval with co-testing.**
- **To maintain protocols** for correct handling of all body fluids (given later).
- **Widespread integrated counseling and testing** (ICT) in the clinic.

Definitive

HIV treatment protocols change frequently.

Antiretroviral therapy: Antiretroviral drugs are grouped into:

A. **Nucleoside reverse transcriptase inhibitors (NRTIs):** Zidovudine, Zalcitabine, Lamivudine, Abacavir.
B. **Non-nucleoside reverse transcriptase inhibitors (NNRTIs):** Delavirdine, Nevirapine, Efavirenz.
C. **Protease inhibitors (PI):** Indinavir, Saquinavir, Ritonavir.
D. **Entry inhibitor:** Enfuvirtide.
E. **Integrase inhibitor:** Raltegravir. The combinations of these drugs are effective in increasing CD4 counts and reducing viral load. Monotherapy is not preferred as it hastens drug resistance. Combination therapy is known by the acronym **HAART** (Highly Active Antiretroviral Therapy).

Drug combinations: Up-to-date treatment recommendations are available at: www.cdcnpin.org.

- Two from Gr A (NRTIs) plus one from Gr B or 2 from Gr A (NRTIs) plus one from Gr C (PI).

Plasma HIV RNA levels indicate the degree of viral replication and CD4+ T cell count indicate level of immune competence.

Important side effects of drugs are: Lactic acidosis, anemia, granulocytopenia, pancreatitis, peripheral neuropathy, hepatic dysfunction and carbohydrate intolerance.

When to start therapy:

- Acute HIV infection syndrome.
- Symptomatic HIV infection.
- Asymptomatic but CD4 cell count <350 cells/mm^3 or with viral load—HIV RNA >50,000 copies/mL.
- Postexposure prophylaxis (given below).
- Patients with CD4 count <200/mm^3 should also receive trimethoprim and sulfamethoxazole combination (*P. carinii* prophylaxis).
- Opportunistic infections (*Mycobacterium*) should be treated simultaneously with specific drugs when CD4+ T cells <50/mm^3.
- Pregnant women or women with HIV associated nephropathy should have HAART therapy.

With effective treatment viral load should reach 'undetectable' levels (<50 copies/mL) and CD4 count should rise.

Efavirenz is the first line therapy in all patients **unless she is planning to conceive and has primary NRTI or NNRTI resistance**.

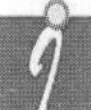

PRECAUTIONS TO PREVENT OCCUPATIONAL TRANSMISSION OF HIV (UNIVERSAL BLOOD AND BODY FLUID PRECAUTIONS)

- All blood and body fluids should be considered potentially infectious for HIV.
- Nonsurgical management whenever possible.
- Barrier precautions: Use of cap, mask, gown, double gloves, eye wear (goggles), and boots.
- Use of blunt tipped needles (risk of HIV infection following needle stick injury is 0.3%).
- Washing of anybody fluid contamination off the skin immediately.
- Use of disposable syringes, needles and anesthetic circuits.
- Resuscitation bags or mouthpieces should be available for emergency resuscitation.
- Thorough theater disinfection after the operation.

When to change therapy: (a) Failure to reduce viral load; (b) Persistently declining CD4+ T cell count; (c) Clinical deterioration; (d) In presence of side effects due to drugs.

Postexposure prophylaxis: A combination of two NRTIs is given for 4 weeks. Prophylactic use of zidovudine (300 mg BID) and lamivudine (150 mg BID) for a period of 4 weeks immediately following an exposure may reduce the risk of seroconversion (CDC – 2001).

Preconception Counseling

It is done about the impact of HIV infection on preganancy, perinatal transmission, side effects of medication and mode of delivery. Patient is advised regarding vaccinations prior conceiving (c.f. HPV vaccine, Ch. 23).

GENITAL WARTS (CONDYLOMA ACUMINATA)

Condylomata are papillary lesions caused by **Human Papilloma Virus (HPV) usually type 6 and 11** (p. 270). These are usually multiple and can be contaminated from other parts of the body. They can be transmitted sexually. Associated vaginal discharge favors their growth and so does pregnancy. Typically, they grow in clusters along a narrow stalk giving it a cauliflower appearance but at times the stalk may be broad and thick (Fig. 12.2).

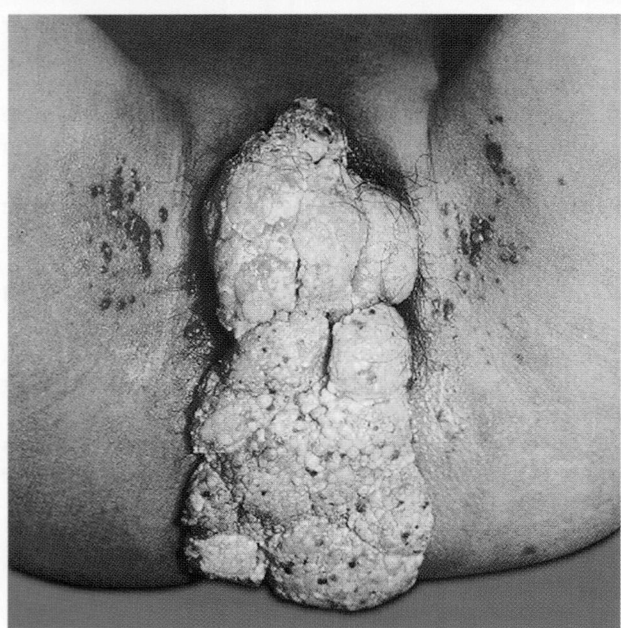

Fig. 12.2: Giant condyloma acuminata of vulva.

The condylomata may at times, spread to the vagina or even the cervix. **Anatomic distribution of anogenital HPV infection is: Cervix 70%, Vulva 25%, Vagina 10%, and Anus 20%.** The lesion should be differentiated from syphilitic condylomata or vulvar carcinoma. Very rarely, it becomes malignant. Conditions known to predispose women to infection with HPV are: Immunosuppression, diabetes, pregnancy, and local trauma.

There may be an **association between HPV infection and malignant epithelial transformation of the cervix, vagina, and vulva. It is usually associated with HPV types 16, 18, 45, 56 (p. 270).**

Treatment

HPV vaccine (Types 6 and 11) can prevent 90% of condyloma (p. 266+). Most low risk and two-thirds of high risk HPV infections are spontaneously eradicated over a 24 months period.

Different treatment modalities used are: Cryotherapy (with liquid nitrogen), laser therapy, surgical excision or topical use of imiquimod cream, trichloro-acetic acid, intralesional interferon or photodynamic therapy.

MOLLUSCUM CONTAGIOSUM

Molluscum contagiosum is caused by a pox virus transmitted by body contact or towels or clothing. It is commonly seen in immunodeficient subject or with HIV infections. They vary in size up to 1 cm, dome-shaped, flesh color and often umbilicated. They are usually multiple and can occur anywhere in the skin and genitalia. Microscopic appearance reveals numerous inclusion bodies (molluscum bodies) in the cytoplasm of the cells with Giemsa stain.

Treatment

It is usually self-limiting and resolves spontaneously in immunocompetent subjects. However, treatment will decrease sexual transmission and autoinoculation of the virus. Immunocompromised individuals are treated with HAART.

Evacuation of caseous material from the nodule under local anesthetic is done. The floor of the nodule is then treated chemically with ferric subsulfate or trichloroacetic acid (85%) solution.

Cryotherapy with liquid nitrogen is applied until a halo of ice is formed around the lesion. Repeat application may be necessary.

PEDICULOSIS PUBIS

The infective agent is a crab louse (*Phthirus pubis*) which affects the coarse hair of the pubis. The louse alongwith its eggs are attached to the hair. It is transmitted by sexual contact or infected clothes encouraged by inadequate hygiene. It produces intense pruritis → scratching → secondary infection → suppuration.

Treatment

Permethrin cream (1%) is applied over the affected area and washed off after 10 minutes. Lindane 1% is used as a shampoo. Ivermectin 200 mg/kg orally is given and is repeated in 2 weeks.

Treatment may also be done by application of 1% gamma-benzene hexachloride or malathion (0.5%) cream. After rubbing the preparation, the area should not be washed after 12 hours. The application may be repeated after 4 days, if necessary. It is mandatory to treat the contact and sterilize the clothings by boiling.

SCABIES

This is caused by *Sarcoptes scabiei*. It produces intense itching and often excoriation of skin. It is often associated with poor local hygiene.

Treatment

Permethrin cream 5% or malathion 0.5% aguan solution is applied to all areas of the body below the neck and washed off after 8–14 hours.

The treatment is also done by local application of 25% benzyl benzoate emulsion for the entire body below the neck. Single application is often enough. The clothings should be boiled. The family members are also to be treated simultaneously to prevent reinfection.

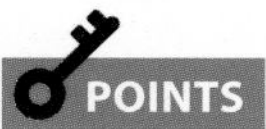

POINTS

- **Sexually transmitted infections (STIs)** includes those diseases which are predominantly transmitted through sexual contact from an infected partner. A patient with a STI is likely to have another one. *Chlamydia trachomatis* is now on the top in the list of the organisms causing STIs, the other common diseases are bacterial vaginosis, gonorrhea, syphilis, herpes genitalis and trichomonas vaginitis.
- ***Neisseria gonorrhoeae*** commonly invades the columnar and transitional epithelium of the genitourinary tract (endocervix, urethra, Bartholin's gland). Infertility, ectopic pregnancy, and chronic pelvic pain are the long-term complications (p. 121). Investigations should include for other STIs also.
- **Herpes genitalis** is caused by herpes simplex virus (HSV) type 1 and 2. Acyclovir orally in doses of 200 mg 5 times a day for 7 days is effective in reducing the constitutional symptoms, duration of viral shedding, and helps rapid healing.
- **Syphilis** is caused by *Treponema pallidum*. The hard chancre of primary syphilis is painless with an indurated base. VDRL and TPHA tests are used for screening and FTA-abs is used for confirmation. Treatment according to CDC recommendation includes Benzathine-penicillin IM (p. 124).
- **Chancroid** (soft sore) is caused by a gram-negative *Haemophilus ducreyi* and is always painful. Unilateral inguinal lymphadenitis may occur which may suppurate to form abscess. Demonstration of ducreyi bacillus from the discharge of the ulcer or aspirated pus from the lymph gland is confirmatory. Ceftriaxone 250 mg IM single dose is effective.
- **Granuloma inguinale** is caused by gram-negative *Donovania granulomatis*. There is localized ulcer formation without lymph node suppuration and abscess formation. Diagnosis is confirmed by demonstrating *Donovan bodies* within the mononuclear cells (p. 125). Doxycycline, 100 mg BID for at least 3 weeks is effective.
- **Lymphogranuloma venereum** is caused by L serotype *Chlamydia trachomatis*. The inguinal glands are involved early, become necrosed and abscess forms. Healing occurs with intense fibrosis and lymphatic obstruction (p. 125). Doxycycline 100 mg BID for atleast 21 days is effective.
- **AIDS** is caused by human immunodeficiency virus (HIV). The methods of transmission are by sexual intercourse, transfusion of contaminated blood or blood products, use of contaminated needles, and vertical transmission to the baby (25–35%) during pregnancy and childbirth. Male condom is protective. It suppresses the immune system (depletion of CD4+ T lymphocytes) so that the opportunistic organisms flare up.
- **Plasma HIV-RNA levels** indicate the degree of viral replication and CD4+ T cell count indicate level of immune competence (p. 128). Viral DNA amplification and detection by PCR is gold standard. Any HIV infected individual with CD4 + T cell count <200/ µL has AIDS.
- **HIV related other diseases are:** Recurrent vaginal candidiasis, PID, CIN, VIN, atypical tuberculosis, and others as observed in an immunocompromised patient. Preventive measures (p. 128) and infection control during surgery must be rigorous.
- **HAART** inhibits reverse transcriptase and slows down the progress of the disease. For HIV treatment protocols (p. 129). HAART increases CD4 count and reduces viral load. Monotherapy hastens development of drug resistance.
- **Barrier method of contraception** (condom) is effective to reduce the risk of HIV transmission and to prevent unwanted pregnancy. In addition, another contraceptive may be used to increase the contraceptive efficiency. LNG-IUS with condoms give excellent benefit.
- **High-risk factors for AIDS** (Table 12.4) and preventive measures (p. 127) must be considered in controlling AIDS.
- **Condyloma accuminata** is viral (HPV) in origin. **HPV vaccine** can prevent 90% of condyloma (p. 130).
- **Molluscum contagiosum** is caused by pox virus. It is commonly seen with immunodeficient subjects (p. 130).
- **Bacterial vaginosis** is caused by *Gardnerella vaginalis*. The vaginal discharge is homogeneous, adherent to vaginal wall with pH >4.7 and has an fishy odor when mixed with KOH solution (Whiff test). Presence of **clue cells** (stippled epithelial cells) on the wet smear of vaginal discharge is diagnostic. Oral metronidazole is highly effective.
- **Trichomona vaginalis** is a common STI in women. It is highly contagious. Bacterial vaginosis is involved in 50%; candidiasis and trichomonias are involved in 25% each, amongst all cases of vaginitis. Differentiation of vaginal discharge is helpful for the clinical diagnosis and management (Table 13.1).

CHAPTER

13 Infections of the Individual Pelvic Organ

CHAPTER OUTLINE

VULVAR INFECTION

The vulvar and perineal skin is usually resistant to common infection. But the defense is lost following constant irritation by the vaginal discharge or urine (urinary incontinence). Furthermore, there may be atrophy or degenerative changes, either in disease or following menopause when the infection is more likely. The vulvar infection can thus occur de novo or may be affected secondarily. The primary site may be elsewhere in the adjacent structures. **In this section, only the lesions affecting primarily—the vulva will be discussed.**

It is indeed difficult to classify the vulvar infection but the following etiological classification is of help.

I. Due to specific infection.
II. Due to sensitive reaction.
III. Due to vaginal discharge or urinary contamination.

VULVITIS DUE TO SPECIFIC INFECTION

Bacterial

- Pyogenic (nongonococcal)
- Sexually transmitted diseases (p. 121)
  - Gonorrhea (p. 121)
  - Syphilis (p. 123)
  - Chancroid (p. 124)
  - Lymphogranuloma venereum (p. 125)
  - Granuloma inguinale (p. 125)
- Tubercular (p. 113)

Viral

- Condylomata accuminata (p. 129)
- Herpes genitalis (p. 126)
- Molluscum contagiosum (p. 130)
- Herpes zoster.

Fungal

- Moniliasis (p. 135)
- Ringworm.

Parasitic

- Pediculosis pubis (p. 130)
- Scabies (p. 130)
- Threadworm.

INFECTIONS OF BARTHOLIN'S GLAND

Bartholin's glands are the two pea sized (2 cm) glands, located in the groove between the hymen and the labia minora at 5 o'clock and 7 o'clock position of the vagina.

Causative organisms: Although *Gonococcus* is always in mind but more commonly other pyogenic organisms such as *Escherichia coli, Staphylococcus, Streptococcus, Chlamydia trachomatis, Bacteroides, Peptostreptococcus* or mixed types (polymicrobial) are involved.

Pathology: Both the gland and the duct are involved. The epithelium of the gland or the duct gets swollen. The lumen of the duct may be blocked or remains open through which exudates escape out.

Fate: The infection may resolute completely or an abscess is formed. In others, the infection subsides only to recur in future. In such cases, the gland becomes fibrotic. Too often, the duct lumen heals by fibrosis with closure of the orifice → pent up secretion of the gland → formation of Bartholin cyst. **Thus, the end results of acute bartholinitis are:** (a) Complete resolution; (b) Recurrence; (c) Abscess; (d) Cyst formation.

Clinical Features

Initially, there is local pain and discomfort even to the extent of difficulty in walking or sitting. Examination reveals tenderness and induration of the posterior half of the labia when palpated between thumb outside and the index finger inside the vagina (Fig. 9.6). The duct opening looks congested and secretion comes out through the opening when the gland is pressed by fingers. The secretion should be collected with a swab for bacteriological examination.

Treatment

Hot compress over the area and analgesics to relieve pain are instituted. Systemic antibiotic like amoxicillin-clavulanate orally 8 hourly is effective or else appropriate antibiotic according to the bacteriological sensitivity should be instituted.

Recurrent bartholinitis: Periodic painful attacks cause problems in 5–10% women. Excision of the gland with the duct may have to be done in the quiescent phase.

BARTHOLIN'S ABSCESS

Bartholin's abscess is the end result of acute bartholinitis. The duct gets blocked by fibrosis and the exudates pent up inside to produce abscess. If left uncared for, the abscess may burst through the lower vaginal wall. A sinus tract may remain open with periodic discharge through it.

Clinical Features

The local pain and discomfort become intense. The patient cannot walk or even sit. Fever is often associated.

On examination, there is an unilateral tender swelling beneath the posterior half of the labium majus expanding medially to the posterior part of the labium minus. The overlying skin appears red and edematous.

Treatment

Rest is imposed. Pain is relieved by analgesics and daily sitz bath. Systemic antibiotic—ampicillin 500 mg orally 8 hourly or tetracycline in chlamydial infection is effective. Abscess should be drained at the earliest opportunity before it bursts spontaneously.

In case of recurrent Bartholin's abscess, excision should be done in the quiescent phase after the infection is controlled.

BARTHOLIN'S CYST

There is closure of the duct or the opening of an acinus. The cause may be infection or trauma followed by fibrosis and occlusion of the lumen.

Pathology

It may develop in the duct (common) or in the gland. **Commonly, it involves the duct**; the gland is adherent to it posterolaterally. Cyst of the duct or gland can be differentiated by the lining epithelium. The content is glairy colorless fluid—secretion of the Bartholin's gland.

Clinical Features

A small size often remains unnoticed to the patient or escapes attention to the physician even following internal examination. If it becomes large (size of hen's egg), there is local discomfort and dyspareunia. Examination reveals an unilateral **swelling on the posterior** half of the labium majus which opens up at the posterior end of the labium minus. Its medial projection makes the vulvar cleft 'S'-shaped. The overlying skin is thin and shiny. The cyst is fluctuant and not tender (Fig. 13.1).

Treatment

Marsupialization is the gratifying surgery for Bartholin's cyst. An incision is made on the inner aspect of the labium minus just outside the hymenal ring. The incision includes the vaginal wall and the cyst wall. The cut margins of the either side are to be trimmed off to make the opening an elliptical shape and of about 1 cm in diameter. The edges of the vaginal and cyst walls are sutured by interrupted catgut, thus leaving behind a clean circular opening.

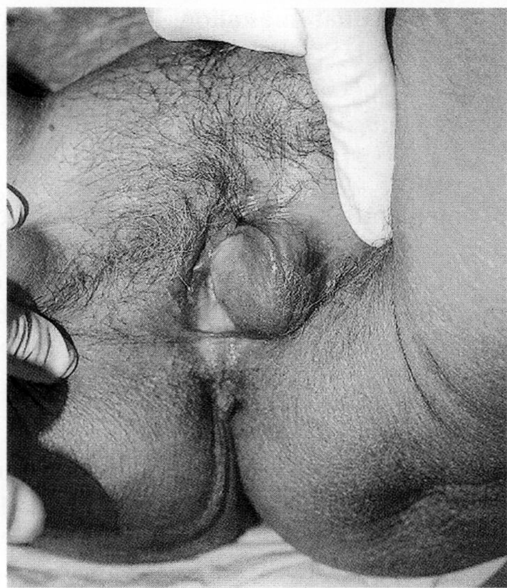

Fig. 13.1: Bartholin's cyst (*left*).

Ciprofloxacin or second generation cephalosporin are used to control infection.

The advantages of marsupialization over the traditional excision operation are: (a) Simple; (b) Can be done even under local anesthesia; (c) Shorter hospital stay (24 hours); (d) Postoperative complication is almost nil; and (e) Gland function (moisture) remains intact.

Catheter drainage of the abscess cavity following incisional drainage has also been done.

VAGINAL INFECTION (VAGINITIS)

- Vulvovaginitis in childhood
- Trichomoniasis
- Moniliasis
- Vaginitis due to *Chlamydia trachomatis*
- Atrophic vaginitis
- Nonspecific vaginitis
- Toxic shock syndrome.

VULVOVAGINITIS IN CHILDHOOD

Inflammatory conditions of the vulva and vagina are the most common disorders during childhood. Due to lack of estrogen, the vaginal defense is lost and the infection occurs easily, once introduced inside the vagina.

Etiology

- Nonspecific vulvovaginitis
- Presence of foreign body in the vagina

- Associated intestinal infestations—threadworm being the most common.
- Rarely, more specific infection caused by *Candida albicans* or *Gonococcus* may be implicated.

Clinical Features

The chief complaints are pruritus of varying degree and vaginal discharge. There may be painful micturition.

Inspection reveals soreness of the vulva. The labia minora may be swollen and red. If a foreign body is suspected, a vaginal examination with an aural or nasal speculum may help in diagnosis.

Investigations

The vaginal discharge is collected with a platinum loop and two smears are taken, one for direct examination and the other for Gram stain.

A small amount may be taken with a pipette for culture in Stuart's media. To exclude intestinal infestation, stool examination is of help.

Vaginoscopy is needed to exclude foreign body or tumor in a case with recurrent infection.

Treatment

In most cases, the cause remains unknown. Simple perineal hygiene will relieve the symptoms. In cases of soreness or after removal of foreign body, estrogen cream is to be applied locally, every night for two weeks. When the specific organisms are detected, therapy should be directed to cure the condition.

TRICHOMONAS VAGINILIS

Vaginal trichomoniasis is the most common and important cause of vaginitis in the childbearing period.

Causative Organism

It is caused by *Trichomonas vaginalis*, a pear-shaped unicellular flagellate anaerobic protozoa. It measures 20 μ long and 10 μ wide (larger than a WBC). It has got four anterior flagellae and a spear-like protrusion at the other end with an undulating membrane surrounding its anterior two-third. It is actively motile (Fig. 13.2).

Mode of Transmission

The organism is predominantly transmitted by sexual contact, the male harbors the infection in the urethra and prostate. It is a highly contagious STI. The transmission may also be possible by the toilet articles from one woman to the other or through examining gloves. The incubation period is 3–28 days.

Pathology

In about 25% of women in the reproductive period, the parasites harbor in the vagina is in asymptomatic state. When the local defense is impaired—during and after menstruation, after sexual stimulation, and following illness, the pH of the vagina is raised to 5.5–6.5. At this level of pH, the trichomonads thrive. The organisms usually lie in between the rugae and produce surface inflammatory reaction when the defense is lost. In about 75% cases, the organism can be isolated from the urethra, Skene's tubules or even from the Bartholin's glands.

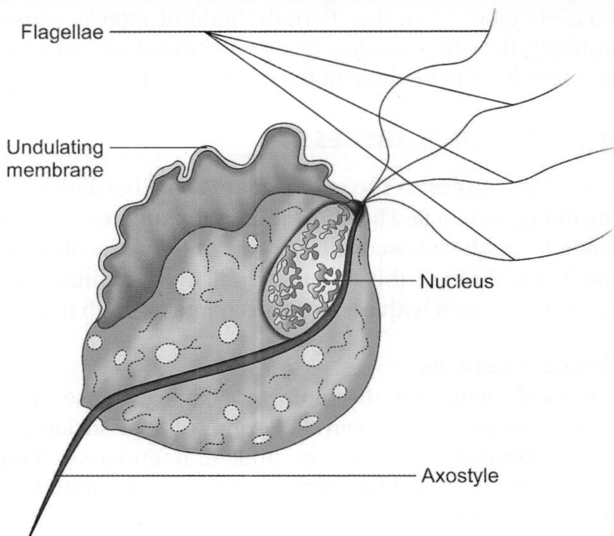

Fig. 13.2: Physical appearance of *Trichomonas vaginalis*.

Clinical Features

- **Sudden profuse and offensive vaginal discharge** often dating from the last menstruation.
- **Irritation and itching** of varying degrees within and around the introitus are common.
- **Urinary symptoms**: Dysuria and frequency of micturition.
- **History** of previous similar attacks.

Women with trichomoniasis should be evaluated for other STDs including *N. gonorrhoea, C. trachomatis,* and HIV (Table 13.1).

On Examination

- **Vaginal discharge: Thin, gray, greenish-yellow, frothy and offensive.**
- **The vulva** is inflamed with evidences of pruritus.
- **Vaginal examination** may be painful. The vaginal walls become red and inflamed with multiple punctate hemorrhagic spots. Similar spots are also found over the mucosa of the portio vaginalis part of the cervix on speculum examination. This gives the appearance of a **'strawberry'** (Fig. 13.3). The sign of a strawberry appearance of the upper vagina and the cervix is the classic but rare (10%).

Diagnosis

- Identification of the trichomonas is done by **hanging drop preparation**. If found negative even on repeat examination, the confirmation may be done by culture.
- NAATs are 3–5 times more sensitive than wet preparation. NAAT can be done with vaginal discharge or urine.

TABLE 13.1: Differential diagnosis of vaginal discharge.

Characteristics	*Trichomoniasis*	*Candidiasis*	*Bacterial vaginosis*	*Chlamydia*	*Normal vaginal discharge*
Color	Gray, yellow or green	Curdy white	Gray white to green yellow white	Mucopurulent	White, clear
Consistency	Thin, frothy, adherent	Thick	Thin, adherent homogeneous	Thick	Thin
Whiff test (p. 125)	Negative Has unpleasant odor	Negative	Positive (Fishy amine)	Negative	Negative
pH	≥4.5	<4.5	≥4.5	<4.5	<4–4.5
Pruritus	+++, dysuria	++	Nonirritating	—	—
Diagnosis (Wet mount microscopy)	Motile trichomonas (p. 89)	Hyphae and buds, spores	Clue cells (>20%) (p. 126), amine odor after adding KOH to wet mount; ↓ lactobacilli	Chlamydia NAAT (p. 124)	—
Treatment	Metronidazole 500 mg PO BID × 7 days Or 200 mg TID × 7 days	▪ Clotrimazole intravaginal 1–3 days ▪ Fluconazole 150 mg PO weekly for 6 weeks	Metronidazole 500 mg PO BID × 7 days	Azithromycin 1 g orally single dose	—

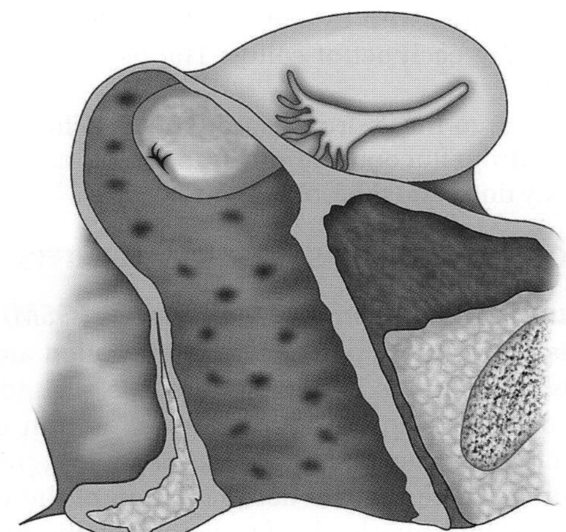

Fig. 13.3: Punctate hemorrhagic spots and 'strawberry' appearance on vaginal walls in trichomonas negatives.

In suspected cases, gonococcal or monilial infection should be excluded.

Treatment

The treatment is very much effective with nitroimidazole. **Metronidazole** 200 mg thrice daily by mouth is to be given for 1 week. A single dose regimen of 2 g is an alternative. Tinidazole single dose 2 g PO is equally effective. The husband should be given the same treatment schedule for 1 week. Resistance to metronidazole is extremely rare. Metronidazole is safe in all trimesters of pregnancy. Women should not take alcohol for 24 hours after metronidazole to avoid disulfiram like reaction. Patients should be screened with NAAT in 3 months due to high reinfection rates. The **husband** should use condom during coitus irrespective of contraceptive practice until the wife is cured.

CANDIDA VAGINITIS (MONILIASIS)

Causative Organism

Moniliasis is caused by *Candida albicans*, a gram-positive yeast-like fungus (Fig. 13.4). The risk factors for candida vaginitis are listed in Table 13.2.

Clinical Features

The patient complains of vaginal discharge with intense vulvovaginal pruritus. **The pruritis is out of proportion to the discharge**. There may be dyspareunia due to local soreness.

On Examination

- The discharge is thick, curdy white and in flakes, (cottage cheese type) often adherent to the vaginal wall (Fig. 13.5).

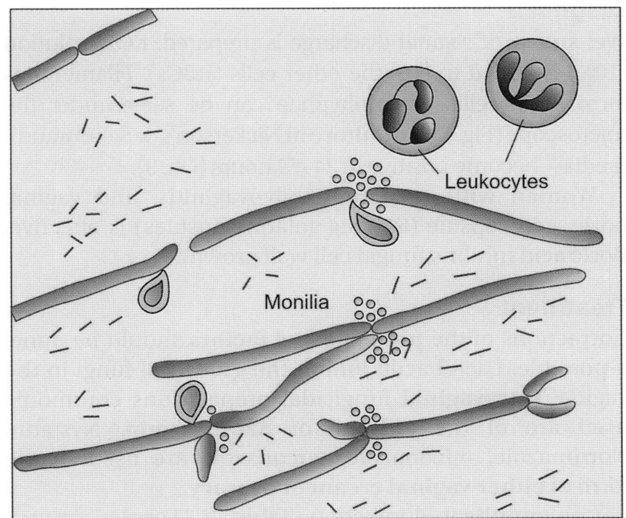

Fig. 13.4: Physical appearance of *Candida albicans* dimorphic features (yeast buds and hyphal forms) are seen.

TABLE 13.2: Risk factors for candida vaginitis.

Diabetes:	↑ Glycogen in the cells, glycosuria
Pregnancy:	↑ Vaginal acidity, glycosuria ↑ Glycogen in the cells *lactobacillus*
Broad-spectrum antibiotics: ↓ Acid forming *lactobacillus*	
Combined oral pills **Immunosuppression**—HIV **Drugs**—steroids **Thyroid, parathyroid disease** **Obesity**	

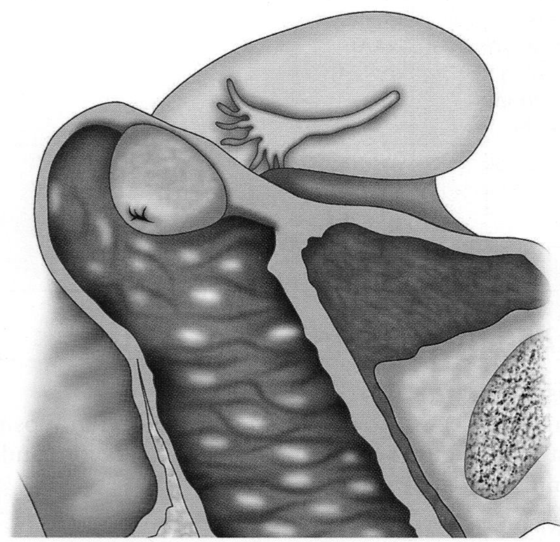

Fig. 13.5: Curdy white flakes adherent to the vaginal wall.

- Vulva may be red and swollen with evidences of pruritus.
- Vaginal examination may be tender. Removal of the white flakes reveals multiple oozing spots.
- Atrophy of the vulvovaginal structures are common in menopause due to deficiency of estrogen.

Diagnosis

Wet smear of vaginal discharge is prepared. KOH solution (10%) is added to lyse the other cells (RBCs). Filamentous form of mycella, pseudohyphae can be seen under the microscope (Fig. 13.4). **Culture** in Nickerson's or Sabouraud's media—become positive in 24–72 hours (Ch. 9).

Women with recurrent vulvovaginitis, and vaginal boric acid capsule (600 mg gelatin capsules) is effective. Boric acid inhibits fungal cell wall growth.

Treatment

Corrections of the **predisposing factors** should be done, if possible. Lactobacilli inhibit the growth of fungi in the vagina. **Intravaginal** fungicidal preparations commonly used are of the polyene or **azole group**. Nystatin, clotrimazole, miconazole, terconazole are used in the form of **either vaginal cream** or **pessary**.

For **uncomplicated** infection (Table 13.3) azoles are very effective.

- **Uncomplicated vulvovaginal candidiasis:**

TABLE 13.3: Classification of vulvovaginal candidiasis (CDC – 2015).

Uncomplicated	*Complicated*
Sporadic or infrequent Mild to moderate in severity Likely to be *C. albicans* Nonimmune compromised women	Recurrent Severe Non-albicans candidiasis Women with uncontrolled diabetes, debilitation or immunosuppression

  - Topical antifungal agents for 1–3 days. OR
  - A single oral dose of fluconazole or itraconazole.
- **Complicated vulvovaginitis (Table 13.3):**
  - Topical azoles 2 doses for 7–14 days.
  - Oral therapy—a second dose of fluconazole 150 mg, 72 hours after the first dose.
  - Vaginal boric acid capsules (600 mg in gelatin capsule) is the other option.

The treatment should be continued even during menstruation.

Associated **intestinal moniliasis** should be treated by fluconazole 50 mg daily orally for 7 days. Husband should be treated with nystatin ointment locally for few days following each act of coitus. The use of condom is preferred.

Resistance to these drugs is not known. The systemic antifungal drugs fluconazole and itraconazole are effective in a weekly dose oral therapy.

ATROPHIC VAGINITIS (SENILE VAGINITIS)

Genitourinary Syndrome of Menopause (GSM)

Vaginitis in postmenopausal women is called atrophic vaginitis. The term is preferable to senile vaginitis. The vaginal defense is lost. Vaginal mucosa is thin due to deficiency of estrogen and is more susceptible to infection and trauma. There may be desquamation of the vaginal epithelium which may lead to formation of adhesions and bands between the walls.

Clinical Features

- Yellowish or blood stained vaginal discharge
- Discomfort, dryness, soreness in the vulva
- Dyspareunia.

On Examination

- Evidences of pruritus vulvae.
- Vaginal examination is often painful and the walls are found inflamed.

Diagnosis

Senile endometritis may coexist and **carcinoma body or the cervix should be excluded prior to therapy**.

Treatment

Improvement of general health and treatment of infection if present should be done. Systemic estrogen therapy may be considered if there is no contraindication. This improves the vaginal epithelium, raises glycogen content, and lowers vaginal pH.

Intravaginal application of estrogen cream by an applicator is also effective. About one-third of the vaginal estrogen is systemically absorbed.

TOXIC SHOCK SYNDROME

Toxic shock syndrome (TSS) is a febrile illness with abrupt onset following infection caused by *Staphylococcus aureus*. It is commonly seen about 2 days after the surgery or onset of menstruation. Due to the bacterial exotoxin (TSS-1), it may have a fulminating course with multiorgan dysfunction. These days menstruation related TSS are less common compared to severe postoperative infections. **It is characterized by several features with abrupt onset.**

Diagnostic Criteria of TSS

- **Major criteria**
  - **Hypotension** (systolic BP <90 mm Hg)
  - **Temperature** ≥38.8°C
  - **Late skin desquamation** (palms, hands, soles)
  - **Diffuse macular erythroderma**
- **Minor criteria**
  - **Gastrointestinal:** Diarrhea, vomiting
  - **Hematologic platelets:** Count ≤100,000 mm^3
  - **Renal:** ↑BUN, creatinine (>twice the normal)
  - **Respiratory:** ARDS
  - **Hepatic:** ↑SGOT, ↑SGPT, ↑Bilirubin (>twice the normal)
  - **Muscular:** Myalgia
  - **Mucous membrane:** Hyperemia (oral, pharyngeal, vaginal)
  - **CNS:** Altered consciousness, disorientation

It may lead to multiorgan system failure. Blood cultures are negative.

Treatment is supportive. Correction of hypovolemia and hypotension with intravenous fluids and dopamine infusion is done in an intensive care unit. Parenteral corticosteroids may be used. Blood coagulation parameters and serum electrolytes are checked and corrected.

Mechanical ventilation is required for women with ARDS.

- **Cases with methicillin-susceptible *S. aureus*:** Clindamycin 600 mg IV 8 hourly plus oxacillin 2 g IV 4 hourly is given for 10–14 days.
- **Methicillin-resistant *S. aureus* (MRSA):** Clindamycin plus vancomycin (30 mg/kg/day) IV in two divided doses or linezolid 600 mg IV every 12 hours is recommended. Therapy should not wait for the culture report.
- Death has been reported (5%) despite treatment due to complications like ARDS, DIC or persistent hypotension as myocardial failure.

CERVICITIS

The term cervicitis is reserved to **infection of the endocervix including the glands and the stroma.** The infection may be acute or chronic. Cervical mucus is a physical barrier to infection. Moreover, it exerts a bacteriostatic effect. Cervical mucous contains antibodies and inflammatory cells that prevent many STTs.

ACUTE CERVICITIS

The **endocervical infection** usually follows child-birth, abortion, or any operation on cervix. The responsible organisms are pyogenic (p. 106). Other common pathogens are: ***Gonococcus, Chlamydia trachomatis, Trichomonas, bacterial vaginosis, Mycoplasma, HSV and HPV***, the first one being less common nowadays.

The organisms gain entry into the glands of the endocervix and produce acute inflammatory changes. The infection may be localized or spread upwards to involve the tube or sidewards involving the parametrium.

Clinical Features

The vaginal examination is painful. The cervix is tender on touch or movements. Cervix looks edematous and congested. **Mucopurulent discharge** is seen escaping out through the external os.

Prognosis

Prognosis may include: (a) It may resolve completely; (b) The infection may spread to involve the adjacent structures or even beyond that; (c) Becomes chronic.

Treatment

High vaginal and endocervical swabs are taken for bacteriological identification and drug sensitivity test. Appropriate antibiotics should be prescribed. General measures are to be taken as outlined in acute pelvic infection (Ch. 11).

CHRONIC CERVICITIS

Chronic cervicitis is the most common lesion found in women attending gynecologic outpatient. It may follow an acute attack or usually chronic from the beginning. **The endocervix is a potential reservoir for *N. gonorrhoea, Chlamydia*, HPV, *Mycoplasma* and bacterial vaginosis.**

Pathology

The mucosa and the deeper tissues are congested, fibrosed, and infiltrated with leukocytes and plasma cells. The glands are also hypertrophied with increased secretory activity. Some of the gland opening mouths are closed by fibrosis or plugs of desquamated epithelial cells to cause retention cyst—**nabothian follicles** (Fig. 19.4). There is associated lacerated and everted endocervix, the so-called **eversion or ectropion.**

Clinical Features

There may not be any symptom. Excessive **mucopurulent discharge**, is the predominant symptom. History of contact bleeding may be present.

On Examination

(a) The cervix may be tender to touch or on movement; (b) Speculum examination reveals—**mucoid or mucopurulent discharge escaping out through the cervical os.** Associated tear in cervix may be present (Fig. 13.6).

Treatment

Cervical scrape cytology to exclude malignancy is mandatory prior to any therapy.

- There is a need of antimicrobial therapy in cases with *C. trachomatis*, gonococcal or proved cases of bacterial vaginosis.

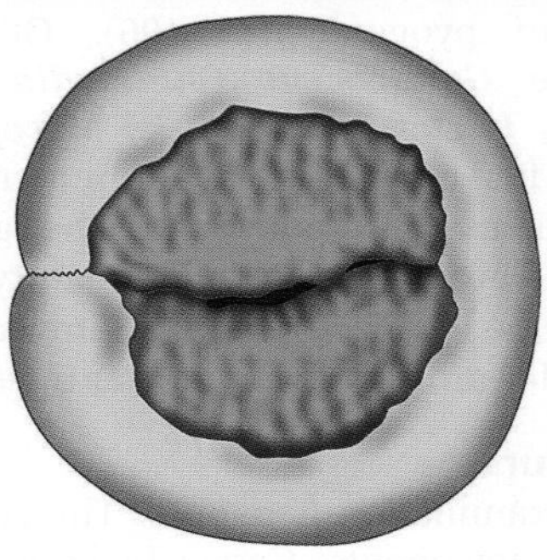

Fig. 13.6: Ectropion with unilateral tear of the cervix.

- For presumptive cervicitis, therapy includes azithromycin 1 g orally, a single dose of doxycycline 100 mg orally BID for 7 days.
- The diseased tissue may be destroyed by electro or diathermy cauterization or laser or cryosurgery. The ectropion is corrected by deep linear burns and the coincidental ectopy may be coagulated.
- **Mucopurulent cervicitis,** is characterized by observation of yellow mucopurulent material on a white cotton swab and presence of ≥10 polymorphonuclear leukocytes per microscopic field on Gram-stained smear. On clinical examination there is cervical ectopy with erythema and edema associated with bleeding. There is endocervical ulceration also. *C. trachomatis* and *N. gonorrhoea* are the causes of mucopurulent cervicitis. Treatment includes empirical therapy for *C. trachomatis* or *N. gonorrhoea*.

ENDOMETRITIS

During childbearing period, infection hardly occurs in the endometrium except in septic abortion or puerperal sepsis and acute gonococcal infection.

Endometrium is protected from infection due to vaginal and cervical defense and also due to periodic shedding of endometrium.

ACUTE ENDOMETRITIS

It almost always occurs after abortion or childbirth. The details of such infection has been dealt on page 110. For details see author's Textbook of Obstetrics, Chapter 30. Treatment of acute endometritis is similar to acute salpingitis (p. 139) for 14 days.

CHRONIC ENDOMETRITIS

It is indeed rare for chronic endometritis to occur during reproductive period even following acute pelvic inflammatory disease (PID) and endometritis. This is because of cyclic shedding of endometrium. Ascending infection due to *C. trachomatis, N. gonorrhoea* or both may be there.

The infection can gain foothold, however, when there is **persistent source of infection** in the uterine cavity. Such conditions are IUCD, infected polyp, retained products, uterine malignancy, and endometrial burns due to radium. Tubercular endometritis is chronic from the beginning and has been described on page 114.

Elderly women presents with purulent or seropurulent vaginal discharge. **Diagnosis** is made by cervical smear, culture of the discharge, transvaginal ultrasonography and **histology of the endometrium**.

Treatment

The offending cause is to be removed or eradicated. Levofloxacin 500 mg PO daily for 14 days with metronidazole 400 mg PO twice daily for 14 days are given.

ATROPHIC ENDOMETRITIS (SENILE ENDOMETRITIS)

Following menopause, due to deficiency of estrogen, the defense of the uterocervicovaginal canal is lost. There is no periodic shedding of the endometrium. As a result, organisms of low virulence can ascend up to infect the atrophic endometrium. There is intense infiltration of the endometrium with polymorphonuclear leukocytes and plasma cells. The endometrium becomes ulcerated at places and is replaced by granulation tissues. The purulent discharge either escapes out of the uterine cavity or may be pent up inside producing pyometra. It is a common genitourinary symptom of manopause.

Clinical Features

The postmenopausal women complain of vaginal discharge, at times offensive or even blood-stained. Pelvic examination reveals features of atrophic vaginitis. Purulent discharge may be seen escaping out through the cervix. In presence of pyometra, the uterus is enlarged; feels soft and tender.

Diagnosis

Ultrasonography (TVS) is helpful to the diagnosis. Diagnostic curettage should be done and the endometrium is subjected to histological examination. **Carcinoma of the endometrium must be excluded prior to treatment.** In fact, pyometra may be present both in atrophic endometritis and endometrial carcinoma.

If **pyometra is present, drainage of pus by simple dilatation should be done first.** After 1–2 weeks, diagnostic curettage is to be done under cover of antibiotics.

Treatment

In women with recurrent attacks, hysterectomy should be done and **the specimen should be subjected to histological examination.**

PYOMETRA

Collection of pus in the uterine cavity is called pyometra. **The prerequisites for pyometra formation are**:

- Occlusion of the cervical canal
- Enough sources of pus formation inside the uterine cavity
- Presence of low-grade infection.

CAUSES

- **Obstetrical:** The only condition is following infection of lochiometra
- **Gynecological:** The conditions which are associated with pyometra are:
  - Carcinoma in the lower part of the body of uterus
  - Endocervical carcinoma
  - Senile endometritis
  - Infected hematometra following amputation, conization or deep cauterization of cervix
  - Tubercular endometritis.

PATHOLOGY

There is abundant secretion of pus from the offending sites. The cervical canal gets blocked due to senile narrowing by fibrosis or due to debris. The accumulated pus distends the uterine cavity.

The organisms responsible are coliforms, streptococci or staphylococci. Rarely, it may be tubercular. Except in tubercular (caseous), the fluid is thin, offensive, at times purulent or blood stained. The pus may be sterile on culture or the offending organism can be detected.

CLINICAL FEATURES

The patient complains of intermittent blood stained purulent offensive discharge per vaginam. There may be occasional pain in lower abdomen. Systemic manifestation is usually absent.

- **Per abdomen:** An uniform suprapubic swelling may be felt of varying size. **Pelvic ultrasonography** reveals distended uterine cavity with accumulation of fluid within.
- **Internal examination reveals:** The swelling is uterine in origin. The offensive discharge is seen escaping out through the cervix.

DIAGNOSIS

Investigations are to be made to exclude malignancy of the body of the uterus and endocervix.

TREATMENT

Once malignancy is excluded, the pyometra is drained by simple dilatation of the cervix. Diagnostic curettage should be withheld for about 7–14 days. This will minimize such complications such as perforation of the uterus and spreading peritonitis. During the interval period, antibiotics should be prescribed. Even in nonmalignant cases or in cases of recurrence, hysterectomy may be indicated. Definite surgery for malignancy is to be done following drainage of pus.

SALPINGITIS

Infection of the fallopian tube is called salpingitis. The details of salpingitis has already been described in the Chapter of pelvic infection (Ch. 11). The pathogenesis of salpingitis (acute and chronic) will be described in this section. **The following facts are to be borne in mind while dealing with salpingitis.**

TABLE 13.4: Organisms responsible for salpingitis.

Sexually transmitted: • *Gonococcus* • *Chlamydia trachomatis* • *Mycoplasma* (rarely)
Pyogenic: • Aerobes—*Streptococcus, Staphylococcus, E. coli* • Anaerobes—*Bacteroides fragilis, Actinomycosis* (rarely), *Peptococcus*
Tubercular: *Mycobacterium tuberculosis*

- The infection is usually polymicrobial in nature (Table 13.4)
- Both the tubes are usually affected
- Ovaries are usually involved in the inflammatory process and as such, the terminology of salpingo-oophoritis is preferred
- Tubal infection almost always affects adversely the future reproductive function.

Etiology

- **Ascending infection from the endometrium, cervix, and vagina**
  - ***Pyogenic organisms*** (Table 13.4).
  - ***Sexually transmitted infections*** (STIs) (Table 12.1).
- **Direct spread from the adjacent infection**
  One or both the tubes are affected in appendicitis, diverticulitis, or following pelvic peritonitis. The organisms are usually *E. coli* or *Streptococcus faecalis*. *Bacteroides fragilis* is too often involved whenever abscess is formed.
- **Tubercular (p. 113)**

Modes of spread to the tubes (p. 107).

ACUTE SALPINGITIS

Pathology

- **Pyogenic**
- **Gonococcal**

Acute Pyogenic

The pathological changes in the tubes depend on the virulence of the organisms and the resistance of the host.

There is intense hyperemia with dilated vessels visible under the peritoneal coat. The wall is enormously thickened and edematous. The mucopurulent or purulent exudate can be expressed out through the abdominal ostium.

Microscopically, the epithelium looks normal or the mucosa slightly edematous. The muscularis shows marked edema and acute inflammatory reaction. **As the outer coat is involved, adhesions are likely and are dense.**

If the infection is very severe, the endosalpinx is destroyed in part or whole and pus is formed. If the fimbrial end is open, the pus escapes out to cause pelvic peritonitis and abscess (Table 13.5).

TABLE 13.5: Clinical diagnostic criteria for acute salpingitis.

▪ Abdominal tenderness ▪ Rebound tenderness (±) ▪ Cervical and uterine motion tenderness ▪ Adnexal tenderness	Box-A
▪ Temperature (>38°C) ▪ Leukocytosis (>10,000/mm^3) ▪ Purulent material from peritoneal cavity by laparoscopy or by culdocentesis (p. 108) ▪ Pelvic abscess or tubo-ovarian mass on bimanual examination or on sonography	Box-B

Presence of all the features from Box-A and any one or more from Box-B are required for diagnosis.

Acute Gonococcal

Like pyogenic infection, there is hyperemia and the tube is swollen and edematous. As the pathology is principally endosalpingitis, **adhesions are less and flimsy**.

The purulent exudate may escape in the peritoneal cavity and produces pelvic peritonitis and pelvic abscess. The ovaries may be involved in the process.

More often, the fimbriae get edematous, phymotic with closure of the abdominal ostium. The uterine opening is closed by congestion. The exudate is pent up inside the lumen producing **pyosalpinx**. The pus becomes sterile by 6 weeks and become hydrosalpinx.

Complications of Acute Salpingitis

- Pelvic or generalized peritonitis
- Pelvis cellulitis
- Pelvic thrombophlebitis
- Pelvic abscess
- Tubo-ovarian abscess
- Endotoxic shock (rare)

Fate of Acute Salpingitis

- **Complete resolution:** Provided the tissue destruction is not appreciable, the tube returns to its normal structure and function.
- But severe endosalpingitis too often produces loss of cilia which is responsible for **infertility.**
- Delay in transport of the fertilized ovum, resulting in **ectopic pregnancy (10%)**.
- **Chronic:** The infection may be chronic due to reinfection or flaring up of the infection at the site.
- **Recurrent acute PID** is observed in about 25% cases.

CHRONIC SALPINGITIS

Pathology

- Hydrosalpinx
- Pyosalpinx
- Chronic interstitial salpingitis
- Salpingitis isthmica nodosa.

Hydrosalpinx

Collection of mucus secretion into the fallopian tube is called hydrosalpinx.

Pathogenesis

It is usually due to the end result of repeated attacks of mild endosalpingitis by pyogenic organisms. The organisms involved are *Staphylococcus, E. coli, Gonococcus, Chlamydia trachomatis,* etc. (Table 13.6).

TABLE 13.6: Comparative features of gonococcal and pyogenic salpingitis.

Gonococcal	***Pyogenic***
Sexually transmitted	Endogenous organisms
Infection occurs usually during and following menstruation	Following abortion and childbirth
Mode of infection—by continuity and contiguity (Fig. 11.1)	Through lymphatics and veins → pelvic cellulitis → tubal affection (Fig. 11.2)
Always bilateral affection	May be unilateral
Pathology: ▪ Endosalpingitis ▪ Intraluminal exudation ++ ▪ Closure of the abdominal ostium by indrawn fimbriae → pyosalpinx ▪ Peritoneal coat is less involved, adhesions—scanty and flimsy	Pathology: ▪ Perisalpingitis (predominantly) ▪ Less ▪ Closure by adhesions. May remain patent ▪ More involvement and as such adhesions are more and dense
Pus becomes sterile by 6 weeks → hydrosalpinx	Takes longer time (≥1 year), may have recurrent attack
Restoration of reproductive function is unlikely	May be possible

During initial infection, the fimbriae are edematous and indrawn with the serous surface, adhering together to produce closure of the abdominal ostium. The uterine ostium gets closed by congestion. The secretion is pent up to make the tube distended. The distension is marked on the ampullary region than the more rigid isthmus. As the mesosalpinx is fixed, the resultant distension makes the tube curled and **looks 'retort-shaped'**. The wall is smooth and shiny containing clear fluid inside, which is usually sterile (Fig. 13.7).

The uterine ostium is not closed anatomically, thus favors repeated infection. At times, there is intermittent

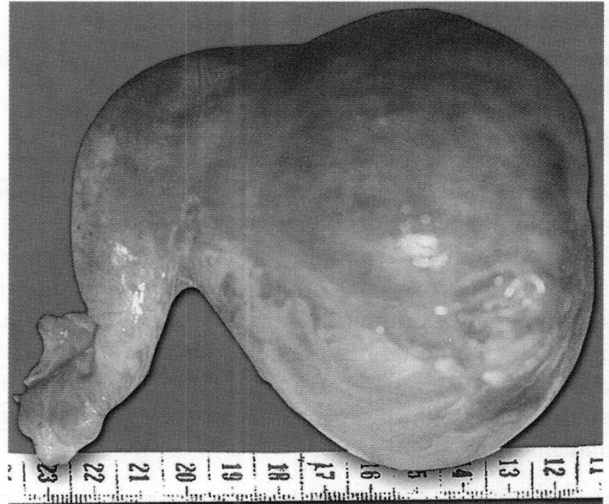

Fig. 13.7: Hydrosalpinx. Note the retort shape of the tube. Depending on tubal diameter **hydrosalpinx** may be mild <15 mm; **moderate** 15–30 mm; **severe** >30 mm.

Classification of Tubal Disease with Distal Fimbrial Obstruction

Mild: Small hydrosalpinx <15 mm diameter, inverted fimbriae, patency is present, no significant peritubal or periovarian adhesions. Tubal rugae pattern is present on HSG.
Moderate: Hydrosalpinx 15–30 mm in diameter. Fimbriae not readily identified, periovarian or tubal adhesion present without fixation, minimal cul-de-sac adhesion. Tubal rugae pattern is absent on HSG.
Severe: Hydrosalpinx >30 mm in diameter no fimbriae. Dense pelvic, adnexal adhesions with fixation of the ovary and tube. Obliteration of the cul-de-sac. Frozen pelvis: Pelvic organs are difficult to define.

discharge of the fluid into the uterine cavity (**intermittent hydrosalpinx or hydrops tubal profluens**).

Hydrosalpinx is also considered as the end stage of pyosalpinx when the pus becomes liquefied to make the fluid clear.

Ultrasonography Including Color Doppler (TVS)

Hydrosalpinx appears as a sausage shaped complex, cystic, hypoechoic, adnexal mass. There may be incomplete septa and multiple small hyperechoic mural nodules that give the appearance of "beads on a string".

The nodules represent the fibrotic endosalpingeal folds. When the distended tube is seen in cross-section, it may give the "cogwheel sign" appearance due to the endosalpingeal folds.

Dilated and fluid filled tubes, free peritoneal fluid and adnexal masses may be seen. TVS has got high positive predictive value.

Color and power Doppler show increased blood flow (reduced RI) due to hyperemia of the inflamed tubes (Fig. 13.8).

Complications

The following may happen: (a) Formation of tubo-ovarian cyst; (b) Torsion; (c) Infection from the gut; (d) Rupture.

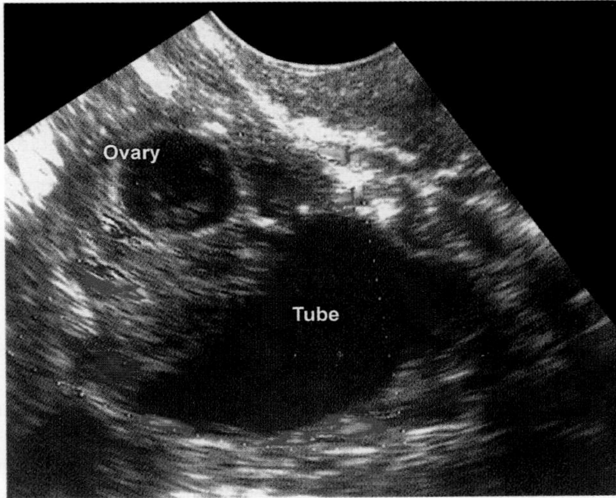

Fig. 13.8: Color Doppler scan (TVS) showing ovary and the tube with hydrosalpinx change.

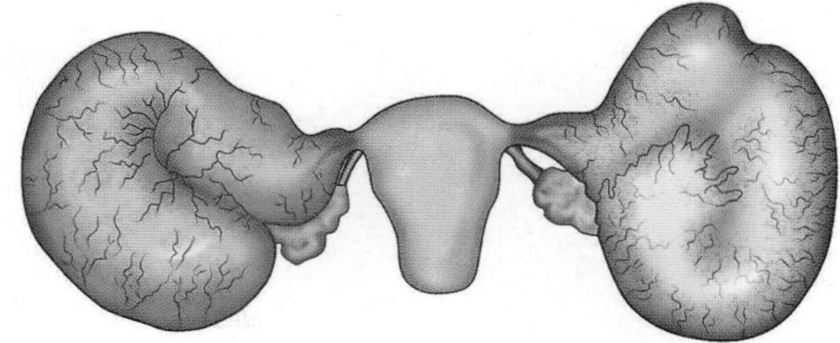

Fig. 13.9: Bilateral pyosalpinx.

Pyosalpinx

The pyogenic organisms, if become virulent, produce intense inflammatory reaction with secretion of pus. The tube becomes closed at both ends; the abdominal ostium by adhesions of the fimbriae and the uterine end by exudate. Because of intense inflammatory reaction and/or escape of pus into the peritoneal cavity, there is dense adhesions with the surrounding structures like ovaries, intestines, omentum, and pelvic peritoneum (Fig. 13.9). Thus, a tubo-ovarian mass is formed. The inner wall of the tube is replaced in part by granulation tissue.

Chronic Interstitial Salpingitis

The tube enlarges mainly due to great thickness of the wall. The distension of the tube by the exudate is unusual. The abdominal ostium may be closed or partially open. The adjacent organs are adherent to the tube. Microscopically, there is extensive infiltration of plasma cells and histiocytes in all the myosalpinx layers. There is intense fibrosis of the muscle coat along with inflammatory changes. This hinders the tubal motility and favors ectopic pregnancy.

Salpingitis Isthmica Nodosa

Pathogenesis

The exact nature still remains unclear.

The following are the probabilities:

- It is related to tubercular infection, although it may be the residue of any form of chronic interstitial salpingitis.
- There is infiltration of the tubal mucosa directly into the muscularis resembling adenomyosis of the uterus.
- It is one form of endometriosis of the tube.

Naked eye examination reveals one or two nodules in the isthmus of the tube, often involving the uterine cornu. The nodule is small but may be as large as 2 cm.

Microscopically, there is thickening of the muscularis in which the tubal epithelium lined spaces are scattered, giving an adenomatous picture. There may be inconsistent mild inflammatory reaction (Fig. 13.10).

The clinical features and investigations of **salpingitis** **have already been described in p. 139 and 140 (Tables 13.5 and 13.6)**.

Laparascopy is useful for both diagnosis and therapy.

Treatment of Acute Salpingitis/Peritonitis (CDC)

- **Outpatient therapy**: Levofloxacin 500 mg PO once daily for 14 days plus metronidazole 500 mg PO twice

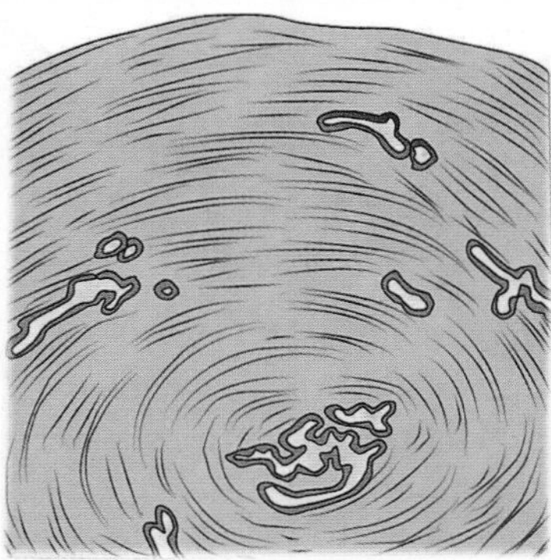

Fig. 13.10: Histology of salpingitis isthmica nodosa. Note the tubal epithelial lined spaces inside the muscularis.

daily for 14 days are given. Patient is admitted for inpatient therapy if there is no response by 72 hours.

- **Inpatient therapy** (Temp >39°C, toxic look, lower abdominal guarding, and rebound tenderness). Clindamycin 900 mg IV 8 hourly, plus gentamicin 2 mg/kg IV, then 1.5 mg/kg IV every 8 hours are given. This is followed by doxycycline 100 mg twice daily orally for 14 days. Intravenous fluids to correct dehydration and nasogastric suction in the presence of abdominal distension or ileus are maintained. Laparotomy is done if there is clinical suggestion of abscess rupture.

Prognosis of Salpingitis

With early diagnosis and therapy with potent antibiotics, the immediate risk is markedly reduced. With effective therapy, the prospect of future reproductive function of the tube is not so gloomy. But once the cilia is damaged, commonly with gonococcal infection or pyogenic infection (repeated), the prospect of future fertility is very much poor even with reconstructive surgery. Even if pregnancy occurs, chances of ectopic is more (10–15%). Salpingectomy is recommended before consideration of ART.

OOPHORITIS

Isolated infection to the ovaries is a rarity. The ovaries are almost always affected during salpingitis and as such the nomenclature of salpingo-oophoritis is preferred. **The affection of the ovary from tubal infection occurs by the following routes:**

- Directly from the exudates contaminating the ovarian surface producing perioophoritis.
- Through lymphatics of the mesosalpinx and mesovarium producing interstitial oophoritis.
- Blood-borne—mumps.
- Through the rent of the ovulation producing interstitial oophoritis.

If the organisms are severe, an abscess is formed and a tubo-ovarian abscess results. In others, the ovaries may be adherent to the tubes, intestine, omentum, and pelvic peritoneum producing tubo-ovarian mass (TO mass). Such a mass is usually bilateral (Fig. 13.11).

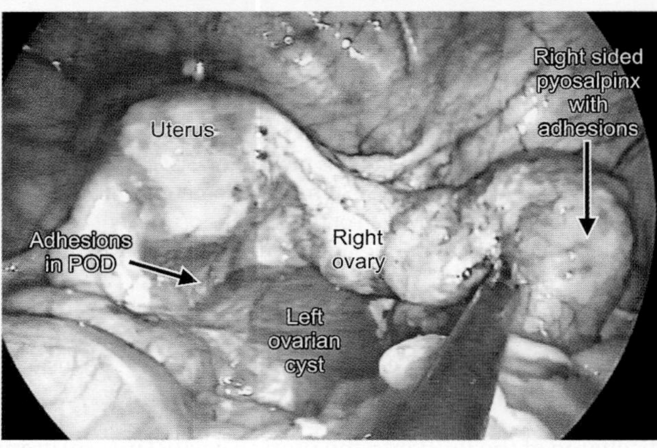

Fig. 13.11: Laparoscopic view of bilateral tubo-ovarian mass (TO mass) with extensive adhesions.

(POD: pouch of Douglas)

Direct affection of the ovaries without tubal involvement may be due to mumps or influenza. Patients need admission for IV antibiotic to cover polymicrobial infections for gram positive, negative and the anerobes. The symptomatology and treatment are like those of salpingitis.

PARAMETRITIS

Inflammation of the pelvic cellular tissue is called parametritis.

Etiology of Parametritis

- Delivery and abortion through placental site or from lacerations of the cervix, vaginal vault, or lower uterine segment.
- Acute infections of the cervix, uterus, and tubes.
- Cesarean section
- Hysterectomy—abdominal or vaginal (cuff cellulitis).
- Secondary to pelvic peritonitis.
- Carcinoma cervix or radium introduction.

PATHOLOGY

The causative organisms are anaerobic *Streptococcus, Staphylococcus, E. coli, Bacteroides* species (fragilis, fusobacteria), etc. There is intense hyperemia with exudation of serous fluid, lymph, and polymorphonuclear leukocytes.

CLINICAL FEATURES

- **Acute**
- **Chronic**

Acute

The onset is usually insidious and appears about 5–7 days following initial infection.

The temperature rises to about 102°F. Pain is not a prominent feature, may be dull aching deep in the pelvis.

On examination, the pulse rate is raised proportionate to the temperature. There is generalized deep tenderness on lower abdomen. Rigidity is absent because the lesion is extraperitoneal. Pelvic examination reveals hot and tender vagina. There is an indurated tender mass usually unilateral, which extends to the lateral pelvic wall and to which the uterus is firmly fixed. The uterus is pushed to the contralateral side.

Rectal examination confirms the indurated tender mass or horseshoe-shaped induration of the uterosacral ligaments surrounding the rectum. **Ultrasonograhy** can localize any collection with its site and extent.

Tubo-ovarian Abscess

Ultrasonography is helpful to the diagnosis. Normal adnexal anatomy is altered. On the other hand multiseptated cystic mass with multiple internal echoes are seen. Computed tomography when done with intravenous (IV)/ oral contrast may provide improved images.

TREATMENT

The outline of management protocol is the same like that of acute salpingitis of pyogenic origin.

Patient needs hospitalization for IV antibiotics. Antibiotics should cover a wide range of polymicrobial infections including the anaerobics.

PELVIC ABSCESS

Encysted pus in the pouch of Douglas is called pelvic abscess.

ETIOLOGY

Pelvic Causes (Common)

- Postabortal and puerperal sepsis
- Acute salpingitis
- Perforation of an infected uterus such as attempted uterine curettage in septic abortion or pyometra
- Infection of pelvic hematocele usually following disturbed tubal pregnancy
- Postoperative pelvic peritonitis following abdominal or vaginal hysterectomy
- Irritant peritonitis following contamination of urine, bile, vernix caseosa, meconium (spilled during cesarean section), iodine containing dye used in hysterosalpingography or contents of ruptured ovarian cyst (sebum in dermoid cyst), etc.

Extrapelvic Causes (Rare)

Appendicitis, diverticulitis, ruptured gallbladder, perforated peptic ulcer usually produce generalized peritonitis. The condition may ultimately settle to the dependent pouch of Douglas and produces pelvic abscess.

CLINICAL FEATURES

Patient can be ill from any of the causative factors mentioned earlier. **But the localization of pus in the pouch of Douglas is evidenced by**:

Symptoms

- Spiky rise of high temperature with chills and rigor
- Rectal tenesmus—frequent passage of loose mucoid stool
- Pain lower abdomen—variable degrees
- Urinary symptoms—difficulty or even retention of urine.

Signs

General: Pulse rate is raised out of proportion to temperature.

Per abdomen

- Tenderness and rigidity in lower abdomen
- A mass may be felt in the suprapubic region—tender, irregular, soft, and resonant on percussion.

Per vaginam

- The vagina is hot and tender
- The uterus is pushed anteriorly; the movement of the cervix is painful
- A boggy, fluctuant, and tender mass is felt in the pouch of Douglas
- A separate mass may be felt through the lateral fornix.

Rectal examination defines precisely the mass in the pouch of Douglas.

INVESTIGATIONS

- **Blood:** There is high leukocytosis with increased polymorphs.
- **Bacteriological study:** Swabs are taken from high vagina, endocervical canal and from the pus. Culture is done for both aerobic and anaerobic microorganisms. Sensitivity of the microorganisms to antibiotics is also to be detected.
- **Confirmation of diagnosis:** The diagnosis is easy in most of the cases but at times confusion arises between pelvic hematocele and pelvic abscess.

  Pelvic ultrasonography reveals accumulation of fluid in the pouch of Douglas. Large amounts (normal amount is 10 mL) of anechoic free fluid suggests inflammatory etiology.

TREATMENT

General: Systemic antibiotics should cover anaerobic as well as aerobic microorganisms (broad spectrum): Cefoxitin 1–2 g IV every 6–8 hours and gentamicin 2 mg/kg IV per 24 hours and metronidazole 500 mg IV 8 hourly are started. Antibiotic regimen may have to be changed depending upon the sensitivity report.

Surgery: Posterior colpotomy is the definitive surgery to drain the pus through posterior fornix. The loculi should be broken with finger.

Laparotomy is done when the patient's condition deteriorates despite aggressive management. In patients with recurrent infection and with loss of reproductive function total abdominal hysterectomy with bilateral salpingo-oophorectomy is the preferred treatment.

The pus should be sent for culture and drug sensitivity test.

SYNDROMIC MANAGEMENT OF SEXUALLY TRANSMITTED INFECTIONS (WHO-1991)

PRINCIPLE

Treatment of STIs should be initiated at the patient's first visit to a clinic. At the same time, the couple is counseled about the importance of condom use and **prevention of STIs.**

Syndromic managements are based on epidemiological studies all over the world. Syndromic diagnosis and laboratory assisted diagnosis have been found similar in terms of accuracy.

METHOD

Management is done by criteria for syndromic diagnosis of pelvic inflammatory disease (PID) (Table 13.7). These include:

- Medical history including detail of sexual history.
- Physical examination including pelvic examination: (a) speculum and (b) bimanual examination to detect any vaginal discharge (Table 13.1), abdominal pain, cervical motion tenderness, adnexal tenderness, and to exclude cervical cancer and pregnancy.
- VCT (Voluntary Counseling and Testing for HIV) is promoted.
- Counseling with education is done as regard the preventive issues of STIs.
- Promotion of condom use is done:
  - To refer all patients to ICTC
  - To treat the partner. Follow-up after 7 days for all patients with STI's
  - To advice immunisation against hepatitis B.

STI/RTI Syndromic case management includes:

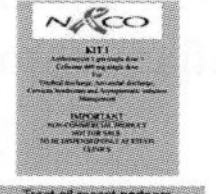

Treatment of:
(a) Uretheral discharge
(b) Cervical discharge.
(c) Painful scrotal swelling

KIT 1/Grey

Tab Azithromycin 1 gm OD stat + tab Cefixime 400 mg OD stat

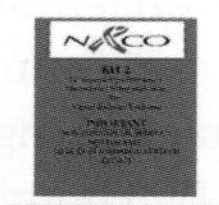

(d) Vaginal discharge **KIT 2/Green**

Tab Secnidazole 2 gm OD stat + Cap Fluconazole 150 mg OD stat

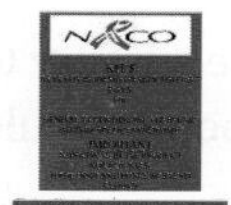

(e) Genitial ulcer herpetic **KIT 5/Red**

Tab Acyclovir 400 mg TDS X 7 days

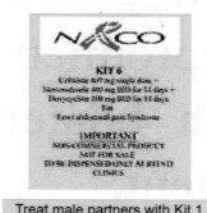

(f) Lower Abdominal Pain **KIT 6/Yellow**

Tab Cefixime 400 mg OD stat + Tab Metronidazole 400 mg BD X 14 days + Tab Doxycylline 100 mg BD X 14 days

TABLE 13.7: Management of STIs based on syndromic approach (WHO).

Syndrome	Treatment options
Vaginal discharge	Vaginitis: ▪ Trichomoniasis ▪ Bacterial vaginosis ▪ Candidiasis
Cervicitis	Chlamydia, Gonorrhea
Lower abdominal pain	Chlamydia, Gonorrhea, others pyogenic
Genital ulcers	▪ Genital herpes (p. 126) ▪ Chancroid (p. 126) ▪ Syphilis (p. 123)

Healthcare providers are trained up to follow a standardized protocol (flowcharts) for treatment such a patient. This is particularly suitable in a healthcare set up in developing countries.

ADVANTAGES OF SYNDROMIC MANAGEMENT

- It gives an opportunity for counseling and treating simultaneously.
- Patient education is a standard care for all types of STIs.
- Use of standardized protocols (flowcharts) allow diagnosis, treatment and disease surveillance in a better way.
- It avoids delay of treatment, where laboratory facilities are limited.
- It avoids loss of patient follow up, where referral system is not well-structured.
- Continued transmission of infection is prevented.
- It is a simple, inexpensive, cost-effective and rapid management for sexually transmitted infections (STIs).
- High cure rate is observed once treated appropriately.

LIMITATIONS

- Prediction is poor as it is based on symptoms rather than investigations.
- Over diagnosis and treatment is a known hazard.
- Not useful for patients who are asymptomatic.
- Syndromic approach for vaginal discharge predicts poorly with the infection of Chlamydia and Gonorrhea.
- Over treatment of women's partners is there who may not have an STIs.

OTHER GYNECOLOGIC INFECTIONS

POSTOPERATIVE INFECTIONS

Necrotizing Fasciitis

It is due to polymicrobial synergistic infection. It is seen in cases following surgical infections or following minor injuries.

Organisms commonly involved are: *E. coli, E. faecalis, Bacteroides, Clostridium perfringens, Peptostreptococcus, S. aureus* and group A and B hemolytic streptococci. Patients present with pain, erythema, fascial tissue necrosis and myonecrosis. Crepitus, and edema are present. Tissue destruction is more extensive. Patient may become severely toxic.

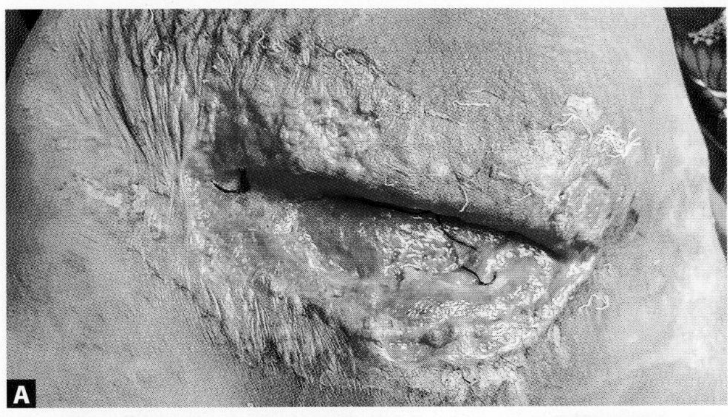

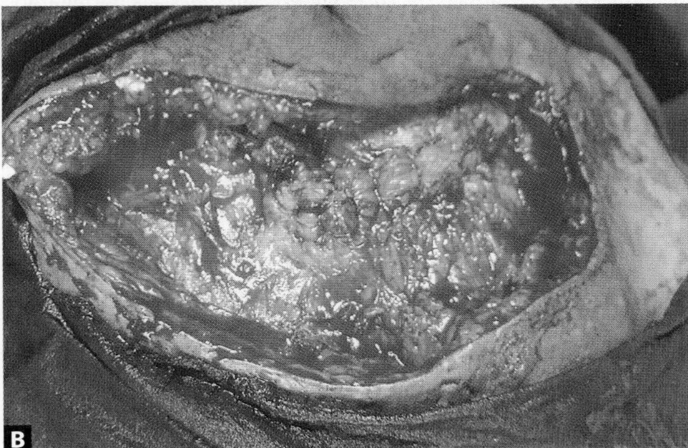

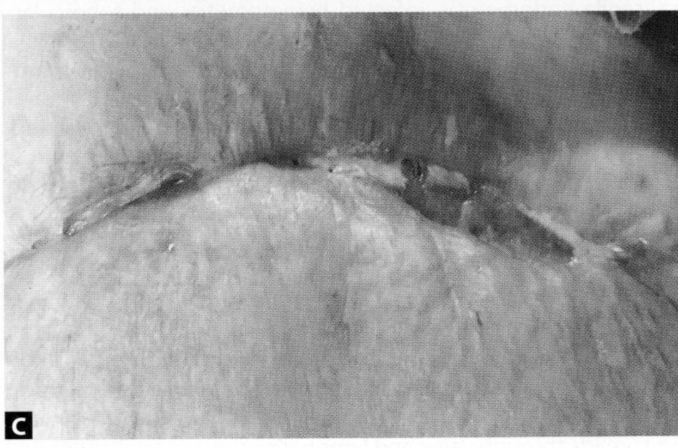

Figs. 13.12A to C: (A) Necrotizing fasciitis of the lower abdominal wall following abdominal hysterectomy operation. Extensive necrosis of the adjoining skin, subcutaneous tissue, rectus sheath and the muscles (myofascitis); (B) Appearance of the same wound after debridement of wide areas of gangrenous and necrotic tissues; (C) The same wound in the phase of healing, following secondary suture.

Features of Necrotising Infections

- Wound of edema and crepitius
- Skin blistering
- Extensive tissue destructions
- Focal skin gangrene
- Myonecrosis
- Greyish wound discharge

Management: Broad spectrum antibiotics to cover the MRSA are used: Clindamycin 600–900 mg IV, 6–8 hourly PLUS second generation cephalosporin or vancomycin 15–20 mg/kg/dose IV 8 hourly is given. Urgent surgical wound debridement is needed. Supportive care therapy (IV fluids, crystalloids, blood transfusion) to be given as needed.

Surgical Site Infections (SSIs)

Postoperative infections cause significant patient morbidity and even mortality. Extent of surgical site wound contamination during the surgery is important. Depending upon the degree of bacterial contamination of the operative site at the time of surgery, wounds are classified as below:

1. **Clean wounds:** Characterized by— (a) No acute inflammation; (c) No entry to genitourinary, alimentary or respiratory tract; (d) No break in aseptic technique; (e) *Infection risk is* <5%.
2. **Clean contaminated wound:** Characterized by—(a) Entry to GU, alimentary or respiratory tract was there but no significant spillage of contents; (b) No evidence of infection or major break in aseptic technique; (c) *Infection risk is* <15%.
3. **Contaminated wounds:** (a) Entry to internal organs with inflammation or spillage of contents; (b) Major breaks in sterile technique; (c) *Chance of infection is* 15–20%.
4. **Dirty wounds:** (a) Purulent, inflammation present, intraperitoneal abscess formation or visceral perforation; (b) *Infection is risk* 30–100%.

Important Risk Factors for Postoperative SSIs

- Pre-existing anemia
- Older age
- Pre-existing sepsis
- Excessive blood loss
- Immunocompromised status
- Low socioeconomic status
- Obesity
- Prolonged surgical procedure (>3.5 hours)
- Foreign body placement (catheter, drain)
- Diabetes
- Smoking
- Post operative HbA1C >7% or CBG >250 mg/dL.

Criteria for defining SSIs (CDC - 2014)

1. **Superficial incisional:** Develops within 30 days of surgical procedure .
   Features (at least one): (a) Purulent drainage from the superficial incision; (b) Bacteria in culture obtained; (c) Signs and symptoms: pain, tenderness, heat/redness, local swelling. Stitch abscess and cellulitis, do not meet the criteria for SSI.
2. **Deep incisional:** Develops within 30 days of surgical procedure.
   Features (at least one): Purulent discharge, wound dehiscence; signs/symptoms: localised pain/tenderness, temperature $\geq$ 38°C, formation of abscess.
3. **Organ/space:** Occurs within 30 days of surgical procedure. Purulent discharge from a drain placed into the organ/space, abscess found by reoperation or radiology.

Management

Empiric therapy with broad spectrum antibiotics is started before the culture report is available. Therapy may be given orally or parenterally. Some patients may need hospitalisation and treatment with IV broad spectrum antibiotics. Patients with MRSA need to be treated with parenteral therapy of Clindamycin or Vancomycin. General management of IV fluids and electrolytes are to be maintained. Surgical intervention like drainage of abscess or exploratory laparotomy may be needed for cases with involvement of organ or the spaces.

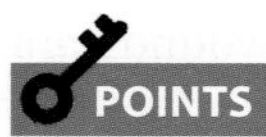

POINTS

- **In recurrent vulvitis** due to fungal infection, diabetes is to be excluded.
- **Bartholin's cyst** usually develops in the duct. The gratifying treatment is marsupialization under local anesthesia. A normal Bartholin's gland cannot be palpated.
- **Excision of Bartholin's duct and gland** is indicated for persistent and/or recurrent infections especially when it occurs beyond the age of 40.
- **During childbearing period, vaginal trichomoniasis** is the most common STD caused by *Trichomonas vaginalis*—a flagellated parasite. Hanging drop preparation with identification of *Trichomonas* is diagnostic. Treatment is specific with metronidazole to both partners. The husband is to use condom during treatment. Vaginitis may be due to other causes also (p. 134).
- **A vaginal discharge** with pH >5.0 indicates atrophic vaginitis, bacterial vaginosis, or *Trichomonas* infection whereas a vaginal discharge with pH <4.5 may be either physiologic or due to fungal infection. Vaginal discharge needs to be differentiated before treatment (Table 13.1).
- **Moniliasis** is caused by *Candida albicans*—a gram-positive fungus. The infection is more likely related to diabetes, pregnancy, or amongst 'pill' users (p. 135). Diagnosis is by identification of the mycelia by direct smear and stained by methylene blue or cultured in Sabouraud's media.
- **Toxic shock syndrome** is a febrile illness of acute onset. It caused by the exotoxin following infection. The causative organism is *Staphylococcus aureus*. Dysfunction of multiple organ system is due to the bacterial exotoxin (p. 137). Treatment is supportive. β-lactamase resistant anti-staphylococcal penicillin (cloxacillin, methicillin) should be the choice.
- **Necrotizing fasciitis** is due to microvascular thrombosis causing extensive necrosis of the superficial fascia. There is infiltration of WBC. **High-risk factors are:** Older age, diabetes, obesity, smoking or previous radiation therapy. The patient needs wound debridement and broad-spectrum antibiotics that cover MRSA also.
- **The feature of senile endometritis** may simulate endometrial carcinoma which should be ruled out prior to treatment. Common causes of pyometra are endometrial and endocervical carcinoma, senile endometritis, infected hematometra, and tubercular endometritis.
- **Pyogenic nongonococcal organisms** affect the tubes by producing perisalpingitis; gonococcal produces endosalpingitis and tubercular infection produces interstitial salpingitis.
- **The organisms producing hydrosalpinx** are *Staphylococcus, Streptococcus, E. coli, Gonococcus, Cl. trachomatis,* etc. Hydrosalpinx is the end result of repeated attacks of mild endosalpingitis. It may also be the end stage of pyosalpinx when the pus becomes liquefied. Prognosis of salpingitis in terms of reproductive function depends on the type of infection, severity, and number of episodes. When the cilia is damaged and or motility is impaired (adhesion), prospect is very poor.
- **Salpingitis isthmica nodosa** may be one variety of endometriosis or related to tubercular infection. Tube is nodular and thickened. There is proliferation of tubal epithelium within the muscle layer (myosalpinx).
- **Pelvic abscess** is the encysted pus in the pouch of Douglas. The common causes are acute salpingitis, postabortal sepsis, infected pelvic hematocele and postoperative pelvic peritonitis, etc.
- Confirmation of diagnosis is by culdocentesis and the definitive surgery is drainage of pus through posterior colpotomy.
- **Endocervix** is the major reservoir of pathogenic organisms. Most common site of *Chlamydia* infection in the female genital tract is the columnar cells of the endocervix.
- **Mode of spread of infection to the tubes are : Pyogenic infection** spreads through veins and lymphatics causing perisalpingitis and endosalpingitis. Cornual block following postabortal or puerperal sepsis may occur.
- **Gonococcal infection** ascends through continuity and contiguity causing endosalpingitis.
- **Tubercular infection** spreads through bloodstream (hematogenous) causing interstitial salpingitis.
- **Clinical diagnostic criteria for acute salpingitis include:** Abdominal tenderness, cervical or uterine motion tenderness, adnexal tenderness plus one or more other features (p. 140).
- **Indication of surgery** for pelvic inflammatory disease (PID) are restricted to life-threatening infection, not responding to medical therapy (e.g. tubo-ovarian abscess, pelvic abscess, or any clinical suspicion of abscess rupture).
- **Syndromic management** of STIs (WHO) includes: Risk assessment of a patient from medical including sexual history and physical examination (pelvic), to detect the pathology (including cancer cervix) and to organize treatment of the patient following a standardized protocol. The patient is also counseled and educated for the prevention of recurrence of STI. Syndromic management of STIs has many benefits (p. 144).
- **Surgical site infection may be:** (a) Superficial incisional; (b) Deep incisional; or (c) Involving organ/space. Often the patient has got risk factors for SSIs (p. 145). Management depends on extent and severity of the infection.

CHAPTER

14 Dysmenorrhea and Other Disorders of Menstrual Cycles

CHAPTER OUTLINE

- Dysmenorrhea
  - Primary Dysmenorrhea
  - Secondary Dysmenorrhea
  - Pelvic Congestion Syndrome
- Premenstrual Syndrome

DYSMENORRHEA

Dysmenorrhea literally means painful menstruation. But a more realistic and practical definition includes cases of **painful menstruation of sufficient magnitude so as to incapacitate day to day activities**.

Types:

- **Primary**
- **Secondary**

PRIMARY DYSMENORRHEA (SPASMODIC)

The primary dysmenorrhea is one where there is no identifiable pelvic pathology.

Incidence

The incidence of primary dysmenorrhea of sufficient magnitude with incapacitation is about 15–20%. With the advent of oral contraceptives and nonsteroidal anti-inflammatory drugs (NSAIDs), there is marked relief of the symptom.

Causes of Pain

The mechanism of initiation of uterine pain in primary dysmenorrhea is difficult to establish. **But the following are too often related**:

- Mostly confined to adolescents
- Almost always confined to ovulatory cycles
- The pain is usually cured following pregnancy and vaginal delivery
- The pain is related to dysrhythmic uterine contractions and uterine hypoxia.
  - **Psychosomatic factors** of tension and anxiety during adolescence; lower the pain threshold.
  - **Abnormal anatomical and functional aspect of myometrium.**

    Uterine myometrial hyperactivity has been observed in cases with primary dysmenorrhea.

    The outer myometrium and the subendometrial myometrium are found to be different structurally and functionally. The subendometrial layer of myometrium is known as junctional zone (JZ). There is marked hyperperistalsis of the JZ in women with endometriosis and adenomyosis. In women with dysmenorrhea significant changes in JZ are seen. These include irregular thickening and hyperplasia of smooth muscle and less vascularity. This is known as **junctional zone hyperplasia. Dysperistalsis and hyperactivity of the uterine JZ are the important mechanisms of primary dysmenorrhea.**
  - **Imbalance in the autonomic nervous control of uterine muscle**: There is overactivity of the sympathetic nerves → hypertonicity of the circular fibers of the isthmus and internal os. The relief of pain following dilatation of the cervix or following vaginal delivery may be explained by the damage of the adrenergic neurons which fail to regenerate.
  - **Role of prostaglandins:** In ovulatory cycles, under the action of progesterone; prostaglandins ($PGF_2\alpha$, PGE_2) are synthesized from the secretory endometrium. Prostaglandins are released with maximum production during shedding of the endometrium. $PGF_2\alpha$ is a strong vasoconstrictor, which causes ischemia (angina) of the myometrium.

    Either due to increased production of the prostaglandins or increased sensitivity of the myometrium to the normal production of prostaglandins, there is increased myometrial contraction with or without dysrhythmia. The possible cause of pain owing to JZ change is discussed (Flowchart 14.1).
  - **Role of vasopressin:** There is increased vasopressin release during menstruation in women with primary dysmenorrhea. This explains the persistence of pain in cases even treated with antiprostaglandin drugs. The mechanism of action is yet to be explored.

Flowchart 14.1: Primary dysmenorrhea: Etiopathogenesis.

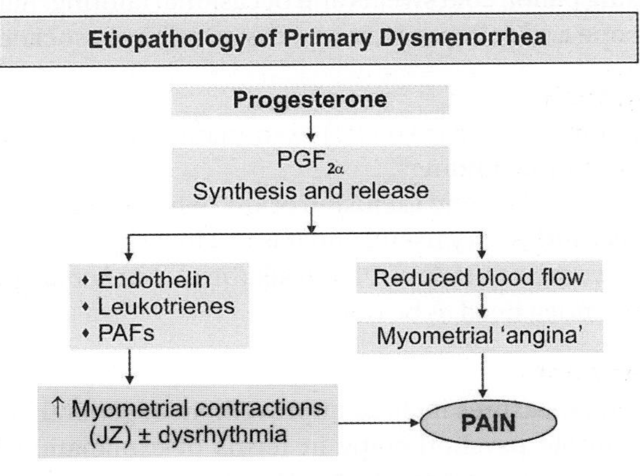

(JZ: junctional zone; $PGF_{2\alpha}$: prostaglandin $F_{2\alpha}$; PAFs: platelet activating factors)

Vasopressin increases prostaglandin synthesis and also increases myometrial activity directly. It causes uterine hyperactivity and dysrhythmic contractions → ischemia and hypoxia with which causes pain.

- **Endothelins** causes myometrial smooth muscle contractions, especially in the endomyometrial JZ. Endothelins in endometrium can induce $PFG_{2\alpha}$. Local myometrial ischemia caused by **endothelins and $PGF_{2\alpha}$ aggravate uterine dysperistalsis and hyperactivity**.
- **Platelet activating factor (PAF)** is also associated with the etiology of dysmenorrhea as its concentration is found high. Leukotrienes and PAFs are vasoconstrictors and stimulate myometrial contractions.

Patient Profile

Primary dysmenorrhea is predominantly confined to adolescent girls. It usually appears within 2 years of menarche. The mother or her sister may be dysmenorrheic. It is more common amongst girls from affluent society.

CLINICAL DIFFERENTIATING FEATURES BETWEEN PRIMARY AND SECONDARY DYSMENORRHEA

Primary	*Secondary*
▪ No identifiable pelvic pathology ▪ Mostly in adolescents ▪ Confined to ovulatory cycle ▪ Starts with the onset or just before the mens	▪ Secondary to pelvic pathology (p. 149) ▪ Elderly/parous women ▪ Pain starts 7–10 days before the onset of menstruation ▪ No systemic discomfort ▪ Intermenstrual period not completely free of pain

Clinical Features

The pain begins a few hours before or just with the onset of menstruation. The severity of pain usually lasts for few hours, may extend to 24 hours but seldom persists beyond 48 hours. The pain is spasmodic and confined to lower abdomen; may radiate to the back and medial aspect of thighs. Systemic discomforts like nausea, vomiting, fatigue, diarrhea, headache and tachycardia may be associated. It may be accompanied by vasomotor changes causing pallor, cold sweats and occasional fainting. Rarely, syncope and collapse in severe cases may be associated.

Diagnosis

Abdominal or pelvic (rectal) examination does not reveal any abnormal findings.

For detection and exclusion of any pelvic abnormalities, **ultrasound** is very useful and it is not invasive.

In women at risk of PID, tests for *C. trachomatis* and Gonorrhoea need to be done.

Treatment

General measures include improvement of general health and simple psychotherapy in terms of explanation and assurance (Flowchart 14.2). Usual activities including sports are to be continued.

During menses, bowel should be kept empty; mild analgesics and antispasmodics may be prescribed. **Habit forming drugs such as pethidine or morphine must not be prescribed**. With these simple measures, the pain is relieved in majority.

Severe Cases

- **Expectant management**
- **Drugs**
- **Surgery**

Expectant management

- Assurance
- To keep bowels empty
- Weight reduction
- Encourage activities

Drugs

The drugs used are:

- Prostaglandin synthetase inhibitors (Table 14.1).
- Oral contraceptives (combined estrogen and progestogen).

Prostaglandin synthetase inhibitors (PSI)

These drugs reduce the prostaglandin synthesis (by inhibition of cyclooxygenase enzyme) and also have a direct analgesic effect. Intrauterine pressure is reduced significantly. Any of the preparations listed under medical management can be used orally for 2–3 days starting with the onset of period. The drug should be continued for 3–6 cycles.

Newer drugs: Nonsteroidal anti-inflammatory drugs (NSAIDs) (Table 14.1) inhibit two different isoforms of the enzyme cyclooxygenase: COX-1 and COX-2. Selective inhibitors of the enzyme COX-2 may have similar analgesic efficacy but fewer side effects.

Suitable cases for medical therapy are: Comparatively young age and having contraindications to 'pill'. The contraindications of medical therapy include allergy to aspirin, gastric ulceration and history of asthma.

- ***Oral contraceptive pills:*** The suitable candidates are patients (a) wanting contraceptive precaution; (b) with heavy periods; and (c) unresponsive or contraindications to antiprostaglandin drugs. The pill should be used for 3–6 cycles.
- ***Dydrogesterone (progestogen):*** It does not inhibit ovulation but probably interferes with ovarian steroidogenesis. The drug should be taken from day 5 of a cycle for 20 days. It should be continued for 3–6 cycles.
- ***LNG-IUS*** is very effective (50%) in reducing pain. It is used in women who desires contraception and where estrogen is contraindicated.

If the above protocol fails, laparoscopy is indicated to find out any pelvic pathology to account for pain, the important one being endometriosis.

Surgery

Transcutaneous electrical nerve stimulation (TENS) has been used to relieve dysmenorrhea. Results are not better than that of analgesics.

Surgical procedures: Laparoscopy may be needed for diagnosis and treatment. Laparoscopic uterine nerve ablation (LUNA) for primary dysmenorrhea has not been found beneficial. **Laparoscopic presacral neurectomy**

Flowchart 14.2: Therapeutic approach in a patient with primary dysmenorrhea.

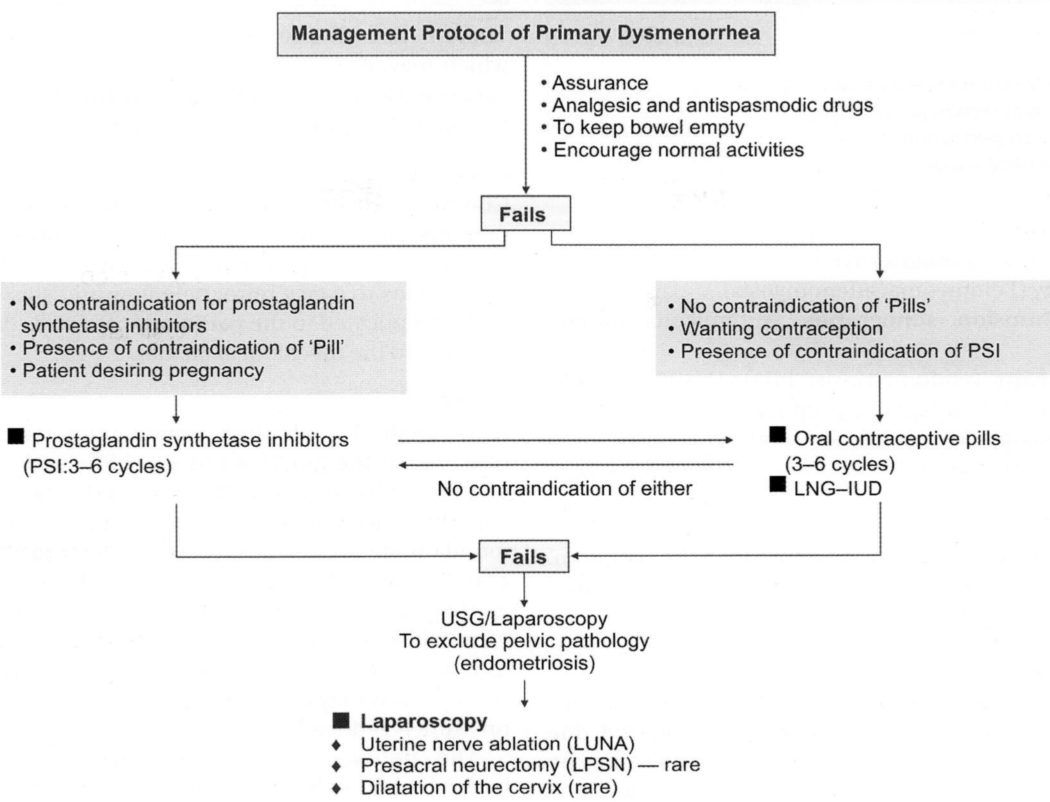

TABLE 14.1: Common treatment modalities for primary dysmenorrhea.

- **Non hormonal**
  - Mefenamic acid: 250–500 mg 8 hourly
  - Ibuprofen 400 mg 8 hourly
  - Naproxen 250 mg 6 hourly
  - COX-2 inhibitors: Celecoxib 200 mg twice daily
- **Hormones**
  - Combined oral contraceptive pills: 1 tablet daily
  - Oral progestins (dydrogesterone): D5-D25
  - LNG-IUS
- **Surgical management**
  - Laparoscopic uterine nerve ablation (LUNA)
  - Laparoscopic presacral neurectomy (LPSN)

is done to cut down the sensory pathways (via T_{11}-T_{12}) from the uterus. It is not helpful for adnexal pain (T_9-T_{10}) as it is carried out by thoracic autonomic nerves along the ovarian vessels. As such its role in true dysmenorrhea is questionable.

Dilatation of cervical canal: It is done under anesthesia for slow dilatation of the cervix to relieve pain by damaging the sensory nerve endings. It is not commonly done.

SECONDARY DYSMENORRHEA (CONGESTIVE)

Secondary dysmenorrhea is normally considered to be menstruation—associated pain occurring in the presence of pelvic pathology.

TABLE 14.2: Common causes of secondary dysmenorrhea.

▪ Endometriosis ▪ Adenomyosis ▪ IUCD in utero ▪ Obstruction due to Müllerian anomalies ▪ Cervical stenosis	▪ Pelvic adhesions ▪ Uterine fibroid ▪ Pelvic congestion ▪ Endometrial polyp ▪ Chronic pelvic infection

Causes of Pain

The pain may be related to increasing tension in the pelvic tissues due to premenstrual pelvic congestion or increased vascularity in the pelvic organs (Table 14.2).

Patient Profile

The patients are usually in their thirties; more often parous and unrelated to any social status.

Clinical Features

The pain is dull, situated in the back and in front without any radiation. It usually appears 3–5 days prior to the period and relieves with the onset of bleeding. There is no systemic discomfort unlike primary dysmenorrhea. The patients may have got some discomfort even in between periods. Patient may present with few other gynecological symptoms like dyspareunia, dysuria, abnormal uterine bleeding and infertility.

Abdominal and vaginal examinations usually reveal the pathology.

TABLE 14.3: Causes of unilateral dysmenorrhea.

- Ovarian dysmenorrhea
- Bicornuate uterus
- Unilateral location of pelvic endometriosis
- Small fibroid polyp near one cornu
- Right ovarian vein syndrome
- Colonic or cecal spasm

Investigations

- **Transvaginal sonography:** Can detect most pelvic pathology (Leiomyoma, adenomyosis).
- **Saline infusion sonography** (submucous fibroid, polyps).
- **Laparoscopy** (endometriosis, PID): Useful for both diagnostic and therapeutic purposes.
- **Hysteroscopy** is useful for both diagnostic and therapeutic purposes.

Treatment

The treatment aims at the cause rather than the symptom. The type of treatment depends on the severity, age and parity of the patient.

Ovarian Dysmenorrhea

Right ovarian vein syndrome: Right ovarian vein crosses the ureter at right angle. During premenstrual period, due to pelvic congestion or increased blood flow, there may be marked engorgement in the vein → pressure on ureter → stasis → infection → pyelonephritis → pain.

This is an important cause of unilateral dysmenorrhea. (Table 14.2).

Other causes of unilateral dysmenorrhea are listed in Table 14.3.

OTHER DISORDERS TO CAUSE MENSTRUAL PAIN

MITTELSCHMERZ'S SYNDROME (OVULATION PAIN)

Ovular pain is not an infrequent complaint. It appears in the midmenstrual period. The pain is usually situated in the hypogastrium or in either of the iliac fossa. The pain is usually located on one side depending upon the side of ovary is ovulating and does not change from side to side. Nausea or vomiting is conspicuously absent. It rarely lasts more than 12 hours. It may be associated with slight vaginal bleeding or excessive mucoid vaginal discharge.

The exact cause is not known. **The probable factors are:** (a) Increased tension of the Graafian follicle just prior to rupture; (b) Peritoneal irritation by the follicular fluid following ovulation; and (c) Contraction of the tubes and uterus.

Treatment

It is effective with assurance and analgesics. In obstinate cases, the cure is absolute by making the cycle anovular with contraceptive pills.

PELVIC CONGESTION SYNDROME

There is disturbance in the autonomic nervous system, which may lead to gross vascular congestion with pelvic varicosities. The patient has a congestive type of dysmenorrhea without any demonstrable pelvic pathology.

Pathogenesis

Chronic pelvic pain, sensation of heaviness and pelvic pressure are due to the congested and tortuous ovarian and pelvic veins. This is mainly due to incompetent valves in the veins to cause retrograde flow and stasis. Estrogen is also implicated in the pathology of venous dilatation in addition to the mechanical factors.

Diagnosis

It is made by physical examination, tenderness is observed at the junction of the middle and lateral third of a line drawn between the symphysis and the anterior superior iliac spine or direct ovarian tenderness may be found. Radiologic study (pelvic venography), Doppler scan, duplex ultrasound scans, CT, MRI or angiography are helpful. Dilated tortuous ovarian vein with diameter ≥6 mm is seen. Laparoscopic diagnosis is difficult, as with intraperitoneal pressure and Trendelenburg position, these vessels may be compressed but will reappear as the pressure is reduced.

The patient complains of vague disorders with backache and pelvic pain with long standing position, at times with dyspareunia. There may be menorrhagia or metrorrhagia. The uterus may feel bulky and boggy.

Treatment

It is often unsatisfactory. Hormonal suppression, ovarian vein embolization or hysterectomy with bilateral salpingo-oophorectomy (BSO) are the options. Medroxyprogesterone acetate (MPA) 50 mg daily for 4 months or with GnRH agonist was found effective. In parous women with advancing age, hysterectomy may relieve the symptoms.

PREMENSTRUAL SYNDROME (SYN: PREMENSTRUAL TENSION)

Premenstrual syndrome (PMS) is a psychoneuroendocrine disorder of unknown etiology, often noticed just prior to menstruation. There is cyclic appearance of a large number of symptoms during the last 7–10 days of the menstrual cycle. Several biological factors like estrogen, progesterone, neurotransmitters—gamma aminobutyric acid (GABA), serotonin and the renin-angiotensin-aldosterone system (RAAS) are thought to be involved.

Diagnosis

According to American Psychiatric Association (2013) Diagnostic and Statistical Manual (DSM) recommends symptoms to be confirmed by prospective patient mood charting for at least two menstrual cycles (Table 14.4).

Common psychiatric conditions like depression and anxiety disorders are excluded. Additionally other medical conditions that have a multisystem presentation

TABLE 14.4: Diagnostic criteria for premenstrual dysphoric disorder (PMDD).

A. **Presence of symptoms (at least 5 or more must occur):** Occur in most cycles during the week before menses and improve within a few days after the onset of menses, and diminish in the week postmenses

B. **One (or more) of the following symptoms must be present:**
- Marked affective lability (mood swings, tearful, rejection)
- Marked irritability or anger or increased interpersonal conflicts
- Marked depressed moods, feelings of hopelessness, or self-deprecating thoughts
- Marked anxiety, tension

C. **One (or more) of the following symptoms must also be present:**
- Decreased interest in usual activities (school)
- Difficulty in concentrating
- Easy fatigability, low energy, lethargy
- Hypersomia or insomnia; over eating, food cravings
- Feelings of being overwhelmed
- Physical symptoms such as breast tenderness, muscle or joint aches, "bloating" or weight gain

Note: Criteria A–C must be present for most menstrual cycles in the preceding year

D. Symptoms are associated with significant distress or interferences with work, school, or relationships

E. The disturbance is not merely an exacerbation of another disorder such as major depression, panic disorder, persistent depressive disorder, or a personality disorder

F. Criterion A should be confirmed by prospective daily ratings in at least two symptomatic cycles

G. The symptoms are not due to physiological effects of a substance (drug abuse) or another medical condition (hyperthyroidism).

(*Courtesy:* American Psychiatric Association: Diagnostic and Statistical Manual of Mental Disorders, 5th edition. DSM-5, Washington, American Psychiatric Association; 2013)

like hypothyroidism, systemic lupus erythematosus (SLE), endometriosis, anemia, chronic fatigue syndrome and migraine are considered.

Pathophysiology

The exact cause is not known but the **following hypothesis are postulated**:

- **Alteration in the level of estrogen and progesterone** starting from the midluteal phase. Either there is altered estrogen: Progesterone ratio or diminished progesterone level.
- **Neuroendocrine factors:**
  - **Serotonin** is an important neurotransmitter in the central nervous system (CNS). During the luteal phase, decreased synthesis of serotonin is observed in women suffering from PMS.
  - **Endorphins:** The symptom complex of PMS is thought to be due to the withdrawal of endorphins (neurotransmitters) from CNS (Ch. 7) during the luteal phase.
  - **γ-aminobutyric acid (GABA)** suppresses the anxiety level in the brain. Medications that are GABA agonist, are effective.
- **Psychological and psychosocial factors** may be involved to produce behavioral changes.
- **Others:** Variety of factors have been mentioned to explain the symptom complex of PMS. These are thyrotrophin releasing hormone (TRH) prolactin, renin, aldosterone, prostaglandins, etc. Unfortunately, nothing is conclusive.

Clinical Features (Table 14.4)

PMS is more common in women aged 30–45. It may be related to childbirth or a disturbing life event.

There are no abnormal pelvic findings excepting features of pelvic congestion.

Treatment

As the etiology is multifactorial and too often obscure, various drugs are used either on speculation or empirically with varying degrees of success. **Lifestyle modification and congnitive behavior therapy are important steps.**

Overall therapy includes: Psychotropic agents, ovulation suppression and dietary modifications.

When the symptoms are severe and/or the treatment fails, psychiatric referral should be done.

General Management of PMS and PMDD (Table 14.5)

- **Nonpharmacological measures:**
  - (a) Assurance, yoga, stress management, diet manipulation; (b) Avoidance of salt, caffeine and alcohol especially in second half of cycle improves the symptoms.
  - Exercises: 30 minutes in most days of the week, including the luteal phase

TABLE 14.5: Management of PMS and PMDD.

Psychoactive drugs	*Indications*	*Drugs*	*Common side effects*
Selective serotonin reuptake inhibitors (SSRIs)	Depression, anxiety, PMS	Fluoxetine, Citalopram, Escitalopram, Sertraline, Paroxetine	Nausea, headache, insomnia, diarrhea, dry mouth, sexual dysfunction
Serotonin noradrenergic reuptake inhibitors (SNRIs)	Depression, anxiety, PMS	Venlafaxine XR, Duloxetine	Dizziness, constipation, dry mouth, anxiety, agitation
Tricyclic and tetracyclic antidepressants	Depression, anxiety disorders	Desipramine, Amitriptyline, Nortriptyline, Doxepin	Drowsiness, dry mouth, dizziness, blurred vision, urinary frequency, retention
Benzodiazepines	Anxiety disorders	Alprazolam, Clonazepam, Diazepam	Drowsiness, impaired memory, ataxia, hypotension

- Lifestyle modification
- Cognitive and behavioral therapy: Group psycho-education and relaxation therapy often benefit patients

■ **Nonhormonal medications:**
- Pyridoxine 100 mg twice daily is helpful by correcting tryptophan metabolism especially following 'pill' associated depression.
- Diuretics in the second half of the cycle—furosemide 20 mg daily for consecutive 5 days a week reduces fluid retention.

■ **Hormones**: Any one of the following drugs is to be prescribed:
- **Oral contraceptive pills (OCPs):** The idea is to suppress ovulation and to maintain an uniform hormonal milieu. The therapy is to be continued for 3–6 cycles. Newer OCPs contain progestin drospirenone. It has antimineralocorticoid and antiandrogenic properties. Drospirenone containing OCPs are found to have better control of symptoms.
- **Progesterone:** It is not effective in treating PMS. **Levonorgestrel intrauterine system (IUS)** had been used to suppress ovarian cycle.
- **Spironolactone:** It is a potassium sparing diuretic. It has antimineralocorticoid and antiandrogenic effects. It is given in the luteal phase (25–200 mg/day). It improves the symptoms of PMDD.
- **Bromocriptine:** 2.5 mg daily or twice daily may be helpful, at least to relieve the breast complaints.

■ **Suppression of ovarian cycle:** Suppression of the endogenous ovarian cycle can be achieved by:
- **Danazol** 200 mg daily is to be adjusted so as to produce amenorrhea. Barrier method of contraception should be advised during the treatment (Side effects of danazol are dose dependent, p. 445).
- **GnRH analog (p. 441):** The gonadal steroids are suppressed by administration of GnRH agonist for 6 months (medical oophorectomy). GnRH analog in PMS are used: (a) To assess the role of ovarian steroids in the etiology of PMS; (b) This can also predict whether bilateral oophorectomy would be of any help or not. The preparations and doses used are as given.
  - Goserelin (Zoladex): 3.6 mg is given subcutaneously at every 4 weeks.
  - Leuprorelin acetate (Prostap): 3.75 mg is given by SC or IM at every 4 weeks.
  - Triptorelin (Decapeptyl): 3 mg is given IM every 4 weeks.

  Results of GnRH agonist therapy are dramatic: GnRH agonist therapy is combined with estrogen progestin 'add-back' to combat the hypoestrogenic symptoms (Side effects are more with the long term use of GnRH, p. 442).

■ **Oophorectomy:** In established cases of primary PMS with recurrence of symptoms and approaching to menopause, hysterectomy with bilateral oophorectomy is a last resort.

MENSTRUAL MIGRAINE

It is characterized by attack of migraine that occurs either perimenstrually or both perimenstrually and also at other times. **Treatment** includes drugs of migraine (triptans)/or others (NSAIDs).

Catamenial seizure is defined as the seizure that occurs around the menstrual cycle. Imbalance of estrogen: Progesterone ratio is thought to be the cause as both the hormones modulate the cerebral excitability.

Treatment: Anticonvulsants are used as in other convulsions, depot medroxyprogesterone acetate (DMPA) has been found to be helpful.

KEY POINTS

- **Dysmenorrhea** is painful menstruation of sufficient magnitude so as to incapacitate the day to day activities. The incidence of primary dysmenorrhea is about 15–20%.
- **Primary dysmenorrhea** is almost always confined to ovulatory cycle and relieved following pregnancy and vaginal delivery. The pain usually appears following painless periods after menarche.
- **Primary dysmenorrhea** usually occurs before the age of 20 and **secondary dysmenorrhea** may occur at any age.
- Uterine junctional zone (JZ) dysperistalsis and hyperactivity are the basic pathological area for primary dysmenorrhea. The biochemical mediators involved are: Progesterone, $PGF_{2\alpha}$, endothelin, PAFs and leukotrienes.
- **Prostaglandin synthetase inhibitors** (NSAIDs), oral contraceptives or dydrogesterone are usually effective to minimize pain. Only cervical dilatation is required in obstinate cases. **Secondary dysmenorrhea** is almost always secondary to other pelvic pathology such as PID, endometriosis or uterine fibroids or obstruction due to Müllerian malformations.
- **Combined oral contraceptives (COCs)** reduce the severity of dysmenorrhea. It is the drug of choice when contraception is required.
- NSAIDs are the treatment of choice for primary dysmenorrhea.
- COCs reduce the severity of dysmenorrhea. This can be used with extended cycles for better relief. This can be used as a reasonable first line treatment especially when contraception is desired.
- *In **ovarian dysmenorrhea**, the pain is referred to the area innervated by T_{10} to L_1 segments.*
- Right ovarian vein syndrome is due to engorgement of right ovarian vein premenstrually so as to compress the right ureter with resultant pyelonephritis and pain.
- **Pain due to pelvic venous congestion** is relieved by continuous high dose para-methoxyamphetamine (MPA).

Contd...

Contd...

- **Mittelschmerz's syndrome** (ovular pain)—is an indirect evidence of ovulation—occurring in the midmenstrual period.\
- **Premenstrual syndrome (PMS)** regularly occurs in the luteal phase of each ovulatory menstrual cycle.
- There is no impairment of corpus luteal function for a woman who suffers from PMS. The symptoms are grouped together and described under the name premenstrual dysphoric disorder (PMDD).
- **Women with PMDD** show no deficit in cognitive function in the luteal phase.
- **Exact etiology** is unknown. Altered estrogen, progesterone ratio; reduced circulatory level of neurotransmitters (serotonin, GABA or endorphins) in the CNS may be responsible for the symptom complex.
- **The symptoms are not specific** (Table 14.4) and there is usually no abnormal pelvic finding.
- **The most useful diagnostic tool** for PMS is patient's symptom diary (Table 14.4).
- **Treatment** is supportive. Patient education, exercise along with dietetic support of calcium, vitamin B_6 may relieve PMS. Bromocriptine is effective in relieving breast tenderness. In obstinate cases, hormones—**LNG-IUS**, danazol are found helpful. Results of GnRH agonist therapy are dramatic. Tranquillizers (alprazolam—0.25 mg) and/or antidepressants (fluoxetine 20 mg daily or sertraline 50 mg/day) significantly improve the symptoms. Oral contraceptive pills suppressing ovulation, calcium, aerobic exercise are helpful in relieving symptoms of PMDD.
- Psychotropic drugs, particularly SSRIs have been accepted in RCTs to relieve PMS and PMDD symptoms. These drugs should be considered first line therapy (Table 14.5).
- Women desiring contraception, COCs can be given to improve the PMS/PMDD symptoms.
- *In proved cases—relief of symptoms, producing amenorrhea either by danazol or GnRH analogs for 3 months can be achieved. Hysterectomy with bilateral salpingo-oophorectomy in patients approaching menopause may be an option.*

CHAPTER

15 Abnormal Uterine Bleeding

CHAPTER OUTLINE

INTRODUCTION

Any uterine bleeding outside the normal volume, duration, regularity or frequency is considered abnormal uterine bleeding (AUB). Nearly 30% of all gynecological outpatient attendants are for AUB.

Normal Menstruation	
Cycle interval	28 days (21–35 days)
Menstrual flow	4–5 days
Menstrual blood loss	35 mL (20–80 mL)

COMMON CAUSES OF ABNORMAL UTERINE BLEEDING

PALM–COEIN (FIGO – 2011)

The acronym PALM-COEIN subdivides all the causes of AUB into nine main categories. The first few causes under the group PALM are structural or histologic causes. These conditions are diagnosed by imaging or by histology. The second group of causes, under "COIEN" are the nonstructural causes (Table 15.1).

This classification according to FIGO is notated in a consistent and systematic manner. The acronym AUB is followed by the letters PALM-COEIN and a subscript 0 or 1 associated with each letter to indicate the absence or presence in respect of the abnormality.

Example: A patient with abnormal uterine bleeding due to adenomyosis would be described as:

AUB: $P_0A_1L_0M_0$-$C_0O_0E_0I_0N_0$

A patient having AUB due to both polyp and anovulation, is described as (Table 15.1):

$P_1A_0L_0M_0$-$C_0O_1E_0I_0N_0$

The leiomyoma category is subdivided into patients with at least one submucosal myoma (LSM) and those with myomas that do not affect the endometrial cavity (L_0).

TABLE 15.1: Classification of AUB (FIGO – 2011).

Structural causes (PALM)		*Nonstructural systemic causes (COEIN)*	
Polyp	AUB–**P**	**C**oagulopathy	AUB–**C**
Adenomyosis	AUB–**A**	**O**vulatory dysfunction	AUB–**O**
Leiomyoma ▪ Submucosal myoma ▪ Other myoma	AUB–**L** AUB–**L SM** AUB–**LO**	**E**ndometrial	AUB–**E**
		Iatrogenic	AUB–**I**
Malignancy and hyperplasia	AUB–**M**	**N**ot yet identified	AUB–**N**

PATTERNS OF ABNORMAL UTERINE BLEEDING

MENORRHAGIA (SYN: HYPERMENORRHEA)

Menorrhagia is defined as cyclic bleeding at normal intervals; the bleeding is either excessive in amount (>80 mL) or duration (>7 days) or both.

Causes

Menorrhagia is a symptom of some underlying pathology—organic or functional.

Organic

Pelvic: The causes are tabulated in Tables 15.2 and 15.3.

Systemic: Liver dysfunction (cirrhosis)—failure to conjugate and thereby inactivate the estrogens.

- Congestive cardiac failure
- Severe hypertension

Endocrinal

- Hypothyroidism
- Hyperthyroidism

Hematological

- Idiopathic thrombocytopenic purpura
- Leukemia

TABLE 15.2: Pelvic pathology to cause menorrhagia.

Due to congestion, increased surface area, or hyperplasia of the endometrium
▪ Fibroid uterus ▪ Adenomyosis ▪ Pelvic endometriosis ▪ IUCD in utero ▪ Chronic tubo-ovarian mass ▪ Tubercular endometritis (early cases) ▪ Retroverted uterus—due to congestion ▪ Granulosa cell tumor of the ovary

TABLE 15.3: Common causes of menorrhagia.

- Fibroid uterus
- Pelvic endometriosis
- Adenomyosis
- Chronic tubo-ovarian mass

- von Willebrand's disease
- Platelet deficiency (thrombocytopenia)
- Deficiency of clotting factor (V, VII, X, XI, XIII)
- Women with anticoagulation therapy (heparin LMWH).

Emotional upset

Functional

Due to disturbed hypothalamo-pituitary-ovarian-endometrial axis. Common causes of abnormal vaginal bleeding includes all the causes of organic, systemic and also the nonmenstrual causes of bleeding.

Diagnosis

Long duration of flow, passage of big clots, use of increased number of thick sanitary pads, pallor, and low level of hemoglobin give an idea about the correct diagnosis and magnitude of menorrhagia.

Treatment

The definitive treatment is appropriate to the cause for menorrhagia.

POLYMENORRHEA (SYN: EPIMENORRHEA)

Polymenorrhea is defined as cyclic bleeding where the cycle is reduced to an arbitrary limit of **less than 21 days** and remains constant at that frequency. If the frequent cycle is associated with excessive and/or prolonged bleeding, it is called epimenorrhagia.

Causes

Dysfunctional: It is seen predominantly during adolescence, preceding menopause and following delivery and abortion. Hyperstimulation of the ovary by the pituitary hormones may be the responsible factor.

Ovarian hyperemia as in pelvic inflammatory disease (PID) or ovarian endometriosis.

Treatment

Persistent dysfunctional type is to be treated by hormone as outlined in DUB (discussed later in this Ch.).

METRORRHAGIA (INTERMENSTRUAL BLEEDING)

Metrorrhagia is defined as irregular, acyclic bleeding from the uterus. Amount of bleeding is variable. While metrorrhagia strictly concerns uterine bleeding but in clinical practice, the bleeding from any part of the genital tract is included under the heading. Then again, irregular bleeding in the form of contact bleeding (Table 15.4) or intermenstrual bleeding (Tables 15.5 and 15.6) in an otherwise normal cycle is also included in metrorrhagia. In fact, it is mostly related to surface lesion in the uterus (Fig. 15.1).

Menometrorrhagia is the term applied when the bleeding is so irregular and excessive that the menses (periods) cannot be identified at all.

TABLE 15.4: Causes of contact bleeding.

- Carcinoma cervix
- Mucus polyp of cervix
- Vascular ectopy of the cervix especially during pregnancy, pill use cervix
- Infections—chlamydial or tubercular cervicitis
- Cervical endometriosis

TABLE 15.5: Causes of acyclic bleeding.

- DUB—usually during adolescence, following childbirth and abortion and preceding menopause
- Submucous fibroid
- Uterine polyp
- Carcinoma cervix and endometrial carcinoma

TABLE 15.6: Causes of intermenstrual bleeding.

Apart from the causes of contact bleeding, other causes are:
- Urethral caruncle
- Ovular bleeding
- Breakthrough bleeding in pill use
- IUCD in utero
- Decubitus ulcer
- Progesterone only contraceptive use

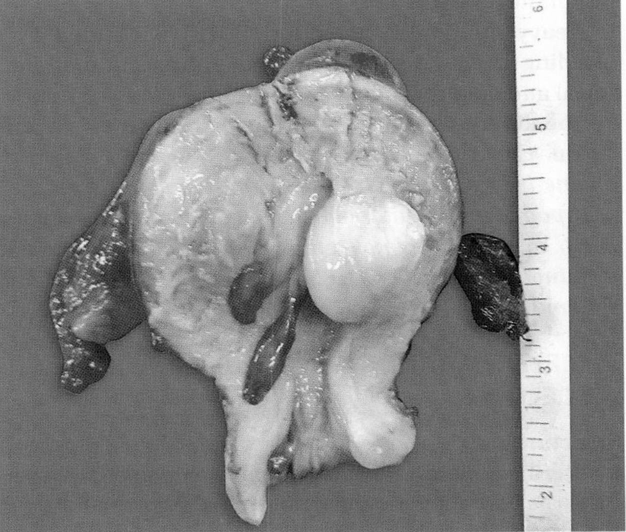

Fig. 15.1: Metrorrhagia due to multiple uterine submucous polyps (endometrial and fibroid).

TABLE 15.7: Common causes of oligomenorrhea.

- **Age-related**—during adolescence and preceding menopause
- **Weight-related**—obesity
- **Stress and exercise** related
- **Endocrine disorders**—PCOS (most common), hyperprolactinemia, hyperthyroidism
- **Androgen producing tumors**—ovarian, adrenal
- **Tubercular endometritis**—late cases
- **Drugs:**
  - Phenothiazines
  - Cimetidine
  - Methyldopa

Treatment

Treatment is directed to the underlying pathology.

Malignancy is to be excluded prior to any definitive treatment.

OLIGOMENORRHEA

Menstrual bleeding occurring **more than 35 days** apart and which remains constant at that frequency is called **oligomenorrhea**. Causes are mentioned in Table 15.7.

HYPOMENORRHEA

When the menstrual bleeding is unduly scanty and lasts for less than 2 days, it is called **hypomenorrhea**.

Causes

The causes may be local (uterine synechiae or endometrial tuberculosis), endocrinal (use of oral contraceptives, thyroid dysfunction, and premenopausal period), or systemic (malnutrition).

DYSFUNCTIONAL UTERINE BLEEDING

Dysfunctional uterine bleeding (DUB) is defined as **a state of abnormal uterine bleeding without any clinically detectable organic, systemic, and iatrogenic cause (pelvic pathology, e.g. tumor, inflammation or pregnancy is excluded).**

Heavy menstrual bleeding (HMB) is defined as a bleeding that interferes with woman's physical, emotional, social and maternal quality of life.

The diagnosis is based with the exclusion of 'organic lesion'. *Currently DUB is defined as a state of abnormal uterine bleeding following anovulation due to dysfunction of hypothalamo-pituitary-ovarian axis* (endocrine origin). ***DUB, so defined, is not currently favored as the newer terminology, PALM-COIEN is more consistent and systematic.***

DIFFERENTIAL DIAGNOSIS OF ABNORMAL BLEEDING

Structural:

- **Uterine:** Leiomyoma, adenomyosis, endometrial hyperplasia or malignancy, arteriovenous malformation
- **Cervix:** Polyp, cancer
- **Vagina:** Cancer
- **Fallopian tube:** Cancer
- **Ovarian tumors:** Granulosa cell tumor.
- **Anovulation**
- Thyroid dysfunction
- Androgen excess: PCOS
- Hyperprolactinemia
- Premature ovarian failure

Pregnancy complications: Miscarriages, gestational trophoblastic disease (GTD).

Iatrogenic: Medications—anticoagulants, heparin, LMWH, IUCD, trauma.

Infections: STIs, endometritis, tuberculosis.

Systemic: Hepatic and renal dysfunction, coagulopathies.

Endometrial polyps (AUB-P) (p. 235)

Adenomyosis (p 264): Diagnosis is made by sonography. MRI is superior to USG.

Leiomyoma: For classification system of fibroids including submucosal, intramural and subserosal (Fig. 20.5).

Malignancy (AUB-M): It includes female genital tract (vulva, vagina, cervix, endometrium, uterus, tubes and ovary) cancers. Malignancy is observed in 4.5% of postmenopausal women when they present with symptoms.

Coagulopathy (AUB-C): Von Willebrand disease, prothrombin deficiency, hemophilias A, B, ITP, leukemia, platelet deficiency, inherited coagulopathies due to deficiency of other clotting factors (V, VII, X, XI, XIII).

Anticoagulation therapy: Women on heparin or LMWH may present with AUB. Nearly 20% of adolescent girls with AUB have been found to suffer from coagulation disorders.

Ovulatory dysfunction (AUB-O): Often seen in the premenarchal and premenopausal women. This is often due to abnormality of neuroendocrine function. It may be due to steady state of anovulation, resulting in continued estrogenic endometrial stimulation without any effect of progesterone.

Causes of anovulation may be: Extremes of reproductive age (adolescent and perimenopausal women), dysfunction of HPO axis.

Iatrogenic (AUB-I): It is mostly due to medications. **Iatrogenic causes are:** Breakthrough bleeding following the use of combined oral contraceptives; erratic use of pills or any contraceptive steroids (vaginal rings), use of IUCDs, or LNG-IUS.

Endometrial (AUB-E): Abnormal endometrial production of PGI_2 and deficiency of $PGF_{2\alpha}$ or excessive production of PGE, explain ovulatory AUB.

Chronic inflammatory changes of the endometrium may also result in AUB. Subclinical infection with *C. trachomatis* also causes AUB.

Not otherwise specified (AUB–N): Trauma and foreign bodies are included in the category. Investigation and treatment are done according to the cause.

Diagnostic Criteria to Detect Coagulopathy

Individuals with heavy menstrual bleeding (HMB) and history evaluation:

One of the following	*Two of the following*
▪ PPH ▪ Surgical bleed ▪ Dental bleed	▪ Bruising >5 cm ▪ Epistaxis 1–2 episodes/month ▪ Gum bleeding ▪ Family history of bleeding

Investigations: (a) CBC; (b) PT/PTT; (c) vWF antigen; (d) Ristocetin cofactor.

PATHOPHYSIOLOGY OF DUB

The physiological mechanism of hemostasis in normal menstruation are: (a) Platelet adhesion formation; (b) Formation of platelet plug with fibrin to seal the bleeding vessels; (c) Localized vasoconstriction; (d) Regeneration of endometrium; (e) Biochemical mechanism involved are: In increased endometrial ratio of $PGF_{2\alpha}$/ PGE_2 and thromboxane. **$PGF_{2\alpha}$ causes vasoconstriction and reduces bleeding.** Progesterone increases the level of $PGF_{2\alpha}$ from arachidonic acid. **Levels of endothelin,** which is a powerful vasoconstrictor is also increased. In anovulatory DUB, there is decreased synthesis of $PGF_{2\alpha}$ and the ratio of $PGF_{2\alpha}/PGE_2$ and the endothelin is low.

Anovulatory cycles are usually not associated with dysmenorrhea as the level of $PGF_{2\alpha}$ is low. Women with menorrhagia have low level of thromboxane in the endometrium.

The endometrial abnormalities may be *primary or secondary* to **incoordination in the hypothalamo-pituitary-ovarian axis.** It is thus *more prevalent in extremes of reproductive period*—adolescence and premenopause or following childbirth and abortion.

The abnormal bleeding (DUB) may be associated with or without ovulation and accordingly grouped into:

- **Ovular bleeding (20%)**
- **Anovular bleeding (80%)**

Ovular bleeding (DUB) may present with: Polymenorrhea or oligomenorrhea or functional menorrhagia.

These conditions usually occur during adolescence and the premenopausal period.

- **Polymenorrhea** is due to speeded follicular growth with hyperstimulation of FSH and/or shortened luteal phase due to premature lysis of corpus luteum. In either situation, the endometrium is secretory type.
- **Oligomenorrhea** is again rare. It may be due to ovarian unresponsiveness to FSH. The proliferative phase is prolonged with normal secretory phase. Endometrium is of secretory type.
- **Functional menorrhagia:**
  - ***Irregular shedding of the endometrium:*** Irregular shedding is continued for a variable period as there is simultaneous failure of endometrial regeneration. This is due to incomplete atrophy of the corpus luteum, leading to serum progesterone level low and persistent. Endometrium reveals a mixture of secretory and proliferative picture.
  - **Irregular ripening of the endometrium**—is clinically manifested as slight bleeding that starts prior to the actual onset of menses. Secretion of both estrogen and progesterone is inadequate to support the endometrium. This is due to poor formation and function of corpus luteum. The plasma level of progesterone is low. Endometrium reveals patchy areas of secretary changes amidst proliferative endometrium.

Anovular Bleeding

- **Menorrhagia:** Anovulatory bleeding is usually excessive. There is absence of progesterone due to anovulation. The endometrial growth is under the influence of estrogen throughout the cycle. There is inadequate structural stromal support and the endometrium remains fragile.

  Thus, with the withdrawal of estrogen due to negative feedback action of FSH, the endometrial shedding continues for a longer period in asynchronous sequences because of lack of compactness.
- **Cystic glandular hyperplasia**

  (Syn: Metropathia hemorrhagica, Schroeder's disease)

  This type of abnormal bleeding is usually met in premenopausal women.

  The basic fault may lie in the ovaries or may be due to disturbance of the rhythmic secretion of the gonadotropins. There is slow increase in secretion of estrogen but no negative feedback inhibition of FSH. The net effect is gradual rise in the level of estrogen with concomitant phase of amenorrhea for about 6–8 weeks. As there is no ovulation, the endometrium is under the influence of estrogen without being opposed by growth limiting progesterone for a prolonged period. After a variable period, however, the estrogen level falls resulting in endometrial shedding with heavy bleeding. Bleeding also occurs when the endometrial growth have outgrown their blood supply. Due to increased endometrial thickness, tissue breakdown continues for a long time. Bleeding is heavy as there is no vasoconstrictor effect of $PGF_{2\alpha}$. Bleeding is prolonged until the endometrium and blood vessels regenerate to control it.

  Changes in the uterus: There is variable degree of myohyperplasia with symmetrical enlargement of the uterus to a size of about 8–10 weeks due to simultaneous hypertrophy of muscles (Fig. 15.2).

Microscopically

- There is marked hyperplasia of all the endometrial components. There is; however, intense cystic glandular hypertrophy rather than hyperplasia with marked disparity in sizes. Some of the glands are small,

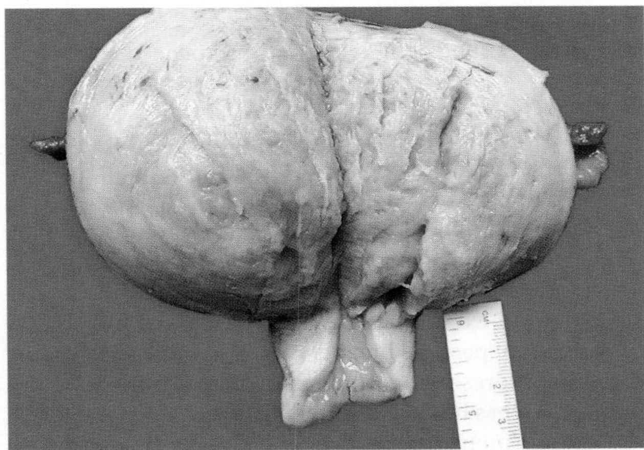

Fig. 15.2: Increased uterine size with significant myohyperplasia and marked hyperplasia of the endometrium.

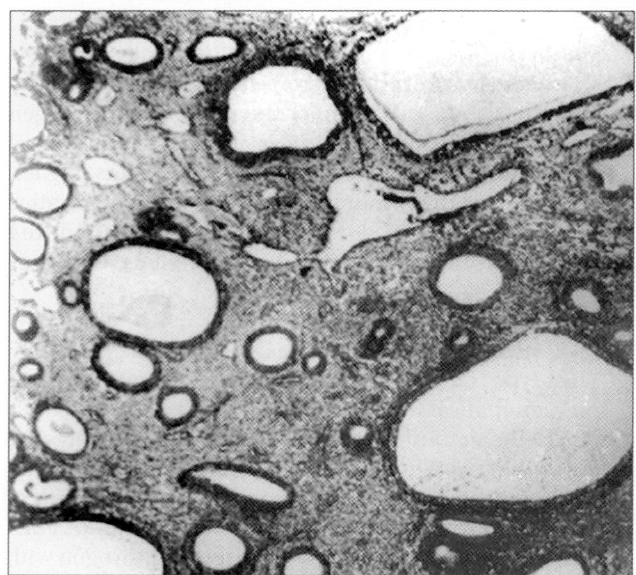

Fig. 15.3: Endometrium showing 'Swiss cheese' appearance.

others are large giving the appearance of 'Swiss cheese' pattern (Fig. 15.3) (small and large holes of Swiss cheese made in Switzerland). The glands are empty and lined by columnar epithelium.

- Absence of secretory changes.
- Areas of necrosis in the superficial layers with small hemorrhages and leukocytic infiltration.

Changes in the ovary: Cystic changes may be observed involving one or both the ovaries. The cyst is of follicular type. There is no evidence of corpus luteum.

In anovulatory DUB, there is decreased synthesis of $PGF_{2\alpha}$ ($PGF_{2\alpha}/PGE_2$ is low) and thromboxane. **Due to this reason, DUB of this type is absolutely painless**.

INVESTIGATIONS

The investigation aims at:

- To confirm the menstrual abnormality as stated by the patient
- To detect the **systemic, iatrogenic or 'organic'** pelvic pathology
- To work out the definite therapy protocol.

History

First, it is to be confirmed that the bleeding is through the vagina and not from the urethra or rectum. Through history is taken as regard the frequency, duration and the amount of bleeding. History is taken to describe the abnormality such as oligomenorrhea, polymenorrhea, heavy menstrual bleeding or intermenstrual bleed. **The statement of excessive bleeding is assessed by** number of pads used, passage of clots (size and number). Among the patients presenting with menorrhagia, only about 50% have got excess blood loss (> 80 mL).

Nature of menstrual abnormality is then to be enquired—cyclic or acyclic, its relation to puberty, pregnancy events and last normal cycle. Use of steroidal contraceptives or IUCD insertion should be enquired. History of abnormal bleeding from the injury site, epistaxis, gum bleeding (p 156), or that suggestive of anticoagulation therapy should be enquired.

A thorough general and relevant systemic examination are to be made in an effort to find out the cause or effect of abnormal bleeding.

Estimation of menstrual blood loss either directly by alkaline hematin or indirectly by pictorial chart is not routinely done.

General and Physical Examination

Pallor, edema, neck glands, thyroid, and systemic examination are done.

Internal Examination

Bimanual examination including speculum examination should be done in all cases except in virgins, where rectal examination is to be done to exclude palpable pelvic pathology. If vaginal examination is required in virgins, it should be done under general anesthesia and along with endometrial curettage.

Special Investigations

- **Blood values:** Hemoglobin estimation is done in every case. In pubertal menorrhagia not responding to usual therapy, platelet count, prothrombin time, bleeding time, partial thromboplastin time are to be estimated. In suspected cases of thyroid dysfunction, serum TSH, T_3, and T_4 estimations are to be done. Direct assessment of menstrual blood loss is not generally always possible.
  - Estimation of hemoglobin concentration, serum iron levels and serum ferritin levels are useful.
  - Additional tests are: Serum β-hCG and prolactin. **Von willebrand factor:** It is responsible for platelet adhesion and protection against degradation of coagulation factors.
  - Family history of bleeding, epistaxis, bruising, gum bleeding, surgical bleeding or PPH are indications for study of coagulation profile (*see* Table above ....).
- **Transvaginal sonography (TVS) and color Doppler** findings of endometrial hyperplasia are: (a) Endometrial thickness >12 mm; (b) Hyperechoic and regular outline; (c) Angiogenesis and neovascular signal study and (d) **Endometrial thickness** ≤4 mm suggests atrophic endometrium. TVS is also very sensitive to detect any anatomical abnormality (fibroid, adenomyosis) of the uterus, endometrium and adnexae.
- **Saline infusion sonography (SIS)** is found superior (p. 99) to diagnose endometrial polyps, submucous fibroids and intrauterine abnormality (septate/subseptate uterus).
- **Ultrasonography and MRI:** Evaluation of the myometrium for other structural uterine or pelvic pathology (leiomyomas, adenomyosis, or ovarian tumor) can be diagnosed.

- **Magnetic resonance imaging (MRI)** is superior in the diagnosis of adenomyosis when compared to ultrasonography (p. 264).
- **Hysteroscopy** is done for better evaluation of endometrial lesion and to take biopsy from the offending site under direct vision. The frequent findings of polyp and submucous fibroid are often missed by blind curettage. **Hysteroscopy and directed biopsy (H and B)** can be performed as an outpatient basis. H and B has replaced conventional D&C (for details p. 492).
- **Endometrial sampling** (p. 94) can be done as an outpatient basis. **Pipelle sampler** is easy to use. As it is a blind procedure, intrauterine pathology (polyps, submucous fibroids) cannot be detected.
- **Laparoscopy:** To exclude unsuspected pelvic pathology such as endometriosis, PID or ovarian tumor (granulosa cell tumor). The indication is urgent, if associated with pelvic pain.
- **Endometrial biopsy (EB)**
  Diagnostic uterine curettage (D&C) is indicated in DUB:
  - To exclude the **organic lesions in the endometrium** (incomplete abortion, endometrial polyp, tubercular endometritis or endometrial carcinoma).
  - To determine the functional state of the endometrium.
  - To have incidental therapeutic benefit.

In adolescent AUB, EB is rarely needed only if bleeding fails to stop with medical therapy or is severe in nature.

During childbearing period (20–40 years), EB should be done, **if the bleeding is acyclic. Risk of endometrial carcinoma in this age group is very low.**

During postmenopausal period, EB is **mandatory** to exclude endometrial malignancy. Thin plastic endometrial tissue samplers (pipelle) are available (Fig. 9.21). It helps to obtain adequate endometrial sample for histological examination. It is done as an OPD procedure without any anesthetic.

SUMMARY OF INVESTIGATIONS

(a) Blood values including coagulation profile; (b) TVS, SIS to exclude uterine structural abnormalities; (c) USG or MRI imaging; (d) Endometrial sampling with pipelle or hysteroscopic guided biopsy; (e) Laparoscopy, for a selected case.

MANAGEMENT

Because of diverse etiopathology of AUB in different phases of woman's life, the management protocols vary. **Management depends on:** (a) Age; (b) Desire for childbearing; (c) Severity of bleeding; (d) Associated pathology.

- **Pubertal and adolescent menorrhagia <20 years (p. 154).**
- **Reproductive period (20–40 years).**
- **Premenopausal (>40 years).**
- **Postmenopausal.**
- **Associated pathology.**

Reproductive Period

- **General**
- **Medical**
- **Surgery**

General

- **Rest** is advised during bleeding phase. Assurance and sympathetic handling are helpful particularly in adolescents.
- **Anemia** should be corrected appropriately by diet, hematinics, and even by blood transfusion.
- **Any systemic or endocrinal abnormality** should be investigated and treated accordingly.

Medical Management of DUB

Dysfunctional uterine bleeding, in majority responds well to conservative treatment during adolescence and early reproductive period. The derivatives of drugs used are listed in the Table 15.8.

Nonhormonal Management

- **Prostaglandin synthetase inhibitors:** All NSAIDs inhibit cyclooxygenase and thus block the synthesis of both thromboxane and prostacyclin pathway. NSAIDs reduce menstrual blood loss in ovulatory DUB by about 25% to 50%. Mefenamic acid is much effective in women aged more than 35 years and in cases of ovulatory DUB. The dose is 150–600 mg orally in divided doses during the bleeding phase. The fenamates inhibit the synthesis of prostaglandins and interfere with the binding of PGE_2 to its receptor. NSAIDs can reduce menstrual blood loss by 25–50%. Improvement of dysmenorrhea headache, or nausea are the added benefits. Side effects GI system are often mild. **NSAIDs may be used as second line medical treatment.**
- **Antifibrinolytic agents (tranexamic acid)** reduces menstrual blood loss by 50%. It counteracts the endometrial fibrinolytic system. It is particularly helpful in IUCD induced menorrhagia. Gastrointestinal side effects are common. **Antifibrinolytic agents can be used as a second line therapy.**

  History of thromboembolism is a contraindication to its use.

Hormones

- With the introduction of potent **orally active progestins, they became the mainstay in the management of DUB in all age groups** and practically replaced the isolated use of estrogens and androgens.
- **Progestins**: The common preparations used are norethisterone acetate and medroxyprogesterone acetate (Table 15.8). The latter one is better than the former as it does not alter the serum lipids. **Mechanism of antiestrogenic action of progestins are**: (a) Stimulates the enzyme (17-β-hydroxysteroid dehydrogenase) that

TABLE 15.8: Medical management of AUB (for further details: p. 159).

Drug class and Name	*Dosage*	*Common side effects*
A. Prostaglandin (p. 157) synthesis inhibitor (PSI)		
Mefenamic acid	500 mg TID x 5 days	GI system: Nausea, vomiting, gastric ulcer, diarrhoea, GI bleed, thrombocytopenia
B. Antifibrinolytic agents		
Tranexamic acid (TA)	500 mg–1 g 6 hourly x 5 days	GI symptoms: Nausea, vomiting, diarrhoea, headache, visual disturbances
C. Hormones		
■ **COCs**	EE: 20–30 μg + Levonorgestrel 0.15 mg: Once a day x 21 days/ Extended use (p. 406)	p. 408
■ **Progestogens**: • Norethisterone acetate (D_5–D_{25}) • Medroxyprogesterone acetate (D_5–D_{25}) • Dydrogesterone (D_5–D_{25})	 5 mg TID 10 mg TID 10 mg TID	Depression, headache, acne, weight gain (p. 450)
■ Gestrinone	1.25–2.5 mg twice a week	Weight gain, acne, hirsuitism, dyslipidemia (p. 445)
• Danazol (19 nor steriod)	200 mg/day	Weight gain, acne, hirsuitism, dyslipidemia (p. 445)
• LNG-IUS (Mirena)	Daily release 20 μg; effective for 5 years	■ Very effective ■ Many other noncontraceptive benefits
• GnRH analogs	(Ch. 32)	■ Hypoestrogenemia, menopausal symptoms, osteoporosis on prolonged use (p. 442)
• Equine conjugated estrogen	10 mg/day in 4 divided doses (for control of acute bleeding	Nausea, vomiting, thrombosis
D. Others		
■ Ormeloxifene ■ Ethamsylate	60 mg twice a weak 500 mg QID	Oligomenorrhea Nausea, vomiting, headache

converts estradiol to estrone (less potent); (b) Inhibits induction of estrogen receptor; (c) Antimitotic effect on the endometrium; (d) Stops endometrial growth; (e) Raises $PGF_{2\alpha}$/PGE and thromboxane ratio in the endometrium; (f) Causes organized endometrial shedding up to the basal layer; (g) Progesterone raises the level of endometrial endothelin and VEGF to generate new vessels. While isolated progestins therapy is highly effective in anovular DUB, in ovular DUB combined preparations of progestogen and estrogen (combined oral pills) are effective.

The preparations are used:

- **Cyclic therapy**
- **Continuous therapy**

To stop bleeding and regulate the cycle:

Norethisterone preparations (5 mg tab) are used thrice daily till bleeding stops, which it usually does by 3–7 days.

Cyclic therapy

- 5th–25th day course
- 15th–25th day course.

5th to 25th day course

In ovular bleeding: **Any low dose combined oral pills are effective** when given from 5th to 25th day of cycle for 3 consecutive cycles. It causes endometrial atrophy. It is more effective compared to progesterone therapy as it suppress the hypothalamo-pituitary axis more effectively.

In anovular bleeding: Cyclic progestogen preparation of medroxyprogesterone acetate (MPA) 10 mg (TID) or norethisterone 5 mg (TID) is used from 5th to 25th day of cycle for 3 cycles.

15th to 25th day course

In ovular bleeding, where the patient wants pregnancy or in cases of irregular shedding or irregular ripening of the endometrium, dydrogesterone 1 tab (10 mg) daily or twice a day from 15th to 25th day may cure the state. This regimen is less effective than 5th to 25th day course. However, it does not suppress ovulation.

Adolescent anovulatory women have immaturity of hypothalamo-pituitary-ovarian (H-P-O) axis. They are ideal for use of short-term cylic therapy until the maturity of the positive feedback system is established.

Continuous progestins

Progestins also inhibit pituitary gonadotropin secretion and ovarian hormone production.

Medroxyprogesterone acetate 10 mg thrice daily is given and treatment is usually continued for at least 90 days.

Various continuous preparations may be used. Oral (Table 15.8), long-acting intramuscular injections, DMPA implants, progestogen only pill are effective to reduce menstrual blood loss. They may also result in oligomenorrhea or amenorrhea.

- **Estrogen:** In situations where the bleeding is acute and severe, conjugated estrogen 25 mg is given intravenously (IV). It helps with rapid growth of the denuded endometrium and promotes platelet adhesiveness.

It controls bleeding by process of healing. It may be repeated every four hours till the bleeding is controlled, when oral therapy is started. Once the bleeding stops, progestin (MPA 10 mg a day) is to be added. Combined oral contraceptive (COC) is used for long-term treatment. Proliferation of endometrium, increase in the level of fibrinogen, factors—V, X, and platelet aggregation are the other mechanisms of action for estrogen therapy. If bleeding continues further, D&C is indicated.

- **Intrauterine progestogen:** Levonorgestrel intrauterine system (LNG-IUS) induce endometrial glandular atrophy, stromal decidualization and endometrial cell inactivation. It is effective for 5 years. It has minimal systemic absorption. Reduction of blood loss is significant (80–100%). It is considered as medical hysterectomy. In addition to its many other health benefits it is an effective contraceptive measure. LNG-IUS is also on alternative to hysterectomy. Women with AUB due to coagulopathy including von Willebrand disease, or due to anticoagulation therapy, are also managed successfully with LNG-IUS. **LNG-IUS is recommended as a first line therapy for a woman with HMB, in the absence of any structural or histological abnormality.**
- **Danazol**: Danazol is suitable in cases with recurrent symptoms and in patients waiting for hysterectomy. The dose varies from 200–400 mg daily in 4 divided doses continuously for 3 months. A smaller dose tends to minimize the blood loss and a higher dose produces amenorrhea. It reduces blood loss by 60%.
- **Mifepristone (RU 486)**: It is an antiprogesterone (19 nor-steroid). It inhibits ovulation and induces amenorrhea and reduces myoma size.
- **GnRH agonists:** The subtherapeutic doses reduce the blood loss, whereas therapeutic doses produce amenorrhea. It is valuable as short-term use in severe DUB, particularly if the woman is infertile and wants pregnancy. The drugs are used subcutaneously or intranasally. It improves anemia, and is helpful when used before endometrial ablation (*see* below). A varying degree of hypoestrogenic features may appear.
- **Ormeloxifene** (estrogen receptor modulator) is used as an oral contraceptive and it reduces the blood loss also. It is given 60 mg twice weekly for 3 months.
- **Desmopressin:** It is a synthetic analog of arginine-vasopressin. It is especially indicated in cases with von Willebrand's disease and factor VIII deficiency. It is given IV (0.3 μg/kg) or intranasally.

Surgical Management of DUB

- Uterine curettage
- Endometrial ablation/resection
- Hysterectomy.

Uterine Curettage

It is done predominantly as a diagnostic tool for elderly women but at times, it has got hemostatic and therapeutic effect by removing the necrosed and unhealthy endometrium (Table 15.9). It should be done following ultrasonography for detection of endometrial pathology. The indication is an urgent one, if the bleeding is acyclic and where endometrial pathology is suspected. **Ideally, hysteroscopy and directed biopsy should be considered both for the purpose of diagnosis and therapy. Presently, dilatation and curettage should be used neither as a diagnostic tool nor for the purpose of therapy.**

TABLE 15.9: Time schedule for uterine curettage.

Cyclic	▪ Menorrhagia ▪ Irregular shedding ▪ Irregular ripening	▪ 5–6 days prior to period ▪ 5–6 days after the period starts ▪ Soon after the period starts
Acyclic	—	Soon after the period starts
Continuous	—	Any time

Endometrial Ablation/Resection (EA/ER)

***Indications are*:** (a) Failed medical treatment; (b) Women who do not wish to preserve menstrual or reproductive function; (c) Uterus—normal size or not bigger than 10 weeks pregnancy size; (d) Small uterine fibroids (<3 cm); (e) Women who want to avoid longer surgery; (f) Woman who prefers to preserve her uterus.

Prior to any EA, endometrial sampling should be done. Uterine cavity should be evaluated for the size and any pathology. Pretreatment with Danazol or GnRH agonist should be given.

- **Uterine thermal balloon (Thermal** for destruction of endometrium is currently used with satisfactory results. Endometrium is destroyed using a thermal balloon with hot normal saline (87°C) for 8–10 minutes. No dilatation of the cervical canal is needed. This procedure is suitable for women who are not suitable for general anesthetic or long duration surgery. The success rate is similar to transcervical resection of the endometrium (TCRE). No pretreatment endometrial thining is required. **This is considered as a first line therapy and is done as a day care basis.**
- **Microwave endometrial ablation** is simple and carried out as an outpatient procedure. Microwave electromagnetic heat energy causes ablation of the endometrium. Probe used is of 8 mm. Endometrial tissue up to a depth of 6 mm is ablated. Temperature in the tissue is 30°C. Treatment time (2–4 minutes) is less compared to TCRE. Results are similar to TCRE.
- **Novasure:** Endometrial ablation is done using bipolar radiofrequency mounted on an expandable probe of 7.2 mm. This creates a confluent lesion on the entire endometrial surface. Time required for global endometrial ablation is 90 seconds approximately.

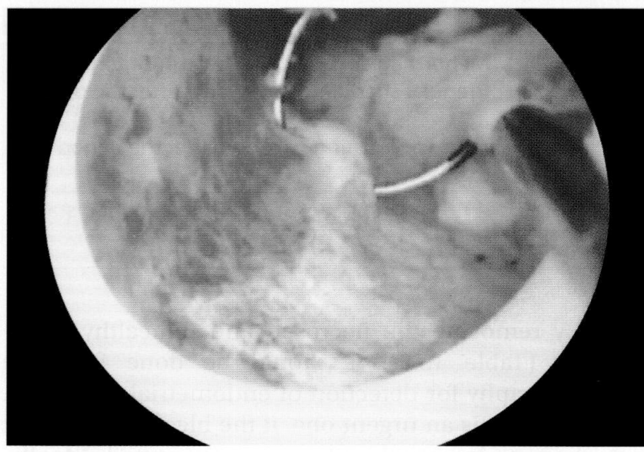

Fig. 15.4: Endometrial resection with the cutting loop.

Radiofrequency energy vaporizes or coagulates the endometrium up to the myometrium. The procedure is quick, simple, and safe. **Women with uterine cavity <4 cm, PID, cesarean delivery are contraindicated.** **Pretreatment** with danazol or GnRH agonists for 3 weeks prior to endometrial ablation is helpful to make the endometrium atrophic.

- **Transcervical resection of the endometrium (TCRE)** through continuous flow resectoscope is quicker and less costlier than laser ablation. It can be carried out even under paracervical block. Resectoscope loop must remove the basal layer of endometrium along with superficial layer of myometrium, otherwise regeneration of endometrium causes failure of operation (Fig. 15.4). Use of bipolar (versa point), is more safe.
- **Laser ablation** of the endometrium using the Nd: YAG laser through hysteroscope is an alternative to hysterectomy. Tissue destruction (coagulation, vaporization, and carbonization) to a **depth of 4–5 mm produces a therapeutic Ashermann's syndrome and amenorrhea**. The method is largely replaced by resection methods.
- **Roller ball ablation** of endometrium is also effective. It coagulates endometrium up to a depth of about 4 mm.

The first generation ablation methods (TRCE and REA) are used when hysteroscopic myomectomy is to be done simultaneously.

Complications: Infection, uterine perforations (<1%), endometritis, tubal pain rarely pregnancy. Fluid absorption may occur during hysteroscopic procedure. After global endometrial ablation procedure, sexually active women should use some form of contraception.

Contraindications of Endometrial Ablation

- Women desiring pregnancy
- Acute PID
- Prior uterine scar (myomectomy, C-section)
- Endometrial hyperplasia/cancer
- Postmenopausal women.

Results of endometrial ablation or resection

Overall success with these methods is 80–90%. About 35–45% women become amenorrheic and another 50% will have significant decrease in blood loss. But 10% of women may need repeat procedure or hysterectomy. For case selection, side effects, contraindications, and complication (p. 522).

Uterine artery embolization is commonly done in women with large uterine fibroid (>3 cm) with heavy bleeding. Polyvinyl alcohol microspheres (p. 99) are injected to block uterine artery under fluoroscopic guidance through a catheter in the femoral artery. This shrinks fibroids and control the bleeding. The procedure is safe and effective (p. 99).

Hysterectomy (p. 181)

It is not recommended as a first line therapy for heavy menstrual bleeding (HMB) or DUB. However, hysterectomy is justified when the conservative treatment fails or contraindicated and the blood loss impairs the health and quality of life. Presence of endometrial hyperplasia and atypia on endometrial histology is an indication for hysterectomy. The decision can be made easily as the patient is approaching 40. **Hysterectomy** may be done depending on the route by vaginal, abdominal, or laparoscopic assisted vaginal method or robotic medthod. In this regard, the factors to consider are: Uterine size, mobility, descent, previous surgery, and presence of comorbidities (obesity, diabetes, heart disease, or hypertension). Healthy ovaries may be preserved at the time of hysterectomy especially those under 45 years of age.

Surgical Treatment of AUB

- Endometrial ablation
  - Thermal balloon
  - Novasure
  - Microwave
- Transcervical resection of endometrium (TCRE)
  - Laser
  - Rollerball
- Uterine artery embolization (p. 99)
- Hysterectomy (abdominal, vaginal, laparoscopic, robotic)

MANAGEMENT OPTIONS FOR A CASE WITH AUB

- Management issues of AUB depend upon the pathology obtained in an individual woman (discussed above).
- Women with AUB with age ≥45 years should have endometrial biopsy (D&C or hysteroscopy directed biopsy) as an initial step of management.
- Adolescent girls with AUB or heavy menstrual bleeding need exclusion of bleeding disorders besides other investigations. Complete hemogram, platelet count, prothrombin time, and partial thromboplastin time need to be done (Flowchart 15. 1).

Flowchart 15.1: Management protocol of abnormal uterine bleeding (AUB).

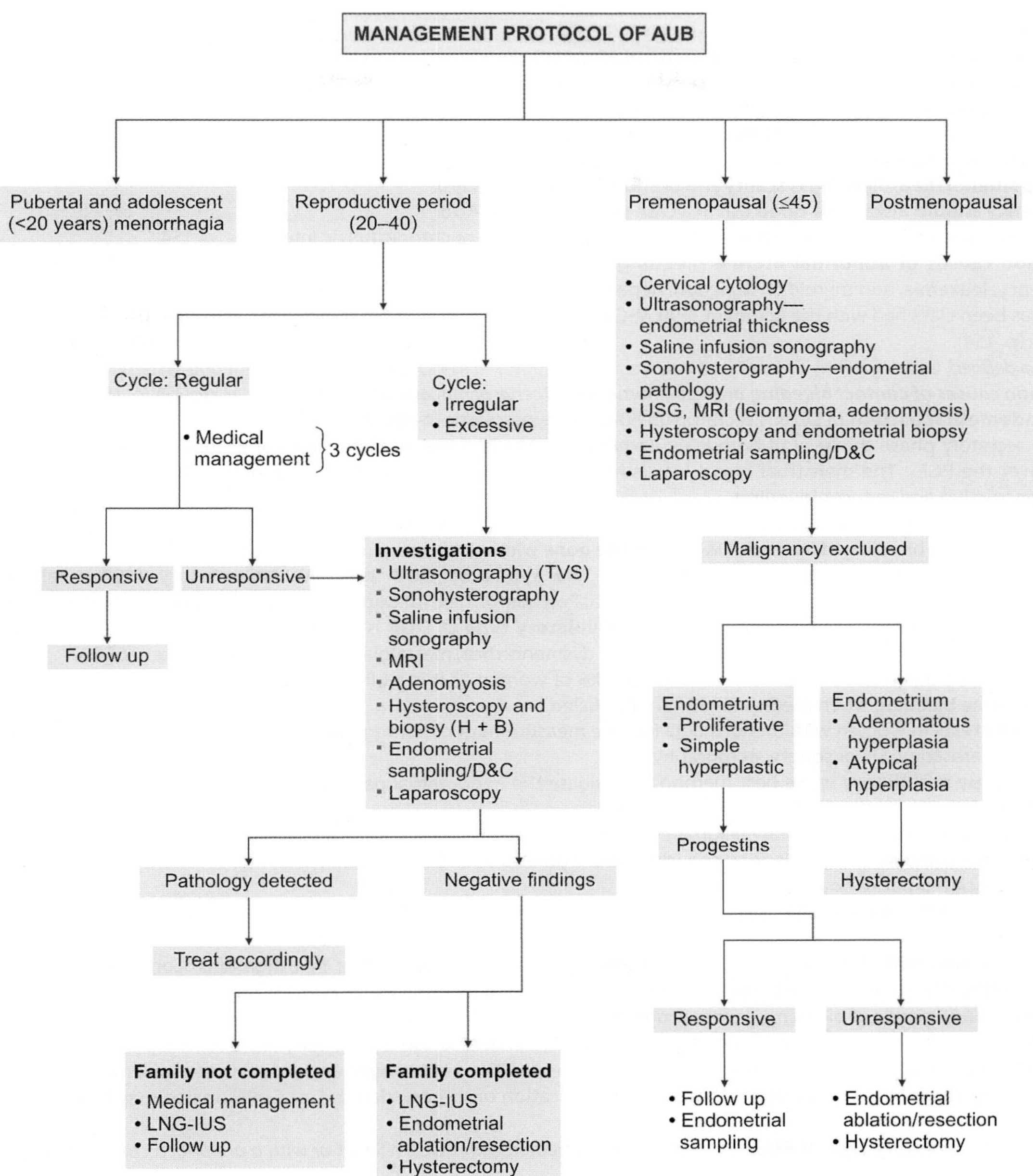

Causes of abnormal vaginal bleeding with relation for age.

Neonate/infant	*Premenarchal*	*Adolescent*	*Reproductive age*	*Menopausal age*
E2 withdrawal effects	Foreign body	DUB	AUB (PALM-COIEN)	Senile endometritis
	Infection	Endocrine dysfunction (thyroid)		Endocrine dysfunction (thyroid)
	Sexual abuse	Coagulation disorders		Ca cervix
	Precoicious puberty	Pregnancy complication		Ca endometrium
	Leech bite	Polyp		Malignancy of vulva and vagina
	Trauma	Sexual abuse		Endometrial hyperplasia/polyps
	Neoplasm	Neoplasm		Estrogen replacement therapy

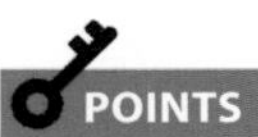

- **The commonly used terminology and the criteria for AUB are:**
  - **Menorrhagia**: Cycle regular; bleeding pattern is excessive in amount or in duration or both.
  - **Polymenorrhea**: Cyclic bleeding, cycle is reduced to <21 days.
  - **Metrorrhagia**: Irregular acyclic bleeding (intermenstrual).
  - **Oligomenorrhea**: Cyclic bleeding, cycle is occurring >35 days apart.
  - **Hypomenorrhea**: Bleeding is scanty and of short duration (<2 days).
- **Pregnancy should always be ruled out** in a case presenting with AUB.
- **Common causes of menorrhagia are:** DUB, fibroid, adenomyosis, or chronic pelvic infections (p. 154.
- **Common causes of abnormal uterine bleeding are:** Uterine fibroid, endometriosis, adenomyosis, IUCD, TO mass, platelet deficiency, leukemia, and thyroid dysfunction, hepatic dysfunction and DUB (p. 154).
- **AUB** has been classified with the acronym. "PALM-COEIN" by FIGO – 2011. It broadly divides AUB into structural and nonstructural causes (p. 154).
- ***DUB**, so defined, is not currently favored as the newer terminology, PALM-COIEN is more consistent and systematic.*
- ***Common causes of contact bleeding are:** Carcinoma cervix, cervical mucous polyp, and vascular erosion (p. 155).*
- **The endometrial pattern in DUB** is secretory in 60% and hyperplastic in about 30%.
- In late secretory phase the level of both PGE_2 and $PGF_{2\alpha}$ in the endometrium increases and during ovulatory cycles $PGF_{2\alpha}$ level rises over the PGE_2. The menstrual blood loss is inversely related to the level of endometrial $PGF_{2\alpha}/PGE_2$ ratio. $PGE_{2\alpha}$ causes vasoconstriction and reduces bleeding.
- **Methods of assessment** of menstrual blood loss are very inaccurate. Alkaline hematin method is a relatively precise method.
- **In acyclic type** of bleeding, diagnostic D&C should be done within 24 hours of menstruation.
- **DUB** is a state of abnormal uterine bleeding. **The types of DUB are:** (A) **Anovulatory (90%):** (a) Menorrhagia; (b) Metropathia hemorrhagica; (B) **Ovulatory (20%):** (a) Polymenorrhea; (b) Oligomenorrhea; (c) Functional menorrhagia (irregular shedding and irregular ripening of endometrium). **Ovulatory type of DUB** is usually characterized by: (a) regular cycle length, (b) heavy bleeding, (c) there may be presence of PMS, dysmenorrhea, mastalgia and the biphasic pattern of BBT.
- **D&C** misses the diagnosis of uterine lesions in 10–20% of women as it is a blind procedure. D&C can stop the acute episode of excess uterine bleeding when medical treatment has failed.
- **Diagnostic tests** in women with menorrhagia include measurement of hemoglobin, serum iron, serum ferritin, TSH, endometrial biopsy, hysteroscopy, SIS or sonohysterography.
- **Hysteroscopy and biopsy** is the best method to evaluate the endometrial pathology in DUB and also to detect lesions such as submucous fibroid or polyp (AUB).
- **In perimenopausal period**, genital malignancy should be ruled out prior to any therapy.
- **Management options** for AUB depends on individual woman's age, desire for child bearing, severity of bleeding, etiopathology and the associated pathology (Flowchart 15.1).
- **Women with AUB with age ≥45 years** should have endometrial biopsy (D&C or hysteroscopy directed biopsy) as an initial step of management.
- **Adolescent girls with AUB** need exclusion of bleeding disorders besides other investigations. Complete hemogram, platelet count, prothrombin time, and partial thromboplastin time need to be done (Flowchart 15. 1).
- **To arrest** acute episode of bleeding, potent progestogens are suitable in all phases of life. However, natural estrogen administered parenterally (conjugated estrogen 25 mg IV) is more effective in hemostasis during early reproductive period.
- **For cycle regulation**, either progestogens or combined preparations of estrogen and progestogen (pill) may be used.
- **In refractory cases** or in cases with temporary contraindication of surgery, danazol, or GnRH analog may be used for short-term therapy.
- ***Women with ovulatory type of AUB,** respond well when treated with COCs, NSAIDs or with a prolonged course of progestins or with LNG -IUS.*
- **Prostaglandin synthetase inhibitors** are effective in ovulatory DUB above the age of 35.
- **Antifibrinolytic agents** are suitable in a case of DUB and also for bleeding following IUCD insertion.
- **In cases with completed family**, endometrial ablation/resection or hysterectomy are the options (p. 161).
- **Endometrial ablation or resection (TCRE)** is done in a woman who is over 35 years, who do not respond to medical therapy, has completed her family and without any significant endometrial pathology (e.g. cancer, submucous fibroid >3 cm in diameter).
- **Ablation of endometrium** up to a depth of 4–5 mm using laser, roller ball, thermal balloon, microwave, is an effective method. Resection of endometrium up to the basal layer is also a quicker and less costlier method. Overall, amenorrhea occurs in 30–40% of women, about 50% have decreased bleeding and 10% may need repeated procedure or hysterectomy.
- **NSAIDs reduces menstrual blood loss** by 20% to 50% in women with ovulatory DUB.
- **LNG-IUS is the first line therapy** for women with HMB due to anticoagulation or with inherited bleeding.

CHAPTER

16 Displacement of the Uterus

CHAPTER OUTLINE

The uterus is not a fixed organ. Minor variations in position in any direction occur constantly with changes in posture, with straining, with full bladder or loaded rectum. Only when the uterus rests habitually in a position beyond the limit of normal variation, should it be called displacement.

RETROVERSION

Definition

Retroversion (RV) is the term used when the long axis of the corpus and cervix are in line and the whole organ turns backwards in relation to the long axis of the birth canal.

Retroflexion signifies a bending backwards of the corpus on the cervix at the level of internal os. **The two conditions are usually present together and are loosely called retroversion or retrodisplacement (Fig. 16.1).**

Degrees

Conventionally, three degrees are described.

- **First degree:** The fundus is vertical and pointing towards the sacral promontory.
- **Second degree:** The fundus lies in the sacral hollow but not below the internal os.
- **Third degree:** The fundus lies below the level of the internal os.

Causes

- **Developmental**
- **Acquired**

Developmental

Retrodisplacement is quite common in fetuses and young children. Due to developmental defect, there is lack of tone of the uterine muscles. The infantile position is retained. This is often associated with short vagina with shallow anterior vaginal fornix.

Acquired

Puerperal: The stretched ligaments caused by childbirth fail to keep the uterus in its normal position. A subinvoluted bulky uterus aggravates the condition.

Prolapse: RV is usually implicated in the pathophysiology of prolapse which is mechanically caused by traction following cystocele.

Tumor: Fibroid, either in the anterior or posterior wall produces heaviness of the uterus and hence, it falls behind.

Pelvic adhesions: Adhesions, either inflammatory, operative or due to pelvic endometriosis, pull the uterus posteriorly.

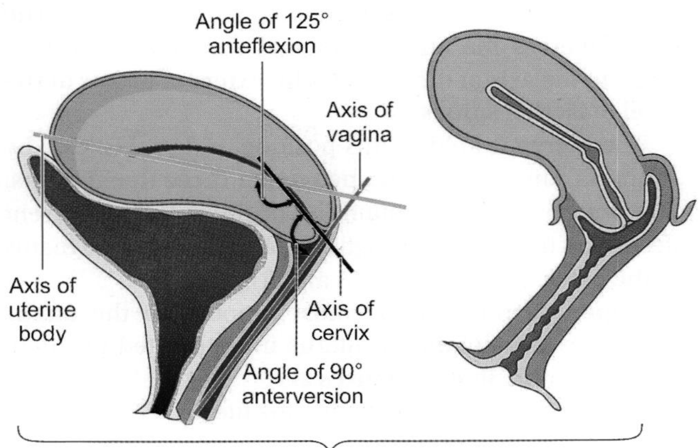

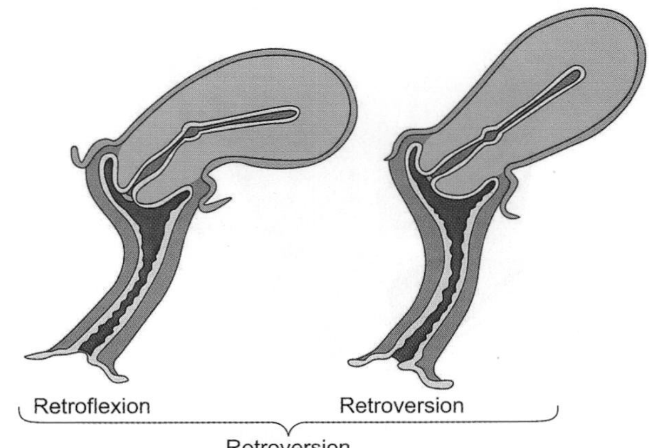

Fig. 16.1: Normal and retroverted uterus.

Incidence

Retroversion is present in about 15–20% of normal women.

Clinical Presentation

The condition is classified either as mobile and fixed or uncomplicated and complicated by pelvic diseases.

Mobile Retroverted Uterus

Mobile retroverted uterus is common and almost always remains asymptomatic. **However, the following symptoms may be present.**

- **Chronic premenstrual pelvic pain:** It is due to varicosities in broad ligament produced by the kinks. The manifestations are those of 'pelvic congestion syndrome'.
- **Backache**
- **Dyspareunia:** Deep dyspareunia may be due to direct thrust by the penis against the retroflexed uterus or the prolapsed ovaries lying in the pouch of Douglas. Retroversion itself is a rare cause.

Signs

- **Bimanual examination reveals**—(a) The cervix is directed upwards and forwards; (b) The body of the uterus is felt through the posterior fornix. The size of the uterus is difficult to assess at times. Bimanual pelvic examination should be done with an empty bladder to maintain the normal relationship of the uterus with the axis of the cervix and the vagina (Fig. 16.2).
- **Speculum examination reveals**—the cervix comes in view much easily and the external os points forwards.
- **Rectal examination** is of help to confirm the diagnosis.

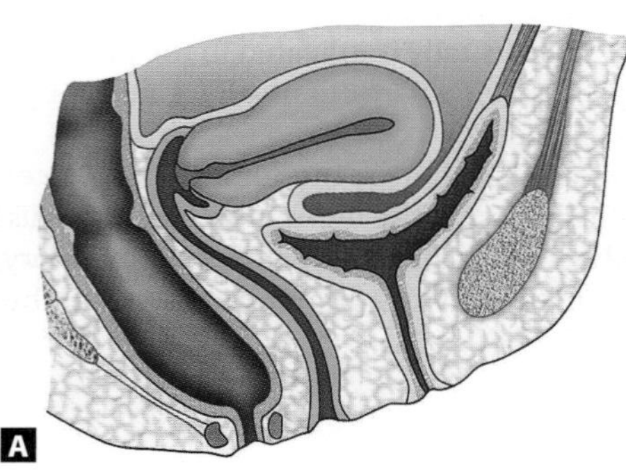

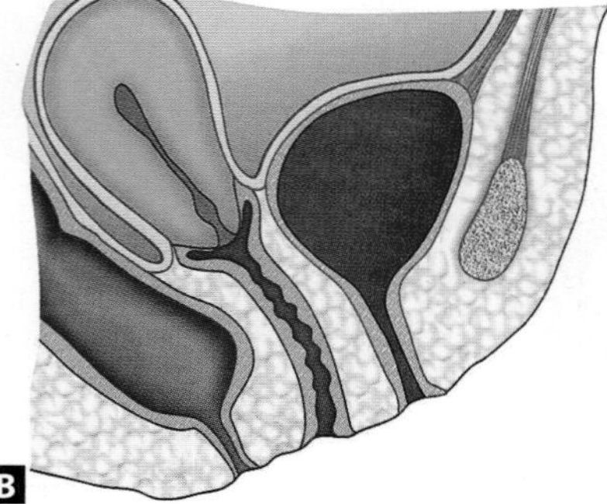

Figs. 16.2A and B: Note the degree of displacement of anteverted uterus: (A) Reason to empty the bladder prior to examination; (B) Due to full bladder.

Pregnancy in Retroverted Uterus

Retroversion *per se* has got practically no adverse effect either on fertility or in early pregnancy. In pregnancy, spontaneous correction usually occurs by 12–14 weeks.

Corrective Treatment

- **Pessary**
- **Surgical**

Prevention: The woman is advised to lie on prone position for half to one hour once or twice a day.

Pessary

It is less commonly used in present day gynecologic practice. However, it may be indicated: (a) for pessary test, in cases where symptoms improve with use of pessary; (b) in subinvolution of uterus; and (c) in pregnancy when spontaneous correction to anteversion fails by 12th week.

Usually, Hodge-Smith pessary is used. The pessary acts by stretching the uterosacral ligaments so as to pull the cervix backwards (Figs. 16.3A to D).

Surgical Treatment

Surgical correction is **rarely** indicated in: (a) Fixed retroverted uterus producing symptoms like backache or dyspareunia; (b) Cases where the 'pessary test' is positive indicating that the symptoms are due to retroversion.

The principle of surgical correction is **ventrosuspension of the uterus** by plicating the round ligaments of both the sides extraperitoneally to the under surface of the anterior rectus sheath. This will pull the uterus forwards and maintains it permanently in the same position.

PELVIC ORGAN PROLAPSE

Pelvic organ prolapse (POP) is one of the common clinical conditions met in day-to-day gynecological practice **especially among the parous women.** The entity includes descent of the vaginal wall and/or the uterus. It is infact a form of hernia.

SUPPORTS OF UTERUS

The uterus is normally placed in anteverted and anteflexed position. It lies in between the bladder and rectum. The cervix pierces the anterior vaginal wall almost at right angle to the axis of the vagina. **The external os lies at the level of ischial spines.**

The uterus is held in this position and at this level by supports conveniently grouped under **three tier systems.** The objective is to maintain the position and to prevent descent of the uterus through the natural urogenital hiatus in the pelvic floor (Figs. 16.4A and B).

- **Upper tier:** The upper most supports of the uterus primarily maintain the uterus in anteverted position. **The responsible structures are:**
  - Endopelvic fascia covering the uterus
  - Round ligaments
  - Broad ligaments with intervening pelvic cellular tissues.

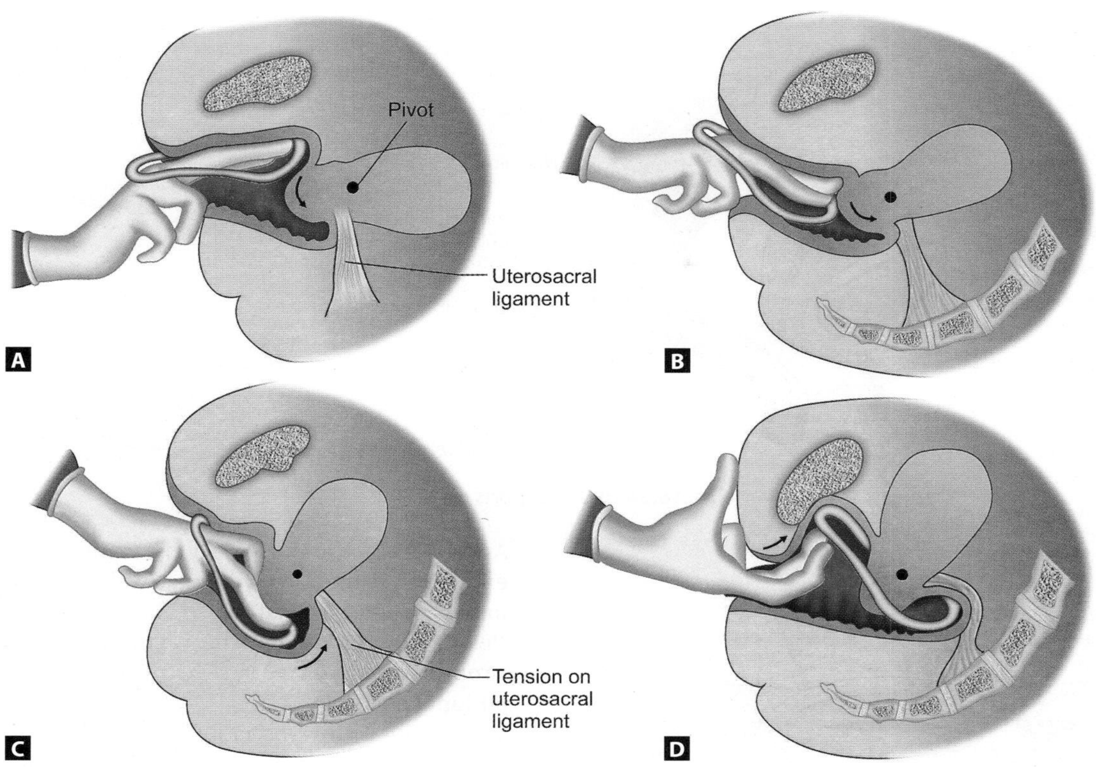

Fig. 16.3A to D: Methods of introduction of pessary to correct the position of a retroversion (RV) uterus.

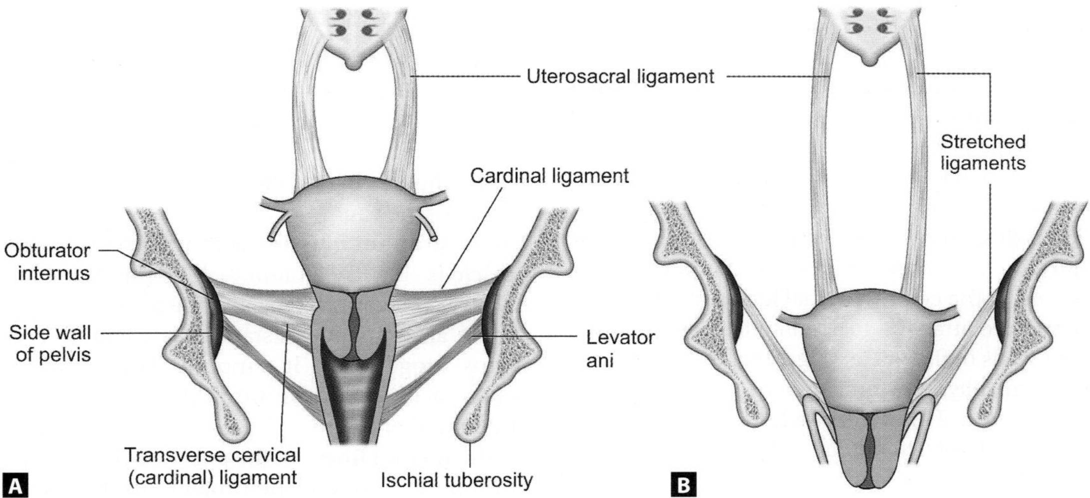

Figs. 16.4A and B: (A) Supports of uterus; (B) Prolapse of uterus due to weakness of the supporting structures. Note all the ligaments are stretched.

The last two are actually acting as a guy rope with a steadying effect on the uterus. **They have no action in preventing descent of the uterus.**

- **Middle tier (Figs. 16.5 and 16.6):** This constitutes the strongest support of the uterus. **The responsible structures are**:
  - **Pericervical ring (Fig. 16.6):** It is a collar of fibroelastic connective tissue encircling the supravaginal cervix. It is connected with the **pubocervical ligaments** and vesicovaginal septum anteriorly, **cardinal ligaments** laterally and **uterosacral ligaments** and **rectovaginal septum posteriorly** (p. 17).
    Function: It stabilizes the cervix at the level of interspinous diameter along with the other ligaments.
  - **Pelvic cellular tissues:** The endopelvic fascia consist of connective tissues and smooth muscles. The blood vessels and nerves supplying the uterus, bladder and vagina pass through it from the lateral

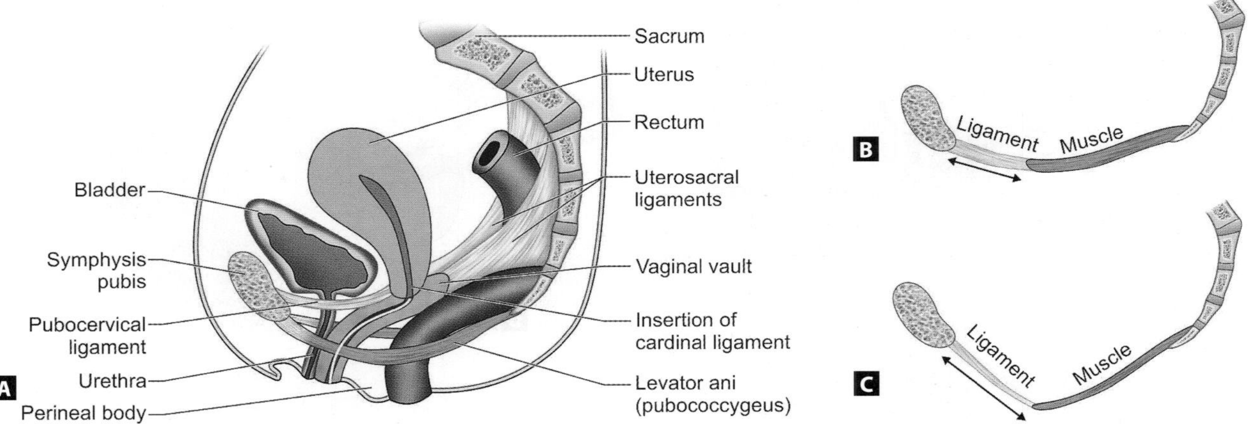

Figs. 16.5A to C: Supports of uterus.

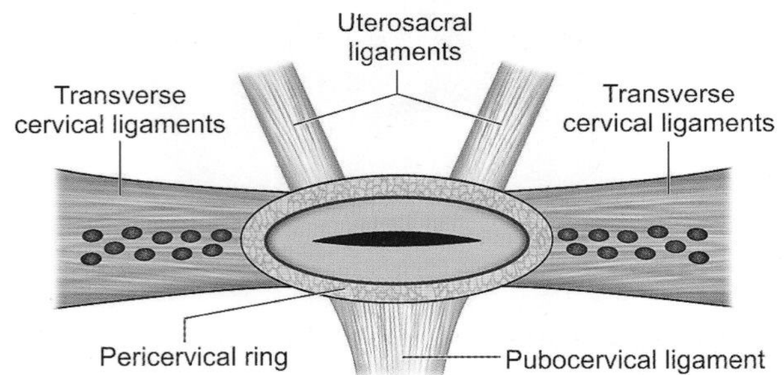

Fig. 16.6: Ligamentous supports of uterus.

pelvic wall. As they pass, the pelvic cellular tissues condense surrounding them and give good direct support to the viscera.

The endopelvic fascia at places is condensed and reinforced by plain muscles to form ligaments—Mackenrodt's, uterosacral and pubocervical. On the medial side, these are attached to the pericervical ring covering the cervicovaginal junction and on the other end are attached to the lateral, posterior and anterior walls of the pelvis (Figs. 16.4 to 16.6). These are anatomically, morphologically and functionally the same unit. This hammock-like arrangement of condensed pelvic cellular tissues is the cardinal support of the uterus.

- **Inferior tier:** This gives the indirect support to the uterus. The support is principally given by the *pelvic floor muscles (levator ani), endopelvic fascia, levator plate, perineal body and the urogenital diaphragm (p. 15).*

SUPPORTS OF VAGINA

Supports of the Anterior Vaginal Wall

- **Positional support:** In the erect posture, the vagina makes an angle of 45° to the horizontal. Normal vaginal axis is horizontal in the upper two-third and vertical in the lower-third (Fig. 16.5A). A well-supported vagina lies on the rectum and the levator plate (Figs. 16.5A and B). Any raised intra-abdominal pressure is transmitted exclusively to the anterior vaginal wall which is apposed to the posterior vaginal wall.
- **Pelvic cellular tissue:** The vagina is ensheathed by strong condensation of pelvic cellular tissue called **endopelvic fascia**.

Traced below, this fascia forms the posterior urethral ligament, which is anchored to the pubic bones giving strong support to the urethra. Traced laterally, this fascia form the pubocervical fascia or ligament which is the anterior extension of the Mackenrodt's ligaments.

Supports of the Posterior Vaginal Wall (Figs. 16.5A to C)

- Endopelvic fascial sheath covering the vagina and rectum.
- Attachment of the uterosacral ligament to the lateral wall of the vault.

The levator ani muscles with its fascial coverings: This muscle is slug like a hammock around the midline pelvic effluents (urethra, vagina and the anal canal). This strong, robust and fatigue-resistant striated muscle guards the hiatus urogenitalis. It supports the pelvic viscera and counteracts the downward thrust of increased intra-abdominal pressure.

The **medial fibers** of the pubococcygeus part of levator ani muscles, are attached mainly to the urethra, vagina and rectum. Few fibrous pass behind the rectum, vagina and the urethra forming a sling. These pubovisceral fibers of the levator ani muscles squeeze the rectum, vagina and urethra and keep them closed by compressing against the pubic bone.

When the levator ani muscles are damaged, the pelvic floor opens and there is **widening of the hiatus urogenitalis**. The vagina is then pushed down by the increased intra-abdominal pressure. Eventually, the genital organs prolapse.

- **The levator plate (Figs. 16.5A to C)**: Clinically, it is a thick band of connective tissue formed by the medial fibers of the two levator ani muscles. Anatomically, it is the anococcygeal raphe that extends between the anorectal junction and the coccyx. Some of the fibers extend anteriorly encircling the anorectal junction and are inserted into the **perineal body**.

The levator plate forms a horizontal supportive shelf upon which the rectum, upper vagina and the uterus rest (Figs. 16.5A and B). The horizontal position of this shelf is maintained by the anterior traction of the fibers of pubococcygeus and the iliococcygeus muscles. Due to its horizontal position, the levator plate can prevent the prolapse of genital organs. **The recto genitourinary hiatus** enlarges and predisposes to prolapse of the genital organs when the levator plate is damaged and sags (Fig. 16.5C). This is due to the loss of tone of the levator ani muscles following injury, overstretching (childbirth process) or attenuation (menopause). Clinically, the levator plate is assessed by palpating the perineum between two fingers inside the introitus and the thumb outside. It is palpable as 2–2.5 cm band of muscle on each lateral side of the distal 1/3 of the vagina.

- **Perineal body** and urogenital diaphragm. **Perineal body** is a solid pyramidal structure at the central point of the perineum. It receives 9 muscles like the hub of a wheel that grasps the spokes. **Damage to perineal body causes loss of normal vaginal axis.**
- **Biomechanical basis of uterovaginal supports** (Delancey, 1992) and development of prolapse have been discussed before (p. 15).

Different levels of uterovaginal support as explained on biomechanical basis (Delancy - 1992), has been discussed in Table 1.1.

ETIOLOGY OF PELVIC ORGAN PROLAPSE (TABLE 16.1)

The genital prolapse occurs due to weakness of the structures supporting the organs in position. These factors may be anatomical or clinical. The clinical factors are grouped as:

- **Predisposing**
- **Aggravating**

Predisposing Factors

- **Acquired**
- **Congenital**

Acquired: Vaginal delivery with consequent injury to the supporting structures is the single most important acquired predisposing factor in producing prolapse. The prolapse is unusual in cases delivered by cesarean section.

The injury is caused by:

- Overstretching of the Mackenrodt's and uterosacral ligaments: (a) Premature bear down efforts prior to full dilatation of the cervix; (b) Delivery with forceps or ventouse with forceful traction; (c) Prolonged second stage of labor; (d) Downward pressure on the uterine fundus in an attempt to deliver the placenta; (e) Precipitate labor.

  In all these conditions, the uterus tends to be pushed down into the flabby distended vagina.
- Overstretching and breaks in the endopelvic fascial sheath.
- Overstretching of the perineum.
- Imperfect repair of the perineal injuries. Poor repair of collagen tissue.
- Loss of levator function.
- Neuromuscular damage of levator ani during childbirth.
- Subinvolution of the supporting structures. This is particularly noticeable in: (a) Ill-nourished and asthenic women; (b) Early resumption of activities which greatly increase intra-abdominal pressure before the tissues regain their tone; (c) Repeated childbirths at frequent intervals.

Congenital: Congenital weakness of the supporting structures is responsible for nulliparous prolapse or prolapse following an easy vaginal delivery. One should exclude an occult spina bifida and associated neurological abnormalities.

TABLE 16.1: Etiology of pelvic organ prolapse.

	Clinical factors	
Anatomical factors	***Predisposing factors***	***Aggravating factors***
▪ Gravitational stress due to human bipedal posture ▪ Anterior inclination of pelvis directing the force more anteriorly ▪ Stress of parturition (internal rotation) causing maximum damage to puborectal fibers of levator ani ▪ Pelvic floor weakness due to urogenital hiatus and the direction of obstetric axis through the hiatus ▪ Inherent weakness (genetic) of the supporting structures	**A. Acquired** Trauma of vaginal delivery causing injury (tear or break) to: • Ligaments • Endopelvic fascia • Levator muscle (myopathy) • Perineal body • Nerve (pudendal) and muscle damage due to repeated child birth **B. Congenital** • **Genetic** (connective tissue disorders), decreased ratio of type I collagen • Woman with Marfan or Ehlers-Danlos syndrome • Spina bifida	▪ Postmenopausal atrophy ▪ Poor collagen tissue repair with age ▪ Increased intra-abdominal pressure as in chronic lung disease (COPD) and constipation ▪ Occupation (weight lifting) ▪ Asthenia and undernutrition ▪ Obesity, smoking ▪ Increased weight of the uterus as in fibroid or myohyperplasia ▪ Multiparity, smoking These factors possibly operate where the supports of the genital organs are already weak

Flowchart. 16.1: Clinical types of genital prolapse.

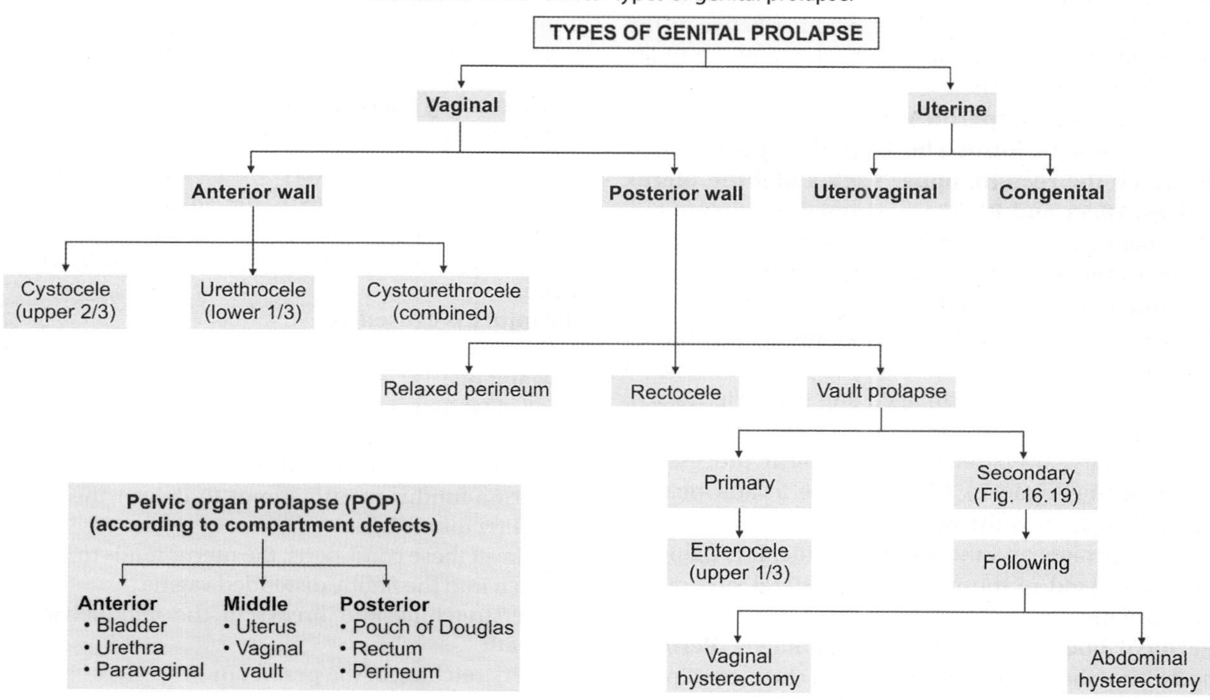

Ultrasonography (3D) with **color thickness mapping** and MRI study of the levator ani muscle revealed loss of levator ani bulk in women with POP and stress incontinence. MRI demonstrate more vertical axis and wider genital hiatus in women with POP.

CLINICAL TYPES OF PELVIC ORGAN PROLAPSE

The genital prolapse is broadly grouped into (Flowchart 16.1):

- **Vaginal prolapse**
- **Uterine prolapse**

While vaginal prolapse can occur independently without uterine descent, the uterine prolapse is usually associated with variable degrees of vaginal descent.

Vaginal Prolapse

Anterior Wall

- **Cystocele:** The cystocele is **formed by laxity and descent of the upper two-thirds of the anterior vaginal wall**. As the bladder base is closely related to this area, there is herniation of the bladder through the lax anterior wall.
- **Urethrocele:** When there is laxity of the **lower-third of the anterior vaginal wall**, the urethra herniates through it. This may appear independently or usually along with cystocele and is called cystourethrocele.

Posterior Wall

- **Relaxed perineum:** Torn perineal body produces gaping introitus with bulge of the lower part of the posterior vaginal wall.
- **Rectocele:** There is laxity of the middle-third of the posterior vaginal wall and the adjacent rectovaginal septum. As a result, there is herniation of the rectum through the lax area.

Vault Prolapse

- **Enterocele:** Laxity of the upper-third of the posterior vaginal wall results in herniation of the pouch of Douglas. It may contain omentum or even loop of small bowel and hence, called enterocele. **Traction enterocele** is secondary to uterovaginal prolapse. Pulsion enterocele is secondary to chronically raised intra-abdominal pressure.
- **Secondary vault prolapse:** This may occur following either vaginal or abdominal hysterectomy. Undetected enterocele during initial operation or inadequate primary repair usually results in secondary vault prolapse (Table 16.2).

TABLE 16.2: Degrees of uterine prolapse (clinical).

- **Normal:** External os lies at the level of ischial spines. No prolapse
- **First degree:** The uterus descends down from its normal anatomical position but the external os still remains above the introitus
- **Second degree:** The external os protrudes outside the vaginal introitus but the uterine body still remains inside the vagina (Fig. 16.7)
- **Third degree** (*Syn: Procidentia, Complete prolapse*): The uterine cervix and body and the fundus descends to lie outside the introitus (Fig. 16.8)
- **Procidentia** involves prolapse of the uterus with eversion of the entire vagina.

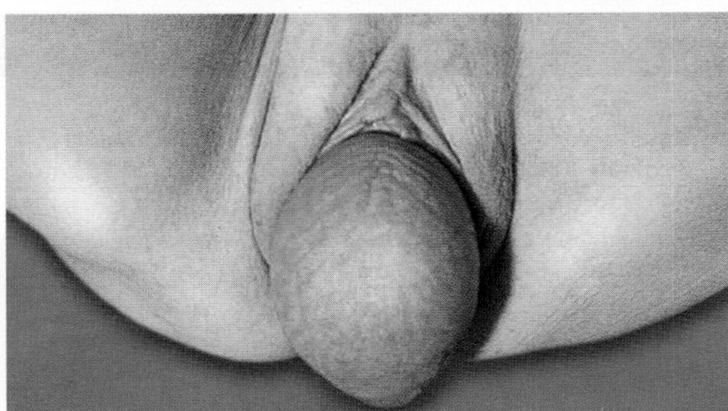

Fig. 16.7: Second degree uterine prolapse with marked cystocele.

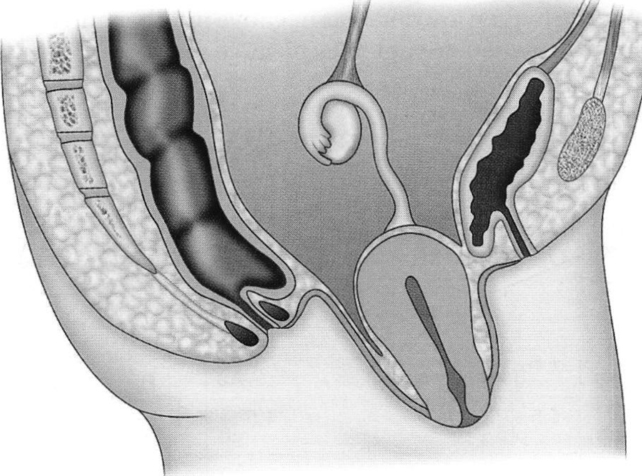

Fig. 16.8: Third degree uterine prolapse.

Uterine Prolapse

There are two types:

- **Uterovaginal prolapse** is the prolapse of the uterus, cervix, and upper vagina.

  This is the most common type. Cystocele occurs first followed by traction effect on the cervix causing retroversion of the uterus. Intra-abdominal pressure has got piston like action on the uterus thereby pushing it down into the vagina.

TABLE 16.3: Baden-Walker Halfway system for the evaluation of pelvic organ prolapse during physical examination.*

Grade	
Grade 0	Normal position for each respective site
Grade 1	Descent halfway to the hymen
Grade 2	Descent to the hymen
Grade 3	Descent halfway past the hymen
Grade 4	Maximum possible descent for each site

(*Descent of the anterior vaginal wall, posterior vaginal wall, or apical prolapse can be graded with this system. From Baden, JB Lippincott, 1992)

- **Congenital prolapse:** There is usually no cystocele. The uterus herniates down along with inverted upper vagina. This is often met in nulliparous women and hence called **nulliparous prolapse**. The cause is congenital weakness of the supporting structures holding the uterus in position.

  Complex prolapse is one when prolapse is associated with some other specific defects. **Complex prolapse** includes the following: Prolapse with urinary or fecal incontinence, nulliparous prolapse, recurrent prolapse, vaginal and rectal prolapse or prolapse in a frail woman.

  Pelvic organ prolapse quantification (POP-Q) system **has been recommended by the International Continence Society as it standardizes terminology and is most objective, site specific and anatomical** (Tables 16.3 and 16.4, Figs. 16.9 and 16.10).

Staging or Pelvic Floor Prolapse Using International Continence Society Terminology.

- **Stage 0:** No prolapse is demonstrated. Points Aa, Ap, Ba and Bp are all at –3 cm, and either point C or D is between total vaginal length –2 cm.
- **Stage I:** Criteria for stage 0 are not met, but the most distal portion of the prolapse is >1 cm above the level of the hymen.
- **Stage II:** The most distal portion of the prolapse is ≤1 cm proximal or distal to the plane of the hymen.
- **Stage III:** The most distal portion of the prolapse is >1 cm below the plane of the hymen but protrudes no farther than 2 cm less than the total vaginal length in centimeters.
- **Stage IV:** Essentially complete eversion of the total length of the lower genital tract

TABLE 16.4: Site specific measurements in pelvic organ prolapse quantification (POP-Q) system.

Site	Description	Range
Aa	Anterior vaginal wall, midline 3 cm proximal to external urinary meatus (point of urethrovesical crease)	–3 cm to + 3 cm
Ba	Anterior vaginal wall, most distal position between Aa and anterior fornix	–3 cm to + TVL
C	Cervix or vaginal cuff	±TVL
D	Posterior fornix or vaginal apex	±TVL
Ap	Posterior vaginal wall, midline 3 cm proximal to hymen	–3 cm to + 3 cm
Bp	Posterior vaginal wall, most distal position, between Ap and posterior fornix	–3 cm to + TVL
Gh	External urinary meatus to posterior midline hymenal ring	2 cm
TVL	Point C or D to the hymenal ring	10 cm
Pb	Posterior hymen to anal opening	3 cm

(TVL: total vaginal length; Pb: perineal body)

TVL is measured with prolapse reduced. All other measurements are done with full straining or valsalva maneuver.

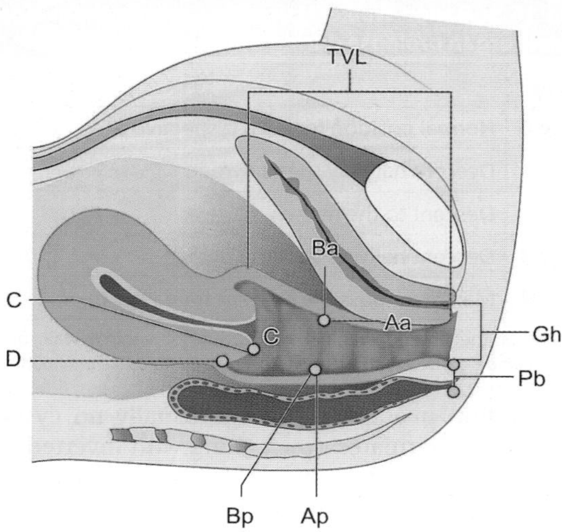

Fig. 16.9: Anatomical points to be taken in quantification of pelvic organ prolapse (POP -Q).

[Aa: anterior wall (–3 cm to +3 cm); Ba: anterior wall (–3 cm to +8 cm); C: Cervix or vaginal cuff (–8 cm to +8 cm) Ap: posterior wall (–3 cm to +3); Bp: Posterior wall (–3 cm to +8 cm); D Posterior fornix (–10); Gh: genital hiatus (2 cm); Pb: perineal body (3 cm); TVL: total vaginal length (10 cm)]; ***TVL is measured with prolapse reduced. All other measurements are done with full straining or valsalva maneuver.***

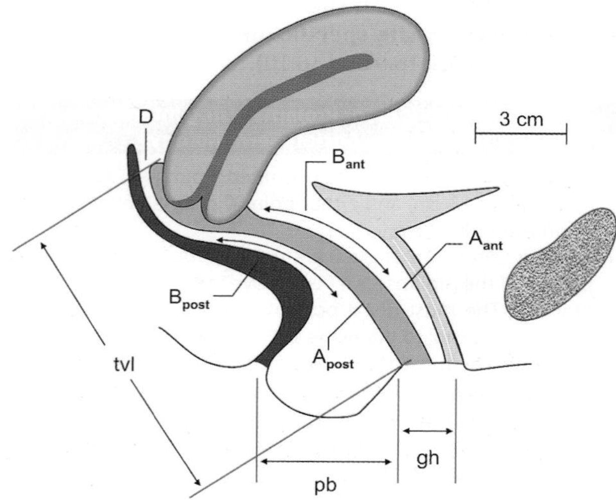

Fig. 16.10: Nine specific sites are considered. Hymen is taken as the fixed point. The plane of hymen is defined as the zero level. Leading point of prolapse may be above (proximal) or below (distal) to the plane of hymen. Prolapse measurements (cm) are recorded as negative (–ve) numbers when above and positive (+ve) numbers when lies below the plane of hymen. Organ prolapse is measured with a wooden PAP spatula with markings. The woman may be examined in lithotomy or standing position (or even under anesthesia). She may be asked to do some maneuvers (Valsalva) to demonstrate the prolapse maximally. TVL is measured after reducing the prolapse while rest of the measurements are done when the prolapse is seen maximally. Measurements are tabulated in the grid as shown in Table 16.5. POP-Q is considered as the objective, site specific and standard system for assessment of POP.

(TVL: total vaginal length; POPQ: pelvic organ prolapse-quantification; POP: pelvic organ prolapse; gh: genital hiatus; pb: perineal body)

TABLE 16.5: Grid used to record measurements in POP-Q system

Aa Anterior wall (– 3 cm to + 3 cm)	Ba Anterior wall (– 3 cm to + 8 cm)	C Cervix or vaginal cuff (– 8 cm to +8 cm)
Gh Genital hiatus (2 cm)	Pb Perineal body (3 cm)	TVL Total vaginal length (10 cm)
Ap Posterior wall (– 3 cm to +3)	Bp Posterior wall (– 3 cm to +8 cm)	D Posterior fornix (–10)

Assessment POP-Q: Grid system charting is to follow (Fig. 16.10). Anatomic position of all the six points are measured from the hymen. Measurement is done in centimetres and hymen is taken as point zero. Points above the hymen are noted as negative number and points below the hymen are noted as positive number.

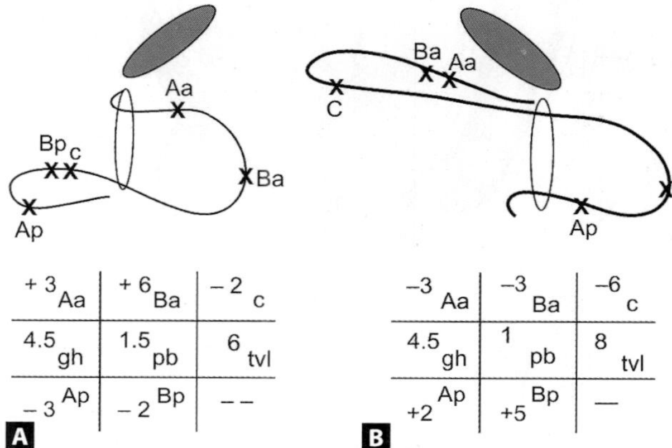

Fig. 16.11: The grid and the drawing of: (a) Anterior support defect; (b) Posterior support defect.

MORBID CHANGES

Vaginal Mucosa

The mucosa becomes stretched and if exposed to air, becomes thickened and dry with surface keratinization. There may be pigmentation.

Decubitus Ulcer

It is a trophic ulcer, always found at the dependent part of the prolapsed mass lying outside the introitus. There is initial surface keratinization → cracks → infection → sloughing → ulceration. There is complete denudation of the surface epithelium. The diminished circulation is due to constriction of the prolapsed mass by the vaginal opening and narrowing of the uterine vessels by the stretching effect.

Management: (a) Cervical cytology to exclude malignancy; (b) Colposcopy and directed biopsy if needed; (c) Manual reduction of prolapse; (d) Vaginal pack with roller bandage soaked with antiseptic lotion glycerin and acriflavine or using estrogen cream (postmenopausal women).

Cervix

- **Vaginal part:** There is chronic congestion which may lead to hyperplasia and hypertrophy of the fibromusculoglandular components. These lead to vaginal part becoming bulky and congested. Addition of infection leads to purulent or at times blood-stained discharge from ulceration.

- **Supravaginal part:** The supravaginal part becomes elongated due to the strain imposed by the pull of the cardinal ligaments to keep the cervix in position, whereas the weight of the uterus makes it fall through the vaginal axis. Chronic interference of venous and lymphatic drainage favors elongation.

Urinary System

- **Bladder:** There is incomplete emptying of the bladder due to sharp angulation of the urethra against the pubourethral ligament during straining. As a result, there is hypertrophy of the bladder wall and trabeculation. Incomplete evacuation also favors cystitis.
- **Ureters:** The ureters are carried downwards along with elongated Mackenrodt's ligaments and thus, mechanically obstructed by the hiatus of the pelvic floor. They may be compressed even by the uterine arteries at their crossing. As a result, hydroureteric changes may occur.

  Infection of the bladder may thus ascend up to produce pyelitis or pyelonephritis. On rare occasions, uremia may occur, especially in long-standing cases of procidentia.

Incarceration

At times, infection of the paravaginal and cervical tissues makes the entire prolapsed mass edematous and congested. As a result, the mass may be irreducible.

Peritonitis

Rarely, the peritoneal infection (pelvic peritonitis) may occur through the posterior vaginal wall.

Carcinoma

Carcinoma rarely develops on decubitus ulcer.

SYMPTOMS

The symptoms are variable. Even with minor degree, the symptoms may be pronounced, paradoxically there may not be any appreciable symptom even in severe degree. However, **the following symptoms are usually associated:**

- **Vaginal:** Feeling of something coming down per vaginam, sensation of pelvic pressure and vaginal bulge. There may be variable discomfort on walking when the mass comes outside the introitus.
- **Pain:** Backache or dragging pain in the pelvis.

  The above two symptoms are usually relieved on lying down.
- **Sexual:** Dyspareunia, loss of sexual activity.
- **Urinary symptoms (in presence of cystocele).**
  - **Difficulty** in passing urine, more the strenuous effort, the less effective is the evacuation. The patient has to elevate the anterior vaginal wall for evacuation of the bladder.
  - **Incomplete evacuation** may lead to frequent desire to pass urine.
  - **Urgency and frequency** of micturition may also be due to cystitis.
  - **Painful micturition** is due to infection.
  - **Stress incontinence** is usually due to associated urethrocele.
  - **Retention** of urine may rarely occur.
- **Bowel symptom (in presence of rectocele).**
  - Difficulty in passing stool, constipation and straining. The patient has to push back the posterior vaginal wall (digital decompression) in position to complete the evacuation of feces and for flatus. Fecal incontinence may be associated.
- Excessive white or blood-stained discharge per vaginam is due to associated vaginitis or decubitus ulcer.

CLINICAL EXAMINATION AND DIAGNOSIS OF POP

- **Composite examination**—inspection and palpation: Vaginal, rectal, rectovaginal or even under anesthesia may be required to arrive at a correct diagnosis.
- **General examination**—details, including body mass index (BMI), signs of myopathy or neuropathy, features of chronic airway disease (COPD) or any abdominal mass should be done.
- **Pelvic organ prolapse** is evaluated by pelvic examination in both dorsal and standing positions. The patient is asked to strain as to perform a Valsalva maneuver during examination. This often helps to demonstrate a prolapse which may not be seen at rest. This "hands off" method displays the true altered anatomy. Now to see whether the protruding mass (a) comes beyond the hymen; (b) leading part of the prolapse [anterior (bladder), apical (cervix), the posterior (rectum) and (c) the extent of gaping of the genital hiatus.
- **A negative finding** on inspection in dorsal position should be reconfirmed by asking the patient to strain on squatting position.
- Usually the patient is examined without emptying of the bladder. To demonstrate SUI patient is asked to cough after the prolapse mass is reduced. Leakage of urine as a spurt suggests stress incontinence and the patient needs appropriate surgery for the same (Table 16.6).
- **Prolapse of one organ (uterus)** is usually associated with prolapse of the adjacent organs (bladder, rectum).
- **Etiological aspect** of prolapse and the high risk factors should be evaluated.

Pelvic examination is done to assess: Staging (POP-Q), levator ani muscle tone, urinary incontinence, decubitus ulcer, uterine size, mobility, perineal body and anal sphincter tone.

Cystocele (Fig. 16.12): There is a bulge of varying degree of the anterior vaginal wall, which increases when the patient is asked to strain. This may be seen on inspection. In others, to elicit this, one may have to separate the labia or depress the posterior vaginal wall with fingers or using Sims' speculum, placing the patient in lateral position (p. 84).

The mucosa over the bulge has got transverse rugosities. The bulge has got impulse on coughing, with diffuse margins and is reducible.

TABLE 16.6: Type of prolapse and the common surgical repair procedures.

Organ descent	*Clinical condition*	*Type of operation*
VAGINAL WALL		
Anterior (upper 2/3) or whole	Cystocele/cystourethrocele Paravaginal defect	▪ Anterior colporrhaphy ▪ Paravaginal defect repair.
Posterior (lower 2/3)	Rectocele	▪ Colpoperineorrhaphy
Posterior (upper 1/3)	Enterocele	▪ Vaginal repair of enterocele with PFR ▪ McCall culdoplasty ▪ Moskowitz procedure
Combined anterior and posterior	Cystocele and rectocele	▪ PFR (combined procedure)
Uterovaginal Uterus along with vaginal walls	Uterovaginal prolapse	▪ Vaginal hysterectomy with PFR (elderly woman, family completed) ▪ Fothergill's operation (preservation of uterus)
Vaginal wall **Following hysterectomy** (vaginal or abdominal)	Vault prolapse (secondary)	**Vaginal:** ▪ Repair of vaginal vault along with PFR ▪ Sacrospinous colpopexy ▪ Colpocleisis (Le Fort) **Abdominal:** Sacral colpopexy
Uterus (without vaginal walls)	Congenital or nulliparous prolapse (young women)	Cervicopexy or Sling (Purandare's) operation
Pelvic organ prolapse (POP)	POP with stress in continence	▪ **Vaginal:** TOT operation ▪ **Abdominal:** Burch operation

(PFR: pelvic floor repair; TOT: transobturator tape procedure)

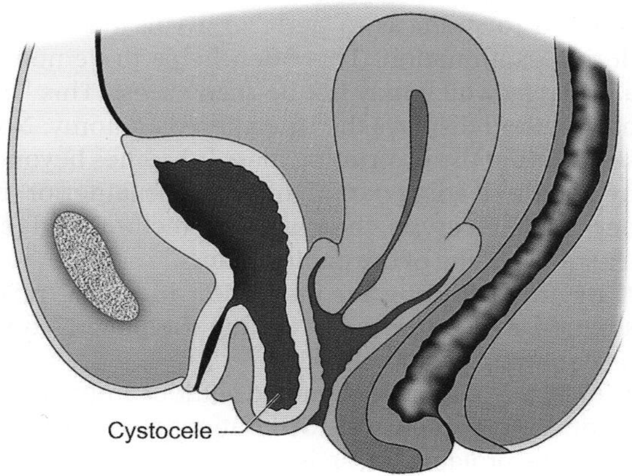

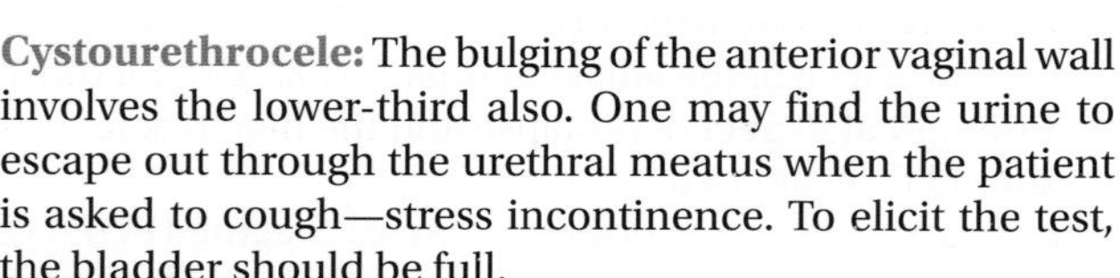

Fig. 16.12: Cystocele (diagrammatic).

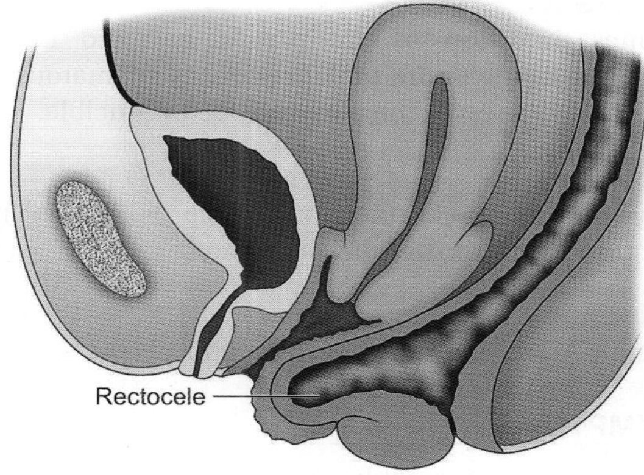

Fig. 16.13: Rectocele (diagrammatic).

Cystourethrocele: The bulging of the anterior vaginal wall involves the lower-third also. One may find the urine to escape out through the urethral meatus when the patient is asked to cough—stress incontinence. To elicit the test, the bladder should be full.

Relaxed perineum: There is gaping introitus with old scar of incomplete perineal tear. The distance between the introitus and the anal verge is decreased. The lower part of the posterior vaginal wall is visible with or without straining.

Rectocele and enterocele: When the two conditions exist together, there is bulging of the posterior vaginal wall with a transverse sulcus between the two. The midvaginal one being rectocele with diffuse margins and reducible. This is visualized by retracting the anterior vaginal wall by Landon's retractor. Ultimate differentiation of the two entities is by rectal or rectovaginal examination. In enterocele, the bulging is close to the cervix and cannot be reached by the finger inside the rectum (Figs. 16.13 and 16.14).

Uterine prolapse: In second or third degree of prolapse, inspection can reveal a mass protruding out through the introitus, the leading part of which is the external os. In first degree of uterine descent, the diagnosis is made through speculum examination when one finds the cervical descent below the level of ischial spines on straining. In others, however, the external os is visible on separating the labia (Fig. 16.7).

To diagnose a third degree prolapse, palpation is essential. Thumb is placed anteriorly and the two fingers (middle and the index fingers) posteriorly above the mass outside the introitus. If the examining fingers could be

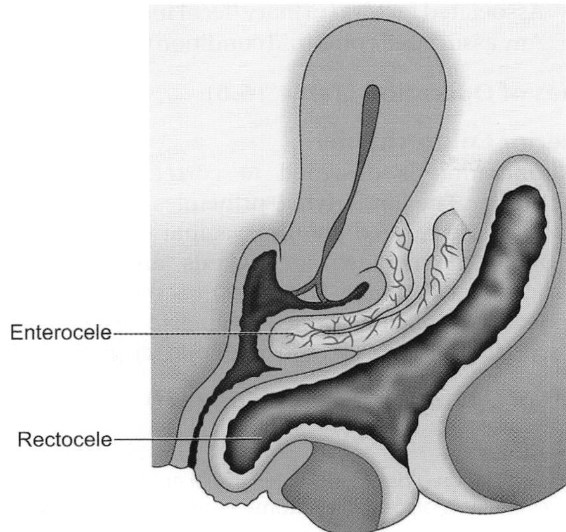

Fig. 16.14: Enterocele and rectocele (diagrammatic).

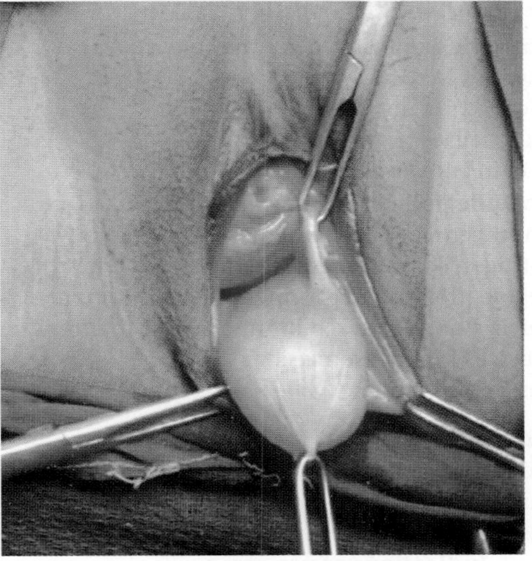

Fig. 16.15: Gartner's cyst.

apposed, it is the third degree (Fig. 16.8). *Degree of prolapse or POP quantification should be done.*

There may be evidences of decubitus ulceration or dark pigmented areas.

Bimanual examination reveals shallow vaginal fornices and normal length of the vaginal cervix with normal size uterine body. The introduction of a sound reveals marked increase in length of the uterine cavity. This signifies elongation of the supravaginal part of the cervix.

Levator ani muscle tone is assessed by placing examining fingers (index and middle) inside the vagina and thumb outside. The muscle (pubococcygeus) is palpated in the lower third of vagina. Patient is asked to squeeze the anus and the muscle tone is felt. Rectal examination helps to detect deficient perineum.

DIFFERENTIAL DIAGNOSIS

Cystocele

The cystocele is often confused with a cyst in the anterior vaginal wall, the most common being Gartner's cyst (retention cyst in remnants of Wolffian duct).

Features of Gartner's cyst (Fig. 16.15) are:

- Situated anteriorly or anterolaterally, and of variable sizes
- Rugosities of the overlying vaginal mucosa are lost
- Vaginal mucosa over it becomes tense and shiny
- Margins are well-defined
- It is not reducible
- There is no impulse on coughing
- The metal catheter tip introduced per urethra fails to come underneath the vaginal mucosa.

Uterine Prolapse

- ***Congenital elongation of the cervix*** **(Fig. 19.6, p. 223)**
  - It is unassociated with prolapse (usually)
  - Vaginal part of the cervix is elongated
  - External os lies below the level of ischial spines
  - Vaginal fornices are narrow and deep
  - Cervix looks conical
  - Uterine body is normal in size and in position.
- ***Chronic inversion***
  - Leading protruding mass is broad
  - There is no opening visible on the leading part
  - It looks shaggy
  - Internal examination reveals—cervical rim is on the top around the mass
  - Rectal examination confirms the absence of the uterine body and a cup-like depression is felt.
- ***Fibroid polyp***
  - The mass is shaggy with a broad leading part
  - No opening is visible on the leading part
  - Internal examination reveals—the pedicle coming out through the cervical canal or arising from the cervix
  - Rectal examination reveals normal shape and position of the uterus.

MANAGEMENT OF PROLAPSE

- **Preventive**
- **Conservative**
- **Surgery**

Preventive

The following guidelines may be prescribed to prevent or minimize genital prolapse.

Adequate antenatal and intranatal care

- To avoid injury to the supporting structures during the time of vaginal delivery either spontaneous or instrumental.

Adequate postnatal care

- To encourage early ambulance.
- To encourage pelvic floor exercises by squeezing the pelvic floor muscles in the puerperium.

General measures

- To avoid strenuous activities, chronic cough, constipation and heavy weight lifting.
- To avoid future pregnancy too soon and too many by contraceptive practice.

Conservative

Indications of conservative management:

- Asymptomatic women
- Old woman not willing for surgery
- Mild degree prolapse
- POP in early pregnancy.

Meanwhile, following measures may be taken:

- Improvement of general measures (*see* above).
- Estrogen replacement therapy may improve minor degree prolapse in postmenopausal women.
- Pelvic floor exercises in an attempt to strengthen the muscles (Kegel exercises).
- Pessary treatment.

Pessary Treatment

It should be emphasized that the pessary cannot cure prolapse but relieves the symptoms by stretching the hiatus urogenitalis, thus preventing vaginal and uterine descent. **Indications of use are**:

- *Early pregnancy*—the pessary should be placed inside up to 18 weeks when the uterus becomes sufficiently enlarged to sit on the brim of the pelvis.
- *Puerperium*—to facilitate involution.
- *Patients absolutely unfit for surgery* especially with short life expectancy.
- *Patient's unwillingness* for operation.
- *While waiting for operation.*
- *Additional benefits*: Improvement of urinary symptoms (voiding problems, urgency).

Complications of Pessary:

- Vaginal bleeding
- Pessary ulcers
- Pelvic pain (with large size pessary)
- Vaginal discharge

Pessary ulcers are treated by local estrogen.

SURGICAL MANAGEMENT OF PROLAPSE

Guidelines for Prolapse Surgery

- Surgery is the treatment of symptomatic prolapse where conservative management has failed or is not indicated.
- Surgical procedures may be: (A) **Restorative**—(i) correcting her own support tissues or (ii) compensatory—using permanent graft material (p. 184). (B) **Extirpative**—removing the uterus and correcting the support tissues. (C) **Obliterative**—closing the vagina (colpocleisis, p. 183).
- Meticulous examination, even under anesthesia, is necessary to establish the correct diagnosis of the organ prolapsed so that effective and appropriate repair can be carried out.
- There is no single procedure for all types of prolapse. **Factors determining the choice of surgery are**:
  - Patient's age
  - Parity
  - Degree of prolapse
  - Type of prolapse (cystocele, enterocele)
  - Any prior surgery for prolapse
  - Associated factors (urinary/fecal incontinence, PID)
  - Any associated comorbid condition (cardiac disease).

Types of Operation (Table 16.6)

Anterior Colporrhaphy

This operation is designed to correct cystocele and urethrocele. The underlying principles are to excise a portion of the relaxed anterior vaginal wall, to mobilize the bladder and push it upwards after cutting the vesicocervical ligament. The bladder is then permanently supported by plicating the endopelvic fascia and the pubocervical fascia under the bladder neck in the midline.

Steps of Operation (Figs. 16.16A to H)

Preliminaries

- The operation is done under general or epidural anesthesia.
- The patient is placed in lithotomy position.
- Vulva and vagina are to be swabbed with antiseptic solution.
- The perineum is to be draped with sterile towel and legs with leggings.
- Bladder is to be emptied by metal catheter.
- Vaginal examination is done to assess the type and degree of prolapse.

Actual Steps

- Sims' posterior vaginal speculum is introduced and the anterior lip of the cervix is held by multiple toothed vulsellum and firmly brought down by assistant (Fig. 16.16B).
- A metal catheter is introduced to know the lower limit of the bladder.
- An inverted 'T' incision is made on the anterior vaginal wall. The horizontal incision is made below the bladder and the vertical incision is made starting from the midpoint of the transverse incision up to a point about 1.5 cm below the external urethral meatus (Fig. 16.16A).
- The triangular vaginal flaps including the fascia on either sides are separated from the endopelvic fascia covering the bladder by knife and gauze dissection. The line of cleavage is vesicovaginal space and, if properly negotiated, the dissection is easy with minimal blood loss (Fig. 16.16B).
- The bladder with the covering endopelvic fascia (pubocervical) is now exposed as the edges of the vaginal wall are retracted laterally.
- The vesicocervical ligament is held up with Allis tissue or toothed dissecting forceps and divided. The bladder is then pushed up by gauze covered finger till the peritoneum of the uterovesical pouch is visible. The vesicocervical space is now exposed (Figs. 16.16C and D).
- The pubocervical fascia is plicated by interrupted sutures with No. 'O' chromic catgut using round body needle. The lower one or two stitches include a bite on the cervix, thus closing the hiatus through which the bladder herniates (Fig. 16.16E).
- The redundant portion of the vaginal mucosa is cut on either side (Fig. 16.16F).
- The cut margins of the vagina are apposed by interrupted sutures with No. 'O' chromic catgut using cutting needle (Figs. 16.16G and H).
- The catheter is reintroduced once more to be sure that the bladder is not injured.
- Toileting of the vagina is done.
- Vagina is tightly packed with roller gauze smeared with antiseptic cream.
- A self-retaining catheter is introduced.
- The last two formalities are optional.

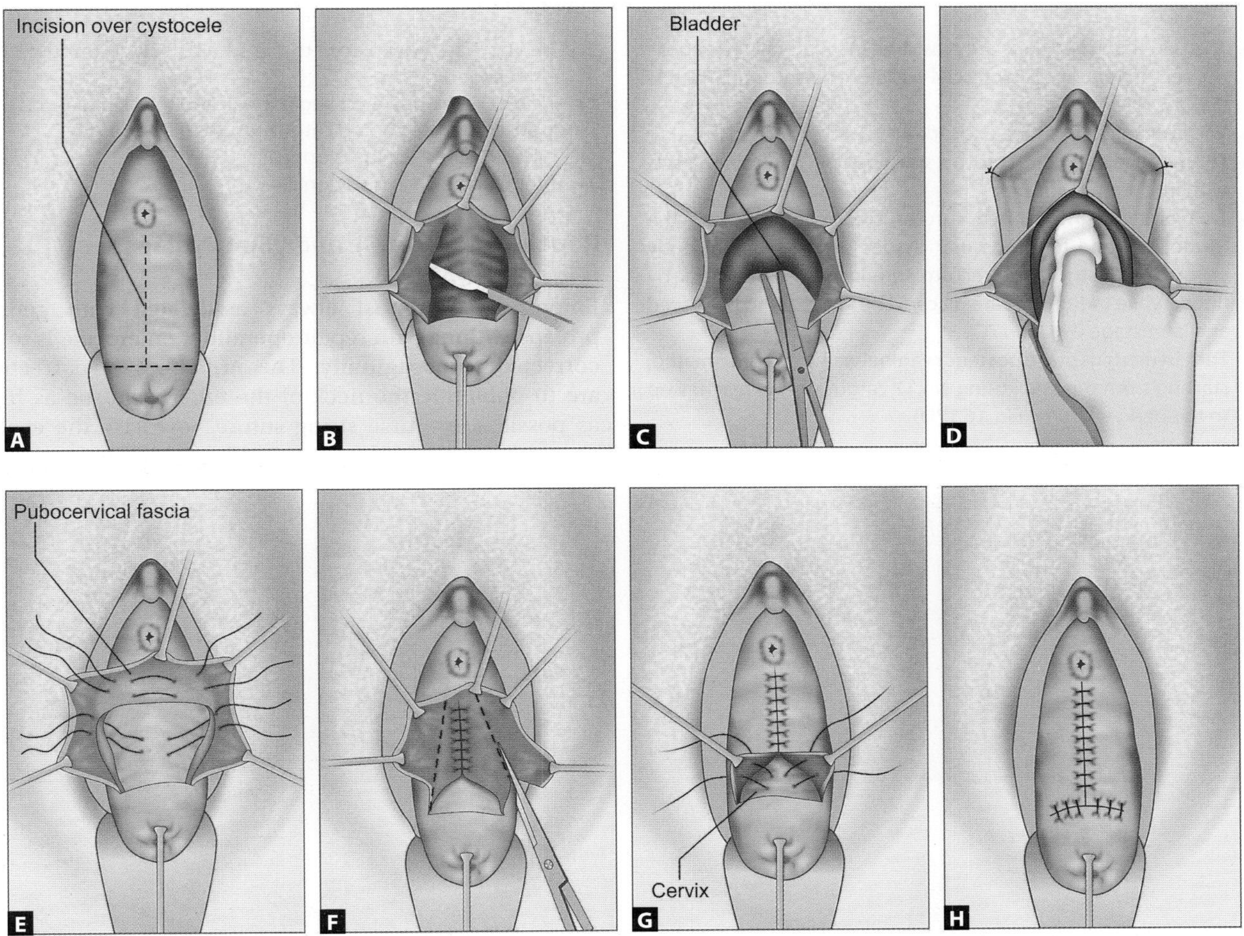

Figs. 16.16A to H: Steps of anterior colporrhaphy.

Paravaginal Defect and its Repair

Paravaginal defect is characterized by presence of rugae on the anterior vagina and absence of sulci on the lateral vagina; whereas in **central defect** (cystocele), rugae are absent and the lateral vaginal sulci is present.

Anterior vaginal wall prolapse (cystocele) is repaired by anterior colporrhaphy and plicating the endopelvic fascia in the midline under the bladder neck. But anterior vaginal prolapse may be due to the detachment of the endopelvic fascia from the lateral pelvic side wall. In that case, repair should be done by fixing (reattaching) the endopelvic fascia to the arcus tendineus fascia (white line) of the pelvis. This may be done retropubically through the space of Retzius or vaginally. This is indicated in cases with recurrent cystocele following repair.

Perineorrhaphy/Colpoperineorrhaphy

It is an operation designed to repair the prolapse of posterior vaginal wall. Its uses and extent of repair are employed in:

- **Relaxed perineum:** The operation is extended to repair the torn perineal body.
- **Rectocele:** The repair is extended to correct rectocele by tightening the pararectal fascia.
- **Enterocele:** High perineorrhaphy is to be done right up to the cervicovaginal junction along with correction of enterocele.

Restoration of perineal body is essential with any form of pelvic floor repair. This maintains the normal vaginal axis.

Steps of Operation (Figs. 16.17A to F)

Preliminaries: The preliminaries are to be followed as in anterior colporrhaphy.

Actual Steps

- A pair of Allis tissue forceps is placed on each side at the lower end of labium minus and a third pair of Allis is placed on the posterior vaginal wall in the midline well above the rectocele bulge (Fig.16.17A).
- A horizontal incision is made on the mucocutaneous junction joining the two Allis tissue forceps (Fig. 16.17A).
- Through this incision, with the help of perineorrhaphy scissors, the posterior vaginal wall is dissected off from the perineal body and rectum up to the third Allis forceps placed on the posterior vaginal wall (Fig. 16.17A).
- A vertical incision is made from the apex to the middle of the horizontal incision (inverted 'T' shaped incision) (Fig. 16.17A).

Contd...

Contd...

- The two triangular flaps are now dissected laterally to expose the rectum and musculofascial structures levator ani muscle (Fig. 16.17B).
- The lax vaginal flaps are excised.
- The rectocele is corrected by suturing the pararectal fascia with interrupted sutures.
- Two or three interrupted sutures are placed through the levator ani and fibromuscular tissues of the perineal body using No. 'I' catgut. The rectum should be pressed back by finger while the sutures are placed. The knots are to be placed at a later stage (Fig. 16.17C).
- The cut margins of the posterior vaginal wall are approximated, starting from the apex using No.'O' catgut until it reaches up to the perineal body (Fig. 16.17D).

Contd...

- The knots are now placed to the sutures passed through the perineal body.
- The rest of the posterior vaginal wall and the skin margins are opposed by interrupted catgut sutures (Fig. 16.17E).
- Toileting of the vagina is done.
- Tight vaginal pack is optional.

Repair of Enterocele and Vault Prolapse (Figs. 16.18A to D)

Enterocele is almost always associated with genital prolapse. Along with repair operation, enterocele is to be corrected **transvaginally**. The principles of correction are to obliterate the neck of the enterocele sac as high as possible by purse string suture, to excise the excess

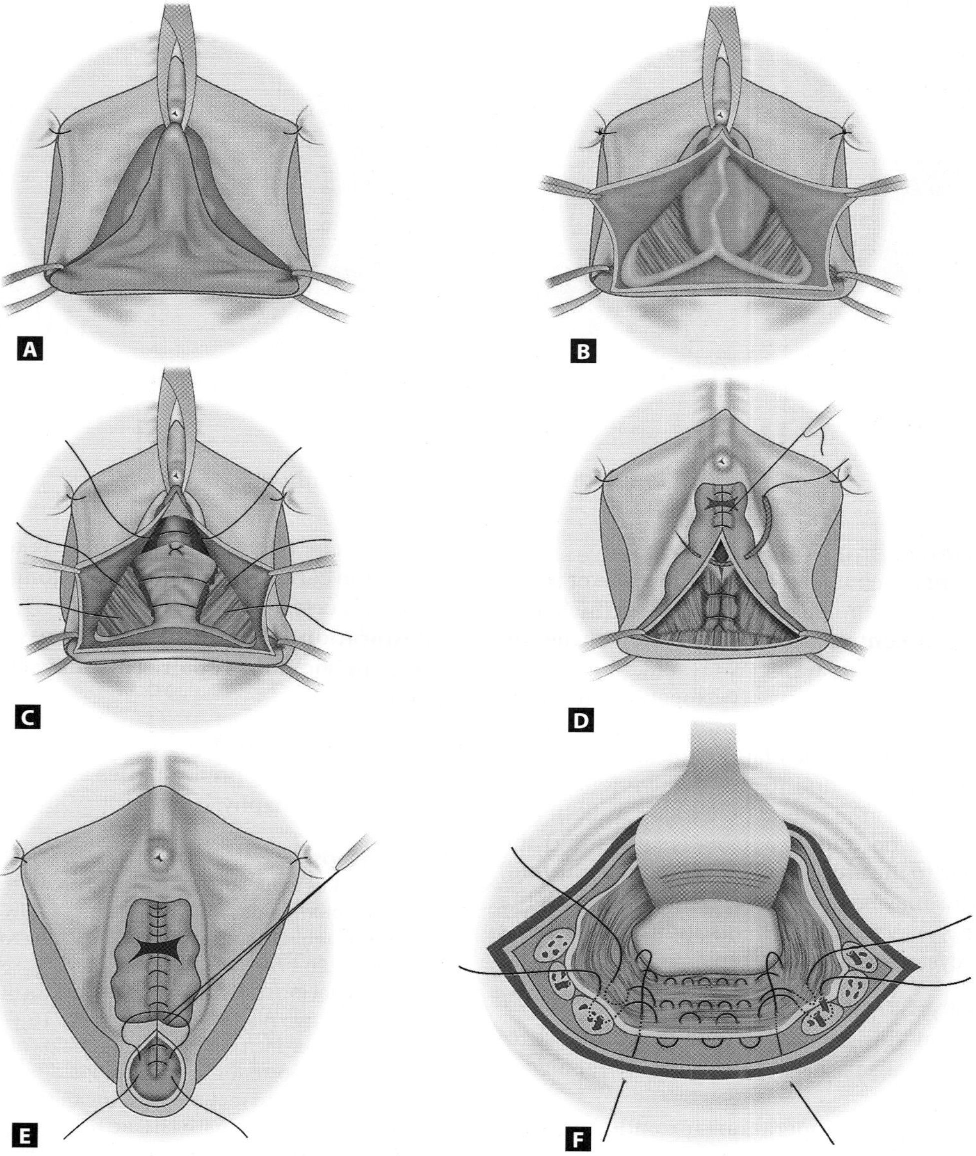

Figs. 16.17A to F: Steps of perineorrhaphy.

peritoneal sac and approximation of the uterosacral ligaments (Figs. 16.18A to D).

Actual Steps

- An inverted 'T' shaped incision is made with the vertical arm of the 'T' extending up to the apex of the vaginal vault and the horizontal arm, along the mucocutaneous border (Fig. 16.18A).
- Dissection is carried out to expose the enterocele sac (Fig. 16.18A).
- The sac is opened, the contents (bowel, omentum) are pushed away (Fig. 16.18B).
- The peritoneum of the posterior *cul-de-sac* is dissected off the anterior surface of the rectum and lower sigmoid and excised.
- A purse string suture (2-0 vicryl) is placed high at the neck of the sac and tied. The excess peritoneum is resected off (Figs. 16.18C and D).
- The cervix is pulled upwards. Two interrupted sutures are now placed around the uterosacral ligaments. These sutures also pass through the posterior aspect of the cervix. These sutures are tied. Rest of the steps are same as that of perineorrhaphy. *Vaginal repair of posthysterectomy enterocele:* The initial steps are the same as described in repair of enterocele (Fig. 16.18).

Contd...

Contd...

When the uterus is absent as in posthysterectomy vault prolapse, a purse string suture is passed high at the neck of the enterocele sac and left untied (Fig. 16.18C). The left-sided uterosacral ligament is picked up with the fingers of the left hand. Suture is passed through this ligament (ureter to be excluded).Fingers are mobilized to pick up the right uterosacral ligament and a bite is taken through this ligament also. This suture is tied. **Depending upon the size of the enterocele one or more such (internal McCall) suture may be placed (Fig. 16.17F).** The purse string suture is now tied and the excess peritoneum is cut away (Fig. 16.18D).

Use of supportive tissue (mesh) is currently advised in cases with complex prolapse.

- The rest of the steps are same as that of perineorrhaphy (Figs. 16.17A to F).

Abdominal repair of enterocele is done by obliterating the pouch of Douglas to prevent herniation of bowel. This is known as **Moskowitz procedure**. Generally three to four concentric sutures are placed incorporating the uterosacral ligaments and peritoneum over the rectosigmoid.

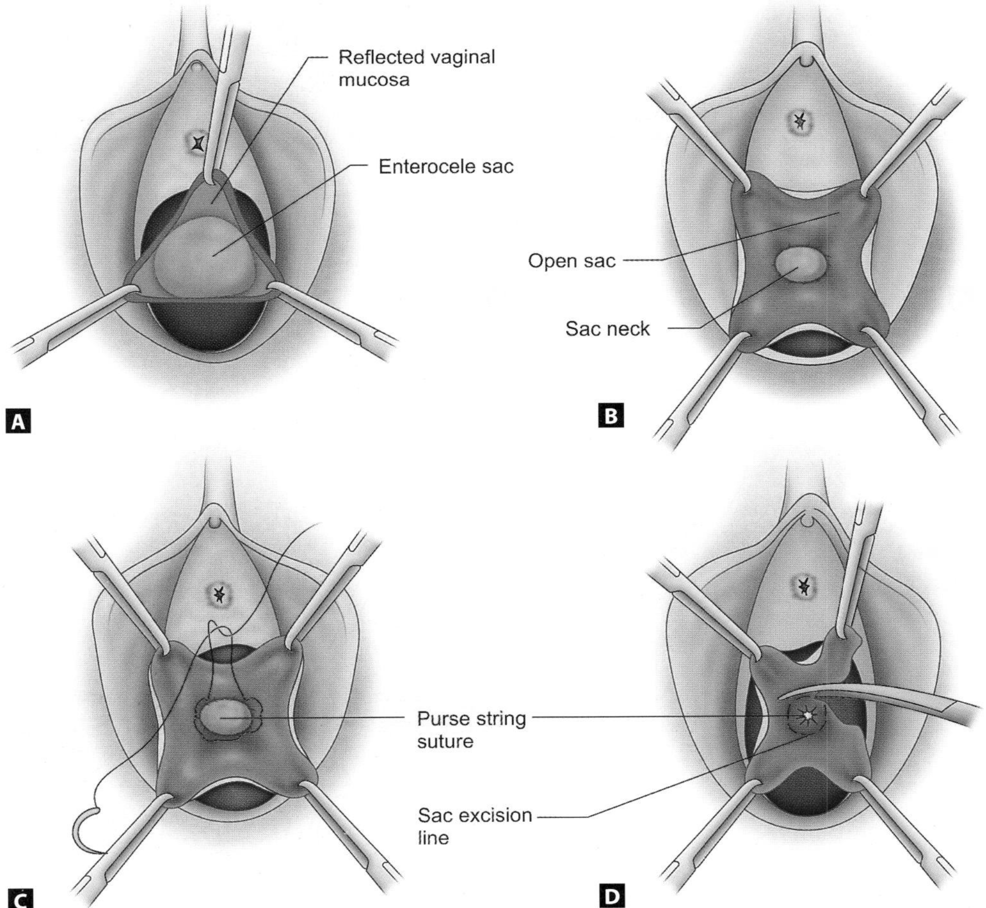

Figs. 16.18A to D: Steps of enterocele repair operation with cervix still present: (A) Dissection to expose the enterocele; (B) To open the sac and reduce the contents if any; (C) A purse string suture is placed at the neck of the sac and tied; (D) The excess peritoneum is resected.

Pelvic Floor Repair (PFR)

Usually, the prolapse of the anterior vaginal wall is associated with any form of posterior wall prolapse and relaxed perineum. As such, the corrective operation is known as pelvic floor repair. **This includes anterior colporrhaphy and colpoperineorrhaphy**. It should be emphasized that the PFR is not the operation for uterine descent. But as the uterine descent is most frequently associated with prolapse of the vaginal wall, PFR has to be done along with operation for uterine descent.

Fothergill's or Manchester Operation (Figs. 16.19A to D)

The operation is designed to correct uterine descent associated with cystocele and rectocele where **preservation of the uterus** is desirable.

The indications are:

- Preservation of reproductive function.
- When the symptoms are due to vaginal prolapse associated with elongation of the (supravaginal) cervix.

The Principal Steps of the Operation (Table 16.7)

- *Preliminary dilatation and curettage*—uterine sound gives the idea about elongation of cervix. **Dilatation** of the cervical canal is done to facilitate the passage of the sutures passing through the cervical canal during covering of the amputated cervix by vaginal flaps. It also ensures adequate uterine drainage and prevents cervical stenosis during healing of the external os. **Curettage is done** to remove the unhealthy endometrium.
- *Amputation of the cervix*—where future reproduction is required, low amputation is to be done.

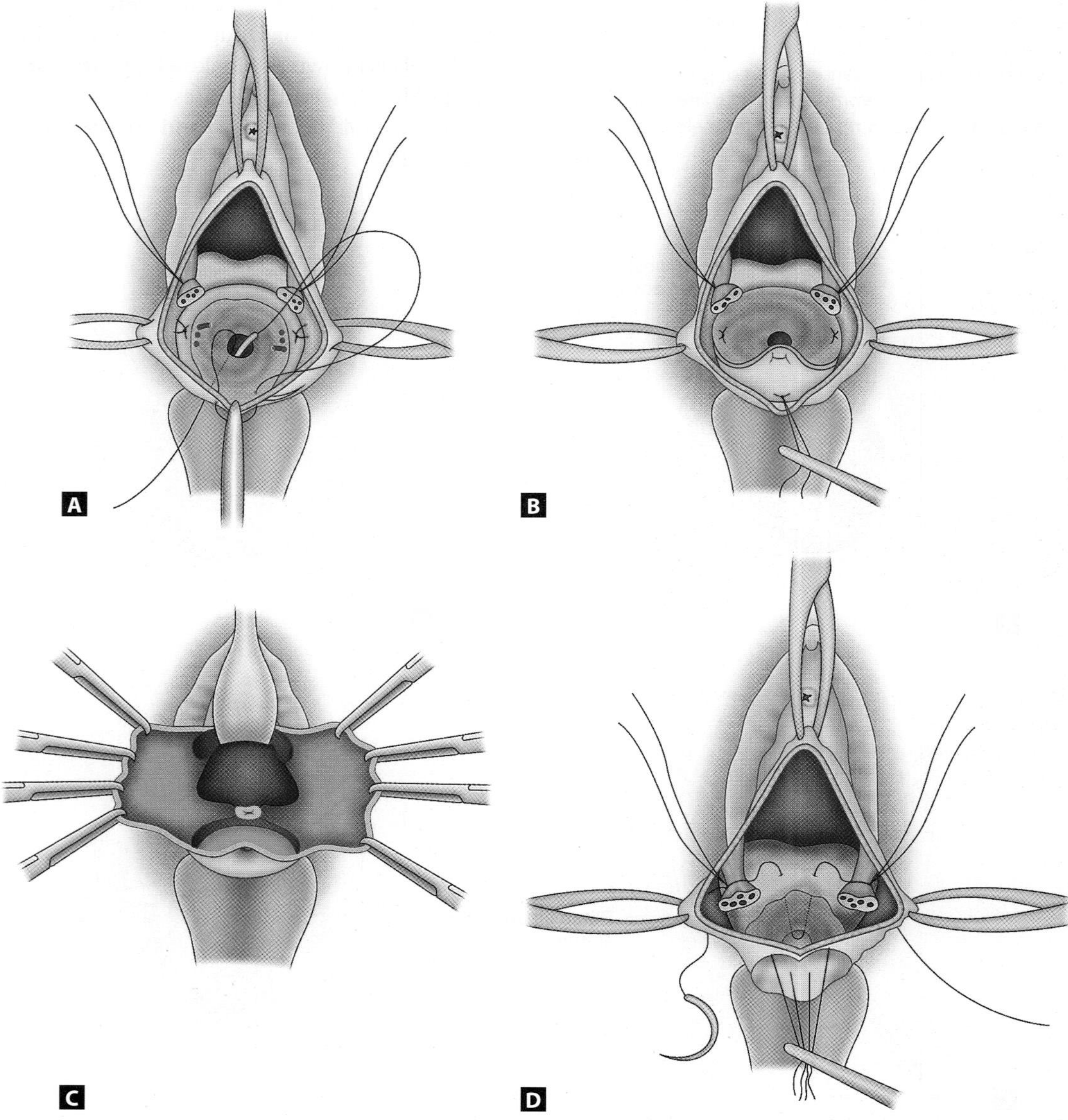

Figs. 16.19A to D: Principle steps of Fothergill's or Manchester operation: (A) After amputation of the cervix, the raw posterior lip of the cervix is covered by the posterior vaginal mucosa using Sturmdorf suture; (B) The knot is tied in the new posterior fornix; (C) Approximation of the cut ends of the Mackenrodt's ligament and fixing them in front of the cervix; (D) Approximation of the cut ends of the Mackenrodt's ligaments in front of the cervix using Fothergill's stitch.

TABLE 16.7: Composite steps of Fothergill's operation.

- Preliminary D&C
- Amputation of cervix
- Plication of Mackenrodt's ligaments in front of cervix
- Anterior colporrhaphy
- Colpoperineorrhaphy.

- *Plication of the Mackenrodt's ligaments* in front of the cervix. This facilitates their shortening and raising the cervix so as to place it in its normal position.
- *Anterior colporrhaphy.*
- *Colpoperineorrhaphy.*

If the family is completed, vaginal sterilization is to be done.

Steps of Operation

Preliminaries

The preliminaries are the same as those followed in anterior colporrhaphy.

- Preliminary D&C.
- The next step is like that of anterior colporrhaphy up to the pushing up the bladder.
- The posterior lip of the cervix is to be held with vulsellum and the cervix is drawn upwards.
- A pair of Allis forceps is placed in the midpoint of the posterior cervicovaginal junction.
- The anterior transverse incision is now extended posteriorly across the posterior cervicovaginal junction. The lateral and posterior vaginal wall is dissected off from the cervix by scissors and finger dissection.
- The Mackenrodt's ligament with descending cervical artery of either side is clamped at a higher level of amputation, cut and replaced by ligature (chromic catgut No.'1').
- The presence of enterocele should be searched for and if detected, to be repaired (Fig. 16.18).
- The cervix is now amputated at the calculated level.
- Anterior lip of the amputated cervix is now held with single-toothed vulsellum.
- The posterior lip of the amputated cervix is covered by the vaginal flap using a **Sturmdorf suture** (Figs. 16.19A and B) or by Bonney's method.

In **Bonney's method**, a catgut stitch is fixed at the apex of the posterior vaginal flap. The ends of the ligature are passed through the cervical canal and are taken out laterally on either side of new posterior fornix. The ends of the ligature are tied in the midline.

- The cut ends of the Mackenrodt's ligament are sutured to the anterior surface of the cervix (Fig. 16.19C). Alternatively, the ligaments are fixed using **Fothergill's stitch** (Fig. 16.19D). Fothergill's stitch is used to make the uterus anteverted. The stitch passes through the following tissues in sequence. Vaginal skin at the level of the Fothergill's lateral point → Mackenrodt's ligament → through the cervical tissue from outside inwards → cervical tissue from inside outwards → Mackenrodt's ligament of the other side → vaginal skin (Fothergill's lateral point) of the other side.
  - Pubocervical fascia is approximated as in anterior colporrhaphy.
  - Redundant portion of the vaginal mucosa is excised.
  - The cut margins of the vagina are opposed by interrupted sutures.
  - Posterior colpoperineorrhaphy is performed.

Contd...

Contd...

- Toileting the vagina is done.
- Vaginal pack is given.
- Self-retaining catheter is introduced.

Complications: Table 16.8.

Vaginal Hysterectomy with Pelvic Floor Repair

The operation is often designated as Ward Mayo's operation named after Mayo (1915) and Ward (1919) both from United States.

Removal of the uterus per vaginam (vaginal hysterectomy) is mostly done in cases of uterine prolapse. It should be emphasized that hysterectomy is not the surgery for the prolapse. It is done for elderly women who have completed their families. It is the associated repair of the pelvic floor repair, which is the corrective surgery for prolapse.

Indications

- Uterovaginal prolapse in postmenopausal women.
- Genital prolapse in perimenopausal age group along with diseased uterus like dysfunctional uterine bleeding (DUB), unhealthy cervix or small submucous fibroid requiring hysterectomy.
- As an alternative to Fothergill's operation where family is completed.
- As an alternative to abdominal hysterectomy in undescended uterus either as a routine or in selected cases where abdominal approach is unsafe. PFR is not done in such cases.
- As an alternative to laparoscopic assisted vaginal hysterectomy (LAVH) in selected cases of undescended uterus. Compared to LAVH, vaginal hysterectomy is less expensive and the perioperative morbidity is no different.

Principles of the Operation in Prolapse

- Removal of the uterus through vaginal route.
- Correction of enterocele, if any.
- Approximation of the pedicles in the midline to have a good buttress.
- Fixation of the uterosacral ligaments to the vault to prevent vault prolapse.
- Bladder support is reconstituted utilizing the broad ligaments and round ligaments as buttress.
- Repair of cystocele.
- Reconstruction of the perineum.

TABLE 16.8: Complications of Fothergill's operation.

During operation	▪ Hemorrhage ▪ Injury to the bladder and rectum
Postoperative	▪ Retention of urine or cystitis ▪ Hemorrhage—primary or secondary ▪ Infection
Late	▪ Dyspareunia ▪ Cervical stenosis—hematometra ▪ Infertility ▪ Cervical incompetency ▪ Cervical dystocia in labor ▪ Recurrence of prolapse

Steps of Operation for Vaginal Hysterectomy (Figs. 16.20A to H) (Indication—Genital Prolapse)

Preliminaries

The preliminaries are the same as in anterior colporrhaphy.

- To proceed as like that of anterior colporrhaphy up to pushing up the bladder (Fig. 16.20A).
- The uterovesical peritoneum is cut open. Landon's retractor is introduced and to be held by an assistant (Fig. 16.20B).

Contd...

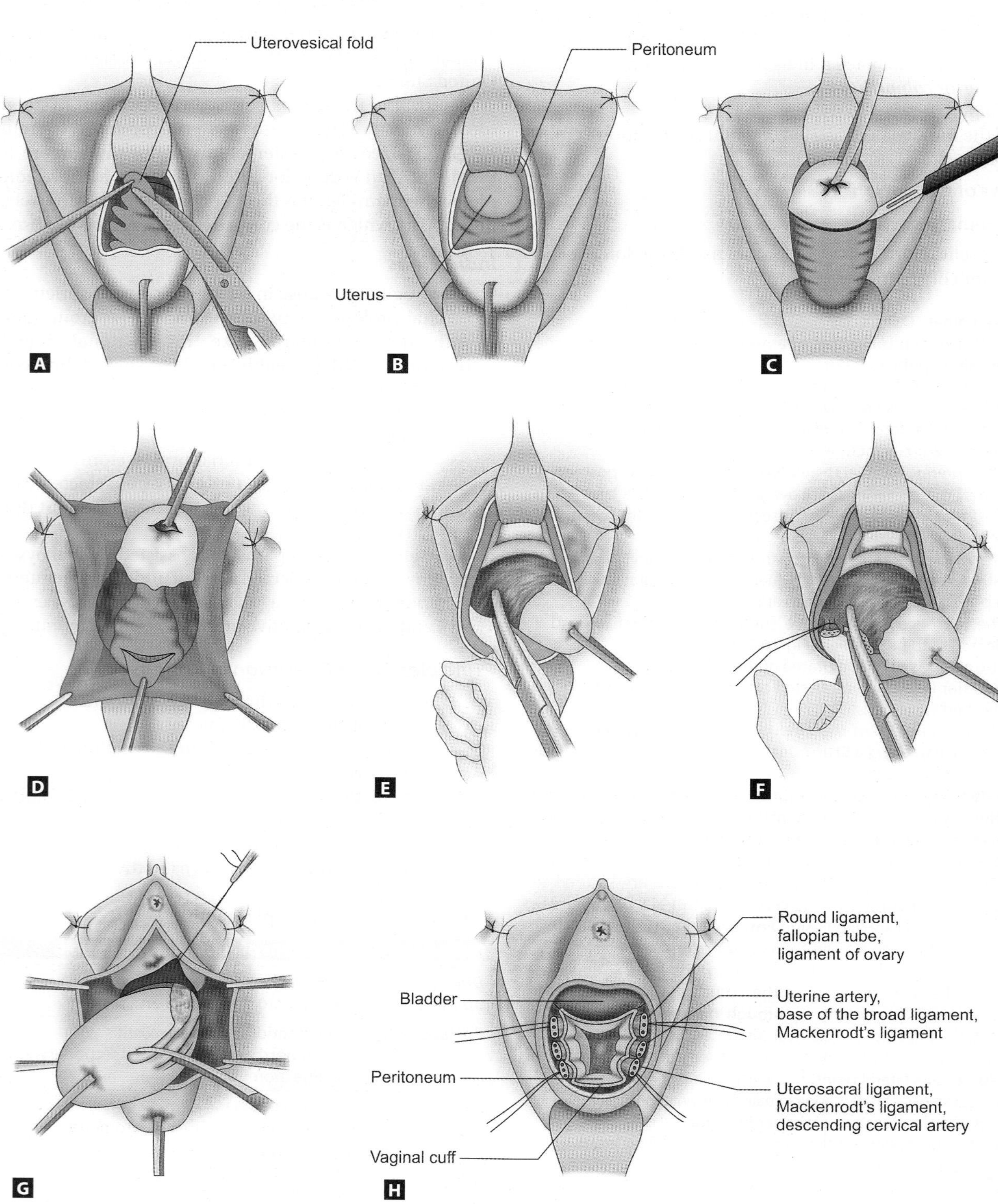

Figs. 16.20A to H: Principal steps of vaginal hysterectomy.

Contd...

- The posterior vaginal wall along the cervicovaginal junction is cut as in Fothergill's operation. The vaginal wall is dissected down till the pouch of Douglas is reached. The peritoneum is cut open (Figs. 16.20C and D).
- **First clamp is placed which includes** uterosacral ligament, Mackenrodt's ligament and descending cervical artery. The tissues are cut as close to the cervix and replaced by Vicryl No. 1. Similar procedures are followed on the other side (Fig. 16.20E).
- **Second clamp includes** uterine artery and base of the broad ligament. The structures are cut as close to the uterus and replaced by ligature (Vicryl No. 1). Same procedures are followed on the other side (Fig. 16.20F).
- The fundus is now brought out through the anterior pouch by a pair of Allis tissue forceps.
- **The third clamp includes** round ligament, fallopian tube, mesosalpinx and ligament of the ovary. The structures are cut and replaced by transfixing suture (Vicryl No. 1). Same procedures are carried out on the other side. The uterus is removed (Fig. 16.20G).
- Correction of the enterocele is to be done at this stage.
- Peritoneum is closed by a purse string suture (Fig. 16.20H).
- The sutures of the uppermost pedicles on either side are tied. The excess sutures of the uterine artery pedicle on each side are cut. The sutures of the pedicle containing the uterosacral and Mackenrodt ligaments are passed through the vault crosswise and are to be held temporarily.
- As in anterior colporrhaphy, the pubocervical fascia is approximated and fixed to the uppermost tied broad ligament pedicles to close the hiatus.
- Redundant portions of the vaginal flaps are excised and the margins approximated by interrupted sutures (Vicryl No.'O').
- Crosswise passed sutures of the lowermost pedicles are now tied, thus fixing the ligaments with the vaginal cuff. Cardinal and uterosacral ligaments to the vaginal cuff is useful to prevent vault prolapse.
- Perineorrhaphy is done.
- Vaginal packing is optional.
- Self-retaining catheter is introduced.

VAULT PROLAPSE (FIG. 16.21)

Posthysterectomy (vaginal or abdominal) vault prolapse is usually accompanied by an enterocele (70%). However, cystocele and/or rectocele may be present. The vault prolapse in such cases may be effectively repaired transvaginally maintaining the same principle of repair of enterocele along with anterior colporrhaphy and colpoperineorrhaphy.

Sometimes, it may require suspension of the vault with the anterior sacral ligament in front of 3rd sacral vertebra (sacral colpopexy) transabdominally using nonabsorbable sutures such as Teflon or Mersilene mesh.

Management of Vault Prolapse

Conservative

Pessary treatment—generally not recommended (p. 176).

Surgical

- Transvaginal approach
  - Repair of enterocele along with PFR (p. 178)
  - Le Fort's operation
  - Colpocleisis (cases following hysterectomy)
  - Sacrospinous colpopexy.
- Abdominal approach
  - Vault suspension (sacral colpopexy).

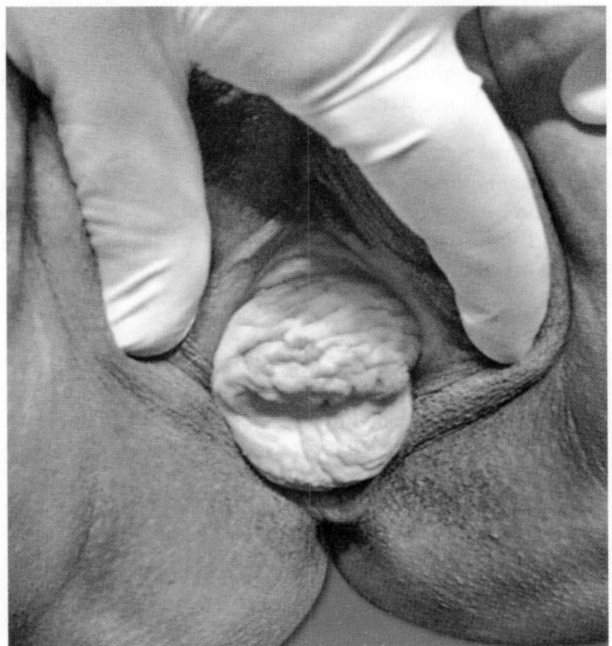

Fig. 16.21: Vault prolapse following vaginal hysterectomy. Scar is seen in the center.

Le Fort operation: The procedure is almost obsolete. It may be done in old age with procidentia when the patient is unfit for longer duration of surgery as vaginal hysterectomy with PFR. There should not be any uterine or pelvic pathology. Cervical cytology (Pap smear) should be normal. The operation can be done under local anesthesia.

The principal steps of the operation are:

- Denudation of rectangular vaginal flap from the anterior and posterior vaginal walls.
- Apposition of the denuded anterior and posterior vaginal walls by chromic catgut. Two small channels are thus left in the vagina one on either side for drainage.

Complications: Pyometra and urinary stress incontinence.

Colpocleisis (after hysterectomy)

Denudation of vaginal mucosa is done all round. Successive purse string absorbable sutures are placed from above downwards to appose the vaginal walls. It is a simple, safe and effective operation for a woman who is no longer interested in coital function.

Sacrospinous colpopexy: The sacrospinous ligament is attached medially to the sacrum and coccyx and laterally to the ischial spine. It is within the body of coccygeus muscle. Vaginal vault is fixed to the coccygeus sacrospinous ligament (CSSL) complex of the right side. This is done under direct vision following dissection of the pararectal space. A special needle (Miya hook) is used. Overall results are good.

Complications: Injury to the rectum, pelvic vessels (internal pudendal, inferior gluteal), stress urinary incontinence, gluteal pain (pudendal or sciatic nerve injury). Risk of recurrence about 3%.

Abdominal Approach for Repair of Vault Prolapse

Vault suspension (sacral colpopexy): Principle of the operation is to suspend the vaginal vault to be anterior longitudinal ligament in front of the 3rd sacral vertebra. Nonabsorbable suture material (Mersilene or Gore-Tex mesh) is used.

Actual Steps

- Abdomen is opened by vertical or transverse incision.
- A vertical incision is made on the posterior peritoneum over the sacral hollow while the rectosigmoid is pulled up laterally.
- Lateral angles of the vagina are identified and grasped with Allis tissue forceps.
- Two strips of Mersilene or Gore-Tex mesh (1.5 cm wide) are fixed to the vaginal angles and are pulled up in the midline. The other ends are fixed to the anterior longitudinal ligament in front of 3rd sacral vertebra with proper tension.
- Posterior peritoneum is sewn over the strips to make them retroperitoneal.

Complications: Stress urinary incontinence is an important one. ***Laparoscopic sacrocolpopexy*** is found to be effective with similar result to open sacrocolpopexy.

CERVICOPEXY OR SLING OPERATION (PURANDARE'S OPERATION)

The operation is indicated in **congenital** or **nulliparous prolapse** without cystocele where the cervix is pulled up mechanically through abdominal route. Strips of rectus sheath of either side passed extraperitoneally are stitched to the anterior surface of the cervix by silk.

Principal Steps of the Operation

- A transverse abdominal incision is made through the skin and fat.
- Two facial strips (rectus sheath) of 1.5 cm wide are dissected off, keeping its lateral attachment at the lateral border of the rectus muscle intact.
- The peritoneal cavity is opened in the midline. Bladder peritoneum is dissected off and the uterine isthmus is exposed mobilizing the bladder.
- The medial ends of the facial strips are now brought down between the leaves of the broad ligament to this site of uterine isthmus. (This procedure is technically similar as described in Gilliam's operation).
- The free edges of the facial strips are now fixed at the uterine isthmus with a sturdy bite using silk. This is done after adjusting the correct position of the uterus.
- Bladder peritoneum is repaired and abdomen is closed in layers. This operation may be combined with **Moskowitz procedure**. Instead of fascial strips, currently nonabsorbable (Marlex or Gore-Tex) tape is used for this purpose.

To know much details and variations of all the operations, the readers are requested to consult books of operative gynecology.

POP with stress urinary incontinence (SUI): The woman is evaluated for SUI (Ch. 25). Urodynamic studies are done with reduction of the prolapsed mass. If SUI present, concurrent surgery is done. Transobturator vaginal tape or Burch colposuspension (abdominal surgery) is commonly done.

MANAGEMENT OF POP USING MESH

Synthetic and biological mesh have been used. They are found to work better compared to traditional method of repair. Some synthetic (polygalactin) and all biological materials (fascia lata, dermis, rectus sheath) are absorbable. Nonabsorbable mesh are synthetic (polypropylene, polytetrafluoroethylene). Graft augments fibroblast proliferation and collagen tissue formation as they have pores. Prolene mesh (synthetic, macroporous 50–200 μg, monofilament) is commonly used. Absorbable mesh or grafts are less likely to cause complications but failure rates are high. In contrast, nonabsorbable mesh has low failure rate but higher rate of complications.

Suitable cases for mesh surgery are: Symptomatic anterior/posterior vaginal wall prolapse, recurrent prolapse, prolapse due to congenital connective tissue disorder prolapse in high risk woman.

Complications are: Mesh erosion, dyspareunia, vaginal pain, chronic sepsis, discharge, urinary incontinence and fistula formation.

Contraindications: Atrophic tissues, active pelvic infection, uncontrolled diabetes, obesity, smoking and history of pelvic radiation.

Owing to the complications, it is recommended that vaginal synthetic mesh for treatment of POP should be used for high risk women in whom benefits outweigh the risks (ACOG – 2011, AUCS – 2012)

COMPLICATIONS OF VAGINAL REPAIR OPERATIONS

Complications of PFR

- **Operative**
  - **Hemorrhage:** The hemorrhage may at times be brisk. The hypovolemic state can be tackled by infusion and blood transfusion.
  - **Trauma:** The bladder in anterior colporrhaphy or rectum in perineorrhaphy may be injured. The injury should be effectively repaired else, either VVF or RVF may develop later on.
- **Postoperative**

  Urinary
  - Retention of urine is a common complication. This is due to:
    - Spasm, edema and tenderness of pubococcygeus muscle.
    - Edema of the urethral wall.
    - Reflex from the wounds.
  - Infection leading to cystitis.

Hemorrhage

Primary hemorrhage occurs within 24 hours. **It is due to** imperfect hemostasis at operation or due to slipping of the ligature.

Along with the resuscitative procedures, the patient is to be brought to the operation theater. Under anesthesia, the suture sites in the vagina, both anterior and posterior are explored and hemostatic sutures are given. The vagina should be packed tightly with dry roller gauze which should be removed after 24 hours without anesthesia.

Secondary hemorrhage occurs usually between 5–10th day but may occur even in the 3rd week. **It is due to sepsis of the wound**. If the hemorrhage is brisk, along with resuscitative procedures, the patient is to be brought to the operation theater and under general anesthesia, the vagina is explored. The clots are removed to find any bleeding point. **If only generalized oozing is found**, tight intravaginal pack using dry roller gauze is enough. **If bleeding point is visible**, hemostatic sutures should be given followed by vaginal packing. The plug should be removed after 24 hours. Antibiotics are to be started again.

Sepsis

Infection occurs on the vaginal or perineal wounds. Rarely, disruption of the perineal wound occurs.

Late:
- **Dyspareunia**
- **Recurrence of prolapse**
- **Vesicovaginal fistula (VVF) following bladder injury (Ch. 26)**
- **Rectovaginal fistula (RVF) following rectal injury (Ch. 26)**

COMPLICATIONS OF VAGINAL HYSTERECTOMY WITH PFR

All the complications mentioned in PFR operation may occur, at times with increased intensity. Additional complications include:

Immediate
- Vault cellulitis
- Pelvic abscess
- Thrombophlebitis.
- Pulmonary embolism.

Late: Vault prolapse

CHRONIC INVERSION

Definition

Inversion is a condition where the uterus becomes turned inside out; the fundus prolapsing through the cervix.

Causes

- Incomplete obstetric inversion unnoticed or left uncared following failure to reduce for a variable period of 4 weeks or more.
- Submucous myomatous polyp arising from the fundus → traction effect (Figs. 16.22 and 16.23).
- Sarcomatous changes of fundal fibroma → infiltration of malignancy into the myometrium → softening of the wall.
- Senile inversion following high amputation of the cervix. It is probably due to cervical atony and incompetence.

Types

Two types are described in chronic inversion.
- **Incomplete:** The fundus protrudes through the cervix and lying inside the vagina.
- **Complete:** Whole of the uterus including the cervix are inverted. The vagina may also be involved in the process.

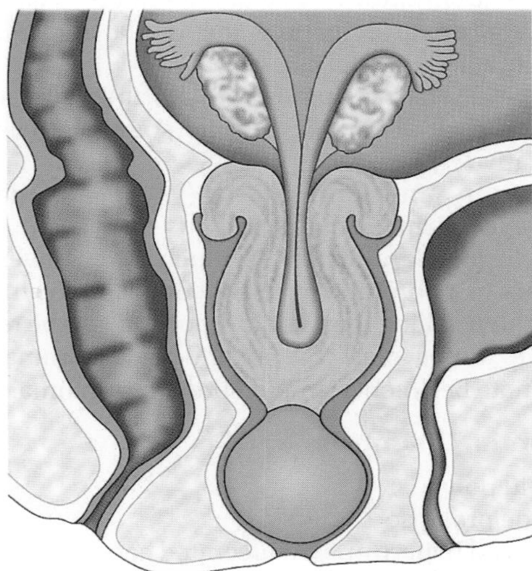

Fig. 16.22: Chronic incomplete inversion due to fundal fibroid (diagrammatic)

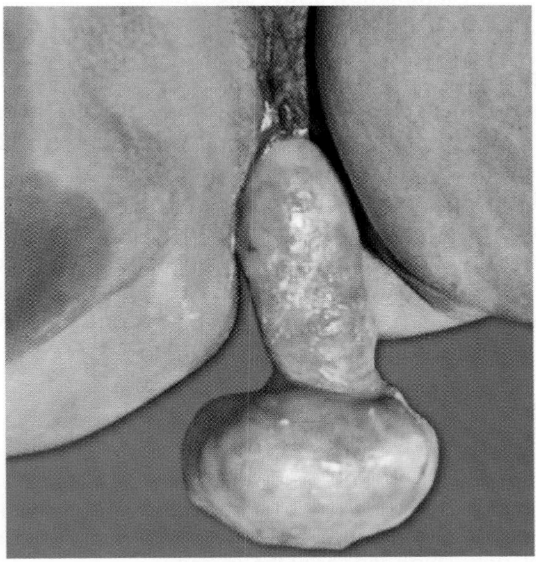

Fig. 16.23: Complete chronic inversion of uterus with a fundal fibroid.

(*Courtesy:* Department of Obstetrics and Gynecology, Government Maternity Hospital, Osmania Medical College, Hyderabad)

Symptoms

- Sensation of something coming down per vaginam
- Irregular vaginal bleeding
- Offensive vaginal discharge.

Signs

Inspection: The protruding mass has got the following features:
(i) Globular, (ii) No opening in the leading part, (iii) Shaggy look, (iv) Tumor may be present at the bottom.

Per vaginam: (a) The cervical rim is felt high up in incomplete variety but not felt in complete one. (b) Cup-shaped depression at the fundus is felt or the uterus is not felt in position.

Rectal examination: Rectoabdominal examination is more informative to note the fundal depression or displacement of the uterus.

Sound test: Demonstration of shortness or absence of uterine cavity using an uterine sound is reasonably confirmative.

Examination under anesthesia (EUA): At times, it is needed to confirm the diagnosis.

The diagnostic difficulty is much when inversion is secondary to a fibroid polyp or sarcoma and the inversion is incomplete, filling the vagina. A portion is to be removed from the tumor mass for histological examination to differentiate between a simple fibroid or sarcoma.

Differential Diagnosis

- Fibroid polyp
- Uterine prolapse
- Prolapsed hypertrophied ulcerated cervix
- Fungating cervical malignancy.

In fibroid polyp—the uterus is in normal position and the uterine sound can be passed into the uterine cavity. In difficulty, examination under anesthesia may be required (Fig. 16.24).

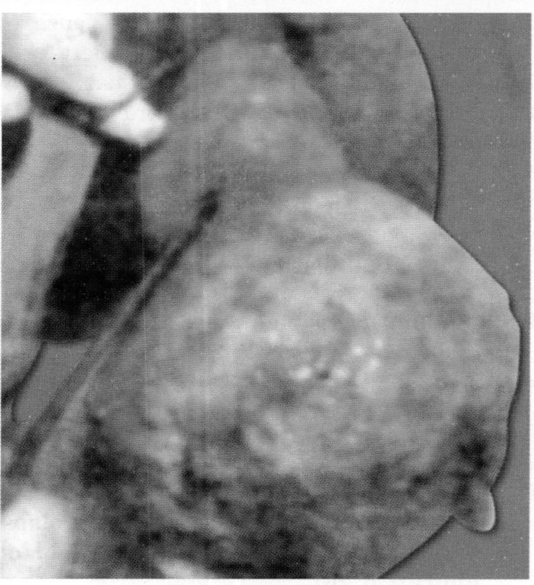

Fig. 16.24: Cervical fibroid polyp confusing diagnosis with chronic inversion. Note the uterine sound into the cervical canal.

Treatment

General measures: The patients are usually anemic. Prior improvement should be made if necessary, by blood transfusion. Local sepsis is to be controlled.

Definitive treatment: There is no place of manipulative replacement by taxis. Rectification should be done by surgery. Preservation or removal of the uterus is determined by such factors like age, parity, associated complicating factors. If hysterectomy is contemplated, it should be done by following rectification.

Conservative surgery: Rectification may be done abdominally (Haultain's operation—after cutting the posterior ring of the cervix) or vaginally (Spinelli's operation—after cutting the anterior ring of the cervix). Following Haultain's operation, some form of suspension operation has to be done to prevent posterior adhesions.

Contemplating polypectomy in suspected inversion, prior confirmation by 'sound test' is mandatory. **It is a sound policy to remove the tumor by shelling from its capsule rather than dividing the pedicle in such cases.**

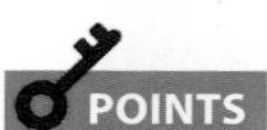

POINTS

- **Retroversion of the uterus** is quite common and is present in about 15–20% of normal women.
- Emptying the bladder prior to its diagnosis is mandatory. Retroversion *per se* has got no adverse effect on fertility or early pregnancy.
- **Pelvic organ prolapse** is the prolapse of the pelvic organs into the vaginal canal. The important risk factors for prolapse is history of vaginal birth and age of the woman.
- **Supports of uterus** are grouped under 3 tier system. Levator ani muscle guards the hiatus urogenitalis. It supports the pelvic viscera as it is a strong, robust and striated muscle.
- **Important support structures of uterus** are the cardinal, uterosacral, pubocervical ligaments, endopelvic fascia, levator ani muscle (pubococcygeus, iliococcygeus, levator plate) and the perineal body.
- **Prolapse** is due to a combination of injury to the neuromuscular as well as supporting structures.
- **Etiology of genital prolapse** includes the anatomical factors, as well as the different clinical factors.
- **The hammock-like arrangements** of levator ani muscle, the condensed endopelvic fascia, especially the Mackenrodt's ligaments are the cardinal support of the uterus. The levator plate and the perineal body maintains the normal vaginal axis.
  - **Cystocele and urethrocele** are more common with a gynecoid pelvis than with android or anthropoid types. In cases of congenital prolapse, occult spina bifida should be looked for. Secondary vault prolapse is more following vaginal hysterectomy than abdominal one. Decubitus ulcer is a trophic ulcer. Malignancy is a rare association. Predominant urinary complaints in genital prolapse are difficulty in passing urine, incomplete evacuation, frequency, stress incontinence and rarely retention. To diagnose a third degree uterine prolapse, digital palpation is mandatory. Cystocele may be confused with Gartner's cyst. Uterine prolapse may be confused with congenital elongation of the cervix, chronic uterine inversion and fibroid polyp.
- **The examination for prolapse** should be done with the patient in dorsal position then standing and using Valsalva's maneuver for correct assessment.
- **Degree of urine prolapse**: ***1st degree***: Uterus descends from its anatomical position but external uterine os remains in the vagina; ***2nd degree***: External os protrudes outside the vagina but uterine body remains inside; ***3rd degree***: Uterine body descends outside the vaginal introitus (procidentia) (p. 171).

Contd...

Contd...

- Newer classifications of **pelvic organ prolapse quantification (POP-Q)** have been introduced for more objective quantification. It is site specific and anatomical. Prolapse must be documented in terms of anterior or posterior vaginal wall and the uterine descent (Table 16.3). In this regard fixed anatomic reference points are used (Fig. 16.9, Table 16.4).
- **Pessary treatment** may be indicated in early pregnancy, puerperium, patient unfit for surgery or while the patients are waiting for operation.
- **The surgical procedures** for the management of prolapse are different. The type of surgery for an individual woman depends on her age, parity, reproductive and sexual function and also the type and degree of prolapse (Table 16.6).
- **The component parts of Fothergill's operation** are D&C, amputation of the cervix, plication of Mackenrodt's ligaments in front of the cervix, anterior colporrhaphy and colpoperineorrhaphy.
- **Posthysterectomy vault prolapse** (0.1–10%) is usually accompanied by an enterocele (70%). Vault prolapse can be repaired either by vaginal or by abdominal route. Colpocleisis is an easy, safe and effective method for a woman who is no longer interested in coital function.
- **When an enterocele is present**, the sac should be dissected high up and ligated at its neck to prevent recurrence. McCall culdoplasty is done. External McCall suture is placed at a higher level than the internal McCall (p. 184). Vicryl (1-0) suture is passed through the left posterior vaginal wall, peritoneum, pararectal fascia (uterosacral ligament) and it is then carried over in front of the sigmoid colon to include the similar points on the right hand side. One or more such sutures may be placed. It is tied after the closure of the peritoneal purse string suture (Fig. 16.17F).
- **Cervicopexy** (sling operation) is the method of repair for a patient with congenital or nulliparous prolapse (p. 184).
- **Use of mesh in** the management of prolapse is found to work better. Synthetic as well as biological materials are used (p. 184). Case should be properly selected to minimize complications. Use of mesh is restricted to selective cases only (ACOG 2011).
- After pelvic floor repair, bladder drainage (transurethral catheter) for 3–5 days is generally necessary before normal voiding starts.
- **The gynecologic inversion** is usually incomplete. Rectal examination is more informative in the diagnosis of chronic inversion. Chronic inversion may be confused with fibroid polyp, uterine prolapse, fungating cervical malignancy or prolapsed hypertrophied ulcerated cervix. There is no place manipulative replacement of chronic inversion. Surgical rectification is done either abdominally (Haultain's) or vaginally (Spinelli's).
- Vaginal vault prolapse is repaired either vaginally or abdominally. Sacral colpopexy is done abdominally using a synthetic mesh.
- Sacrospinous ligament fixation is a vaginal procedure for vaginal vault prolapse. Vaginal vault is fixed to the sacrospinous ligament on the right hand side. Miyazaki hook is used for the procedure. Injury to the pudendal and inferior gluteal vessels and the pudendal and the sciatic nerves are the known complications.

CHAPTER

17 Infertility

CHAPTER OUTLINE

DEFINITION

Infertility is defined as the inability to conceive within one or more years of regular unprotected coitus.

Primary infertility denotes those patients who have never conceived. **Secondary infertility** indicates previous pregnancy but failure to conceive subsequently.

Fecundability is defined as the probability of achieving a pregnancy within one menstrual cycle. In a healthy young couple, it is 20%. **Fecundity** is the probability of achieving a live birth within a single cycle.

INCIDENCE

About 80% of the couples achieve conception if they so desire, within one year of having regular intercourse with adequate frequency (4–5 times a week). Another 10% will achieve the objective by the end of second year. As such, 10% remain infertile by the end of second year.

Factors Essential for Conception

- **Healthy spermatozoa** should be deposited high in the vagina at or near the cervix (male factor).
- The spermatozoa should undergo changes **(capacitation, acrosome reaction)** and acquire motility (cervical factor).
- The **motile spermatozoa** should ascend through the cervix into the uterine cavity and the fallopian tubes.
- There should be **ovulation** (ovarian factor).
- The fallopian tubes should be patent and the oocyte should be picked up by the fimbriated end of the tube **(tubal factor)**.
- The spermatozoa should **fertilize** the oocyte at the ampulla of the tube.

The embryo should reach the **uterine cavity** after 3–4 days of fertilization.

The **endometrium** should be receptive [by estrogen, progesterone, insulin-like growth factor-1 (IGF-l), cytokines, integrins] for **implantation,** and the **corpus luteum** should function adequately.

PHYSIOLOGICAL CONSIDERATION

Due to anovulation, infertility is the rule prior to puberty and after menopause. But it should be remembered that the girl may be pregnant even before menarche and pregnancy is possible within few months of menopause. Conception is not possible during pregnancy as the pituitary gonadal axis is suppressed by human chorionic gonadotropin (hCG) and hence, no ovulation. During lactation, infertility is said to be relative. Despite the fact that the patient is amenorrheic during lactation, ovulation and conception can occur. However, in fully lactating women (breastfeeding 5–6 times a day and spending 60 minutes in 24 hours), pregnancy is unlikely up to 10 weeks postpartum.

CAUSES OF INFERTILITY

Conception depends on the fertility potential of both the male and female partner. **The male is directly responsible in about 30–40%, the female in about 40–55% and both are responsible in about 10% cases.** The remaining 10%, is **unexplained,** in spite of thorough investigations with modern technical know-how. It is also strange that 4 out of 10 patients of unexplained category become pregnant within 3 years without having any specific treatment.

It is also emphasized that the relative subfertility of one partner may sometimes be counterbalanced by the high fertility of the other.

Areas of Male Infertility (Table 17.1)

- Defective spermatogenesis
- Obstruction of the efferent duct system
- Failure to deposit sperm high in the vagina
- Errors in the seminal fluid.

Physiology of Spermatogenesis

Follicle-stimulating hormone (FSH) stimulates spermatogenesis from basal cells of the seminiferous tubules. Sertoli cells envelope the germ cells and support spermatogenesis. Sertoli cell function is controlled by FSH and

TABLE 17.1: Common causes of male infertility.

Pretesticular	*Testicular*	*Post-testicular*
Genetic ■ 47 XXY ■ Y chromosome deletions ■ Single gene mutations **Endocrine** ■ Gonadotropin deficiency ■ Obesity ■ Thyroid dysfunction ■ Hyperprolactinemia **Psychosexual** ■ Erectile dysfunction ■ Impotence **Drugs** ■ Antihypertensives ■ Antipsychotics	■ Immotile cilia (Kartagener) syndrome ■ Cryptorchidism ■ Infection (mumps orchitis) ■ Toxins: Drugs, smoking, radiation ■ Varicocele ■ Immunologic ■ Sertoli-cell-only syndrome ■ Primary testicular failure ■ Oligoasthenoteratozoospermia	**Obstruction of efferent duct** ■ **Congenital:** • Absence of vas deferens (cystic fibrosis) • Young's syndrome ■ **Acquired infection:** • Tuberculosis • Gonorrhea ■ **Surgical** • Herniorrhaphy • Vasectomy **Others** ■ Ejaculatory failure ■ Retrograde ejaculation ■ Hypospadias ■ Bladder neck surgery

testosterone. Scrotal temperature should be 1–2°F less than the body temperature. Luteinizing hormone (LH) is required for the synthesis of testosterone from the Leydig cells. FSH also stimulates the Sertoli cells to produce androgen binding proteins (ABP) and inhibin B. ABP binds to testosterone and dihydrotestosterone to maintain the local high concentration of androgens. Spermatogenesis and sperm maturation need a high androgenic environment. Inhibin B inhibits FSH secretion. Spermatogenesis is controlled predominantly by the genes on Y chromosome. **Approximately 74 days are required to complete the process of spermatogenesis.** Additional 12–20 days are needed for spermatozoa to travel the epididymis.

Common causes of male infertility

The important causes are: (a) Hypothalamic-pituitary disorders (1–2%); (b) Primary testicular disorders (30–40%); (c) Disorders of sperm transport (10–20%); (d) Idiopathic (40–50%).

- **Congenital:**
  - **Undescended testes:** The hormone secretion remains unaffected, but the spermatogenesis is depressed. Vas deferens is absent (bilateral) in about 1–2% of infertile males.
  - **Kartagener syndrome** (autosomal disease)—there is loss of ciliary function and sperm motility.
  - **Hypospadias** causes failure to deposit sperm high in vagina.
- **Thermal factor:** The scrotal temperature is raised in conditions such as varicocele. Varicocele probably interferes with the cooling mechanism or increases catecholamine concentration. However, no definite association between varicoceles and infertility has been established.
- **Infection:** (a) Mumps orchitis after puberty may permanently damage spermatogenesis; (b) The quality of the sperm is adversely affected by chronic systemic illness like bronchiectasis. Bacterial or viral infection of the seminal vesicle or prostate depresses the sperm count; (c) *T. mycoplasma* or *Chlamydia trachomatis* infection is also implicated.
- **General factors:** Chronic debilitating diseases, malnutrition or heavy smoking reduce spermatogenesis. Alcohol inhibits spermatogenesis either by suppressing Leydig cell synthesis of testosterone or possibly by suppressing gonadotropin levels.
- **Endocrine:** Testicular failure due to gonadotropin deficiency **(Kallmann's syndrome)** is rare. FSH level is raised in idiopathic testicular failure with germ cell hypoplasia **(Sertoli-cell-only-syndrome)**. Hyperprolactinemia is associated with impotence.
- **Genetic:** Common chromosomal abnormality in azoospermic male is Klinefelter's syndrome (47 XXY). Gene microdeletion have been detected in the long-arm of Y chromosome (Yq) for patients with severe oligospermia and azoospermia. Nearly 80% of men with congenital bilateral absence of vas deferens (CBAVD) have genetic mutations. About 66% of men with cystic fibrosis have CBAVD.
- **Iatrogenic:** Radiation, cytotoxic drugs, nitrofurantoin, cimetidine, β blockers, antihypertensive, anticonvulsant, and antidepressant drugs are likely to hinder spermatogenesis.
- **Immunological factor:** Antibodies against spermatozoal surface antigens may be the cause of infertility. This results in clumping of the spermatozoa after ejaculation.

Obstruction of the Efferent Ducts

The efferent ducts may be obstructed by infection like tubercular, gonococcal or by surgical trauma (herniorrhaphy) following vasectomy. In **Young's syndrome**, there is epididymal obstruction and bronchiectasis.

Failure to Deposit Sperm High in the Vagina (Coital Problems)

- Erectile dysfunction
- Ejaculatory defect—premature, retrograde or absence of ejaculation
- Hypospadias.

Sperm abnormality: Loss of sperm motility (asthenozoospermia), abnormal sperm morphology (roundheaded sperm, teratozoospermia) are the important factors.

Errors in the Seminal Fluid

- Unusually high or low volume of ejaculate
- **No ejaculate:** Ductal obstruction, retrograde ejaculation, hypogonadism
- **Low volume:** Absence of seminal vesicles, infection, ductal obstruction
- **Abnormal viscocity:** Cause unknown.

Causes of Semen Abnormalities

- **Azoospermia:** Klinefelter's syndrome, Sertoli cell only syndrome, agenesis of seminiferous tubules, hypogonadotropic hypogonadism, Young syndrome.
- **Oligozoospermia:** Genetic disorder, endocrinopathies, maturation arrest, exogenous factors.
- **Abnormal motility:** Immunologic factors, infection, varicocele, sperm structural defects, metabolic abnormalities.

CAUSES OF FEMALE INFERTILITY (FIGO) (FIG. 17.1)

- Ovulatory dysfunction: 30–40%
- Tubal disease: 25–35%
- Uterine factors: 10%
- Cervical factors: 5%
- Pelvic endometriosis: 1–10%.

Ovarian Factors

The ovulatory dysfunctions (dysovulatory) are:

- Anovulation or oligo-ovulation
- Decreased ovarian reserve
- Luteal phase defect (LPD)
- Luteinized unruptured follicle (LUF).

Anovulation or oligo-ovulation

The ovarian activity is totally dependent on the gonadotropins and the normal secretion of gonadotropins depends on the pulsatile release of GnRH from hypothalamus. As such, **ovarian dysfunction is likely to be linked with disturbed hypothalamo-pituitary-ovarian axis either primary or secondary from thyroid or adrenal dysfunction.**

Thus, the disturbance may result not only in anovulation but may also produce **oligomenorrhea** or **even amenorrhea. Other causes of anovulation are:** Polycystic ovarian syndrome, elderly women and women with premature ovarian failure (p. 389). **Possible causes of anovulation** are given schematically (Fig. 17.1).

As there is no ovulation, there is no corpus luteum formation. In the absence of progesterone, there is no secretory endometrium in the second half of the cycle. The other features of ovulation (later in the Ch.) are absent.

Luteal phase defect (LPD)

In this condition, there is inadequate growth and function of the corpus luteum. There is inadequate progesterone secretion. The lifespan of corpus luteum is shortened to less than 10 days. As a result, there is inadequate secretory changes in the endometrium which hinder implantation. LPD is due to defective folliculogenesis which again may be due to varied reasons. Drug-induced ovulation, decreased level of FSH and/or LH, elevated prolactin, subclinical hypothyroidism, older women, pelvic endometriosis, dysfunctional uterine bleeding are the important causes.

Luteinized unruptured follicular syndrome (trapped ovum)

In this condition, the ovum is trapped inside the follicle, which gets luteinized. The cause is obscure but may be associated with **pelvic endometriosis or with hyperprolactinemia.**

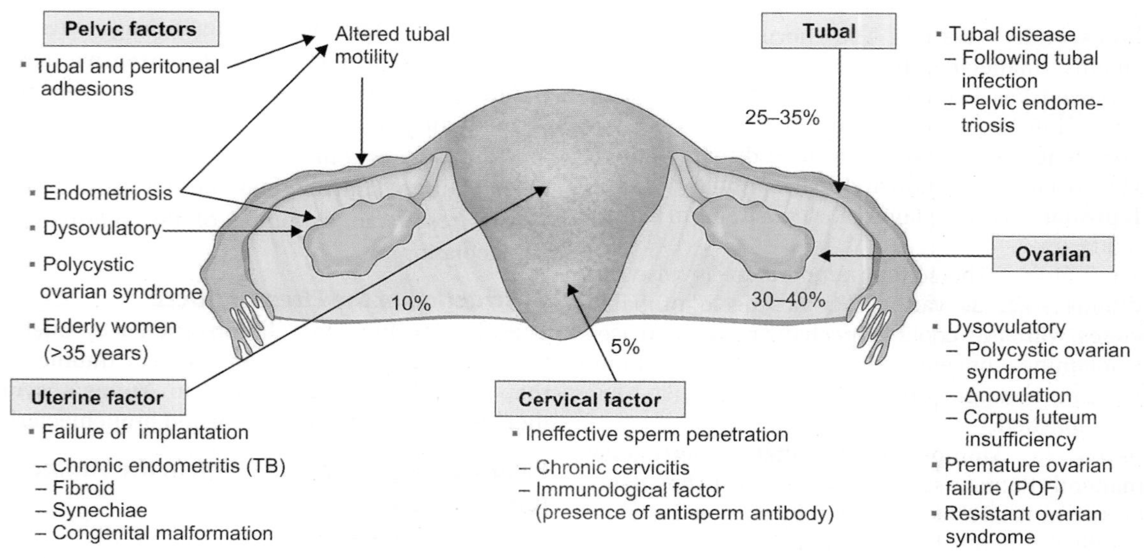

Fig. 17.1: Showing common causes of female infertility.

Resistant ovarian syndrome: The follicles are present but FSH receptor is either absent or resistant.

Tubal Factors

Tubal and peritoneal factors are responsible for about 30–40% cases of female infertility.

The obstruction of the tubes may be due to— (a) **Pelvic infections causing:** (i) Peritubal adhesions, (ii) Endosalpingeal damage; (b) Previous tubal surgery or sterilization; (c) Salpingitis isthmica nodosa (p. 114); (d) Tubal endometriosis and others; (e) Polyps or mucous debris within the tubal lumen; (f) Tubal spasm.

Common infections are: Chlamydia and gonococcus, tuberculosis (postabortal or puerperal).

Peritoneal factors: In addition to peritubal adhesions, even minimal **endometriosis** may produce infertility. Deep dyspareunia too often troubles the patient. The possible multifactorial mechanisms which operate in minimal endometriosis are depicted schematically at Table 17.2.

Uterine Factors

The endometrium must be sufficiently receptive enough for effective nidation and growth of the fertilized ovum. **The possible factors that hinder nidation are** uterine hypoplasia, inadequate secretory endometrium, fibroid uterus, endometriosis, endometritis (tubercular in particular), uterine synechiae or congenital malformation of uterus.

Cervical Factors

Anatomic: Anatomic defects preventing sperm ascent may be due to congenital elongation of the cervix and second degree uterine prolapse.

Physiologic: The cervical mucus may be scanty following amputation, conization or deep cauterization of the cervix. Presence of antisperm or sperm immobilizing antibodies may be implicated as immunological factor of infertility.

Vaginal Factors

Atresia of vagina (partial or complete), transverse vaginal septum, septate vagina, or narrow introitus causing dyspareunia are included in the congenital group. Dyspareunia may be the real problem in such cases.

Combined Factors

- Presence of factors both in the male and female partners causing infertility.
- General factors: Advanced age of the wife beyond 35 years is related but male spermatogenesis continues throughout life although aging reduces the fertility in male also.
- Infrequent intercourse
- Apareunia and dyspareunia (p. 470).
- Anxiety and apprehension.
- Use of lubricants during intercourse, which may be spermicidal.
- Immunological factors.

INVESTIGATIONS OF INFERTILITY

Objectives of Investigation

- To detect the etiological factor(s)
- To rectify the abnormality in an attempt to improve the fertility
- To give assurance with explanation to the couple if no abnormality is detected.

When to investigate? As per the definition, the infertile couple should be investigated after one year of regular unprotected intercourse with adequate frequency. The interval is however, shortened to 6 months after the age of 35 years of the woman and 40 years of the man.

What to investigate? The basic investigations to be carried out are: (a) Semen analysis; (b) Confirmation of ovulation; (c) Confirmation of tubal patency.

It is important that both partners should come at the first visit. Detailed general and reproductive history should be taken in presence of both. However, the clinical examination of each partner is carried out separately.

Clinical Approach to Investigations

- **Male**
- **Female**

Male

History

- Age
- Duration of marriage
- Contraception used
- History of previous marriage
- Sexual dysfunction
- Anosmia.

TABLE 17.2: Possible mechanism of subinfertility in women with pelvic endometriosis.

Ovarian dysfunction	*Tubal dysfunction*	*Uterine and others*
▪ Endocrinopathies • Defective folliculogenesis • Anovulation (PCOS) • Luteal phase defect • Reduced ovarian reserve • Hyperprolactinemia ▪ Oocyte maturation defect ▪ Luteolysis due to ↑ $PGF_{2\alpha}$	▪ Altered tubal motility ▪ Pelvic adhesions, tubal obstruction • Distortion of normal tube and ovarian relationship • Impaired pick-up of oocyte by the fimbria	▪ Impaired fertilization ▪ Implantation failure ▪ Early miscarriage ▪ Abnormal endometrial receptivity ▪ Dyspareunia (poor coital function) ▪ Abnormal peritoneal fluid ▪ Abnormal systemic immune response ▪ Increased sperm phagocytosis by macrophages

A general medical history should be taken with special reference to family history, durgs, history of chemotherapy durgs, radiotherapy, sexually transmitted diseases: (a) Mumps orchitis after puberty; (b) Diabetes; (c) Recurrent chest infection; (d) Bronchiectasis. Enquiry about relevant surgery such as herniorrhaphy, operation on testes, also about the sexual history, erectile dysfunction, social habits, particularly heavy smoking or alcohol.

Examination

A thorough physical examination is performed to determine the general state of health. This includes: Body mass index (BMI), hair, growth and gynecomastia—inspection and palpation of the genitalia. Attention should be paid to the size and consistency of the testicles. **Testicular volume** (measured by an orchidometer) should be at least 20 mL. Presence of varicocele should be elicited in the upright position.

Investigations

- **Routine investigations** include urine and blood examination including postprandial sugar.
- **Semen analysis: This should be the first step in investigation** because, if some gross abnormalities are detected (e.g. azoospermia), the couple should be counseled for the need of assisted reproductive technology.

Collection

The collection is best done by masturbation, failing which by coitus interruptus. The semen is collected in a clean wide mouthed dry glass jar. The sample so collected should be sent to the laboratory as soon as possible so that the examination can be performed within 2 hours. Sperm motility begins to decline 2 hours after ejaculation. The coitus should be avoided for 2–3 days prior to the test (abstinence).

Semen analysis (Table 17.3): Normal reference value WHO (2010).

In selected cases, biochemical tests of creatine phosphokinase and reactive oxygen species are done as sperm function tests. Creatinine phosphokinase helps sperm transport while reactive oxygen species and the peroxides interfere with sperm function.

TABLE 17.3: Semen analysis (WHO – 2010).

Semen analysis	*Normal reference value and lower reference (within parenthesis) limit*
Volume	2.0 mL or more (1.5 mL)
pH	7.2–7.8
Viscosity	<3 (scale 0–4)
Sperm concentration	20 million/mL (15 million/mL)
Total sperm count	>40 million/ejaculate (39 million/ejaculate)
Motility	>50% progressive forward motility (Progressive motility = 32%)
Morphology	>14% normal form (4%)
Viability	75% or more living (58%)
Leukocytes	Less than 1 million/mL
Round cells	<5 million/mL
Sperm agglutination	<10% spermatozoa with adherent particles

Normal male fertility requires a count of over 15 million spermatozoa per mL and a progressive motility of over 32%. Semen values normally vary widely. Two properly performed semen analysis at least 4 weeks apart should be done when one report is abnormal.

In-depth evaluation for the male

These are needed in cases of (a) Azoospermia; (b) Oligospermia; (c) Low volume ejaculate; (d) Problems of sexual potency. Further diagnostic protocols has been appropriately designed (Flowchart 17.1).

NOMENCLATURE

- ***Aspermia:*** Failure of emission of semen (no ejaculate).
- ***Hypospermia:*** Low semen volume (<2 mL).
- ***Oligospermia/oligozoospermia:*** Sperm count is less than 20 million per mL.
- ***Polyzoospermia:*** Count is more than 350 million/mL.
- ***Azoospermia:*** No spermatozoan in the semen.
- ***Asthenozoospermia:*** Reduced sperm motility. Leukocytospermia: Increased white cells in semen.
- ***Necrozoospermia:*** Spermatozoa are dead or motionless.
- ***Teratozoospermia:*** >70% spermatozoa with abnormal morphology.
- ***Oligoasthenoteratozoospermia:*** Disturbance of all 3 variables.

- **Serum FSH, LH, testosterone, prolactin, and TSH:** Testicular dysfunction causes rise in FSH and LH. Low level of FSH and LH suggest hypogonadotropic hypogonadism (Flowchart 17.1). Leydig cell dysfunction causes low testosterone and high LH level. Elevated prolactin due to pituitary adenoma may cause impotency.
- **Testicular biopsy:** Either open or percutaneous testicular biopsy is done to differentiate primary testicular failure from obstructive cause of azoospermia or severe oligospermia. Men with elevated serum FSH, may have adequate sperm on biopsy for use in intracytoplasmic sperm injection (ICSI). The biopsy specimen may be cryopreserved for future use in IVF/ICSI cycle. Thus testicular biopsy may have diagnostic prognostic and therapeutic value.
- **Karyotyping and genetic testing:** Abnormal karyotype has been observed in men suffering from azoospermia (15%) and severely oligospermia (5%). Genetic abnormalities have health risks of patient and the offsprings. Men with sperm concentration between 3 and 10 million/mL are considered for karyotyping and genetic testing. Klinefelter syndrome (47, XXY) are seen 1 in 500 men. Nearly 15% of men with severe oligospermia or azoospermia, will have microdeletion of the Y chromosome. These deletions are inherited by their offspring.
- **Immunological tests:** Two types of antibodies have been described—sperm agglutinating and sperm immobilizing; the latter is probably related to infertility. The antibodies are produced following infection (orchitis), trauma or vasectomy. These antibodies can be detected from the serum by the sperm immobilizing test. Presence of sperm antibodies in the cervical mucus is demonstrated by **postcoital test**.

Flowchart 17.1: Investigation protocol for male factors of infertility.

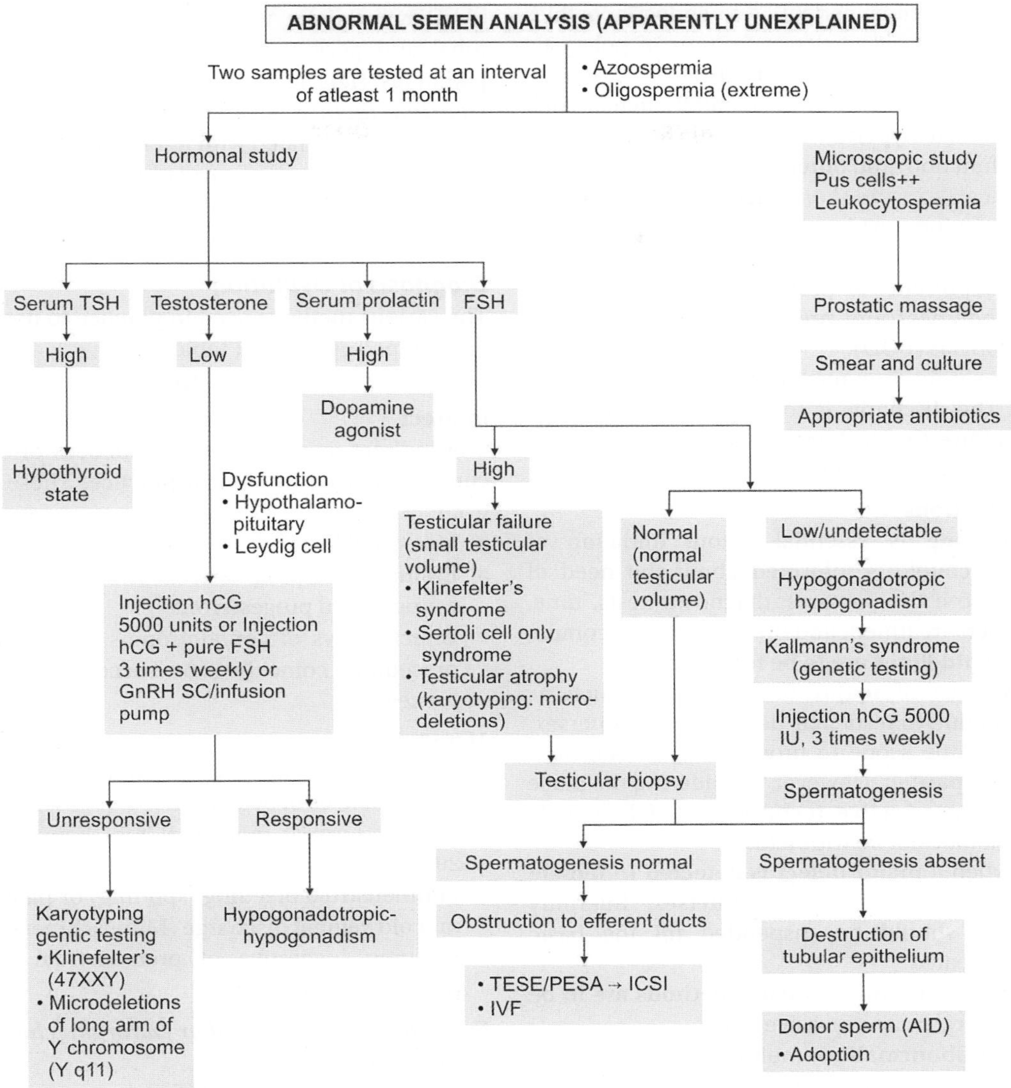

(PESA: percutaneous epididymal sperm aspiration; ICSI: intracytoplasmic sperm injection; TESE: testicular sperm extraction; AID: artificial insemination donor)

- **Presence of plenty of pus cells** requires prostatic massage. The collected fluid is to be examined by staining and culture to detect the organisms and appropriate antibiotic sensitivity.

Female

History

Age, duration of marriage, history of previous marriage with proven fertility if any, are to be noted.

- **A general medical history** should be taken with special reference to tuberculosis, sexually transmitted infections, features suggestive of pelvic inflammation or diabetes.
- **The surgical history** should be directed especially towards abdominal or pelvic surgery.
- **Menstrual history** should be taken in details. Wide spectrum of abnormalities ranging from hypomenorrhea, oligomenorrhea to amenorrhea are associated with disturbed hypothalamo-pituitary ovarian axis. This may be either primary or secondary to adrenal or thyroid dysfunction.
- **Previous obstetric history:** In a case of secondary infertility history of postabortal or puerperal sepsis may be responsible for ascending infection and tubal damage. Uterine synechiae may be due to vigorous curettage.
- **Contraceptive practice** should be elicited. IUCD use may cause PID.
- **Sexual problems** such as dyspareunia, and loss of libido are to be enquired.

Examinations

- **General, systemic and gynecological examinations** are made to detect any abnormality which may hinder fertility.
- **General examination** must be thorough—special emphasis being given to obesity or marked reduction in weight (BMI). Hirsutism, acne, acanthosis nigricans or

underdevelopment of secondary sex characters are to be noted. Physical features pertaining to endocrinopathies are carefully evaluated to detect features of polycystic ovary syndrome (PCOS) and galactorrhea.

- **Systemic examination** may accidentally detect such abnormalities like hypertension, organic heart disease, thyroid dysfunction, and other endocrinopathies.
- **Gynecological examination** includes adequacy of hymenal opening, evidences of vaginal infections (*C. trachomatis, Mycoplasma*), uterine size, position and mobility, presence of unilateral or bilateral adnexal masses—tenderness and presence of nodules in the pouch of Douglas (POD).
- **Speculum examination** may reveal abnormal cervical discharge. The discharge is to be collected for Gram stain and culture. Cervical smear is taken as a screening procedure as a routine or in suspected cases.

Special investigations

Couple counseling is essential before initiation of treatment. The couple is informed about the need of evaluation for both the partners, diagnostic tests, time, needed the cost of treatment and the probable outcome.

The following guidelines are to be followed:

- In the presence of **major fault in male** such as azoospermia due to testicular destruction or intersex, there is very little scope to proceed for investigation for the female partner. However, considering the place of **assisted reproductive technology (ART)** female investigation may not be withheld.
- Similarly, when a **major defect is detected in female** such as Müllerian agenesis or intersex, infertility investigations should be suspended till the basic pathology is treated.
- **Noninvasive or minimal invasive methods** are to be employed prior to major invasive one.
- **Detection of abnormality**—multiple defects may be present in the same case, e.g. tubal defects may be associated with anovulation.
- **Pregnancy following laparoscopy and dye test** or hysterosalpingography is not uncommon. It is presumed that small flimsy adhesions or any mucus plug obstructing the tubal lumen is removed during such procedures.
- **Genital tuberculosis** as a cause of infertility is to be kept in mind especially in the developing countries. The association is as high as 10–15% in contrast to a low figure of 0.5% in the developed countries.
- **Use of ultrasonography:** Ultrasonography (TVS) is helpful to detect pathologies like fibroids, endometriosis, PCOS, or tubo-ovarian mass. Antral follicular count (AFC) can be done to assess the ovarian reserve similar to that of anti-Müllerian hormone AMH. AFC is done on cycle D1 to D4. Ovarian AFC is a reliable predictor of the response to ovulation induction. Antral follicles between 2 and 10 mm are counted in both the ovaries. A count <10 (normal 10–20) predicts poor response to gonadotropin stimulation.

Investigations of the Female Partner

(A) Diagnosis of ovulation (Table 17.4); (B) Diagnosis of tubal and peritoneal factors; (C) Diagnosis of uterine pathology; (D) Diagnosis of cervical pathology.

***Ovarian factors*:** Ovarian dysfunctions (dysovulatory) commonly associated with infertility are:

- Anovulation or oligo-ovulation (infrequent ovulation).
- Luteal phase defect (LPD).
- Luteinized unruptured follicle (LUF).

Diagnosis of Ovulation

The various methods used in practice to detect ovulation are grouped as follows (Table 17.4):

- **Indirect**
- **Direct**
- **Conclusive**

Indirect

The indirect or presumptive evidences of ovulation are commonly used in clinical practice. These are inferred from:

- Menstrual history
- Evaluation of peripheral or endorgan changes due to estrogen and progesterone
- Direct assays of gonadotropins or steroid hormones preceding, coinciding or succeeding the ovulatory process.

Menstrual history

The following features in relation to menstruation are strong evidences of ovulation.

- Regular normal menstrual loss between the age of 20–35.
- Midmenstrual bleeding (spotting) or pain or excessive mucoid vaginal discharge (Mittelschmerz syndrome).
- Features suggestive of premenstrual syndrome or primary dysmenorrhea.

Evaluation of peripheral or endorgan changes (Table 17.4)

Basal body temperature (BBT)

TABLE 17.4: Diagnosis of ovulation.

Indirect ▪ Menstrual history: Regular menstruation suggests ovulatory cycle. ▪ Evaluation of peripheral or endorgan changes • BBT: Biphasic pattern • Cervical mucus study: Disappearance of fern pattern • Vaginal cytology: Shift of MI to the left • Hormone estimation (Table 17.7) – Serum progesterone: Rise in level – Serum LH: Midcycle surge – Serum estradiol: Midcycle rise – Urine LH • Endometrial biopsy ▪ Sonography (TVS)
Direct Laparoscopy
Conclusive Pregnancy

Observation: There is "biphasic pattern" of temperature variation in ovulatory cycle. If pregnancy occurs, the rise of temperature sustains along with absence of the period. In anovulatory cycle, there is no rise of temperature throughout the cycle (monophasic).

Principle

The rise of temperature is secondary to rise in serum progesterone following ovulation. Progesterone is thermogenic. The primary reason for the rise is the increase in the production and secretion of norepinephrine which is also thermogenic.

Procedures: The patient is instructed to take her oral temperature **daily on waking up in the morning before rising out of the bed.** The temperature is recorded on a special chart.

Interpretation: The body temperature is raised to 0.5–1°F (0.2–0.5°C) following ovulation. The rise sustains throughout the second half of the cycle and is called "biphasic pattern" (Fig. 17.2). There may be a drop in the temperature to about 0.5°F before the rise and almost coincides with either LH surge or ovulation. The demonstrable rise actually occurs about 2 days after the LH peak and with a peripheral level of progesterone greater than 5 ng/mL. Optimally timed intercourse during the fertile period increases the chance of conception (20%). "Biphasic temperature" pattern suggests ovulation. Measurement of LH by urinary immunoassays is superior to BBT in determining the optimal time of intercourse or insemination (IUI).

Clinical importance: It helps the couple to determine the most fertile period, if the cycle is irregular.

Limitations of BBT

- BBT indicates ovulation retrospectively
- It cannot predict ovulation precisely with time
- Ovulation may occur over a span of several days in the thermogenic phase
- Rarely, ovulation has been observed though BBT is monophasic.

Cervical mucus study: Disappearance of fern after 22nd day of the cycle is suggestive of ovulation. Persistence of fern pattern even beyond 22nd day suggests anovulation. Progesterone causes dissolution of the sodium chloride crystals. Following ovulation, there is loss of stretchability (spinnbarkeit), which was present in the midcycle (p. 93).

Vaginal cytology: Maturation index shifts to the left from the midcycle to the mid second half of cycle due to the effect of progesterone (p. 92). Single smear on day 25 or 26 of the cycle reveals features of progesterone effect, if ovulation occurs.

Hormone estimation

- **Serum progesterone:** Estimation of serum progesterone is done on day 8 and 21 of a cycle (28 days). An increase in value from less than 1 ng/mL to greater than 6 ng/mL suggests ovulation.
- **Serum LH:** Daily estimation of serum LH at midcycle can detect the LH surge. Ovulation occurs about 34–36 hours after beginning of the LH surge. It coincides about 10–12 hours after the LH peak.
- **Serum estradiol** attains the peak rise approximately 24 hours prior to LH surge and about 24–36 hours prior to ovulation. The serum LH and estradiol estimation is used for in vitro fertilization.
- **Urinary LH:** LH kits are available to detect midcycle LH surge. **Ovulation usually occurs within 14–24 hours of detection of urine LH and almost always within 48 hours.** (The test should be done on a daily basis. It is started 2–3 days before the expected surge depending upon the cycle length).

Endometrial biopsy

Endometrial tissues to detect ovulation (endometrial sampling) can easily be obtained as an outpatient procedure using instruments such as Sharman curette or Pipelle endometrial sampler.

When to do? Biopsy is to be done on 21st–23rd day of the cycle. Barrier contraceptive should be prescribed during the cycle to prevent accidental conception.

Findings: Evidences of secretory activity of the endometrial glands in the second half of the cycle give not only the diagnosis of ovulation but can predict the functional integrity of the corpus luteum.

Subnuclear vacuolation is the earliest evidence appearing 36–48 hours following ovulation.

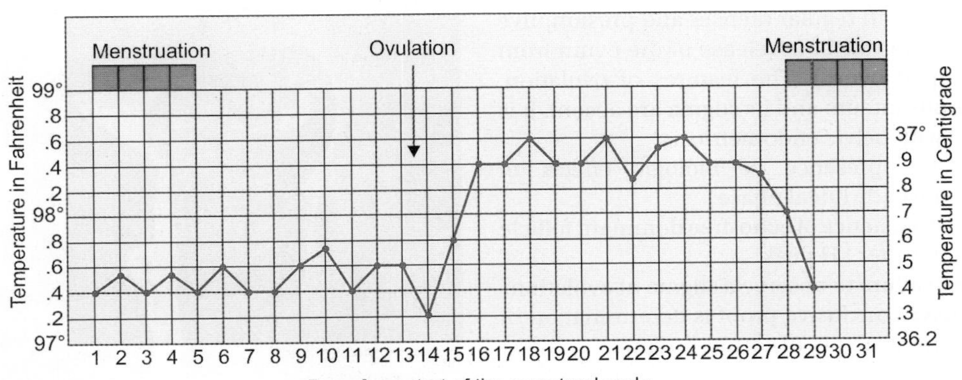

Fig. 17.2: Biphasic BBT chart.

Cause: The secretory changes are due to the action of progesterone on the estrogen primed endometrium. Endometrial biopsy is not done as a routine for detection of ovulation.

Hysteroscopy is useful to exclude intrauterine pathology (polyps, fibroid). It may be done as an OPD procedure.

Sonography

Serial **transvaginal sonography (TVS)** during midcycle can precisely measure the Graafian follicle just prior to ovulation (18–20 mm). It is particularly helpful for confirmation of ovulation following ovulation induction, artificial insemination, and in vitro fertilization. **The features of recent ovulation are:** Collapsed follicle and fluid in the pouch of Douglas. **TVS** can detect endometrial thickness. Trilaminar endometrium with a thickness >8 mm is favorable for implantation.

Direct

Laparoscopy

Laparoscopic visualization of recent corpus luteum or detection of the ovum from the aspirated peritoneal fluid from the pouch of Douglas is the only direct evidence of ovulation.

Conclusive

Pregnancy is the surest evidence of ovulation.

Luteal Phase Defect

Diagnosis of LPD is difficult. However, it is based on the following:

- BBT chart: (a) Slow rise of temperature taking 4–5 days following the fall in the midcycle; (b) Rise of temperature sustains less than 10 days.
- Endometrial biopsy—biopsy done on 25–27th day of the period reveals the endometrium at least 3 days out of phase (***Example***: If the biopsy is done on 25th day of cycle, the endometrial changes observed correspond to the day 22). This lag phase endometrium must be proved in two consecutive cycles. However, it is not conclusive.
- Serum progesterone estimated on 8th day following ovulation is less than 10 ng/mL.

Luteinized Unruptured Follicle

Luteinized unruptured follicle (LUF) syndrome refers to an infertile woman with regular menses and presumptive evidences of ovulation without release of the ovum from the follicle (trapped ovum). The features of ovulation, formation of corpus luteum and its stigma are absent. It is often associated with pelvic endometriosis.

Diagnosis: In the presence of biologic effects of progesterone in the early luteal phase:

- **Sonography:** Persistence of echo-free dominant follicle beyond 36 hours after LH peak.
- **Laparoscopy:** Failure to observe a stigma of ovulation.
- **Ovarian biopsy:** Conclusive proof is determination of ovum amidst the structure of corpus luteum.

Tubal Factors (Table 17.5)

The anatomical patency and functional integrity of the tubes are assessed by the following tests:

TABLE 17.5: Tests to assess tubal patency.

- Dilatation and insufflation test (DI)
- Hysterosalpingography (HSG)
- Saline infusion sonography
- Hysterosalpingo contrast sonography (HyCoSy)
- Sonohysterosalpingography
- Laparoscopy and chromopertubation
- Falloposcopy
- Salpingoscopy

Insufflation Test (Rubin's Test)

Principle: The underlying principle is that the cervical canal is in continuity with the peritoneal cavity through the tubes. As such, entry of air or CO_2 into the peritoneal cavity when pushed transcervically under pressure, suggests of tubal patency (it is not commonly done these days).

When to be done? It should be done in the postmenstrual phase at D7 to D10 of this cycle.

Limitation: It should not be done in the presence of pelvic infection.

Observations: The patency of the tube is confirmed by: (1) Fall in the pressure when raised beyond 120 mm Hg; (2) Hissing sound heard on auscultation on either iliac fossa and (3) Shoulder pain experienced by the patient (irritation of the diaphragm by the air).

Drawbacks: In about one-third of cases, it gives false-negative findings due to cornual spasm. It also cannot identify the side and site of the block in the tube. As such, it is inferior to other methods of tubal study. This test is not commonly done these days.

Hysterosalpingography (HSG) (Fig. 17.3) (*see* detail p. 494)

Principle: The principle is the same like that of insufflation test. Instead of air or CO_2, dye is instilled transcervically.

When to be done?: D7–D10 of the cycle.

Limitation: As in D&I.

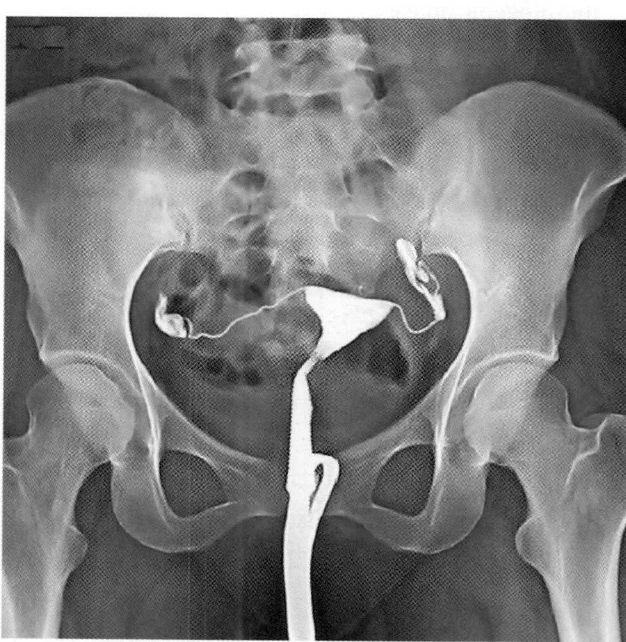

Fig. 17.3: Hysterosalpingogram showing bilateral peritoneal spillage.

Advantages: It has got distinct advantages over insufflation test. It can precisely detect the side and site of block in the tube. It can reveal any abnormality in the uterus (congenital or acquired like synechiae, fibroid). As such, insufflation of the tubes has largely been replaced by HSG (Fig. 17.3).

Disadvantages: It involves radiation risk amongst others.

Laparoscopy and Chromopertubation (Fig. 17.4)

Laparoscopy is the gold standard (definitive method) for evaluation of tubal factors of infertility. The indications of its use are mentioned in Table 17.6.

Drawbacks: Laparoscopy is more invasive than hysterosalpingography (HSG). It cannot detect abnormality in the uterine cavity or tubal lumen. **Thus, the two procedures (HSG and laparoscopy) should be regarded as complementary to each other and not a substitute to the other procedure.**

When to be done? It is commonly done in the proliferative phase.

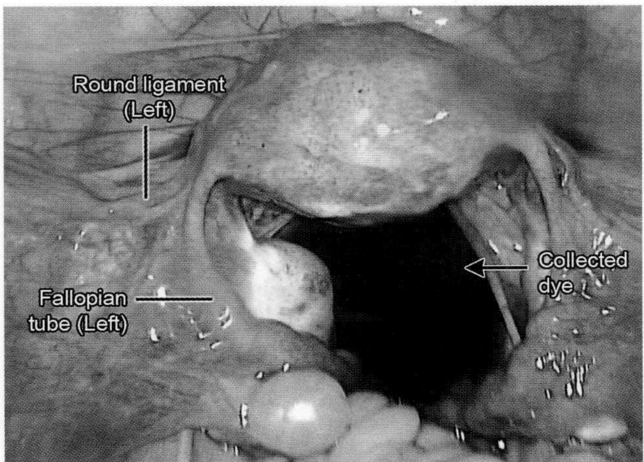

Fig. 17.4: Laparoscopic chromopertubation shows the patency of the tubes with spillage of dye (methylene blue) in the peritoneal cavity and the POD. Dye spillage from both the tubes is seen.
(*Courtesy*: Dr Manoj Samanta)

TABLE 17.6: Indications of laparoscopy in infertility.

Diagnostic	▪ Age >35 years ▪ History of pelvic pain, dyspareunia, pelvic surgery, adhesions ▪ Abnormal HSG ▪ Failure to conceive after reasonable period (6 months) with normal HSG ▪ Women with comorbid pelvic pathology (PID, endometriosis)
Operative (therapeutic)	▪ Unexplained infertility ▪ Reconstructive tubal surgery ▪ Adhesiolysis (Table 17.10) ▪ Fulguration of endometriotic implants ▪ Ovarian drilling in PCOS ▪ GIFT and ZIFT procedures

BENEFITS OF LAPAROSCOPIC EVALUATION

- **Tubes:** For detection of tubal patency, block (site and side), motility, hydrosalpinx change, peritubal adhesions, fimbrial agglutination.
- **Ovaries:** PCOS changes, endometriosis, PID, adhesions
- **Uterus:** Anomalies, fibroids.
- **Peritoneal factors:** Adhesions, PID, endometriosis, tuberculosis.
- **Therapy** at the same sitting (as appropriate).

Sonohysterosalpingography

Principle: Normal saline is pushed within the uterine cavity with a pediatric, Foley catheter. The catheter balloon is inflated at the level of the cervix to prevent fluid leak. Ultrasonography of the uterus and fallopian tubes are done. Ultrasound can follow the fluid through the tubes up to the peritoneal cavity and in the pouch of Douglas.

Advantages: It is a noninvasive procedure. It can detect uterine malformations, synechiae, or polyps (superior to HSG). Tubal pathology could be detected as that of HSG. There is no radiation exposure.

Falloposcopy

It is to study the entire length of tubal lumen with the help of a fine and flexible fiberoptic device. It is performed through the uterine cavity, using a hysteroscope. It helps direct visualization of tubal ostia, mucosal pattern, intratubal polyps, or debris.

Salpingoscopy

Tubal lumen is studied introducing a rigid endoscope through the fimbrial end of the tube. It is performed through the operating channel of a laparoscope.

Uterine factor: Uterine factors commonly associated with subfertility are submucous fibroids, congenital malformations (Ch. 4), and intrauterine adhesions (Asherman's syndrome). They are more likely to cause recurrent pregnancy loss rather than primary infertility.

Ultrasonography, HSG, hysteroscopy, and laparoscopy are needed in the evaluation of uterine factor for subfertility.

Hysteroscopy (p. 520)

It is the gold standard for visualizing the uterine cavity and the tubal ostia. Besides diagnosis, **therapeutic benefits of hysteroscopy are:** (a) Polypectomy for endometrial polyp; (b) Submucous resection of myoma; (c) Hysteroscopic adhesiolysis; and (d) Resection of uterine septum.

Cervical factor (Table 17.7): The cervix functions as a biological valve. This is because in the proliferative phase, it permits the entry of sperm and in the secretory phase, hinders their penetration. As such, dysfunction at this level should be carefully evaluated.

Postcoital test (PCT) (Sims-Huhner test)

Principle: PCT is to assess the quality of cervical mucus and the ability of sperm to survive in it. PCT is rarely done these days. Sperm cervical mucus contact test (SCMCT) not done presently.

Endocrinopathy: In-depth investigations in suspected or overt endocrinopathy with or without menstrual

TABLE 17.7: Infertility work-up calendar.

<table>
<tr><th>Identification of factor</th><th>Methods employed</th><th>Day of cycle</th><th colspan="2">Observation</th></tr>
<tr><td rowspan="7">Ovulation</td><td>■ BBT
■ Cervical mucus
• Nature
• Threadability
• Fern pattern</td><td>Throughout cycle
D 12–14 and D 21–23</td><td>Biphasic pattern
D 12–14
Clear, watery
+
+</td><td>
D 21–23
Thick, viscid
–
–</td></tr>
<tr><td>■ Endometrial biopsy
■ Vaginal cytology</td><td>D 21–23
D 12–14 and D 21–23</td><td>Secretory endometrium
D 12–14
Discrete cells
Pyknotic nuclei
background clear</td><td>
D 21–23
Folded edges, in clumps;
background dirty</td></tr>
<tr><td>■ Serum progesterone</td><td>D 8 and D 21</td><td>D 8 <1 ng/mL</td><td>D 21 >6 ng/mL</td></tr>
<tr><td>■ Serum LH</td><td>Midcycle daily (D 12–14)</td><td colspan="2">Ovulation: About 10–12 hours after LH surge</td></tr>
<tr><td>■ Urinary LH</td><td></td><td colspan="2"></td></tr>
<tr><td>■ Serial transvaginal sonography (TVS)</td><td>D 12–14</td><td colspan="2">Follicular measurements—approaching 20 mm</td></tr>
<tr><td>■ Laparoscopy</td><td>Secretory phase</td><td colspan="2">Recent corpus luteum, fluid in pouch of Douglas</td></tr>
<tr><td rowspan="5">Tubal factor</td><td>■ Insufflation test</td><td>Proliferative phase—2 days after the bleeding stops</td><td colspan="2">■ Drop in pressure when raised to 120 mm Hg
■ Hissing sound on iliac fossa
■ Shoulder pain</td></tr>
<tr><td>■ Hysterosalpingography</td><td>As above</td><td colspan="2">Spillage of dye into the peritoneal cavity</td></tr>
<tr><td>■ Laparoscopy and dye test</td><td>Proliferative phase (7th–10th day of cycle) Royal College of Obstetricians and Gynecologists</td><td colspan="2">■ Peritubal pathology
■ Pelvic pathology (endometriosis)
■ Ovulation
■ Tubal patency by dye spillage from both the tubes</td></tr>
<tr><td>■ Sonohysterosalpingography
■ Hysterosalpingo-contrast sonography (HyCoSy)</td><td>Proliferative phase</td><td colspan="2">Better than HSG for detection of intrauterine pathology</td></tr>
<tr><td>■ Falloposcopy</td><td>Proliferative phase</td><td colspan="2">Tubal luminal pathology</td></tr>
<tr><td rowspan="2">Cervical</td><td>■ Postcoital test (PCT)</td><td>Around ovulation (D 12–14)</td><td colspan="2">Presence of progressive motile sperm (10 per high power field)</td></tr>
<tr><td>■ Sperm cervical mucus contact test (SCMCT)</td><td>As above</td><td colspan="2">Sperm antibodies</td></tr>
</table>

abnormality or ovarian dysfunction include estimation of serum TSH, prolactin, FSH, LH, dehydroepiandrosterone sulfate, testosterone, and progesterone in mid luteal phase. In cases with family history of diabetes, postprandial blood sugar is to be estimated.

Immunological factor: Human sperm has immunologic potential. The antibodies against sperm affect fertility by immobilizing sperm or causing sperm agglutination.

Most common variety of antisperm antibodies are IgG, IgM, and IgA isotypes. IgG may be found in cervical mucus, serum, and semen. Agglutinating antibodies of IgA class are found in cervical mucus and seminal plasma. The IgM (larger) molecules are found exclusively in the serum. **These immunoglobulins can bind to different parts of the sperm (e.g. head, body, or tail) and make them immobile.**

Detection of antisperm antibody has not been found to be helpful in the management of infertility. Treatment of antisperm antibodies has not improved the pregnancy outcome. Such cases are treated with IUI, IVF, or ICSI.

Unexplained infertility is defined when no obvious cause for infertility has been detected following all standard investigations. These include semen analysis, ovulation detection, tubal and peritoneal factors, endocrinopathy, and PCT. Overall incidence is 10–20%. With expectant management about 60% of couples with unexplained infertility will conceive within a period of 3 years. IVF and ET may be an option for those who fail to respond.

TREATMENT OF INFERTILITY

Couple Counseling

Assurance: The infertile couple remains psychologically disturbed right from the beginning, more so as the investigation progresses. The couple in such cases should be tactfully handled to minimize psychologic upset.

Body weight: Overweight or underweight of any partner should be adequately dealt with to obtain an optimum weight. Body mass index of 20–24 is optimum.

Smoking and alcohol: Excess smoking or alcohol consumption is to be avoided.

Coital problems: The coital problems should be carefully evaluated by intelligent interrogation. Advice to have intercourse during the midcycle too often gives good result even prior to investigation. Using LH test kit, one can detect LH surge in urine by getting a deep blue color of dipstick. The test should be performed daily between day 12 and day 16 of a regular cycle. Intercourse should occur for 2 days around the LH surge. Normal sperm retain the fertilizing ability for up to 72 hours. Ovum disintegrates less than 1 day when it reaches the ampulla of the tube.

Management is directed to the problems of:

- **Male**
- **Female**
- **Combined**

Male Infertility

The treatment of male is indicated in: (a) Extreme oligospermia; (b) Azoospermia; (c) Low volume ejaculate; and (d) Impotency. Management is often difficult and unsatisfactory.

To improve spermatogenesis the following measures may be helpful.

- **General care:** Improvement of general health support.
- Medications that interfere spermatogenesis (p. 189) should be avoided.
- In **hypogonadotropic-hypogonadism**, the disorders of spermatogenesis can be treated with the following therapy with varying success.
  - hCG 5000 IU intramuscularly once or twice a week is given to stimulate endogenous testosterone production.
  - hMG or pure FSH (75–150 IU) is added to hCG when there is no sperm in the ejaculate with hCG alone.
  - Dopamine agonist (cabergoline) is given in hyperprolactinemia to restore normal prolactin and testosterone level. This improves libido, potency and fertility.
- Pulsatile GnRH therapy in infertile male with GnRH deficiency (Kallmann's syndrome) is effective. It is administered by minipump infusion.
- **Hypergonadotropic-hypogonadism,** Men with raised FSH may have adequate sperm on biopsy for use in IVF or ICSI (p. 209). Otherwise treatment options available are insemination with donor sperm or adoption when no sperm is available. IVF with ICSI may be done in cases with severe oligospermia.
- Hypergonadotropic hypogonadism indicates testicular failure. Normal spermatogenesis requires high levels of testosterone within the testis. This cannot be achieved with exogenous testosterone. Replacement may help to improve libido, sexual function, maintenance of muscle mass, bone density and a general sense of well being.
- **Presence of antisperm antibodies** in the male and its significance is unclear. Currently intrauterine insemination (IUI) is the choice of treatment for such cases (p. 205).
- **Leukocytospermia:** Genital tract infection needs prolonged course of antibiotics. Generally doxycycline or erythromycin is given for a period of 4–6 weeks, depending on the response.
- **Retrograde ejaculation:** Phenylephrine (α-adrenergic agonist) is used to improve the tone of internal urethral sphincter. Sperm may be recovered from the neutralized urine. Processed spermatozoa could be used for IUI.
- **Teratospermia, asthenospermia:** Specific causes are unknown. Karyotyping and genetic testing are indicated. Generally no treatment is available. Donor insemination (AID) is the option (p. 209).
- **Genetic abnormality:** Artificial insemination with donor sperm (AID) is the option as no other treatment is available.
- **Surgical:**
  - When the patient is found to be azoospermic and yet testicular biopsy shows normal spermatogenesis, obstruction of vas must be suspected. This should be corrected by microsurgery—vasoepididymostomy or vasovasostomy. TESE/PESA and IVF or ICSI is the alternative.
  - Surgery for varicocele for improvement of fertility is not helpful. Hydrocele is corrected by surgery.
  - Orchidopexy in undescended testes should be done between 2–3 years of age to have adequate spermatogenesis in later life.
- **Impotency:** Psychosexual treatment may be of help. Hyperprolactinemia needs further investigation and treatment. For erectile dysfunction sildenafil (25–100 mg) or tadalafil (10–20 mg) is currently advised. A single dose (depending on response) is given orally one hour before sexual activity. In unresponsive cases, artificial insemination is to be thought of use.

Assisted Reproductive Technology for Male Infertility (p. 206)

Prospect of male infertility has improved significantly with the advent of ART. IUI, TESE, PESA, MESA and intracytoplasmic sperm injection (ICSI) are now the treatment preferred for infertile males.

Female Infertility

For convenience, the treatment modalities (Flowchart 17.2) in female infertility are grouped as follows according to the disorders identified:

- Ovulatory
- Tubal
- Associated disorders like endometriosis, infections or endocrinopathy
- Cervical
- Immunological
- Unexplained infertility
- Uterovaginal canal abnormality
- Assisted reproductive technology (ART).

Flowchart 17.2: Management options for female infertility.

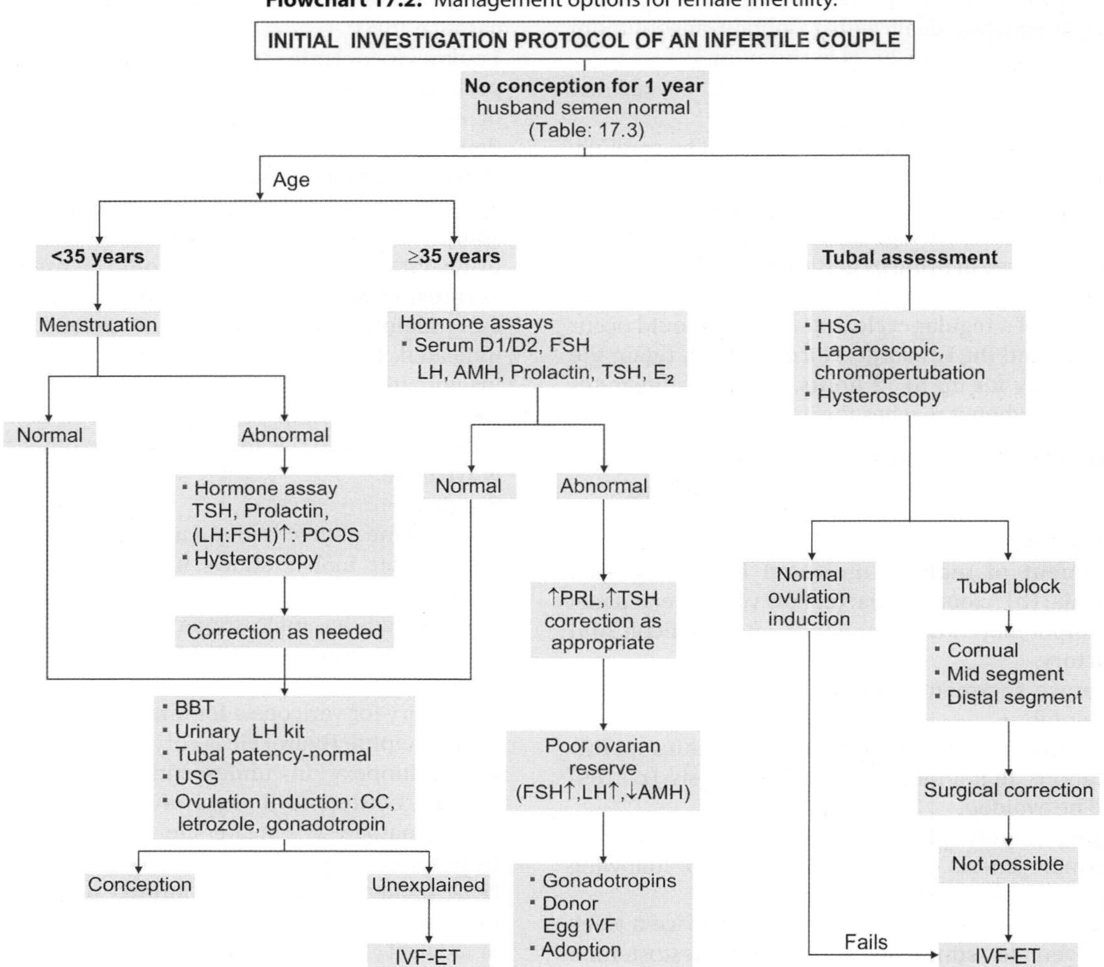

Ovulatory Dysfunction

- **Anovulation**
- **LPD**
- **LUF**

Anovulation

Anovulation is a common factor for female infertility. It may be present in otherwise normal menstrual cycle or may be associated with oligomenorrhea or amenorrhea.

Induction of ovulation—Measures are:

- **General**
- **Drugs**
- **Surgery**

- **General:** Reduction of weight for obesity as in PCOS cases is essential to have a good response of drug therapy for induction.
- **Drugs:** The following drugs are of use either singly or in combination (Table 17.8).

Monitoring during ovulation induction (Table 17.9): For diagnosis of ovulation, BBT estimation serum progesterone level on D21 of the cycle is done.

Monitoring with BBT chart and cervical mucus study are noninvasive, simple and quite informative. Other parameters used are serial estimation of plasma E_2 and ultrasonic measurement of growing follicles (folliculometry). These last two are obligatory in ART.

TABLE 17.8: Drugs used in induction of ovulation.

Stimulation of ovulation ▪ Clomiphene citrate (CC) ▪ Letrozole ▪ hMG (FSH 75 IU + LH 75 IU) ▪ FSH • Purified urinary FSH (uFSH) • Highly purified urinary FSH (HP) • Recombinant FSH (rFSH)—given SC • Recombinant LH (or rLH)—given SC • hCG } to trigger ovulation • Recombinant hCG } to trigger ovulation ▪ GnRH ▪ GnRH analogs
Correction of biochemical abnormality ▪ Hyperinsulinemia (insulin resistance): Metformin (insulin sensitizer) ▪ Androgen excess: Dexamethasone ▪ Prolactin raised: Dopamine agonist
Substitution therapy ▪ Hypothyroidism—thyroxin ▪ Diabetes mellitus—antidiabetic drugs ▪ Congenital adrenal hyperplasia—corticosteroid

TABLE 17.9: Objectives of monitoring for induction of Ovulation.

- To select time for preovulatory administration of hCG
- To prevent ovarian hyperstimulation syndrome
- To select time for intercourse or artificial insemination
- To select time for ovum retrieval in IVF

Clomiphene Citrate: Patient Selection

- Normogonadotropic—normoprolactinemic patients who are having normal cycles with absent or infrequent ovulation.
- PCOS cases with oligomenorrhea or amenorrhea. The estradiol level should be >40 pg/mL.
- Hypothalamic amenorrhea following stress or 'pill' use.

Dose: Clomiphene therapy is simple, safe and at the same time cost-effective. Most centers use an initial dose of 50 mg daily. Dose is increased in 50 mg steps to a maximum 250 mg daily, if ovulation is not induced by the lower dose. The actual starting day of its administration in the follicular phase varies between day 2 and day 5 and therapy is given for 5 days. Ovulation is expected to occur about 5–7 days after the last day of therapy. Therapy for six cycle is generally given.

Mechanism of action: Clomiphene citrate is anti-estrogenic as well as weakly estrogenic. It blocks the estrogen receptors in the hypothalamus. This results in increased GnRH pulse amplitude causing increased gonadotropin (LH and FSH) secretion from the pituitary. Antiestrogenic effects are seen on the endometrium and on the cervical mucus.

Side effects: Hot flashes, nausea, vomiting, headache, visual symptoms and ovarian hyperstimulation (rare). Incidence of abortion and congenital fetal malformations are not increased.

Couple instruction: The couple is advised to have sexual intercourse as per following guidelines:

- Daily or on alternate days beginning 5–7 days after the last dose of clomiphene therapy.
- Several times for 24–48 hours after the color change in urine when tested by LH kit.
- Number of times over 24–36 hours following hCG administration.

Result: Successful induction rate is as high as 80% but cumulative pregnancy rate is about 70% over 6–9 cycles. **The discrepancy is due to** premature luteinization, luteal phase defect PD, cervical mucus hostility and other nonovulatory factors. The incidence of multiple pregnancy is about 7%. **Maximum of 6 cycles may be given.**

Letrozole is an aromatase inhibitor. It is used as a primary drug for ovulation induction.

Mechanism of action: Inhibition of ovarian E_2 production. There is negative feedback on the hypothalamic pituitary axis. Serum FSH levels are increased. Intraovarian androgen levels are increased. These enhances the sensitivity of the ovarian follicles to FSH.

Dose: 2.5 mg or 5 mg daily is given for 5 days between D3 and D7 of the cycle. Antiestrogenic effects of clomiphene on the cervical mucus and the endometrium are not seen with letrozole.

Pregnancy rates are either same or superior when compared to clomiphene citrate.

Side effects: Fetal congenital malformations and multiple pregnancy rates are same to clomiphene citrate.

Letrozole has been used with gonadotropins for controlled ovarian stimulation (COS). This regimen reduces the dose of gonadotropins (p. 440).

- **Adjuvant therapy:** Some adjuvant therapy is often needed.
- **Hyperinsulinemia and insulin sensitizer:** Patients with polycystic ovarian disease with BMI >25 (Ch. 29) are often found insulin resistant. Obese women with PCOS often suffer from impaired glucose tolerance (33%) or type 2 diabetes (10%). Correction of their metabolic abnormality along with weight reduction gives satisfactory result. **Treatment with metformin (insulin sensitizer) is found to reduce hyperinsulinemia and hyperandrogenemia.** Combination treatment with metformin and clomiphene increases ovulation rate significantly. Side effects include GI intolerance, rarely lactic acidosis.
- Pre-existing or induced **elevated androgens** may be suppressed by dexamethasone 0.5 mg daily for 10 days, starting from 1st day of cycle. The drug should be stopped soon after ovulation.
- Eltroxin 0.1 mg may be administered daily during the therapy in obese patients with **subclinical hypothyroidism.**
- **Elevated prolactin level** with or without galactorrhea indicates abnormal GnRH pulse secretion. This causes ovulatory dysfunction, LPD or amenorrhea. **Bromocriptine or cabergoline (dopamine agonist)** therapy increases the ovarian responsiveness to clomiphene. Patients with normal or minimally elevated prolactin when treated with bromocriptine and clomiphene are found to have increased pregnancy.

  Results: Dopamine agonist treatment normalizes prolactin level (80%), restores cyclic menses (80%) and ovulation in majority (70%) of women.

  Side effects: Nausea, dizziness, vomiting and orthostatic hypotension are common. Side effects of cabergoline are less, especially when it is used by the vaginal route.
- **hCG:** In cases of anovulation due to failure of LH surge, hCG 5000 IU is administered usually 7 days after the last dose of clomiphene therapy. Prior monitoring of serum estradiol level and ultrasonic measurement of follicular diameter (18–20 mm) is preferred to get a good result.
- **Growth hormone:** Is combined to the poor responders especially, in the elderly group as it mediates its action via IGF-I.
- Because of the antiestrogenic effect of clomiphene citrate, the cervical mucus becomes thick and viscid and it hinders sperm penetration. Conjugated estrogen 1.25 mg given daily for 10 days starting on first day of cycle may be helpful.

Gonadotropins

Prerequisites for gonadotropin therapy.

- **Ovarian reserve** must be present (p. 442).
- Other (non-ovulatory) factors for infertility must be ruled out.
- Parameters for poor ovarian reserve are
  - Age >36 years
  - Serum FSH on D1/D2 of the cycle ≥10 IU/L
  - Serum AMH <0.5 ng/mL
  - Antral follicular count on TVS: <10
  - Others (Ch. 22)

Indications of gonadotropin use

- Hypogonadotropic hypogonadism (WHO Group I).
- Clomiphene or letrozole failed or resistant cases (WHO Group II).
- Unexplained infertility.
- Sub-fertile women who are elderly.

Dose schedule

- hMG stimulates follicular growth with a variable dose schedule starting with a low dose (75 IU 1M/day). Human menopausal gonadotropin (hMG) is a mixture of FSH and LH.
- Stimulation is started any time from D2 to D5 of the cycle and is continued for 7–10 days depending on the response.
- Follicular growth is monitored with serum estradiol estimation and follicular number and size are measured by transvaginal sonography (TVS).
- Serum estradiol level of 500–1500 pg/mL (150–300 pg/mature follicle) and maximum follicular diameter of 18–20 mm are optimum. Endometrial thickness (TVS) ≥ 8–9 mm (trilaminar) is taken as optimum.
- When these optimum levels are obtained, 5000–10000 IU of hCG is administered IM to induce ovulation.
- Endometrial thickness of 8–10 mm (as measured by TVS) on the day of hCG administration favors successful implantation.
- Ovulation is expected to occur, approximately 36 hours after the hCG administration.

Gonadotropin regimens may be "step up" or "step down" depending upon the response of the woman to exogenous gonadotropin.

Couple instruction: Couple is advised for the timing of intercourse or insemination (ART) accordingly (*see* above).

Patients with PCOS are more sensitive to hMG stimulation. Purified FSH or highly purified FSH or recombinant FSH (Gonal-F, Recagon) have been used successfully with minimal side effects.

In cases of hypergonadotropic hypogonadism, high gonadotropin levels are lowered with the use of combined estrogen and progestogen preparations (oral pill). Use of long-acting GnRH agonist also suppresses high endogenous gonadotropin levels. When the levels reach normal, gonadotropin therapy may be employed to achieve ovulation. The success rate is poor.

Side effects of gonadotropin therapy (p. 440)

Contraindications of gonadotropin therapy

- Primary ovarian failure with raised serum FSH
- Uncontrolled thyroid and adrenal dysfunction
- Sex hormone dependent tumor in the body
- Pituitary tumor
- Ovarian cysts.

Results: Pregnancy rate after six courses of treatment is 90%. Incidence of multiple pregnancy (10–30%), overall incidence of miscarriage (20–25%) and ectopic pregnancy are high. Risks of congenital anomalies are not increased.

GnRH

Exogenous GnRH: Pulsatile GnRH treatment stimulates physiologic levels of pituitary gonadotropin secretion. So development of follicular growth, selection, recruitment and ovulation occurs as in normal menstrual cycle.

Patient selection: Ovulatory dysfunction is due to:

- Hypothalamic amenorrhea
- Hypogonadotropic hypogonadism
- Women with hyperprolactinemia.

GnRH is administered intravenously or subcutaneously with an infusion pump in a pulsatile fashion.

A pulse of 5 μg is used IV at every 90 minutes. Follicular growth is similar to a normal menstrual cycle. Follicular growth monitoring, hCG administration and couple instructions are same as in hMG therapy.

Results: Pregnancy rate is 80% following six courses of treatment. Multiple pregnancy rate is 5%. Overall risk of miscarriage is 30%. The risk of ovarian hyperstimulation is low (p. 444).

GnRH Analogs (p. 441)

Patient selection

- Patients refractory to gonadotropins
- Patients having elevated LH
- Patients with normal gonadotropins.
- Patients with premature follicular luteinization or premature ovulation due to premature LH surge.

GnRH agonist (buserelin, nafarelin) is given subcutaneously or intranasally either maintaining a short or long protocol. GnRH agonist is used for downregulation of pituitary gland by desensitization of pituitary GnRH receptors (p. 56). GnRH agonist initially produce stimulation of gonadotropin secretion known as 'flare' effect. Generally, this flare effect lasts for about 2–3 weeks. Adequate pituitary suppression is achieved when serum estradiol level is less than 10 pg/mL and FSH level is less than 10 mIU/mL. Follicular stimulation is achieved with highly purified or recombinant FSH. Follicular number and growth monitoring is similar as in hMG therapy. hCG is also administered when criteria is fulfilled as discussed with hMG therapy.

Results—ovulation rate is about 75% and pregnancy rate is about 25%.

GnRH antagonists—can block pituitary GnRH receptors completely without any initial stimulation (flare effect). Cetrorelix is currently being tried to prevent premature LH surge.

As with GnRH analogue, gonadotropin stimulation is done (*see* above).

When pregnancy occurs following superovulation with GnRH agonist therapy, **luteal phase support should be maintained** by giving hCG and/or progesterone.

It should be emphasized that the gonadotropins, GnRH and GnRH analogs are costly drugs. **Their uses have to be monitored carefully with sophisticated gadgets** not only to control the regimen but also to minimize the hazards (Table 17.8). Thus, its use is restricted in selected centers and is commonly used in ART.

Luteal phase defect (LPD)

Treatment: The following treatment may be of help in the idiopathic groups:

- Natural progesterone as vaginal suppositories 100 mg thrice daily starting from the day of ovulation is effective. It should be continued until mens begins. If mens fails to appear after 14 days, pregnancy test is to be done. If the test is positive, it should be continued up to 10th week of pregnancy.
- hCG is a potent luteotropic hormone, however, the response of LPD to hCG is unpredictable.
- In unresponsive cases, clomiphene citrate may be tried. It increases FSH which may improve folliculogenesis and normal corpus luteum formation with adequate production of progesterone. In refractory cases, IVF may be tried.

Luteinized unruptured follicle (LUF)

Defective folliculogenesis or inadequate LH surge may be corrected with:

- Optimally timed intramuscular injection of hCG 5000–10,000 IU.
- Administration of ovulation inducing drugs in the follicular phase followed by ovulatory hCG (5000–10000 IU).
- Bromocriptine therapy, if associated with hyperprolactinemia (p. 391).

Surgery

- **Laparoscopic ovarian drilling (LOD) or laser vaporization:** This is done by multiple puncture (4–6 sites) of the cysts in polycystic ovarian syndrome by diathermy or laser. It reduces systemic and intraovarian androgen levels. This procedure is helpful in clomiphene resistant, hyperandrogenic anovulatory women. The woman ovulates spontaneously following LOD.
  - **Benefits:** Risks of OHSS and multiple pregnancy are reduced
  - **Disadvantage:** Excessive destruction of ovarian cortex may cause premature ovarian failure
  - **Complications of LOD:** Adhesion formation, premature ovarian failure (POF)
- **Wedge resection:** This is not done these days. Bilateral wedge resection of the ovaries is done in PCOS as cases where clomiphene citrate fails to induce ovulation. It produces adhesions.
- **Surgery** for pituitary prolactinomas
- **Surgical removal** of virilizing or other functioning ovarian or adrenal tumor
- **Uterovaginal surgery**
- **Bariatric surgery**.

Tubal and Peritoneal Factors

Tubal factors for infertility are corrected only by surgery. The different surgical methods are:

- **Peritubal adhesions:** Correction is done by salpingo-ovariolysis either by laparoscopy (preferred) or by laparotomy.
- **Proximal tubal block:** Salpingography under fluoroscopy may be helpful to remove any block due to mucus plugging. Otherwise proximal tubal cannulation with a guide wire under hysteroscopic guidance is done. In about 85% cases, tubal patency can be restored and over all pregnancy rate of about 45–60% is reported. **Cannulation and balloon tuboplasty can avoid the need of ART which is expensive.**
- **Distal tubal block:** (a) *Fimbrioplasty/fimbriolysis*—release of fimbrial adhesions and/or dilatation of fimbrial phimosis; (b) *Neosalpingostomy*—to create a new tubal opening in an occluded tube.
- **Mid tubal block:** *Reversal of tubal ligation*— pregnancy rates after this procedure varies between 50–82%. Success rate depends on—(a) Age; (b) The method of sterilization (Pomeroy's, Falope rings, diathermy, etc.); (c) Site of anastomosis (isthmic-isthmic or isthmic-cornual); (d) Final length of reconstructed tube (>4 cm optimal). Risk of ectopic pregnancy following tubal reanastomosis is 3–7%.

Considerations for tubal surgery

- **Tubal surgery** may be considered in **young women** after previous tubal sterilization or in women with mild disease at the distal tubal segment.
- Tubal surgery may be tried for mild proximal tubal block.
- **Preoperative assessment** and planning for surgery has to be done by HSG and or laparoscopy and if possible, by falloposcopy to assess the tubal mucosa.
- Prior counseling of the couple about the hazards of surgery and prospect of future pregnancy should be done.
- In tubercular salpingitis, surgery is to be withheld. Following antitubercular therapy, IVF-ET may be employed, when the endometrium becomes free from the disease.
- ***Large hydrosalpinx causing distal tubal disease should be treated by salpingectomy and IVF.***
- IVF is considered as the best treatment option for any complicated tubal occlusive disease.
- Salpingectomy should be done before IVF when hydrosalpinges are present.

Methods of tubal surgery

Tuboplasty is the name given to the finer surgery on the tubes to restore the anatomy and physiology as far as practicable (Table 17.10).

TABLE 17.10: Tuboplasty operation.

Adhesiolysis (Salpingo-ovariolysis)	Separation or division of adhesions
Fimbrioplasty	Separation of the fimbrial adhesions to open up the abdominal ostium (Fig. 17.5)
Salpingostomy	That creates a new opening in a completely occluded tube. It is called **terminal or 'cuff'** at the abdominal ostium. The eversion of the neo-ostium is maintained by few stitches of 6-0 Vicryl
Tubotubal anastomosis	When the segment of the diseased tube following tubectomy operation is resected and end to end anastomosis is done (Fig. 17.6)
Tubocornual anastomosis	When there is cornual block, the remaining healthy tube is anastomosed to the patient's interstitial part of the tube

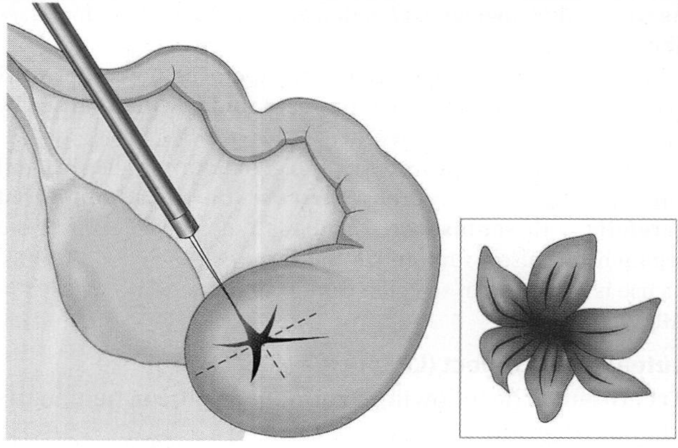

Fig. 17.5: Fimbrioplasty is done laparoscopically to release the agglutinated fimbriae (fimbrial phimosis). Inset: Flaps are created at the end of the procedure. Bleeding vessels are desiccated electrosurgically.

The **operation** can be done by conventional methods, or by microsurgical techniques which may be employed following laparotomy or by laparoscopy.

Microsurgical techniques give better result due to minimal tissue handling and damage, perfect hemostasis and minimal adhesion formation. **Laparoscopic surgery gives the best result.**

Nylon may be used as a temporary splint to facilitate suturing the ends. It should be removed following anastomosis.

Intraoperative instillation of Ringer's lactate mixed with heparin or hydrocortisone may be employed to minimize adhesion formation.

Adjuvant therapy

Adjunctive procedures to improve the result of tubal surgery include prophylactic antibiotics, use of adhesion prevention devices (interceed, seprafilm) and postoperative hydrotubation.

Hydrotubation: Hydrotubation is a procedure to flush the tubal lumen by medicated fluids passed transcervically through a cannula. The fluid contains antibiotic and hydrocortisone (Gentamicin 80 mg and dexamethasone 4 mg in 10 mL distilled water). It should be done in postmenstrual phase.

Results of tuboplasty: The result depends upon the nature of pathology, type of surgery and techniques employed—macro or microsurgery. **Overall pregnancy rate (following laparoscopic surgery) is as follows:** Salpingo-ovariolysis 65%; Fimbrioplasty 32%; Tubotubal anastomosis 75%; Tubocornual anastomosis 55%. The result is better in microsurgical techniques when done laparoscopically. **The result is best in reversal tubal sterilization by tubotubal anastomosis using microsurgical techniques (Fig. 17.6).**

Factors for Poor Outcome Following Tuboplasty

- Dense pelvic adhesions
- Loss of fimbriae

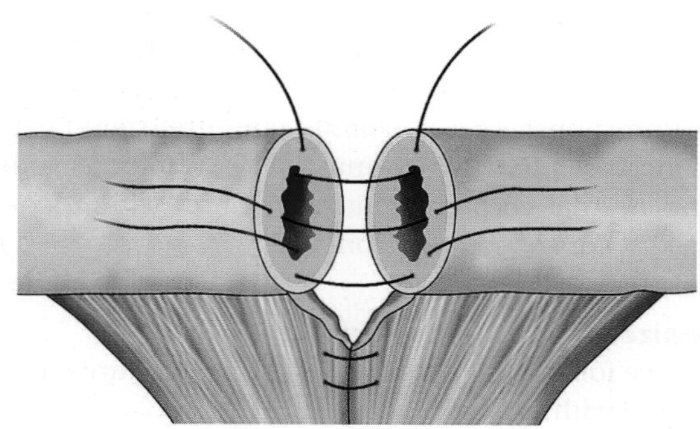

Fig. 17.6: Tubotubal anastomosis. Placement of four to five interrupted sutures using 8–0 polyglactin (under 10 × magnification).

- Bilateral hydrosalpinx >3 cm
- Length of the reconstructed tube <4 cm
- Reversal done after 5 years of sterilization operation
- Presence of other factors for infertility.

Endometriosis

Minimal asymptomatic pelvic endometriosis may be an incidental finding and intensive medical or surgical therapy does not improve the fertility status. Fertility improving surgery is done to control pain and where endometriomas are large. Smaller endometriomas (<4 cm) are managed conservatively. Ovarian cystectomy reduces ovarian reserve. COS with IUI is the preferred treatment. If there is no pregnancy following three to six cycles of therapy, IVF is the next step of treatment.

Cervical factor

Cervical mucus study is less commonly done these day.

In proved cases of *Cl. trachomatis or M. hominis,* doxycycline 100 mg twice daily for 14 days is to be given to both the partners. **Cervical factor when cannot be treated, is overcome by ART procedures like IUI, IVF or GIFT (p. 206).**

Immunological factor

In the presence of antisperm antibodies in the cervical mucus, dexamethasone 0.5 mg at bed time in the follicular phase may be given. As there is no distinct benefit of such treatment in antisperm antibody positive patients, COH and IUI or IVF (p. 206) or ICSI (p. 209) is recommended.

Uterovaginal surgery: The operations in the uterus to improve the fertility includes:

- **Myomectomy** especially in submucous fibroid. Care should be taken to prevent or to minimize adhesions causing tubopathy.
- **Metroplasty (Ch. 4)** either removal of septum or unification operation may be tried when no other cause is detected. This abnormality seldom causes infertility.
- **Adhesiolysis (hysteroscopic)** with insertion of IUCD in uterine synechiae.
- **Enlargement of the vaginal introitus** (Fenton's operation) or removal of vaginal septum causing dyspareunia results in improvement of fertility.
- **Endometrial polyps:** Hysteroscopic polypectomy.

Bariatric surgery

Obesity is associated with hypogonadotrophic hypogonadism. Serum free testosterone concentrations are inversely related to body weight and BMI. Estrogen levels are raised due to increased aromatase activity in adipose tissue.

Obesity reduces fertility. Obese women require higher doses of gonadotropins to achieve pregnancy. Women with BMI >35 kg/m^2 are considered for bariatric surgery.

Method

An adjustable silicone band is placed (laparoscopically) around the upper part of the stomach to create a small upper gastric pouch. This limits hunger and food intake by early feeling of satiety.

Bariatric surgery improves the problems of anovulation, hirsutism, insulin resistance and PCOS.

Unexplained Infertility

Unexplained infertility is defined as the couples who have undergone complete basic infertility work up and in whom no abnormality has been detected (normal semen quality, ovulatory function, normal uterine cavity and bilateral tubal patency) and still remains infertile. It is the diagnosis of exclusion. The incidence is extremely variable and largely dependent on the magnitude of the in-depth investigation protocol extended to the couple. **The reported incidence varies from 10–30%.**

About 40% of these couples become pregnant within 3 years without having any specific treatment.

Therapy: The prospect of spontaneous conception decreases with increasing age of the woman and the duration of infertility. The recommended treatment for unexplained infertility are induction of ovulation, IUI, COS (p. 207) combined with IUI or assisted reproductive technology (*see* below).

Combined factor: The faults detected in both the partners **should be treated simultaneously and not one after the other.**

ARTIFICIAL INSEMINATION

Different methods artificial insemination (AI) are:

- Intrauterine insemination (IUI)
- Fallopian tube sperm perfusion.

INTRAUTERINE INSEMINATION

Intrauterine insemination (IUI) may be either artificial insemination husband (AIH) or artificial insemination donor (AID). Husband's semen is commonly used. **The purpose of IUI** is to bypass the endocervical canal which is abnormal and to place increased concentration of motile sperm as close to the fallopian tubes. The indications are tabulated in Table 17.11.

Technique

Common methods to extract sperm from the seminal plasma are: Washing, swim-up and density gradient double centrifugation. Swim-up method allows most motile sperm to swim-up into the supernatant. This increases sperm motility and capacitation. Compared to washing method it contains no dead sperm and cellular debris. About 0.3 mL of washed and concentrated sperm is injected through a flexible polyethylene catheter within the uterine cavity around the time of ovulation. Washing in culture media removes the proteins and prostaglandins from semen that may cause uterine cramps or anaphylactoid reactions. Density gradient centrifugation recovers most highly motile as well as morphologically normal sperm. The processed motile sperm count for insemination should be at least 1 million. Best results are obtained when the motile sperm count exceeds 10 million. Normal sperm survive in this female reproductive tract and can fertilize an egg for at least 3 days but an oocyte survives only for 12–24 hours. The procedure may be repeated 2–3 times over a period of 2–3 days. To increase sperm motility, pentoxifylline (phosphodiesterase inhibitor) has been used. Generally 4–6 cycles of insemination with superovulation is advised.

Timing of IUI: In cervical insemination, timing is not so much vital because the sperm can survive in the cervical canal for a day or two. As the reservoir function is not available in IUI, some form of controlled ovarian hyperstimulation (COH) is required (Table 17.12).

Insemination is done on the day or just prior to the day of ovulation.

Urinary LH kit may be used to detect the urinary LH peak (the day prior to ovulation). Timing may be adjusted with hCG injection. This is used for trigging ovulation.

TABLE 17.11: Indications of IUI.

- Hostile cervical mucus
- Cervical stenosis
- Oligospermia or asthenospermia
- Immune factor (male and female)
- Male factor—impotency or anatomical defect (hypospadias) but normal ejaculate can be obtained
- Unexplained infertility

TABLE 17.12: Timing of IUI.

- Natural cycles
  Cervical mucus study, BBT chart, urine LH surge
  IUI × 2, likely on day 12 and 14
- Clomiphene-induced cycles
  IUI—hand 7 days after completion of CC
- Urinary LH detection
  IUI—24 hours after color change
- Use of hCG and sonography
  hCG at 18 mm diameter of the follicle
  IUI × 2, following 34–40 hours of hCG administration

Results

Cumulative conception rates after 12 insemination cycles is 75–80%. The best results are obtained in the treatment of cervical factor and unexplained infertility and in stimulated cycle. IUI along with superovulation (induction of ovulation with hMG/FSH, hCG) gives higher result.

ARTIFICIAL (THERAPEUTIC) INSEMINATION DONOR

When the semen of a donor is used for insemination it is called artificial (therapeutic) insemination donor (AID). **The indications are:**

- Untreatable azoospermia, asthenospermia
- Genetic disease
- Rh-negative donor insemination—for woman with Rh-sensitization.

The donor should be healthy and of the same ethnic group as husband. He should be serologically and bacteriologically free from venereal diseases including AIDS and hepatitis. The recipient and donor must be matched for blood grouping and Rh typing. Either fresh or frozen semen is used. Sperm specimen should only be used when it is kept sequestered for at least 180 days and thereafter it has been found negative for HIV. The legal, psychological and religious aspects should be counseled before its application.

Results: A total of 3–6 cycles may have to be utilized to get a success. The success rate is about 50–60%. Insemination when combined with superovulation, enhances success rate.

FALLOPIAN TUBE SPERM PERFUSION

Indications are same as that of IUI.

Technique

Large volume of washed and processed sperm is injected within the fallopian tube laparoscopically around the time of ovulation. This causes perfusion of the fallopian tubes with spermatozoa. In conjunction with ovulation induction pregnancy rate is 25–30% per cycle. Currently PROST or ZIFT or TET are done (Table 17.13).

ASSISTED REPRODUCTIVE TECHNOLOGIES

The ART encompasses all the procedures that involve manipulation of gametes and embryos outside the body for the treatment of infertility (Table 17.13).

TABLE 17.13: Assisted reproductive techniques (ART).

IVF-ET	: In vitro fertilization and embryo transfer
GIFT	: Gamete intrafallopian transfer
ZIFT	: Zygote intrafallopian transfer
POST	: Peritoneal oocyte and sperm transfer
PROST	: Pronuclear stage tubal transfer
TET	: Tubal embryo transfer zone
SUZI	: Subzonal insemination
ICSI	: Intracytoplasmic sperm injection
AH	: Assisted hatching
IVM	: In vitro maturation of oocyte
PGD/s	: Preimplantation genetic diagnosis/screening
Cryopreservation: Embryo/oocyte/ovarian tissue/sperm	
Gestational surrogacy	
Sperm retrieval techniques	
TESE	: Testicular sperm extraction
MESA	: Microsurgical epididymal sperm aspiration
PESA	: Percutaneous epididymal sperm aspiration

IN VITRO FERTILIZATION AND EMBRYO TRANSFER

The field of reproductive medicine has changed forever with the birth of Louise Brown in 1978 by in vitro fertilization and embryo (IVF-ET). **Patrick Steptoe and Robert Edwards of England are remembered for their revolutionary work.**

The past decade has witnessed two more dramatic changes in the technique protocol of IVF-ET. One such change was from natural cycle to superovulation protocol and the other one was replacement of laparoscopy by vaginal sonography for ovum retrieval. The indications of IVF are used in Table 17.14.

TABLE 17.14: Indications of IVF.

- Fallopian tubes block or absent
- Unexplained infertility
- Endometriosis
- Oligospermia or azoospermia requiring TESE
- Advanced reproductive age
- Fertility preservation
- Multiple factors (female and male)
- Failed ovulation induction
- Ovarian failure (donor oocyte IVF)
- Women with normal ovaries but no functional uterus (Müllerian agenesis)
- Women with genetic risk (IVF and PGD)

Patient Selection (Ideal)

- Age <35 years
- Presence of ovarian reserve (D3, serum FSH <10 IU/L)
- Husband—normal seminogram
- Couple must be screened negative for HIV and hepatitis
- Normal uterine cavity as evaluated by hysteroscopy/ sonohysterography.

Principal Steps of an ART Cycle

- Downregulation using GnRH agonist
- Controlled ovarian stimulation (COS)
- Monitoring of follicular growth
- Oocyte retrieval
- Fertilization in vitro (IVF, ICSI)
- Transfer of gametes or embryos
- Luteal support with progesterone.

GnRH Analog for Downregulation

Currently most ART procedures involve the use of GnRH agonists (p. 441).

- GnRH agonist therapy used for downregulation of pituitary to prevent premature LH surge. It gives higher pregnancy rates.
- GnRH agonist therapy is continued either subcutaneously or intranasally during the gonadotropin treatment phase.
- GnRH antagonists are currently tried along with gonadotropin stimulation to prevent premature LH surge or premature ovulation. Cetrorelix and Ganirelix are the available drugs.
- Different schedules for GnRH agonist are available.
- *Long follicular downregulation*—when therapy is started in the follicular phase of previous cycle.
- *Long luteal downregulation* (most commonly used) therapy is begun on D-21 of the previous cycle. Gonadotropin stimulation is started following the menses.
- *Short 'flare' protocol*—GnRH therapy is started in the follicular phase (0-1) along with gonadotropin stimulation. This is also called flare protocol, as gonadotropin can work over the stimulatory effect of GnRH agonist. In short ('flare') protocol, GnRH agonist (leuprolide acetate 1.0 mg daily) is given on cycle day 2–4, continuing thereafter at a reduced dose (0.5 mg daily). Gonadotropin stimulation begins on cycle D3. Adjustments of gonadotropin dose is done depending upon the response.

Natural Cycle

In the first case, Steptoe and Edwards (1978) achieved success from collecting the oocyte from a **natural cycle**, 36 hours after the onset of LH surge. Compared to stimulated IVF cycles, **it has few advantages**. It requires no medication, less cost, minimizes complication [multiple pregnancy, ovarian hyperstimulation syndrome (OHSS)].

Disadvantages: High cycle cancelation rates due to premature LH surge. It has a low success rate.

Advantages of induction of superovulation: Improved quality of the oocyte, timing of ovulation can be controlled, suited to the personnel involved and extended to all cases of ovulatory dysfunction (Fig. 17.7).

Controlled Ovarian Stimulation (COS)

Gonadotropin stimulation is begun once pituitary down regulation is achieved (serum E_2 <40 pg/mL and no ovarian follicles are seen >10 mm on TVS). Exogenous gonadotropins for (uFSH, rFSH, HMG) ovarian stimulation are used. The drug regimens used differ in each center. Following drugs or combination of drugs are commonly used (Table 17.15).

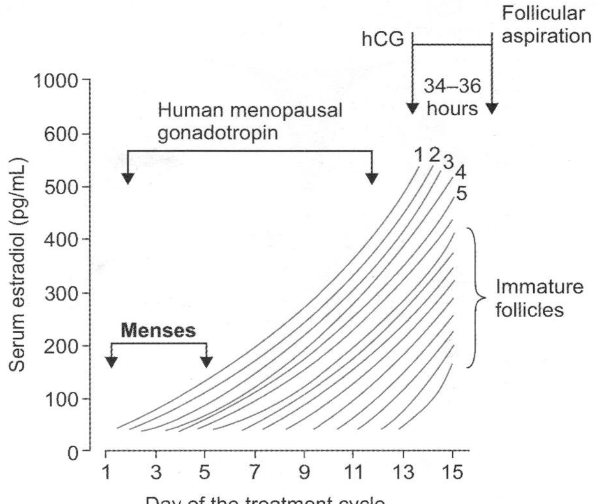

Fig. 17.7: Example of stimulated cycle in ART.

TABLE 17.15: Ovarian stimulation regimen.

▪ Clomiphene citrate (CC)
▪ CC + human menopausal gonadotropin (hMG)
▪ Letrozole + pure FSH
▪ Letrozole + recombinant FSH
▪ hMG
▪ FSH (Table 17.8)
▪ GnRH analogs + hMG or pure FSH

hCG is administered in each regimen (Table 17.8)

Monitoring of Follicular Growth

The follicular growth response is monitored by sonographic measurement of the follicles and serum estradiol estimation, commencing on the 8th day of treatment cycle. The endometrial thickness (stripe) ≥8–9 mm (trilaminar) is optimum. When two or more follicles are 17–18 mm in diameter and serum E_2 levels >250 pg/mL/per follicle, 5,000–10,000 IU of hCG (250 µg of recombinant hCG) is given intramuscularly. Oocyte is retrieved 36 hours after the hCG is given. hCG induces oocyte maturation. The individual woman may be a **high responder or a poor responder**. Depending upon the response, management is done.

Oocyte Retrieval

Oocyte retrieval is done aseptically through vaginal route under ultrasound guidance (Fig. 17.8). With the use of vaginal transducers, vaginal needle aspiration is done about 36 hours after hCG administration but before ovulation occurs (Fig. 17.8). Intravenous analgesia and sedation (propofol) is adequate in most of the cases. The oocyte is readily recognizable as a single cell surrounded by a mass of cumulus cells. After recovery, the oocytes are maintained in culture in vitro for 4–6 hours.

Complications of aspiration of follicles (oocyte retrieval) are: Infection, internal bleeding and ovarian torsion.

Fertilization (in vitro)

The sperm used for insemination in vitro is prepared by the wash and swim-up or density gradient centrifugation (preferred) technique. Approximately 50,000 to 100,000 capacitated sperm

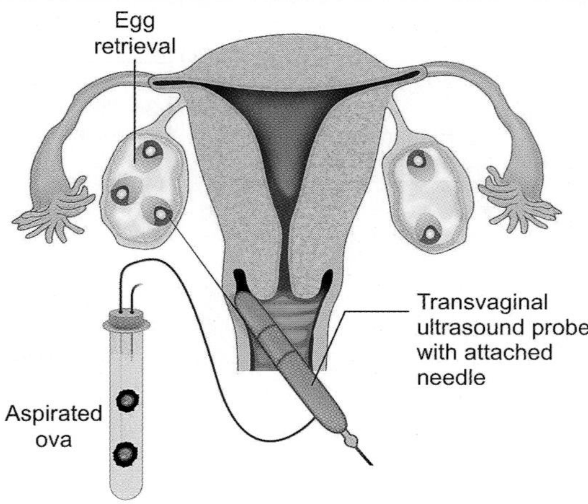

Fig. 17.8: Oocyte retrieval.

are placed into the culture media containing the oocyte within 4–6 hours of retrieval. The eggs may demonstrate signs of fertilization when examined 16–18 hours after insemination (presence of two pronuclei in the presence of a second polar body). **Sperm density and motility are the two most important criteria for successful IVF.** The semen is collected just prior to ovum retrieval.

Embryo Transfer (Day 3 embryo)

The fertilized ova at the 6–8 blastomere stage are placed into the uterine cavity close to the fundus about 3 days (Fig. 17.9) after fertilization through a fine flexible soft catheter transcervically. Usually two and **not more than three embryos are transferred** per cycle to minimize multiple pregnancy. D5 blastocyst transfer is also done (Fig. 17.10).

The process of transfer should be accurate, atraumatic and aseptic. Small volume transfer using soft catheter under ultrasound guidance gives the best result. Trial transfer is beneficial. The number of embryos to be transferred depends mainly on maternal age and the embryo quality.

Excess oocytes and embryos can be **cryopreserved** for future use. This will reduce the cost of ovulation stimulation as well as the risk of ovarian hyperstimulation.

Luteal phase support is maintained with progesterone. It is started on the day after oocyte retrieval. hCG is given in supplemental doses (1,500–2,500 IU). Micronized progesterone 200 mg thrice a day oral or as vaginal suppository (preferred) or progesterone in oil injection 50 mg IM daily is continued for about 14 days. By this time diagnosis of pregnancy by estimation of β–hCG (quantitative value) is possible.

Result: The overall **live birth rate varies from 40% in women of age <35 years to 4.5% at age >42 years per cycle oocyte retrieval.**

There is increased risk of miscarriage (18%), multiple pregnancy (31%), ectopic (0.9%), low birth weight baby and prematurity. The risk of congenital malformation of the baby remains similar to general population.

Prognostic Factors for IVF-ET

- **Maternal age**—there is age related decline in response to ovarian stimulation, less oocytes, poor oocyte quality, less embryos and implantation rate.
- **Ovarian reserve**—declines with age (Ch. 17).
- **Indication of IVF and past reproductive success.** Women with tubal or ovulatory factors, endometriosis, or unexplained factor—have higher success rate compared to women with poor ovarian reserve.

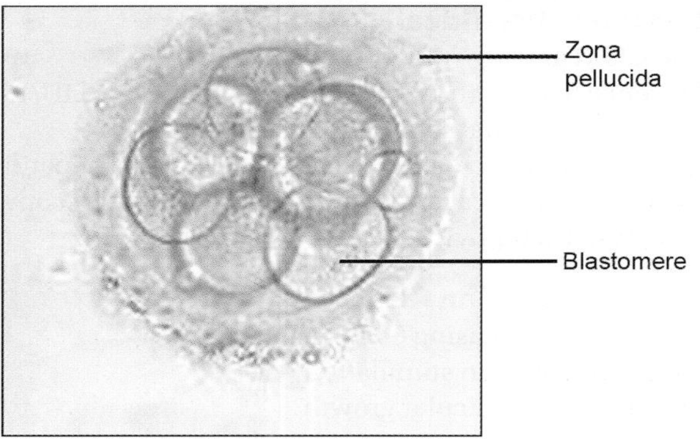

Fig. 17.9: Day 3 embryo.

(*Courtesy:* Professor BN Chakravorty, Director, Institute of Reproductive, Medicine, Kolkata)

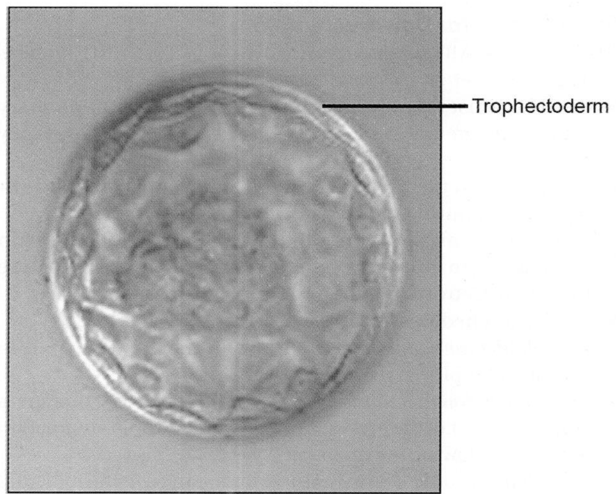

Fig. 17.10: Blastocyst (day 5 or day 6 embryo).

(*Courtesy:* Professor BN Chakravorty, Director, Institute of Reproductive, Medicine, Kolkata)

- **Presence of hydrosalpinges**—affect the outcome adversely.
- **Fibroid uterus**—especially the submucous or interstitial variety have adverse outcome.
- **Smoking**—poor outcome.
- **Endometriosis** (Ch. 22).

GAMETE INTRAFALLOPIAN TRANSFER

Gamete intrafallopian transfer (GIFT) was first described by Asch and colleagues in 1984. It is a more invasive and expensive procedure than IVF but the result seems better than IVF. In this procedure, both the sperm and the unfertilized oocytes are transferred into the fallopian tubes. Fertilization is then achieved in vivo.

The prerequisite for GIFT procedure is to have normal uterine tubes. The indications are the same as that of IVF except the tubal factor. Best result is obtained in unexplained infertility and the result is poor in male factor abnormality.

The superovulation is done as in IVF. Two collected oocytes along with approximately 200,000–500,000 motile sperm for each fallopian tube are placed in a plastic tube container. It is then passed through laparoscope and inserted 4 cm into the distal end of the fallopian tube where the combination is injected.

Result: The overall delivered pregnancy rate is as high as 27–30%.

ZYGOTE INTRAFALLOPIAN TRANSFER

Zygote intrafallopian transfer (ZIFT) was first described by Devroey et al. (1986).

The placement of the zygote (following one day of in vitro fertilization) into the fallopian tube can be done either through the abdominal ostium by laparoscope or through the uterine ostium under ultrasonic guidance.

This technique is a suitable alternative of GIFT when defect lies in the male factor or in cases of failed GIFT. *Results* (29–30%) are similar to that of IVF. GIFT or ZIFT is avoided when tubal factors for infertility are present.

The risk of ectopic pregnancy is high for GIFT and ZIFT compared to IVF.

MICROMANIPULATION

INTRACYTOPLASMIC SPERM INJECTION

Intracytoplasmic sperm injection (ICSI) was first described by van Steirteghem and colleagues in Belgium (1992).

Indications

- Severe oligospermia (5 million sperm/mL)
- Asthenospermia, teratospermia
- Presence of sperm antibodies
- Obstruction of efferent duct system (male)
- Congenital absence of vas (bilateral)
- Failure of fertilization in IVF
- Fertilization of cryopreserved oocytes (with hardened zona pellucida)
- Unexplained infertility.

Sperm is recovered from the ejaculate. Otherwise sperm is retrieved by testicular sperm extraction (TESE) or by microsurgical epididymal sperm aspiration (MESA) procedures.

Technique: One single spermatozoon or even a spermatid is injected directly into the cytoplasm of an oocyte by micropuncture of the zona pellucida. This procedure is carried out under a high quality inverted operating microscope. The oocyte is stabilized at 6 or 12 O'clock position and entered at the 3 O'clock position. The injecting pipette pierces the zona and oolemma and the sperm is injected directly into the ooplasm (Fig. 17.11).

ICSI is found to be very effective compared to other micromanipulation methods like subzonal insemination (SUZI). ICSI is very effective to reduce the need of AID.

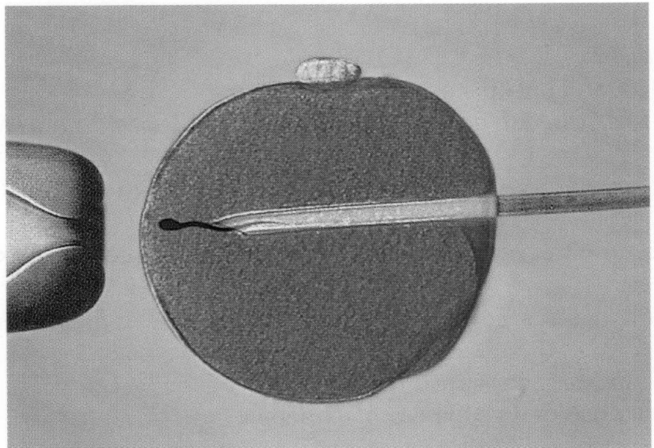

Fig. 17.11: Technique of intracytoplasmic sperm injection (ICSI).

Presently, ICSI is utilized in all cases of male infertility and for all couples where IVF produces have failed. Pregnancy rate after ICSI is ≥15% even if the retrieved sperm by TESE or PESA remain immotile.

Results: Fertilization rate is about 60–70%. Pregnancy rate is 20–40% per embryo transfer.

EMBRYO OR OOCYTE DONATION

Ovum donation and IVF can help women with successful pregnancy. The essential requirements for successful outcome are: (a) Successful ovum donation and IVF; (b) Embryo-endometrial synchronization; (c) Exogenous hormonal support until luteal-placental shift.

Indications

- Women with premature ovarian failure
- Women with removed ovaries
- Older women (poor oocyte quality)
- Failure to respond with superovulation regimen (poor ovarian reserve)
- Women with repeated failure of ART cycles
- Genetic disease.

The oocytes are collected from:

- Sister or a friend (age between 21 and 34 years).
- Those for IVF candidates, excess oocytes following retrieval and cryopreservation (*see* above).
- One undergoing laparoscopic sterilization (with financial compensation).
- The oocyte donor like the semen donor must be screened for infection and genetic diseases.

Successful implantation needs a perfect coordination of embryo and the endometrium. Estrogen therapy (in the recipient) is started at the same time when the donor gets cycle stimulation. Progesterone treatment in the recipient generally begins on the day the donor undergoes ovum retrieval. Generally, third day embryos are transferred on the fourth day of progesterone therapy.

Luteal Support

As the recipient has no corpus luteum, exogenous luteal support is needed. Exogenous estrogen and progesterone treatment should therefore be continued until 10 weeks of gestation. Oocytes and embryos can be cryopreserved (at –196° under liquid nitrogen) for restoration of fertility in future. Survival of cryopreserved embryo is more than that of oocytes.

Results: Live birth rate is approximately 55%.

GESTATIONAL CARRIER SURROGACY

A woman without a functional uterus can be a mother with the help of ART.

In this procedure of ART (IVF), a fertilized egg is placed into the uterus of a surrogate (gestational carrier) but not into "intended mother".

Indications are: (a) Irrepairable uterine factor; (b) When pregnancy may cause significant health risks; (c) Women with recurrent unexplained miscarriage; (d) Prior hysterectomy.

Cryopreservation of ovarian tissue: Restoration of reproductive function of a woman undergoing chemotherapy or radiotherapy is possible these days with the help of cryobiology. Cryopreservation of ovarian tissue or autotransplantation may allow natural pregnancy later on. Surgical removal of whole or part of the ovary for cryopreservation is done. The frozen tissue can be thawed and transplanted orthotopically or heterotopically back to the patient's body. With this method, ovulation using exogenous gonadotropins can be achieved.

Oocyte/embryo cryopreservation: By freezing is an alternative method. Vetrification, using high concentration of cryoprotectant can solidify cells without ice formation. Human pregnancies and deliveries from vetrified mature oocytes have been done.

Indications:

- Young women with cancer about to have chemotherapy
- Young healthy women desiring to delay child bearing
- Women with her husband/partner—desiring use of sperm to fertilize the oocyte and to freeze embryo rather than oocytes. This is more successful for the higher pregnancy rates.

Preimplantation genetic diagnosis (PGD)/screening: Can be performed on polar bodies removed from oocytes before fertilization. It can also be done by blastomere biopsy from a D3 embryo.

Risks for PGD: Results may be false positive (due to mosaicism) or false negative. Patient still need antenatal genetic testing (CVS or amniocentesis). Genetic screening can avoid transferring embryos with aneuploidy and autosomal recessive (cystic fibrosis) or autosomal dominant gene mutation.

Frozen embryo transfer: Endometrium is primed with estrogen therapy (oral, transdermal or IM) over a period of 2 weeks. Endometrial thickness is measured with TVS and also the level of serum estradiol. Progesterone supplement is given once the endometrial thickness is of 6–8 mm. Embryos are thawed on the day of scheduled transfer. Depending upon the age of the woman at the time of freezing, number of embryo transfer is decided. One or two embryo are transferred when the age is ≤35. Three or more embryos are transferred with age ≥40. Blastocyst (D5/6) stages are preferred. Frozen embryo transfer observed to have improved pregnancy rates.

Three-day old embryos are assessed with the following criteria: (a) Blastomere morphology; (b) Symmetry; (c) Degree of embryo fragmentation (Fig. 17.10). Embryos with a high degree of fragmentation (>10%) have lower implantation and pregnancy rates.

Assisted hatching (AH) is the drilling to create a small hole in the zona pellucida of the embryo. It is done at the time of D3 embryo transfer. AH improves implantation and clinical pregnancy rates specifically in older women (>37 years) and in women with prior unexplained IVF failures.

Excess embryos of good quality may be cryopreserved by slow cooling or vetrification.

Result: Live birth rates per cycle range from 40.1% in women <35 years of age to 4.5% at age >42 years. Overall pregnancy rates after 6 cycles of IVF is 72%.

Health Hazards of ART

- **Birth defects: Most of the ART procedures are not associated with any increased risk of fetal congenital malformations or birth defects.** ICSI is often done due to male factors for infertility and it eliminates the natural process of sperm selection. It is not yet certain whether ICSI is associated with increased chromosomal abnormalities of the offspring.
- **Increased** miscarriage, multiple pregnancy, ectopic and heterotrophic pregnancy, placenta praevia and low birth weight babies have been observed.
- **Perinatal mortality** and morbidity are high.
- **Ovarian hyperstimulation syndrome (p. 444)** though rare but is a known health risk.
- **Fertility drugs and cancer**—no association have been found between ovulation induction drugs and ovarian cancer.
- **Psychological stress** and anxiety of the couple are severe. It is especially so when there is failure in the treatment or with a pregnancy loss.

PROGNOSIS OF INFERTILITY

The pregnancy rate within 2 years after the start of investigation, ranges between 30–40%. The rate is however, increased to about 72% when repeated cycles of ART procedures are included.

Adoption: In spite of excellent advances in the field of infertility management, expectations are not always fulfilled. Couple must understand the infertility factors, cost and risk of management. End point of management must be realistically understood. Adoption is an alternative for many couples.

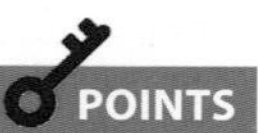

- **Infertility** is defined as a failure to conceive within 1 year of regular unprotected coitus. 10% remain infertile by the end of 2nd year. The **incidence increases** further after the age of 30 years.
- In fully lactating women, pregnancy is unlikely up to 10 weeks postpartum.
- **Male factor** is responsible in 30–40%, the female in 40–50%, both in 10% and unexplained in 10%.
- **Common causes** of male infertility include defective spermatogenesis, obstruction of efferent duct, failure to deposit sperm high in vagina and error in seminal fluid (Table 17.1).
- **Important causes** of female infertility are tubal factor (25–35%), ovulatory factor (20–25%) and endometriosis (0–10%) (Flowchart 17.2).
- **Ovulatory dysfunction** is likely to be linked with disturbed hypothalamo-pituitary-ovarian axis either primary or secondary from thyroid or adrenal dysfunction.
- **Luteal phase defect** is observed in older women, drug-induced ovulation, elevated prolactin, patients with repeated pregnancy wastage, pelvic endometriosis, DUB and subclinical hypothyroidism.
- **Serum progesterone** more than 10 ng/mL on 8th postovulatory day indicates adequate luteal function.
- **Luteinized unruptured follicle** is often associated with pelvic endometriosis or with hyperprolactinemia.

Contd...

Contd...

- **Tubal factors** are related to tubal infection, peritubal adhesions or endometriosis. The most common peritoneal factor is endometriosis.
- **Investigation of an infertile couple** should be started after 1 year. The initial investigations of an infertile couple include: Semen analysis (male factor), hysterosalpingography (tubal factor), BBT and/or serum progesterone (evidence of ovulation) (Flowchart 17.2).
- **BBT** increases when circulating level of progesterone is increased following ovulation.
- **Diagnosis of ovulation** is from indirect, direct and conclusive evidences (Table 17.4).
- **Subnuclear vacuolation** of the endometrial glandular epithelium is the earliest evidence of ovulation (36–48 hours).
- **A persistent rise in BBT** and/or a serum progesterone more than 5 ng/mL is the presumptive evidence of ovulation. Sonographic evidences of ovulation are collapsed follicle and fluid in the pouch of Douglas. Pregnancy is the surest evidence of ovulation.
- **A thorough investigation** following an abnormal semen analysis, is needed to find out the specific cause of male infertility (Flowchart 17.1).
- **Tubal factor** is assessed by HSG and laparoscopy both of these two are complimentary. Sonohysterosalpingography has got no radiation exposure. Falloposcopy and salpingoscopy are used to study the tubal mucosa (Table 17.7).
- **Postcoital test (PCT)** is done in late proliferative phase. The examination is done 8–12 hours after coitus. The presence of active motile sperm numbering at least 10 per HPF is satisfactory. Routine PCT is not recommended.
- **Presence of antisperm antibodies** may not be the cause of infertility.
- **Of all the etiological factors**, greatest success is obtained following treatment of anovulation.
- **For induction of ovulation**, the commonly used drugs are clomiphene citrate, hMG, FSH, hCG, GnRH analogs, bromocriptine (Table 17.8).
- ***The suitable patients*** *for clomiphene citrate (CC) are—normogonadotropic-normoprolactinemic, PCOS with amenorrhea or hypothalamic amenorrhea.*
- ***Following CC therapy****, incidence of multiple gestation is about 5% and all being twins. The incidence of miscarriage, ectopic pregnancy or congenital malformation is not increased.*
- ***Women with PCOS*** *who do not ovulate with CC, insulin sensitizers (metformin) and/or LOD (p. 247) is effective in inducing ovulation.*
- *Women with unexplained infertility, therapy with COS and IUI yield better pregnancy rates. After 3 to 6 cycles, IVF should be next course of treatment.*
- Treatment of infertility due to anovulation has got maximum success with ovulation induction.
- Large hydrosalpinx causing distal tube disease should be treated by salpingectomy and IVF.
- The rate of pregnancy is inversely related to the age of the female patient.
- **Gonadotropin therapy** is indicated in cases with hypogonadotropic-hypogonadism and clomiphene failure.
- **GnRH is used** in a pulsatile manner for cases with hypothalamic amenorrhea and hypogonadotropic hypogonadism.
- **GnRH analogs** are used in patient's refractory to gonadotropins, with elevated LH, with normal gonadotropins or in cases with premature LH surge.
- **Gonadotropins**, GnRH analog and hCG are mostly used in ART with careful monitoring.
- **Hyperprolactinemia** and anovulation (5–10%) are due to inhibition of gonadotropin secretion. Serum FSH, estradiol levels are low. Women suffer from oligomenorrhea or amenorrhea. Bromocriptine is indicated in cases of hyperprolactinemia with or without galactorrhea.
- **Corpus luteum insufficiency** can be treated by progesterone as vaginal suppositories or by hCG. LPD is currently thought to be a normal biologic variant and not a true cause of infertility.
- **Unruptured luteinized follicle** is treated by intramuscular injection of hCG 5000–10,000 IU or ovulation inducing drugs, or bromocriptine if associated with hyperprolactinemia.
- **Tuboplasty** is the surgical procedure performed to restore the anatomy and physiology of the tube (Table 17.6). Endoscopic surgery gives the best result. Prognosis for fertility depends upon the extent and the site of damage to the tube. Tubal reconstructive surgery may be considered for mild proximal tubal block. For any complicated tubal occlusive disease, IVF is the best therapy.
- **Proximal tubal obstruction** is usually treated by cannulation through tubes with catheters under hysteroscopic visualization. No tubal surgery should be attempted in women with pelvic tuberculosis. IVF may be considered once endometrium is free from the disease.
- **Overall result** in terms of pregnancy following tuboplasty ranges between 15–60%. The pregnancy rate after salpingolysis and fimbrioplasty is about 65%. The result is best in reversal of tubal sterilization by tubotubal anastomosis.
- **Any form of therapy for minimal endometriosis** does not improve fertility status. Unexplained infertility is observed in about 10–15% cases. Women with mild endometriosis can be treated with COH and IUI to improve fertility.
- **Assisted reproductive technology (ART)** includes different methods (Table 17.13). These are expensive and need sophisticated laboratory facilities.
- **The best results of IUI** are obtained in the treatment of cervical factor and unexplained infertility (Table 17.11) and in stimulated cycle (controlled ovarian stimulation). Overall pregnancy rate ranges between 20–40%.
- **Controlled ovarian stimulation (COS)** and IUI (Table 17.12) are the options for women with unexplained infertility and for women whose male partner (husband) suffers from oligospermia.
- **Donor insemination (AID)** should be performed with frozen sperm, stored at least for 6 months. The donor should be retested and should be negative for antibodies to HIV during the time of insemination. This is because antibodies to HIV may take several months to develop after the infection.

Contd...

Contd...

- **IVF-ET** (Steptoe and Edwards–1978)—overall pregnancy rate varies from 20 to 35 per oocyte retrieval. Take baby home rate is about 15–20% per procedure.
- **GIFT** (Asch, 1984) procedure needs normal fallopian tubes. In some centers the success rate of GIFT and IVF-ET is the same.
- **ICSI** (Van Steirteghem, 1992) is an effective method for male infertility (severe oligospermia or sperm dysfunction). It reduces the need of AID.
- **Pregnancy** following donor oocyte or embryo is the option for women with ovarian failure, removed ovaries or with genetic disease.
- **The pregnancy rate** within 2 years after the start of investigations for infertility is 30–40%. The rate is however increased to 50–60%, if AID cases are included. When the couple fails to conceive after 2 years of therapy, the chance of conception is remote.
- IVF with and without ICSI, the delivery rate per cycle is 50%
- ***Health hazards of ART*** *include psychological stress of the couple, increased number of pregnancy loss, multiple pregnancy and ectopic pregnancy. Risk of fetal congenital malformations is not increased. Ovarian hyperstimulation syndrome is rare but a known health hazard.*
- ***Ovarian hyperstimulation syndrome (OHSS)*** *is a complication of ovulation induction. Basic pathology is increased capillary permeability (VEGF) leading to ascites, hypovolemia, oliguria and electrolyte imbalance. Management is conservative. Abdominal paracentesis, to relieve respiratory distress and human albumin (IV), to correct hypovolemia may be needed.*
- **According to WHO, ovulatory disorders are grouped into**:
  Group I: Hypothalamic-pituitary failure—women in this group have hypogonadotrophic hypogonadism, low gonadotropin and low estradiol level, normal prolactin and negative progesterone challenge test. **Included in this group are:** Stress-related amenorrhea, Sheehan's syndrome, Kallmann's syndrome, anorexia nervosa. These women are treated with hMG or GnRH with or without ARTs.
  Group II: Hypothalamic-pituitary dysfunction—women are normogonadotrophic, normoestrogenic, anovulatory and oligomenorrheic. Women with PCOS are in this group. These women are treated with clomiphene citrate.
  Group III: Ovarian failure—women are hypergonadotrophic and hypogonadal with low estrogen level. Women with Turner's syndrome, premature ovarian failure, ovarian radiation or chemotherapy belong to the group. These women are treated with ovum donation (ART).

CHAPTER

18 Benign Lesions of the Vulva and Vagina

CHAPTER OUTLINE

VULVAR EPITHELIAL DISORDERS

TERMINOLOGY, DEFINITION AND TYPES

Nonneoplastic epithelial disorders of vulvar skin and mucosa have been classified according to International Society for the Study of Vulvovaginal Diseases (ISSVD) in 2006. Vulvar intraepithelial neoplasia (VIN) lesions have been excluded from the classification (p. 266). Presently, a broader group of dermatologic disorders are considered. These include dermatoses, infections and neoplasias with similar clinical presentations.

ISSVD Classification of Vulvar Dermatoses: Pathological Subsets and their Clinical Correlates

Spongiotic pattern
- Atopic dermatitis
- Allergic contact dermatitis
- Irritant contact dermatitis

Acanthotic pattern
- Psoriasis
- Lichen simplex chronicus
  - Primary (idiopathic)
  - Secondary (superimposed on lichen sclerosus, lichen planus, etc.)

Lichenoid pattern
- Lichen sclerosus
- Lichen planus

Dermal homogenization/sclerosis pattern
- Lichen sclerosus

Vesiculobullous pattern
- Pemphigoid, cicatricial type
- Liner IgA disease

Acantholytic pattern
- Hailey-Hailey disease
- Darier disease
- Papular genitocrural acantholysis

Granulomatous pattern
- Crohn disease
- Melkersson-Rosenthal syndrome

Vasculopathic pattern
- Aphthous ulcers
- Behcet disease
- Plasma cell vulvitis

ETIOLOGY

Multiple factors such as trauma (scratching), autoimmune, allergy (atopic), irritation, nutritional (deficiency of folic acid, vitamin B_{12}, riboflavin, or achlorhydria, etc.), infection (fungus), metabolic or systemic (hepatic, hematological), etc. are implicated. **Autoimmune disorders** like thyroid disease, pernicious anemia and diabetes are often associated. About 40% women are either having or going to develop an autoimmune condition. **Patient's personal or family history of atopic conditions** (asthma, eczema, hay fever) should be taken. **Drugs**: β-blockers, angiotensin-converting enzyme (ACE) inhibitors, may be associated. **Common allergens are** cosmetics, synthetic underwears and fragrances.

DIAGNOSIS OF VULVAR EPITHELIAL DISORDERS

Details of history is essential to reach the accurate diagnosis. History should cover:

- **Symptoms:**
  - Itching, irritation, pain or vulvar discharge
  - Associated symptoms if any—oral, ocular or intestinal
  - Relationship with menstruation
  - Association with cervical smear, cell abnormality or CIN.
- **Sexual history**: Dyspareunia, discharge, sexually transmitted infections (STIs), human immunodeficiency virus (HIV); use of medications to cause allergy or irritation (latex, soaps, shampoos, bubble bath).
- **Others**: Smoking, alcohol intake.

Examination should be done with good light and using magnifying lens or colposcope. Global skin examination of the vulva includes hair, skin color, and pigmentation. Skin thickening ulceration, discharge or nodularity.

Specific anatomical sites for examination are: (a) Mons pubis; (b) Labia majora; (c) Labia minora; (d) Interlabial sulci; (e) Clitoris; (f) Vestibule; (g) Perianal skin; (h) Vagina; (i) Cervix; (j) Inspection of the oral mucosa, eyes and the scalp.

Skin biopsy may not be needed when a diagnosis can be made on clinical examination. **Biopsy is required** if the woman fails to respond to treatment or there is clinical suspicion of VIN or cancer.

The sites for biopsy are from the margins of cracks and fissures and the sky blue areas left behind after applying 1% aqueous toluidine blue to the vulva and washing it off after 1 minute with 1% acetic acid.

LICHEN SCLEROSUS

It is an autoimmune mediated dermotosis. It occurs in postmenopausal women. It affects the skin of the anogenital region. The epithelium is metabolically active. It usually occurs following menopause, may occur even in childhood but in that case, it resolves after menarche.

Pathophysiology

Autoimmune disorders [diabetes, achlorhydria with or without pernicious anemia, systemic lupus erythematosus (SLE)] are associated in 20–30% cases. Levels of dihydrotestosterone (DHT) and androstenedione are low in these women.

Distribution of Lesion

The entire vulva is involved. Lesion encircles the vestibule. It involves clitoris, labia minora, inner aspects of labia majora and the skin around the anus. It is usually bilateral and symmetrical in a figure of eight distribution. It may even extend to the perineum and beyond the labiocrural folds to the thighs. It may also affect other parts of the body (trunk and limbs—18%).

Clinical Features

Pruritus is more than soreness. There is dyspareunia (excluding childhood), sleeplessness, and dysuria. Dyspareunia is due to stenosis of the vulvar outlet (Fig. 18.1). The skin is thin and looks white. Inflammatory adhesions of the labia minora and fusion may cause difficulty with micturition and even retention of urine. There may be narrowing of vaginal introitus. Pruritus is related to active inflammation with erythema. Scratching results in subepithelial hemorrhages (ecchymosis).

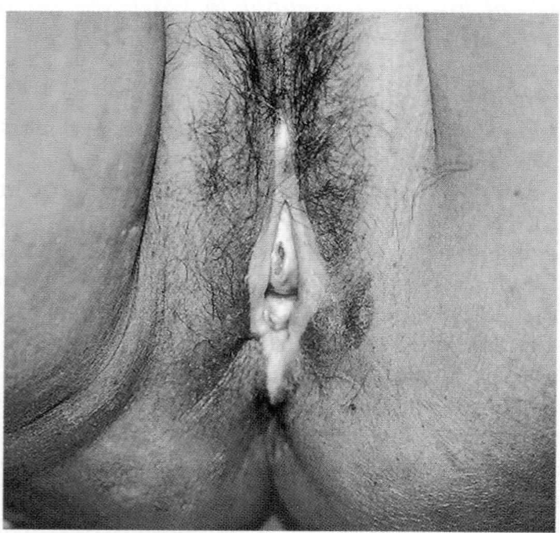

Fig. 18.1: Vulvar lichen sclerosus. Vulvar skin—thin and pale; fusion of labia minora beneath the clitoris. Lesion extends below to involve the perineum and anus. Clitoris is concealed. Introital stenosis is there.

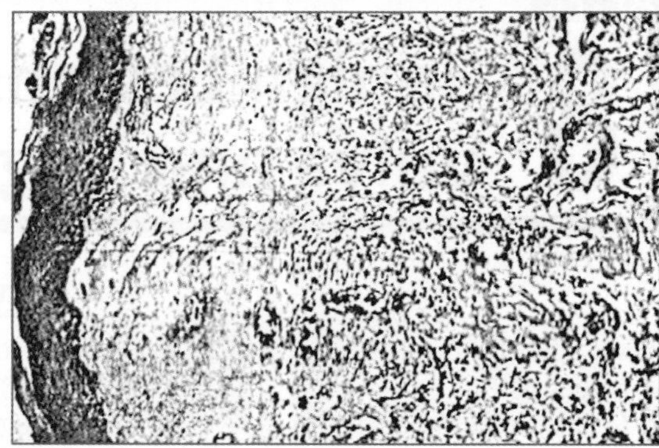

Fig. 18.2: Histologic picture of lichen sclerosus showing atrophic and flat epithelium with loss of rete ridges. There is presence of hyalinized collagen tissue and chronic inflammatory cells.

Diagnosis

The diagnosis should be confirmed by biopsy. Biopsy can be taken with a punch biopsy forceps (Keyes) under local anesthesia as an outpatient procedure. Monsel's solution (ferric subsulfate) is applied to control bleeding.

Histology

The epithelium is thin with epidermal atrophy. At times, there is hyperkeratosis, parakeratosis, acanthosis and elongation of rete ridges with evidence of collagen hyalinization. Fibroblasts are absent. There is presence of inflammatory cells including lymphocytes and plasma cells (Fig. 18.2).

The **risk of malignancy is less than 5%**.

Treatment

Patient education is important. She should avoid chemical or mechanical irritants on the vulvar skin. Ultrapotent topical corticosteroid preparation such as clobetasol propionate 0.05% (or 0.05% halobetasol propionate) is effective. Phototherapy following pretreatment with 5-aminolevulinic acid improved symptoms on short-term basis.

Lesions resistant to corticosteroids need treatment with tacrolimus and pimecrolimus. These are immunosuppressants (calcineurin inhibitors).

Surgery: Women, nonresponsive to topical steroids or having hyperkeratotic lesion on biopsy, needs excision.

Perineoplasty: Vaginal dilatation, surgical release of adhesions may be needed. This chronic disease often has the episodes of spontaneous remissions and exacerbations.

LICHEN PLANUS

It affects the skin, oral and genital mucosa. It is seen between 30 and 60 years of age. T cell autoimmunity directed against the basal keratinocytes, is thought to be the cause. The lesion may be any of three types: (1) erosive, (2) papulosquamous and (3) hypertrophic. Erosive type is most common. It involves the vulva, vagina and gingival margins. It may be drug induced [methyldopa, β blockers, nonsteroidal anti-inflammatory drugs (NSAIDs)]. The woman presents with vulvovaginal pruritus, burning pain, dyspareunia and postcoital bleeding. Vaginal erosions can produce adhesions. **Management** needs multidisciplinary team involvement. Ultrapotent topical corticosteroid (clobetasol 0.05%) is effective. Vaginal lichen planus is treated with corticosteroid, vaginal suppositories containing 25 mg of hydrocortisone. Surgical adhesiolysis is the last option. **The risk of malignancy is low**.

LICHEN SIMPLEX CHRONICUS

It presents with severe intractable pruritus, especially at night. Nonspecified inflammation involves the labia majora, mons pubis and the inner thighs. There may be erythema, swelling and lichenification. Symptoms may be exacerbated by chemicals or low body iron stores.

Investigations are done to look for thyroid dysfunction, diabetes, STIs, serum ferritin as 20% women suffer iron deficiency anemia. Autoimmune disorders (asthma, eczema) may be present. Skin biopsy may be needed for confirmation.

Mainstay of treatment is to avoid any irritants, antihistamines, ultrapotent topical steroids (clobetasol) are helpful to break the itch-scratch cycle. Corticosteroid suppository may be used.

EXTRAMAMMARY PAGET'S DISEASE

Extramammary Paget's disease of the vulva is a rare condition, seen in postmenopausal women. It presents with pruritus. On examination, the lesion appears florid eczematous with erythema and excoriation. **It can be associated with underlying adenocarcinoma.** The gastrointestinal (GI), urinary tract and the breasts should be checked.

Surgical excision is recommended to exclude adenocarcinoma of a skin appendage. Photodynamic therapy and topical imiquimod have been used with some success. Recurrence is common.

Vulvar intraepithelial neoplasia (VIN)—presents as vulvar skin disorders (p. 266).

VULVAR CROHN'S DISEASE

Crohn's disease affecting the intestine may involve the vulva in late stage of the disease in about 25% of cases. It may be precede GI symptoms. **Vulvar lesions are commonly metastatic.** It presents with typical granulomatous inflammation. It affects the inguinal, genitocrural and interlabial folds. The vulva is swollen, edematous with granulomas, abscesses, draining sinuses or ulceration. There may be classic **'knife-cut' fissures** in the interlabial sulci. Surgery may cause sinus and fistula formation and tissue breakdown. Therefore, it should be avoided. Histology shows nonspecific granulomatous inflammation.

Treatment

Multidisciplinary team involvement is needed. Potent topical steroids along with systemic steroids may be needed. Other medications include prolonged courses of metronidazole and oral immunomodulators (corticosteroids). Use of tumor necrosis factor (TNFα) blockers (infliximab) is found to be effective. Despite treatment recurrences are common.

PSORIASIS

It is a common and generalized skin disease of multifactorial origin. It is a T-cell mediated autoimmune disease. There is proliferation of proinflammatory cytokines, keratinocytes and endothelial cells. Vulvar skin is affected in about 20% of these affected women. The lesions are present on labia majora, genitocrural and inguinal folds. Often the lesions are symmetrical. The disease is chronic and has phases of remissions and exacerbations. **Skin changes are** silvery scale appearance and bleeding on gentle scraping. Vulvar psoriasis may resemble candidiasis. Psoriasis usually does not involve in the vaginal mucosa.

Treatment

Emollients, topical corticosteroid and calcipotriene are used to control the symptoms.

Oral therapy with methotrexate, cyclosporine may be used in resistant cases. Phototherapy gives short-term, relief. Severe cases may be treated with immune modulating agents like infliximab or ustekinumab.

RELATION WITH MALIGNANCY

About 50% of all invasive carcinomas of the vulva arise in an area of chronic vulvar epithelial disorder. **The malignant potential of VIN disorders is about 10–15%.** The chance is more with hyperplastic variety with cellular atypia (Fig. 18.3).

Vulvar Care in General

- Patients should avoid irritants, as the use of deodorants, spermicides, depilatory creams and perfumes (allergic or irritant dermatitis). Aqueous creams may be used.

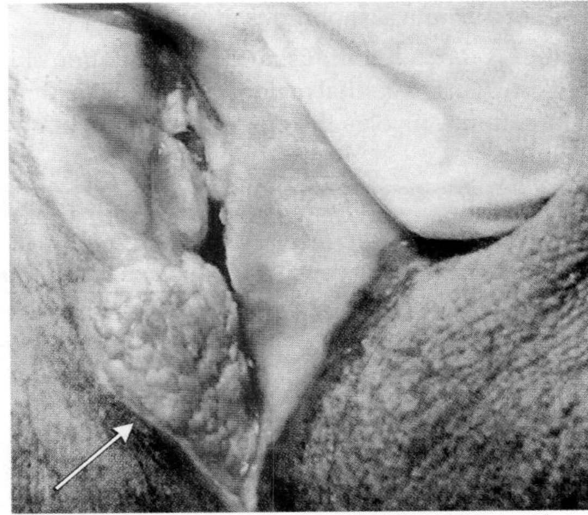

Fig. 18.3: Vulvar dystrophy associated with malignancy.

- A nonirritant soap should be used in the area and dried carefully without much rubbing.
- To avoid wearing tight-fitting pants.
- The patient should use either cotton underwear or nothing at all (at home).
- Histopathological diagnosis has to be made by biopsy prior to institution of any therapy.

Dermatitis, Eczema

Allergic contact dermatitis in the anogenital area may develop due to exposure with irritant agents. Patients present with burning, itching or with local erythema, edema or vesicle formation. Scaly patches and skin fissuring are seen. Patch testing is done to detect the allergen.

MANAGEMENT

All allergens or irritants should be avoided. Use of potent topical corticosteroids and immunomodulator (tacrolimus), bland emollients are effective and also control flares. For dry skin moisturizing with emollients are helpful. Antihistamines at night may be helpful to reduce scratching.

VULVAR ULCERS

Vulvar ulcers are predominantly due to sexually transmitted diseases (STDs). Rarely, it may be due to nonspecific causes. Malignant ulcer may be present. The various etiological factors related to vulvar ulcers are given in the Table 18.1.

All are described in appropriate Chapters. **Other systemic diseases with vulvar manifestation** are mentioned below.

Crohn's disease: See above (vulvar Crohn's disease).

Behçet's disease: This is a rare chronic autoinflammatory disease characterized by recurrent oral and genital ulcers (cervix, vulva or vagina) with ocular ulcer (anterior uveitis). It may be the manifestation of an underlying autoimmune process with systemic vasculitis. It may affect the brain, GI tract, lungs, joints and the vessels. Monoarticular arthritis may also be associated. The vulvar ulceration may be extensive and leaving behind dense scar after healing.

Treatment is similar to aphthous ulcer.

Vitiligo: It is a condition of skin depigmentation (loss of melanocytes) in the genital region. Genetic factory may be the cause. It may involve the other parts of the body also. It is usually observed as a patchy and symmetrical lesion. It is an autoimmune disorder that destroys the melanocytes. Autoimmune diseases like thyroiditis, Graves disease, diabetes, rheumatoid arthritis, psoriasis, vulvar lichen sclerosus are often associated.

There is no specific treatment. Narrow band ultraviolet B, phototherapy, excimer laser therapy and topical immune modulators have been used. **Topical and systemic corticosteroids are used for relief of the symptoms.** Systemic immunomodulators are found useful.

Reiter's disease: It is an ulcerative lesion of the vulva. It is an inflammatory response of the vulva following infections of the bowel or lower genital tract. It manifests with arthritis, uveitis and skin lesions. The histological picture is similar to pustular psoriasis.

Aphthous ulcer: It is seen over oral mucosa and also on the vulvar and vaginal surfaces. Ulcers are painful. Etiology is unknown and is thought to be immune-mediated. Stress, infections, nutritional deficiencies of vitamin B_{12}, folic acid, iron and zinc have been found to be related.

Treatment: HIV needs to be excluded. High potency topical corticosteroids are found useful. Oral corticosteroids may be needed in few cases.

Lipschutz ulcer: The lesion affects mainly the labia minora and introitus. In acute state, there may be constitutional upset with lymphadenopathy. The causative agent may be Epstein-Barr virus. Treatment is with antiseptic lotions and ointment.

Acanthosis nigricans: It is characterized by valvety to warty brown to black, poorly marginated plaques.

Sites: It is seen on the flexures of the neck, axillae and the genitocrural folds.

It is commonly associated with polycystic ovarian syndrome, obesity and diabetes. The skin thickness of acanthosis nigricans is due to insulin resistance. The resultant hyperinsulinemia causes dermal fibroblast proliferation.

Treatment: Weight loss improves insulin resistance. Metformin—improves the condition. Topical keratolytics may be helpful.

Leukemia: Rarely may cause nodular infiltration and ulceration of the vulva.

Dermatological disorders: Disseminated lupus erythematosus may cause recurrent ulcerations of the vulva and mucous membrane of the mouth and vagina.

TABLE 18.1: Ulcers of the vulva.

Sexually transmitted infections (STIs) related	*Autoimmune*	*Tuberculosis*	*Malignancy*	*Systemic disease related or dermatoses*
▪ Syphilis ▪ Herpes genitalis ▪ Chancroid ▪ Granuloma inguinale ▪ Lymphogranuloma venereum	▪ Behçet's disease ▪ Reiter's disease ▪ Aphthous ulcers ▪ Lipschutz ulcers	Tubercular infection	**Primary** ▪ Squamous cell carcinoma ▪ Malignant melanoma ▪ Basal cell carcinoma **Secondary** ▪ Leukemia ▪ Choriocarcinoma	▪ Lupus erythematosus ▪ Crohn's disease ▪ Lichen planus ▪ Lichen sclerosus ▪ Sjogren's syndrome ▪ Acanthosis nigricans

VULVAR MANIFESTATIONS OF SYSTEMIC DISEASES

Vulvar manifestations of systemic illness may occur on vulvar or vaginal mucosa in the form of bullous, nodular or ulcerative lesions. Diseases are SLE, sarcoidosis, or Stevens-Johnson syndrome.

- **Dermatologic disorders:** (a) Contact dermatitis—due to agents that may be locally irritant; (b) Psoriasis; (c) Ulceration due to disseminated lupus erythematosus.
- **Vulvar ulceration or deposits** due to **leukemia**.
- **Acanthosis nigricans:** The characteristic skin changes are thickened, hyperpigmented and velvety areas over the labia majora and perianal region. Similar skin changes are observed in the region of the neck and axilla.

  It is commonly observed in women with obesity, diabetes and polycystic ovarian syndrome (PCOS) (p. 384). Specific skin changes are due to insulin resistance (hyperinsulinemia).

  Treatment is mainly weight reduction. Other managements are similar to that of PCOS.
- **Behçet's syndrome** see above.
- **Chronic vulvovaginal candidiasis:** Due to diabetes, obesity and antibiotic use. Correction of basic pathology and prolonged topical antifungal therapy clears the infection.
- **Sjogren's syndrome:** Patients present with vaginal dryness and pain associated with ocular or oral dryness. There may be arthralgia, myalgia due to presence of autoantibodies. **Management** is symptomatic. Hydroxychloroquine is helpful. Corticosteroids may be needed.

MISCELLANEOUS SWELLINGS

VULVAR CYSTS

Bartholin's cyst: Ch. 12.

Sebaceous cyst: These are usually multiple and are formed by accumulation of the sebaceous material due to occlusion of the ducts. These are located in the labia majora. If infected, treatment is done by antibiotics and surgical drainage.

Cyst of the canal of Nuck: Part of the processus vaginalis, which accompanied the round ligament and got obliterated prior to birth may persist to form a cyst. It invariably occupies the anterior part of the labium majus.

Inguinolabial hernia: When the entire processus vaginalis remains patent, there may be herniation of the abdominal contents along the tract. The hernia may be limited to the inguinal canal or may extend up to the anterior part of the labium majus. The contents of the sac may be intestine or omentum. The swelling is reducible and impulse on straining can be elicited. **One should be conscious of the entity as casual surgical incision on labial swelling may cause inadvertent injury to the gut.**

Vulvar varicosities: These are met predominantly during pregnancy and subside following delivery. Sometimes, they may produce intolerable aching on standing. Support pads and tights or T-bandage may be tried to relieve the symptoms.

Elephantiasis vulva: It is mainly due to consequence of lymphatic obstruction by microfilaria (filariasis). Plastic surgery may be tried to restore the normal anatomy along with antifilarial treatment. There is a chance of recurrence.

Ectopic breast tissue: It may rarely be present in the embryological milk lines that extend from the axilla to the mons pubis. This breast tissue may be hormonally sensitive and may enlarge during pregnancy.

BENIGN TUMORS OF THE VULVA

- **Fibroma, lipoma, neurofibroma:** These are all benign tumors of varying sizes. Fibroma or leiomyoma is the most common benign solid tumor of the vulva. It arises from deeper connective tissues of the labia majora (dermatofibroma). Vulvar fibroma grow slowly. It may be small but **malignant change is very low**. *These tumours need study with USG including doppler to differentiate from any vascular tumour like hemangioma.* Surgical removal is necessary as they produce discomfort (Figs. 18.4 and 18.5).

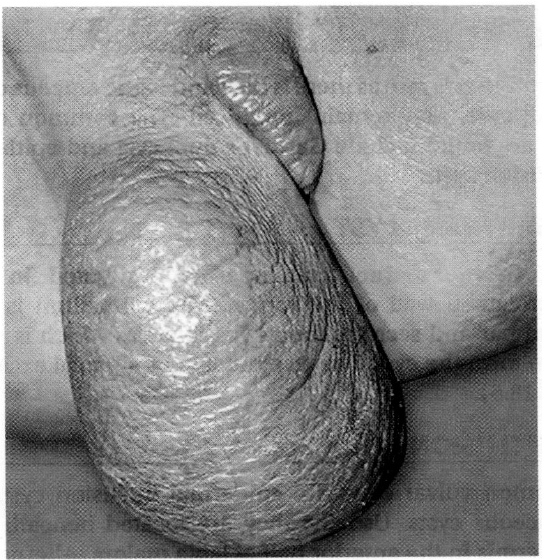

Fig. 18.4: Vulvar fibroma.

(*Courtesy:* Dr Chandana Das, Professor and Head, Department of Obstetrics and Gynecology, NRS Medical College, Kolkata, India).

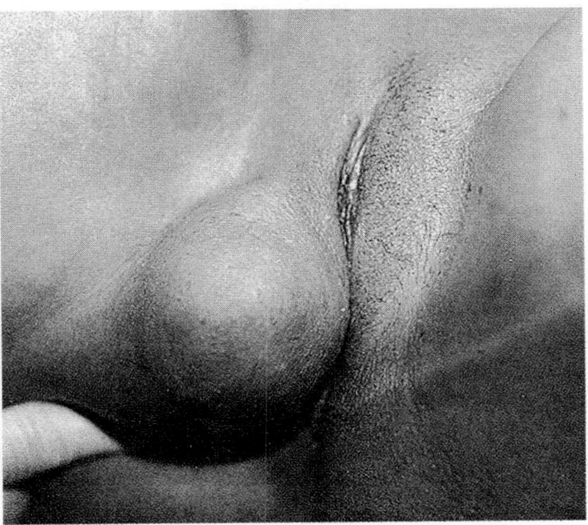

Fig. 18.5: Vulvar lipoma.

- **Hydradenoma:** Hydradenoma arises from the sweat gland in the vulva, usually located in the anterior part of the labia majora (38%). It rarely exceeds 1 cm. It is a benign lesion but its reddish look and complex adenomatous pattern on histology may be confused with adenocarcinoma. Simple excision and biopsy is adequate.

VULVAR ENDOMETRIOSIS

Vulvar endometriosis is usually found at the site of old obstetric laceration, episiotomy or area of excised Bartholin's duct cyst. It may appear as a swelling near the insertion of the round ligaments in the anterior part of the labia majora. It may be associated with pelvic endometriosis. Its presence is limited only during reproductive period and becomes enlarged and tender during menstruation. Treatment is surgical excision and *confirmation by biopsy* (endometrial glands and stroma with hemosiderin-laden macrophages).

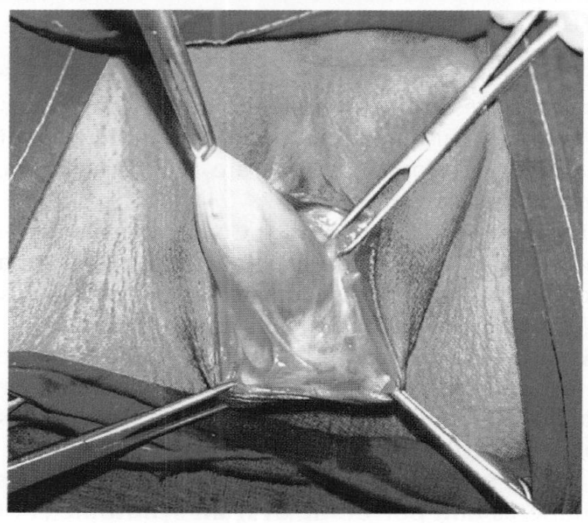

Fig. 18.6: Gartner's duct cyst.

VAGINAL WALL CYSTS

Vaginal cyst is rare as there is no gland in the mucous coat. Small cysts may remain unnoticed. The common cysts that are found include Gartner's duct cyst and epithelial inclusion cyst.

GARTNER'S CYST

The Gartner's duct cyst is usually situated in the anterolateral wall of the vagina. The epithelium is low columnar and secretes mucinous material which is pent up to form the cyst. The treatment is by surgical excision (Fig. 18.6).

INCLUSION CYST

Common vulvar cysts are epidermal inclusion cysts or sebaceous cysts. Usually, they are located beneath the epidermis in the anterior half of labia majora. Alternative histogenesis is embryonic remnants or occlusion of pilosebaceous ducts of sweat glands.

The vaginal epithelial inclusion (epidermoid) cysts arise from the epithelium buried under the mucosa during healing from a traumatic injury following childbirth or surgery. They are usually located in the lower-third of the vagina on the posterior or posterolateral wall. The lining epithelium is stratified squamous (epidermoid cyst). The content is a thick cheesy or viscous material. **The treatment** in symptomatic cases is by surgical excision (Figs. 18.7A and B).

VULVAR PAIN SYNDROME

Vulvar pain (Table 18.2) sensation may be burning, stinging or irritation. It may be due to several reasons:

- Aphthous ulcer
- Vulvar dermatoses
- Herpes genitalis
- Pudendal or genitofemoral nerve neuralgia

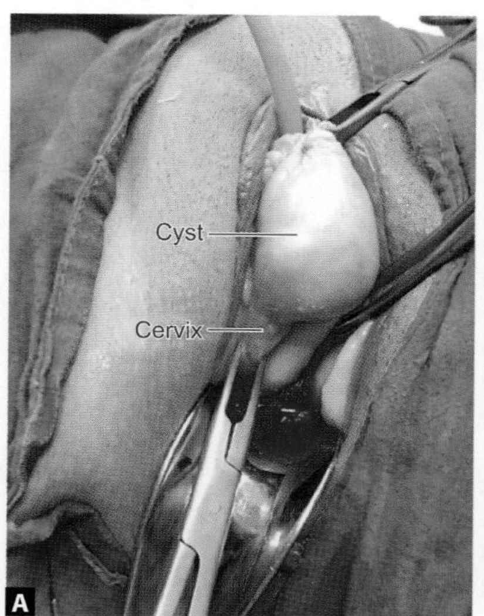

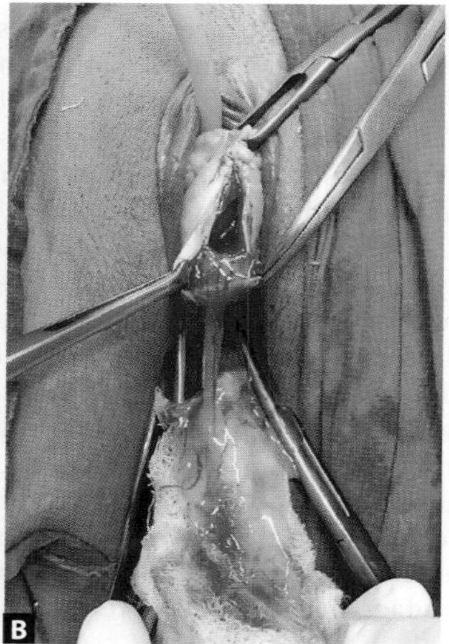

Figs. 18.7A and B: (A) Vaginal wall inclusion cyst; (B) Same cyst is being excised.

TABLE 18.2: Classification of vulvar pain (ISSVD).

A. Vulvar pain with specific disorders	B. Vulvodynia generalized	C. Vulvodynia localized (vestibulodynia, clitorodynia, etc.)
▪ Infections ▪ Inflammations ▪ Neurogenic ▪ Neoplastic	▪ Provoked ▪ Unprovoked ▪ Mixed	▪ Provoked ▪ Unprovoked ▪ Mixed

- Vulvodynia (burning vulva syndrome)
- Vulvar vestibulitis syndrome (VVS)
- Referred pain from urethral or vagina
- Psychological.

VULVODYNIA

It is a severely painful socially debilitating disease where infection, invasive disease or inflammation have been excluded. There is absence of any relevant visible finding and clinically identified neurological disorders. It is **characterized by burning sensation over the vulva (burning vulva syndrome)**. It is often seen in perimenopausal or postmenopausal women. Exact etiology is not known. Patient may have associated other chronic pain disorders (irritable bowel, interstitial cystitis). Clinical examination does not reveal any abnormality in most of the cases. It is a diagnosis of exclusion (ACOG). Cotton swab test to detect the tender area (pain mapping) may be helpful. **Treatment is unsatisfactory**. There is no specific therapy. Behavioral therapy (vulvar care treatment) to be followed.

Medications: Topical agents used: 5% lidocaine applied over the vestibule found to relief dyspareunia. Tricyclic antidepressant (amitriptyline) is found helpful. A dose of 60 mg/day for 3–6 months is given. Carbamazepine or gabapentin is also found beneficial. Yeast culture is done from the positive cotton swab test. Antifungal therapy may be helpful in that case. Psychosexual counseling, biofeedback and physical therapy are needed for some cases.

Surgery: Resection of the vestibule (vestibulectomy) and or perineoplasty may be done.

Vulvar vestibulitis syndrome is a condition of hyperesthesia (allodynia), pain without any painful stimuli. It is characterized by pain around the ducts of Bartholin gland and the introitus. There may be superficial dyspareunia and vestibular tenderness on touch.

TREATMENT

Treatment needs sympathetic approach. Considering the various, etiologies, numerous treatment options are available. Improvement of vulvar local hygiene, control of infective agents and allergens, diet modification (low oxalate) are the initial steps. Psychological **tricyclic antidepressants, gabapentin, biofeedback**, behavioral treatment and even surgery (vestibulectomy, perineoplasty, laser vaporization) have been tried. Surgery is done in women only who have failed with conservative management. Treatment results are often unsatisfactory.

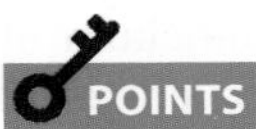

POINTS

- **Etiology** of vulvar epithelial disorders are multiple.
- Infection, inflammation, trauma (scratching), autoimmune, allergy (atopic), nutritional (deficiency of folic acid, vitamin B_{12}, riboflavin, or achlorhydria) are implicated.
- **Diagnosis of vulvar epithelial disorders** needs details of history, symptoms, including sexual history.
- **Lichen sclerosus** usually occurs following menopause. It is an autoimmune disease. The lesion can extend beyond the labiocrural folds to the thighs. Pruritus is more than soreness. The risk of malignancy is 4–6%. Ultrapotent topical corticosteroid (clobetesol 0.05%) is effective.
- **Vulvar Crohn's disease** present with classic 'Knife-cut' fissures in the interlabial sulci. Such a patient needs multidisciplinary team involvement.
- **Ulcers of the vulva** may be: (a) STI related; (b) Idiopathic; (c) Tubercular; (d) Malignancy; (e) Systemic disease related.
- Women with lichen sclerosus or planus should be investigated for autoimmune conditions
- **About 50%** of all invasive carcinomas of the vulva arise in an area of chronic vulvar epithelial disorder. Only 10–15% of VIN may develop malignancy. Multiple biopsies are to be taken from the sky blue areas left behind after applying 1% aqueous toluidine blue and washed off with 1% acetic acid. Cases with atypia have got increased chance of malignancy. Considering the risk, local vulvectomy is justified specially when associated with atypia (p. 281).
- **Vulvar cyst** may be—Bartholin's cyst, sebaceous cyst or cyst of canal of Nuck.
- **Vulvar ulcers** are predominantly STI related but other pathology may be there (Table 18.1).
- **Vulvodynia** is a painful condition of the vulva of unknown etiology. Psychosexual counseling, behavioral therapy, tricyclic antidepressants (amitriptyline) are helpful.
- **Vulvar vestibulitis syndrome**—may be a generalized or focal painful condition of unknown etiology. Topical agents (steroids, antifungal creams), vestibulectomy, behavioral therapy, have been tried.
- **Vaginal ulcer** is rare. Common vaginal cysts are Gartner's cyst and epithelial inclusion cyst.

CHAPTER

19 Benign Lesions of the Cervix

CHAPTER OUTLINE

- Cervical Ectopy (Erosion)
- Eversion (Ectropion)
- Cervical Tear
- Cervical Cysts
- Elongation of the Cervix

CERVICAL ECTOPY (EROSION)

Definition

Cervical ectopy is a condition where the squamous epithelium of the ectocervix is replaced by columnar epithelium, which is continuous with the endocervix. It is not an ulcer (Figs. 19.1A and B).

Etiology

- **Congenital**
- **Acquired**

Congenital

At birth, in about one-third of cases, the columnar epithelium of the endocervix extends beyond the external os. This condition persists only for a few days until the level of estrogen derived from the mother falls. Thus, the congenital ectopy heals spontaneously.

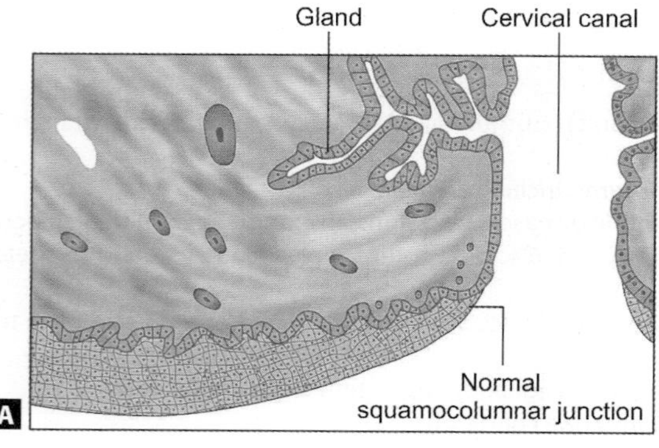

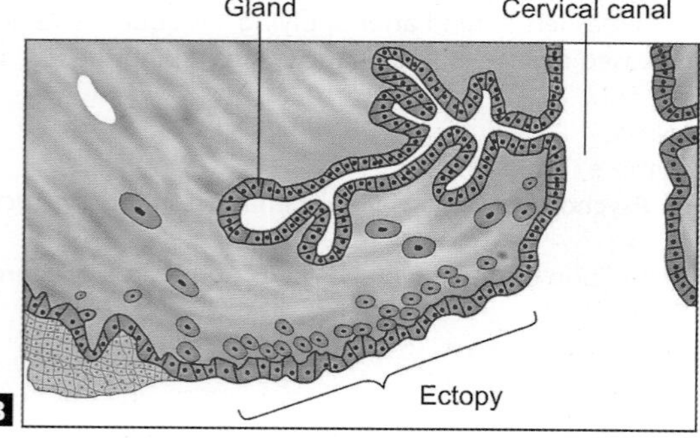

Figs. 19.1A and B: (A) Normal squamocolumnar junction; (B) Ectopy.

Acquired

Hormonal: The squamocolumnar junction (SCJ) is not static and its movement, either inwards or outwards is dependent on estrogen. When the estrogen level is high, it moves out so that the columnar epithelium extends onto the vaginal portion of the cervix replacing the squamous epithelium. **This state is observed during pregnancy and amongst 'pill users'.** The squamocolumnar junction returns back to its normal position after 3 months following delivery and little earlier following withdrawal of 'pill'.

Infection: The role of infection as the primary cause of ectopy has been discarded. However, chronic cervicitis may be associated or else the infection may supervene on an ectopy because of the delicate columnar epithelium which is more vulnerable to trauma and infection.

Pathogenesis

In the active phase of ectopy, the squamocolumnar junction moves out from the os. The columnar epithelium of the endocervix maintains its continuity while covering the ectocervix replacing the squamous epithelium. The replaced epithelium is usually arranged in a **single layer (flat type)** or may be so hyperplastic as to fold inwards to accommodate in the increased area—**a follicular ectopy.** At times, it becomes heaped up to fold inwards and outwards—**a papillary ectopy** (Fig. 19.2). Underneath the epithelium, there are evidences of round cell infiltration and glandular proliferation. The features of infection are probably secondary rather than primary. The columnar epithelium is less resistant to infection than the squamous epithelium.

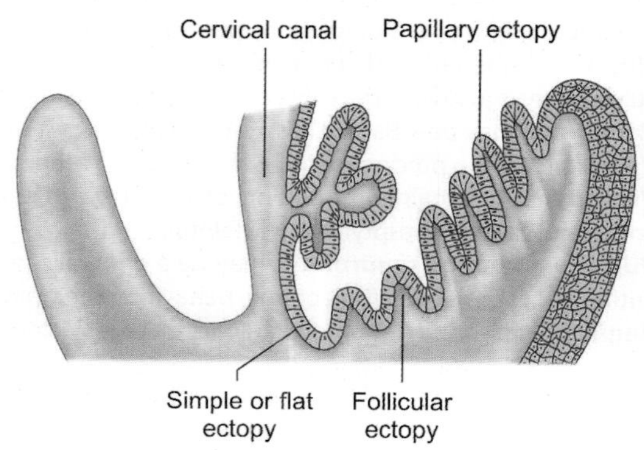

Fig. 19.2: Different types of ectopy.

During the process of healing, the squamocolumnar junction gradually moves up towards the external os. The squamous epithelium grows beneath the columnar epithelium until it reaches at or near to its original position at the external os. Alternatively, the replacement is probably by squamous metaplasia of the columnar cells. The possibility of squamous metaplasia of the reserve cells is also likely (details in Ch. 23).

During the process, the squamous epithelium may obstruct the mouth of the underlying glands (normally not present in ectocervix) → pent up secretion → retention cyst → **nabothian follicle**. Alternatively, the epithelium may burrow inside the gland lumina. **This process of replacement by the squamous epithelium is called epidermidization**.

Clinical Features

Symptoms: The lesion may be asymptomatic. However, the following symptoms may be present.

- Vaginal discharge—the discharge may be excessively mucoid. It may be mucopurulent, offensive and irritant in presence of infection; may be even blood-stained.
- Contact bleeding especially during pregnancy and 'pill use' either following coitus or defecation may be associated.
- Associated cervicitis may produce backache, pelvic pain and at times, infertility.

Signs: Internal examination reveals (Figs. 19.3A to D):

- Per speculum—there is a bright red area surrounding and extending beyond the external os in the ectocervix. The outer edge is clearly demarcated. The lesion may be smooth or having small papillary folds. It is neither tender nor bleeds to touch. On rubbing with a gauze piece, there may be multiple oozing spots (sharp bleeding in isolated spots in carcinoma).

  The feel is soft and granular giving rise to a grating sensation.

Differential Diagnosis

The diagnosis is confused with:

Ectropion: The lips of the cervix are curled back to expose the endocervix. This may be apparent when the lips of the cervix are stretched by the bivalve speculum.

Early carcinoma: It is indurated, friable and usually ulcerated which bleeds to touch. Confirmation is by biopsy (Ch. 23).

Primary lesion (chancre): The ulcer has a punched-out appearance (Ch. 12).

Tubercular ulcer: There is indurated ulcer with caseation at the base. Biopsy confirms the diagnosis.

Management

Guidelines: All cases should be subjected to cytological examination from the cervical smear to exclude dysplasia or malignancy (p. 90).

Symptomatic cases

- Detected during pregnancy and early puerperium, the treatment should be withheld for at least 12 weeks postpartum. In pill users, the 'pill' should be stopped and barrier method is advised.
- Persistent ectopy with troublesome discharge should be treated surgically by—(a) thermal cauterization; (b) cryosurgery; and (c) laser vaporization (Ch. 23).

All the methods employed are based on the principle of destruction of the columnar epithelium to be followed by its healing by the squamous epithelium.

EVERSION (ECTROPION)

In chronic cervicitis, there is marked thickening of the cervical mucosa with underlying tissue edema. These thickened tissues tend to push out through the external os along the direction of least resistance. The entity is most marked where the cervix has already been lacerated. In such conditions, the longitudinal muscle fibers are free to act unopposed. Due to this, the lips of the cervix curl upwards and outwards to expose the red looking endocervix so as to be confused with ectopy (Figs. 19.3A to D). As a result the SCJ lies external to the cervical os.

CERVICAL TEAR

Varying degrees of cervical tear is invariable during vaginal delivery. One or both the sides may be torn or the tear may be irregular (stellate type). If there is no superimposed infection and the tear is small, the torn surfaces may appose leaving behind only a small notch. However, if infection supervenes, eversion occurs confusing the diagnosis of ectopy (Figs. 19.3A to D).

Nonobstetric causes of cervical lacerations are during operative procedures of dilatation of the cervix. Postmenopausal atrophy or chronic cervicitis predisposes to tear.

CERVICAL CYSTS

Nabothian Cysts (Fig. 19.4)

These are usually multiple. They are formed due to blocking of the cervical gland mouths usually as a result of healing of ectopy by metaplastic squamous epithelium.

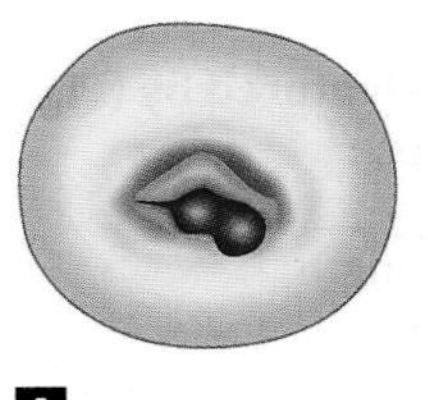

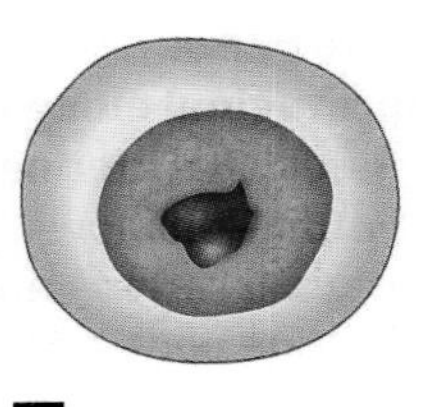

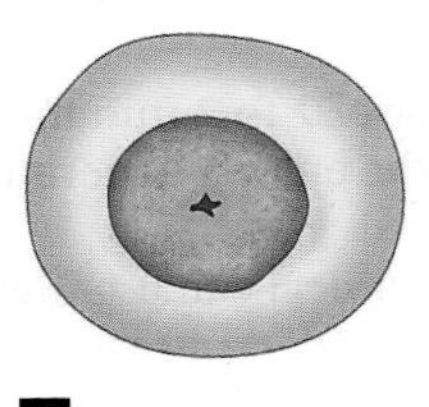

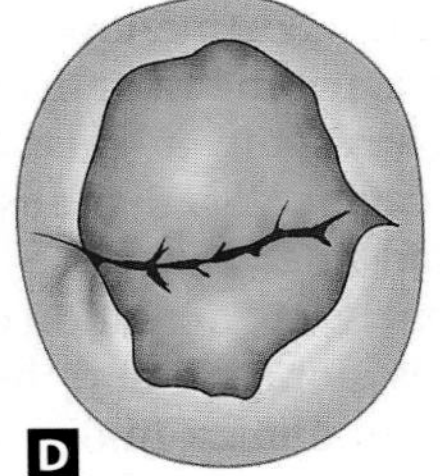

Figs. 19.3A to D: Common benign lesions in the cervix: (A) Polyp; (B) Polyp with ectopy; (C) Ectopy; (D) Eversion.

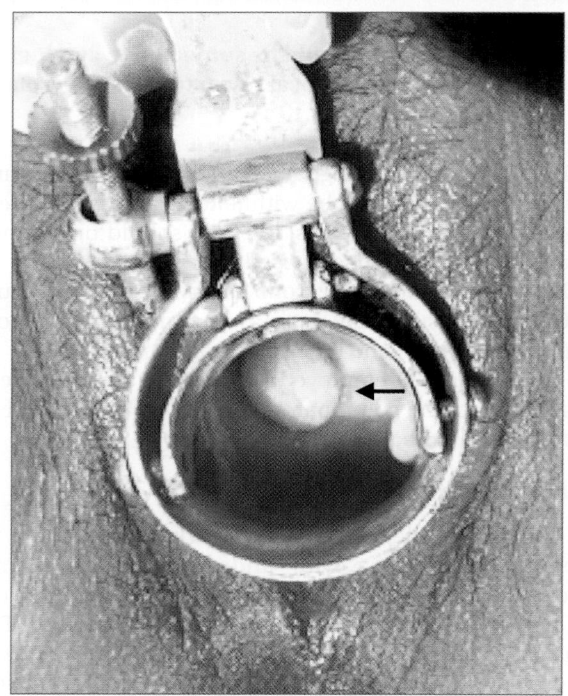

Fig. 19.4: Nabothian cyst of cervix (arrow).

The pent up secretion produces cysts of varying sizes from microscopic to pea. **The presence of the cysts furthest from the external os indicates the extent of transformation zone**. The lining epithelium is columnar. The treatment is to open up the cyst for drainage.

Endometriotic Cysts

These are situated in the portio vaginalis part of the cervix. The cyst is small and reddish and of less than 1 cm in diameter. It is more explained by the implantation theory. The implantation of the endometrium occurs during delivery or surgery. The lining epithelium shows endometrial glands and stroma.

Symptoms include intermenstrual or postcoital bleeding, deep dyspareunia and dysmenorrhea. Speculum examination reveals a small reddish cyst. The treatment is destruction by cauterization and rarely by excision.

Cervical Stenosis

It is due to narrowing of the cervical canal. It may be congenital or acquired. Congenital is due to hypoplasia of the lower part of Müllerian ducts. Acquired may be due operative trauma (forceps delivery), LLETZ, D/E, cervical amputation, infection, neoplasia, radiation or cone biopsy.
Symptoms: Dysmenorrhea, pelvic pain, amenorrhea and infertility. Postmenopausal women may develop hematometra, pyometra or hydrometra.
Diagnosis: Resistance to pass a dilator of 1 to 2 mm into the uterine cavity. USG demonstrates the enlarged uterine size with fluid-filled cavity.
Management: Slow dilatation of the cervical canal under anesthesia is done. It may be done under ultrasound guidance to minimize injury. Misoprostol may be used to soften the cervix. A latex tube may be kept in the cervical canal for sometime to maintain the patency. In postmenopausal women endometrial biopsy when needed, should be done after 7 days following drainage of the pyometra or hematometra.

Cervical Polyps

Polyps are the most common benign neoplastic growth of the cervix. Polyps may arise from the endocervical canal (common) or from the ectocervix. Polyps develop secondary to the effect of chronic inflammation or due to hormonal stimulation. Endocervical polyps are usually reddish in color whereas the cervical polyps are grayish white.
Symptoms: Most patients present with intermenstrual bleeding, postcoital bleeding, vaginal discharge. Sometimes it remains asymptomatic and often diagnosed incidentally during routine speculum examination.
Histology: (a) Surface epithelium is columnar or squamous epithelium (squamous metaplasia); (b) The pedicle is composed of vascular connective tissue which is loose, inflamed and edematous.

Histologic subtypes are: (a) Adenomatous; (b) Fibromyomatous; (c) **Malignant change of an endocervical polyp is rare (0.5%)**.
Treatment: Avulsion of the polyp with a sponge forceps and removal on twisting mostly is done. The specimen is sent for histological examination. The pedicle of the polyp when present may be treated with electrodiathermy. Endometrial curettage may be done following polypectomy in women older than 40 years to rule out any coexisting pathology.

ELONGATION OF THE CERVIX

The normal length of the cervix is about 2.5 cm. The vaginal and the supravaginal parts are of equal length. The elongation may affect either part of the cervix.

Causes

Elongation of the supravaginal part is commonly associated with the uterine prolapse. The mechanism has been described in page 175.

Vaginal part is always elongated congenitally. Chronic cervicitis may produce some hypertrophy and makes the **cervix bulky**.

Symptoms

There is no specific symptom for supravaginal elongation. However, congenital elongation of the vaginal part may present the following:
- Sensation of something coming down
- Dyspareunia
- Infertility.

Pelvic Examination

Supravaginal elongation is featured by (Fig. 19.5):
- Associated uterine prolapse
- Fornix—shallow
- Vaginal cervix—normal length
- Uterine body—normal in size.
- Uterocervical canal—increased in length evidenced by introduction of an uterine sound. This indirectly proves that the increase is in the supravaginal part.

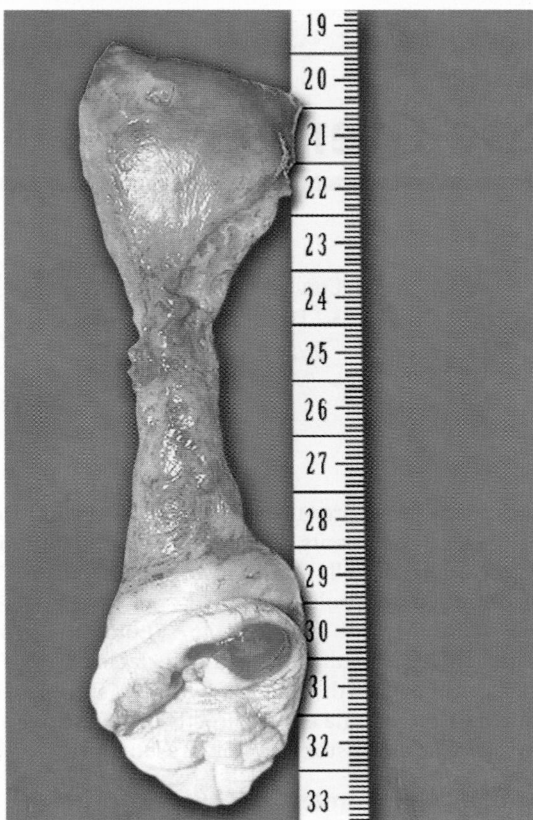

Fig. 19.5: Supravaginal elongation of cervix in prolapse.

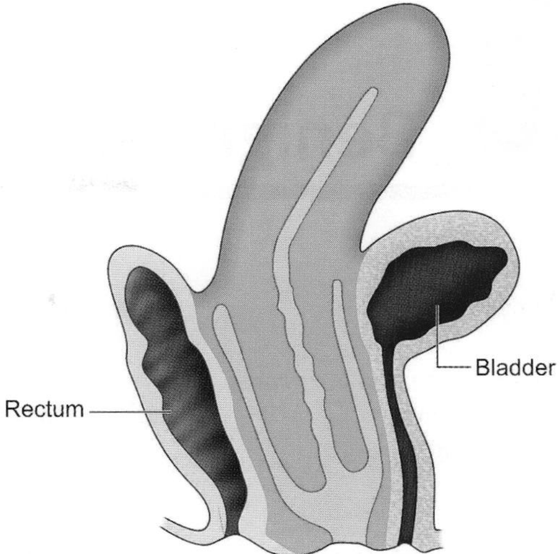

Fig. 19.6: Congenital elongation of cervix.

Congenital elongation is featured by (Fig. 19.6):

- Fornix—deep
- Vaginal cervix—elongated
- Uterine body—normal in size
- Uterocervical canal—increased in length, evidenced by uterine sound.

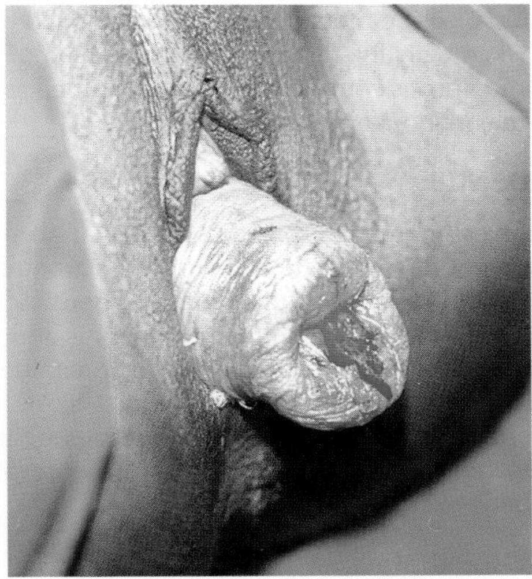

Fig. 19.7: Congenital elongation of cervix with prolapse.

Treatment

- **Supravaginal elongation (Fig. 19.5):** As it is associated with uterine prolapse, its treatment protocol will be the same as that for prolapse.
- **Congenital elongation (Fig. 19.7):** The excess length of the cervix is amputated (cervical amputation). In presence of congenital prolapse, some form of cervicopexy has to be done (p. 180).

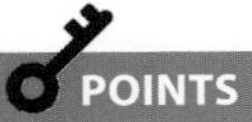

POINTS

- **Chronic cervicitis and cervical ectopy** are the two most common cervical lesions encountered in gynecological practice.
- **Cervical ectopy (erosion)** may be congenital (circumoral) or acquired due to hormonal effect as observed during pregnancy and 'pill users'. The role of infection as the primary cause has been discarded.
- **Histologically**, the erosion is either flat, papillary or of follicular variety.
- **Healing of the ectopy** occurs through replacement of the columnar epithelium by downgrowth of the squamous epithelium or by squamous metaplasia of the columnar cells or the reserve cells. This process of replacement is called epidermidization. Ectopy is not a precancerous state.
- **Ectopy** is not an ulcer as it is entirely lined by columnar epithelium.
- All cases should be subjected to cytological examination to exclude dysplasia or malignancy.
- **In asymptomatic cases**, treatment should be withheld.
- **Detected during pregnancy**, treatment should be withheld for at least 12 weeks postpartum.
- **Persistent ectopy** with troublesome discharge should be treated surgically by thermal cauterization, cryosurgery or best by laser vaporization.
- **Cervical cysts** may be nabothian, endometriotic or mesonephric. The confirmation of diagnosis is by histology.
- **Supravaginal elongation** of the cervix is associated with uterine prolapse and elongation of the vaginal part of the cervix is congenital in origin. Supravaginal elongation needs to be differentiated from congenital elongation of the cervix.

CHAPTER

20 Benign Lesions of the Uterus

CHAPTER OUTLINE

- Leiomyomas
- Types
- Secondary Changes in Fibroids
- Clinical Features
- Investigations
- Management
  - Asymptomatic
  - Symptomatic
  - Medical
  - Surgical
- Cervical Fibroid
  - Treatment
- Polyps
  - Management

LEIOMYOMAS

Leiomyomas are **the most common benign tumors of the uterus** and also the most common benign solid tumor in female. Histologically, this tumor is composed of smooth muscle and fibrous connective tissue, so named as uterine leiomyoma, myoma or fibromyoma.

INCIDENCE

It has been estimated that at least 20% of women at the age of 30 have got fibroid in their wombs. Fortunately, most of them (50%) remain asymptomatic. The incidence of symptomatic fibroid in hospital outpatient is about 3%. A high incidence of 70% prevails in white women. In African-American women, the incidence is higher (80%).

These are more common in nulliparous or in those having one child infertility (Table 20.1). The prevalence is highest between 35 and 45 years.

TABLE 20.1: Risk factors for leiomyomas.

Risk factors	*Protective factors*
▪ Increasing age ▪ Early menarche ▪ Nulliparity ▪ Obesity, ↑ body mass index (BMI) ▪ Polycystic ovary syndrome (PCOS) ▪ Hyperestrogenic state ▪ Black women ▪ High fat diet ▪ Family history	▪ Late menarche ▪ Multiparity ▪ Menopause ▪ Combined oral contraceptives (COCs) use ▪ Smoking

HISTOGENESIS

Origin

The etiology still remains unclear. The prevailing hypothesis is that, it arises from the neoplastic single smooth muscle cell (myocyte) of the myometrium. Thus each myoma is monoclonal. The stimulus for initial neoplastic myocyte transformation is not known. The following are implicated:

- **Chromosomal abnormality:** In about 40% of cases, there is a varying type of chromosomal abnormality, particularly the chromosome seven (17%) or twelve (12%) (rearrangements, deletions). Somatic mutations in myometrial cells may also be the cause for uncontrolled cell proliferation.
- **Role of polypeptide growth factors:** Epidermal growth factor (EGF), insulin-like growth factor-1 (IGF-1), transforming growth factor-β (TGF-β), stimulate the growth of leiomyoma either directly or via estrogen.

  A positive family history is often present.

Growth of Leiomyomas

Leiomyoma-predominantly an Estrogen-dependent Tumor

- Both estrogen and progesterone receptors are found in higher concentrations in myomas.
- Myomas cells have higher levels of the enzyme aromatase. This increases the high local levels of estrogen.
- Are rare before menarche and majority decreases in size following menopause.
- They often enlarge during pregnancy.
- Hypoestrogenic conditions (GnRH agonist use) reduces the size of myomas.
- Hypercellularity of myomas (cellular leiomyomotas) are less common (<5%). Cellular myomas are often larger in size. Clinical presentation is more close to a sarcoma (leiomyosarcoma).
- However, most cellular leiomyomata have a benign course and prognosis.
- Myoma cell contains more estrogen receptors than the adjacent myometrium.
- Frequent association of anovulation.

The growth potentiality is not squarely distributed amongst the fibroids which are usually multiple, some grow faster than the others. On the whole, **the rate of growth is slow and it takes about 3–5 years for the fibroid to grow sufficiently to be felt per abdomen (c.f.—ovarian tumor grows in months).**

However, **the fibroid grows rapidly** during pregnancy. Rapid growth may also be due to degeneration or due to malignant change.

The newer low dose oral contraceptives may reduce the size.

TYPES

- **Body**
- **Cervical (Flowchart 20.1)**

Body

The fibroids are mostly located in the body of the uterus and are usually multiple (Flowchart 20.1, Figs. 20.1 and 20.2).

Interstitial or Intramural (75%)

Initially, the fibroids are intramural in position but subsequently, some are pushed outward or inward. Eventually, in about 70%, they persist in that position.

Subperitoneal or Subserous (15%)

In this condition, the intramural myoma is pushed outwards towards the peritoneal cavity. The fibroids are either partially or completely covered by peritoneum. When completely covered by peritoneum, it usually attains a pedicle—called pedunculated subserous myoma. On rare occasion, the pedicle may be torn through; the fibroid gets its nourishment from the omental or mesenteric adhesions and is called '**wandering**' or '**parasitic**' fibroid. Sometimes, the intramural fibroid may be pushed out in between the layers of broad ligament and is called broad ligament myoma (false or pseudo). **These myomas are difficult to differentiate from a solid ovarian tumor. These myoma may cause hydroureter. Leiomyomas may cause pseudo-Meig's syndrome (p. 245).**

Submucous (5%) (Fig. 20.3)

The intramural fibroid when pushed toward the uterine cavity, and is lying underneath the endometrium, it is called

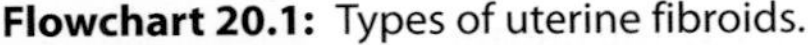

Flowchart 20.1: Types of uterine fibroids.

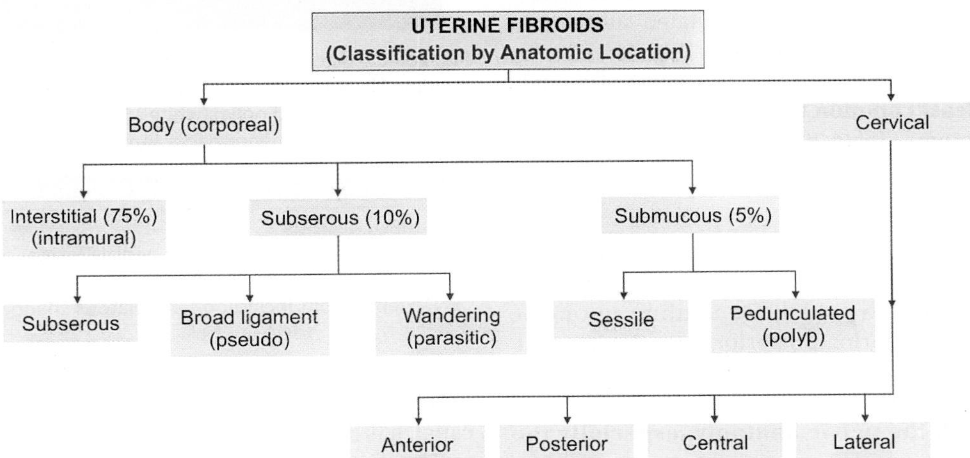

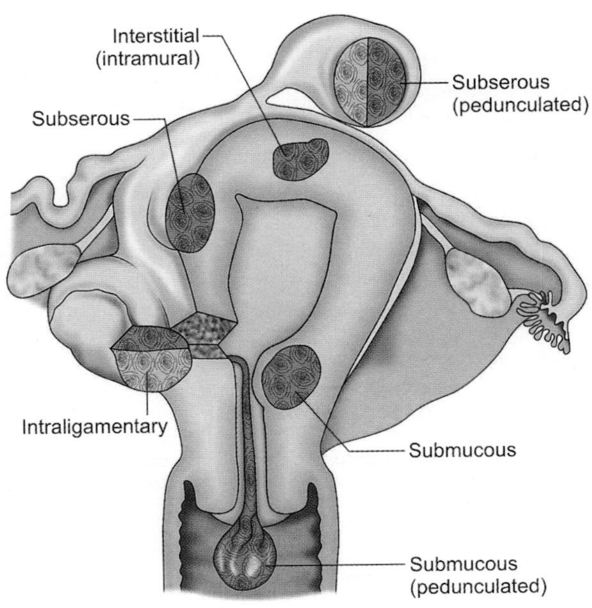

Fig. 20.1: Various types of uterine fibroids.

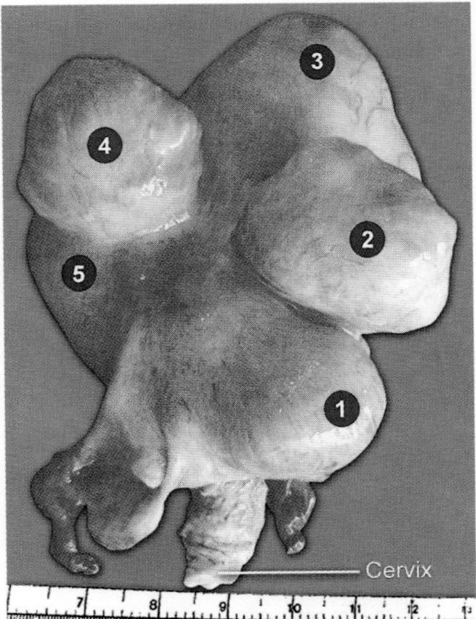

Fig. 20.2: Multiple fibroids causing marked distortion of the uterus. The uterine corpus is almost completely replaced by multiple myomas in subserous, intramural, and submucous positions (Multiple myomas, marked as 1 to 5).

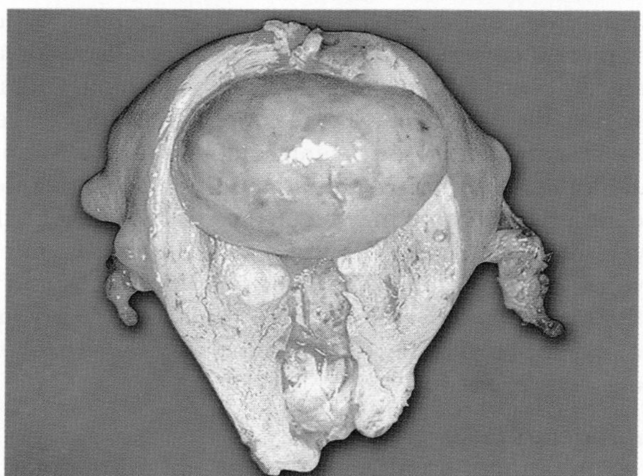

Fig. 20.3: Cut section of a uterus showing a submucous fibroid.

submucous fibroid. Submucous fibroid can make the uterine cavity irregular and distorted. Pedunculated submucous fibroid may come out through the cervix (Fig. 20.4). It may be infected or ulcerated to cause metrorrhagia. Although, **this variety is least common (about 5%)** but it produces maximum symptoms (Table 20.2) including infertility and miscarriage.

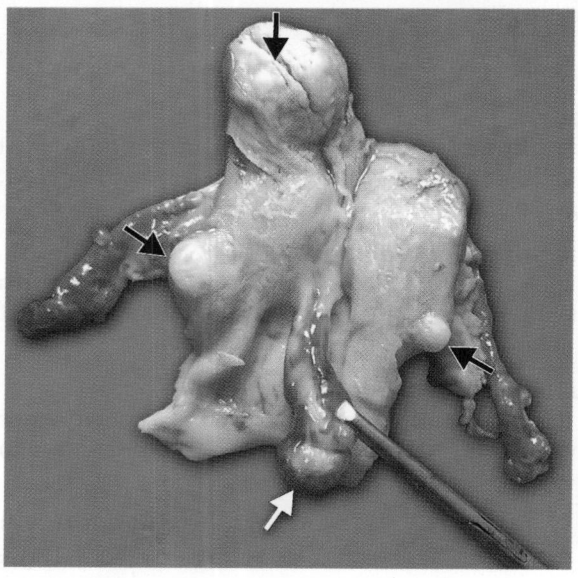

Fig. 20.4: Postoperative specimen of a uterus, cut opened to show multiple fibroids in the body (black arrows) and a long submucous pedunculated fibroid polyp (white arrow). This 45-year-old woman suffered from both menorrhagia and intermenstrual bleeding.

Cervical

Cervical fibroid is rare (1–2%). In the supravaginal part of the cervix, it may be interstitial or subperitoneal variety and rarely polypoidal. Depending upon the position, it may be anterior, posterior, lateral or central. Interstitial growths may displace the cervix or expand it so much that the external os is difficult to recognize. **All these disturb the pelvic anatomy, especially the ureter.**

In the vaginal cervix, the fibroid is usually pedunculated and rarely sessile.

TABLE 20.2: The eventual fate of a submucous fibroid.

- Surface necrosis
- Polypoid change—following pedicle formation
- Infection
- Degenerations including sarcomatous change

Pseudocervical fibroid: A fibroid polyp arising from the uterine body when occupies and distends the cervical canal, it is called pseudocervical fibroid.

The leiomyoma subclassification system proposed by FIGO useful for clinical investigation is shown in Figure 20.5.

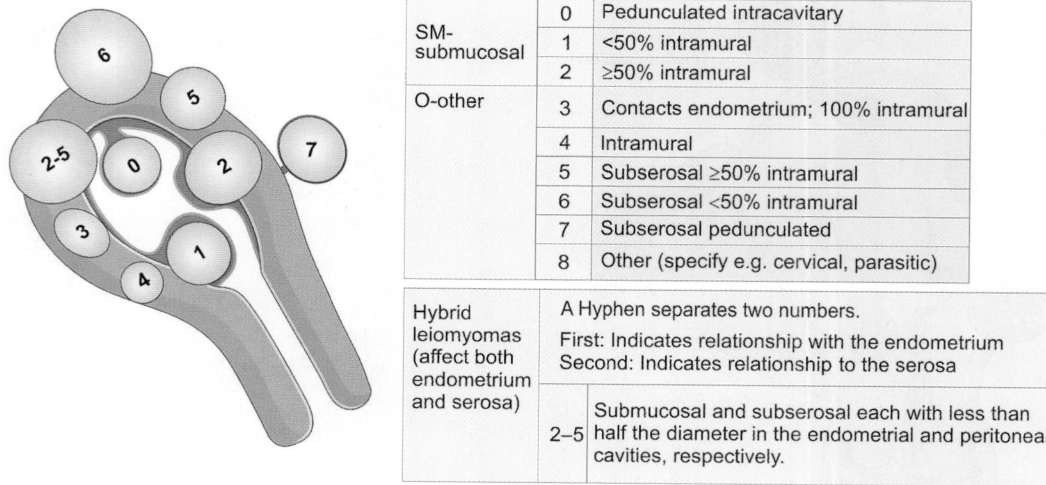

SM-submucosal	0	Pedunculated intracavitary
	1	<50% intramural
	2	≥50% intramural
O-other	3	Contacts endometrium; 100% intramural
	4	Intramural
	5	Subserosal ≥50% intramural
	6	Subserosal <50% intramural
	7	Subserosal pedunculated
	8	Other (specify e.g. cervical, parasitic)
Hybrid leiomyomas (affect both endometrium and serosa)		A Hyphen separates two numbers. First: Indicates relationship with the endometrium Second: Indicates relationship to the serosa
	2–5	Submucosal and subserosal each with less than half the diameter in the endometrial and peritoneal cavities, respectively.

Fig. 20.5: Leiomyoma subclassification system.

Source: Modified from M.G. Munro et al. FIGO classification system (PALM-COEIN) for causes of abnormal uterine bleeding in nongravid women of reproductive age. *International Journal of Gynecology and Obstetrics* 113 (2011) 3–13.

BODY OR CORPOREAL FIBROIDS

PATHOLOGY

Naked Eye Appearance

The uterus is enlarged; the shape is distorted by multiple nodular growth of varying sizes. Occasionally, there may be uniform enlargement of the uterus by a single fibroid. The feel is firm (Fig. 20.3).

Cut surface of the tumor is smooth and whitish. The cut section, in the absence of degenerative changes, shows features of whorled appearance and trabeculation. These are due to the intermingling of fibrous tissues with the muscle bundles.

The false capsule is formed by the compressed adjacent myometrium. They have more parallel arrangement and are pinkish in color in contrast to whitish appearance of the tumor. The capsule is separated from the growth by a thin loose areolar tissue. The blood vessels run through this plane to supply the tumor. It is through this plane that the tumor is shelled out during myomectomy operation. The periphery of the tumor is more vascular and have more growth potentiality. **The center of the tumor is least vascular and likely to degenerate.** It is due to contraction of the false capsule that makes the cut surface of the tumor to bulge out.

Microscopic Appearance (Fig. 20.6)

The tumor consists of smooth muscles and fibrous connective tissues of varying proportion. Originally, it consists of only muscle element but later on, fibrous tissues intermingle with the muscle bundles. As such, the nomenclature of 'fibroids' although commonly used, is inappropriate and should better be called either myomata or fibromyomata.

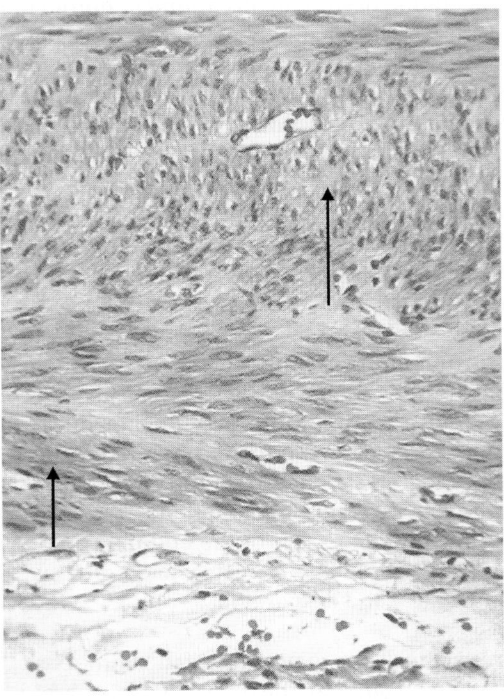

Fig. 20.6: Histological picture of fibroid.

SECONDARY CHANGES IN FIBROIDS (TABLE 20.3)

DEGENERATIONS

The arterial supply of myomas is less compared to a same sized area of normal myometrium. Degenerations occur as the tumor out grows its blood supply.

- **Hyaline degeneration is the most common (65%)** type of degeneration affecting all sizes of fibroids except the tiny one. It is common especially in tumors having more connective tissues. The central part of the tumor which is least vascular is the common site.

  Naked eye examination on the cut surface shows irregular homogeneous areas with loss of whorl-like appearance.

  Microscopic examination reveals hyaline changes of both the muscles and fibrous tissues. Cellular details are lost.
- **Cystic degeneration** usually occurs following menopause and is common in interstitial fibroids. It is formed by liquefaction of the areas with hyaline changes. The cystic spaces are lined by irregular ragged walls. The cystic changes of an isolated big fibroid may be confused with an ovarian cyst or pregnancy.

  Myxomatous degeneration (15%) is common. It occurs mainly in the central part of the myoma. Smooth muscle cells undergo myxomatous degenerations.
- **Fatty degeneration** is usually found at or after menopause. Fat globules are deposited mainly in the muscle cells.
- **Calcific degeneration (10%)** usually involves the subserous fibroids with small pedicle or myomas of postmenopausal women. It is usually preceded by fatty degeneration. There is precipitation of calcium carbonate or phosphate within the tumor. When whole of the tumor is converted into a calcified mass, it is called **"womb stone"** (p. 549).
- **Red degeneration** (carneous degeneration) occurs in a large fibroid mainly during second half of pregnancy and puerperium (5–10%). Partial recovery is possible and as such called necrobiosis. The cause is not known but is probably vascular in origin. Infection does not play any part.

  Naked eye appearance of the tumor shows dark areas with cut section revealing raw-beef appearance often containing cystic spaces. The odor is often fishy due to fatty acids. Color is due to the presence of hemolyzed red cells and hemoglobin.

  Microscopically, evidences of necrosis are present. Vessels are thrombosed but extravasation of blood is unlikely.
- **Atrophy:** Atrophic changes occur following menopause due to loss of support from estrogen. There is reduction

TABLE 20.3: Secondary changes in a fibroid.

▪ Degenerations	▪ Infection
▪ Atrophy	▪ Vascular changes
▪ Necrosis	▪ Sarcomatous change

in the size of the tumor. Similar reduction also occurs following pregnancy enlargement.

- **Necrosis:** Circulatory inadequacy may lead to central necrosis of the tumor. This is present in submucous polyp or pedunculated subserous fibroid.
- **Infection:** The infection gains access to the tumor core through the thinned and sloughed surface epithelium of the submucous fibroid. This usually happens following delivery or abortion. Intramural fibroid may also be infected following delivery.
- **Vascular changes:** Dilatation of the vessels (telangiectasia) or dilatation of the lymphatic channels (lymphangiectasis) inside the myoma may occur. The cause is not known.
- **Sarcomatous changes:** Sarcomatous change may occur **in less than 0.1% cases**. The usual type is leiomyosarcoma. Recurrence of fibroid polyp, sudden enlargement of fibroid or fibroid along with postmenopausal bleeding raises the suspicion.

Associated Changes in the Pelvic Organs

Uterus: The shape is distorted; usually asymmetrical but at times, uniform. Myohyperplasia is almost a constant finding. It may be due to hyperestrinism or work hypertrophy in an attempt to expel the fibroid.

The endometrium may be of normal type. In others, there are features of anovulation with evidences of hyperplasia. There is dilatation and congestion of the myometrial and endometrial venous plexuses. The endometrium as a result becomes thick, congested, and edematous. The endometrium overlying the submucous fibroid may be thin and necrotic with evidences of infection.

The uterine cavity may be elongated and distorted in intramural and submucous varieties.

Uterine tubes: The frequent tubal infection (about 15%) detected in association with fibroid seems coincidental.

Ovaries: The ovaries may be enlarged, congested, and studded with multiple cysts. The cause may be due to hyperestrinism.

Ureter: There may be displacement of the anatomy of the ureter in broad ligament fibroid. The compression effect results in hydroureter and or hydronephrosis.

Endometriosis: There is increased association of pelvic endometriosis and adenomyosis (30%).

Endometrial carcinoma: The incidence remains unaffected.

CLINICAL FEATURES

Patient Profile

The patients are usually nulliparous or having long period of secondary infertility. However, early marriage and frequent childbirth make its frequency high even amongst the multiparous women. The incidence is at its peak between 35–45 years. There is a tendency of delayed menopause.

Symptoms

The majority of fibroids remain asymptomatic (75%). They are accidentally discovered by the physician during routine examination or at laparotomy or laparoscopy.

The symptoms are related to anatomic type and size of the tumor. **The site is more important than the size.** A small submucous fibroid may produce more symptoms than a big subserous fibroid.

SYMPTOMS OF FIBROID UTERUS

- Asymptomatic—majority (75%)
- Abnormal uterine bleeding (AUB) (30%): Menorrhagia, metrorrhagia
- Dysmenorrhea
- Dyspareunia
- Subfertility
- Pressure symptoms (bladder, ureter, and rectum)
- Recurrent pregnancy loss (miscarriage, preterm labor)
- Lower abdominal or pelvic pain
- Abdominal enlargement

Menstrual abnormalities

a. **Menorrhagia (30%) is the classic symptom of symptomatic fibroid.**
The menstrual loss is progressively increased with successive cycles. It is conspicuous in submucous or interstitial fibroids. **The causes are:**
   - Interference with normal uterine contractility due to interposition of fibroid
   - Congestion and dilatation of the subjacent endometrial venous plexuses caused by the obstruction of the tumor
   - Endometrial hyperplasia due to hyperestrinism (anovulation)
   - Pelvic congestion
   - Role of prostanoids—imbalance of thromboxane (TXA_2) and prostacyclin (PGI_2) with relative deficiency of TXA_2.
   - Increased surface area of the endometrium (normal is about 15 cm^2) may be a cause.

b. **Metrorrhagia or irregular bleeding**:
   - Ulceration of submucous fibroid or fibroid polyp
   - Torn vessels from the sloughing base of a polyp
   - Associated endometrial carcinoma.

Dysmenorrhea: The congestive variety may be due to associated pelvic congestion or endometriosis. Spasmodic type is associated with extrusion of polyp and its expulsion from the uterine cavity.

Subserous, broad ligament or cervical fibroids are usually unassociated with menstrual abnormalities.

Infertility: Infertility (30%) may be a major complaint. **The probable known attributing factors are:**

Uterine

- Distortion and/or elongation of the uterine cavity → difficult sperm ascent
- Preventing rhythmic uterine contraction due to fibroids during intercourse → impaired sperm transport
- Congestion and dilatation of the endometrial venous plexuses → defective implantation
- Atrophy and ulceration of the endometrium over the submucous fibroids → defective nidation
- Menorrhagia and dyspareunia.

Tubal

- Cornual block due to position of the fibroid
- Marked elongation of the tube over a big fibroid
- Associated salpingitis with tubal block.

Ovarian: Anovulation
Peritoneal: Endometriosis
Unknown—majority

Pregnancy-related problems like abortion, preterm labor and intrauterine growth restriction are high. The reasons are defective implantation of the placenta, poorly developed endometrium, reduced space for the growing fetus and placenta. **Red degeneration** and torsion of subserous pedunculated fibroid is common in pregnancy. Labor dystocia, increased operative delivery postpartum hemorrhage are also more.

Pain lower abdomen

The fibroids are usually painless. Pain may be due to some complications of the tumor or due to associated pelvic pathology.

Due to tumor

- Degeneration
- Torsion subserous pedunculated fibroid
- Extrusion of polyp.

Associated pathology

- Endometriosis
- Pelvic inflammatory disease (PID).

Abdominal swellings (lump)

The patient may have a sense of heaviness in lower abdomen. She may feel a lump in the lower abdomen even without any other symptom.

Pressure symptoms

Pressure symptoms are rare in body fibroids. The fibroids in the posterior wall may be impacted in the pelvis producing constipation, dysuria or even retention of urine. A broad ligament fibroid may produce ureteric compression → hydroureteric and hydronephrotic changes → infection → pyelitis.

Signs

General examination reveals varying degrees of pallor depending upon the magnitude and duration of menstrual loss.

Abdominal examination

The tumor may not be sufficiently enlarged to be felt per abdomen (Table 20.4). But if enlarged to 14 weeks or more, the following features are noted.

Palpation

- Feel is firm, more toward hard; may be cystic in cystic degeneration
- Margins are well-defined except the lower pole which cannot be reached suggestive of pelvic in origin
- Surface is nodular; may be uniformly enlarged in a single fibroid

TABLE 20.4: Causes of symmetrical enlargement of uterus (differential diagnosis).

▪ Pregnancy ▪ Submucous or intramural (solitary) fibroid ▪ Adenomyosis ▪ Myohyperplasia ▪ Pyometra	▪ Hematometra ▪ Lochiometra ▪ Malignancy • Carcinoma body • Choriocarcinoma • Sarcoma

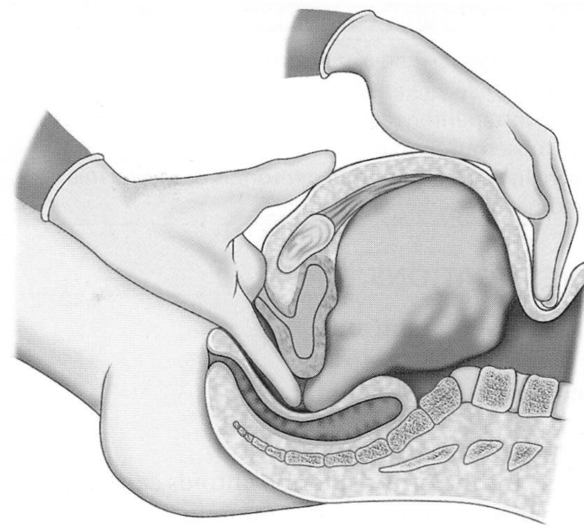

Fig. 20.7: Bimanual examination in a case of uterine fibroid.

- Mobility is restricted from above downwards but can be moved from side to side.

Percussion

The swelling is dull on percussion.

Pelvic examination

Bimanual examination reveals the uterus irregularly enlarged by the swelling felt per abdomen, **the swelling is uterine is evidenced by:**

- Uterus is not felt separated from the swelling and as such a groove is not felt between the uterus and the mass (Fig. 20.7).
- The cervix moves with the movement of the tumor felt per abdomen.

The only exception of these two findings is a subserous pedunculated fibroid. As such, such type is too often confused with an ovarian tumor. However, a submucous fibroid may produce symmetrical enlargement of the uterus and at times, it is difficult to diagnose accurately.

COMPLICATIONS

These are listed in Tables 20.5 and 20.6.

TABLE 20.5: Complications of leiomyomas.

	Types of degenerations
▪ Degenerations ▪ Necrosis ▪ Infection ▪ Sarcomatous change (rare) ▪ Torsion of subserous pedunculated fibroid ▪ Hemorrhage • Intracapsular • Ruptured surface vein of subserous fibroid → intraperitoneal hemorrhage (Table 20.6)	▪ Hyaline (65%) ▪ Cystic ▪ Fatty ▪ Calcific ▪ Red (rare) ▪ Necrosis
▪ Polycythemia due to • Erythropoietic function by the tumor • Altered erythropoietic function of the kidney through ureteric pressure	

TABLE 20.6: Life-threatening complications of leiomyomas.

- Persistent menorrhagia, metrorrhagia or continued vaginal bleeding → severe anemia
- Severe intraperitoneal hemorrhage due to rupture of veins over subserous fibroid
- Severe infection leading to peritonitis or septicemia
- Sarcoma (rare)

INVESTIGATIONS

The investigations aim at:
- To confirm the diagnosis
- Preoperative assessment.

To Confirm the Diagnosis

Although, the majority of uterine fibroids can be diagnosed from the history and pelvic examination but at times pose problems in diagnosis.

- ***Ultrasound and color Doppler (TVS) findings***—(a) Uterine contour is enlarged and distorted; (b) Depending on the amount of connective tissue or smooth muscle proliferation, fibroids are of different echogenicity-hypoechoic or hyperechoic; (c) Vascularization is at the periphery of the fibroid and (d) Central vascularization indicates degenerative changes. **Ultrasound** is an useful diagnostic tool to confirm the diagnosis of fibroid. **Transvaginal ultrasound** can accurately assess the myoma location, dimensions volume, number and also any adnexal pathology. Hydroureter or hydronephrotic changes can be diagnosed. **Three-dimensional** ultrasonography can locate fibroids accurately. Serial ultrasound examination is needed during medical or conservative management (Fig. 20.8).
- ***Saline infusion sonography (SIS)*** is helpful to detect any submucous fibroid or polyp (p. 99).
- ***Hysteroscopy*** is of help to detect submucous fibroid in unexplained infertility and repeated pregnancy wastage. The presence and site of submucous fibroid can be diagnosed by direct visualization during hysteroscopy (Fig. 20.9). Submucosal fibroid can be resected at the same time using a resecting hysteroscope.

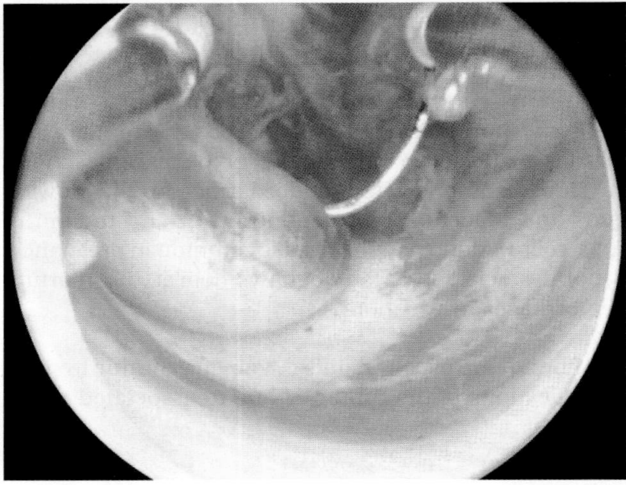

Fig. 20.9: Hysteroscopic view of a submucous fibroid. Endoscopic resection is possible.

- ***HSG*** when done, a filling defect can be seen.
- ***Magnetic resonance imaging (MRI)***—is more accurate compared to ultrasound. **It helps to differentiate adenomyosis from fibroids** (p. 98). MRI is not used routinely for the diagnosis. It is expensive and not widely available (Fig. 20.10).
- ***Laparoscopy***—is helpful, if the uterine size is less than 12 weeks and associated with pelvic pain and infertility. Associated pelvic endometriosis and tubal pathology can be revealed. It can also differentiate a pedunculated fibroid from ovarian tumor, not revealed by clinical examination and ultrasound.
- ***Uterine curettage***—in the presence of irregular bleeding, to detect any coexisting pathology and to study the endometrial pattern, curettage is helpful. It additionally helps to diagnose a submucous fibroid by

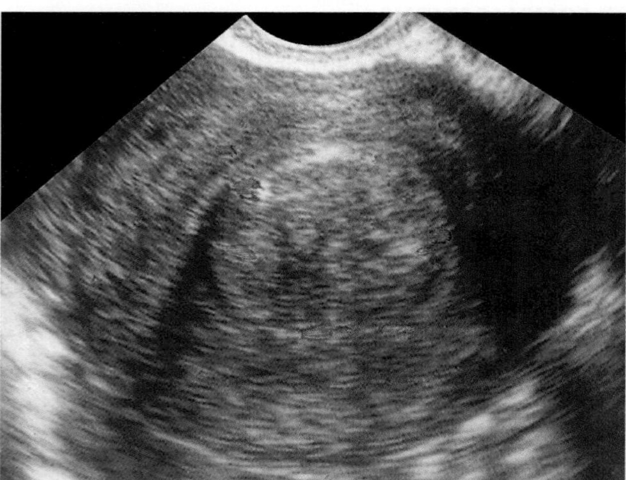

Fig. 20.8: Ultrasonographic view of a uterine fibroid.

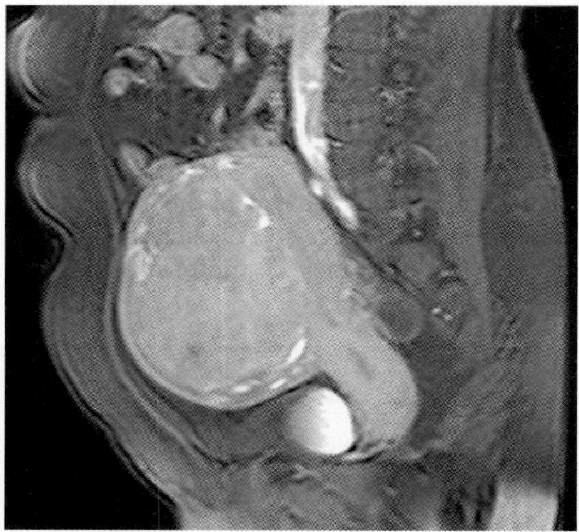

Fig. 20.10: Magnetic resonance image of a fairly large size fibroid arising from the body of the uterus.

feeling a bump. However, hysteroscopy and biopsy is a better alternative.

Preoperative Assessment

Apart from routine preoperative investigations, intravenous pyelography to note the anatomic changes of the ureter may be helpful.

DIFFERENTIAL DIAGNOSIS

The fibroid of varying sizes may be confused with: (a) Pregnancy; (b) Adenomyosis; (c) Myohyperplasia; (d) Ovarian tumor; (e) TO mass; (f) Full bladder.

MANAGEMENT OF FIBROID UTERUS (FLOWCHART 20.2)

- **Asymptomatic**
- **Symptomatic**

ASYMPTOMATIC LEIOMYOMAS (75%)

Fibroids detected accidentally on routine examination for complaints other than fibroids are dealt with as follows:

- **Observation**
- **Surgery**
- **Observation: A certain diagnosis of fibroid should be a must, prior to contemplating expectant management.** The risk of sarcomatous changes is so insignificant (0.1%) that prophylactic removal of fibroid is unjustified in asymptomatic cases.
- **Indications of expectant management:**
  - Size <12 weeks (of pregnancy size), Myoma size >8 cm
  - Diagnosis certain
  - Follow up possible.

Periodic examination at interval of 6 months and ultrasound evaluation annually is needed. If the symptoms of fibroid appear and or it grows and increases in size, surgery is indicated.

Flowchart 20.2: Therapeutic options in a patient with uterine fibroids.

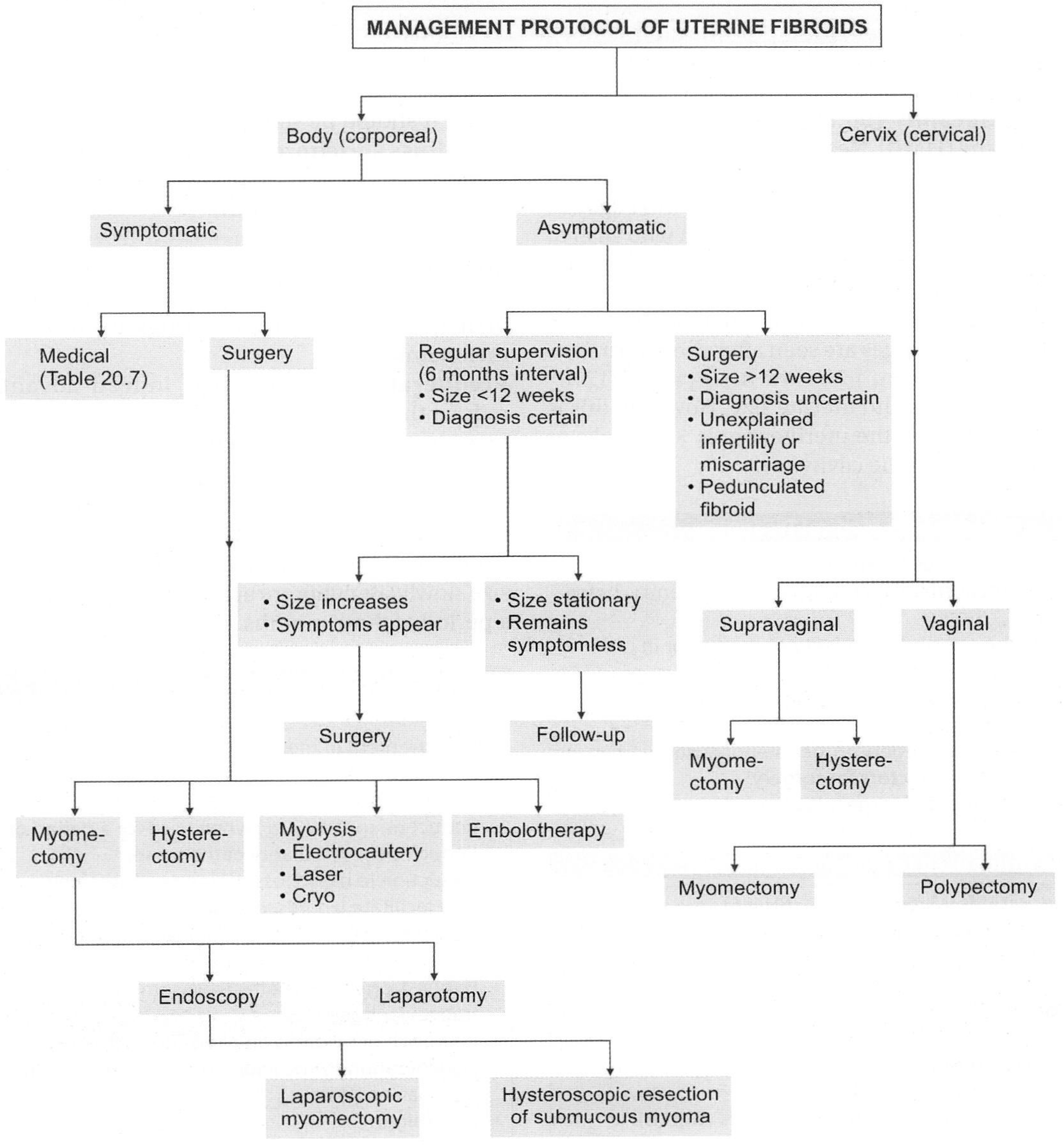

SYMPTOMATIC LEIOMYOMAS

Medical Management

Drug therapy has established a firm place in the management of symptomatic fibroids. The drugs are used either as a temporary palliation or may be used in rare cases, as an alternative to surgery. **Prior to drug therapy, one must be certain about the diagnosis.**

To Minimize Blood Loss

As a temporary palliation, various drugs are used to minimize blood loss and to correct anemia when a definite surgery cannot be undertaken for certain periods (Table 20.7).

Antiprogesterones: Mifepristone (RU486) is very effective to reduce fibroid size and also menorrhagia. It may produce amenorrhea. It reduces the size of the fibroid significantly. A daily dose of 5–10 mg is recommended and is found effective to reduce the size (50%) and bleeding significantly. Long-term therapy is avoided as it causes endometrial hyperplasia.

Selective progesterone receptor modulator (SPRM): Ulipristal is used with success. It is a SPRM. It does not cause endometrial hyperplasia. Ulipristal acetate reduces blood loss significantly (90%) in women with heavy menstrual bleeding (HMB). Nearly 70% of women became amenorrhea after 10 days of treatment. There is reduction in size of myoma. It is as effective as that of GnRH agoinst (leuprolide acetate). It may be used in women who wish to avoid surgery; to reduce the size (53%) before surgery and the HMB (98%). It is used for 3 months.

Side effects: Long-term endometrial safety is unknown. Benign endometrial changes are seen after short-term use.

Levonorgestrel-releasing intrauterine system (LNG-IUS) reduces blood loss and uterine size. However, this is not recommended when the uterine size is >12 weeks or there is distortion of uterine cavity.

Objectives of Medical Treatment

- Young women desirous of pregnancy.
- To improve menorrhagia and to correct anemia before surgery.
- To minimize the size and vascularity of the tumor in order to facilitate surgery.
- In selected cases of infertility to facilitate hysteroscopic or laparoscopic surgery (Ch. 36).
- As an alternative to surgery in perimenopausal women or women with high-risk factors for surgery.
- Where postponement of surgery is planned temporarily.

TABLE 20.7: Drugs used to minimize blood loss.

- Antiprogesterones (Mifepristone)—(RU486)
- Antigonadotropins: Danazol, gestrinone
- GnRH analogs:
  - Agonists
  - Antagonists
- LNG-IUS
- Combined oral contraceptives (COCs)
- Prostaglandin synthetase inhibitors
- Selective progesterone receptor modulators (SPRMs)

Danazol can reduce the volume of a fibroid slightly. Because of androgenic side effects, danazol is used only for a period of 3–6 months. Danazol administered daily in divided doses ranging from 200–400 mg for 3 months minimizes blood loss or even produce amenorrhea by its antigonadotropin and androgen agonist actions.

GnRH agonists: Drugs commonly used are goserelin, leuprorelin, buserelin or nafarelin. **Mechanism of action is sustained pituitary down regulation and suppression of ovarian function.** Optimal duration of therapy is 3 months. Add-back therapy may be needed to combat hypoestrogenic symptoms.

GnRH antagonists: Cetrorelix or ganirelix causes immediate suppression of pituitary and the ovaries. They do not have the initial stimulatory effect. Benefits are same as that of agonists (Table 20.8). Onset of amenorrhea is rapid.

Nonhormonal Options

Tranexamic acid (TXA) is an antifibrinolytic agent. Use of TXA for myoma related bleeding is found useful.

Aromatase inhibitors (AIs) for the treatment of leiomyomas are effective as the aromatase levels are higher in myomas. It is found to reduce the volume (10–70%) and the HMB. It should be started in the luteal phase. Commonly used drugs are letrozole and anastrazole. Similar to GnRH agonists it induces systemic hypoestrogenism. It is used for 2–3 months to reduce HMB.

Prostaglandin synthetase inhibitors (PSI): These are used to relieve pain due to associated endometriosis or degeneration of the fibroid. They cannot improve menorrhagia due to fibroids. Drugs used are: Naproxen, mefenamic acid.

Preoperative therapy: It is indeed advantageous to reduce the size and vascularity of fibroid prior to either myomectomy or hysterectomy. While operation will be technically easier in broad ligament or cervical fibroid, in myomectomy, there may be little difficulty in enucleation of the tumor from its pseudocapsule. However, with the stoppage of the therapy, the tumor will attain its previous size slowly. Benefits are achieved when therapy is given for a period of three months.

TABLE 20.8: Advantages and disadvantages of GnRH analog.

Advantages
- Improvement of menorrhagia and may produce amenorrhea
- Improvement of anemia
- Relief of pressure symptoms
- Reduction in size (50%) when used for a period of 6 months
- Reduction in vascularity of the tumor
- Reduction in blood loss during myomectomy
- May facilitate laparoscopic or hysteroscopic surgery
- May facilitate nondescent vaginal hysterectomy

Disadvantages
- Hypoestrogenic side effects (vasomotor symptoms, trabecular bone loss)
- Regrowth of myomas on cessation of therapy
- Degeneration (some leiomyomas)—causing difficulty in myoma enucleation
- Cost (high)

Surgical Management of Fibroid Uterus

- **Myomectomy** (may be done by)
  - Laparotomy
  - Laparoscopy
  - Hysteroscopy
  - Robotic
- **Embolotherapy**
- Laparoscopic uterine artery ligation
- Myolysis
- Endometrial ablation
- Hysterectomy

Myomectomy (p. 506, Tables 20.9 to 20.12)

Myomectomy is the enucleation of myomata from the uterus leaving behind a potentially functioning organ capable of future reproduction.

As such, the surgeon should be satisfied with the operation designed to serve the objective. It is indeed useless to perform a hectic surgery to remove such myomata only to leave behind an uterus which is unlikely to conceive in future.

Among the contraindications few are relative rather than absolute. Restoration of anatomy and function of the uterus, tubes, and ovaries following myomectomy are important, not only for future reproductive function but also to avoid the future hazards (Table 20.9).

However, the final decision as to whether to perform myomectomy or hysterectomy is to be taken following laparotomy. As such, it is prudent on the part of surgeon to declare the operative decision as '**myomectomy to be tried**' and if the conditions arise, it may end in hysterectomy.

Pretreatment with GnRH analogs may be used to reduce the size and vascularity of the uterus. Steps of myomectomy and complications of myomectomy have been discussed (p. 498).

Vaginal myomectomy: Submucous pedunculated myoma can be removed vaginally. **Morcellation** (removal by piecemeal) is needed if the tumor is large. A moderate size fibroid can be removed by twisting. In that case, fibroid is grasped with a sponge forceps.

TABLE 20.9: Important considerations prior to myomectomy.

- It should be done mainly to preserve the reproductive function
- The wish to preserve the menstrual function in parous women should be judiciously complied with
- Myomectomy is a more risky operation when the fibroid(s) is too big and too many
- Risk of recurrence and persistence of fibroid is about 30–50%
- Risk of persistence of menorrhagia is about 1–5%
- Risk of relaparotomy is about 20–25%
- Pregnancy rate following myomectomy is about 40–60%
- Pregnancy following myomectomy should have a mandatory hospital delivery, although the chance of scar rupture is rare (little more when the cavity is open)

TABLE 20.10: Indications of myomectomy.

- **Persistent uterine bleeding** despite medical therapy
- **Excessive pain or pressure** symptoms
- **Size >12 weeks,** woman desirous to have a baby
- **Distortion of the uterine cavity** without any other cause
- **Recurrent pregnancy loss** due to fibroid
- **Rapidly growing myoma** during follow-up
- **Subserous pedunculated fibroid**

TABLE 20.11: Prerequisites to myomectomy.

- Hysteroscopy or hysterosalpingography—to exclude any submucous fibroid or a polyp or any tubal block
- Hysteroscopy/endometrial biopsy—in cases of irregular cycles, not only to remove a polyp but also to exclude endometrial carcinoma
- Examination of the husband from fertility point of view (semen analysis)

TABLE 20.12: Contraindications of myomectomy.

- Infected fibroid
- Growth of myoma after menopause
- Suspected malignant change (sarcoma)
- Parous women where hysterectomy is safer and is a definitive treatment (Table 20.9)
- Functionless fallopian tubes (bilateral hydrosalpinx, tubo-ovarian mass)—decision must be judicious with the advent of microsurgery and assisted reproductive technology (ART)
- Pelvic or endometrial tuberculosis
- During pregnancy or during cesarean section (relative)

Endoscopic Surgery (Ch. 36)

- ***Hysteroscopy:*** Generally, a fibroid of 3–4 cm in diameter or a polyp is resected with a hysteroscope. Pedicle or the base of the fibroid is coagulated using electrocautery (Fig. 20.10). Nd:YAG laser can also be used.

  Complications of hysteroscopic surgery are uterine perforation, fluid overload, hemorrhage and others .
- ***Laparoscopy:*** Subserous and intramural fibroids could be removed laparoscopically. Electro-diathermy, harmonics, laser and extracorporeal sutures are used for hemostasis. Laparoscopic surgery is not suitable when the fibroid is large, deep intramural, multiple or technically inaccessible. Myoma specimens following MIS, are removed using power morcellater, in a bag.
- Other MIS methods are: Myolysis, done in women who want to preserve the uterus but not the fertility. Women with small size fibroids (<10 cm) are considered. Principles of surgery are to destroy the fibroids and/or the blood supply with high frequency ultrasound, laser, cryotherapy or bipolar diathermy.

  Complications of laparoscopic surgery, contraindications others are discussed in Chapter 36.

Other approaches: Laparoscopic uterine artery occlusion (LUAO) causes myoma devascularization. It is done by sealing both the uterine arteries near its origin from the internal iliac artery and the ovarian arteries. It needs advanced surgical skill.

Magnetic Resonance Guided Focused Ultrasound (MRgFUS)

Focussed high-energy ultrasound waves induce coagulative necrosis in myomas. It causes localized thermal ablation of the fibroid tissue. It may need multiple treatments. It causes less pain compared to uterine artery embolization (UAE).

It has less postoperative complications. It is safe, feasible and minimally invasive.

Contraindications of MRgFUS

Abdominal wall scars, uterine size >24 weeks, myoma size >10 cm, desire for future fertility are the contraindications to MRI.

Embolotherapy

Uterine artery embolization (UAE) (p. 99)

It causes avascular necrosis followed by shrinkage of fibroid. Uterine arteries are occluded by injecting polyvinyl alcohol particles through percutaneous femoral catheterization. This may be an option for women with symptomatic fibroid where surgery is not preferred.

Result: Improvement of menorrhagia is observed in 80–90% with 60% reduction in size. **Others:** Relief of pressure symptoms.

Complication of UAE: Postembolization syndrome: Pain, fever, sepsis, myometrial infarction and necrosis, amenorrhea and ovarian failure. **Complications related to the procedure:** Femoral artery injury.

Contraindications of UAE

Hysterectomy

Hysterectomy in fact, is the operation of choice in symptomatic fibroid when there is no valid reason for myomectomy. The patients over the age of 40 years and in those not desirous of further child are the classic indications.

Total hysterectomy is performed. However, a subtotal hysterectomy may have to be done in few conditions (p. 499).

Removal of the ovary: It is preferable to remove the ovaries in postmenopausal women and to preserve the same in earlier age, if they are found healthy (For details Ch. 24). Prophylactic salpingectomy during hysterectomy is an option to prevent ovarian cancer.

Advantages of hysterectomy

- There is no chance of recurrence.
- Adnexal pathology and the unhealthy cervix, if any, are also removed.

Place of vaginal hysterectomy

Fibroids with size of 10–12 weeks of pregnancy associated with uterine prolapse are better dealt by the vaginal route. Vaginal hysterectomy with repair of pelvic floor is the operation of choice. Pretreatment with GnRH analog may facilitate vaginal hysterectomy.

Emergency Surgery

The indications for emergency surgery in a fibroid are listed in Table 20.13.

TABLE 20.13: Indications of emergency surgery in a fibroid.

- Torsion of a subserous pedunculated fibroid
- Massive intraperitoneal hemorrhage following rupture of veins over subserous fibroid
- Uncontrolled infected fibroid
- Uncontrolled bleeding fibroid

CERVICAL FIBROID (FIGS. 20.11 AND 20.12)

SYMPTOMS

In nonpregnant state, the symptoms are predominantly due to pressure effect on the surrounding structures.

Anterior cervical: Bladder symptoms like frequency or even retention of urine are conspicuous. The retention is more due to pressure than elongation of urethra.

Posterior cervical: Rectal symptom is in the form of constipation.

Lateral cervical: Vascular obstruction may lead to hemorrhoids and edema legs (rare). The ureter is pushed laterally and below the tumor.

Central cervical (Fig. 20.12): Central fibroid produces predominantly bladder symptoms. The cervix is expanded on all sides. The uterus sits on the top of the expanded cervix (lantern on the dome of St Paul's).

In pregnancy, it remains asymptomatic but produces insuperable obstruction during labor.

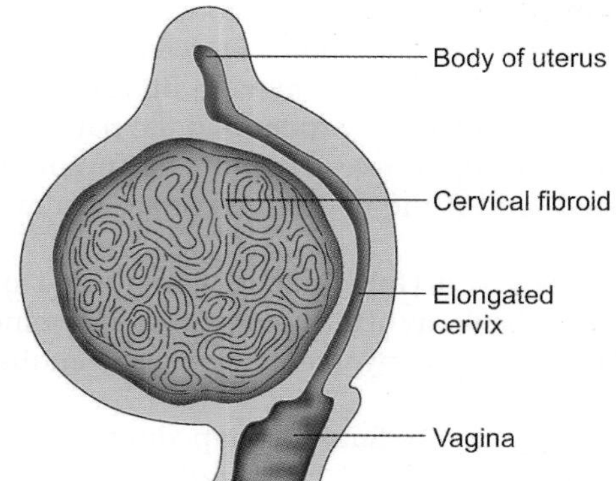

Fig. 20.11: Cervical fibroid.

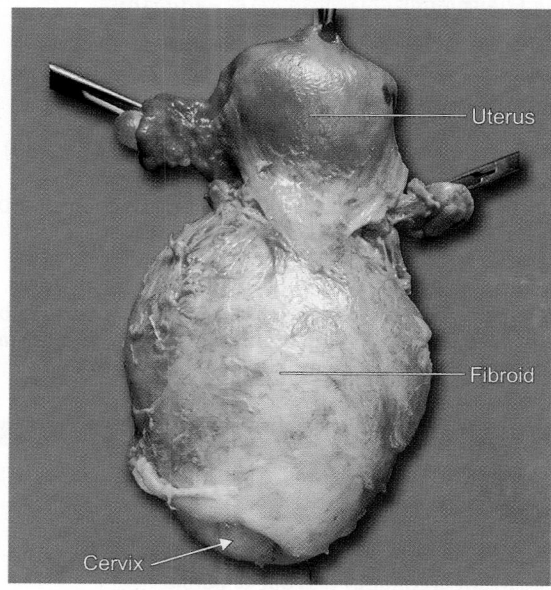

Fig. 20.12: Central cervical fibroid (huge).
(*Courtesy*: Dr Biswajit Ghosh, Burnpur)

Fibroids arising from the vaginal part of the cervix may remain asymptomatic during nonpregnant state but produces obstruction during labor. If pedunculated, there may be a sensation of something coming down or if infected a foul smelling discharge per vaginam.

TREATMENT

Supravaginal fibroids: Myomectomy may be tried if the patient is young and desirous of having a baby. But, it is not only technically difficult—but the anatomic and functional restoration of the cervix may not be adequate to achieve the objective of future reproduction.

As such, mostly it is dealt with by hysterectomy. **The principle to be followed is enucleation followed by hysterectomy** to minimize the injury to the ureter. Preoperative GnRH analogs administration for 3 months facilitates surgery.

Vaginal part fibroids: If the tumor is sessile, myomectomy and if pedunculated, polypectomy is done.

POLYPS

Polyp (Table 20.14) is a clinical entity referring a tumor attached by a pedicle.

ENDOMETRIAL POLYPS

The most common type of benign uterine polyp is endometrial one. It may arise from the body of the uterus or from the cervix (Figs. 20.13 and 20.14).

Risk factors: Hormone replacement therapy, tamoxifen therapy, diabetes, hypertension, obesity, and increased patient age are the important risk factors.

TABLE 20.14: Different types of polyp.

Benign	*Malignant*
▪ Endometrial ▪ Endocervical ▪ Fibroid ▪ Placental	▪ De novo ▪ Secondary changes of benign polyp

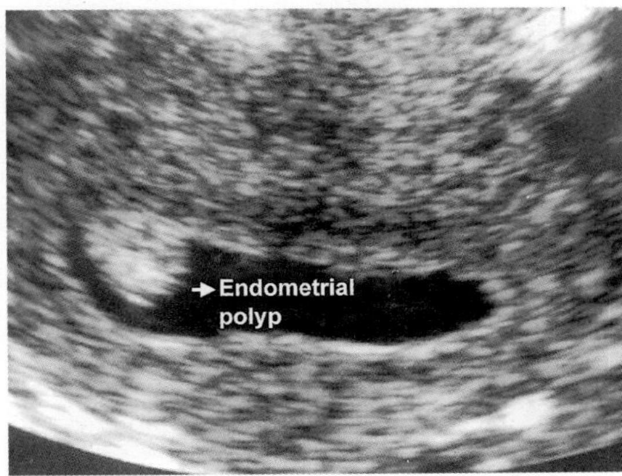

Fig. 20.13: Sonogram (TV) of the uterus showing an echogenic area within the endometrial cavity—submucous polyp.

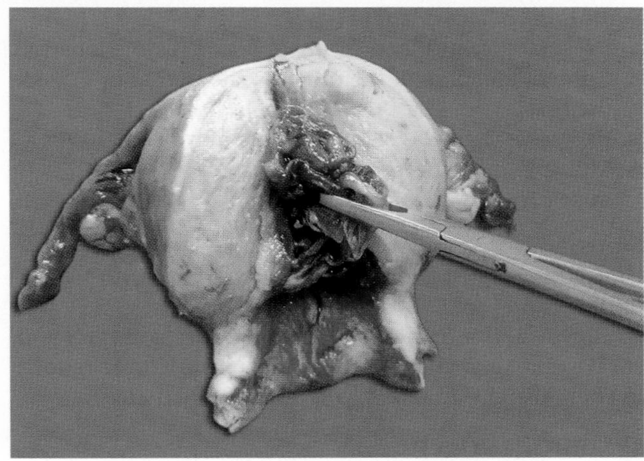

Fig. 20.14: Multiple polyps are seen within the endometrial cavity.

Pathogenesis

Body

A part of the thick endometrium projects into the cavity and ultimately attains a pedicle.

Naked eye appearance: It shows a small polyp size of about 1–2 cm, looks reddish and feels soft. The pedicle may at times be long enough to make the polyp protruded from the cervix.

Microscopically: The core contains stromal cells, glands and large thick-walled vascular channels. The surface is lined by epithelium. The tip may undergo squamous metaplasia. Malignant change is rare but may coexist with endometrial carcinoma. The pedicle contains thin fibrous tissue with thin blood vessels. Rarely, smooth muscles invade the polyp and is then called adenomyomatous polyp.

***Predictors of malignancy are*:** (a) Size >10 mm; (b) Postmenopausal status; (c) Abnormal uterine bleeding.

Cervical

The polyp mainly arises from the endocervix and rarely from the ectocervix. The stimulus of epithelial overgrowth is probably due to hyperestrinism, chronic irritation by infection or localized vascular congestion.

Naked eye appearance: It shows the polyp of usually small size rarely exceeding 1–2 cm, single and red in color. The pedicle may at times be long enough to reach the vaginal introitus.

Microscopically: The stroma consists of fibrous connective tissues with numerous small blood vessels and occasional cervical glands. The lining epithelium is tall columnar like that of endocervix. The tip may undergo squamous metaplasia. Malignant change is rare and usually of squamous cell carcinoma.

Clinical Features

Symptoms

There may not be any symptom. The entity is accidentally discovered during speculum examination, following hysterosalpingography (filling defect) or hysteroscopy.

Symptoms of a cervical polyp

- Irregular uterine bleeding, either pre or postmenopausal.
- Contact bleeding, if the polyp is situated at or outside the cervix.
- Excessive vaginal discharge which may be offensive.
- Multiple endometrial polyps may cause infertility or miscarriage in young women.

Signs

Unless the polyp is at or outside the external os, no positive finding is present.

However, if it protrudes out of the cervix, it feels soft, slippery and is small in size. Per speculum, it looks reddish in color, usually attached with a slender pedicle.

FIBROID POLYP

The fibroid polyp may arise from the body of the uterus or from the cervix.

Pathogenesis

Body (Fig. 20.15)

Fibroid polyp is almost always due to extrusion of a submucous fibroid into the uterine cavity. During this process, it attains a pedicle which is often broad and usually attached to the posterior wall. The torn ends of the pseudocapsule are retracted in the base of the pedicle. The uterus contracts to expel the polyp out and as a result, the polyp may be pushed out through the cervix to lie even in the vagina.

Naked eye: The polyp is usually single, of varying sizes. There may be evidences of necrosis, infection and hemorrhage especially at the tip. The pedicle is broad. There may be associated other varieties of fibroids in the uterus.

Microscopically: The polyp including the pedicle is covered by endometrium. In the tip, there may be squamous metaplasia. The core of the polyp is composed of fibromuscular structures. The pedicle is composed of fibrous tissues with slender blood vessels.

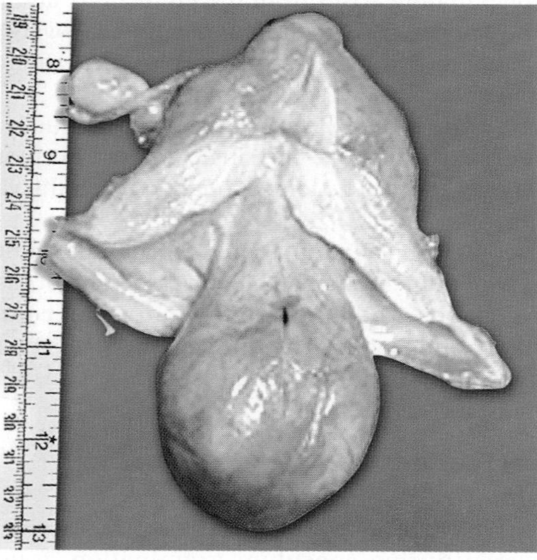

Fig. 20.15: Fibroid polyp. Note the wide pedicle and thinning out of the cervix.

Cervical (Fig. 20.16)

Cervical fibroid polyp usually arises from the ectocervix and from its posterior lip. It may be small and usually single. At times, it is big enough to distend the vagina or even comes out of the introitus confusing the diagnosis of uterine inversion.

Symptoms

The patients are usually in reproductive period. The chief complaints are:

- Intermenstrual bleeding, often continuous, especially in fibroid polyp arising from the body
- Colicky pain in the lower abdomen due to uterine contraction in an effort to expel the polyp out of the uterine cavity
- Excessive vaginal discharge which may be offensive
- Sensation of something coming down when the polyp becomes big distending the vagina
- It may remain asymptomatic also.

Signs

General examination reveals varying degrees of anemia.

Per vaginam

- The uterus may be bulky.
- The cervix may be patulous and the tip of the polyp is felt or else, the polyp is felt distinctly outside the external os.

Speculum examination: It reveals the size and color of the polyp which is usually pale; may be hemorrhagic. Whereas, the attachment of the pedicle to the cervix can be visualized but attachment higher up may be at times difficult to locate.

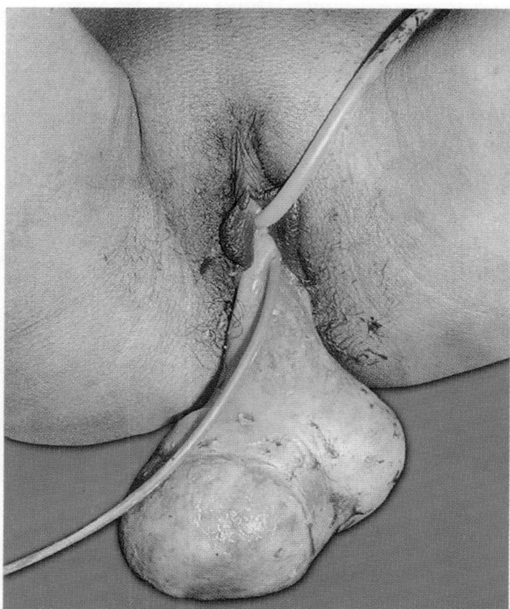

Fig. 20.16: Cervical fibroid polyp may be confused with inversion. Catheters: One in urethra and the other in the cervical canal.
(*Courtesy*: Prof S Mitra, MMCH)

Investigations

- **Transvaginal sonography (TVS)**, the polyp is seen as an echogenic mass.
- **Saline infusion sonography** (gold standard), the polyp is seen as a echogenic mass much better compared to TVS.
- **Hysteroscopy**—to visualize the uterine polyp and simultaneously polypectomy could be done.
- **Hysterography**—to detect the filling defect in a fibroid polyp.
- **Examination under anesthesia** and exploration of the uterine cavity by curette or ovum or ring forceps can help in diagnosis of an uterine polyp. In all cases, following polypectomy histological examination should be done.
- **Sound test**—to differentiate a fibroid polyp from chronic inversion, sound test is done. If an uterine sound is passed all round between the pedicle and the dilating cervical canal, it is a polyp. In complete chronic inversion, the sound cannot be passed (Fig. 16.21).

Polyps could be seen when hysterectomy specimens are cut opened postoperatively.

Placental Polyp

A retained bit of placental tissue when adherent to the uterine wall gets organized with the surrounding blood clots.

Clinical Features

There is history of recent childbirth or abortion. Irregular bleeding per vaginam and offensive vaginal discharge are present dated back to the pregnancy events.

Endometrial Mucous Polyps

These are the localized outgrowth of endometrium projecting into the cavity of the uterus. Polyps contain the endometrial glands and stroma. Polyps may be single or multiple; sessile or pedunculated or may be small or large to occupy endometrial cavity.

Polyps are commonly seen at all age groups of women but more common between the ages of 40 to 50 years. Overall prevalence is 20%.

Etiology of polyp is unknown. Common causes are uncontrolled endometrial hyperplasia due to the effect of unopposed estrogen. It could be associated with prolonged therapy with tamoxifen.

Common symptoms are: Abnormal uterine bleeding in the form of intermenstrual, premenstrual bleeding, menorrhagia, postmenstrual spotting, pedunculated polyp may come out through the external os to be seen in the vagina. Rarely, an endometrial polyp may cause subfertility. Often it may remain asymptomatic.

Risks of malignancy in an endometrial polyp is low (3–5%). It depends on the age of the women and other associated pathology. Prolonged therapy with tamoxifen may result in endometrial hyperplasia (2–4%) and carcinoma (1–2%).

Diagnosis: Discussed above.

Differential diagnosis: Submucous leiomyoma, retained products of conception, endometrial hyperplasia, polypoid endometrial hyperplasia and endometrial carcinoma.

Histology: *See* below.

MANAGEMENT

Removal of polyp(s) hysteroscopially is the best option. D/C and polypectomy may be done. During curettage routine use of a narrow polyp forceps helps to remove any polyp that often eludes during blind curettage. Patients who have completed the family, hysterectomy may be an option. Histologically examination of the polyp and the endometrium should be done.

The causes of recurrence of polyps are: (a) Incomplete removal; (b) Persistence of the cause leading to polyp formation; (c) Malignancy. Cervical polyps are removed by twisting of the pedicle. The base of the pedicle should be cauterized to prevent recurrence.

Place of Hysteroscopy, is useful to locate the position, size, and the base of the polyp. Submucous fibroid polyps can be resected out hysteroscopically as an outpatient basis (Fig. 20.9). **Endometrial polyps that cause infertility, postmenopausal bleeding or abnormal uterine bleeding should be removed hysteroscopically under direct vision.** It is superior to blind avulsion. After the polyp is removed, endometrium is curetted to rule out coexisting pathology (5%).

Histology

Histologically, the polyp may be adenomatous (80%), cystic, fibrous, vascular and fibromyomatous. There may be ulceration of the dependent portion of the polyp. Malignant change of an endometrial polyp is extremely rare (0.5%).

Big Fibroid Polyp Lying in the Vagina

One should be sure that it is a polyp and not uterine inversion or fibroid with inversion (*see* above).

- **Diagnosed polyp:** Removal of polyp by **morcellement** (piecemeal) followed by transfixation suture on the pedicle and removal of the redundant pedicle distal to the ligature.
- **Associated with chronic uterine inversion:** The incision is made close to the fibroid and to enucleate it.

When hysterectomy is indicated, the polyps of such type are expected to be infected and are to be removed first. Antibiotics are to be administered. The general condition of the patient is to be improved and hysterectomy should be done at a later date.

The polyps should be sent for histological examination after its removal.

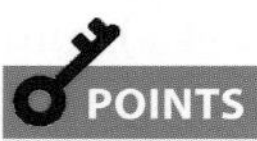

KEY POINTS

- **Fibroid** is the most common pelvic tumor. The incidence of symptomatic fibroid varies from 3–10%. It is common in nulliparous and the prevalence is highest between 35–45 years.
  Fibroid arises from the smooth muscle elements of the myometrium, could be genetically determined and the growth is dependent on the polypeptide growth factors (EGF, IGF-1, TGF) and estrogen. It is slow growing compared to ovarian neoplasm.
  Fibroids may affect the reproductive outcome adversely by enlargement and distortion of the uterus, anovulation, cervical or cornual black or poor endometrial vascularity.
- There are certain factors that, on the other hand reduces the risk of fibroid (p. 224).
- **Types of fibroid** depend on their anatomical location (p. 225).
- **Corporeal fibroid** is common and often multiple. All fibroids are interstitial but later on become submucous or subserous. Cervical fibroid is rare (1–2%).
  Fibroid has got a false capsule formed by the compressed myometrium. The center is least vascular and degeneration is common. Fibroids often undergo **secondary changes** (*see.* p. 227).
  Hyaline degeneration is the most common secondary change and sarcoma is rare 0.1%. Red degeneration occurs mainly in pregnancy and puerperium.
  Associated endometriosis and adenomyosis is found in 30% and pelvic infection in 15%.
  Majority of fibroids remain asymptomatic (75%). Menorrhagia is the classic symptom of fibroid. Pelvic examination is supportive—the tumor of uterine origin. For **confirmation of diagnosis**, the help of sonography, laparoscopy, hysteroscopy or HSG or rarely CT, MRI may be useful in selected cases.
  Life-threatening complications include—severe anemia, intraperitoneal hemorrhage from ruptured veins over the subserous fibroid, severe infection and sarcomatous changes.
  There is definite place of **observation in asymptomatic fibroid** provided one is certain of diagnosis and follow-up is possible.
- **Medical management** aims mostly as palliative and the drugs used are antiprogesterones, danazol, GnRH analogs (agonists and antagonists) and LNG-IUS. Benefits of preoperative GnRH analog therapy are many (Table 20.8).
- **MR guided focused ultrasound (MRgFUS)** is safe feasible and minimally invasive. It has certain contraindications also (p. 233).
  The surgical treatment of fibroid may be hysterectomy or myomectomy, depending upon the age of the patient and need for preservation of reproductive function. **Indications of myomectomy** may be either due to a symptomatic or due to an asymptomatic fibroid (Table 20.10). **Contraindications** must be carefully judged (Table 20.12).
  Laparoscopic or hysteroscopic procedures can be done with reduced morbidity.
  Myomectomy is a risky operation. Prior to myomectomy, there are many important considerations (Tables 20.9 to 20.12). There is chance of recurrence (30–50%), persistence of menorrhagia (1–5%) and relaparotomy (20–25%). Pregnancy rate following myomectomy is about 40–60%. Subserous and interstitial fibroids could be removed laparoscopically. Hysteroscopic resection of the submucous fibroid can be done in selected cases (Fig. 20.10).
  Uterine artery embolization (UAE) and myolysis are the other methods of treatment (p. 99). The newest modality of management is uterine artery embolization which is an ambulatory and nonsurgical management. UAE has got certain contraindications and complications also.
- The most common type of **benign uterine polyp** is a mucous one. Risk factors for polyps are: Hormone replacement therapy, tamoxifen therapy or increased patient age. A big polyp may be confused with chronic uterine inversion or may be associated with it. Malignant transformation of endometrial polyps is about 0.5%. Hysteroscopic removal of endometrial polyps is superior to blind avulsion.
- Intravenous leiomyomatosis (IL) and leiomyomatosis peritonealis disseminata (LPD).
- Intravenous leiomyomatosis is a rare condition where smooth muscle fibers slowly grow into the venous channels and the pelvis. It may grow within the vena cava and the right heart. Antiestrogen therapy with aromatase inhibitors after the resection of leiomyomatosis is found effective.
- LPD is a benign condition with multiple small nodules over the surface of the pelvis and abdominal peritoneum. LPD mimics disseminated carcinoma. Use of power morcellation increases the risk of LPD. Therapy with SPRMs or aromatase inhibitors found to be useful.

CHAPTER

21 Benign Neoplasms of the Ovary

CHAPTER OUTLINE

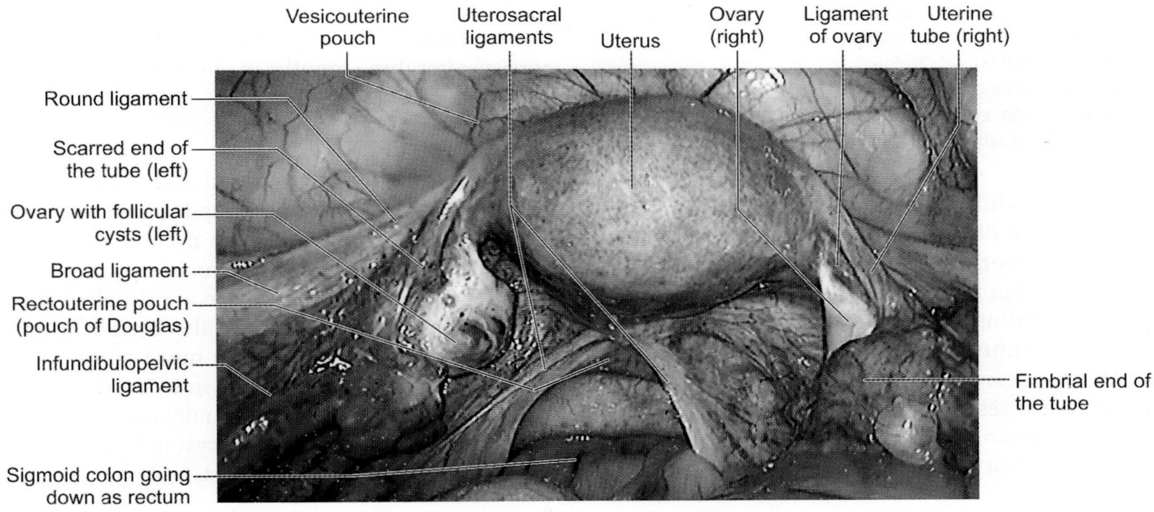

Fig. 21.1: Laparoscopic view of the pelvis of a 33-year-old parous woman. Laparoscopy was done for chronic pelvic pain. She had tubectomy operation done in the past.

NORMAL OVARY (FIG. 21.1)

Measurement (average) of a normal ovary

- Neonate—1.3 cm × 0.6 cm × 0.4 cm
- Reproductive—4 cm × 2 cm × 3 cm
- Menopause—2 cm × 1.5 cm × 0.5 cm

  Volume: 10 cm^3 (maximum 18 cm^3)

OVARIAN ENLARGEMENT

- **Non-neoplastic**
- **Neoplastic (benign)**

NON-NEOPLASTIC

The non-neoplastic enlargement of the ovary is usually due to accumulation of fluid inside the functional unit of the ovary.

Follicular Cysts

Follicular cysts are the most common functional cysts (Fig. 21.2). They are usually multiple and small as seen in

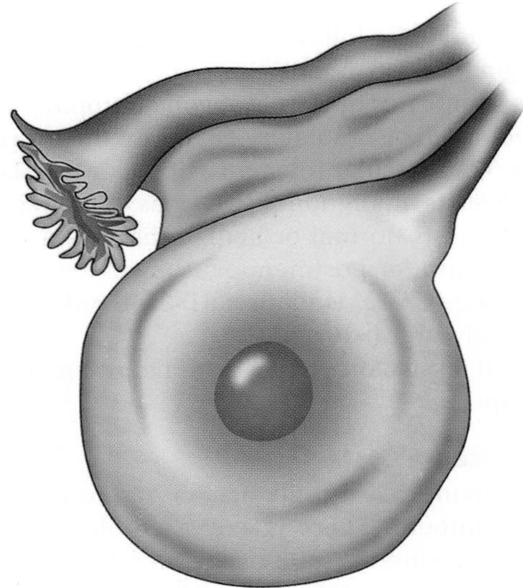

Fig. 21.2: Follicular cyst.

Causes of Non-neoplastic Cysts of the Ovary

- Follicular cysts
- Corpus luteum cyst
- Theca lutein and granulosa lutein cysts
- Polycystic ovarian syndrome
- Endometrial cyst (chocolate cyst)

Except the last one, all are functional cysts of the ovary and are loosely called cystic ovary.

Clinical Features of a Functional Cyst

- Related to temporary hormonal disorders
- Rarely becomes complicated
- Sometimes confused with neoplastic cyst but can be distinguished by the following features:
  - Usually ≤7 cm in diameter
  - Usually asymptomatic
  - Spontaneous regression occurs following correction of the temporary hormonal dysfunction
  - Unilocular (on USG)
  - Usually contains a clear fluid
  - Lining epithelium corresponds to the functional epithelium of the unit from which it arises.

cases of cystic glandular hyperplasia of the endometrium or in association of fibroid. Hyperestrinism is implicated as its cause. However, an isolated cyst may be formed in unruptured Graafian follicle, which may be enlarged but usually not exceeding 5 cm. The cyst is lined by typical granulosa cells without lutein cells or the cells may be flattened due to pressure.

In majority of cases, the detection is made accidentally on bimanual examination, sonography, laparoscopy or laparotomy. The cyst may remain asymptomatic or may cause vague pain.

Management

A follicular cyst ≤3 cm requires no further investigations. A simple cyst <7 cm, unilocular, echo free without solid areas or papillary projections, with normal serum cancer antigen (CA 125) should be followed up with repeat ultrasound (endovaginal) in 3–6 months time.

COCs suppresses the levels of gonadotropins. Thereby COCs reduces the stimulatory effects on the ovaries and the cysts. Low vascular resistance on color flow Doppler study suggests malignancy whereas high resistance usually suggests normal or benign disease. A cyst in a perimenopausal or postmenopausal women should be removed when CA 125 is abnormal (>35 IU/mL) or the cyst is persistently large (>10 cm).

Removal (cystectomy) may be done by laparotomy or laparoscopy.

Corpus Luteum Cysts

Corpus luteum cyst usually occurs due to overactivity of corpus luteum. There is excessive bleeding inside the corpus luteum. In spite of the blood filled cyst, the progesterone and estrogen secretion continues. As a result, the menstrual cycle may be normal or there may be amenorrhea or delayed cycle. Most corpus luteum cysts are small. Rarely, a cyst may be 11–15 cm in diameter. It is usually followed by heavy and/or continued bleeding. It is then confused with a case of **threatened abortion** or else, if the intracystic bleeding is much, it may rupture producing features of acute **intraperitoneal hemorrhage** with clinical picture simulating disturbed **tubal ectopic pregnancy**.

It may often be associated with pregnancy and persists for about 12 weeks. Unless complicated, spontaneous regression is expected.

If features of acute abdomen appears, laparoscopy/laparotomy with enucleation of the cyst (cystectomy) is to be done along with resuscitative measures as in disturbed tubal pregnancy. Cut section looks yellowish-orange in color.

These two types of cysts are rather uncommon in women taking oral contraceptive pills. As such, if the cyst persists after three months of observation, it is more likely to be neoplastic.

Lutein Cysts (Fig. 21.3)

Lutein cysts are usually bilateral and caused by excessive **chorionic gonadotropin** secreted in cases of **gestational trophoblastic tumors**. These may also develop with administration of **gonadotropins or even clomiphene** to induce ovulation (OHSS). These are usually bilateral and asymptomatic. Leutin cysts are also seen in latter months of pregnancy. These cysts are more common in cases where placenta is large such as in twins, diabetes and Rh alloimmunization. They are usually lined either by theca lutein cells, called theca lutein cyst or by granulosa lutein cells, called granulosa lutein cyst.

Treatment

Spontaneous regression is expected within few weeks following effective therapy of the tumors with the gonadotropin level returning back to normal.

Combined oral contraceptives (COCs) suppress ovarian activity and protect against ovarian cyst development. Progestin only contraceptives including levonorgestrel-intrauterine system (LNG-IUS) have been associated with development of functional cyst. Tamoxifen use have an increased risk of ovarian cyst formation.

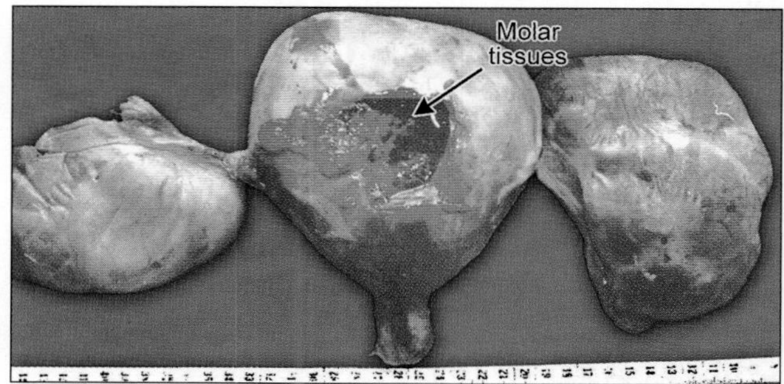

Fig. 21.3: Bilateral lutein cysts in association with hydatidiform mole. Window is made in the uterus to show the molar tissues.

BENIGN OVARIAN NEOPLASMS

Incidence

The incidence of ovarian tumor amongst gynecologic admission varies from 1 to 3%. About 75% of these are benign.

Classification of Ovarian Neoplasms (WHO)

The classification along with the frequency of occurrence is given in Table 21.1. Epithelial tumors are the most common. Germ cell tumors are the second most frequent are most common among the younger age. Sex cord stromal tumors are the third most frequent ovarian neoplasm. Lipid (lipoid) cell tumors are extremely rare. These tumors histologically resembles the adrenal gland. Gonadoblastoma occurs in individuals with dysgenetic gonads where Y chromosome is present.

The principal ovarian tissue components are:

- Epithelial cells derived from the **coelomic epithelium**.
- Oocytes derived from the primitive **germ cells**.
- Mesenchymal elements from the **gonadal stroma**.

The classification given in the text is based on **WHO classification (Table 21.1)**.

Although full classification of the ovarian neoplasms has been presented, **only the benign ovarian tumors and that too, only the common varieties** will be presented in this Chapter. These are:

- Mucinous cyst adenoma
- Serous cyst adenoma
- Brenner tumor
- Dermoid cyst
- Endometrioid tumors
- Clear cell tumors.

These tumors constitute about 80% of the primary ovarian tumors and are called ovarian tumors as opposed to cystic ovaries in functional ones.

The cell types of ovarian epithelial tumors recapitulate the Müllerian duct epithelium (serous from endosalpinx, mucinous from endocervix, endometrioid from endometrium).

Mucinous Cyst Adenoma

Origin

Mucinous tumors arise from the surface epithelial cells. Cells are filled with mucin. **These cells resemble the cells of the endocervix or that of intestinal cells.**

Pathology

These are quite common and account for about 20–25% of all ovarian tumors. The tumors are **bilateral** in about 10% cases. **The chance of malignancy is about 5–10%.**

Naked Eye Appearance

It may attain a huge size if left uncared for. In fact, **it is the largest benign ovarian tumor.**

The wall is smooth, lobulated with whitish or bluish-white hue. At places, it is thin so as to be translucent.

On Cut Section

The content inside is thick, viscid, mucin—a glycoprotein with high content of neutral polysaccharides. It is colorless unless complicated by hemorrhage. The cyst is frequently multiloculated, sometimes with papillary growth arising from the septum (Fig. 21.4).

Microscopic Examination

The cyst is lined by a single layer of tall columnar epithelium with dark staining basal nucleus but without any cilia. The epithelial characteristics are like those of endocervix (Figs. 21.5 and 21.6).

TABLE 21.1: Classification of ovarian tumor (WHO).

A. Epithelial tumor (60–70%) These tumors may be benign, borderline malignant or malignant. ▪ Serous tumor ▪ Mucinous cyst adenoma ▪ Endometrioid tumors ▪ Mesonephroid or clear cell tumors ▪ Transitional cell: Brenner tumors ▪ Squamous cell tumors ▪ Mixed epithelial tumors ▪ Undifferentiated carcinoma
B. Germ cell tumors of the ovary (20–25% of all primary ovarian neoplasms) ***Germ cell tumors*** a. Dysgerminoma b. Endodermal sinus tumor (yolk sac tumor) c. Embryonal cell carcinoma d. Polyembryoma e. Choriocarcinoma f. Teratoma: – Immature – Mature (dermoid cyst) – Monodermal: Struma ovarii, carcinoid g. Mixed forms (combinations of types a to f)
C. Sex cord stromal tumors (6–10%) ▪ Granulosa cell tumors ▪ Tumors of thecoma-fibroma group • Thecoma • Fibroma • Unclassified ▪ Androblastoma • Sertoli cell tumor • Sertoli-Leydig cell tumor • Hilus cell tumor
D. Lipid cell tumor (<0.1%)
E. Tumors composed of germ cells and sex cord stromal derivatives (<0.1%) • Gonadoblastoma • Mixed germ cell—sex cord stromal tumor • Others
F. Unclassified tumors: These are the tumors that cannot be placed in any of the categories as mentioned above. Soft tissue tumors are not specific to ovary such as hemangioma or lipoma.
G. Secondary metastasis
H. Tumor like conditions include the conditions that are associated with ovarian enlargement: These are—massive ovarian edema, pregnancy luteoma, luteal cysts, endometriomas. These are not true neoplasms.

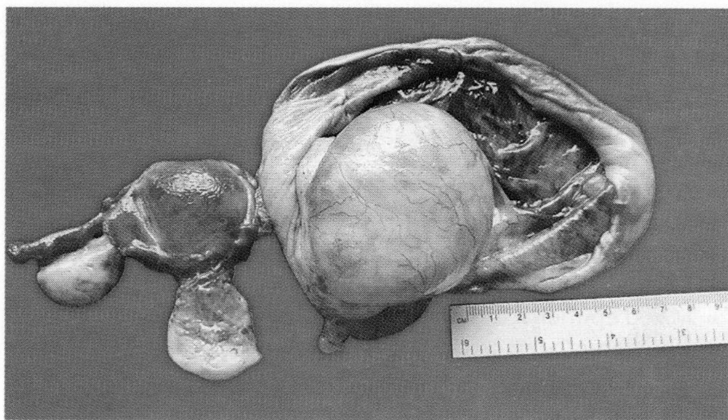

Fig. 21.4: Cut section showing mucinous cyst adenoma. Multilocularity of the tumor is seen. Cyst wall is thick and there was intracystic hemorrhage.

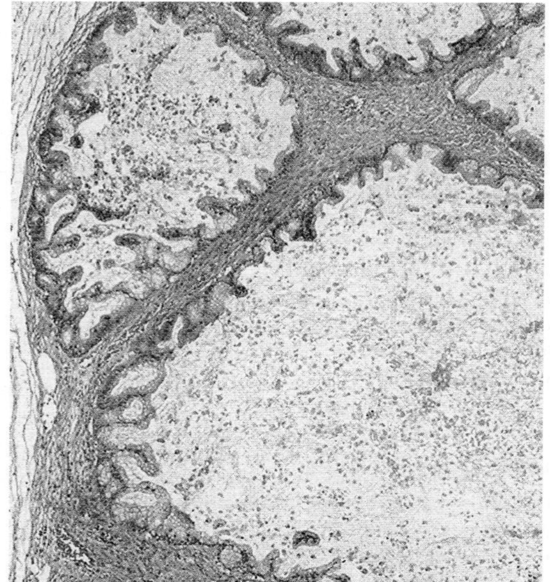

Fig. 21.5: Microphotograph showing the lining epithelium of mucinous cyst adenoma. The epithelium does not invade the wall and the serosa is intact.

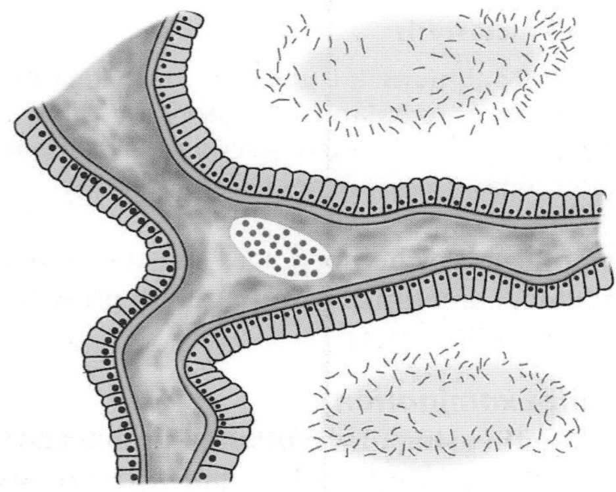

Fig. 21.6: Diagrammatic picture showing a single layer of tall columnar epithelial cells with basal nuclei. These cells secrete mucin—mucinous cyst adenoma.

IMPORTANT FEATURES OF A MUCINOUS CYST ADENOMA

- Epithelial ovarian tumor
- Second common (20–25%) epithelial tumor
- Bilateral in 5–10%
- Cut section multilocular
- Cyst fluid is thick, viscid and mucinous
- Risk of malignancy 5–10%
- *Histology:* Single layer tall columnar cells with basal nuclei.

Serous Cyst Adenoma

Origin

It is quite common and **accounts for about 40%** of ovarian tumors. It is **bilateral in about 40%** and **chance of malignancy is about 40%.**

Pathology

The cysts are not so big as that of mucinous type. As the secretion is not abundant, there is more chance of proliferation of the lining epithelium to form papillary projection. As such, intracystic hemorrhage is more likely. **Often, the papillary growth projects outwards perforating the cyst wall in about 15% cases.**

Naked Eye Appearance

The wall is smooth, shiny and grayish white. At times, there are exuberant papillary projection. It may be multilobulated on cut section. The content fluid is clear, rich in serum proteins—albumin and globulin.

Microscopic Examination

It is lined by a single layer of cubical epithelium.

The papillary structures consist of broad dense fibrous stroma covered by single or multiple layers of columnar epithelium. There may be presence of ciliated, secretory and peg cells resembling tubal epithelium (Fig. 21.7).

Psammoma bodies: These are tiny, spherical, laminated calcified structures which are most often found in areas of cellular degeneration (15%). Its presence per se does not denote malignancy. It is not present in slow growing tumor.

IMPORTANT FEATURES OF A SEROUS CYST ADENOMA

- Epithelial ovarian tumor
- Common (40%) ovarian tumor
- Bilateral in up to 20%
- May be multilocular or unilocular
- Surface papillary projections are often present
- Psammoma bodies may be present (15%)
- *Histology:* Columnar epithelial cells single/multiple layers
- Risk of malignancy up to 40%.

Endometrioid Tumors

Endometrioid tumors are rare (5%) and consists of epithelial cells resembling those endometrium. Endometroid carcinomas (malignant variety) may occur.

Clear Cell (Mesonephroid) Tumors

Clear cell (mesonephroid) tumors contain cells with abundant glycogen and are called **hobnail cells.** The nuclei of the cells protrude into the glandular lumen. They occur in women 40–70 years of age and are highly aggressive.

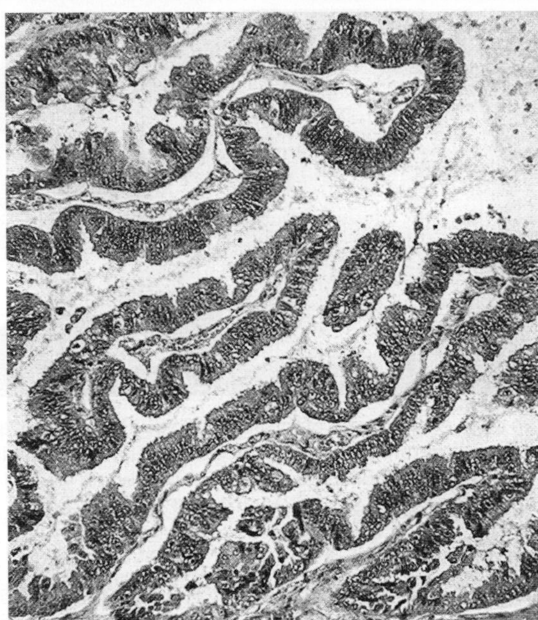

Fig. 21.7: Microphotograph showing the lining epithelium of papillary serous cyst adenoma. The cells from long papilliform processes.

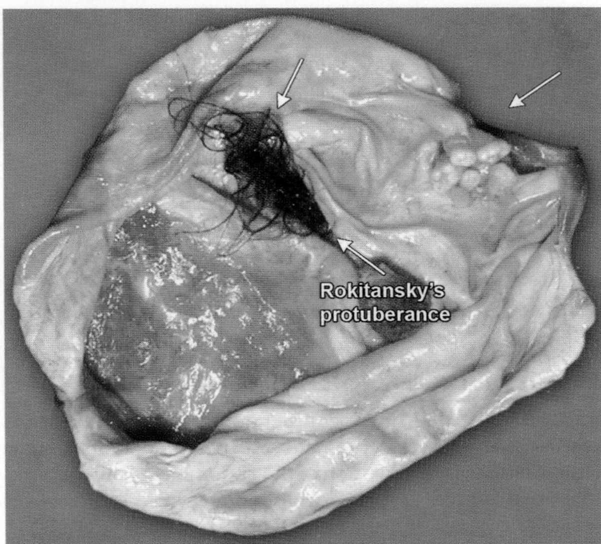

Fig. 21.8: Cut section of a dermoid cyst showing hair teeth.

Brenner Tumor

Brenner tumor account for 2–3% of all ovarian tumors, **8–10% are bilateral** and **usually seen in women above the age of 40**. Majority are solid and are less than 2 cm in diameter. **It usually arises from squamous metaplasia of surface epithelium**. Gross picture of Brenner is similar to that of fibroma. **Histologically islands of transitional epithelium (Walthard nests) in a compact fibrous stroma are seen. The cells look like 'coffee bean' as the nuclei have longitudinal grooves**. They are usually benign in nature. **Estrogen is secreted by the tumor** and the woman may present with abnormal vaginal bleeding. Unilateral oophorectomy in a young woman and total hysterectomy and bilateral salpingo-oophorectomy in elderly women is the treatment choice.

Dermoid Cyst (Mature Teratoma)

Origin

Dermoid cyst **arises from a single germ cell** arrested after the first meiotic division. Karyotype in majority is 46XX.

Pathology

Dermoid cyst constitutes about 97% of teratomata. Its incidence is about **30–40%** amongst ovarian tumors. The tumor is **bilateral in about 15–20%**. It constitutes about **20–40%** of all ovarian tumors in pregnancy. **Torsion is the most common (15–20%) and rupture is an uncommon (1%) complication. The chance of malignancy is about 1–2%**. Squamous cell carcinoma is the most common.

Naked Eye Appearance (Fig. 21.8)

The cyst is of moderate size and usually <10 cm. The capsule is tense and smooth. On cut section, the content is a predominantly sebaceous material with hair. There may be clear fluid (cerebrospinal fluid) derived from the neural tissues (choroid plexus). There is one area of solid projection called **Rokitansky's protuberance** which is covered by skin with sweat and sebaceous glands. It is here that teeth and bones are found. This prominence can be seen with USG as an echogenic region. **Histological section should be made from this area**. A rare one consists predominantly of thyroid tissue—called **struma ovarii,** which may be associated with hyperthyroidism. Other medical diseases associated with dermoid cysts are: carcinoid syndrome, and autoimmune hemolytic anemia. It is diagnosed with raised serum serotonin levels and urinary 5-OH indole acetic acid.

Characteristic sonographic diagnostic features are: (a) Fat-fluid or hair fluid levels are seen as distinct linear demarcation; (b) Accentuated lines and dots of floating hair could be seen; (c) Rokitansky protuberance is seen as echogenic region; (d) The sign "tip of the iceberg" is created by amorphous echogenic interfaces of fat, hair and tissues in the foreground of that shadow and obscure structures behind it.

Microscopic Examination

The wall is lined by stratified squamous epithelium and at places by granulation tissue. The epithelium may be transitional or columnar. **The most common tissue elements are ectodermal.**

IMPORTANT FEATURES OF A DERMOID CYST

- Germ cell ovarian tumor
- 40% of all ovarian tumors
- Bilateral: 15–20%
- Contains elements of three germ cell layers
- Many contain thyroid tissues (struma ovarii)
- Symptomatic (50%)
- Torsion is common (15–20%)
- Risk of malignancy is low (1–2%).

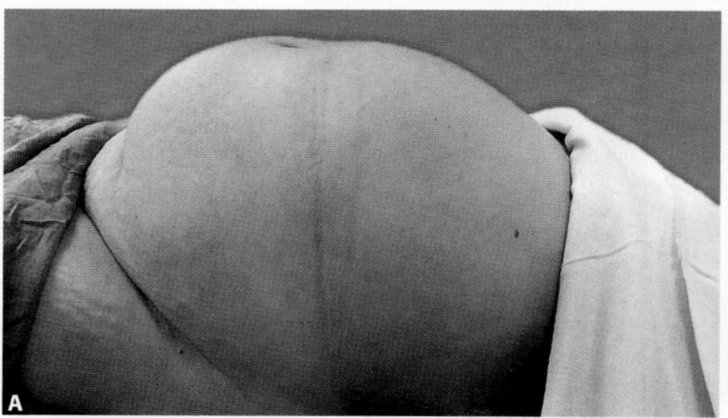
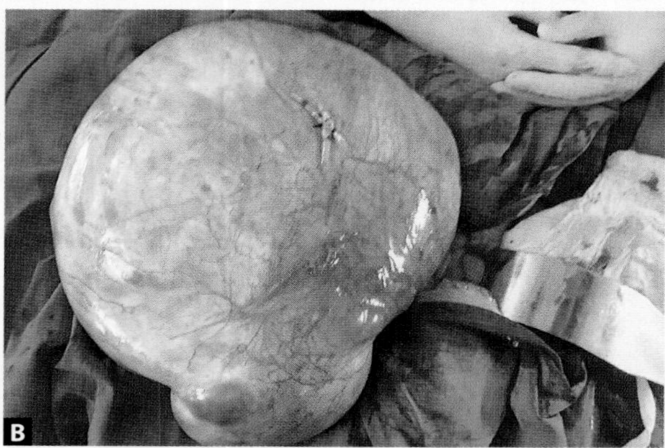

Figs. 21.9A and B: (A) Preoperative photograph of a 67-year-old woman with huge enlargement of the abdomen due to a large ovarian mass that remained asymptomatic; (B) The intraoperative finding was a huge ovarian tumor. It was a mucinous cyst adenoma arising from the left ovary. Exploration of the abdominal cavity followed by total hysterectomy with bilateral salpingo oophorectomy was done. Patient had uneventful recovery. Histology revealed mucinous ovarian tumour with Low Malignant Potential (LMP) (p. 250).

The terminology of 'dermoid cyst' is misnomer, as apart from **ectodermal element, there may be endodermal and mesodermal tissues as well**.

Tissue components are:

- **Ectodermal**: Skin, hair, teeth, nerve tissue, sebaceous material, glial tissue.
- **Mesodermal**: Bone, cartilage, muscle.
- **Endodermal**: Thyroid, salivary gland, bronchus, intestine.

Struma Ovarii and Strumal Carcinoids

Rarely ovarian teratomas contain a specialized tissue type. **Struma ovarii is composed of thyroid tissue.** This accounts for less than 3% of **mature teratomas. Malignant changes in a struma ovarii is extremely rare. Strumal carcinoids** are also rare teratomas. Primary carcinoid tumors of the ovary account for less than 5% of ovarian teratomas. These tumors may be **hormonally active with secretion of serotonin, bradykinin and other peptide hormones from the argentaffin cells** as found in gastrointestinal tract or bronchial tissues.

Carcinoid syndrome is characterized by episodic facial flashing, abdominal pain, diarrhea, and bronchospasm. **Metastatic carcinoid tumors are often bilateral.** Carcinoid syndrome is more common in metastatic carcinoid than in ovarian primaries.

Operative treatment of benign cystic teratoma is cystectomy with preservation of normal healthy ovarian tissue. Laparoscopic surgery may be done using endo bag. **Copious pelvic irrigation with normal saline is essential.**

Clinical Features of Benign Ovarian Tumors

Age

Benign tumors predominantly manifest in the late childbearing period. However, dermoid (90%), mucinous cyst adenoma, is common in the reproductive period. As such, the dermoid is more common during pregnancy (10%).

Parity

There is no correlation with parity of the patient (c.f. fibroid—more related with nulliparity).

Symptoms

Most tumors are asymptomatic (Figs. 21.9A and B). These are detected accidentally by a general physician to find a lump in the lower abdomen during routine abdominal palpation or by a gynecologist to find a tumor during pelvic examination, laparoscopy or laparotomy.

However, the patient may present the following symptoms:

- Heaviness in the lower abdomen.
- A gradually increasing mass in lower abdomen (ovarian tumor grows in months—c.f. fibroid).
- Dull aching pain in lower abdomen.
- In few cases, the tumor may be big enough to fill whole of the abdomen. It then produces cardiorespiratory embarrassment or gastrointestinal symptoms like nausea or indigestion.
- **Menstrual pattern remains unaffected unless associated with hormone producing tumor**—menorrhagia or postmenopausal bleeding or precocious puberty in feminizing tumor-like granulosa cell tumor or amenorrhea in masculinizing tumor-like Sertoli-Leydig cell tumor is observed.

Signs

- **General condition** remains unaffected. However, in huge mucinous cyst adenoma, the patient may be cachetic due to protein loss (Fig. 21.10).
- **Pitting edema** of legs may be present when a huge tumor presses on the great veins.

Abdominal examination: An ovarian tumor which is enlarged sufficiently so as to occupy the lower abdomen presents with the following:

- ***Inspection***: There is bulging of the lower abdomen over which the abdominal wall moves freely with respiration. The mass may be placed centrally or in one side. At times, the mass fills the entire abdominal cavity everting the umbilicus with visible veins under the skin; the flanks remain flat (c.f. flanks are full with ascites) (Figs. 21.11A and B).

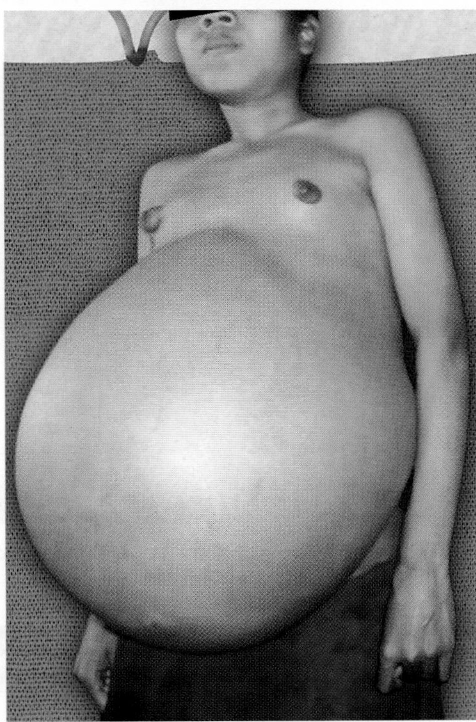

Fig. 21.10: Marked enlargement of the abdomen due to a huge mucinous cyst adenoma.
(*Courtesy:* Prof. S Pati; Dr A Halder, Assistant Professor, NB Medical College, Sushrutnagar, Darjeeling).

- ***Palpation:***
  - **Feel** is cystic or tense cystic. Benign solid tumors such as fibroma, thecoma, and Brenner tumor are rare.
  - **Mobility:** Freely mobile from side to side but restricted from above down unless the pedicle is long. Too big a tumor or adhesions make its mobility restricted.
  - **Borders:** Upper and lateral borders are well-defined but the lower pole is difficult to reach suggestive of pelvic origin. However, with long pedicle, the tumor may be displaced upwards so as to reach the lower pole.
  - **Surface** over the tumor is smooth but often grooved in lobulated tumor.
  - **Tenderness:** It is usually not tender.
- ***Percussion*** (Figs. 21.11A and B): Percussion note is dull in the center and resonant in the flanks (c.f. in ascites—just the opposite). A fluid thrill may be elicited when the walls are thin and the content is watery. Coexisting ascites may be present even in a benign solid tumor (fibroma) and is called Meigs' syndrome.

Meigs' Syndrome

Ascites and right side hydrothorax in association with fibroma of the ovary, Brenner, thecoma and granulosa cell tumor is called Meigs' syndrome. There is spontaneous remission of ascites and hydrothorax on removal of the tumor. Ascites and hydrothorax when present in conditions other than those mentioned above, are called pseudo-Meigs' syndrome (*c.f. leiomyoma*).

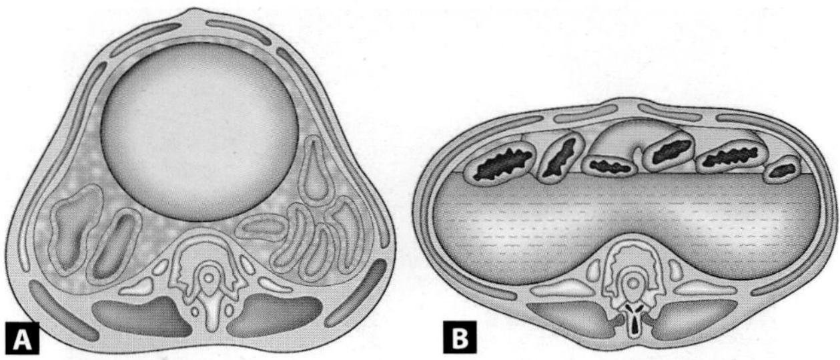

Figs. 21.11A and B: Note the contour of the abdomen in ovarian tumor (A) and ascites (B).

- ***Auscultation:*** A friction rub may be present over the tumor (hissing sound over a vascular fibroid, gargling sound in ascites and FHS over a pregnant uterus).

Pelvic examination

- **Bimanual examination**
  - The uterus is separated from the mass.
  - A groove is felt between the uterus and the mass.
  - Movement of the mass per abdomen fails to move the cervix.
  - On elevation of the mass per abdomen, the cervix remains in stationary position.
  - The lower pole of the cyst can be felt through the fornix.

It is indeed difficult to identify a huge cyst even by bimanual examination as the findings are all obscured. It is also difficult to foretell from which side the tumor arises. However, with elevation of the tumor per abdomen, the stretched pedicle may be felt through the corresponding fornix. **If a cyst is felt lying anterior to the uterus, it is more likely to be dermoid.**

Special Investigations

If the clinical features are equivocal, the following may be employed to substantiate the diagnosis.

- **Sonography (Fig. 21.12):** It can identify the uterus and the tumor in the same scan. Transvaginal sonography with color flow **Doppler** study gives information about the tumor volume, cyst wall, septa, and the vascularity.

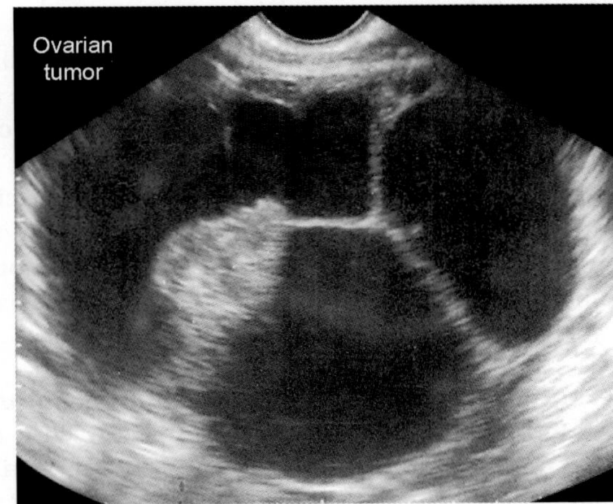

Fig. 21.12: Sonography transvaginal (TV) of a benign ovarian cyst—multilocular with thin septum.

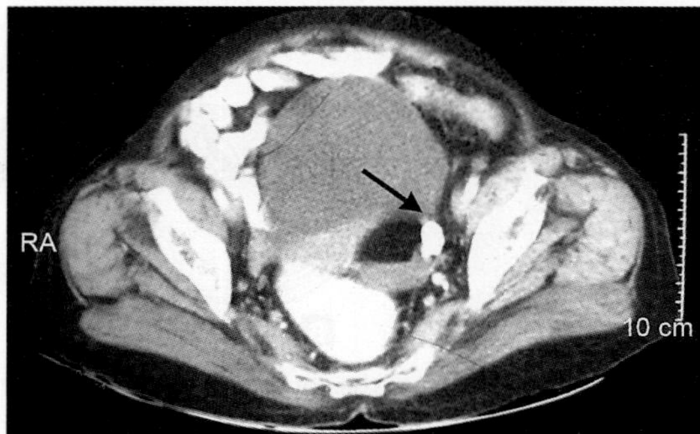

Fig. 21.13: CT scan shows a typical benign cystic teratoma containing fat, dental elements (arrow) and a fat-fluid level.

Presence of the following ultrasonographic features suggest the high risk of malignancy: (a) Multilocular cyst; (b) Presence of solid areas; (c) Metastasis; (d) Ascites; (e) Bilateral tumors; (f) High blood flow.

- **CT (Fig. 21.13):** The presence of an adnexal mass with mixed attenuation due to the presence of large amount of fat, calcification and tooth.
- **MRI:** It is helpful to determine whether the cyst is likely to be benign or malignant. It is not done as a routine (p. 100).
- **Serum Tumour Markers (p. 438):** (a) **Serum CA 125**; (b) **α-fetoprotein**; (c) **β-hCG**
- **Examination under anesthesia (EUA):** In doubtful diagnosis especially in virgins, EUA is helpful.
- **Cyst aspiration**: It is usually avoided due to the risk of tumor spill and spread of malignancy. Cyst aspiration and cytologic evaluation is mostly nondiagnostic. False positive and false negative results are common. Sometimes aspiration may be done to reduce the size of the tumor during operation.
- **Straight X-ray of the abdomen over the tumor:** The finding of a shadow of teeth or bones is a direct evidence of a dermoid cyst. An outline of a soft tissue shadow may also be visible (Fig. 21.14).
- **Laparoscopy:** This is of help to differentiate a painful cystic mass with disturbed ectopic pregnancy.
- **Laparotomy:** If the clinical and ancillary aids fail to diagnose the mass, laparotomy is justified to arrive at a diagnosis. This is especially indicated when a suspected functional cyst fails to regress in follow up.
- **Cytology:** When the patient presents with ascites or pleural effusion, cytological examination of the aspirated fluid is done for malignant cells. Ultrasound guided cyst aspiration for cytological diagnosis of malignancy is not recommended.

Differential Diagnosis of a Benign Ovarian Tumor

Full bladder: Always examine the patient with the bladder empty; if necessary following catheterization. One should not be confused with overflow incontinence in chronic retention as normal urination, as stated by the patient.

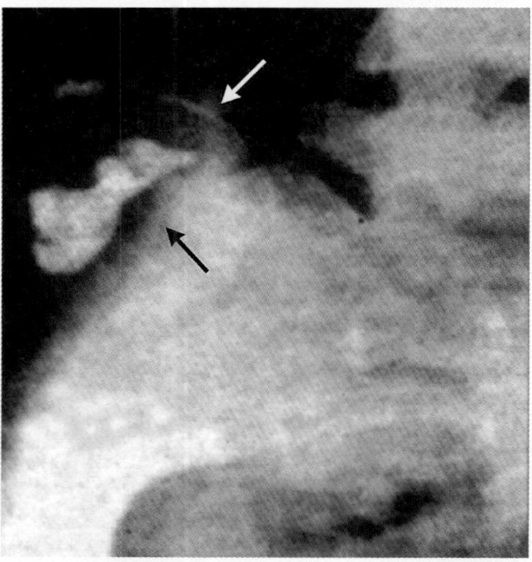

Fig. 21.14: Plain X-ray of the abdomen over a tumor showing shadow of a tooth in dermoid (arrows).

Differential Diagnosis of a Benign Ovarian Tumor

An ovarian tumor, apparently uncomplicated, may be confused (depending upon its size) with the following:
- Full bladder
- Pregnancy
- Fibroid
- Ovarian endometrioma (chocolate cyst)
- Functional ovarian cyst (theca lutein cysts)
- Pregnancy with fibroid
- Encysted peritonitis
- Ascites

Pregnancy: It should be excluded in a woman with child-bearing age. Ultrasonography is helpful for the diagnosis.
Fibroid: Confusion arises especially in cases subserous fibroid more so, if degeneration occurs. Ultrasonography or laparoscopy helpful.
Chocolate cyst of the ovary: For detail p. 249.

Sometimes, the ovarian tumor is so big as in mucinous cyst adenoma, that it is difficult to differentiate by clinical examination alone. In such cases, USG or MRI is helpful.

Functional cyst: These cysts are usually small. Ultrasonography or re-examination after 4–6 weeks solves the diagnosis in most cases. The follicular or corpus luteum cyst usually regresses, while neoplastic cyst usually increases in size. Laparoscopy is of help.
Pregnancy with fibroid: In such condition, the pregnant uterus feels more soft and cystic but the fibroid feels little firm. As such, the former is confused as ovarian cyst and the latter one as uterus. USG is useful to differentiate.
Encysted peritonitis: There may be features of tubercular infection. The encysted mass is usually irregular, not movable with ill-defined margins and usually situated high up. Pelvic examination usually gives a negative finding.
Ascites: There is fullness of the flanks. On percussion, flanks are dull with resonance in the center. There may be presence of fluid thrill and positive shifting dullness on auscultation.

Complications of Benign Ovarian Tumors

- Torsion of the pedicle (axial rotation)
- Intracystic hemorrhage
- Infection
- Rupture
- Pseudomyxoma peritonei
- Malignancy.

Torsion of the Pedicle (Axial Rotation)

The axial rotation is found in about 10–15% cases at operation. It is common in tumor having:

- Moderate size, preferably with round contour.
- Moderate weight as *dermoid cyst* (due to high fat content)
- Free mobility
- Long pedicle.

As such, **the complication is more common in dermoid or serous cystadenoma. The etiology of torsion of the pedicle is obscure.**

Predisposing Factors for Torsion

- Trauma
- Violent physical movements
- Contractions of pregnant uterus
- Pulsation of pelvic major vessels
- Intestinal peristalsis.

CASE SUMMARY

A sixteen year young girl, admitted as emergency with acute lower abdominal pain. Clinical examination revealed a fairly large size pelvic abdominal mass with severe tenderness. Ultrasonography showed a large ovarian tumor with internal septations. Emergency laparotomy revealed this left sided ovarian tumor (18 cm × 12 cm) that has undergone two and half turns of torsion on its pedicle (Figs. 21.15A and B).

These probably initiate axial rotation. Torsion of right ovary is 2–3 times more that the left as mobility of left ovary is limited by the sigmoid colon.

The clinical presentation depends on the extent of interference with ovarian blood supply. With complete vascular occlusion, the pain will be severe. The lump may be present before or manifested with pain.

Abdominal examination reveals a tender, tense cystic mass, with restricted mobility, situated in the hypogastrium and arising from the pelvis.

Pelvic examination reveals the mass felt per abdomen is separate from the uterus.

Diagnosis: Sonography is helpful to the diagnosis in about 50–70% of cases. Doppler study may show disruption of normal adnexal flow.

Treatment

To control pain, morphine 15 mg IM is given. Laparoscopy/laparotomy is to be done at the earliest. In most situations the involved ovary may be salvaged.

Detorsion of adnexa is recommended where vascularity is maintained. Risk of embolism is too low (0.2%). Detorsion followed by cystectomy is done (Figs. 21.15A and B). Oophoropexy is done to prevent repeat torsion. The definitive surgery may be ovariotomy (salpingo-oophorectomy) when the structures become gangrenous (Fig. 21.17). Structures forming the ovarian pedicle need to be identified (Table 21.2).

TABLE 21.2: Structures forming the ovarian pedicle (Fig. 21.16).

Laterally Infundibulopelvic ligament containing structures therein, (ovarian vessels, nerves, and lymphatics)
Medially ▪ Ovarian ligament ▪ Medial end of the fallopian tube ▪ Mesosalpinx containing utero-ovarian anastomotic vessels
Middle Broad ligament

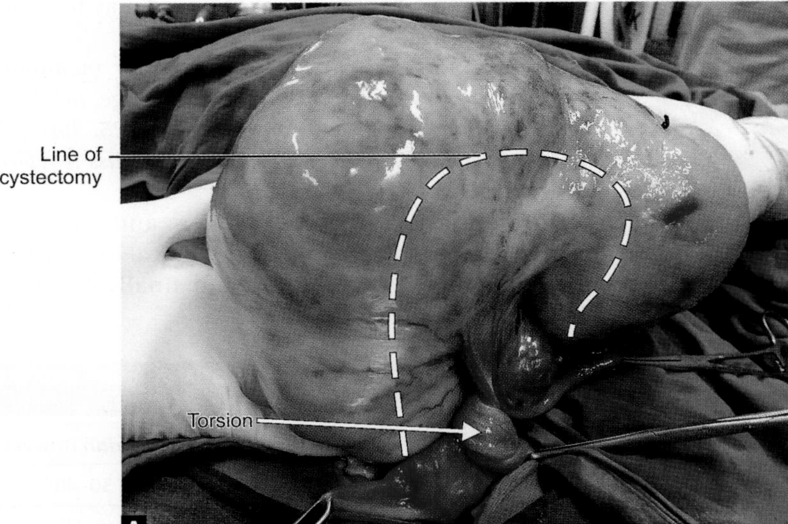

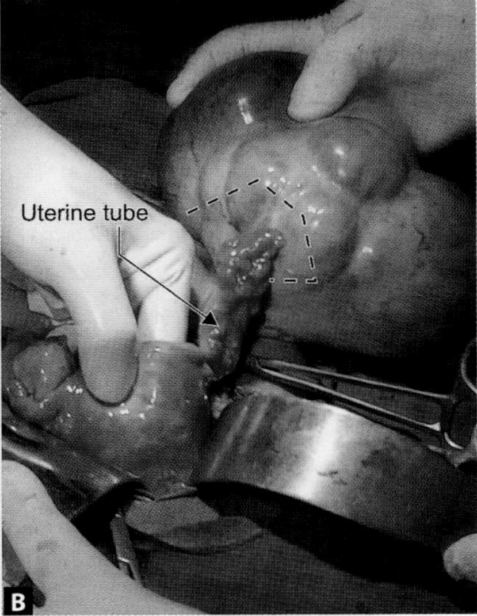

Figs. 21.15A and B: (A) Torsion of the pedicle of an ovarian tumor; (B) The same patient, detorsion of the pedicle was done; normal look of the uterine tube and the ovary following detorsion. Ovarian cystectomy was done.

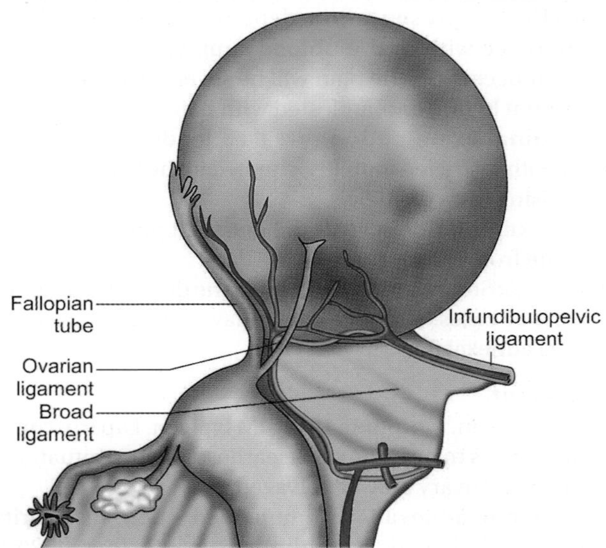

Fig. 21.16: Structures forming the ovarian pedicle.

Summary of Torsion of Ovarian Pedicle

- Common in dermoid or simple serous cyst
- Partial axial rotation followed by complete torsion
- Symptoms: Acute hypogastric pain with a lump
- General condition remains unaffected
- Abdominal examination: A tense cystic tender mass in the hypogastrium arising from the pelvis
- Pelvic examination: Mass is separate from the uterus
- Treatment: Conservative where possible. Laparotomy/laparoscopy and detorsion cystectomy/ovariotomy

Intracystic hemorrhage: It is more common in serous cyst adenoma with papillary varieties. Intracystic hemorrhage also occurs following venous congestion due to axial torsion of the pedicle and also in malignant changes (Fig. 21.17).

Infection: Infection is common following torsion. The organisms are derived from the intestines or uterine tubes when they are adherent to the cyst.

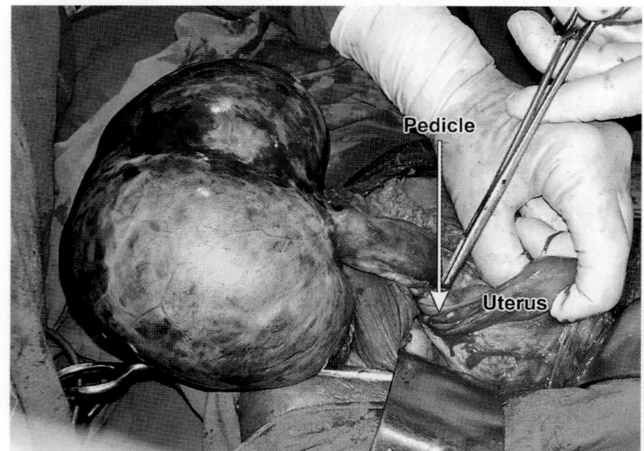

Fig. 21.17: Intracystic hemorrhage following ovarian torsion (see arrow) with gangrenous change. Ovariotomy (salpingo-oophorectomy) was done in this case.

Rupture: Rupture of the cyst usually follows in big and tense cysts with degeneration of a part of cyst wall. The rupture also occurs following intracystic hemorrhage or direct trauma, in papillary variety or in malignancy.

Pseudomyxoma peritonei: It is a condition of mucinous ascites usually secondary to mucinous tumor of intra-abdominal organ. Its exact nature of origin is not known. But **it is often associated with** mucinous cyst adenoma of the ovary, mucocele of the appendix and gallbladder and intestinal malignancy.

Spontaneous leakage of mucinous cyst may lead to implantation of the cells of low-grade malignancy on the peritoneum. Or else, the mesothelium of the peritoneum is converted to high columnar epithelium with secretory activity. The cell type is similar to mucinous cyst adenoma.

Even after removal of the ovarian tumor, these cells continue to secrete mucin. There is a tendency of recurrence. **The prognosis is poor** due to inanition, infection, and intestinal obstruction. Treatment remains unsatisfactory.

Hysterectomy, bilateral salpingo-oophorectomy with removal of mucin, peritoneal implants along with appendicectomy is recommended. Recurrence is high unless implants are removed entirely.

Malignancy: The malignancy rate varies (Table 21.3). The malignant potentiality is maximum in serous cyst adenoma especially of papillary variety and least in dermoid. The former gives rise to adenocarcinoma and the latter to squamous cell carcinoma.

Management of a Benign Ovarian Tumor

Once an ovarian tumor is diagnosed, the patient should be admitted for operation—sooner the better. This is because, **the complication can occur at any time and the nature of the tumor cannot be assessed clinically**. A clinically benign tumor may turn into a malignant one at operation. In others, even a benign tumor removed may be proved malignant on histological examination.

Ovarian mass >8 cm in diameter after menopause or before puberty or a solid tumor at any age, need to be evaluated by MRI/TVS and serum CA 125. Based on guidelines (RCOG), women with ovarian mass is referred to a gynecologic oncology center.

Differentiation between benign and malignant ovarian tumors could be made by clinical examination, ultrasonography, laparotomy and finally by biopsy (Table 21.4).

TABLE 21.3: Common epithelial ovarian tumors and their frequency (%).

Type	*All ovarian neoplasm*	*Ovarian cancers*
Serous	20–40	30–40
Mucinous	20–25	5–10
Endometrioid	5	15–20
Brenner	1–2	Rare

TABLE 21.4: Differentiation between benign and malignant ovarian tumors.

Clinical Presentation		
Characters	***Benign***	***Malignant***
Age	Younger	Older (menopausal transition)
Family history	—	Present (10–25%)
Feel	Cystic	Solid/variegated
Laterality	Unilateral	Bilateral
Mobility	Mobile	Fixed
Surface	Smooth	Irregular
Growth rate	Slow	Rapid
Ascites	Absent	Present
Nodules in POD	Absent	Present
Serum CA 125	Not raised	Raised (>200 IU/mL)
Risk of malignancy-index (RMI) p. 311	<25: Low risk	>250: 75% risk

Laparotomy Findings		
Characters	***Benign***	***Malignant***
Ascites	Absent	Present, often hemorrhagic
Exophytic growth on surface	Absent	Present
Adhesions	Absent	Present
Peritoneal nodules	Absent	Present
Metastatic deposits to other organs	Absent	Present
Cut section	Cystic	Solid and hemorrhagic areas

- **Family history:** Approximately 10–25% of ovarian cancers are hereditary.
- Mutations in *BRCA1* are responsible for 50% and *BRCA2* for 25% of all inherited ovarian cancers. P-53 gene mutations are seen in 100% of cases.
- High-grade serous ovarian cancers (HGSOC) are commonly associated (p. 305)

Diagnostic Differentiation of a Ovarian Tumor on Ultrasonography
International Ovarian Tumor Analysis (IOTA) Group Rules

Benign tumors (B-Rules)		***Malignant tumors (M-rules)***	
B-1:	Unilocular cyst	**M-1:**	Irregular solid tumors
B-2:	Presence of solid components with largest solid component diameter <7 mm	**M-2:**	Presence of ascites
B-3:	Presence of acoustic shadows	**M-3:**	At least four papillary structures
B-4:	Smooth multilocular tumor with largest diameter <100 mm	**M-4:**	Irregular, multilocular, solid tumor with largest diameter ≥100 mm
B-5:	No blood flow (color score-1) (Doppler study)	**M-5:**	Very strong blood flow (color score-4)

Guidelines for surgery in an apparently benign tumor

- **Incision** should be vertical paramedian sufficiently big enough to deliver the cyst intact. An attempt to tap a cyst to minimize its size and to deliver it with a small incision is not suggested. The content may be mucinous, sebaceous material, infective or malignant fluid which contaminates the peritoneal cavity. The longitudinal incision also allows adequate exposure in the upper abdomen.
- **To inspect** the nature of the peritoneal fluid—clear, straw color, hemorrhagic or infective. A sample of the fluid or peritoneal washings should be sent for cytological examination.
- **To deliver the tumor** intact and to note it carefully about its nature (Table 21.4).
- **Cyst aspiration** is not preferred.
- **To inspect and to palpate** the other ovary, pelvic organs, omentum, liver, under surface of diaphragm and para-aortic group of lymph nodes.
- **To proceed** for the definitive surgery.
- **To cut the tumor** and inspect the inner side for any evidence of malignancy. In suspected cases, the facility of frozen section is invaluable (Table 21.4).
- It is not prudent to bisect the contralateral ovary, if it looks absolutely normal.

Definitive Surgery: Laparotomy/Laparoscopy

In young patients desirous of fertility

- **Ovarian cystectomy** leaving behind the healthy ovarian tissue is the operation of choice.
- **Ovariotomy** (salpingo-oophorectomy) is reserved for a big tumor that has destroyed almost all the ovarian tissues or for a gangrenous cyst.
- **If both the ovaries** are involved, ovarian cystectomy may be attempted at least in one ovary.
- **Preservation of the uterus** for possible ART may be considered when bilateral ovariotomy has to be done.

In parous women with age ≥40 years

- Total hysterectomy with bilateral salpingo-oophorectomy is to be done (Fig. 21.18).

In between these two extremes of age

Individualization is to be done as regard the nature of surgery. Due consideration is to be given about the reproductive and menstrual function.

In all cases, the entire tumor is to be sent for histological examination. If a part is to be sent, **a small piece from the comparatively solid or thick capsule is to be selected.**

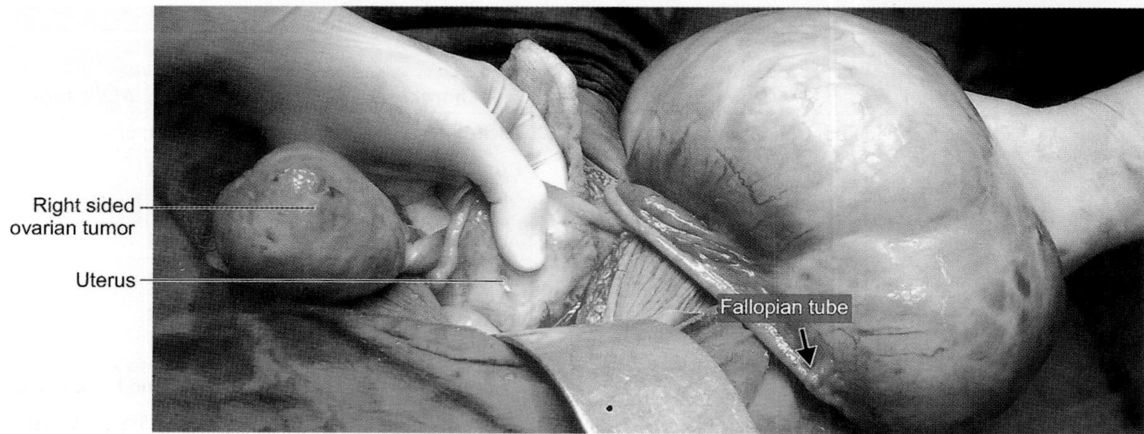

Fig. 21.18: Intraoperative photograph of a 49-year-old woman showing bilateral ovarian tumor (mucinous cyst adenoma). The left sided tumor is fairly large and has undergone torsion. The left fallopian tube is seen stretched out (*see* arrow). She was treated by total hysterectomy with bilateral salpingo-oophorectomy.

BORDERLINE EPITHELIAL TUMORS OF THE OVARY

Borderline malignant epithelial tumors have got some but not all the features of malignancy. They are of low malignant potential. The characteristic features are:

- They constitute 10–20% of all epithelial tumors of the ovary.
- These tumors are intermediate in position between benign and the malignant in term of histology and prognosis.
- Formation of microscopic papillary projections.
- There is stratification of epithelial cells of the papillae.
- There is epithelial cell pleomorphism.
- Presence of papillary projection on the external surface.
- Detachment of cellular clusters from the sites of origin.
- Increased cellular mitotic activity.
- Presence of nuclear atypia of varying degrees.
- No invasion of ovarian stroma.
- Generally found in the younger age group and carry good prognosis.

Treatment

The objectives of surgery are: (a) Confirmation of diagnosis; (b) Fertility sparing surgery in women who are young and desire for it; (c) Thorough surgical staging; (d) Peritoneal washings and frozen section evaluation following ovarian mass removal for reconfirmation; (e) Patients with advanced stage disease, cytoreductive surgery is done; (f) MIS (laparoscopic or robotic) is feasible and safe; (g) Fertility sparing surgery includes ovarian cystectomy or unilateral adnexectomy; (h) LMP tumors are staged with same FIGO criteria, as in invasive ovarian cancer; (i) Prognosis is excellent. 5 year survival rate is around 96 to 99%; (j) Recurrence may occur even after decades.

PAROVARIAN CYST (FIG. 21.19)

Parovarian cyst may **arise either from the vestigial remnants of Wolffian duct in the mesosalpinx or from the peritoneal inclusions or from tubal epithelium (Fig. 21.19).**

The ovary is separated and the uterine tube is stretched over the cyst. The cyst is unilocular; the wall is thin and contains clear fluid. The wall consists of connective tissue lined by a single layer of cuboidal or flat epithelium. There may be a thin muscle tissue along with secretory epithelium suggesting tubal origin.

The cysts are always benign. The **presenting features are like those of benign ovarian tumor. It can undergo torsion like that of ovarian tumor** (Fig. 38.6).

Removal of the tumor, when it burrows in the broad ligament, needs a cautious approach as the ureter is either placed at the bottom or on the top of the cyst. An incision is made anterior and parallel to the round ligament. Enucleation of the tumor is done leaving behind the ovary. Hemostasis at the base is achieved by ligature taking care not to injure the ureter.

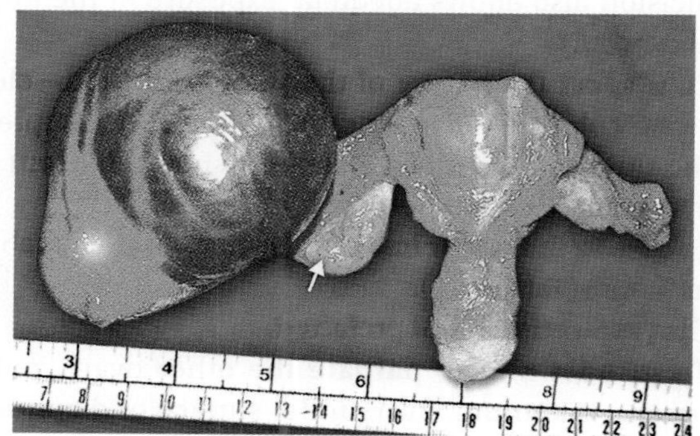

Fig. 21.19: Parovarian cyst (right). The ovary is seen separated (*see* arrow) and the uterine tube is stretched over the cyst.

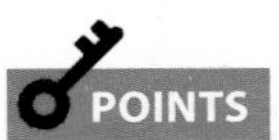

POINTS

- **The functional cysts** of the ovary are predominantly follicular cyst and corpus luteum cyst. Follicular cysts are the most common and the initial management is conservative. Treatment of unruptured corpus luteum cyst is conservative.
- **Ovarian cystic mass 8 cm or more** after menopause or before puberty or a solid tumor at any age indicates thorough investigations. Laparotomy when needed should be done in an oncology center.
- **Theca lutein cysts** are due to excessive gonadotropin (endogenous or exogenous) stimulation of the ovaries. 50% of molar pregnancies and 10% of choriocarcinomas have associated bilateral theca lutein cysts. They usually regress spontaneously with normalization of serum hCG level.
- Theca lutein cysts arise from excessive stimulation of gonadotropins. This condition is termed as hyperreactio luteinalis. Nearly 50% of molar pregnancy and 10% of choriocarcinoma have bilateral theca lutein cysts.
- **The following criteria** must be fulfilled for conservative management of an ovarian cyst: (a) Asymptomatic; (b) Unilateral; (c) Size <8 cm; (d) Unilocular cyst without any solid area; (e) Normal CA 125; (f) No ascites. It should be followed up by—ultrasound re-examination at 3–6 months time.
- **Mucinous cyst adenoma** accounts for 20–25% of all ovarian tumors. They are bilateral in 10% and chance of malignancy is 5–10%. The content is **mucin—a glycoprotein** with high content of neutral polysaccharides. It is lined by tall columnar epithelium with deep stained basal nucleus without cilia, the structure like that of endocervix (p. 241).
- **Serous cyst adenoma** accounts for 40% of ovarian tumors. It is bilateral in 40% and chance of malignancy is about 40%. It is lined by cubical epithelium. In papillary type, the lining epithelium is like that of fallopian tube (p. 242).
- **Dermoid cyst** accounts for 15–20% amongst ovarian tumors. It is bilateral in 15–20%. Chance of malignancy is least 1–2%. If an ovarian cyst is lying anterior to uterus, it is likely to be dermoid. Rokitansky's protuberance is the solid area of the cyst. Rarely dermoid cyst contains thyroid tissues and strumal carcinoids (p. 243).
- **Fibromas** are most common benign, solid tumors of the ovary. They have low malignant potential (Table 21.5)
- **Meigs' syndrome** is ascites and hydrothorax in association with fibroma of the ovary.
- *Nearly 50% of patients with ovarian fibroma have ascites when the tumor is >6 cm.*
- **Ovarian tumor** is commonly confused with full bladder, pregnancy, fibroid, chocolate cyst or ascites.
- **Torsion of pedicle** is the most common complication of benign cystic ovarian tumor and the rarest one is malignancy.
- **Definitive treatment** of torsion is ovariotomy when there is gangrenous changes. However, **detorsion of the adnexa** may be done and the ovary could be salvaged in most of the situations or possibly by cystectomy. Risk of embolism is low (0.2%). Oophoropexy is done to prevent repeat torsion.
- **Pseudomyxoma peritonei** is usually associated with mucinous cyst adenoma of the ovary, mucocele of the appendix and gallbladder and intestinal malignancy.
- **The malignancy** is highest in papillary variety of serous cyst adenoma being adenocarcinoma and lowest one in dermoid being squamous cell carcinoma (Table 21.4).
- **Cyst aspiration** is not preferred due to the risk of tumor spill and spread of malignancy. Cytologic evaluation following cyst aspiration is associated with false-positive and false-negative results.
- **In young women**, conservative surgery, either ovarian cystectomy or ovariotomy (oophorectomy) is to be done. In patient around 40 years and above, total hysterectomy with bilateral salpingo-oophorectomy is justified.
- **Borderline epithelial tumors** of the ovary are of low malignant potential. Though there is cellular mitotic activity and nuclear atypia (p. 250), stromal invasion is absent. Ovarian cystectomy or unilateral oophorectomy is the optimum treatment especially for a young woman. In elderly women total hysterectomy, bilateral salpingo-oophorectomy, and omentectomy are done. Chemotherapy is not usually considered following surgery.
- **5 years survival rate** for patients with borderline epithelial ovarian cancer (grade O) is close to 100%.
- In all cases, the tumor is subjected to histopathological study to note the nature of the tumor and to exclude invasive cancer.

CHAPTER

22 Endometriosis and Adenomyosis

CHAPTER OUTLINE

ENDOMETRIOSIS

DEFINITION

Presence of functioning endometrium (glands and stroma) in sites other than uterine mucosa is called endometriosis. It is not a neoplastic condition, although malignant transformation is possible.

These ectopic endometrial tissues may be found in the myometrium when it is called endometriosis interna or **adenomyosis**. Most commonly, however, these tissues are found at sites other than uterus and are called endometriosis externa or generally referred to as endometriosis.

Endometriosis is a disease of contrast. Although it is a benign but it is locally invasive and disseminates widely. Cyclic hormones stimulate growth but continuous hormones suppress it.

Women with extensive disease may remain asymptomatic whereas a patient with minimal disease may have incapacitating chronic pelvic pain and other symptoms. Endometriosis is an aggressive, progressive and invasive disease.

PREVALENCE

During the last couple of decades, the prevalence of endometriosis has been increasing both in terms of real and apparent. **The real one** is due to delayed marriage, postponement of first conception and adoption of small family norm. **The apparent one** is due to increased use of diagnostic laparoscopy as well as heightened awareness of this disease complex amongst the gynecologists.

The prevalence is about 10–15%. However, prevalence is high amongst the infertile women (30–45%) as based on diagnostic laparoscopy and laparotomy.

SITES (TABLE 22.1)

- **Abdominal**
- **Extra-abdominal**
- **Remote**

Abdominal

It can occur at any site but is usually confined to the abdominal structures below the level of umbilicus.

TABLE 22.1: Sites of endometriosis (Fig. 22.1).

Common sites	*Rare and remote sites*
▪ Ovaries	▪ Umbilicus
▪ Pelvic peritoneum	▪ Abdominal scar
▪ Pouch of Douglas	▪ Episiotomy scar
▪ Uterosacral ligaments	▪ Lungs
▪ Rectovaginal septum	▪ Pleura
▪ Sigmoid colon	▪ Ureter
▪ Appendix	▪ Kidney
▪ Pelvic lymph nodes	▪ Arms
▪ Fallopian tubes	▪ Legs
	▪ Nasal mucosa

Risk Factors for Endometriosis

- Low parity
- Delayed child bearing
- Family history of endometriosis
- Genital (outflow) tract obstruction
- Environmental toxins (dioxins)
- Peritoneal fluid abnormalities (Table 22.2)

TABLE 22.2 Peritoneal fluid: Cytokines and growth factors

Concentration increased	*Concentration decreased*	*Concentration unchanged*
Complement, glycodelin	Interleukin (IL-13)	EGF
Interleukins: IL-1, IL-6, IL-8	TGFβ, VEGF	Basic FGF
PDGF, RANTES, TGFβ, VEGF	FGF	Interleukins: IL-2, IL-4, IL-12

(TGFβ: transforming growth factor β; VEGF: vascular endothelial growth factor; FGF: fibroblast growth factor; PDGF: patelet derived growth factor)

Extra-abdominal

The common sites are abdominal scar of hysterotomy, cesarean section, tubectomy and myomectomy, umbilicus, episiotomy scar, vagina and cervix.

PATHOGENESIS

It still remains unclear and is full of theories (Table 22.3). **The principal ones are:**

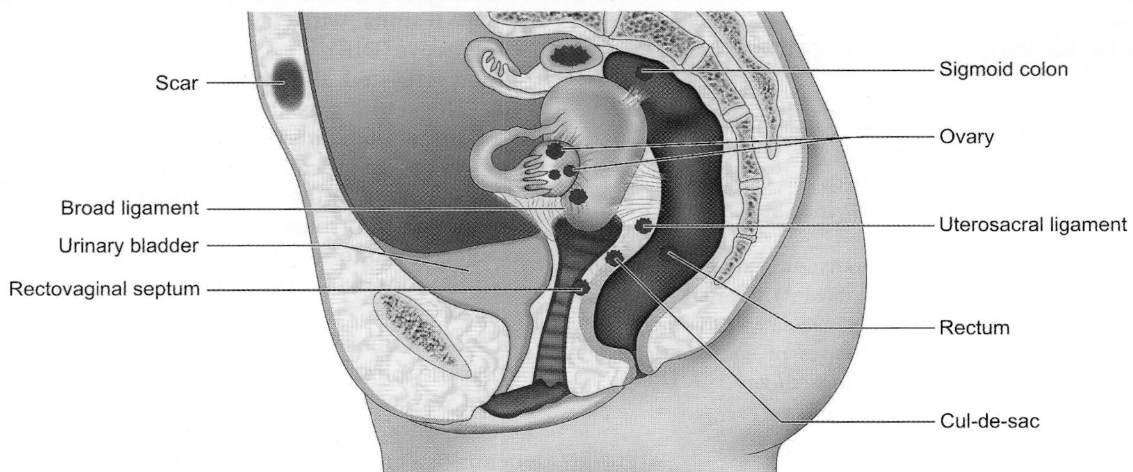

Fig. 22.1: Common sites of endometriosis.

TABLE 22.3: Theories to explain endometriosis at different sites.

Sites	Theory
▪ Pelvic endometriosis	▪ Retrograde menstruation
▪ Pelvic peritoneum	▪ Coelomic metaplasia
▪ Abdominal viscera ▪ Rectovaginal septum ▪ Umbilicus	▪ Coelomic metaplasia
▪ Abdominal scar ▪ Episiotomy scar ▪ Vagina, cervix	▪ Direct implantation
▪ Lymph nodes	▪ Lymphatic spread
▪ Distant sites (lungs, pleura, skin, lymph nodes, nerves)	▪ Vascular spread ▪ Genetic ▪ Immunologic

Retrograde Menstruation (Sampson's Theory, 1927)

There is retrograde flow of menstrual blood through the uterine tubes during menstruation. The endometrial fragments get implanted in the peritoneal surface of the pelvic organs (dependent sites, e.g. ovaries, uterosacral ligaments). **Outflow tract obstruction** in the genital tract is frequently found in women with endometriosis. This is due to the expression of adhesion molecules on the peritoneal surfaces. Subsequently, cyclic growth and shedding of the endometrium at the ectopic sites occur under the influence of the endogenous ovarian hormones. Probably, a genetic factor or favorable hormonal milieu is necessary for successful implantation and growth of the fragments of endometrium. While this theory can explain pelvic endometriosis, it fails to explain the endometriosis at distant sites.

Coelomic Metaplasia (Meyer and Ivanoff)

Chronic irritation of the pelvic peritoneum by the menstrual blood may cause coelomic metaplasia which results in endometriosis. Otherwise, implantation of endometrial based adult stem cells and mesenchymal cells may explain the theory. Coelomic epithelium retains the ability for multipotential development.

This theory can explain endometriosis of the abdominal viscera, rectovaginal septum and umbilicus.

Direct Implantation Theory

According to the theory, the endometrial or decidual tissues start to grow in susceptible individual when implanted in the new sites. Iatrogenic dissemination explains the development of endometriotic implants at the scar tissues. Such sites are abdominal scar following hysterotomy, cesarean section, tubectomy, and myomectomy. Endometriosis at the episiotomy scar, vaginal or cervical site can also be explained with this theory.

This theory, however, fails to clarify endometriosis at sites other than mentioned.

Lymphatic and Vascular Theory (Halban, 1925)

It may be possible for the normal endometrium to metastasize the pelvic lymph nodes (30%) through the draining lymphatic channels of the uterus. This could explain the lymph node involvement.

Vascular Theory

This is sound at least to explain endometriosis at distant sites such as lungs, arms or thighs.

Genetic and Immunological Factors

Autoimmune basis of Endometriosis: Abnormalities both in the cellular and humoral component show involvement of various cytokines and growth factors in its pathogenesis. Peritoneal fluid of women with endometriosis have larger macrophages. These large hyperactive macrophages secrete multiple growth factors and cytokines that promote the development of endometriosis (Table 22.3).

Basis of Autoimmune Theory of Endometriosis

- Failure of destruction of normally extruded endometrial cells in a woman with endometriosis.
- Proliferative activity of endometriotic lesions is increased with the presence of intraleukins and growth factors.
- **Upregulation of local tissue aromatase activity, increased COX-2 expression, dysregulation of 17β dehydrogenase results in high level of local estradiol and PGE2.**
- **There is tissue resistance to progesterone.**

Genetic basis and familial predisposition have been observed. The risk of endometriosis in first degree relatives of a woman with severe endometriosis is about 7%. Deletion of genes in chromosome 17 and aneuploidy have been observed. However, the expression of the disease depends on the environmental and epigenetic factors. Several aberrantly expressed genes and gene products have been expressed in endometriosis (*see* below). Certain ethnic groups particularly Asian women have increased risk (nine-fold) of endometriosis.

Aberrant Expression of Gene and Gene Products in Endometrium for Women with Endometriosis

- Aromatase
- Hepatocyte growth factor
- HOX 10
- Matrix metalloproteinases (MMP) (3,7,11)
- Complements (C3)
- Progesterone receptor isoforms
- VEGF
- Glycodelin

Environment theory suggests somatic mutations of cells due to environmental factors (pollutants, dioxins). Ovarian and deep infiltrating endometriotic lesions are explained with this theory.

Thus, it is certain that, not all cases of endometriosis at different sites can be explained by a single theory.

Summary of etiopathogenesis of endometriosis

- *Genetic mutations (familial clustering)*
- *Immunological*
- *Molecular defects*
- *Mechanical (outflow tract obstruction)*
- *Environmental toxins (dioxins)*
- *Others as described above.*

PATHOLOGY

General Considerations

- **The endometrium (glands and stroma) in the ectopic sites** has got the potentiality to undergo changes under the action of ovarian hormones.
- **Proliferative changes** are constantly evidenced, the secretory changes are conspicuously absent. It may be due to deficiency of steroid receptors in the ectopic endometrium.
- **Cyclic growth and shedding** continue till menopause. The periodically shed blood may remain encysted or else, the cyst becomes tense and ruptures.
- **Blood is irritant and it causes** dense tissue reaction surrounding the lesion with ultimate fibrosis. If it happens to occur on the pelvic peritoneum, it produces adhesions and puckering of the peritoneum.
- **Deep lesions** with penetration >5 mm are more progressive (DIE).
- **When encysted, the cyst enlarges with cyclic bleeding.** The serum gets absorbed in between the periods and the content inside becomes chocolate colored. Hence, the cyst is called **chocolate cyst** which is commonly located in the ovary. **Chocolate cyst may also** be due to hemorrhagic follicular or corpus luteum cyst or bleeding into a cystadenoma. For this reason, the term **endometrial cyst or endometrioma (Fig. 22.2) is preferred** to chocolate cyst.
- **In spite of dense adhesions** amongst the pelvic structures, the **fallopian tubes remain patent**. However the tubo-ovarian anatomic relationship may be disturbed.

Naked eye appearance: The appearance of the lesion depends to a great extent on the organ(s) involved, extent of the lesion and reaction of the surrounding tissues. Early lesions look papular or vesicular.

Pelvic endometriosis: Typically, there are small black dots, the so called **'powder burns'** seen on the uterosacral ligaments and pouch of Douglas (Fig. 22.3). Fibrosis and scarring in the peritoneum surrounding the implants is also a typical finding. Other subtle appearances are: *red flame-shaped areas, red polypoid areas, yellow brown patches, white peritoneal areas, circular peritoneal defects* or *subovarian adhesions*. These lesions are thought to be more active than the '**powder burn**' areas.

The ovaries are frequently involved usually bilaterally. The endometriomas (chocolate cysts) are of varying sizes and are visible as bluish colorations. **The ovaries get adherent to the pelvic structures including rectum and sigmoid colon.**

Microscopic appearance: There is presence of endometrial tissue—**both glands and stroma**. Due to pressure effect, the lining epithelium of the cyst may be absent or flattened (cuboidal) or replaced by granulation tissue. Adjacent to the lining epithelium, there may be presence of large polyhedral **phagocytic cells, laden with blood pigment—hemosiderin** (pseudoxanthoma cells). The cyst wall is composed of fibrous tissue and compressed ovarian cortex.

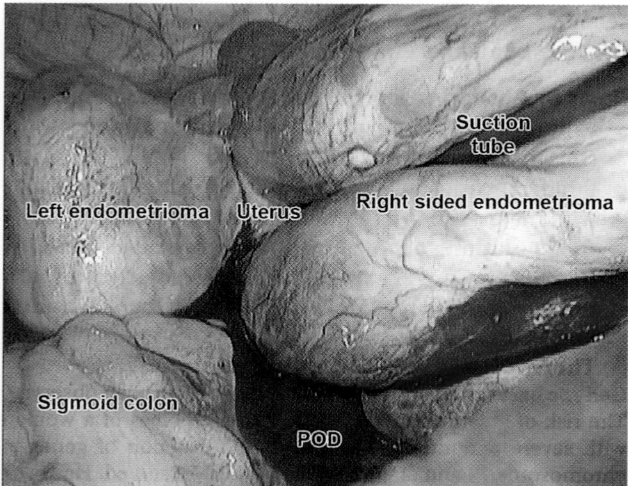

Fig. 22.2: Laparoscopic view of bilateral endometrioma in a 17 year old girl. She remained mostly asymptomatic. She had some pelvic heaviness and pian for last 3 weeks that she sought medical consultation.

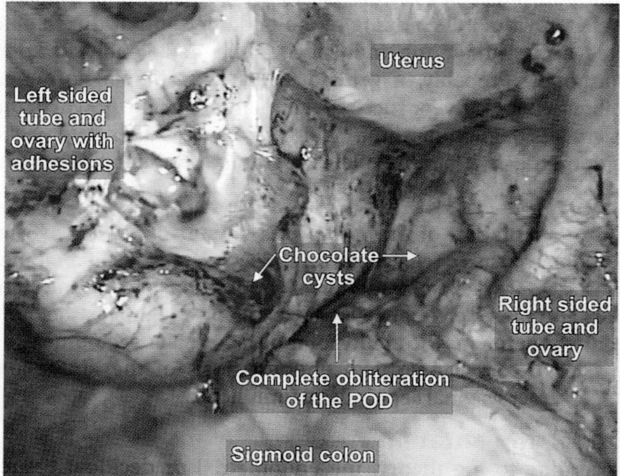

Fig. 22.3: Laparoscopic view of an advanced pelvic endometriosis with bilateral chocolate cysts. *There is extensive pelvic adhesions.*

CLINICAL FEATURES OF PELVIC ENDOMETRIOSIS

Patient Profile

The age is between 30 and 45. The patients are mostly nulliparous or have had one or two children, long years prior to appearance of symptoms. Infertility, voluntary postponement of first conception until at a late age and higher social status are often related. There is often family history of endometriosis. Outflow tract obstruction is an important cause when it is seen in teenagers (10%). **Pelvic endometriosis** may be (a) Minimal or mild; (b) Moderate; (c) Severe or deeply infiltrating endometriosis (DIE).

Symptoms

- **About 25% of patients** with endometriosis have no symptom, being accidentally discovered either during laparoscopy or laparotomy.
- **Symptoms are not related with extent of lesion.** Even when the endometriosis is widespread, there may not be any symptom; conversely, there may be intense symptoms with minimal endometriosis.
- **Depth of penetration** is more related to symptoms rather than the spread. Lesions penetrating more than 5 mm are responsible for pain, dysmenorrhea, and dyspareunia.
- **Nonpigmented endometriotic lesions** compared to the classic pigmented 'powder burns' lesions produce more prostaglandin F (PGF) and hence are more painful.
- **The symptoms are mostly related to the site** of lesion and its ability to respond to hormones. Midline lesions are more symptom producing.
- **Degree of pain is not related to the severity of endometriosis.**

Dysmenorrhea (70%): There is progressively increasing secondary dysmenorrhea. The pain starts a few days prior to menstruation; gets worsened during menstruation and takes time, even after cessation of period, to get relief of pain (co-menstrual dysmenorrhea). Pain usually begins after few years pain-free menses. The site of pain is usually deep seated and on the back or rectum.

Increased secretion of PGF 2α, thromboxane β_2 from endometriotic tissue is the cause of pain.

Abnormal uterine bleeding (AUB) (15–20%): Menorrhagia is the predominant abnormality. If the ovaries are also involved, polymenorrhea or epimenorrhagia may be pronounced. There may be premenstrual spotting.

Infertility (40–60%): Endometriosis is found in 30–45% of infertile women, whereas in about 40–50% patients with endometriosis suffer from infertility. The multiple factors involved in producing infertility have been depicted in page 189 (Table 17.2). Miscarriage may be due to implantation failure.

Dyspareunia (20–40%): The dyspareunia is usually deep. It may be due to stretching of the structures of the pouch of Douglas or direct contact tenderness. As such, it is mostly found in endometriosis of the rectovaginal septum or pouch of Douglas and with fixed retroverted uterus.

Chronic pelvic pain: The pain varies from pelvic discomfort to lower abdominal pain or backache. The causes of pain is multifactorial.

Causes of pain in endometriosis (see keypoint)

- *Peritoneal inflammation (PGF, cytokines)*
- *Tissue necrosis*
- *Adhesion formation*
- *Nerve irritation due to deep penetration*
- *Release of local inflammatory mediators (p. 252)*
- *Endometrioma formation*

The pain aggravates during the period.

Abdominal pain: There may be variable degrees of abdominal pain around the periods. Sometimes, the pain may be acute due to rupture of chocolate cyst.

Other Symptoms

The symptoms are related to the organ involved.

- **Urinary**—frequency, dysuria, hydronephrosis (Fig. 22.4) back pain or even hematuria.

Case History

Mrs CR, 43 years, seen with the complaints of persistent pelvic pain, worsening during menstruation. Severity of pain gradually deteriorated even with the use of medications. She gradually had pain radianting to the back and the loin. She developed features of recurrent pyelonephritis. Investigations (USG, MRI) revealed deep infiltrating endometriosis, involving both the ovaries. Ureteric obstruction was observed at the level of the pelvic floor.

MRI revealed gross hydronephrotic and hydroureteric changes in the right side (Fig. 22.4). Laparotomy was done. Total hysterectomy with bilateral salpingo-oophorectomy with removal of bilateral endometriomas was done. Adhesiolysis and ureterolysis was done. Resection of the cicatrized ureteric segment (4 cm) had to be done (Fig. 22.4). Ureter was implanted in the bladder following mobilization. She had uneventful recovery.

- **Sigmoid colon and rectum**—painful defecation (dyschezia), diarrhea, constipation, rectal bleeding or even melena. Patient may also present with symptom s/o IBS.
- **Chronic fatigue**, perimenstrual symptoms (bowel, bladder).
- **Hemoptysis** (rarely), catamenial chest pain.
- **Surgical scars**—cyclical pain and bleeding bloody pleural fluid (described later).

Abdominal examination: Abdominal palpation may not reveal any abnormality. A mass may be felt in the lower abdomen arising from the pelvis—enlarged chocolate cyst or tubo-ovarian mass due to endometriotic adhesions. The mass is tender with restricted mobility.

Pelvic examination: Bimanual examination may not reveal any pathology. **The expected positive findings are**—pelvic tenderness, nodules in the pouch of Douglas, nodular feel of the uterosacral ligaments, fixed retroverted uterus or unilateral or bilateral adnexal mass of varying sizes.

Speculum examination may reveal bluish spots in the posterior fornix.

Rectal or rectovaginal examination is often helpful to confirm the findings.

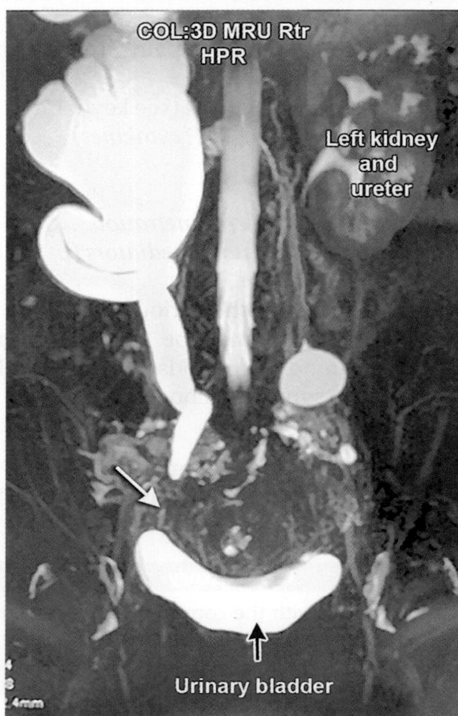

Fig. 22.4: Right ureter showing gross hydroureteric and hydronephrotic changes in a case with advanced (stage IV) deep infiltrating endometriosis (History of the patient as described above p. 255).

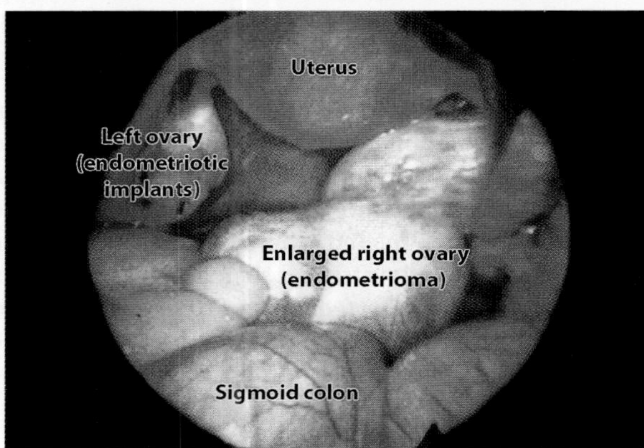

Fig. 22.5: Laparoscopic view of pelvic endometriosis: Left ovary—endometriotic implants, right ovary—chocolate cyst.

DIAGNOSIS

Clinical Diagnosis

It is made often by the classic symptoms of progressively increasing secondary dysmenorrhea, dyspareunia, and infertility. This is corroborated by the **pelvic findings.**

Speculum examination: Bluish powder-burn lesions may be seen on the cervix or the posterior fornix of the vagina. These are tender and sometime may bleed.

Bimanual examination: Reveal nodularity in the pouch of Douglas, nodular feel of the uterosacral ligaments, fixed retroverted uterus, and unilateral or bilateral adnexal mass (chocolate cysts).

However, physical examination has poor sensitivity and specificity. Many patients have no abnormal findings on examination.

Serum marker: Cancer antigen (CA) 125—a moderate elevation of serum CA 125 is noticed in patients with severe endometriosis. It is not specific for endometriosis, as it is significantly raised in epithelial ovarian carcinoma. However, it is helpful to assess the therapeutic response and in follow-up of cases and to detect any recurrence after therapy. **Monocyte Chemotactic Protein (MCP-1)** level is increased in the peritoneal fluid of women with endometriosis.

Glycodelin (placental protein 14) is elevated in endometriosis. Levels also decrease with removal of the disease. However, the levels vary widely, it is not used as a routine. Other predictive markers are interleukin-1 (1L-1) and interferon gamma.

Imaging

Ultrasonography: Transvaginal scan (TVS) can detect ovarian endometriomas. TVS and endorectal ultrasound (ERUS) are found better for rectosigmoid endometriosis specially for diagnosis in endromosis (DIE).

Magnetic resonance imaging (MRI): It is the best diag-nostic tool (Fig. 22.4). There is a characteristic hyperintensity on T1-weighted images and a hypointensity on T2 weighted images. Sensitivity and specificity of MRI is 91–95%. It is superior compared to TVS and CT with much better resolution and soft tissue interfaces. MRI is better to diagnose DIE, and deep seated endometrioma.

Computed tomography (CT): It is better compared to ultrasonography in the diagnosis. MRI is useful for deep infiltrating endometriosis.

Colonoscopy, **rectosigmoidoscopy**, and **cystoscopy** are done when respective organs are involved.

Laparoscopy: It is the gold standard (Fig. 22.5). Confirmation is done by double puncture laparoscopy or by laparotomy.

Other benefits of laparoscopy are:

- *Assessment of the lesion with site, size, and extent*
- *Biopsy can be taken at the same time*
- *Staging (p. 257) can be done*
- *Extent of adhesions could be recorded*
- *Opportunity to do laparoscopic surgery if needed.*

The classic lesion of pelvic endometriosis is described as *'powder burns'* or *'match stick'* spots on the peritoneum of the pouch of Douglas. Findings may be recorded on video or DVD (RCOG - 2006). Microscopically some of these lesions contain endometrial glands, stroma, and hemosiderin-laden macrophages.

Biopsy confirmation of excised lesion is ideal but negative histology does not exclude it. None of the imaging techniques including ultrasound, can diagnose specifically the peritoneal endometriosis. Empiric medical treatment is usually not recommended except for pain relief and to reduce menstrual flow.

Intravenous urography (IVU): It is useful in cases with deep infiltrating endometriosis (DIE) and suspected ureteric involvement.

DIFFERENTIAL DIAGNOSIS

Ovarian endometrioma (chocolate cyst): Ovary is the most common site for endometriosis (60–70%). It starts with a

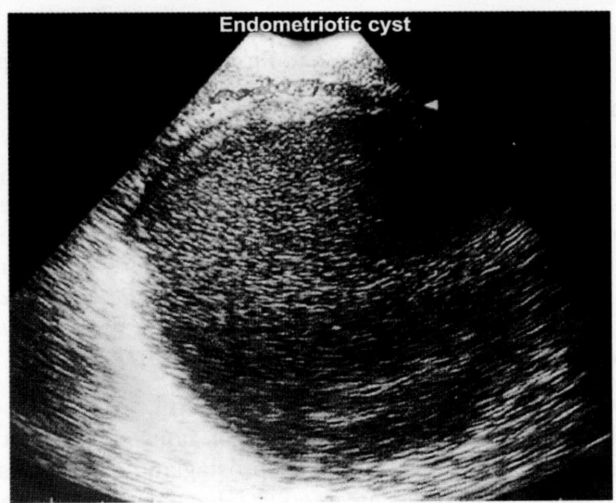

Fig. 22.6: Color Doppler scan (TV) of an ovarian endometrioma (chocolate cyst). Internal echoes are homogeneous. Increased vascularity is seen at the ovarian hilus.

superficial endometriotic implant over the ovarian surface. The endometriotic tissue gradually invades the ovarian stroma. Cyst formation is due to periodic shedding and bleeding from the implant.

Leakage of this altered blood along with inflammation, leads to adhesion formation with the adjacent structures. Fallopian tubes may be affected. Epithelial lining of the cyst contain endometrial glands and stroma. Due to pressure effect the lining epithelium may be flattened. When the cyst ruptures the characteristic thick, tarry fluid (chocolate material) escapes.

If asymptomatic, may be confused with **benign ovarian tumor** and in symptomatic one, with **malignant ovarian**. Presence of nodules in the pouch of Douglas further confuses the diagnosis. **Ultrasonography** showing homogeneous internal echoes may be helpful (Fig. 22.6). **Laparoscopy** differentiates one from the other. Too often, the diagnosis is made only during laparotomy.

On pelvic examination the ovaries are tender, immobile due to inflammation and adhesions. Histological findings: presence of endometrial glands, endometrial stroma and large phagocytic cells containing hemosiderin are seen.

Ultrasound reveals—thick wall cyst with homogeneous echo pattern.

Management is done either medically or surgically depending upon the factors like: (a) Age; (b) Desire of fertility; (c) Severity of symptoms; (d) Size (p. 255).

Excision of endometrioma reduces ovarian reserve and future fertility.

Rupture of the chocolate cyst: During operation, while separating the adhesions, the cyst invariably ruptures with escape of chocolate colored blood. The rupture of the cyst can occur spontaneously causing acute abdomen with clinical features suggestive of acute ectopic. Acute abdomen **is confused with** torsion or rupture of the ovarian tumor, disturbed ectopic pregnancy, appendicitis or diverticulitis.

Chronic pelvic infection: It is most often confused with symptomatic endometriosis. The clinical presentation is almost similar. Laparoscopy is helpful in actual diagnosis.

TABLE 22.4: Causes of subfertility with endometriosis.

- **A. Pelvic cavity:** (a) Peritoneal fluid: Inflammatory changes; (b) Proliferation of microphages, and release of proinflammatory factors (Table 22.2); (c) Changes in peritoneal fluid that alters sperm oocyte interaction; (d) Distorted pelvic anatomy (failure of ovum pickup).
- **B. Ovaries:** (a) Anovulation; (b) oligo-ovulation; (c) Luteal phase defect; (d) Reduced ovarian reserve (destruction by endometriosis and/or surgery); (e) Adhesions covering ovaries and tubes; (f) Poor response to ovulation induction, COS and ART.
- **C. Uterus:** (a) Reduced endometrial receptivity; (b) Implantation failure; (c) Resistance to progesterone.
- **D. Others:** Pelvic pain, dyspareunia.

COMPLICATIONS OF ENDOMETRIOSIS

- **Endocrinopathy**—this may be responsible for **infertility** (Table 22.4).
- **Rupture** of chocolate cyst.
- **Infection** of chocolate cyst.
- **Obstructive features:**
  - Intestinal obstruction
  - Ureteral obstruction → hydroureter → hydronephrosis (Fig. 22.3) → acute pyeloniphiritis.
- **Malignancy risk of ovarian cancer in women with endometriosis four fold (c.f. endometroid variety).**

STAGING

The diagnosed endometriosis should be appropriately staged based on laparoscopic findings (Table 22.5).

TABLE 22.5: American Fertility Society (AFS) scoring system of endometriosis (revised).

	Endometriosis	*<1 cm*	*1–3 cm*	*>3 cm*
Peritoneum	Superficial	1	2	4
	Deep	2	4	6
Ovary	R Superficial	1	2	4
	Deep	4	16	20
	L Superficial	1	2	4
	Deep	4	16	20
	Posterior cul-de-sac obliteration	Partial 4	Complete 40	
	Adhesions	<1/3 Enclosure	1/3–2/3 Enclosure	>2/3 Enclosure
Ovary	R Filmy	1	2	4
	Dense	4	8	16
	L Filmy	1	2	4
	Dense	4	8	16
Tube	R Filmy	1	2	4
	Dense	4*	8*	16
	L Filmy	1	2	4
	Dense	4*	8*	16

* If the fimbriated end of the fallopian tube is completely enclosed, change the point assignment to 16.

- ***Stage I*** (minimal) = 1–5
- ***Stage II*** (mild) = 6–15
- ***Stage III*** (moderate) = 16–40
- ***Stage IV*** (severe) = >40

The findings are depicted in a pictorial chart

- To predict prognosis
- To choose therapy
- To evaluate the treatment protocol.

The scoring (revised) by the American Fertility Society (AFS) is presented in Table 22.5. **The stage is determined by adding specific points given to each**.

Limitations of AFS Staging

- Laparoscopy or laparotomy has to be done
- Interobserver and intraobserver variation
- No correlation between the extent of disease and the degree of symptoms
- Staging has not been correlated with fertility outcome
- Staging has not been correlated with optimum mode of therapy.

TREATMENT OF ENDOMETRIOSIS

Endometriosis needs to be treated as it is a progressive disease (30–60%).

- **Preventive**
- **Curative**

Preventive

The following guidelines may be prescribed to prevent or minimize endometriosis:

- To avoid tubal patency test immediately after curettage or around the time of menstruation.
- Forcible pelvic examination should not be done during or shortly after menstruation.
- Married women with family history of endometriosis are encouraged not to delay the first conception but to complete the family.

Curative

The objectives are:

- To abolish or minimize the symptoms—pelvic pain and dyspareunia
- To improve the fertility
- To prevent recurrence.

The results of treatment are difficult to evaluate because of lack of uniform staging or grading. **The following facts are to be borne in mind.**

- Asymptomatic in good number of cases.
- Subjective symptoms are not proportionate to objective signs.
- Frequent association with infertility.
- Remission during pregnancy and menopause.

Prerequisites prior to therapy are accurate diagnosis with the help of laparoscopy along with staging and pictorial documentation.

TREATMENT OPTIONS FOR PELVIC ENDOMETRIOSIS (FLOWCHART 22.1)

- **Expectant management** (observation only)
- **Medical therapy:** • Hormones • Others
- **Surgery:** • Conservative • Definitive
- **Combined therapy:** • Medical • Surgical

Determinants of Treatment Options

- Age of the patient
- Location of disease
- Size and extent of lesions
- Desire for fertility
- Severity of symptoms
- Results of previous therapy

Expectant Treatment

Endometriosis is a progressive disease in about 30–60% of women. It is not possible to predict in which woman it will progress. Some form of treatment is often needed to arrest the progress of the disease. However, in women with minimal to mild endometriosis role of any treatment is controversial. *Cumulative pregnancy rate is similar when expectant treatment is compared with conservative surgery. Case selection is important (Table 22.6).*

Protocols for Expectant Management

Observation with administration of nonsteroidal anti-inflammatory drugs (NSAIDs) or prostaglandin synthetase inhibiting (PSI) drugs are used to relieve pain. Ibuprofen 800–1200 mg or mefenamic acid 150–600 mg a day is quite effective.

The married women are encouraged to have conception. Pregnancy usually improve the condition. This is due to absence of shedding and decidual changes in the ectopic endometrium causing its necrosis and absorption.

Hormonal Treatment

Endometriosis is an estrogen dependent disease. It regresses with natural and surgical menopause. However recurrence may occur (5%) with use or exogenous estrogen.

The aim of the hormonal treatment is **to induce atrophy of the endometriotic implants**. It should be considered suppressive rather than curative because of high recurrence rate (Table 22.7).

The mechanism of endometrial atrophy is either by producing *'pseudopregnancy'* (combined oral pills) or by *'pseudomenopause'* (danazol) or by *'medical oophorectomy'* (GnRH agonists). The recurrence rate following medical therapy increases from 5% to 15% in the first year to 40% to 50% in 5 years.

The drugs used are combined estrogen and progestogen (oral pill), progestogens, dienogest, danazol, and GnRH agonists. Other are gestrinone, LNG-IUS, aromatase inhibitors (Letrozole) and few SPRMS. *All the drugs are used continuously to produce amenorrhea and as such individualization of the dose is required.*

Combined Estrogen and Progestogen

The low dose contraceptive pills may be prescribed either in a cyclic or continuous fashion with advantages in young patients with mild disease who want to defer pregnancy. It causes endometrial decidualization and atrophy. It may induce amenorrhea. It relieves dysmenorrhea. There is improvement of symptoms in 80% of women. **Anastrozole**, an aromatase inhibitor is found to reduce the growth and pain of endometriosis.

TABLE 22.6: Case selection for expectant treatment.

- Minimal endometriosis with no other abnormal pelvic finding
- Unmarried
- Young married who are ready to start family
- Approaching menopause.

Flowchart 22.1: Therapeutic approach to a patient with pelvic endometriosis.

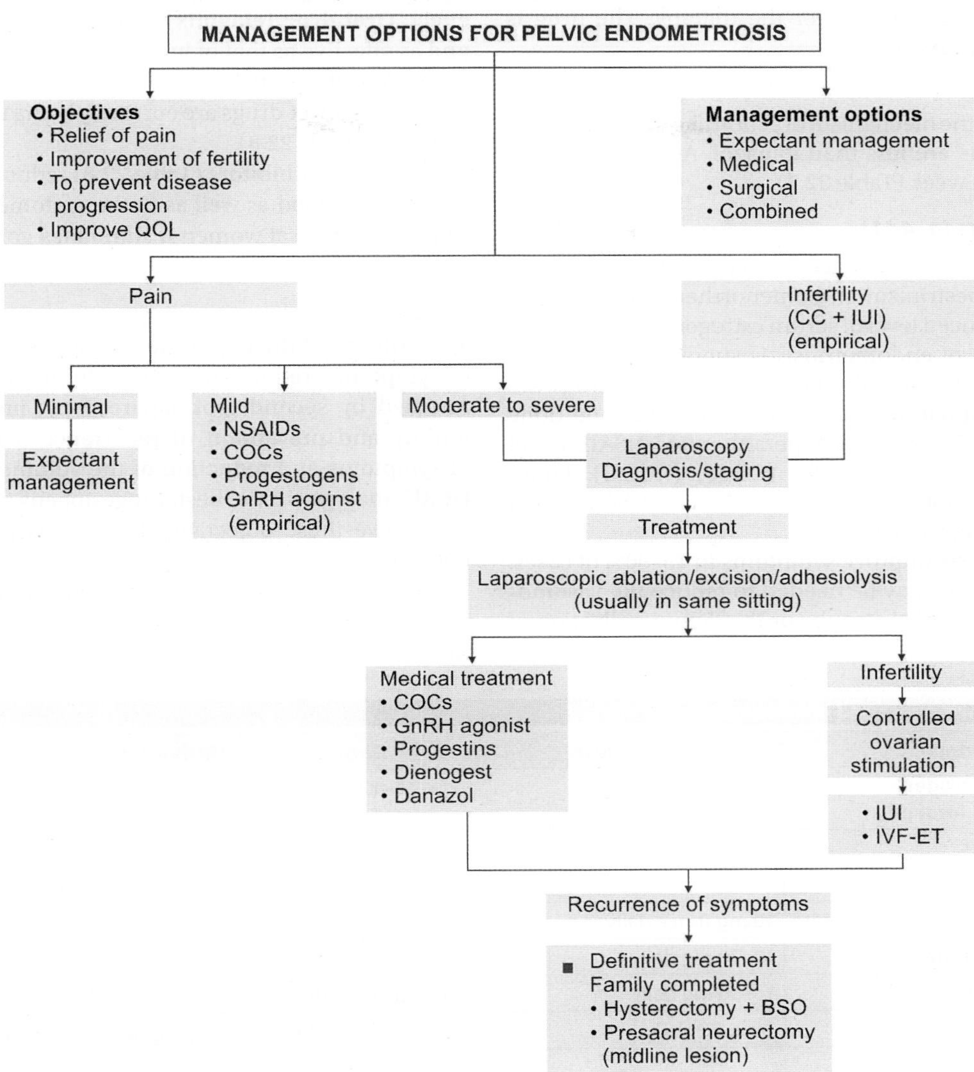

(CC: clomiphene citrate; IUI: intrauterine insemination; NSAIDs: nonsteroidal anti-inflammatory drugs; COCs: combined oral contraceptives; GnRH: gonadotropin-releasing hormone; IVF-ET: in vitro fertilization and embryo transfer; BSO; bilateral salpingo-oophorectomy)

Progestogens

It causes decidualization of endometrium and atrophy. High doses may suppress ovulation and induce amenorrhea.

Oral route is commonly used. Injectable preparations as depot form should be withheld in patients wishing to conceive. Ovulation may remain suspended for several months following withdrawal of the therapy. The side effects (Ch. 34) are well-tolerated. The drug is comparatively cheaper than danazol. **Progesterone antagonists** (mifepristone 50–100 mg/day) has also been found effective.

Dienogest

It is a 19-nortestosterone derivative. It is a selective progesterone that causes anovulation. It has antiproliferative effect on endometrial cells. It inhibits cytokine secretion (Table 22.3). It decreases the nerve fiber density in endometriosis to relieve pain. Dose: 2 mg/day orally is found as effective as GnRH agonists.

Levonorgestrel-releasing-IUCD (IUD)

When used, is found to reduce dysmenorrhea, pelvic pain, dyspareunia, and menorrhagia significantly. It is especially useful for rectovaginal endometriosis.

Danazol (p. 445)

Danazol therapy is to be started from the day 5 of the menstrual cycle. The dose (400–600 mg daily) is variable and depends upon the extent of the lesions but should be adequate enough to produce amenorrhea. **The patient should use barrier methods of contraception** to avoid virilization of a female fetus in accidental pregnancy. **Resolution of endometriotic lesions has been seen in about 80% of cases but the recurrence rate is high (15–30%)**. The side effects are at times intense and intolerable to the extent of discontinuation of the therapy. A few often persist even after the therapy. The drug is costlier than progestogen.

Gestrinone

It has got the same mechanism of action like that of danazol. The side effects are less than danazol. Administration is simple, twice a week (Table 22.7).

GnRH Analogs (p. 441)

When used continuously act as medical oophorectomy, a state of hypoestrinism and amenorrhea. The goal is to maintain a reduced level of serum estrogen (30–45 pg/mL) so that growth of endometriosis is suppressed. The side effects are more tolerable than danazol. The drugs are expensive. **Empiric use** of GnRH agonist may be done in women >18 years if pain persists after NSAIDs and combined oral contraceptives (COCs) (ACOG). Long-term therapy (more than 6 months) should be avoided (add-back therapy page 441).

GnRH agonists improve symptoms in 75–90% of cases. Add-back therapy may be needed to reduce the vasomotor symptoms, vaginal atrophy or the demineralization of bones.

GnRH antagonist can also be used. It has no "flare" effect. **Oral drug (elagolix)** at 150–250 mg is found safe and as effective as that of luprolide acetate. Bone loss and other side effects are less.

Several newer drugs are currently being used with good response (Table 22.8).

Aromatase inhibitors (Table 22.8) reduces the levels of estrogen in blood as well as in the endometriotic tissues. In premenopausal women it stimulates gonadotropins. It induces ovulation.

Results

The efficacy of the hormone therapy is judged by relief of symptoms, reduction of the volume of the lesions as revealed by second look laparoscopy, improvement of fertility and prevention of recurrence. For quick relief of symptoms and reduction of the volume of the lesion, GnRH analogs are the best. Progestogens take some time to achieve these objectives. Danazol is placed midway between the two.

Taking every aspect together (pain relief, pregnancy rates, recurrence rates, costs, and side effects), no single medical treatment is superior to others.

TABLE 22.7: Hormones used in endometriosis.

Drugs	*Dose*	*Duration*	*Mechanism*	*Side effects*
▪ **Combined estrogen progestogen (oral pill)**	1 daily	6–12 months	Pseudopregnancy	Tolerated
▪ **Progestogens**	"	"	"	"
Oral				
• Medroxyprogesterone acetate	10 mg thrice daily	6–9 months	"	"
• Dydrogesterone	10–20 mg daily	6–9 months	"	"
• Norethisterone	10–30 mg daily	6–9 months	"	"
• Dienogest	2 mg PO daily	3–6 months	Pseudopregnancy	Tolerated
IM				
• Depot medroxyprogesterone	150 mg 3 months interval	6–9 months	Pseudopregnancy	Tolerated
IUCD				
• Levonorgestrel-releasing-IUCD (LNG-IUS)	LNG-IUS having 52 mg with 20 µg/day release of LNG	5 years		
▪ **Danazol (p. 445)**	400–600 mg orally in 4 divided doses	6–9 months	Pseudomenopause	Less tolerated
▪ **Gestrinone**	1.25 or 2.5 mg twice a week	6–9 months	Pseudomenopause	Well tolerated
▪ **GnRH analogs (p. 441)**				
• Leuprolide	11.5 mg IM every 3 months	6 months	Medical oophorectomy	Well tolerated
• Triptorelin	3 mg every 4 weeks	6 months		
• Goserelin	3.6 mg depot IM monthly	6 months		

TABLE 22.8: Other medications used for the management of endometriosis.

- **Progesterone antagonists** (mifepristone): 50 mg/day PO; may cause endometrial hyperplasia
- **Selective progesterone-receptor modulators (SPRMs):** Asoprisnil induces endometrial atrophy and amenorrhea
- **GnRH antagonists:** Oral (elagolix): 150–200 mg/day as effective as leuprolide acetate, less demineralization of bones, no hypoestrogenic symptoms
- **Aromatase inhibitors:** Anastrozole (1 mg) or letrozole (2.5 mg) reduces pain symptoms
- **Simvastatin** inhibits cell proliferation: **Rosiglitazone** reduces pain symptoms

Following medical suppression or other conservative surgery, residual endometriotic lesions may regenerate once the ovarian function is re-established. **Overall recurrence rate is about 40% after 5 years.**

SURGICAL MANAGEMENT OF ENDOMETRIOSIS

Indications

- Endometriosis with severe symptoms unresponsive to hormone therapy.
- Severe and deeply infiltrating endometriosis (DIE) to correct the distortion of pelvic anatomy.
- Severe endometriosis with pelvic adhesive disease.
- Endometriomas of more than 1 cm.

Surgery may be conservative or definitive.

Conservative Surgery

Conservative surgery is planned to destroy the endometriotic lesions in an attempt to improve the symptoms (pain, subfertility) and at the same time to preserve the reproductive function.

Laparoscopy: It is commonly done to destroy endometriotic lesions by excision or ablation by electrodiatherapy or by laser vaporization.

Conservative surgical treatment in minimal to mild endometriosis (ablation plus adhesiolysis) improves the fertility outcome. Presacral neurectomy (PSN), reduces pain in midline lesions. **Laparoscopic uterosacral nerve ablation (LUNA)** is done when pain is very severe. The advantage of laser is to cut the tissues precisely with least chance of damage to the underlying vital structures. *Great deal of technical expertize is essential to avoid injury to the ureters.*

Surgical treatment improves fertility and symptoms in women with moderate and severe endometriosis.

TYPES OF SURGERY IN ENDOMETRIOSIS

Conservative surgery	*Definitive surgery*
▪ **Laparoscopic method** • Cauterization • Laser vaporization • Laparoscopic uterosacral nerve ablation (LUNA) • Adhesiolysis • Excision of rectovaginal nodules ▪ **Endometrioma** • Aspiration and irrigation • Cyst wall vaporization • Cystectomy (size ≥4 cm) • Peeling off the cyst wall	▪ **Laparoscopy/ Laparotomy** ▪ Hysterectomy with bilateral salpingo-oophorectomy ▪ Resection of bowel or ureter may be needed for complete removal of endometriosis (p. 355)

Ovarian Endometriomas (Fig. 22.6)

- **Small endometrioma (<3 cm)** is aspirated laparoscopically. The cyst cavity is irrigated with normal saline. Cyst wall epithelium may be peeled off or destroyed by laser vaporization.
- **Large endometrioma (≥4 cm)** is often associated with extensive adhesion to other pelvic structures. Laparoscopy is necessary for ovarian cyst drainage and adhesiolysis.

Results

Laparoscopic cystectomy is effective in relieving pain in about 74% cases of mild to moderate disease. Pregnancy rate is observed in about 60% cases with moderate and 35% cases with severe disease. Restoration of normal pelvic anatomy improves fertility in cases with severe endometriosis. High pregnancy rate is observed within first 6 months of conservative surgery. **However, destruction of ovarian cortex reduces ovarian reserve and reduces the prospect of fertility.**

Definitive Surgery

It is indicated in women with advanced stage endometriosis where there is: (a) No prospect for fertility improvement; (b) Other forms of treatment have failed; (c) Women with completed family.

Definitive surgery means hysterectomy with bilateral salpingo-oophorectomy along with resection of the endometriotic tissues as complete as possible. Improvement of symptoms is seen in 91% of cases.

Combined Medical and Surgical

Preoperative hormonal therapy aims at reduction of the size and vascularity of the lesion which facilitate surgery. The idea of **postoperative hormonal therapy** is to destroy the residual lesions left behind after surgery and to control the pain. But it does not improve fertility. It is generally avoided.

Duration of therapy is usually 3–6 months preoperatively and 3–6 months postoperatively. The **cumulative probability of pregnancy at 3 years following laparoscopic surgery was 47%** (51% for stage I, 45% of stage II, 46% of stage III and 44% for stage IV). **Overall risk of recurrence is 40% by 5 years time.**

Empirical treatment of pelvic pain with the presumptive diagnosis of pelvic endometriosis may be given with combined oral contraceptives, if pain persists after NSAIDs.

Moderate to severe endometriosis need to be treated with surgery to restore normal anatomy and tubal function. Laparoscopic surgery is preferred.

Infertility associated with endometriosis: When there is no improvement of infertility due to endometriosis with the usual treatment, couple should be counseled for ART (p. 204). Controlled ovarian hyperstimulation with IUI, IVF, GIFT, and ICSI are the different methods (p. 206).

Women with extensive pelvic disease (Grade: III–IV) removal of endometriomas is of no benefit and may be harmful. The ovarian reserve is further reduced. Prior suppressive therapy has been shown to be helpful. IVF-ET is a management approach instead removal of endometriomas.

ENDOMETRIOSIS AT SPECIAL SITES

- **Abdominal scar**
- **Bladder and ureter**
- **Cervix and vagina**
- **Umbilicus**
- **Gut**
- **Lung**

Scar endometriosis (Fig. 22.7): It usually manifests following abdominal hysterotomy, cesarean section, myomectomy or even tubectomy. Implantation theory can explain its entity.

The patient complains of painful nodular swelling over or adjacent to the scar which increases in size and often bleeds during periods. The size is variable, nodular feel, tender with restricted mobility. Associated pelvic endometriosis is usually absent. The same type of nodular swelling can be found over episiotomy scar. **Treatment** is by excision. Hormone therapy is ineffective.

Umbilicus: There is nodular painful swelling which increases in size and becomes tender during period. At times, bleeding may also occur. Coelomic metaplasia theory can explain its origin.

Treatment is by excision.

Bladder: The patient complains of dysuria, frequency, hematuria and lower abdominal pain especially during periods. Cystoscopic examination reveals blue area of the mucosa. Intravenous pyelogram (IVP) may reveal ureteric stricture and hydroureteric or even hydronephrotic changes on the affected side.

Treatment is not much effective with hormones. Local excision of the bladder wall and repair should be done. In ureteric involvements, the segment of the ureter is to be excised followed by implantation of the ureter to the bladder.

Bowels: The rectum, sigmoid colon or even the small intestine are the common sites. **The mucosa is not involved, a differentiating feature from malignancy**.

The patient complains of periodic colicky pain on defecation or at times bleeding per rectum especially during periods. Associated pelvic endometriosis is a constant feature. There may be even features of subacute intestinal obstruction.

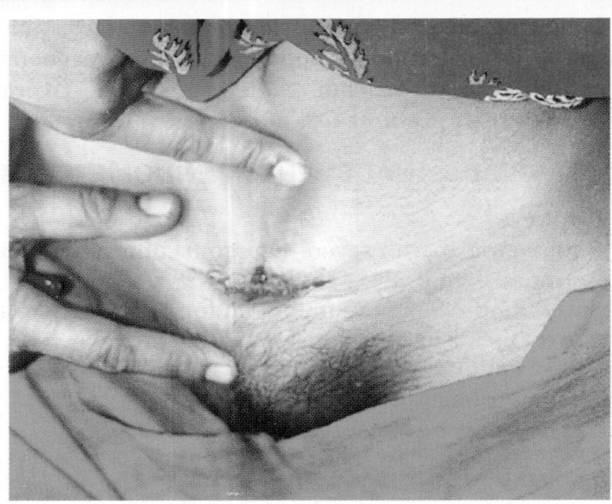

Fig. 22.7: Bleeding from a scar endometriosis. The patient was examined during her menstruation.

Rectal examination and investigations like sigmoidoscopy and barium enema confirm the diagnosis.

Lung, pleura, and **brain** are the rare sites. This may cause catamenial pneumothorax or seizures during menses.

Treatment: Hormone treatment may be effective. If it fails, surgery may have to be done. In young patients, resection anastomosis and in patients above 40, removal of the ovaries may help regression of the lesions.

Cervix and vagina: The lesions are usually due to implantation of the endometrium over the trauma inflicted at operation or following delivery. The only complaint may be dyspareunia. The lesion is revealed by speculum examination. Confusion may arise with carcinoma cervix. There is, bleeding on touch in carcinoma. Confirmation is done by biopsy. **Treatment** by hormone is ineffective. Surgical excision may be required.

ADENOMYOSIS

DEFINITION

Adenomyosis is a condition where there is ingrowth of the endometrium, both the glandular and stromal components, directly into the myometrium. It may be diffuse or focal. It is also defined as endometriosis interna.

CAUSES

The cause of such ingrowth is not known. It is commonly seen in elderly woman with increased parity. It may be related to repeated childbirths, vigorous curettage or excess of estrogen effect. Pelvic endometriosis coexists in about 40%.

PATHOGENESIS

Histologically, it is characterized by the extension of endometrial glands and stroma beyond the endometrial-myometrial interface (EMI). As the submucosa is absent, endometrial glands lie in direct contact with the underlying myometrium. It forms nests, deep within myometrium. Subsequently, there is myometrial hyperplasia around the endometriotic foci. Myometrial zone anatomy is observed by MRI. A junctional zone (with low signal intensity on T2-weighted images) is defined at the innermost layer of myometrium. It is thought that the disturbance of normal junctional zone (JZ) predisposes to secondary infiltration of endometrial glands and stroma to inner myometrial zone. The disturbance of JZ may be due to the endometrial factors, genetic predisposition or altered immune response. Trauma to the deeper endometrium (repeated curettage), causing breakdown of EMI is also taken as an important etiologic factor.

PATHOLOGY

It may affect both the anterior and posterior wall. The posterior wall is commonly affected.

Nearly 60% of woman with adenomyosis, have coexistent pathology like myoma, endometriosis or endometrial hyperplasia.

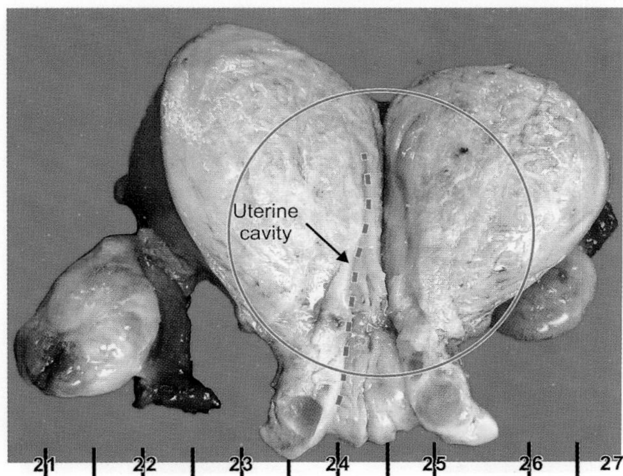

Fig. 22.8: Postoperative specimen of a 41-year-old parous lady. The uterus is cut opened to show characteristic features adenomyosis. Disproportionate thickening of the uterine walls with blood spots are seen. Uterine cavity is shown (*see* arrow).

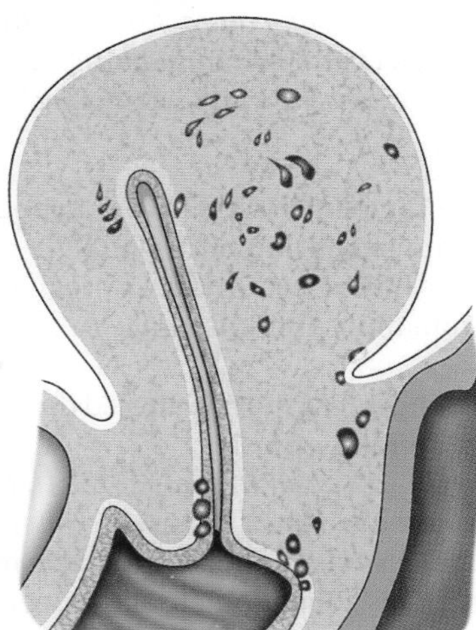

Fig. 22.9: Adenomyosis. Note the absence of capsule and presence of dark blood spots.

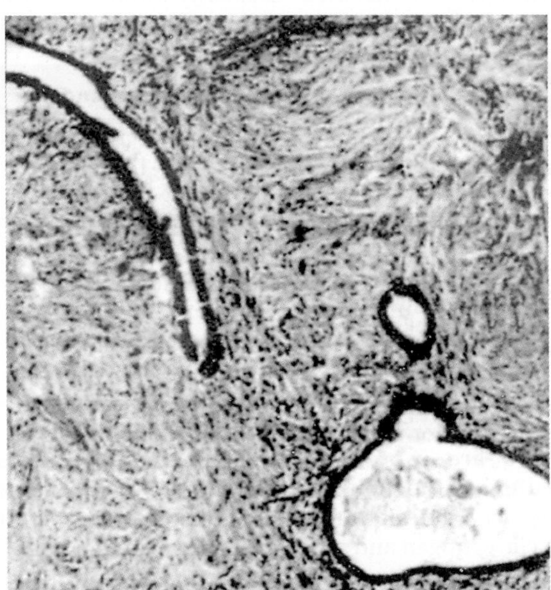

Fig. 22.10: Histologic picture of adenomyosis.

The growth and tissue reaction in the endometrium depend on the response of the ectopic endometrial tissues to the ovarian steroids. *If the basal layer is only present, the tissue reaction is much less, as it is unresponsive to hormones. But, if the functional zone is present which is responsive to hormones, the tissue reaction surrounding the endometrium is marked.* There is hyperplasia of the myometrium producing diffuse enlargement of the uterus, sometimes symmetrically but at times, more on the posterior wall. The growth may be localized or may invade a polyp (adenomyomatous).

Naked eye appearance: There is diffuse symmetrical enlargement of the uterus; the posterior wall is often more thickened than the anterior one. The size usually does not increase more than a large orange (12–14 weeks pregnant uterus). On cut section, it is darker in appearance (c.f. myoma with white surface) there is thickening of the uterine wall. The cut surface presents characteristic trabeculated appearances. Unlike fibroid, there is no capsule surrounding the growth. There may be visible cystic dark spaces and blood spots at places (Figs. 22.8 and 22.9).

Histological examination: Histological examination reveals glandular tissue like that of endometrium surrounded by stromal cells in the myometrium (Fig. 22.10).

CLINICAL FEATURES

In about 50%, it remains asymptomatic being discovered on histological examination.

Patient Profile

The patients are usually parous (90%) with age usually above 40 (80%).

Symptoms

Menorrhagia (70%): The excessive bleeding is due to increased uterine cavity, associated endometrial hyperplasia and inadequate uterine contraction. *During normal menstruation, there are antegrade propagation of subendometrial contractions from the fundus to the cervix. In adenomyosis with distorsion of JZ myometrial contractions are abnormal and inadequate (see below).*

Dysmenorrhea (30%): Progressively increased colicky pain during period is due to retrograde pattern of uterine contractions. It also depends on the number and depth of adenomyotic foci in the myometrium. When the depth of penetration is ≥80% of the myometrium, the pain is severe. Other causes of pain are—local tissue edema and prostaglandins.

Dyspareunia or frequency of urination are due to enlarged and tender uterus.

Infertility: Women with adenomyosis have a higher incidence of infertility and miscarriage. ***The reasons are:*** *(a) Abnormal function of the subendometrial myometrium;*

(b) Retrograde myometrial contractions; (c) Interference in sperm transport and blastocyst implantation; (d) Abnormal endometrial immune respose and nitric oxide level.

Signs

Abdominal examination may reveal a hypogastric mass arising out of the pelvis and occupying the midline. The size usually does not exceed 14 weeks pregnant uterus.

Pelvic examination—reveals uniform enlargement of the uterus.

The findings, however, may be altered due to associated fibroid or pelvic endometriosis.

Ultrasound (3D) and color Doppler (TVS): Myometrium normally has three distinct zones of different echogenecity. The inner layer is hypoechoic relative to the middle and outer layer. This subendometrial hypoechoeic zone is characteristic in adenomyosis. Other features are: (a) Heterogeneous echogenicity; (b) *Hypoechoeic myometrium with multiple small cysts in the myometrium (honeycomb appearance)*; (c) Increased vascularity within the myometrium (Fig. 22.11); (d) Ill-defined endometrial echo.

Diagnostic Criteria of Adenomyosis (Based on MRI) (Fig. 22.8)

- Asymmetrical thickness of the uterine walls (posterior > anterior)
- Heterogeneous myometrial echotexture
- Small myometrial hypoechoic cysts (honey comb appearance
- Striated projections extending from endometrium to myometrium
- Endometrial echo poorly defined
- Uterus is globally enlarged
- J–Z thickening ≥12 mm.

TREATMENT

NSAIDs are commonly used to control pain and bleeding. The definitive treatment is surgical. There is little place of hormone therapy. Treatment with progestins or cyclic estrogen and progestin have got little benefit.

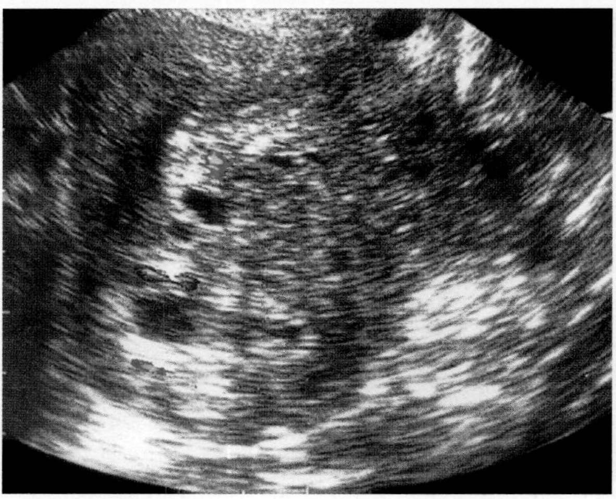

Fig. 22.11: Transvaginal color Doppler scan showing diffusely enlarged uterus with an echoic cysts. 'Swiss cheese' pattern with increased vascularity in the myometrium is suggestive of adenomyosis.

LNG-IUS is found to improve the menorrhagia and dysmenorrhea. **Danazol**—loaded (300–400 mg) intrauterine device (IUD) is also found to improve the symptoms of menorrhagia and dysmenorrhea. Serum danazol levels were not detectable and the side effects were minimal.

Surgical Management

(A) **Conservative surgery:** (a) Adenomyomectomy; (b) Uterine mass reduction (laparotomy or laparoscopy); (c) Uterine artery embolization

Or

(B) **Definitive surgery:** Hysterectomy (parous and aged women).

Medical treatment for adenomyosis is unsatisfactory. Hysterectomy is the definitive treatment provided, it is appropriate to the woman. UAE has been done to relieve symptoms.

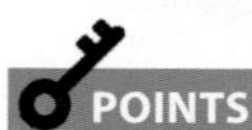

POINTS

- **Endometriosis** is the presence of functioning endometrium (stroma and glands) in sites other than uterine mucosa. **Endometriosis** is a disease seen in the reproductive years of a woman as its growth depends on estrogen. The incidence is about 10% but incidence is high (30–40%) amongst infertile women as based on diagnostic laparoscopy and laparotomy. The most common abdominal site is ovary followed by pouch of Douglas and uterosacral ligaments (organs on the dependent part of the pelvis).
- ***Biochemical mediators and the associated pathology in endometriosis are:***
  - ***Cytokines, interleukin-I, TNFα*** → • *Growth of ectopic endometrial cells* • *Prevention of cell apoptosis* • *Adhesion formation*
  - ***VEGF—A*** → *neoangiogenesis* • ***Matrix metalloproteinase*** → *invasion* • ***Estrogens*** → *cell proliferation*
  - ***Macrophages*** → *Sperm phagocytosis* • ***Prostaglandin and cytokines*** → *Inflammation.*
  - ***Causes of pain in endometriosis is due to:*** *Peritoneal inflammation, tissue necrosis, adhesions formation, nerve irritation due to deep penetration, release of local inflammatory mediators and/or endometrioma formation.*
- **Endometriosis is a disease of contrast**. It is a benign disease but it is locally invasive, disseminates widely and proliferates in the lymph nodes. **Minimal disease** may have severe pain whereas large endometriosis may remain asymptomatic. Cyclic hormones stimulates growth whereas continuous hormones suppress it.
- ***Endometriotic tissues*** *produce estrogen and many inflammatory cytokines locally. Estrogen causes proliferation and growth of endometriotic tissues. Whereas the cytokines and prostaglandins are the causes of pain and the infertility. The endometriotic tissues are resistant to progesterone.*
- ***Endometriotic lesions*** *may appear as red, brown, black, yellow, pink or in the form of vesicles, or subovarian adhesions. Red and the blood filled lesions are the most active.*
- **Abdominal scar** is the most common site of endometriosis following hysterectomy, hysterotomy, cesarean section, tubectomy or myomectomy (Fig. 22.6).

Contd...

Contd...

- **The disease is full of theories** and no one single theory can explain endometriosis at all sites. Genetic basis and defect of local cellular immunity may be implicated (Table 22.3). In spite of dense adhesions amongst the pelvic structures, the fallopian tubes are usually patent. In pelvic endometriosis, typically there are small black dots—'powder burns' or 'gunshot' seen on uterosacral ligaments and pouch of Douglas. Other lesions are flame-shaped polypoidal, hemorrhagic and white patches.
- **Etiopathogenesis** of endometriosis is not well understood. Factors involved are genetic mutations, immunological, molecular defects, mechanical factors and environmental toxins (dioxins).
- **Symptoms:** About 25% have got no symptom. **Symptoms** are not related to the extent of lesion. Severity of endometriosis and the degree of pelvic pain are not always proportional. Unlike primary dysmenorrhea, the pain lasts for many days before and after the menstruation.
- ***Pain from the ovary,*** *outer 2/3rd of the fallopian tube and upper ureter are carried via throracic sympathetics, coeliac and superior mesenteric plexus to the* T_9–T_{10} *spinal segments.*
- **Dysmenorrhea** is associated in 50%, menorrhagia in 60% and infertility in 40–60%. Endometriosis is found in 30–40% of infertile women.
- **Clinical diagnosis** is by the classic symptoms of progressively increasing dysmenorrhea, dyspareunia, infertility and feel of nodules in the pouch of Douglas. Confirmation is by laparoscopy or laparotomy.
- **Histologic diagnosis** of endometriosis is ideal. Microscopic diagnostic features are: Presence of endometrial glands, stroma and hemosiderin-laden macrophages.
- **Double puncture laparoscopy** is considered the **'gold standard'** for the diagnosis.
- **The natural course of the disease** is ill understood. It is progressive in about 30–60% patients and for the remainder it is either static or resolve spontaneously. Unfortunately, it is impossible to predict in which patient it will progress. Red blood filled lesions are the most active phase of endometriosis. Serum marker CA 125 is helpful in follow up cases of proved endometriosis.
- **Endometriosis is often associated** with tubal and ovarian damage (Table 22.5). These combined factors along with endocrinopathy (Table 22.4) may be responsible for infertility. However, the association of minimal to mild endometriosis and infertility is controversial.
- ***Infertility:*** *Common causes of infertility in endometriosis are—changes in the peritoneal fluid, ovulation disorders, reduced endometrial receptivity, implantation failure, or pelvic pain.*
- ***The complications*** *include endocrinopathy (LPD, anovulation, LUF or elevated prolactin level) rupture chocolate cyst, infection of the cyst or obstructive features (intestinal or ureteric).*
- **Other complications** of endometriosis are acute abdomen due to rupture of chocolate cyst, infection of the cyst, colorectal obstruction and ureteral obstruction.
- **The short-term goals of treatment** for endometriosis are: (a) relief of pain and (b) improvement of fertility. The long-term goal is to prevent progression or recurrence of the disease.
- **Expectant treatment** is extended to unmarried or young married with no abnormal pelvic findings. Endometriosis causes pelvic inflammation. So the drugs used are nonsteroidal anti-inflammatory drugs (NSAIDs) or prostaglandin synthetase inhibitors.
- **The hormonal treatment** should be considered suppressive rather than curative. The mechanism of atrophy can be explained by pseudopregnancy or by pseudomenopause or by medical hypophysectomy. The commonly used hormones are given in the Table 22.7.
- **The objective of medical therapy** is to create amenorrhea (hypoestrogenic state). Aromatase inhibitors (letrozol 2.5 mg daily) are used to inhibit aromatase which converts androgens to estrogens. Estrogen promotes its growth. The overall fertility rate and the recurrence rate is about 40%.
- ***The effect of danazol*** *is by its 'pseudomenopause' response. The side effects are due to its androgenic and anabolic properties. GnRH agonists produce 'medical oophorectomy' and the side effects are due to the estrogen deprivation. 'Add-back' therapy is suggested with chronic use of GnRH agonists.*
- **Other medications used are:** Progesterone antagonists (mifepristone), SPRMs (asoprisnil), dienogest and GnRH antagonists.
- **Conservative surgery** in endometriosis includes removal of all macroscopic endometriosis, lysis of adhesions and restoration of normal pelvic anatomy. The surgery is preferably done by laparoscopy (diathermy, laser vaporization). Endoscopic laser surgery is the best in selected cases for the treatment of pain and to prevent the disease progress.
- ***Ovarian endometriosis*** *(<3 cm) is treated by laparoscopic cyst aspiration. Large ovarian endometrioma (>3 cm) is treated by laparoscopic ovarian cystectomy. Laparoscopic adhesiolysis should be done at the same time. Laparoscopic ovarian cystectomy improves pain.*
- *Destruction of ovarian cortex reduces the ovarian reserve and further reduces the prospect of fertility.*
- **Preoperative medical treatment** with GnRH analog may reduce the vascularity and the extent of the disease. Postoperative medical treatment should not prevent pregnancy as the chance of pregnancy is highest during the first 6–12 months after the conservative surgery.
- **Infertility associated with endometriosis:** When there is no improvement of infertility due to endometriosis with usual treatment, ART is the option. Controlled ovarian stimulation with IUI, IVF, GIFT, or ICSI are the different methods.
- **Definitive surgery** includes total hysterectomy with bilateral salpingo-oophorectomy. Laparotomy is done for advanced stage disease or in women who has completed her family.
- **Postoperative estrogen replacement therapy** after total hysterectomy and bilateral oophorectomy may be given 3 months after surgery. The risk of recurrence is very low.
- **Adenomyosis** primarily occurs in parous women over the age of 35. It is associated with pelvic endometriosis in 40%. Menorrhagia (70%) and dysmenorrhea are the chief complaints. Uterus is diffusely enlarged (2–3 times). Uterine size >14 weeks gestation is rare.
- **Adenomyosis** is due in growth of endometrium directly into the myometrium. It is due to the dysfunctions of the junctional zone (JZ) as revealed by MRI.
- **Pathology of adenomyosis** includes hyperplasia of myometrium. Unlike fibroid, there is no capsule surrounding the growth.
- **Women with adenomyosis** presents with: Menorrhagia, dysmenorrhea, dyspareunia or infertility.
- **Hormone treatment** is often ineffective. Levonorgestrel-releasing IUS is found to improve menorrhagia and dysmenorrhea. Hysterectomy is the effective treatment in a parous and aged women.

CHAPTER

23 Premalignant Lesions

CHAPTER OUTLINE

PREMALIGNANT VULVAR LESIONS

Premalignant vulvar lesions include:

- Vulvar intraepithelial neoplasia (VIN)
- Paget's disease (p. 267)
- Lichen sclerosus (p. 214)
- Squamous cell hyperplasia
- Condyloma accuminata (p. 129)
- Melanoma in situ.

VULVAR INTRAEPITHELIAL NEOPLASIA

Earlier classification: VIN I—Mild cellular atypia, limited to the deeper one-third of the epithelium. This category is now eliminated. **VIN II**—Moderate cellular atypia involving up to middle-third of the epithelium. **VIN III**—Severe cellular atypia involving more than 2/3 of epithelium and carcinoma in situ (CIS). There are multinucleated cells, abnormal mitosis and an increase in the nuclear to cytoplasmic ratio. There is no stromal invasion.

International Society for Study of Vulvar Diseases (ISSVD, 2004) introduced a simplified classification. VIN I has been eliminated. VIN II and III are combined. **VIN now encompasses only those lesions having high grade squamous cell abnormalities**. This combines the previous categories of VIN II and III (*see* above).

Special Features of VIN:

- ***VIN is more frequent*** *in patients in the age group 20–40 years, i.e. at a younger age group compared to vulvar carcinoma.* ***The average age is as low as 33 years.***
- It is often **related with STIs** such as condyloma accuminata, herpes simplex virus II, gonorrhea, syphilis or *Gardnerella vaginalis*.
- **HPV** associated VIN is seen more in young women. HPV 6 and 11 are associated with vulvar condylomas. HPV 16, 18, 31, 33, 35 are associated with VIN and invasive lesions.
- There is increased prevalence of **associated CIN (10–80%)**.
- **Regression** frequently occurs in young woman, during pregnancy or when it is caused by viral infection.
- **Progression** to invasive carcinoma high in high grade VIN (VIN 2 and 3) lesions. It takes 20–30 years (for CIN 10–15 years).
- *Treatment of VIN is based on histologic findings and not on the presence or absence of HPV infection or any specific HPV types. HPV-16 frequently associated with vulvar neoplasia (c.f. vaginal intraepithelial neoplasia).*

Pathophysiology

HPV DNA has been found in 80% of VIN lesions. However, of all vulvar cancer specimens only 40% are positive for HPV DNA.

Diagnosis

Symptoms of VIN

- May be symptomless
- Pruritus, burning
- Pain
- Dysuria
- Discharge/bleeding
- Vulvar ulcer
- Difficult sexuality
- Warty growth/lump

Local examination reveals a lesion in the vulva with white, gray, pink or dull red color. Lesions look rough, raised from the surface and often multifocal. *Application of 5%* ***acetic acid*** *turns VIN lesions white with punctuation and mosaic patterns. These changes are seen with a* ***colposcope****.* Toluidine blue test is discarded as it is nonspecific.

A complete pelvic examination is to be done. **To exclude vaginal or cervical neoplasia, cytologic evaluation has to be performed.**

Biopsy: Confirmation of diagnosis is done by biopsy. Usually 3–5 mm diameter dermal punch is taken under local anesthetic using a Keye's punch biopsy forceps. The small amount of bleeding is controlled using Monsel's paste (ferrous subsulfate). Larger biopsy when required may be taken using a scalpel. Multiple site biopsies are useful.

Histology

The cells exhibit features of malignancy. There is complete loss of polarity and stratification. Cellular immaturity, nuclear abnormalities and mitotic activity vary depending upon the grade of VIN. There is hyperkeratosis, acanthosis (hyperplasia of epidermis) and chronic inflammatory cell infiltration. **Koilocytes (Fig. 23.3) may be present.** The rete ridges are large and elongated. **Basement membrane remains** intact. There is no evidence of involvement of the dermis.

Treatment of VIN

The progression of VIN 1 to VIN 3 is rare. Some cases of VIN regress spontaneously. Therefore, VIN 1 should not be treated and is followed up. All high grade VIN (VIN 2 and 3) lesions should be treated (ACOG - 2011).

Medical

Topical therapy: Commonly used agents are—imiquimod 5% cream, cidofovir emulsion, or 5% fluorouracil cream. Photodynamic therapy (PDT) with 5 aminolevulinic acid (5-ALA) is used in cases with VIN or vulvar CIS (carcinoma in situ).

Whatever therapy is employed, it is mandatory for regular follow up. Biopsies to be taken freely whenever an abnormal area is detected.

Surgery

The following are the types of surgery:

- **Local excision: Wide local excision** (WLE) with 1 cm of normal tissue margin and depth of 3–4 mm is reserved in young patient with localized VIN 3 lesion.
- **Laser ablation therapy** using CO_2 laser is done with better cosmetic results. Presence of invasive carcinoma must be excluded beforehand as no specimen is available for histological evaluation following laser ablation.
- **Cavitational ultrascan and surgical aspiration (CUSA)** is used in cases with high grade VIN. This method causes less scarring and pain than WLE.
- **Simple vulvectomy:** It is employed in diffuse type especially in postmenopausal women. Long-term follow-up is needed as the risk of recurrence is high (40–70%). Patient may need skin grafting if there is disfigurement.

Prognosis

Women with high grade VIN, need colposcopic evaluation of the cervix and vagina regardless of normal cervical cytology. Post-treatment follow up consists of vulvar evaluation at 6th and 12th month and then annually (ACOG, ASCCP—2011).

Prevention

Prophylactic HPV vaccination against types 16 and 18 can prevent about one-third of vulvar cancers. Cessation of smoking and optimization immune status are important (p. 274).

PAGET'S DISEASE

This is a special type of VIN (intraepithelial disorder). The lesion grows horizontally within the epidermis. The rete ridges tend to push into the dermis without actually penetrating it.

The characteristic histologic picture is presence of Paget cells in the epidermis. The cells are large—round or oval in shape with abundant pale cytoplasm, this often occur in nests. There may be presence of mucopolysaccharides in most of the cells. Nuclear mitotic figures are rare.

Associated adenocarcinoma of apocrine gland (adenocarcinoma in situ) is present in about 10% of the cases. **There is high incidence (30%) of associated carcinomas of other organs (breast, cervix, ovary, stomach, GI tract and bladder).**

Symptoms

They are mainly pruritus, vulvar soreness, pain or bleeding.

Local examination reveals—labia majora appear red, scaling, with elevated lesion. There may be associated white lesions. The skin is usually thickened.

Diagnosis: Biopsy of the vulva is taken using a Keye's dermal punch biopsy. Usually a 3–5 mm diameter punch is taken. Sometimes a large biopsy is needed.

Treatment

Simple vulvectomy is done. **Local recurrence is a risk.** Multiple biopsies are to be taken to exclude associated adenocarcinoma of the apocrine glands. If it is found positive, bilateral lymph node dissection should be done at a second stage. **Patients should be under routine follow-up annually. Examination of the breasts, cervical cytology, and screening for GI disease is important.**

Topical use of imiquimod cream may be done for women following surgery and those are not fit for repeat surgery.

VAGINAL INTRAEPITHELIAL NEOPLASIA

The etiologic agent is oncogenic HPV infection. In 70% cases of vaginal intraepithelial neoplasia (VaIN) there is associated CIN or VIN.

Risk Factors

- Infection with HPV type 16, 18
- Associated cervical and vulvar neoplasia.

Pathology

VaIN I: There is minimal loss of stratification and polarity of the cells.

VaIN II: Epithelial abnormality extends onto the middle-third of the epithelium.

VaIN III: CIS—there is loss of polarity and stratification through all layers. Basement membrane remains intact.

Diagnosis: Patient presents with postcoital discharge or bleeding.

- **Vaginal scrape cytology**
- **Colposcopy (vaginoscopy)**
- **Biopsy** (Tischler biopsy forceps)

Management

Management of VaIN is done after physical, colposcopic, histologic examination of the lesion and with patient counseling.

VaIN I: Spontaneous regression is common (88%) as it is often due to transient HPV infection. Patient needs to be followed up at an interval of every 6–12 months with cytology with or without colposcopy.

VaIN (II-III): It may be treated with:

- Wide local excision or partial vaginectomy.
- Laser ablation for multifocal lesion (CO_2 laser).
- Medical ablation using 5% fluorouracil (5-FU) cream or imiquimod 5% cream.
- **Radiation therapy:** Very rarely used for cases with carcinoma in situ.

Complications: Vaginal stenosis, adhesions, ulcerations and fistula formation.

Prognosis: Patients with high grade VaIN need long-term follow up with vaginal cytology and vaginoscopy. Recurrence risk for VaIN is 2/3 (20–30%).

CERVICAL INTRAEPITHELIAL NEOPLASIA

NOMENCLATURE

The terminology has been changed over the years. The terminology, carcinoma in situ (CIS) was introduced by Rubin (1910), 'Dysplasia' by Walters and Regan (1956) and cervical intraepithelial neoplasia (CIN) by Richart (1967). WHO (1975) redefined CIN into three categories. **The Bethesda System** (TBS) in 1988 and modified on 2014, introduced a uniform terminology for reporting Pap test results (Table 23.1).

The cytologic and histologic correlation of mild, moderate and severe dysplasia, CIS, CIN and the Bethesda's system have been mentioned in Table 23.1.

The newer terminology CIN, is intended to emphasize that the **disease is a continuum and reflects the prognostic significance, if left untreated** (Figs. 23.1A and B).

TABLE 23.1: Correlation of dysplasia, CIN (WHO) and Bethesda system.

Dysplasia	*CIN*	*Limit of histologic changes*	*Bethesda (p. 91)*
▪ **Mild**	CIN I	Basal one-third	**LSIL**
▪ **Moderate**	CIN II	Basal half to two-third	**HSIL**
▪ **Severe**	CIN III	▪ Whole thickness except one or two superficial layers	
▪ **CIS**		▪ Whole thickness	

Squamocolumnar junction (SCJ) is the meeting point of columnar epithelium, that lines the endocervical canal, with squamous epithelium that lines the ectocervix (Fig. 23.2). **Transformation zone** is the metaplastic squamous epithelium between the original squamocolumnar junction (OSCJ) and the active squamocolumnar junction (ASCJ). The OSCJ is the junction between the stratified squamous epithelium of the vagina and ectocervix and

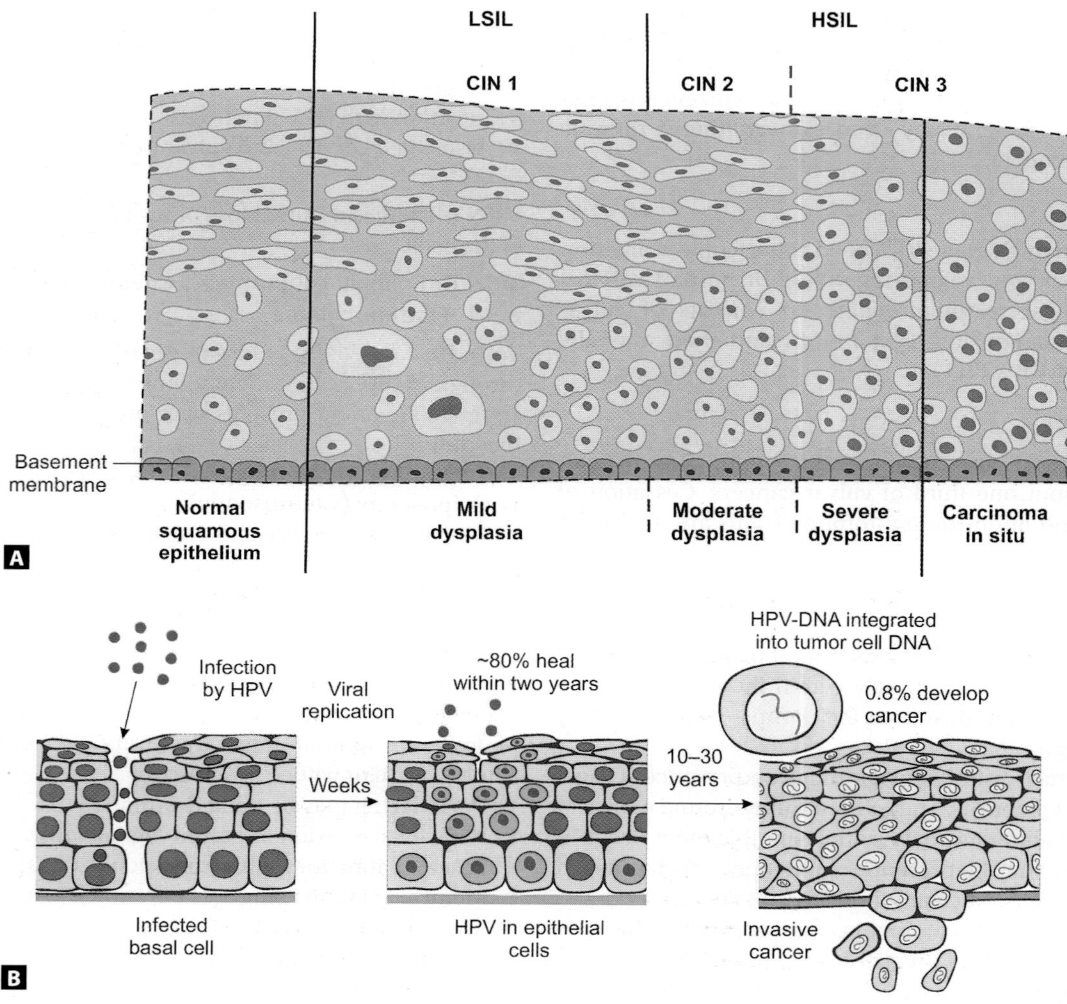

Figs. 23.1A and B: (A) Normal stratified squamous epithelium of the ectocervix on the left is progressed to CIN/CIS on the right through progressive degrees of dysplastic changes; (B) Pathogenesis of HPV infection.

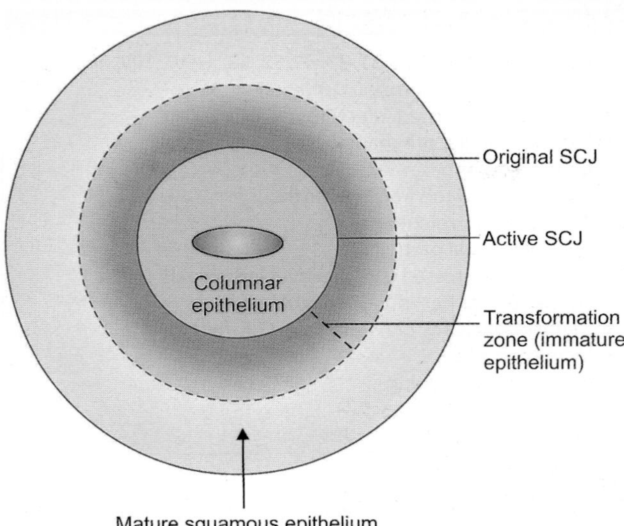

Fig. 23.2: Before puberty, the ectocervix is covered with squamous epithelium. Heightened estrogenic activity exposes the columnar epithelium onto the ectocervix. New squamocolumnar junction is situated at or slightly outside the external os during reproductive period. Replacement of columnar epithelium by squamous epithelium is to form TZ. This squamocolumnar junction is a dynamic point and it changes with phases of life. Indrawing of the squamocolumnar junction and the TZ well into the cervical canal occurs following menopause.

the columnar epithelium of the endocervical canal. **SCJ is a dynamic point**. It moves up and down in relation to different phases of life. This is due to ovarian hormonal and environmental influences. Following menarche, the OSCJ is seen on the ectocervix, with further eversion during pregnancy. In postmenopausal women the SCJ moves up within endocervical canal. Cervical neoplasia originates almost always from the transformation zone. Cervical reserve and the immature metaplastic cells are vulnerable to the oncogenic effects of HPV and other carcinogens. **Metaplastic change is most active during adolescent and pregnancy. With this reason, early age of sexual activity is a high risk factor for cervical cancer.**

PATHOGENESIS

The process of carcinogenesis starts at the '**transformation zone**' **(TZ)**. The zone is not static but in a dynamic state. Two mechanisms are involved in the process of replacement of endocervical columnar epithelium by squamous epithelium.

- By squamous metaplasia of the subcolumnar reserve cells.
- Squamous epidermalization by ingrowth of the squamous epithelium of the ectocervix under the columnar epithelium.

In presence of estrogen the vaginal epithelium accumulates glycogen. The lactobacilli act on glycogen to produce the lactic acid (acidic pH) of vagina. **The acidic pH probably is an important trigger for the metaplastic process.** These metaplastic cells have got the potentiality to undergo atypical transformation by trauma or infection (Flowchart 23.1).

The prolonged effect of carcinogens can produce continuous changes in the immature cells which may progress to malignancy. Early age sexual activity and multiple sexual partners are the most consistent risk factors. HPV infection is transmitted through sexual activity. Microtrauma (sexual intercourse) causes viral entry to the epithelium (basal or parabasal cells) of the transformation zone adjacent to the SCJ (Fig. 23.1B). HPV-DNA positivity is strongly related with the number of sexual partners. Women with multiple partners have high HPV-DNA positivity rate (60%) compared to women with single partner (21%). **The important factors in the genesis of**

Flowchart 23.1: Pathogenesis of CIN and invasive carcinoma.

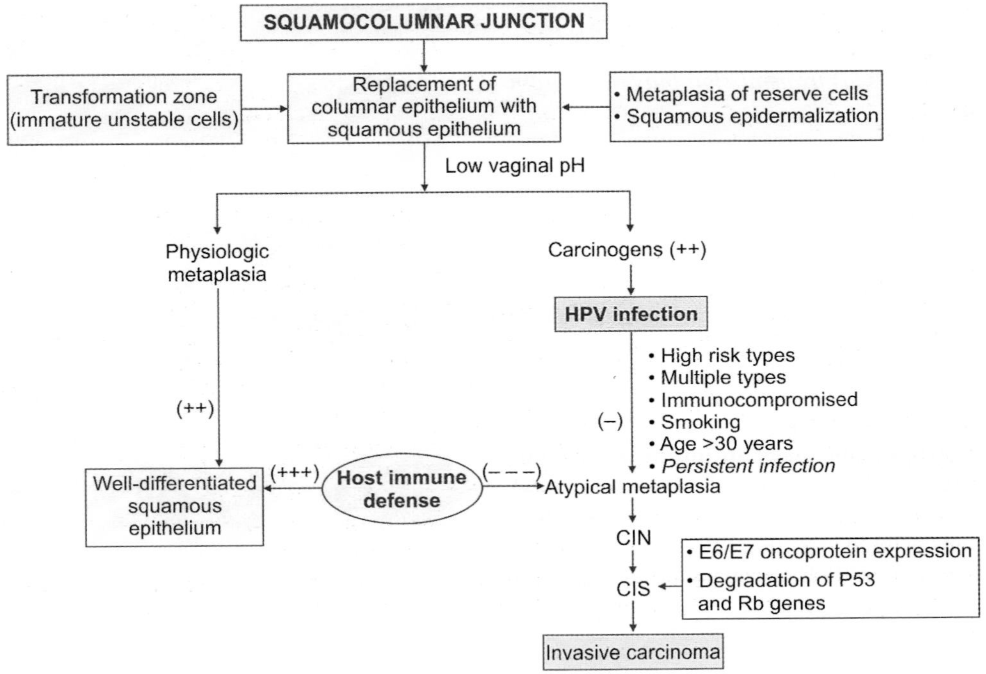

TABLE 23.2: Life cycle of unstable cervical epithelium.

Cervical epithelium	*CIN I*	*CIN II*	*CIN III/CIS*
Regression to normal (%)	60	40	30
Persistence (%)	30	35	50
Progression to CIN III/CIS (%)	10	20	—
Progression to invasion (%)	<1	5	30–40

Duration of disease progression (years)	Normal	CIN I, II	CIN III/CIS	Invasion
	0	5	10	20
Age of the patient (year)		25–30	30–35	40–45

cervical cancer are: (a) Infection with high-risk HPV; (b) Multiple types of HPV; (c) Persistence of infection; (d) Age >30 years; (e) Smoking; (f) Compromised host immunodefense.

Life Cycle of Unstable Cervical Epithelium (Table 23.2)

The cases of CIN I or II are most often related to infection and may revert back normal. Some, however, either remain static or progress to CIN III.

CIN III, however, is more susceptible to progress into invasive carcinoma. This is more so in cases of CIS.

Thus, it is apparent that some of these epithelial atypia either remain stationary, regress or even progress to invasive carcinoma.

The real problem, at least to a clinician, to ascertain which one and how long the mild or moderate dysplasia takes to proceed to invasive carcinoma without passing through CIS. As such, even a CIN I or II should not be ignored, but to be followed up carefully.

EPIDEMIOLOGY

Prevalence: *CIN is commonly seen around the age of 20 years, CIS is around the age of 25–35 years, whereas the incidence of cervical cancer rises significantly by the age of 40 years.*

Condoms may not be 100% protective in HPV infection, as against in others STIs, as transmission may occur from labial-scrotal contact.

More than 90% of immune competent women will have spontaneous resolution of their HPV infection by 2 years. About 10% have a persistent high risk HPV infection which ultimately leads to CIN and invasive cancer.

CIN like invasive carcinoma is most often related to some risk factors (Table 23.3).

Infectious agents: The causative agents appear to be transmitted to the susceptible women during intercourse. Two viruses are implicated as casual agents.

Human Papillomavirus (HPV)

HPV is epitheliotropic and plays an important role in the development of CIN. HPV infected cells **(koilocytes)** are characterized by enlarged cells with perinuclear halos. The nucleus is large, irregular and hyperchromatic (Fig. 23.3). Depending on their oncogenic potential, HPV types are broadly grouped into two. More than 150 HPV types have been identified.

TABLE 23.3: Risk factors for CIN and cervical cancer.

- Infection: HPV (16, 18, 31, 33, 45, 52, 58), HSV2, HIV, *Chlamydia*
- Early sexual intercourse (≤16 years)
- Sexually transmitted infections
- Early age of first pregnancy
- Multiparity
- Too many and too frequent births
- Poor genital hygiene
- Multiple sexual partners
- Immunosuppressed (HIV positive) individuals
- Husband who has multiple sexual partners
- Dietary deficiency of (vitamins A, C, E, folic acid)
- Increasing age
- Inadequate screening
- Oral pill users
- Smoking habit

- High oncogenic risk—types 16, 18, 31, 33, 35, 45, 56, 58, 59, 68.
- Low oncogenic risk—types 6, 11, 42, 43, 44.

Over 99.7% of patients with CIN and invasive cancer are found to be positive with high risk HPV-DNA. HPV-DNA detection in cervical tissues may be a screening procedure as that of Pap smear. Polymerase chain reaction or southern blot or **hybrid capture-2 (HC-2)** technique is used for HR HPV-DNA **detection**.

Pathogenesis of HPV Infection

HPV is epitheliotropic. Cervical epithelium → infection (latent/active with virus replication) → oncogenic HPV-DNA integration to human genome → upregulation of viral oncogenes → expression of E6 and E7 oncoproteins → interference of tumor suppressor genes (p53 and Rb) → host cell immortalization and HPV induced neoplastic transformation.

Viral DNA activates host cell p53 proteins. Activated p53 causes cell apoptosis (cell death) and thus stop the viral multiplication. But HPV E6 and E7 oncoproteins

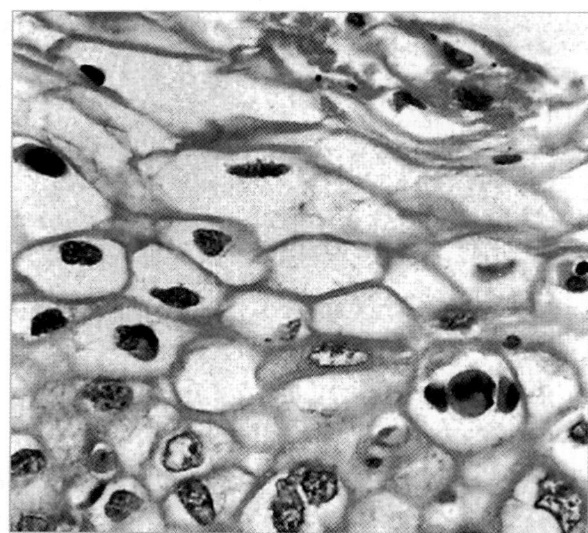

Fig. 23.3: Koilocyte is the hallmark of cellular changes in HPV infection. Koilocytes are large, vacuolated squamous cells with a clear perinuclear halo. The nuclei are hyperchromatic, irregular with multinucleate forms.

cause proteolytic degradation of p53. This causes host cell immortalization and viral multiplication.

HPV triage strategy includes: (a) Pap smear test (LBC, p. 89) → An atypical smear (HSIL, ACS-H) (after exclusion of infection); (b) HPV testing → high-risk HPV positive; (c) Colposcopy. This triage strategy can detect CIN II and III lesions effectively and reduces the load of colposcopy clinic.

Triage Screening

A. Liquid-based thin layer cytology evaluation → atypical squamous cells (HSIL, ASC-H).
B. Hybrid capture 2 for HPV DNA (16, 18).
C. HPV-DNA Test:
- Positive (high-risk viruses) → colposcopy → biopsy
- Negative → repeat smear after 5 years.

DIAGNOSIS OF CIN

- *Cytologic screening (Flowchart 23.2): Exfoliative cytology (Papanicolaou and Traut, 1943) has become the gold standard for screening. The smear should contain cells from SCJ, TZ, and the endocervix. Ayre's spatula and an endocervical brush is used for the purpose. Cells are spread on a single slide and fixed immediately (p. 90).*
  a. Dyskaryotic cells (p. 90) are atypical cells with hyperchromatic large nuclei having abundant cytoplasm (Fig. 23.4 and Table 23.4).
  b. CIS cells contain hyperchromatic nuclei, coarse chromatin and lesser cytoplasm. There may be multiple nuclei and abnormal mitotic figures (Table 23.5 and Fig. 23.5).

Flowchart 23.2: Evaluation of cervical cytology screening.

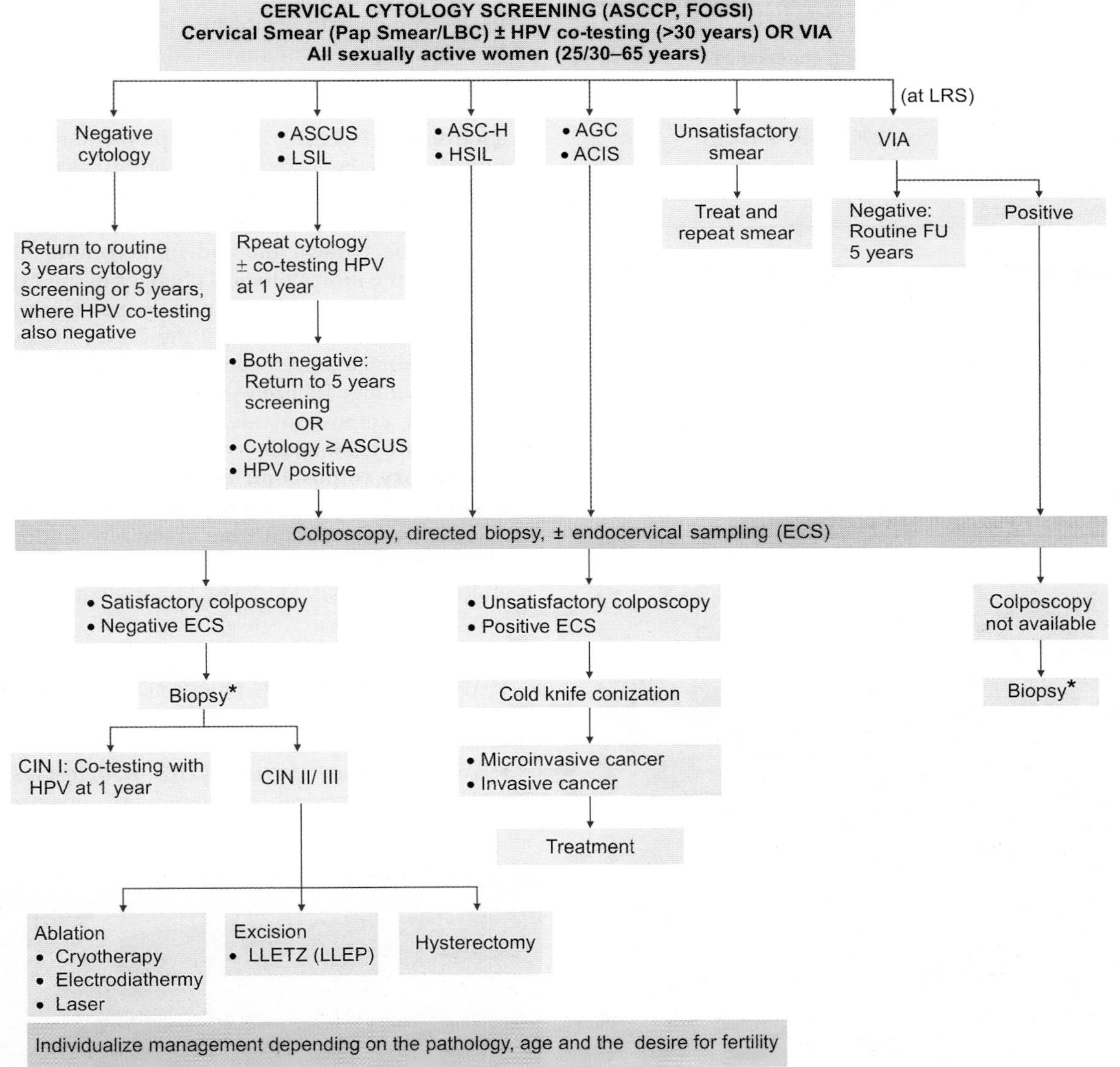

(ASCUS: Atypical squamous cells of undetermined significance; LSIL: Low-grade squamous intraepithelial lesion; HSIL: High-grade squamous intraepithelial lesion; VIA: Visual inspection with acetic acid; AGC: Atypical glandular cells; FU: Follow up; LRS: Low resource setting; ACIS: Adenocarcinoma in situ; LBC: Liquid-based cytology; ASCCP: American Society of Colposcopy and Cervical Pathology; FOGSI: Federation of Obstetric and Gynaecological Societies of India)

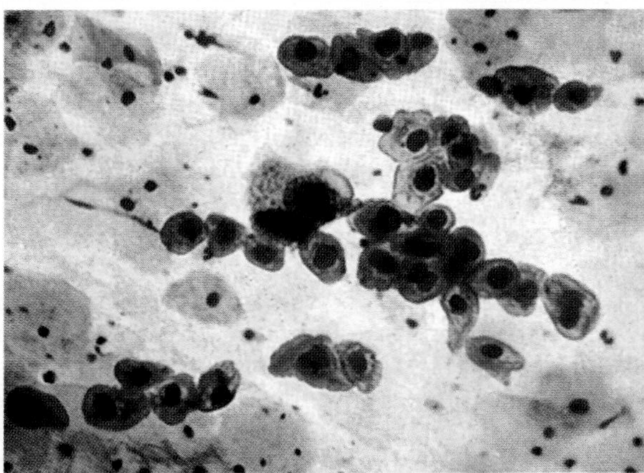

Fig. 23.4: Smear showing dyskaryotic cells.

TABLE 23.4: Features of a dyskaryotic cell.

- Increased cell size
- Pleomorphism—different staining appearance
- Cells vary in their size and shape
- Multinucleation
- Clumping of chromatin—varying degree
- Aneuploidy
- Alteration in nuclear membrane
- Perinuclear halo

TABLE 23.5: Histologic picture of CIS (Fig. 23.5).

- The entire epithelial layer is affected
- There is loss of stratification and polarity
- The cells vary in size and shape
- The nuclei stain deeply with presence of frequent mitosis and abnormal chromatin pattern
- The nuclei are larger and hyperchromatic with scanty cytoplasm
- The basement membrane remains intact
- Abnormal mitotic figures are present.

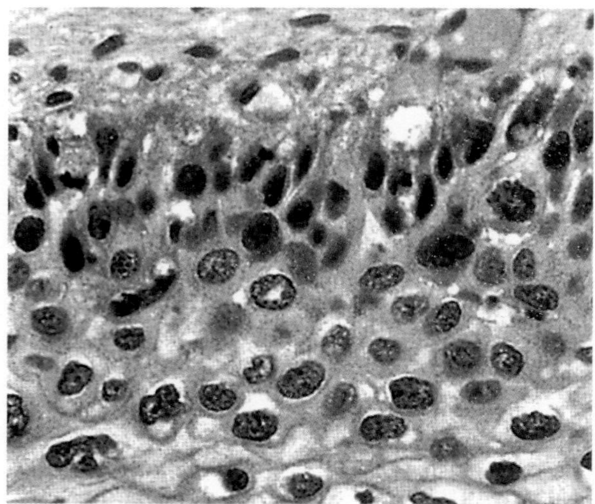

Fig. 23.5: Histology of carcinoma-in-situ of cervix. Marked nuclear abnormalities are seen throughout most of the thickness. Abnormal mitotic figures are present.

Mild dyskaryotic smear is correlated with CIN II/III lesion in about 50% of cases. Severe dyskaryosis is correlated with about 90% of CIN II/III or CIS.

- **High risk HPV-DNA (HR HPV-DNA) testing is useful in cervical screening:** Hybrid capture method can reliably detect the high-risk HPV types within hours. However, **only about 2–5% of women diagnosed with HPV-DNA will ever develop CIN.** Nearly 80% test positive women will clear the infection (HPV) by their own immune defense. Positive test result in elderly women (>30 years) suggests colposcopic examination. **HR HPV-DNA testing is an adjunct to cytology.** Quantitative HPV testing is more important compared to qualitative result. Use of **HR HPV-DNA testing along with genotyping for HPV 16 and 18 may be used as primary method of screening.**
- **Visual inspection with acetic acid (VIA):** A speculum is introduced and acetic acid is applied to the cervix. Those women with acetowhite lesions are considered for colposcopic examination and/or biopsy.
- **Colposcopy: Colposcopy** is in situ examination of the cervix with a low magnification (6–16 times) microscope (Fig. 9.20). It is complementary and not a substitute for cytology. Colposcopy is recommended for women with persistently positive HPV-DNA test results. Cytology is the laboratory method while colposcopy is the clinical method of detection. Cytology evaluates the morphological changes of the exfoliated cells. Colposcopy evaluates mainly the changes in the terminal vascular network of the cervix which reflect the biochemical and metabolic changes of the tissue. In fact, cytology identifies the patient having cervical neoplasm, colposcopy identifies the site where from biopsies are to be taken.

  Satisfactory colposcopic examination includes visualization of the original SCJ, columnar epithelium, and the transformation zone in entirety. Endocervical speculum may be used to see the SCJ that is in the endocervical canal (Fig. 23.6). For procedure of colposcopy, *see* page 93.

  Indications of colposcopy
  - Women with cytology report: HSIL, ASC-H, ASCUS with HPV +ve.
  - Clinically abnormal cervix despite normal cytology.
  - Women with persistent HR HPV-DNA test result.
  - Abnormal cervical cytology with positive HPV testing

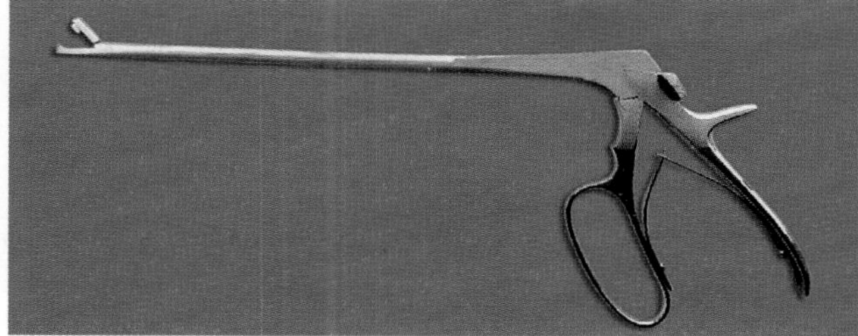

Fig. 23.6: Biopsy forceps used in colposcopy guided procedure.

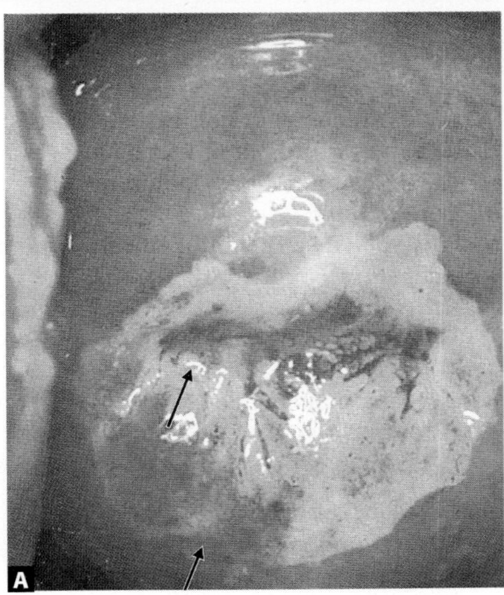

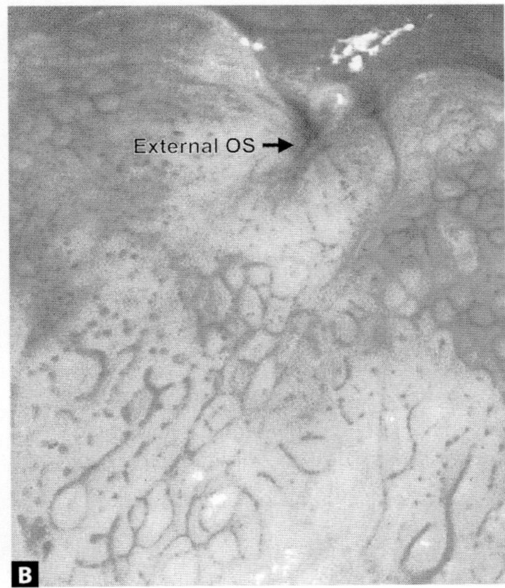

Figs. 23.7A and B: Colposcopic view of acetowhite epithelium (Schiller's negative) around the external os is seen: (A) Squamocolumnar junction is clearly seen (arrow); (B) Colposcopic view of the posterior tip of the cervix showing typical mosaic pattern. Biopsy revealed carcinoma in situ.

- Unexplained postcoital bleeding
- Vulvar or vaginal neoplasia.

■ **Abnormal colposcopic findings**
- **White epithelium**—leukoplakia
- **Acetowhite epithelium**—turning white following application of 5% acetic acid due to cell protein coagulation (Fig. 23.7A).
- **Punctuation**—dilated capillaries which appear on the surface as dots (end on view of vessels).
- **Mosaic**—capillaries encircling polygonal-shaped blocks of epithelial cells (Fig. 23.7B).
- **Atypical blood vessels** with irregular diameter and branching are suggestive of invasive carcinoma (Fig. 23.8).
- **Irregular surface contour** with ulceration and friability.

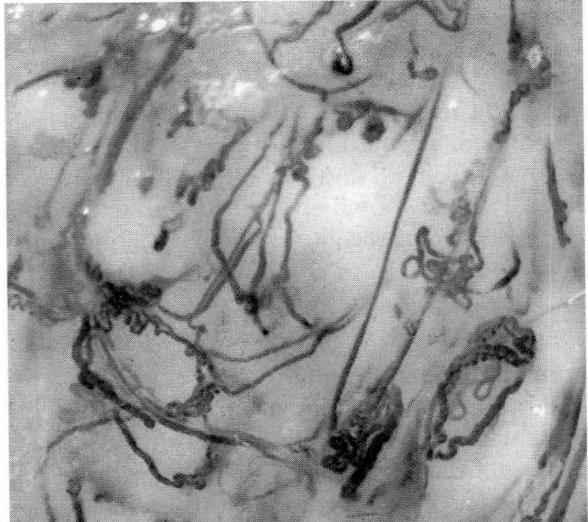

Fig. 23.8: Colposcopic view showing atypical blood vessels in invasive carcinoma.

■ **Cervicography:** Photographs are taken from the cervix. Film is viewed by an expert colposcopist. Similar to colposcopy, cervix is treated with 5% acetic acid before photography. It is complementary to cytology and colposcopy.

■ **Biopsy with or without colposcopy**

A. Colposcopy available (p. 93): Colposcopy detects an abnormal area → biopsy is taken under its guidance (targeted biopsy).

B. Colposcopy not available
- **Schiller's test:** Employing iodine solution (Schiller's 0.3% or Lugol's 5%), multiple punch biopsies are taken from the **unstained areas**. Stained areas (normal) appear brown due to presence of glycogen.
- Alternatively, ring biopsy is taken from the squamocolumnar junction and subjected to serial sections.
- **Endocervical curettage** (ECC) is mandatory whether or not the entire transformation zone can be seen (Table 23.6).

Cervical glandular intraepithelial neoplasia (CGIN): Screening with cytology and even colposcopy are unsatisfactory. Cone biopsy is both diagnostic and therapeutic for young women with high-grade CGIN.

TABLE 23.6: Indications of endocervical curettage (ECC).

■ Unsatisfactory colposcopy ■ Satisfactory colposcopy but abnormal cytology ■ Presence of glandular cell abnormalities ■ Before ablative treatment is done ■ Surveillance after excisional/conization for adenocarcinoma in situ.
However, there is no randomized trial to support the routine use of ECC. Brushing the endocervical canal with a cytobrush may be done alternatively.

TABLE 23.7: Indications of diagnostic conization.

- ***Colposcopy available***
  - Unsatisfactory colposcopy
  - Entire limits of the lesion not seen
  - Transformation zone not seen
  - Evidences of microinvasion on biopsy, colposcopy or cytology
  - CIN on endocervical curettage
  - Discrepancy in observation: Normal colposcopic findings with abnormal cytology/biopsy
  - High grade CGIN lesion
- ***Colposcopy not available***
  - Abnormal smear with apparently healthy cervix
  - Positive diagnosis of CIS to exclude invasive carcinoma
  - Biopsy report is inconsistent with cytologic findings

  Advantages and disadvantage of conization are discussed in page 488.

Diagnostic Conization

In fact, the need for diagnostic cone biopsy has been reduced at least 80% by the use of colposcopically directed biopsies (Table 23.7).

TREATMENT OF CIN

- **Preventive**
- **Definitive**

Preventive

- **HPV vaccines** has been developed from the capsid coat of the virus (HPV). It has high immunogenicity. **Bivalent vaccines** (cervarix) against HPV types 16, 18, and **quadrivalent (Gardasil) vaccines** against HPV types 6, 11, 16, 18 are effective in prevention of about 90% cervical cancer. Currently **nonavalent vaccines are available**. Nine valent vaccines (Gardasil 9) protect against all the HPV types 6,11,16,18,31,33,45,52 and 58. This vaccine can prevent CIN II by 96%. **The vaccines are prophylactic and not therapeutic.** HPV vaccines are not harmful in pregnancy but are not recommended as yet. It is safe during lactation. All the vaccines have some cross protection against other HPV types. **Vaccines are given ideally to girls aged 9–26 years, in three doses IM over the deltoid muscle.** The impact of vaccines is greatest when it is given to females who are not already infected. **This is the reason it is recommended to adolescent girls (9–13 years).** Vaccines are safe and well tolerated.

  Vaccine induced neutralizing antibodies (IgG, IgA) works locally (cervix) by preventing the attachment of the virus to the cervical epithelium. Currently **vaccination schedule (WHO)**: Females <15 years a 2 dose (0, 6 months) and females ≥15 years a 3 dose schedule (0, 1 to 2, 6 months) is recommended. **Immunocompromised** women should be given 3 dose schedule. **Immune defense is type specific and is effective only when given prophylactically.**

  Vaccines are effective for at least 7.5 years. However, screening with Pap test should be continued as the vaccines are type specific and do not protect against the other types of HPV.

Prevention of HPV Infection

- **Behavioral interventions**
  - Delaying sex until the cervical epithelium, in the TZ, has attained physiological maturity.
  - Limiting number of sexual partners
  - Limiting number of children
- **Condom use**
- **HPV vaccines:** To produce local and humoral immunity against HPV infection.
- **Other measures**
  - To maintain local hygiene and to treat vaginal infections.
  - To maintain penile hygiene as it may be the reservoir for high risk HPV.
  - Reducing or quitting smoking reduces CIN.

Definitive Treatment

The treatment modalities depend on:

- Age of the patient
- Desire for reproduction
- Risk factors present
- Degree of dysplasia
- Facilities available for follow up such as colposcopy and/or cytology.

Treatment options are as follows:

- *Observation with repeat smear, HPV testing and/or colposcopy every at an interval of 6 months to 1 year.*
- *Local ablative methods*
  - Cryotherapy
  - Electrodiathermy
  - Cold coagulation
  - Laser vaporization
- *Excisional methods*
  - Large loop (electrosurgical) excision of transformation zone (LLETZ).
  - Cone excision—using a knife or laser.
- *Hysterectomy*—abdominal or vaginal, MIS.

CIN I with LSIL cytology: These patients are managed with observation, as the rates of spontaneous regression are high. These patients are advised co-testing with HPV at 12 months or repeat cytology alone at 12 months. Persistent CIN I lesion and/or positive cotesting with HPV needs treatment.

CIN II/III—Differentiation between CIN II and III is difficult. So CIN II and CIN III are taken as a group and managed similarly. Considering rates of progression (12%–40%) for CIN III and CIN II (5%) to invasive cancer (Table 23.2) most women are treated with either ablative or an excisional procedure. Careful follow up with cytology and colposcopy 6 monthly is to be done for a young women desiring fertility.

Women need long-term (20 years) follow up.

Ablation of the local lesion

The following criteria should be fulfilled:

- The entire lesion is to be seen within the transformation zone.
- No evidence of microinvasion or invasion.
- No endocervical glandular involvement.
- No discrepancy in cytology, colposcopy, and biopsy report.

There are advantages and disadvantage of local ablation (see below).

Methods of local ablation

- **Cryotherapy:** It works on the principle of crystallizing the intracellular water at temperature of –90°C (p. 488). It uses either nitrous oxide or carbon dioxide. **Depth of tissue destruction is 5 mm.** This method is ideal for minor degree and localized CIN lesions. Double freeze technique (freeze-thaw-freeze) increases the effectiveness of cryotherapy (p. 488). Vaginal discharge for 2–3 week is seen. Cryotherapy (N_2O cryo) is commonly used.
- **Cold coagulation** destroys cervical tissue at a temperature of 100–120°C. It does not need any anesthesia. **Depth of tissue destruction is about 4 mm.**
- **Electrodiathermy** destroys cervical tissue up to a depth of 8–10 mm using a unipolar needle electrode. It is done under general anesthesia.
- **Carbon dioxide laser** through colposcopic guidance—can **destroy the epithelium by vaporization up to a depth of 7 mm.** The method is of choice when CIN extends onto the vaginal fornices.

Advantages of laser vaporization: (a) Preservation of transformation zone for subsequent follow up; (b) Precision control technique in depth and breadth; (c) Rapid healing.

Ablative method (cryotherapy, electrodiathermy or laser)	*Excisional method LLETZ or conization*
Indications ▪ Simple procedure ▪ Used to treat CIN ▪ Needs satisfactory colposcopy evaluation ▪ Entire TZ must be seen ▪ Lesion should not involve the endocervical canal ▪ Endocervical curettage should be negative **Disadvantages** ▪ No pathologic specimens for further evaluation **Contraindications** (See below)	**Indications** ▪ CIN II/III ▪ Suspected microinvasion ▪ Unsatisfactory colposcopy in which the TZ is not fully visualized ▪ Discrepancy between cytology, colposcopy and biopsy ▪ Lesion extending into the endocervical canal ▪ ECC showing CIN or glandular abnormality ▪ Recurrence after ablative or excisional method **Advantage** ▪ Pathologic specimens are obtained for further evaluation

Contraindications of ablation treatment

- Suspected invasive lesion or adenocarcinoma in situ (AIS)
- SCJ not clearly seen
- Discrepancy in smear/colposcopy/biopsy finding
- High grade recurrent AGC cytology.

Excision methods

Conization (p. 495): While cold knife conization is commonly done but laser excision cone biopsy is preferable, as it can be done as outpatient under local anesthesia with colposcopic guidance. Blood loss is also less. Conization for CIN is as effective as hysterectomy provided the cone margins are free of disease. ***Complications** such as hemorrhage, infection, cervical stenosis or incompetence depend on the length of cone excised.*

Large loop excision of the transformation zone (LLETZ) or loop electrosurgical excision procedure (LEEP)

A loop (2–3 cm) of very thin stainless-steel wire is used for excision of the TZ. Blended current (cutting and coagulation), low voltage output is used. It is a simple and quicker procedure. It is done under local anesthesia. Tissue up to a depth of 10 mm or more can be removed and sent for histological examination. Complications are minimal as compared to cone excision.

Follow up after treatment of CIN

The rate of recurrence or persistence of disease following ablative or excisional method for CIN II/III is 5–17%. The reasons for recurrence or persistence are: Large size lesion, endocervical involvement and positive margins.

Follow-up recommendations (ASCCP) for cases with CIN II/III with negative margins are: Cotesting with cervical cytology and HPV at 12 and 24 months. If both tests are negative; follow up is done as a routine. In cases with abnormality, colposcopy and endocervical sampling are done.

Hysterectomy

Hysterectomy is only considered in elderly women where fertility is no longer desired. Other associated indications are:

- Recurrent high-grade CIN lesion (elderly women)
- CIN extends into the vagina
- Persistent dyskaryotic smear even with treatment
- CIN associated with other gynecologic problems such as prolapse, fibroid, pelvic inflammatory disease or endometriosis
- High grade CGIN in elderly women
- Patients with CIN III when family completed
- Patients with poor compliance for follow up
- Cancer phobia.

Removal of vaginal cuff is done, if the lesion extends to the vaginal fornices.

Prevention of cervical cancer in low and middle income countries (LMICs)

Considering the need of high level of infrastructure, well trained personnel and above all the huge expense involved in the screening and diagnosis of cervical pathology, alternative approach of management has been suggested. Visual inspection with acetic acid (VIA) and treatment with cryotherapy can be an alternative approach (see and treat) to reduce the cervical cancer mortality by more than 30% in the unscreened communities of the LMICs (Shastri, 2014).

PREMALIGNANT ENDOMETRIAL LESION

There is ample evidence that both endometrial hyper-plasia and carcinoma are estrogen-dependent. Long-term unopposed estrogen, particularly around the

TABLE 23.8: Classification of endometrial hyperplasia and progression rate (WHO).

Type of hyperplasia	*Progression to cancer (%)*
Simple hyperplasia	1
Complex hyperplasia (without atypia)	3
Atypical complex hyperplasia	29
European working group (EWG – 1999) classification: ▪ Endometrial hyperplasia/benign hyperplasia ▪ Endometroid neoplasia (EN)	

time of menopause, often leads to various types of endometrial hyperplasia.

Risks: A significant number of such cases will develop invasive carcinoma during the period of 2–8 years (Table 23.8). *It has been estimated that about 25% of adenomatous hyperplasia, 50% of atypical hyperplasia and 100% of CIS will develop endometrial carcinoma, if left untreated.*

Etiology: Endometrial hyperplasia develops in women of 40–50 years (Table 23.9). Amongst numerous factors (Table 23.10), unopposed estrogen appears to be the primary factor. Premenopausal persistent anovulation is almost a constant factor. In the postmenopausal women with obesity, peripheral conversion of androgens into estrogen is a risk factor. Long-term estrogen stimulation in condition of polycystic ovarian syndrome or feminizing ovarian tumor may predispose to endometrial cancer (Flowchart 23.3).

TABLE 23.9: Protective factors for endometrial hyperplasia.

- Multiparity
- Normal weight
- Combined oral contraceptive use
- Progestogen therapy
- Levonorgestrel-intrauterine system (LNG-IUS) use
- Menopause <49 years.

TABLE 23.10: Risk factors for endometrial hyperplasia.

▪ Unopposed estrogen stimulation ▪ Delayed menopause (>52 years) ▪ Polycystic ovary syndrome (PCOS) ▪ Nulliparity ▪ Family history of endometrial carcinoma, carcinoma of breast, ovary or colon ▪ Tamoxifen therapy	▪ Previous radiation therapy ▪ Diabetes ▪ Obesity (BMI >30) ▪ Hypertension ▪ Insulin resistance ▪ Estrogen secreting ovarian tumors

Diagnosis

- There is no classic symptom of premalignant lesions. But the constant feature is abnormal perimenopausal uterine bleeding and ultimate diagnosis is ideally by hysteroscopy and endometrial biopsy or by uterine curettage and histology.
- TVS is an adjunct to the diagnosis. *In postmenopausal women even with bleeding, an endometrial stripe of <4 mm had a 100% negative predictive value for endometrial pathology.* However, persistent vaginal bleeding should have endometrial sampling regard less of TVS findings.
- Endometrial sampling in OPD is done using a thin plastic Pipelle cannula. It provides accurate information.
- Otherwise diagnosis is made by hysteroscopy and endometrial biopsy may be done.

Histology

Simple hyperplasia: Endometrium is thick. The glands are dilated and some have outpouching and invaginations. They are crowded and have irregular outlines. The stroma is abundant and cellular. Simple hyperplasia with atypia is rarely malignant. Epithelial pseudostratification is present.

Complex hyperplasia (without atypia) (Fig. 23.9): Endometrium is thicker. The glands are crowded and arranged back to back with reduced stroma. Most glands have irregular outpouching. There is adenomatous hyperplasia with moderate to severe degree of architectural atypia but no cytologic atypia. These groups have a low malignant potential.

Flowchart 23.3: Prolonged unopposed estrogen stimulation on endometrium.

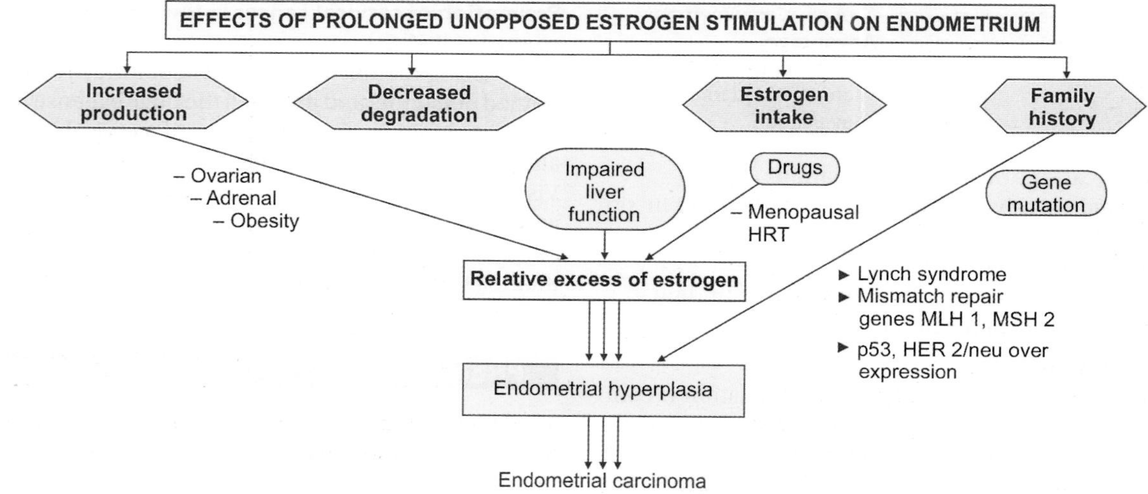

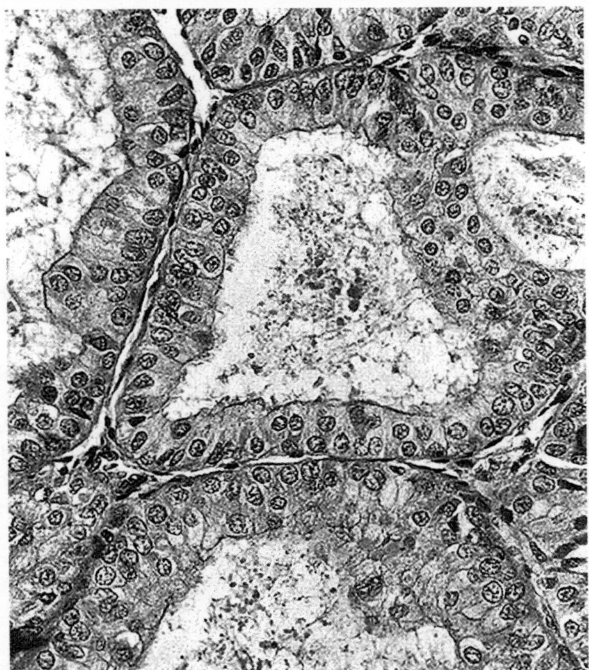

Fig. 23.9: Complex endometrial hyperplasia with nuclear stratification and cytological atypia. The glands are dilated, mitosis is present in stroma also.

Atypical complex hyperplasia: The endometrial glands have cytologic atypia. The gland outlines are of complex hyperplasia in type. The nuclei of the glands show enlargement, irregular size and shape, hyperchromasia, and coarse chromatin. Complex atypical hyperplasia has greatest malignant potential.

Carcinoma in situ (CIS): Commonly describes a lesion with severe cytologic as well as architectural abnormalities of the glands.

Management

- **Preventive**
- **Definitive treatment**

Preventive

- To maintain ideal body weight.
- Estrogen use in nonhysterectomized women should be restricted. The combined estrogen-progestogen preparations reduce the risks than estrogen alone.
- Screening of 'at risk' women mentioned earlier should be done by periodic endometrial sampling.

Definitive Treatment

Treatment depends on:

- **Age of the patient**
- **Desire for fertility**
- **Histologic type of hyperplasia**
- **Degree of atypia**
- **Risks of surgery**

Women in reproductive age (fertility desired)

A. No cytologic atypia:

a. Simple, b. Complex }
- Continued high dose progestin therapy: MPA (high dose)—20–40 mg, 3 to 4 times/day continuous
- Local LNG-IUD

Endometrial sampling at interval of 3–6 months.

B. With cytologic atypia:

a. Simple, b. Complex }
- Continued high dose progestin therapy
- Local LNG-IUD

- **Once atypical hyperplasia is cleared, therapy with intermittent progestin to start until the woman is ready to conceive**

Women in postreproductive years (fertility not desired)

A. No cytologic atypia, B. With cytologic atypia }
- Medical therapy (as above) or hysterectomy (Laparotomy/Laparoscopy)

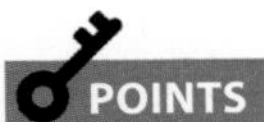

POINTS

- **The premalignant lesions of the vulva** include vulvar intraepithelial neoplasia (VIN), Paget's disease, lichen sclerosus, squamous hyperplasia, and condyloma accuminata.
- **Currently VIN I** has been eliminated. VIN II and III are combined (ISSVD, 2004). Now VIN covers lesions that have high grade squamous cell abnormalities. HPV associated VIN is seen more in young women.
- **Multicentric disease** should be considered when VIN is diagnosed. VIN needs long-term follow up as the recurrence risk is high. Women with VIN presents commonly with complaints of itching, soreness, or burning or may remain asymptomatic. Invasive potential of VIN is less (<10%) compared to CIN (40%). For confirmation of carcinoma in situ, 3–5 mm diameter dermal punch biopsy is taken under local anesthetic. Alternatively, colposcopic examination and biopsy may be done after application of 5% acetic acid.
- **Surgery for carcinoma in situ** includes—simple excision, wide local excision, CUSA, simple vulvectomy, and laser therapy. Regular follow up is mandatory. Paget's disease is often associated with carcinoma breast. Simple vulvectomy is the surgery.
- **Predisposing factors for VaIN** include infection with HPV, herpes virus II, immunosuppression or radiation. VaIN is diagnosed by exfoliative cytology, colposcopy, and biopsy. High grade VaIN is treated with local excision, 5-fluorouracil cream or by ablation therapy, by cryosurgery or laser.
- **Cryosurgery in the treatment of CIN has the following advantages**: Simple and low cost, outpatient procedure, no anesthetic needed, minimal complications, improved cure rate. **The disadvantages are**: No tissue for histopathological evaluation, postoperative vaginal discharge, not suitable for CIN III.
- **CIN is** a spectrum of premalignant changes in the cervical epithelium showing varying degree of cellular atypia. It is a continuum of changes that begin with mild atypia and may progress to CIS. There is no sharp boundary between them.

Contd...

Contd...

- **Pap smear (cytology)** is the gold standard for screening and has reduced the incidence of invasive carcinoma of cervix by about 80% and the mortality by 70%. The false-negative rate of Pap smear is about 5–15%. Liquid-based cytology is found to be superior (p. 89).
- **Combined testing of HPV-DNA and cervical cytology** should preferably be done in women older than age >30.
- **Squamous intraepithelial lesion (SIL)** is a cytologic term, used in Bethesda classification (1988). LSIL corresponds to HPV infection and CIN I whereas HSIL corresponds to CIN II, CIN III, and CIS.
- **The squamocolumnar junction (SCJ)** is a dynamic level that lies near the external os during the reproductive life. It moves further down during pregnancy and recedes up into the endocervical canal after menopause.
- **The process of pathogenesis** starts at the 'transformation zone'. The acid pH is probably an important trigger for the metaplastic process. This metaplastic cells can undergo atypical transformation by trauma or infection, if the host response is poor.
- **The exact cause of CIN** is unknown. HPV infection is an increased risk factor. Human papillomavirus (HPV) types having high oncogenic risk are: 16, 18, 31, 33, 58, and 68. Not all women with HPV infection progress to CIN as HPV infection may regress (80%) spontaneously.
- **HPV vaccines** against HPV types 16, 18 (bivalent) or HPV types 6, 11, 16, 18 (quadrivalent) are effective in prevention of 90% of cervical cancer. Nonvalent vaccines are available. Gardasil-9 is to prevent all types of HPV: 6, 11, 16, 18, 31, 33, 45, 52 and 58. Vaccines are given to girls aged 12–26 years in two to three doses. Both the vaccines have some cross protection against other HPV types 31, 33, and 45. Vaccines are type specific and effective only when given prophylactically. Vaccines are safe and well-tolerated.
- **The risk of progression of CIN** to invasive carcinoma is variable. The risk of malignant progression is lowest with CIN I is <1% with CIN II—5% and highest with CIN III—30–40%. It is indeed difficult to ascertain which type of CIN and with what time, CIN lesions will proceed to invasive carcinoma. CIN should be observed as it usually regresses spontaneously.
- **The mean age of developing CIN** is about 30 years. Some of the documented risk factors are early sexual intercourse, early age of first pregnancy, too many and too frequent births, low socioeconomic status, multiple sexual partners, immunosuppressed (HIV positive) individuals, STIs, husband with multiple partners, oral pill users, smoking habits, etc.
- **Cytologic and colposcopic findings** are aids to the diagnosis but biopsy is only confirmatory.
- **The triage strategy** (p. 271) includes liquid based cytology → atypical smear → HPV-DNA assay using hybroid capture 2 → high-risk HPV → colposcopy. This strategy eliminates the need for unnecessary colposcopic examinations and also frequently repeated Pap smears, when it is negative.
- **Colposcopy** is the examination of the cervix with magnification (6–16 times). Colposcopy is done when the Pap smear is abnormal. Biopsy is indicated when the colposcopic findings (p. 272) are abnormal. Conization of the cervix is performed when there is any discrepancy of cytology, colposcopy, and biopsy reports.
- **CIN I** should be observed rather than treated as it regresses spontaneously. Ablation or LLETZ (LEEP) is used to treat CIN II and III. Cone excision should be done to detect cervical glandular disease when cytology and colposcopy are not reliable.
- **The aim of therapy** is to destroy all the abnormal (CIN) areas. Cryotherapy, cold coagulation, electrodiathermy, laser and LLETZ (LEEP), all can destroy the lesion. In cases with completed family, hysterectomy is the preferred treatment. In conservative surgery, long-term follow-up should be done.
- **LEEP (LLETZ) procedure—The advantages are:** Simple and low cost, done with local anesthetic, tissue specimen is available for histopathology evaluation. **The disadvantages are:** Risk of postoperative hemorrhage, specimen margins are lost due to thermal damage, may have adverse effects on future pregnancy (miscarriage, preterm labor).
- **Conization of the cervix (cold knife)—The advantages are:** Done under anesthesia, tissue specimens are available for histopathological evaluation, suitable for high grade CIN lesions extending into the canal, suitable for CIN recurrent cases, to exclude invasive disease. **The disadvantages are:** Increased risk of hemorrhage, large volume of tissue removed, increased risk of subsequent pregnancy complications (cervical incompetence).
- **Microinvasive carcinoma** requires a conization specimen. Conization is as effective as hysterectomy for CIN, provided the cone margins are free of disease.
- **Follow up of patients** treated for CIN is cytology at 6 months and then repeated at 12 months. Thereafter cytology is repeated at 3 yearly intervals. The risk of recurrence of CIN following initial therapy is about 3–5%.
- **CIN lesions** detected during pregnancy needs to be evaluated in puerperium as such a lesion may regress spontaneously.
- **Endometrial hyperplasia is classified as (WHO):** (a) Simple hyperplasia; (b) Complex hyperplasia; (c) Atypical simple hyperplasia; and (d) Atypical complex hyperplasia.
- ***The endometrial lesions*** *in young patients with cystic or glandular hyperplasia, cyclic or continued progestogen therapy for 6–9 months may be helpful. If regression fails to occur or in perimenopausal women, hysterectomy with bilateral salpingo-oophorectomy should be done.*
- ***Complex atypical hyperplasia*** *contains glands with cytologic atypia. It is considered as a premalignant condition. It has highest malignant potential (29%), compared to simple hyperplasia (1%), and complex hyperplasia without atypia (3%).*
- **Atypical hyperplasia** in peri or postmenopausal women is considered for hysterectomy.
- VaIN is associated with CIN in 70% of cases. VaIN is caused by oncogenic HPV. Other risk factors are similar to CIN.

CHAPTER

24 Genital Malignancy

CHAPTER OUTLINE

GENERAL CONSIDERATIONS

There is wide range of geographical variation in the incidence of major genital malignancies, the reason is far from clear. In US (1985), cancer of the breast, ovary, and uterus accounts for 51% of all cancers among females. These sites accounted for 28% of all deaths caused by cancer. In most of the developed countries, cancer of the breast tops the list in female malignancies; **whereas in the developing countries, including India, genital malignancies top the list (Table 24.1).**

VULVAR CARCINOMA

INCIDENCE

The lesion is rare, about 1.7 per 100,000 females. The distribution varies from 3–5% amongst genital malignancies.

ETIOLOGY

The etiology remains unclear. But the following factors are often related.

- **Advanced age:** Postmenopausal women with a median age of 60.
- More common amongst whites.
- Increased association with obesity, hypertension, diabetes, and nulliparity.
- Associated vulvar epithelial disorders (lichen sclerosus) (4–7%).
- **Infection** with high risk oncogenic HPV (type 16, 18, 31, 33, and 45) has been detected (20–50%) in patients with invasive vulvar cancer.

TABLE 24.1: Lifetime risk of pelvic malignancy.

	Carcinoma cervix	*Carcinoma body*	*Carcinoma ovary*
US			
▪ Black	1.9	1.2	1.0
▪ White	0.9	2.7	1.4
UK (Scotland)	1.2	0.8	1.3
Japan	1.8	0.3	0.5
India (Mumbai)	2.2	0.2	0.8

- **Others:** Smoking, immune deficiency, other STIs, syphilis, and lymphogranuloma venereum.
- Other primary malignancies have been observed in about 20% of cases with vulvar cancer. Cervix is most commonly affected; other sites are breast, skin or colon.

RISK FACTORS FOR VULVAR CANCER

- Infection with high risk oncogenic HPV
- Non-neoplastic chronic epithelial disorders (lichen sclerosis 4–7%)
- Immunocompromised state
- Smoking
- Advanced age
- Immune deficiency
- Presence of cervical neoplasia
- Melanoma
- Paget's disease
- Presence of VIN (5–96%)

PATHOLOGY

Sites

The most common site is labium majus followed by clitoris and labium minus. Anterior two-thirds are commonly affected. Malignant ulcer on the contralateral side may be multifactorial (Figs. 24.1 and 24.2).

Naked Eye

- **Ulcerative:** The features are raised everted edges, sloughing base with surrounding induration. This is common.
- **Hypertrophic:** The overlying skin may be intact or it ulcerates sooner or later. This is rare.

HISTOLOGICAL TYPES OF VULVAR CANCERS

- Squamous cell carcinoma—90% (Fig. 24.3)
- Melanoma—8–10%
- Adenocarcinoma (Bartholin's gland)
- Basal cell carcinoma
- Sarcoma (leiomyosarcoma)
- Metastatic cancers to vulva
- Yolk sac tumors

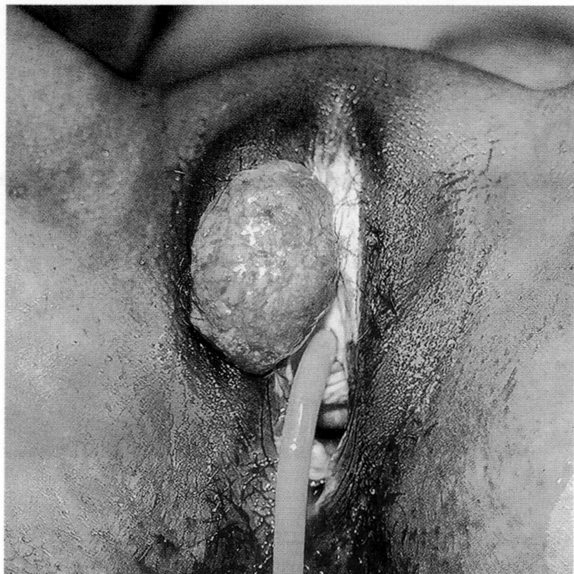

Fig. 24.1: Vulvar carcinoma on labium majus (most common site).

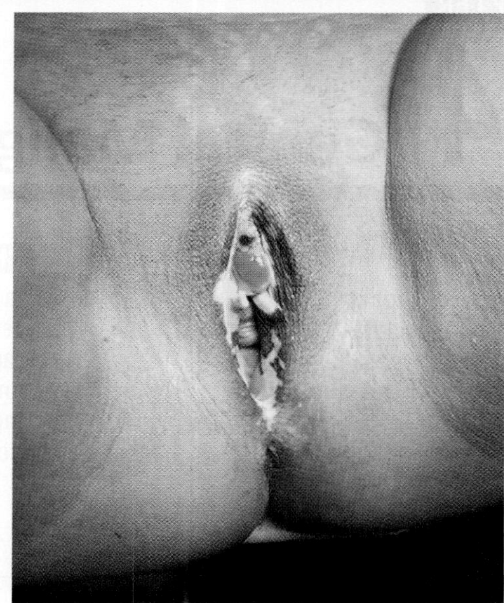

Fig. 24.2: Carcinoma clitoris (second common site of vulvar malignancy).

(*Courtesy:* Prof SN Banerjee Dept. IPGME & R, Kolkata)

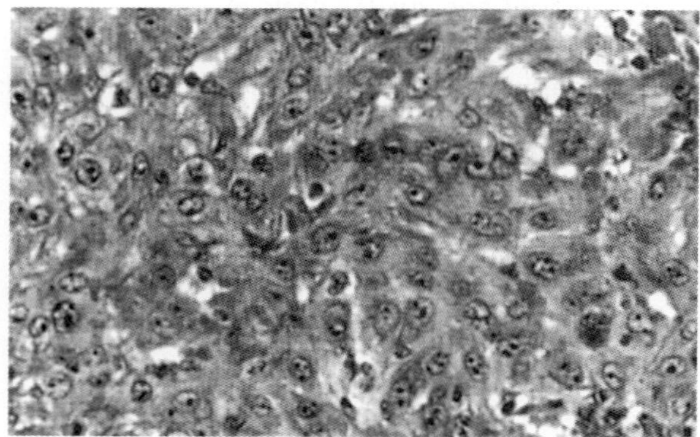

Fig. 24.3: Histological picture of vulvar squamous cell carcinoma.

SPREAD

Direct

The direct spread occurs to the urethra, vagina, rectum and even to pelvic bones. As the disease progresses, other sites in the vulva may develop neoplasia, so that multifocal sites do occur.

Lymphatics

It is the most common method of spread of lesion. It is estimated that in about 50%, the lymph glands are involved by the time the patient consults the physician. **The following facts are to be borne in mind:**

- The lymphatic spread is primarily by embolization and only at a later stage, the spread is by permeation to fill the lymphatic channels.
- Contralateral metastases are not infrequent (25%) as the lymphatics of the vulva cross the midline.
- When the ipsilateral nodes are not involved from a lesion located on one side, spread to the contralateral groin node is very unlikely.
- The lymph node involvement follows a sequential pattern. The lymphatics of labia → superficial inguinal lymph nodes → deep inguinal lymph nodes → pelvic nodes.
- Pelvic nodes are secondarily involved in about 20% with affected inguinal nodes. The **nodes involved are** obturator, external iliac, hypogastric, and common iliac.
- Lymphatics of the clitoris, anus, and rectovaginal septum may drain directly into the pelvic lymph nodes.
- Involvement of pelvic nodes, bypassing the inguinal lymph nodes, is less than 3%.
- Incidence of lymph node involvement is directly related to the site, size of the lesion, and the depth of stromal invasion (Table 24.2). Chance of bilateral lymph node involvement also increases when the midline structures (clitoris, perineum) are involved.
- Histologically proved groin node involvement is present in 25% when missed on clinical assessment. In almost 25%, the nodes are histologically negative when clinically thought to be involved. Approximate incidence of lymph node involvement is given in Table 24.2.
- **Regional lymph nodes** are assessed clinically and also by using MRI (p. 100), **sentinel node lymphoscintigraphy** (p. 285), ultrasound, and PET (p. 101).

TABLE 24.2: Depth of stromal invasion and groin lymph node involvement in squamous cell carcinoma of vulva.

Depth of invasion (mm)	*Percent with positive nodes*
<1	0
1–2	7.5
2.1–3	10.0
3.1–5	30

Hematogenous

This is rare but may occur in advanced cases.

CLINICAL FEATURES

Patient profile: The patients are usually postmenopausal, aged about 60 years often with obesity, hypertension, and diabetes.

Symptoms

- Asymptomatic
- Pruritus vulvae
- Swelling with or without offensive discharge
- Difficulty in urination
- Vulvar ulceration
- Bleeding
- Inguinal mass
- Pain

Signs

- Vulvar inspection reveals an ulcer or a fungating mass on the vulva. The ulcer has a sloughing base with raised, everted, and irregular edges and it bleeds to touch. Surrounding tissue may be edematous and indurated.
- Associated vulvar lesions mentioned earlier may be present.
- Inguinal lymph nodes of one or both the sides may be enlarged and palpable. The enlargement may also be due to infection.
- Clinical examination of the pelvic organs, including the cervix, vagina, urethra, and rectum must be done. This is due to the coexistence of other primary cancers in the genital tract.

Diagnosis

The diagnosis is confirmed by **biopsy**.

- When a definite growth is present, the biopsy is to be taken from the margin.
- Cystourethroscopy, proctoscopy CT/MRI scan (for regional nodes and metastatic disease) may be needed.
- **Colposcopic examination** of the vulva (vulvoscopy) is done by the following application of 3% acetic acid for 5 minutes. Biopsies from the most suspicious aceto-white areas are taken.
- In cases of vulvar dystrophy, the biopsy sites are from multiple areas usually from the persistent red areas or from stained areas following toluidine blue test.

DIFFERENTIAL DIAGNOSIS

The lesion needs differentiation from:

- Condyloma accuminata
- Syphilitic ulcer
- Tubercular ulcer
- Lymphogranuloma venereum
- Soft sore.

STAGING

The staging is based on clinical examination **and includes only the primary carcinoma, excluding melanoma**. The FIGO classification is widely used (Table 24.3).

TABLE 24.3: FIGO staging of carcinoma of the vulva (modified 2009).

STAGE I	**$T_{1/2}$, N_0, M_0. Tumor confined to the vulva**
IA	Tumor confined to the vulva or perineum, ≤2 cm in size with stromal invasion ≤1 mm*, negative nodes
IB	Tumor confined to the vulva or perineum, >2 cm in size or with stromal invasion >1 mm*, negative nodes
STAGE II	**T_3, N_0, M_0. Tumor of any size with adjacent spread (1/3 lower urethra, 1/3 lower vagina, anus), negative nodes**
STAGE III	**T_{1-3}, $N_{1/2}$, M_0. Tumor of any size with or without extension to adjacent perineal structures (1/3 lower urethra, 1/3 lower vagina, anus) with positive inguinofemoral lymph nodes**
IIIA	Tumor of any size with positive inguinofemoral lymph nodes ▪ With 1 lymph node metastasis (≥5 mm) or ▪ With 1–2 lymph node metastasis(es) (<5 mm)
IIIB	▪ With 2 or more lymph nodes metastases (≥5 mm) or ▪ 3 or more lymph nodes metastases (<5 mm)
IIIC	With positive node(s) with extracapsular spread
STAGE IV	**Any T, any N, MI. Tumor invades other regional (2/3 upper urethra, 2/3 upper vagina), or distant structures**
IVA	Tumor invades any of the following: ▪ 2/3 upper urethra, 2/3 upper vagina, bladder mucosa, rectal mucosa, or fixed to pelvic bone or ▪ Fixed or ulcerated inguinofemoral lymph nodes
IVB	Any distant metastasis including pelvic lymph nodes

*The depth of invasion is defined as the measurement of the tumor from the epithelial-stromal junction of the adjacent most superficial dermal papilla to the deepest point of invasion.

CAUSES OF DEATH

- Uremia from ureteric obstruction due to enlarged common iliac and para-aortic nodes.
- Rupture of the femoral vessels by the overlying involved inguinal lymph node.
- Sepsis.

MANAGEMENT

Prophylactic

- Adequate therapy for non-neoplastic epithelial disorders of the vulva (Ch. 18).
- Adequate therapy for persistent pruritus vulvae in postmenopausal women.
- Multiple biopsies in conservative treatment of vulvar intraepithelial neoplasia (VIN).
- Simple vulvectomy in postmenopausal women with VIN where follow-up facilities are not available.

Definitive Treatment

- **Microinvasive lesion (Stage IA):** The invasion is less than 1 mm (stage IA), wide local excision with or without ipsilateral groin lymphadenectomy may be done with follow up. Generally, there is no lymph gland involvement (Table 24.2). Tumor free surgical margin should be 1–2 cm to prevent local recurrence.

There is increased incidence of lymph node involvement in lesion of more than 1 mm invasion. It is thus prudent to perform **radical vulvectomy with bilateral groin node dissection in all cases of stromal invasion more than 1 mm.**

- **Early invasive stage:** Stage IB and II of vulva and clinically negative nodes. Radical resection (1-2 cm surgical margin) of the primarily tumor and ipsilateral inguinofemoral lymphadenectomy is done. Occasionally, a radical complete vulvectomy may be needed, depending on tumor size and location (midline) (p. 501).

  Three separate incision (one for radical vulvectomy and one each for groin node dissection) approach is currently preferred instead of en-block approach (Fig. 35.17).

  Pelvic node metastases are rare unless inguinofemoral nodes are involved. Pelvic lymphadenectomy in cases of positive deep node involvement is omitted in preference to external radiation on the groin and pelvis—in the form of 4500–5000 cGy, usually 4–6 weeks after surgery.

  Negative **sentinel lymph node** biopsy for micrometastasis may avoid extensive lymphadenectomy. Radical vulvectomy is often associated with major long-term morbidity, sexual dysfunction and loss of body image. Radical local excision of the vulva with wide margins (1–3 cm) is considered to be an alternative to radical vulvectomy with equal result.
- **Advanced vulvar cancer (stage III to IV) or if the general condition is poor and/or in presence of comorbid conditions.**

The following principles may be adopted:

- Two stage operation is preferred. Total vulvectomy followed by at a later date, bilateral inguinofemoral lymphadenectomy.
- Total vulvectomy followed by full pelvic and groin irradiation (megavoltage therapy).
- **Stage III** cases with resectable tumors may undergo radical vulvectomy with inguinofemoral lymphadenectomy (nodal debulking) and postoperative pelvic and inguinal growth irradiation. Platinum-based concurrent chemotherapy with radiation therapy is found to be effective. Radical vulvectomy may be done 5 weeks after the completion of chemoradiation therapy.
- **Neoadjuvant chemotherapy**—followed by surgery, radiotherapy or both.
- ***Technically inoperable or recurrent lesion***

  Multimodal approach is made to provide palliation.
  - **Chemotherapy** (cisplatin, gemcitabine bleomycin, 5-FU) can be used as radiation sensitizer.
  - **Chemoradiation therapy** may be combined as primary therapy or following surgical excision of the tumor.
  - **Radiotherapy:** Intensity modulated radiotherapy (IMRT) offers greater sculpting art of covering of radiation delivery to minimize toxicity.
  - **RESULTS**
- **With negative groin nodes**, the 5-year survival rate for invasive carcinoma ranges from 90–100%.

TABLE 24.4A: 5-year survival rate of vulval carcinoma by stage.

Stage	Survival (%)
I	90–100
II	65–75
III	35–45
IV	20–30

TABLE 24.4B: 5-year survival rate by node status.

Nodes	Survival (%)
Negative nodes	80–100
Positive inguinal femoral nodes	30–50
Positive pelvic nodes	10–20

- **With positive groin nodes**, the survival rate falls to 20–55%.
- **With positive pelvic nodes**, the survival rate falls even below 20%.

PROGNOSIS

Approximate 5-year survival rate in squamous cell carcinoma is tabulated in Tables 24.4A and B.

Prognostic Factors

- Clinical stage of the disease
- Site of the tumor
- Depth of stromal invasion
- Lymphovascular space involvement
- Lymph node involvement (inguinofemoral and pelvic)
- Tumor diameter and differentiation (grade)
- DNA ploidy status.

MELANOMA

It is the second most common vulvar cancer. The common sites are the clitoris and labia minora. It may arise from a junctional nevus. Radical vulvectomy and bilateral regional lymphadenectomy (en-block) is the preferred treatment. Pelvic lymph adenectomy does not alter the prognosis. Radiation therapy, adjuvant chemotherapy, or immunotherapy (α interferon) are of limited benefit. Overall prognosis is poor.

BARTHOLIN'S GLAND CARCINOMA

Primary malignancy can be adenocarcinoma, squamous cell carcinoma or transitional cell carcinoma. The surgery is like that of squamous cell carcinoma of the vulva. The surgery is radical vulvectomy with inguinofemoral lymphadenectomy. Postoperative radiation reduces the recurrence. In addition, part of the lower vagina, levator ani, and the ischiorectal fat are to be removed. Prognosis in a case of Bartholin gland carcinoma is similar to squamous cell carcinoma when compared to stage of the disease.

Basal cell carcinoma of the vulva is rare (2%) of all vulvar carcinomas. It is generally ulcerated. Wide local excision of the lesion with wide surgical margin (2–3 cm) is the treatment and the disease is cured.

VAGINAL CARCINOMA

PRIMARY VAGINAL CARCINOMA

Incidence

The incidence of primary vaginal carcinoma is very rare (about 0.6 per 100,000 women). It constitutes about 1% of genital malignancies. **The primary vaginal carcinoma should fulfill the following criteria.**

- The primary site of growth is in the vagina.
- The cervix and the vulva must not be involved.
- There must not be clinical evidence of metastatic disease.
- Carcinoma of vagina is mostly metastatic.

Etiology

Exact etiology is unknown. Following factors are often related:

- HPV may have a causal relationship.
- Progression from VaIN.
- Women with history of cervical cancer (multicentric neoplasia).
- Diethylstilbestrol (DES) is related with clear cell adenocarcinoma of the vagina. This is found in those who had history of intrauterine exposure to diethylstilbestrol.
- Previous irradiation therapy to the vagina or immunosuppression.
- Prolonged use of pessary.
- More common amongst whites than blacks.

Pathology

Site: The most common site is in the upper-third of the posterior wall (Fig. 24.4).

Naked eye: The growth may be ulcerative or fungative.

Histopathology: **Squamous cell carcinoma** accounts for more than 90% of the cases. The rest are adenocarcinoma (8–10%), melanoma, fibrosarcoma, sarcoma botryoides and malignant mixed mullerian tumors.

Spread is by direct continuity, by lymphatics (p. 13 anatomy) and rarely, blood borne. Inguinofemoral lymph nodes and pelvic lymph nodes are commonly involved. Lymphatics spread of upper vagina drain to the pelvic and para-aortic nodes, mid vagina, to the pelvic and groin nodes and the lower vagina to the inguinofemoral nodes. Imaging studies, MRI or PET-CT can assess the extent of spread and the lymph node metastasis. Hematogenous spread involves the lungs, liver or the bones.

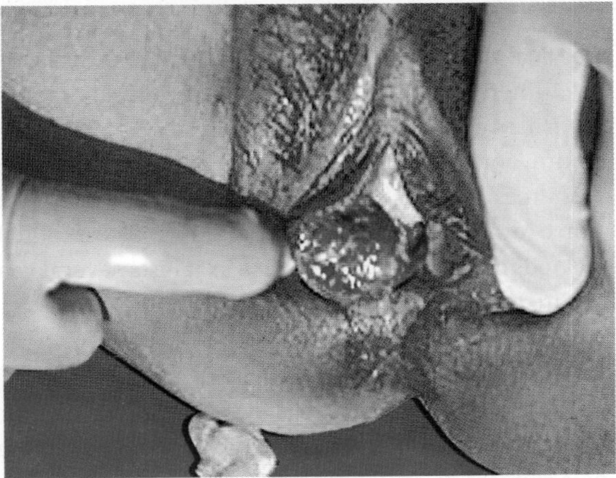

Fig. 24.4: Vaginal carcinoma.

Clinical Features

The mean age of the patient is about 55 years.

Symptoms

- May be asymptomatic, being accidentally discovered during routine screening procedures.
- Abnormal vaginal bleeding including postcoital bleeding is conspicuously present as an early symptom.
- Foul smelling discharge per vaginum.

Signs

- Speculum examination reveals an ulcerative, nodular or exophytic growth.
- The cervix looks apparently normal.

Diagnosis

- During cytology, screening procedure to detect abnormal cells.
- Colposcopic examination and targeted biopsy are helpful for patients with abnormal cytology or unexplained vaginal bleeding.
- Cystourethroscopy, proctosigmoidoscopy, CT/MRI/PET (for nodes and metastases), are done.
- Biopsy from clinically suspected lesion.

Staging

The clinical staging as outlined by FIGO is tabulated on Table 24.5.

Treatment

Primary prevention: Primary vaccination against HPV 16, 18 is effective.

Secondary prevention: Vault smear following hysterectomy due to persistent high-grade squamous intraepithelial lesions (HSIL), is to be done.

Tertiary prevention: Management of precancerous lesion of the vagina is to be done.

Radiotherapy or surgery or the combination is the accepted modality of therapy for invasive primary

TABLE 24.5: Staging of vaginal carcinoma FIGO (1995).

Stage	Description
Stage 0	Carcinoma in situ
Stage I	Carcinoma is limited to the vaginal wall
Stage II	Carcinoma has involved subvaginal tissue but has not extended to the pelvic wall
Stage III	Carcinoma has extended to the pelvic wall
Stage IV	Carcinoma has extended beyond the true pelvis or has involved the mucosa of the bladder or rectum. a. Adjacent organs are involved (bladder, rectum) b. Distant organs are involved

carcinoma of the vagina. Choice depends on the age, clinical stage, anatomical location, and size of the lesion.

Stage I:

- **Growth limited to the upper-third:** Radical hysterectomy, partial vaginectomy, and bilateral pelvic lymphadenectomy is the treatment of choice (as that of stage IB carcinoma cervix).
- **Growth limited to the lower-third:** Radical vulvectomy with removal of bilateral inguinofemoral lymph nodes along with vaginectomy.

Stage II–IV: Radiation, chemoradiation is done by external beam therapy with intracavity or interstitial radiation. Concurrent cisplatin based chemoradiation is thought to have higher efficacy. Care is to be taken to prevent bladder or rectal injury.

Pelvic exenteration operation (p. 293) is done when there is failure with radiation therapy.

Cure Rate

Overall 5-year survival rate ranges from 80% for stage I disease to 10% for stage IV disease.

SECONDARY CARCINOMA OF THE VAGINA

Secondary vaginal malignancy follows carcinoma vulva, cervix or urethra by direct spread. Metastases in the lower-third of the anterior vaginal wall or vault occur in cases of choriocarcinoma (Fig. 24.16) or endometrial carcinoma.

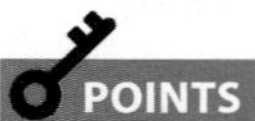

POINTS

- In most of the developed countries, cancer of the breast tops the list in female malignancies, whereas in the developing countries including India, genital malignancies (cancer cervix) top the list.
- **Vulvar cancer** usually occurs in postmenopausal women with median age of 60 years. Vulvar cancer accounts for 3–5% of all genital malignancies.
  The most common site is labia majora followed by clitoris and labia minora. Ulcerative type is more common than the hypertrophic type. In 90%, it is well-differentiated squamous cell carcinoma. The spread is predominantly by lymphatics both ipsilateral and contralateral (25%). Involvement of pelvic nodes bypassing the inguinal is less than 3%.
  Causes of death are due to uremia, rupture of the femoral vessels and sepsis.
  Microinvasive lesion of less than 1 mm requires wide local excision and follow up as metastasis to regional nodes are rare. Invasion of more than 1 mm requires radical vulvectomy with bilateral groin node dissection.
  Frank invasive carcinoma should be dealt with by radical vulvectomy with bilateral inguinofemoral lymphadenectomy. Pelvic lymphadenectomy is omitted in preference to radiation to the groin and pelvis—4500 to 5000 cGy 4–6 weeks after operation. With negative groin nodes, the 5-year survival ranges from 90–100%; with positive groin nodes, the survival rate falls to 20–55% and with positive pelvic nodes, the survival rate is only 20%.
- **Prognosis of vulvar carcinoma** depends on many factors. HPV positive younger patients tend to have a better prognosis.
- **Melanomas** comprise 5% of vulvar cancer and overall 5-year survival is about 50%. **Basal cell vulvar carcinoma** is treated by wide local excision.
- **Primary carcinoma of vagina** is rare and most vaginal cancers are metastatic. It constitutes 2% of gynecological cancers. The most common site is in the upper-third of the posterior wall. The mean age is 55 years. Squamous cell carcinoma accounts for 90% of the cases. 5-year survival rate is about 40–45%.
  Clear cell adenocarcinoma is seen in adolescent girls, who have had history of intrauterine exposure to diethylstilbestrol. Radical hysterectomy, vaginectomy with pelvic lymphadenectomy is the surgery.
- **Surgery** is the treatment of choice for upper vaginal, low stage tumor in younger patients. However, chemoradiation is used widely as a primary therapy. Ideally, 7000–7500 cGy is administered in less than 9 weeks.

CARCINOMA CERVIX

MAGNITUDE OF THE PROBLEM

- Cancer cervix is the lead cause of cancer and the cancer related deaths in women worldwide. More than 5,27,600 new cases and 2,65,700 deaths are recorded annually. More than 85% of these cases and deaths occur in low and middle income countries (LMICs).
- In India cervical cancer is a major public health problem. In India, carcinoma cervix is the second most common gynecological malignancy.
  It is expected to improve with organized screening program.
- Pap smear has reduced the incidence of cervical cancer by nearly 80% and death by 70%.
- HPV vaccine is safe and effective. It is expected to reduce the incidence of cervical cancer by 90–100%. Cervical cancer is an entirely preventable disease as the different screening, diagnostic and therapeutic measures are effective.
- Improvement is needed in the areas of economic resources. It needs changes in culture and implementation of organized screening programs. Disease could be treated in the preinvasive phase as it lasts several years before it becomes invasive and incurable.

Incidence

In India, twelve population-based cancer registries (PBCRs) showed cancer breast was the most common followed by cancer of the cervix (ICMR - 2004). Amongst female cancers, relative proportion of cancer breast varied between 24% and 28% whereas that of cancer cervix was between 14 and 24%. In India, an overall incidence of 23.5/100,000 has been observed (WHO - 2008).

EPIDEMIOLOGY

In India, the prevalence is more amongst the comparatively younger age group (45 years). Carcinoma cervix is rare in women who are sexually not active (nuns, virginal women). Male circumcision is partially protective against cervical carcinogenesis.

GROSS PATHOLOGY

The site of the lesion is predominantly in the ectocervix (80%) and the rest (20%) are in the endocervix.

Naked Eye

- **Exophytic:** These arise from the **ectocervix** and form friable masses almost filling up the upper vagina in late cases. It has a cauliflower like appearance.
- **Ulcerative:** The lesion excavates the cervix and often involves the vaginal fornices (Fig. 24.5).
- **Infiltrative (endophytic):** These are found in **endocervical** growth. They cause expansion of the cervix, so that it becomes barrel-shaped. Diagnosis is often late.

Histopathology

The most common variety is squamous cell carcinoma (80–85%) either well-differentiated or moderately or poorly differentiated (Fig. 24.6). These arise from the ectocervix. **The sources of the squamous epithelium which turn into malignancy are**—squamocolumnar junction, squamous metaplasia of the columnar epithelium.

Squamous cell carcinomas (80–85%)	*Adenocarcinomas (15–20%)*
▪ Large cell (keratinizing or nonkeratinizing) ▪ Small cell (poor prognosis) ▪ Verrucous (warty tumor) ▪ Neuroendocrine tumor (highly aggressive) ▪ Glassy cell carcinoma (virulent variety)	▪ Endocervical ▪ Endometrioid ▪ Clear cell ▪ Adenoma malignum (good prognosis) ▪ Adenosquamous ▪ Mixed carcinomas ***Others*** Large cell, nonkeratinizing are common, sarcomas, lymphomas are rare

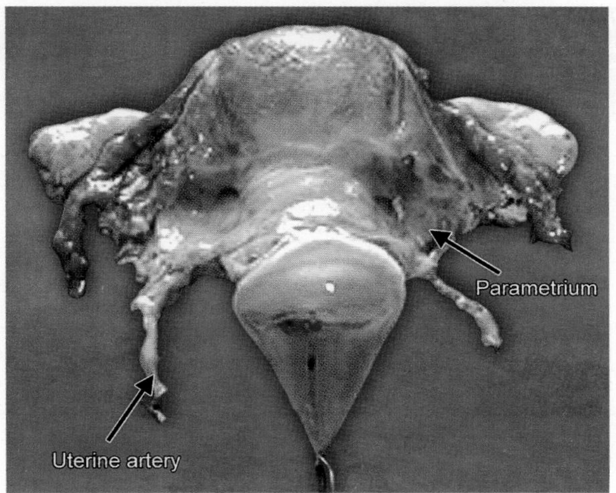

Fig. 24.5: Ulcerative type of cervical malignancy with a friable growth on the posterior lip. Radical hysterectomy done. Uterine arteries are ligated at origin (p. 507).

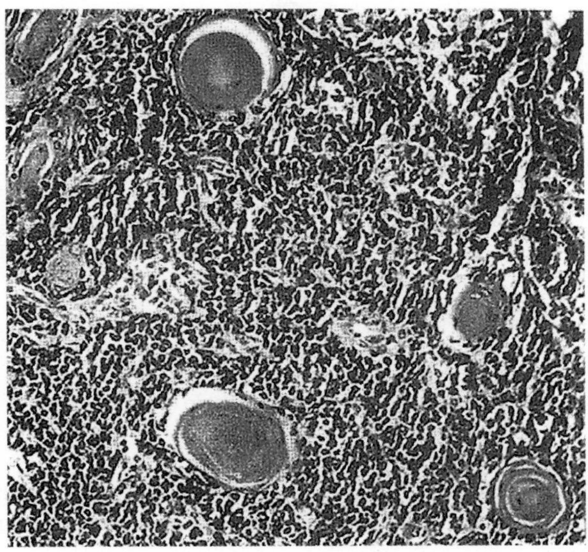

Fig. 24.6: Histology of squamous cell carcinoma of the cervix (small cell type). Keratin pearls within the nests of malignant cells are seen.

MODE OF SPREAD

Direct Extension

The growth spreads directly to the adjacent structures, to the vagina and to the body of the uterus. It extends laterally to the parametrium, paracervical and paravaginal tissues. Here, the tumor cells surround and compress the ureter. It may spread backwards along the uterosacral ligament, to involve the rectum or forwards to involve the base of the bladder, especially in endocervical growth.

Lymphatic

The primary group involved are—parametrial nodes, internal iliac nodes, obturator, external iliac nodes, rectal and sacral nodes. The secondary nodes involved are—common iliac group, the inguinal nodes, and para-aortic nodes (Table 24.6 and Fig. 24.7). Obturator nodes are commonly involved (19%). Left supraclavicular nodes (scalene nodes) are involved after the para-aortic nodes.

Sentinel lymph node (SLN) is the first node that drains the primary tumor. In most cases (85%) there is a single sentinel lymph node (Ch. 38). This node can be detected by intraoperative lymphatic mapping injecting methylene blue dye into the tumor or lymphoscintigraphy using technetium 99.

Hematogenous

Blood-borne metastasis is late and usually by veins rather than the arteries. Lungs, liver or bone are usually involved.

TABLE 24.6: Involvement of lymph nodes in different stages (Approximate).

Stage	*Pelvic nodes (%)*	*Para-aortic nodes (%)*
0	0	0
Ia_1 (<3 mm)	0–0.5	0
Ia_2 (3–5 mm)	5	<1
Ib	16	2
II	30	15
III	44	30
IV	55	40

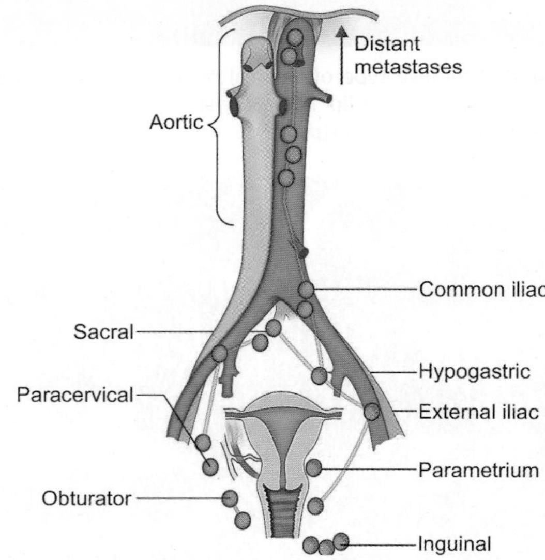

Fig. 24.7: Lymph node involvement in cervical cancer.

Direct Implantation

Direct implantation of the cancer cells at operation on the vault of the vagina or abdominal or perineal wound is very rare.

The risk of ovarian metastases in stage I squamous cell carcinoma of the cervix is 0.5% and it is 1.7% for adenocarcinoma.

STAGING

The purposes of staging are to determine the prognosis, to formulate the line of treatment and to compare the results of one to the other.

- **Staging of cervical cancer is based principally on clinical examination.** In cases with suspected pelvic inflammation, a course of antibiotic should be given prior to clinical staging.
- **Final staging cannot be changed once therapy has begun.**
- When doubt exists as to the correct stage, the lower stage should be assigned.
- **CT, MRI, positron emission tomography (PET), lymphangiography (p. 100 and 101)** can detect involvement of the pelvic parametrial or periaortic lymph nodes. MRI is helpful to detect parametrial extension and to define the tumor volume (Table 24.7).

TABLE 24.7: Staging procedures allowed by FIGO.

- Inspection of cervix and vagina (speculum examination)
- Pelvic examination (vaginal, rectovaginal) under anesthesia

PROCEDURE USED	DETECTION
• Lymph node palpation	Enlargement and site
• Colposcopy • Hysteroscopy • Cystoscopy • Biopsy • Endocervical curettage • Conization	(*see* above) Extension and depth of tumor spread
• Chest X-ray	Pulmonary metastasis
• Skeletal X-ray	Bone metastasis
• Intravenous urogram/USG	Hydronephrosis
• Barium enema	Large bowel involvement
• Proctoscopy	Rectal involvement
• CT	Lymph node, metastasis, tumor size, depth of stromal invasion
• MRI	Lymph node metastases, tumor size, depth of stromal invasion, vaginal and parametrial extension
• FDG-PET	Lymph node (FDG-PET)—superior to CT/MRI
• PET-CT	Metabolic and anatomic spread of the disease

Imaging and pathology can be used where available, to supplement the clinical findings. Notations are to be added: r (imaging) and p (pathology) to indicate the findings. The type of imaging modality or pathology technique used should always be documented.

The clinical staging as recommended by FIGO is tabulated in Table 24.8 and shown in Figure 24.8.

PROGNOSIS

Poor prognostic indicators:

- Tumor size (≥4 cm), involvement of the lymph nodes and positive lymph vascular invasion (LVSI)
- Extra cervical spread (≥10 mm), deep stromal invasion (>70%).
- Adenocarcinoma patients have poorer prognosis compared to patients with squamous cell carcinoma.
- Patients with higher serum values of squamous cell carcinoma antigen (SCA) have poorer survival rate.
- Poor prognosis with the presence of HPV mRNA in the blood of the patient.

Lymph node involvement (pelvic and para-aortic) reduces the survival rate by 50%.

TABLE 24.8: FIGO staging of carcinoma of the cervix uteri (2018).

Stage	Description
I	The carcinoma is strictly confined to the cervix (extension to the uterine corpus should be disregarded)
IA	Invasive carcinoma that can be diagnosed only by microscopy with maximum depth of invasion <5 mm[a]
IA1	Measured stromal invasion <3 mm in depth
IA2	Measured stromal invasion ≥3 mm and <5 mm in depth
IB	Invasive carcinoma with measured deepest invasion ≥5 mm (greater than stage IA), lesion limited to the cervix uteri[b]
IB1	Invasive carcinoma ≥5 mm depth of stromal invasion, and <2 cm in greatest dimension
IB2	Invasive carcinoma ≥2 cm and <4 cm in greatest dimension
IB3	Invasive carcinoma ≥4 cm in greatest dimension
II	The carcinoma invades beyond the uterus, but has not extended onto the lower third of the vagina or to the pelvic wall
IIA	Involvement limited to the upper two-thirds of the vagina without parametrial involvement
IIA1	Invasive carcinoma <4 cm in greatest dimension
IIA2	Invasive carcinoma ≥4 cm in greatest dimension
IIB	With parametrial involvement but not up to the pelvic wall
III	The carcinoma involves the lower third of the vagina and/or extends to the pelvic wall and/or causes hydronephrosis or nonfunctioning kidney and/or involves pelvic and/or para-aortic lymph nodes[c]
IIIA	The carcinoma involves the lower third of the vagina, with no extension to the pelvic wall
IIIB	Extension to the pelvic wall and/or hydronephrosis or nonfunctioning kidney (unless known to be due to another cause)
IIIC	Involvement of pelvic and/or para-aortic lymph nodes, irrespective of tumor size and extent (with r and p notations)[c]
IIIC1	Pelvic lymph node metastasis only
IIIC2	Para-aortic lymph node metastasis
IV	The carcinoma has extended beyond the true pelvis or has involved (biopsy proven) the mucosa of the bladder or rectum. (A bullous edema, as such, does not permit a case to be allotted to stage IV)
IVA	Spread to adjacent pelvic organs
IVB	Spread to distant organs

When in doubt, the lower staging should be assigned.

[a]Imaging and pathology can be used, where available, to supplement clinical findings with respect to tumor size and extent, in all stages.

[b]The involvement of vascular/lymphatic spaces does not change the staging. The lateral extent of the lesion is no longer considered.

[c]Adding notation of r (imaging) and p (pathology) to indicate the findings that are used to allocate the case to stage IIIC. Example: If imaging indicates pelvic lymph node metastasis, the stage allocation would be stage IIIC1r, and if confirmed by pathologic findings, it would be stage IIIC1p. The type of imaging modality or pathology technique used should always be documented.

SURGICAL STAGING OF CANCER CERVIX

There are often discrepancies between clinical staging and surgicopathological findings. Assessment of the pelvic and para-aortic nodes is done by laparoscopy.

DIAGNOSIS

- Early carcinoma (stage IA, IB, IIA)
- Advanced carcinoma (stage IIB–IVB).

The stage once made after all the imaging and pathology report cannot be altered later.

Histopathology grades

1. GX: Cannot be assessed
2. G1: Well differentiated
3. G2: Moderately differentiated
4. G4: Undifferentiated.

Early Carcinoma

Nomenclature: The concept of early carcinoma of the cervix is not well-defined. Presumably, it should include those lesions which have got minimal morbidity and deaths with the best available therapy and a maximal 5-year survival rate. With these criteria, the following stages as per FIGO classification are included in the category of early carcinoma.

Preclinical

There may not be any symptom nor any pelvic finding to raise any suspicion. The cervix may look apparently healthy. The diagnosis is made by the following:

- During screening procedures.
- Incidental on histological examination of tissues removed by biopsy, portio amputation or removal of the uterus.

Stage IA (microinvasive carcinoma)

Microinvasive carcinoma is one which is predominantly intraepithelial carcinoma, except that **there is disruption of the basement membrane**. The mean age is 38–42 years.

In majority, the entity is asymptomatic. There may be blood stained discharge, intermenstrual, postcoital or postmenopausal bleeding. The cervix may look abnormal like ectopy, eversion or cervicitis.

The diagnosis is made only on biopsy of the cervix. Initial screening may be done with cytology, colposcopy, and directed biopsy along with endocervical curettage (ECC).

Clinical

Stage IB (overt)

Symptoms

The duration of symptoms is not proportionate to the stage of the disease.

- Menstrual abnormalities in the form of contact bleeding or bleeding on straining (during defecation), intermenstrual bleeding are very much suspicious, especially over the age of 35.
- Excessive white discharge which may be at times offensive. This is often detected during the screening procedure.

Signs

Speculum examination reveals

- Either a red granular area which looks like an ectopy (erosion) extending from the external os or a **nodular**

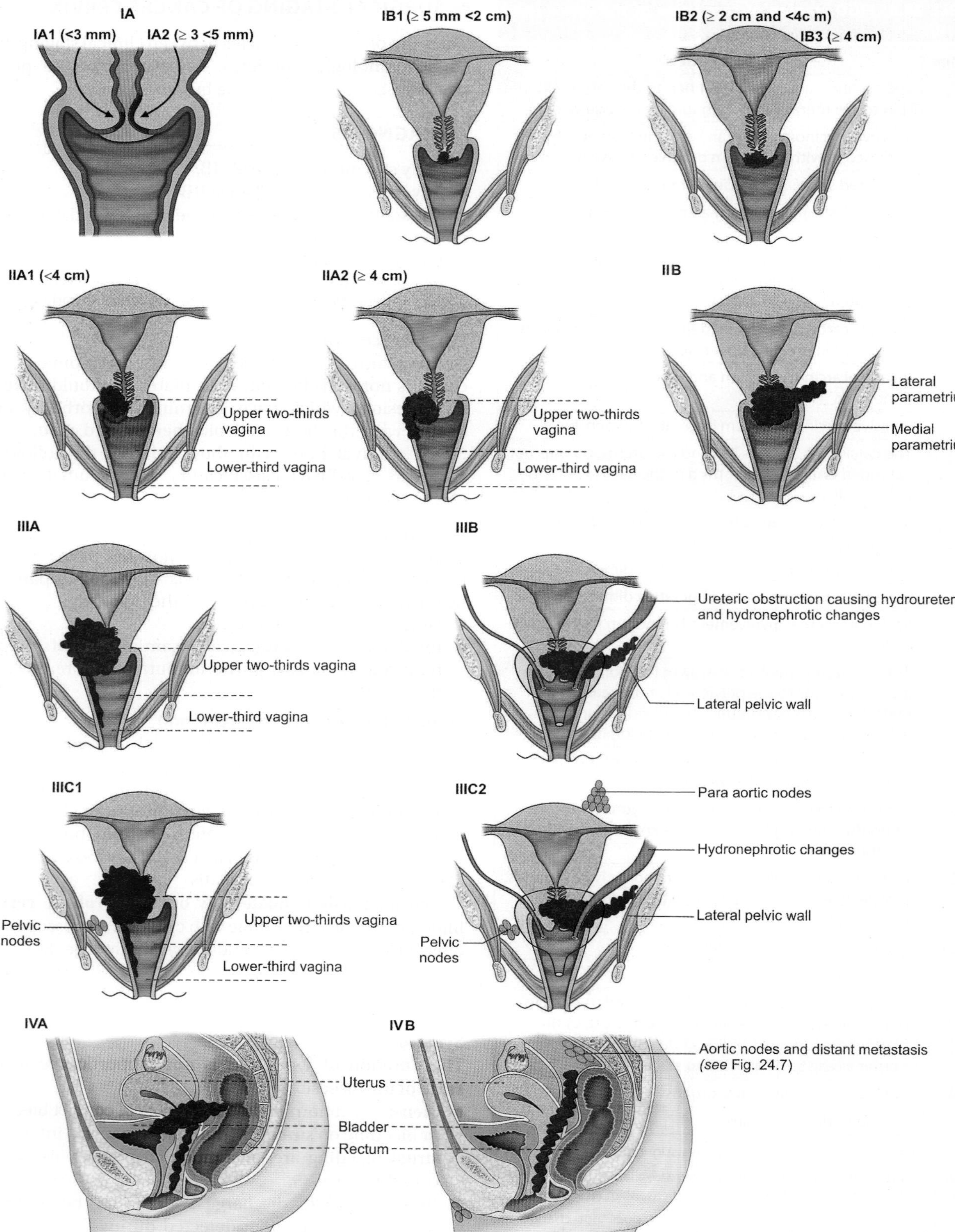

Fig. 24.8: Diagrammatic representation of staging of carcinoma cervix according to FIGO.

growth or an ulcer. The lesion bleeds on friction. **Speculum examination should be done prior to bimanual examination.** The cervical lesion may not be visible due to bleeding from the friable lesion caused by digital examination.

Bimanual examination reveals the lesion is indurated, friable, and bleeds to touch. Cervix is freely mobile.

Rectal examination reveals the parametrium absolutely free.

Confirmation of diagnosis is by biopsy

Ancillary aids for confirmation of staging:

- Cystoscopy
- X-ray chest
- Intravenous pyelography
- Proctoscopy
- USG, CT or MRI, PET-CT.

All these give usually a negative finding and as such, the clinical staging of IB is thereby confirmed.

Other investigations permitted to use for FIGO staging

- **MRI:** Useful to measure tumor size, tumor extent, bladder, rectum, parametrium, and lymph node involvement.
- **CT** is commonly used to detect nodal involvement and distant metastasis. However CT, MRI, PET may be used for FIGO staging.
- **PET (p. 101):** FDG-PET is superior to CT or MRI for detection of node metastasis (size > 5 mm). PET is used for planning the field of radiation, or planning palliative chemotherapy.

Advanced/Late Carcinoma

All cases of carcinoma with stage II B and onwards are arbitrarily called advanced carcinoma considering the reduced 5-year survival rate compared to earlier stages. In fact, in India, this group comprises about 80% of the total cervical carcinoma patients attending the hospitals for treatment.

PATIENT PROFILE

The patients are usually multiparous, in premenopausal age group. They have previous history of postcoital or intermenstrual bleeding which they ignored. Most of them do not have Pap smear screening.

Symptoms

- **Irregular or continued vaginal bleeding** which may at times be brisk.
- **Offensive vaginal discharge.**
- **Pelvic pain** of varying degree: This may be either due to involvement of uterosacral ligament leading to backache or deep seated pain due to involvement of sacral plexus.
- **Leg edema** is due to progressive obstruction of lymphatics and/or iliofemoral veins by the tumor.
- **Bladder symptoms** include frequency of micturition, dysuria, hematuria or even true incontinence due to fistula formation.
- **Rectal involvement** is evidenced by diarrhea, rectal pain, bleeding per rectum or even rectovaginal fistula.
- **Ureteral obstruction** is due to progressive growth of tumor laterally. There may be frequent attacks of pyelonephritis due to ureteric obstruction.

Ultimately, the patient may be **cachectic, anemic with edema legs. Ultimately uremia develops.**

Speculum examination reveals the nature of the growth, ulcerative or fungating which bleeds to touch.

Bimanual examination reveals the induration and extent of the growth to the vagina and to the sides. The induration of the bladder base may be felt through the anterior fornix in advanced cases.

Rectal examination is invaluable to note the involvement of the parametrium and its extent in relation to the lateral pelvic wall. Nature of induration is to be noted carefully. **If it is smooth**, the possibility of inflammation has to be excluded and antibiotics has to be given prior to final assessment for staging. **In malignancy, the induration is nodular**. Incidental involvement of the rectum has to be noted.

For confirmation of diagnosis, *biopsy* is mandatory. If the lesion is small, wedge biopsy is taken which should include a portion of the healthy tissue as well. If it is big, a bit may be taken (punch biopsy) from a comparative non-infective area. There may be brisk hemorrhage which can be effectively controlled by plugging.

Sentinel lymph node mapping and excision can be done. Lymphazurin or isosulfan blue is injected in the cervix (3 and 9 o'clock position). The radioactive blue nodes are identified. Serial node sectioning and immune histochemistry stains identifies the disease volume.

For staging of the disease—procedures (*see* above).

DIFFERENTIAL DIAGNOSIS

The growth needs to be differentiated from:

- Cervical tuberculosis
- Syphilitic ulcer
- Cervical ectopy
- Products of conception in incomplete abortion
- Fibroid polyp.

COMPLICATIONS

The following complications may occur sooner or later, as the lesion progresses.

- **Hemorrhage.**
- **Frequent attacks** of ureteric pain, due to pyelitis and pyelonephritis and hydronephrosis.
- **Pyometra** especially with endocervical variety.
- **Vesicovaginal fistula.**
- **Rectovaginal fistula:** This is comparatively rare because of the interposition of the pouch of Douglas. The rectum may be involved either through the uterosacral ligament or through rectovaginal septum.

CAUSES OF DEATH

The patient may die of:

- **Uremia:** This is due to ureteric obstruction following parametrial involvement. There is hydroureter and hydronephrosis. Infection supervenes, thereby further compromising kidney functions.

- **Hemorrhage:** The vaginal bleeding from the growth may be brisk or continuous. This leads to anemia and ill health.
- **Sepsis:** Localized pelvic or generalized peritonitis may occur which may be fatal.
- **Cachexia:** The cumulative effect of the factors mentioned leads to cachectic condition. The cancerous tissues have got depressant action on general metabolism.
- **Metastases** to the distant organs commonly observed are—lung (36%), lymph nodes (30%), bone (16%) and abdominal cavity (7%). These may be fatal.

MANAGEMENT OF CARCINOMA CERVIX

- **Preventive**
- **Curative**

Preventive

Primary Prevention

It involves identifying the causal factors and eliminating or preventing those from exerting their effects. Initiation of population based, organized screening program [cervical cytology, primary HPV testing or visual inspection with acetic acid (VIA)] is urgently needed.

- **Identifying 'high-risk' female**
  - Women with high-risk HPV infection (p. 270)
  - Early age of first pregnancy
  - High parity
  - Too many births/too frequent birth
  - Long-term use of combined oral contraceptives (COCs)
  - Low socioeconomic status
  - Poor maintenance of genital hygiene.
- **Sexual behavior**
  - Early sexual intercourse
  - Multiple sexual partners
  - Previous wife died of cervical carcinoma.
- **Prophylactic HPV vaccine** (p. 274) is approved to all school girls (12–18 years) and women (16–25 years). Two or three doses are usually to be given (bivalent 0–2–6 month or quadrivalent 0–1–6 month).
- **Use of condom** during early intercourse, raising the age of marriage and of first birth, limitation of family, maintenance of local hygiene, and effective therapy of sexually transmitted infections (STIs) are the positive steps in prevention.
- **Removal of cervix during hysterectomy** as a routine for benign lesion is a definite step in prevention of stump carcinoma. The incidence may be as high as 1%.

Secondary Prevention

It involves identifying and treating the disease earlier in the treatable stage.

This is done by screening procedures. The details have been described in Ch. 9 and 23. It takes 10–15 years for progression of premalignant condition to the invasive carcinoma. The abnormal cervical pathology likely to progress to invasive carcinoma can be detected. Its effective therapy reduces dramatically the incidence of invasive carcinoma. Early detection and treatment of cervical carcinoma can improve the 5-year survival rate by 80–100%.

Downstaging Screening (WHO, 1986)

Downstaging for cervical cancer is **defined as** "the detection of the disease at an earlier stage when it is still curable. Detection is done by nurses and other paramedical health workers using a simple speculum for visual inspection of the cervix".

Compared to cytological screening it is suboptimal. But in places where prevalence of cancer is high and cytological screening is not available, "downstaging screening" is useful. **The strategy is, however, not expected to lower the incidence of cancer cervix, but it can certainly minimize the cancer death through early detection.**

Once the abnormality is suspected, the case is referred to a center where diagnosis and treatment of premalignant and malignant lesions are done.

Curative

Ideally, the management of the patient with cervical cancer is a team approach. Due consideration should be given to:

- General condition of the patient
- Stage of the disease
- Facilities available—surgical and radiotherapy
- Involvement of a gynecologic oncologist
- Radiation oncologist
- Wish of the patient to be judiciously complied with.

Pretreatment Evaluation

Irrespective of the treatment modalities (surgery or radiotherapy) the following evaluations are to be made apart from those already done (Table 24.7) for staging purposes.

Serum Marker (p. 438)

Commonly used serum tumor markers are: Squamous cell carcinoma antigen (SCCA), cancer antigen 125 (CA-125), and carcinoma embryonic antigen (CEA). Elevated levels of SCCA correlate with tumor size, stage, stromal invasion, and lymph node status. This antigen is not specific. However, it has been used as a means to monitor treatment response and to predict tumor recurrence.

Pretreatment Preparations

Irrespective of the methods of treatment, general health of the patient must be improved. Due attention is to be paid to correct anemia and malnutrition. This not only makes the patient sufficiently fit to withstand surgery but rise in hemoglobin percentage improves the tissue oxygenation needed for effective ionizing effect of irradiation.

Perioperative use of leg stockings, prophylactic doses of heparin or low-molecular-weight heparin (LMWH) are used to reduce thromboembolism. Prophylactic antibiotics are to be used.

TREATMENT MODALITIES OF CARCINOMA CERVIX

Management of Cervical Cancer

Modalities: (A) Surgery; (B) Radiation therapy; (C) Chemotherapy; (D) Combination therapy (Tables 24.9A and B).

Surgery is suitable for early stage disease. Types of surgery depending on stages are: (a) Cervical conization; (b) Trachelectomy; (c) Simple hysterectomy; (d) Radical hysterectomy; (e) Pelvic exenteration.

Surgery

The types of surgery employed in invasive carcinoma are:

Radical Hysterectomy and Pelvic Node Dissection (Fig. 24.9)

John Clark (1898) first did the operation while working as a resident in Johns Hopkins Hospital. This operation is commonly done abdominally and is known by different names (**Wertheim** of Viena—1898, **Okabayashi** of Japan—1921, **Meigs** of USA—1944). **Extensive vaginal operation** was subsequently developed to minimize the mortality and morbidity from abdominal approach. Pelvic lymph nodes are removed by bilateral extraperitoneal approach. This operation is also popularly known by different names (**Schauta** of Viena—1902, and **Mitra** of India—1957). There have been several modifications of the techniques of radical hysterectomy and bilateral pelvic lymphadenectomy at present.

Radical hysterectomy as defined by Piver and Rutledge are followed. Type I, II and the III are commonly done compared to type IV and V (Table----). Class II is usually known as Meigs Wertheim hysterectomy. It is done for stage IB and rarely for stage IIA carcinoma cervix. For class III radical hysterectomy, uterine artery is ligated at its origin from the anterior division of the hypogastric artery. In class IV, complete dissection of the ureter from its bed is done. Superior vesical artery is sacrificed. Querleu and Morrow described another classification that is based on lateral dissection with nerve preservation to reduce bladder dysfunction (Ch. 38).

The surgery includes (Fig. 38.68) removal of the uterus, tubes and ovaries of both the sides (ovaries may be spared in young women), upper half of vagina, parametrium (most of cardinal and uterosacral ligaments), and the draining primary cervical lymph nodes (parametrial, obturator, internal and external iliac groups, and sometimes common iliac. **Sacral group is not removed**). **Ovarian function may be preserved in younger patients. Ovariopexy to be done when postoperative radiation is needed.** Para-aortic lymph node evaluation is done. Any enlarged para-aortic lymph node is sampled and sent for frozen section biopsy. Para-aortic lymphadenectomy is done when found positive. Postoperative radiation therapy is to be considered if lymph nodes are found involved. Generally, **negative sentinel lymph nodes may allow omission of lymphadenectomy of the nodal basin.**

Surgery for pelvic and para-aortic lymphadenectomy can detect metastatic spread of the disease more accurately. It is superior to radiologic imaging. Lymph node dissection can avoid unnecessary over treatment or under treatment of radiation therapy. It is expected that with optimum assessment of disease spread, can have a significant survival benefit from subsequent therapy with chemotherapy and/or extended field of radiation. Laparoscopic procedure of lymphadenectomy is superior

TABLE 24.9A: Management options of carcinoma cervix.
Microinvasive (Stage IA), Early Invasive (Stage IB, IIA) and Advanced (Stage IIB–IV) Carcinoma.

Stage	*Patient characters*	*Management option*
IA1 (microinvasive carcinoma) (<3 mm, –LVSI <3 mm, +LVSI)	▪ Young women, fertility preservation desired: LVSI present/absent	▪ Cervical conization and close follow up with cytology screening Or ▪ Mod Rad Trachel
	▪ Elderly women, family completed • LVSI—absent • LVSI—present	• Total extra-fascial hysterectomy • Mod Rad Hyst + Pelvic Lymph Or SLNB
	Method and route of surgery: Abdominal, vaginal, laparotomy, laparoscopy	
IA2 (microinvasive carcinoma) (≥3 mm, <5 mm)	▪ Low risk cases	▪ Mod Rad Trachel Or Mod Rad Hyst + Pelvic Lymph Or SLNB
	▪ Others— • LVSI-present • Young patient, fertility desired	• Mod Rad Hyst or more radical surgery, pelvic lymphadenectomy • Cervical conization and laparoscopic extraperitoneal pelvic lymphadenectomy Or • Radical abdominal, vaginal or Lap Trachel with Pelvic Lymph
	▪ Post-treatment follow-up with cytology (Ch. 23)	
Invasive carcinoma IB1, IB2, IIA1	▪ **Surgical treatment is preferred** ▪ **Routes:** Open or MIS (laparoscopic or robotic)	▪ Rad Trachel Or Type III Rad Hyst + Pelvic Lymph Or SLNB ▪ For stage with IB3 (≥ 4 cm)—chemoradiation (pelvic field) is the option.
IB1 (≥5 mm, < 2 cm)	▪ **Low risk:** Largest diameter <2 cm, stromal invasion <50%, no node on imaging	▪ As above or modified Rad Hyst and Pelvic Lymph
	▪ Young women, desiring fertility	▪ Rad Trachel (stage IA2-IB1)
	Route: Open-abdominal, vaginal or MIS	
	Node negativity to confirm with Lap Pelvic Lymph Or SLNB prior to Rad Trachel.	

Contd...

Contd...

TABLE 24.9B: Management options of carcinoma cervix.

Stage	*Management options*
IB2–IIA1 **IB2: ≥2 cm <4cm;** **IB3: ≥4 cm;** **IIAI: <4 cm + upper vagina**	**Primary modality: Surgery or radiotherapy, both have similar result.** Type III radical hysterectomy (Uterus + parametrium + upper vagina + part of para colpium + pelvic lymph nodes)
IB3 and IIA2 **IB3: ≥4 cm** **IIAI: <4 cm + upper vagina** **IIA2: ≥4 cm + upper vagina**	▪ **Surgery is discouraged due to high morbidity** ▪ Concurrent platinum based chemoradiation therapy (CCRT) ▪ Neoadjuvant chemotherapy (NACT) can be used where radiotherapy facilities are scarce ▪ Advantages
IIB–IVA	▪ CCRT is the standard treatment for patients with locally advanced cervical cancer (LACC). ▪ Radiation therapy to cover Pelvic and the extended field for stages IIIB and above. Systemic chemotherapy is given for cases stage IIIC2 and above.
Stage IVA	▪ Only central disease without pelvic or side wall recurrence or distant spread: Pelvic exenteration. It has poor prognosis ▪ Advanced diseases: Radiotherapy with modern development, can provide improved outcome and reduced toxicity
Stage IVB + Distant organs	CCRT may have better response with overall disease free survival (69%). Carboplatin-paclitaxel combination or cisplatin—topotecan, gemcitabine or vinorelbine found to be effective ▪ Palliative chemotherapy ▪ And/or Radiotherapy/supportive care (hospice)

(LVSI: lymphovascular space invasion; Modi: Modified; Rad: Radical; Trachel: Trachelectomy Hyst: Hysterectomy; SLNB: sentinel lymph node biopsy; lymph: lymphadenectomy)

Management is individualized based on the patient's disease stage, health condition and the available resources

to laparotomy. This has less morbidity with subsequent radiation therapy. However, survival benefit of extensive surgical debulking of retroperitoneal modes are 4–6%.

Limitation

It is ideally limited to early stage disease. **Radical hysterectomy** could be done by abdominal or vaginal route or by laparoscopic, robotic assisted method, depending upon the patient's fitness and surgeon's experience.

Advantages of Surgery over Radiotherapy

- Spread of the disease can be determined more thoroughly by surgicopathological staging.
- Surgical staging (laparotomy or laparoscopy) and assessment of para-aortic and pelvic nodes, can predict the survival rate accurately.

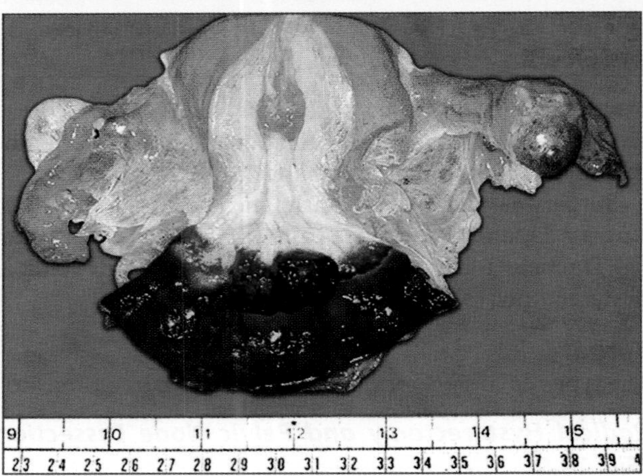

Fig. 24.9: Exophytic type of cervical squamous cell carcinoma—radical hysterectomy done.

- Preservation of ovarian function, if desired, especially in a young woman.
- Ovaries may be transposed out of the radiation field if radiation is considered in the postoperative period.
- Retention of more functional and pliable vagina for sexual function.

Psychologic benefit to the patient in that her cancer bearing organ has been removed.

Special indications: As previously mentioned, there is no superiority of surgery over radiotherapy when the patients are placed in ideal circumstances. But, there are conditions where **radiotherapy is contraindicated** and only the surgical treatment has to be provided.

Contraindication of Radiotherapy

- Associated pelvic inflammatory disease (PID)—acute or chronic, diabetes, inflammatory bowel disease, pelvic kidney.
- Associated myoma, prolapse (procidentia), ovarian tumor or genital fistula, adnexal mass.
- Young patient (to preserve ovarian function).
- Vaginal stenosis—placement of radiation source is inadequate.
- Cases with adenocarcinoma or adenosquamous carcinoma—surgery is preferred.

Complications of Surgery

See complications (below). Women with comorbidities (obesity, heart disease) are at risk for surgery.

Postoperative complications

Major postoperative complications as observed following total abdominal hysterectomy have been discussed (p. 498). **Other complications include:** Ureteric fistula (about 1%), vesicovaginal fistula (0.5%), bladder dysfunction, cystitis pyelonephritis, small bowel obstruction and rectal dysfunction. There may be lymphocyst in the pelvis, lymphedema of one or both the legs, dyspareunia, and recurrence. The mortality rate of the procedure is less than 1%.

Bladder dysfunction (atony) is a known complication. This is due to damage of the sympathetic and parasympathetic fibers to and from the bladder and urethra. Continuous catheterization for bladder drainage is maintained for a period of 6–10 days.

Neuropathies due to nerve injuries (femoral, obturator, sciatic, genitofemoral, ilioinguinal, lateral femoral cutaneous, and pudendal nerves).

Lymphocyst formation is a frequent complication. Tissue fluid, lymph and blood are collected to form the cyst following radical hysterectomy. Lymphocyst is best diagnosed by ultrasound. Rarely, it may be of large size to cause pain and ureteral or venous obstruction. Adequate suction drainage of the retroperitoneal space postoperatively is an important preventive measure. Majority resolve spontaneously. Sometimes, it may drain through vagina. Rarely, needle aspiration is needed when the size is large or it produces symptoms.

Pelvic Exenteration

This type of ultraradical surgery is named after **Brunschwig**. This procedure is done in a very selective cases only:

- Stage IVA disease.
- Central pelvic recurrent carcinoma (biopsy proven) without any metastasis as established by PET/CT scan.
- Completely resectable tumor mass.

Contraindications of pelvic exenteration are extra-pelvic spread of disease with distant metastasis to liver, lungs or bones.

Types

- **Anterior exenteration:** It consists of radical hysterectomy, removal of urinary bladder, and implantation of ureters either in the sigmoid colon or into an artificial bladder made from an ileal loop (ileal bladder).
- **Posterior exenteration:** It consists of radical hysterectomy, removal of rectum and a permanent colostomy.
- **Complete or total:** It consists of combination of anterior and posterior exenteration with a permanent colostomy and an ileal bladder.

  The operative mortality of such type of operation is about 10–20% and with a 5-year survival rate of about 50%.
- **Laparoscopic radical hysterectomy (LRH) with pelvic and aortic lymphadenectomy** is done for early invasive disease (stage I, IIA). The specimen is removed vaginally. Vaginal cuff is closed by endostitch. Pelvic and aortic lymphadenectomy is done.

Primary Radiotherapy

Cancer of the cervix was the first cancer of an internal organ to be treated with ionizing radiation using radium by Margaret Cleves in 1903. **Primary therapy (chemoradiation)** is given in locally advanced (stage IIB to IVA) disease.

External photon beam radiation and brachytherapy are the two main methods (p. 426 and 427).

Both external beam radiation therapy (EBRT) and brachytherapy are delivered. External beam radiation usually proceeds intracavitary therapy (brachytherapy). EBRT is commonly given in 25 fractions during 5 weeks (40–50 Gy).

Hormone replacement therapy following radiation or surgery can be used for women with menopausal symptoms following counseling.

Advantages of Primary Radiotherapy

- Wider applicability in all stages of carcinoma cervix.
- Survival rate 85%, comparable with that of surgery in early stages.
- Less primary mortality and morbidity.
- Individualization of dose distributions/requirement possible.

Principles of Brachytherapy

Technique (Table 24.10) (discussed in Ch. 31): External beam radiation therapy (EBRT) is given in fractions usually 180 cGY/day, 5 days/week to destroy the tumor without affecting the normal tissues. This covers entire pelvis including the regional pelvic nodes. The local implant (brachytherapy) delivers radiation locally to the cervix, vagina, paravaginal and paracervical tissues. Usually tandem and ovoids or a tandem and ring are inserted in the vagina. A pack is placed in the vagina to stabilize the apparatus.

After the position of the application is confirmed by imaging, The radioactive source, such as Cesium 137 or Iridium 192 is inserted (after loading technique). Intracavitary radiation therapy ICRT may be low dose rate or a high dose rate. Both have similar survival rate and toxicity. High dose rate is commonly used and is given as on OPD basis. It is done for 3 to 4 hours.

The container is made up of platinum, gold or alloy steel to absorb alpha and beta particles and allowing the gamma rays to sterilize the cancer cells. In carcinoma cervix, the tandems are inserted in the uterine cavity and the ovoids and colpostats are placed in the vaginal vault under anesthesia. Different methods of brachytherapy are in vogue (Figs. 24.10A to C). High dose **brachytherapy** is safe and effective (NICE - 2010).

In Paris and Manchester techniques, the source strength is smaller but exposure time is increased. The vaginal source is away from the cervix. They are used with either preloaded or afterloaded special applicators. One treatment period in Paris technique is 96–200 hours as compared to Stockholm technique where each application is 24–28 hours in duration. Manchester system, which is a modification of the Paris technique, delivers

TABLE 24.10: Brachytherapy techniques.

Technique	*Amount of radium placement*	*No. of application*	*Duration*
Paris	Intrauterine tandem 33.3 mg—one Vaginal ovoid 13.3 mg—two or three	One	120 hours
Manchester	Intrauterine tandem 30–50 mg Vaginal colpostat 30–50 mg	Two	72 hours each at interval of 7 days
Stockholm	Intrauterine tandem 50 mg—one Vaginal plaque—65–80 mg	Three	24 hours each at weekly interval

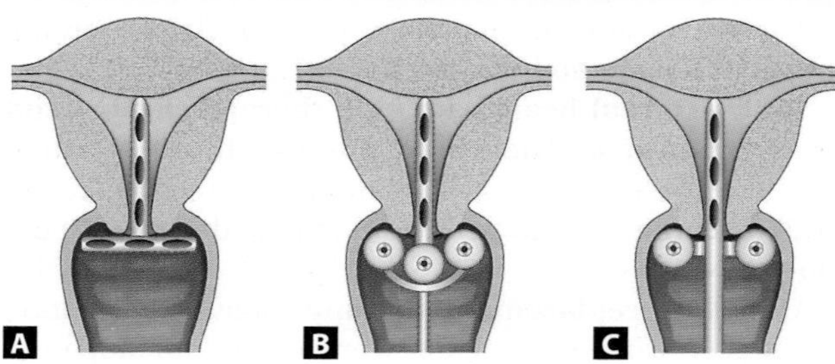

Figs. 24.10A to C: Different methods of brachytherapy: (A) Stockholm technique; (B) Paris technique; (C) Manchester technique.

constant isodose at different depths, regardless of the size of the uterus and vagina.

In Stockholm technique (Fig. 24.10A), large high intensity source with less exposure time is given, but the vaginal source is closer to the cervix.

These three basic techniques are followed all through the world in the brachytherapy for carcinoma cervix. After loading remote control technique is used for calculated dose distribution and to prevent radiation hazard. Fletcher-Suit afterloading modification system is widely used these days.

Disadvantages of Radiotherapy

Intestinal and urinary strictures, fistula formation (2–6%), vaginal fibrosis and stenosis causing dyspareunia, radiation menopause, fibrosis of bowel and bladder. **Ovarian transposition (ovariopexy)** well out of the range of pelvic irradiation may be done to avoid radiation menopause. For other complications of radiation (p. 428).

Calculation of the dose (p. 427): In calculating the doses, two reference points A and B are used (Ch. 31). Total dose calculation depends on tumor stage. Normal cervix is resistant to radiation. It can tolerate doses up to 200 to 250 Gy over 2 months. However for bladder maximum radiation is 80 Gy, rectum is 65 Gy and bowels 45 to 50 Gy. **Point A** is 2 cm cephalic and 2 cm lateral to the external os and is the point of crossing of the uterine artery and ureter. **Point B** is 2 cm cephalic and 5 cm lateral at the same plane and is approximately the site of obturator gland (Fig. 31.3).

It has been calculated that point A gets about 7000–8000 cGy and point B 2000 cGy. Taking into consideration that cancerolytic dose is approximately 7000–7500 cGy, the rest of the dose at point B is supplemented by external beam irradiation of 4000 cGy spreading over another three weeks. For external irradiation, linear accelerator with energy of 4 million electron volts or more is commonly used.

In the immediate vicinity of the source, the vagina and cervix get and tolerate about 20,000–30,000 cGy. Bladder, ureter, and rectum can tolerate up to 7000 cGy. Small gut on the other hand has a tolerance limit of only 4500 cGy.

With the advent of computer dosimetry, exact calculation of the doses on each patient for each application is being provided. **Intensity modulated external radiation therapy (IMRT),** based on computer generated algorithms can distinguish accurately the target tissue volume and normal tissue. IMRT can preferentially limit the dose of radiation to normal tissues and can deliver higher doses to tumor tissues. Treatment planning is done on 3D imaging using CT, MR, and PET to determine the tumor volume. Linear acceletors or conformational radiotherapy techniques (CRT) with 3D-CRT and IMRT are more effective. Normal tissues are spared. Toxicity is reduced. ICRT is given using a tandem and ovoids or tandem and ring. Dose system may be low dose rate (LDR), high dose rate (HDR) or pulsed dose rate (PDR). All the system results in comparable survival rate. Interstitial brachytherapy should be used when ICRT is not feasible due to distorted anatomy. It consists of insertion of multiple needles into the primary tumor and parametrium through the perineum. It is done under USG guidance. It is recommended that entire radiotherapy treatment (EBRT) should be completed within 8 weeks.

- **Advanced cases:** As the blood supply is poor, the resultant anoxia may be overcome by irradiating these cases in a special chamber under condition of hyperbaric oxygenation.
- **Recurrent cervical carcinoma:** Incidence of recurrence or persistent disease after therapy is about 35%. Cases following surgery, whole pelvic irradiation with external beam radiotherapy or chemoradiation has been advocated.
- **Carcinoma cervix detected after simple hysterectomy:** Subsequent management of such patient depends upon the following factors: (a) Microinvasive cancer; (b) Tumor confined to the cervix and the margins are negative; (c) Positive surgical margins but no gross residual tumor; (d) Gross residual tumor by clinical examination and documented by biopsy or patient with recurrent disease.
- **Treatment options are:** (a) To perform radical operation and to remove all the tissues including the pelvic lymph nodes. This may be done especially in younger women; (b) Radiation therapy—(i) No residual disease—brachytherapy to the vaginal apex, (ii) Gross residual disease—full intensity radiotherapy.
- Patients with gross residual disease have poor survival outcome.
- ***Surgery Followed by Radiotherapy***
- This is indicated in cases with **positive lymph nodes** detected following surgery.
- **Accidental discovery of invasive carcinoma cervix** of a uterus removed by simple hysterectomy.
- When **positive tissue resection margin** is present.
  The objective of this form of therapy is to sterilize the cancer cells in the pelvic lymph nodes. The fact remains that even by pelvic lymph node dissection it is not possible to remove all the positive nodes. Radiation dose is reduced to 4500 cGy in 24 fractions over 5 weeks.
- **Postoperative adjuvant chemoradiation therapy** (extended field radiation and platinum-based chemotherapy) significantly improved the survival rate when given following radical hysterectomy.

Radiotherapy Followed by Surgery

- **Endocervical carcinoma** with barrel-shaped cervix.
- **Bulky tumor:** Radiotherapy controls sepsis, the growth shrinks and the tumor resectability is improved.

Neoadjuvant chemotherapy (NACT)

NACT has the following advantages: (a) Reduces tumor volume; (b) Reduces micrometastatic disease; (c) Improves in tumor resectability; (d) It is an alternative therapy when access to radiotherapy is limited or absent; (e) Improved survival rate when compared to radiotherapy alone; (f) It improves survival rate when NACT is combined with surgery. It is especially useful in young women with bulky stage IB–IIB disease desiring for FSS. Neoadjuvant chemotherapy is followed by radiotherapy.

Three cycles of platinum-based combination chemotherapy with radiation therapy followed 3–6 weeks by radical hysterectomy and lymphadenectomy is done. This has improved the resectability of the bulky ≥4 cm (stage IB2 and bulky IIA) disease. This regimen had shown better overall disease free survival rate and reduced recurrence. Due to fibrosis, surgery may be difficult. Risk of ureteric fistula may be more. **The drugs used are in combination of cisplatin, ifosfamide or paclitaxel.**

Concurrent chemoradiation includes radiation and weekly cisplatin-based combination (cisplatin and paclitaxel) chemotherapy. **Cisplatin-based concurrent chemoradiation** is used as a treatment of choice in: (a) Early stage (IA2, IB, IIA) disease after radical hysterectomy; (b) As a primary treatment for patients with bulky (≥4 cm) tumor (stage IB and IIA); (c) Locally advanced (stage IIB to IVA) disease as a primary therapy. Chemotherapy sensitizes the cancer cells to radiation and improves the survival rate.

Fertility Sparing Surgery

- **Laparoscopic assisted vaginal radical trachelectomy with pelvic and aortic lymphadenectomy (LARVT)** was designed (Daniel Dargent, 1987) to treat early invasive cervical cancer. This is done in a **young woman where childbearing function is to be preserved** (fertility sparing surgery). Initially, pelvic and aortic lymph node dissection is done. **Vaginal radical trachelectomy is done only when these nodes are negative**. Laparoscopic approach is similar to LARVH. Vaginal part includes resection of cervical, vaginal, paracervical, and paravaginal tissues. Vaginal cuff is resected circumferentially about 2 cm below the cervicovaginal junction. Ideally, the resected cervical tissue margins should be free of disease as evaluated by frozen section. Cervical permanent cerclage operation is done to prevent miscarriage and preterm labor.

Indications of Trachelectomy

- Preservation of fertility
- Early stage disease (stage IA1, A2, IB1)
- Small tumor volume (<2 cm)
- No pelvic node metastasis
- Cancer margin is at 1 cm below the internal os on MRI

PLANNING OF TREATMENT MODALITIES

A. **Early stage disease:** *See* Tables 24.9A and B.

For **early stage disease**, the survival rate following treatment by either radical hysterectomy and pelvic lymphadenectomy or with primary radiation with concurrent chemoradiation are almost equal.

B. **Advanced stage disease (Table 24.11)**

COMPREHENSIVE PALLIATIVE CARE

Principles of management are: (a) Control of symptoms; (b) Care focused on individual basis; (c) To maintain dignity and quality of life.

Common symptoms of a patient with advanced cervical cancer: (a) Pain; (b) Hemorrhage; (c) Features due to renal failure and uremia with ureteric obstruction; (d) Vaginal discharge (malodorous); (f) Problems related to fistula formation (RVF/VVF); (e) Lymphedema.

Pain control to be done as tiered approach basis. Oral morphine need to be given. Involvement of NGOs, hospice is needed.

Palliative radiotherapy may be used for uncontrolled vaginal bleeding, pelvic pain and metastatic disease pain. Usually, a dose of 20 Gy in five fractions over a week is given. ICRT may be used when EBRT fails.

CARCINOMA OF CERVIX AND PREGNANCY

Incidence of invasive carcinoma of the cervix is about one in 2,500 pregnancies.

Diagnosis is often late. Cone biopsy may be necessary for confirmation. **Complications of cone biopsy include:** Hemorrhage, abortion, preterm labor, and infection. LEEP has no superiority over cone biopsy.

Management

The following points are taken into consideration before actual management: (A) Period of gestation; (B) Survival of the fetus; (C) Wishes of the patient; (D) Histology.

A. **Patient with microinvasive carcinoma** may be followed up to term. Patient is re-evaluated following delivery and treated as in the nonpregnant state.

B. **Advanced stage:** Before 20 weeks, treatment modality is the same as in the nonpregnant state: Either surgery or chemoradiation. In late pregnancy, following maturity, fetus is delivered by classical cesarean section. Subsequent treatment with either radical surgery or radiotherapy or chemoradiation is the same as in the nonpregnant state.

Prognosis

Clinical stage (FIGO) of the disease is the single most important prognostic factor. Stage for stage survival outcome appears to be no different between pregnancy and nonpregnant state (for details see author's Textbook of Obstetrics, Ch. 21).

RESULTS OF THERAPY FOR CARCINOMA CERVIX

The result of therapy is expressed in terms of 5-year survival rate. The overall 5-year survival rate is tabulated in Table 24.11.

TABLE 24.11: 5-year survival rate.

Stage	5-year survival rate (%)
IA	95.01
IB	80.1
II	64.2
III	38.3
IV	14

Recurrent Cervical Cancer

Risk factors for recurrent disease are: Large tumor size, lymphovascular space invasion, positive lymph nodes, advanced stage disease. Over all recurrence is about 30% after 5-years. A patient is declared cured if she remains well even after 10 years following initial therapy.

Most common site of recurrence is central pelvis and the pelvic side wall. Features of disease recurrence are: Pain in the pelvis, back, unilateral leg edema, ureteral obstruction, vaginal bleeding, palpable tumor in the pelvis, and lymphadenopathy. Single agent or multiagent chemotherapy with cisplatin, paclitaxel or ifosfamide is used. Palliative radiation therapy may be used to those who have been treated initially with surgery.

Follow up: The majority of the recurrences occur in the first 2 years. As such, the follow up protocols should be at 3–4 months interval for the first 2 years then at 6 months interval for next 2 years and thereafter annually. Thorough physical examination is done including examination of supraclavicular and inguinal lymph nodes. Cervical or vaginal cytology is performed. Chest X-ray is done annually. Imaging studies (CT/MRI) are done as needed.

Stump Carcinoma

When the carcinoma develops in the cervical stump left behind after subtotal hysterectomy, it is called stump carcinoma. **In true stump carcinoma**, malignancy develops 2 years after primary surgery. If it occurs earlier to that, it is presumed that the carcinoma was present at the time of primary surgery and, as such it is called coincidental, residual or false stump carcinoma.

The incidence may be as high as 1%. It is difficult to stage the disease.

There is also difficulty in the **treatment.** Dense adhesions of bladder, rectum and also ureters with the stump make the operation difficult and risky. The radiation therapy is also technically difficult, because of absence of uterus and close proximity of bladder and rectum to the radiation source. Radical parametrectomy, removal of cervix, upper vagina and pelvic lymphadenectomy is done in early stage disease.

External beam radiation therapy is given when the cervix is short. Vaginal radium application (vaginal cone) is also used. The prognosis is unfavorable. The 5-year survival rate varies from 30–60%.

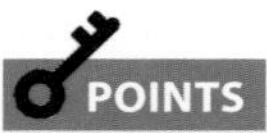

POINTS

- In most of the developing countries, **carcinoma of the cervix is the most common malignancy** in females. It ranks first, the second being breast carcinoma. The site of lesion is predominantly ectocervix (80%). The most common histologic type is squamous cell carcinoma (85–90%) and about 10–15% are adenocarcinomas.
  Squamous cell carcinomas have a viral (HPV) and veneral association unlike that of adenocarcinomas.
  The primary groups of lymph node involvement are parametrial, internal iliac, obturator, external iliac and sacral nodes.
  Preclinical invasive carcinoma is diagnosed by cytology, colposcopy and directed biopsy. If positive lesion is found, diagnostic conization and serial section has to be performed to establish the diagnosis.
  Definitive diagnosis of microinvasive carcinoma is made by cervical conization. The cone margins must be free of disease when conservative therapy is undertaken.
  Clinical presentation of early carcinoma includes menstrual abnormalities—intermenstrual bleeding or contact bleeding or excessive white discharge. Speculum examination reveals the lesion on the ectocervix which bleeds on friction.
  Causes of death are uremia, hemorrhage, sepsis, cachexia and metastases to the lung.
  Primary prevention includes identifying 'high risk' women, and 'high risk' males, sexual behavior, prophylactic **HPV vaccine**, use of condom, and removal of cervix during hysterectomy. **Secondary prevention** involves screening program and identifying the precancerous lesions or invasive lesion at its treatable stage.
- **The prognosis of carcinoma** cervix depends on many factors of which stage of the disease is important. Cancer cervix is a locally invasive tumor. It spreads primarily to pelvic tissues, then to pelvic and para-aortic lymph **nodes.** Rarely hematogenous spread to liver, lungs and bones may occur. Currently, radiation is combined with chemotherapy **(chemoradiation)** to optimize the results. Cisplatin 40 mg/m^2 weekly is used along with radiation (teletherapy and brachytherapy). **Complications** of radiotherapy may occur more than 1 year after therapy.
  Microinvasive carcinoma when treated by total hysterectomy gives 5-year survival rate of almost 100%.
  Radical hysterectomy can be performed up to stage IIA. This is especially used for a younger patient to preserve her ovarian function and to avoid vaginal fibrosis.
  Survival outcome of treatment following surgery or radiation for stage IB/IIA is the same (85%). Extraperitoneal lymphadenectomy has improved survival advantage.
  Results of therapy in terms of 5-year survival is gratifying in early stages—95% in stage Ia, reduced to 70% in stage II and 50% in stage III and 20% in stage IV (Table 24.11). HPV positive younger patients have better prognosis.
  Radical trachelectomy can be done in young women to preserve fertility as an alternative to radical hysterectomy. The disease must be in early stage (IA2 or small IB1 ≤2 cm). A therapeutic lymphadenectomy is also performed.

Contd...

Contd...

Radical trachelectomy can be done through vaginal or abdominal route. It can be done by open surgery, laparoscopic or robotic methods.
- **Leg pain** along the distribution of sciatic nerve and unilateral leg swelling are suggestive of pelvic recurrence of carcinoma cervix.
- The incidence of **stump carcinoma** is about 1%. The 5-year survival rate is 30–60%.
- For women with **carcinoma cervix during pregnancy**, survival rate is not different stage for stage when compared with the non-pregnant state.

ENDOMETRIAL CARCINOMA

INCIDENCE

The incidence is higher amongst the white population of the United States and lowest in India and Japan. In North America, amongst the whites, carcinoma body is the leading site of genital malignancy followed by ovary and cervix. In India, it ranks third amongst genital malignancy next to cervix and ovary.

While in the western countries, there has been increased incidence of carcinoma body relative to cervical one and the ratio becomes almost 1:1 in India, the incidence still remains low and the ratio ranges *between 1:8 and 1:15.*

The higher incidence in the western countries may be real or apparent. **The real one** is due to high expectation of life, rising obesity and use of estrogen in postmenopausal women and the **apparent one** is due to its detection, out of increased awareness amongst the gynecologists.

ETIOLOGY

The following are found to be related to carcinoma body of the uterus:
- **Estrogen**—persistent stimulation of endometrium with unopposed estrogen is the single most important factor for the development of endometrial cancer.
- **Age**—about 75% are postmenopausal with a median age of 60 (c.f. carcinoma cervix is more common in perimenopausal period). About 10% of women with postmenopausal bleeding have endometrial cancer.
- **Parity**—it is quite common in unmarried and in married, nulliparity is associated in about 30% (c.f. carcinoma cervix is associated more with multiparae).
- **Late menopause**—the chance of carcinoma increases, if menopause fails to occur beyond 52 years.
- **Corpus cancer syndrome**—encompasses obesity, hypertension, and diabetes.
- **Obesity** leads to high level of free estradiol as the sex hormone binding globulin level is low.
- **Unopposed estrogen stimulation** in conditions such as functioning ovarian tumors (granulosa cell) is associated with increased risk of endometrial cancer. **Unopposed estrogen replacement therapy in postmenopausal** women is associated with increased risk of endometrial cancer. Use of cyclic progestin reduces the risk. Prior use of combined oral contraceptives reduces the risk significantly (50%).
- **Polycystic ovarian disease** increases the risk due to the persistent hyperestrogenic state.
- **Tamoxifen** is antiestrogenic as well as weakly estrogenic. It is used for the treatment of breast cancer. Increased risk of endometrial cancer is noted when it is used for a long time due to its weak estrogenic effect.
- **Family history:** Hereditary nonpolyposis colorectal cancer (HNPCC) (AD syndrome) is due to the mutations in mismatch repair genes (MLH1, MSH2). Mutation carriers have the risk of developing endometrial cancer (40–60%). *BRCA1* and *BRCA2* mutation carriers have a slight increased risk.
- **Fibroid** is associated in about 30% cases.
- **Endometrial hyperplasia** precedes carcinoma in about 25% cases (Type 1).

PATHOLOGY

Naked Eye

The uterus may be smaller, normal or even enlarged (due to myohyperplasia, myometrial involvement, pyometra or associated fibroid). Two varieties are found: **Localized and diffuse.**

1. **Localized:** The usual site is on the fundus. It is either sessile or pedunculated. Myometrial involvement is late.
2. **Diffuse:** The spread is through the endometrium. The myometrium is commonly invaded; may invade to reach the serosal coat (Fig. 24.11).

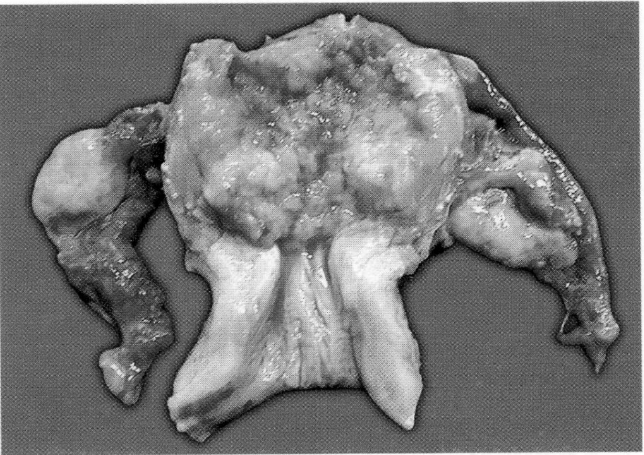

Fig. 24.11: Diffuse type of endometrial carcinoma.

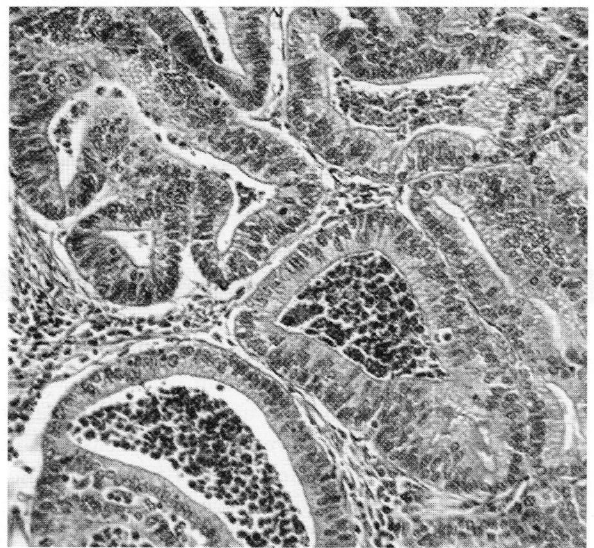

Fig. 24.12: Adenocarcinoma of the endometrium, the most common histologic type. There is significant cellular mitotic activity. The glands are arranged back-to-back.

Microscopic Appearances

The following varieties are noted:

- Adenocarcinoma [endometrioid (80%)] (Fig. 24.12)
- Adenocarcinoma with squamous elements
- Papillary serous carcinoma (5–10%) (virulent)
- Mucinous adenocarcinoma (1–2%)
- Clear cell adenocarcinoma (<5%)
- Secretory carcinoma (1%)
- Squamous cell carcinoma
- Mixed cell carcinoma
- Undifferentiated carcinoma (1–2%).

Endometrial carcinoma are of two types based upon biological and histological behavior (Table 24.12).

TABLE 24.12: Differentiating features of type I and II endometrial carcinoma.

Clinical characters	*Type I*	*Type II*
Risk factor	Unopposed estrogen	Age
Age	Perimenopause	Postmenopause
Endometrial hyperplasia	Present	Absent
Tissue differentiation	Well	Poor
Myometrial invasion	Minimal	Deep
Histology	Endometrioid	Serous, clear
Molecular characters		
Ploidy	Polyploid	Aneuploid
Her2/neu over expression	No	Yes
P-53	No	Yes
PTEN mutations	Yes	No
Prognosis	Favorable	Not favorable

SPREAD

Direct

Common modes of spread are (Type 1): (a) Lymphatic; (b) Direct; (c) Hematogenous; (d) Intraperitoneal exfoliation.

As it is slow growing, it is confined to the stroma for a long time but eventually, it spreads in all directions. Thus, it may infiltrate the myometrium and spread to the parametrium or into the peritoneal cavity through the tubes. It may spread downwards to **involve the cervix in about 15%.**

Lymphatic

Most common mode of spread is through lymphatic route. Lymphatics from the (a) Tubes and the ovaries (infundibulo pelvic ligaments) all drain in the para-aortic nodes; (b) Few lymphatics run along the round ligament drain in the inguinal and femoral nodes; (c) The lymphatics from the broad ligament drain in the pelvic nodes. The pelvic and the para-aortic nodes are the most important clinically.

Lymph node metastasis depends on the degree of tumor differentiation, myometrial invasion, tumor size, and the surgical pathological stage of the disease. Pelvic lymph node involvement in stage I disease varies from about 4% in grade 1 and 2 disease with superficial myometrial involvement to about 40% with grade 3 tumor with deep myometrial invasion. Approximately, 50% of the patients with pelvic lymph nodes will have para-aortic lymph node metastasis. In stage II disease incidence of pelvic lymph node metastasis increases to 30–45%. Lymph node metastasis is the most important prognostic factor.

The **tubes and ovaries** are involved (3–5%) either by direct spread or by lymphatics.

The vagina is involved in about 10–15% cases. The metastasis to the lower-third of the anterior vaginal wall is probably through lymphatic or by retrograde venous flow. The vault metastasis following hysterectomy may be due to direct implantation or may be explained by previous lymphatic or venous embolism.

Hematogenous

Blood borne spread occurs late. The common sites of metastases are lungs, liver, bones, and brain.

Port site metastasis is a rare type of cancer spread (0.33%).

The extent of lymph node metastases (pelvic and para-aortic) varies with histologic grade of the tumor and also with depth of myometrial invasion. Higher the grade and depth of invasion the more is the lymph node metastasis and the risk of recurrence.

Staging: The staging is based on endometrial histology and surgical evaluation, adopted by FIGO (2009). Approximately 75% patients present with stage I disease.

CLINICAL FEATURES

Patient profile: The patient is usually a nullipara, likely to be postmenopausal. There may be history of

TABLE 24.13: 'High-risk' factors for endometrial cancer.

- Late menopause (RR: 2–4)
- Nulliparity (RR: 2–3)
- Unopposed estrogen therapy (RR: 4–8)
- History of persistent anovulation (PCOS)
- History of irregular and excessive premenopausal bleeding
- Obesity (RR: 2–10), diabetes, hypertension
- Personal or family history of breast, ovary, colon or endometrial cancer (Lynch syndrome) (RR: 20)
- Atypical endometrial hyperplasia (RR: 8–29)
- Tamoxifen therapy
- Radiation menopause

(RR: relative risk)

delayed menopause. She may be obese—likely to have hypertension or diabetes (Table 24.13).

Symptoms

- Postmenopausal bleeding (75%) which may be slight, irregular or continuous. The bleeding at times may be excessive.
- In premenopausal women, there may be irregular and excessive bleeding.
- At times, there is watery and offensive discharge due to pyometra.
- Pain is not uncommon. It may be colicky due to uterine contractions in an attempt to expel the polypoidal growth.
- Few patients (< 5%) remain asymptomatic.
- In late cases there may be pelvic pressure, pain or abnormal bleeding.

Signs

The patient presents with the features as mentioned in patient profile. There may be varying degrees of pallor.

Pelvic examination: Speculum examination reveals the cervix looking healthy and the blood or purulent offensive discharge escapes out of the external os.

Bimanual examination reveals—the uterus is either atrophic, normal or may be enlarged due to spread of the tumor, associated fibroid or pyometra. The uterus is usually mobile unless in late stage, when it becomes fixed.

Rectal examination corroborates the bimanual findings.

Regional lymph nodes and breasts are examined carefully.

DIAGNOSIS OF ENDOMETRIAL CARCINOMA

The following guidelines are prescribed:

- **A case of postmenopausal bleeding** is considered to be due to endometrial carcinoma unless proved otherwise.
- Finding a benign condition to account for post-menopausal bleeding does not negate a thorough investigation to rule out carcinoma. **The two lesions may coexist.**
- **History and clinical examination** are to be recorded, as mentioned earlier.
- **Tumor marker:** Serum CA 125, elevated level indicates advanced disease. In cases with uterine papillary serous carcinoma (UPSC), it is helpful to monitor therapy and post-treatment follow up.
- **Papanicolaou smear** is not a reliable diagnostic test for endometrial carcinoma. It is positive only in 30% cases of endometrial cancer. LBC or ECC may detect glandular abnormalities.
- **Endometrial biopsy**—using a Sharman curette or **aspiration biopsy**, using a soft, flexible, plastic suction cannula (Pipelle) has been done with reliability (>90%). This is done as an outpatient procedure (Fig. 9.21). Histology is the definitive diagnosis.
- **Ultrasound and color Doppler (TVS):** Findings suggestive of endometrial carcinoma are—(a) Endometrial thickness $\geq$4 mm; (b) Hyperechoic endometrium with irregular outline; (c) Increased vascularity with low vascular resistance; (d) Intracavitary fluid. However, it cannot replace definitive biopsy.
- **Hysteroscopy:** It helps in direct visualization of endometrium and to take target biopsy.
- **Fractional curettage: It is the definite method of diagnosis** and can detect the extent of growth. This is done under anesthesia with utmost gentleness to prevent perforation of the uterus. If pyometra is detected, the procedure is withheld for about 1 week to avoid perforation and systemic infection.

The orderly steps for fractional curettage:

- Endocervical curettage.
- To pass an uterine sound to note the length of the uterocervical canal.
- Dilatation of the internal os.
- Uterine curettage at the fundus and lower part of the body. The endometrial tissue is usually profuse and often dark color.
- Finally, a polyp forceps is introduced in case any endometrial polyp has escaped the curette.

The specimens, so obtained, should be placed in **separate containers**, labeled properly and submitted for histological examination.

The results of **endometrial biopsy** (EB) correlate well with endometrial curettings. EB is accurate to detect cancer in 91-99%. For these reasons, cases where endometrial biopsy cannot be obtained (cervical stenosis) or results are nondiagnostic should be followed up by dilatation and curettage (fractional curettage).

- **Chest radiography** to detect spread of the disease.
- **Computed tomography (CT) scan** of pelvis and abdomen may be used to detect lymph node metastases (p. 100).
- **Magnetic resonance imaging (MRI)** can detect myometrial invasion, lymph node status and endocervical spead (Fig. 38.88). It is useful for women desiring fertility sparing surgery (to exclude myometrial invasion).
- **Positron emission tomography (PET-CT) (p. 101)** is the best imaging method for assessment of the spread of the disease.

SURGICAL STAGING

Cases with endometrial cancer are staged on surgical pathological basis (FIGO, 2018) following laparotomy (hysterectomy and BSO). MIS staging is safe, feasible and is now recommended (Tables 24.14 and 24.15).

PROTECTIVE FACTORS

- Weight reduction
- Exercise
- Long-term use of COCs (50%)
- Use of progestins
- LNG-IUS
- Smoking (RR: 0.5)

TABLE 24.14: FIGO staging of carcinoma of the endometrium (2008).

Stage[a]	Characteristics
Stage I	**Tumor confined to the corpus uteri**
Stage[a] IA	No or less than half myometrial invasion[a]
Stage[a] IB	Invasion equal to or more than half of the myometrium[a]
Stage II	**Tumor invades cervical stroma, but does not extend beyond the uterus[b]**
Stage[a] III	**Local and/or regional spread of the tumor[a]**
Stage IIIA	Tumor invades the serosa of the corpus uteri and/or adnexae[c, a]
Stage IIIB	Vaginal and/or parametrial involvement[c, a]
Stage IIIC	Metastases to pelvic and/or para-aortic lymph nodes[c, a]
Stage IIIC1	Positive pelvic nodes[a]
Stage IIIC2	Positive para-aortic lymph nodes with or without positive pelvic lymph nodes
Stage IV	**Tumor invades bladder and/or bowel mucosa, and/or distant metastases[a]**
Stage IVA	Tumor invasion of bladder and/or bowel mucosa[a]
Stage IVB	Distant metastases, including intra-abdominal metastases and/or inguinal lymph nodes[a]

Histopathologic criteria for assessing grade:
G1: ≤5% of a nonsquamous a nonmorular solid growth pattern
G2: 6–50% of nonsquamous a nonmorular solid growth pattern
G3: >50% of nonsquamous a nonmorular solid growth pattern
[a]Either G1, G2, or G3
[b]Endocervical glandular involvement only should be considered as stage I and no longer as stage II
[c]Positive cytology has to be reported separately without changing the stage

TABLE 24.15: Distribution of endometrial cancer (FIGO – 2006).

FIGO stage	Percentage
I	73
II	11
III	13
IV	3

MANAGEMENT OF ENDOMETRIAL CARCINOMA

- **Preventive**
- **Curative**

Preventive

Primary Prevention Includes

- **Strict weight control** beginning early in life.
- **To restrict** the use of estrogen after menopause in nonhysterectomized women. If at all it is needed, cyclic administration of progestogen preparations are added and continued under supervision.
- **Prophylactic surgery:** Women with Lynch syndrome (HNPCC) may be considered for prophylactic hysterectomy to reduce the risk from 60% to nil. Bilateral salpingo-oophorectomy should be done to reduce the risk of ovarian cancer (10–12%).
- **Education** as regard the significance of irregular bleeding per vaginam in perimenopausal and postmenopausal period and to report to the physician.

Secondary Prevention

Screening of '**high risk**' women at least in menopausal period to detect the premalignant or early carcinoma is a positive step. There is no role for routine screening. Annual screening in high risk women (p. 275) at age >35 years is recommended.

Methods

- The cytologic specimens are obtained by either endometrial aspiration or endometrial lavage. If suspicious cells are detected, histological specimen is obtained by uterine curettage.
- The presence of abnormal endometrial cells in vaginal pool cytology requires a diagnostic curettage.
- Judicious hysterectomy in premalignant lesions of the corpus (p. 275).

Curative

Pretreatment Work up

As the patients are usually aged, obese and often complicated with medical disorders, careful systemic examination and necessary investigations are mandatory before formulating the line of treatment. Along with a gynecologic oncologist, a physician's help may be needed.

Pretreatment Preparations (Table 24.16)

The same protocol as mentioned in cases of carcinoma cervix is to be followed.

TABLE 24.16: Preoperative evaluation.

- Blood examination—complete hemogram, postprandial sugar, urea, creatinine, and electrolytes
- Liver and renal function tests
- Urine—routine examination for protein, sugar, and pus cells
- ECG and X-ray chest for cardiopulmonary assessment
- Abdominal and pelvic ultrasonography for ascites, metastasis (liver), pelvic/para-aortic nodes
- MRI/CT imaging (optional) to assess the extrauterine spread of the disease and the degree of myometrial invasion
- Steroid receptor status

TREATMENT MODALITIES OF CARCINOMA ENDOMETRIUM

- **Surgery**
- **Radiotherapy**
- **Chemotherapy**
- **Combined therapy**

Surgery

Extrafascial hysterectomy is the preferred treatment for endometrial carcinoma confined to the body. The surgery includes removal of the uterus, tubes, and ovaries of both the sides and cuff of vagina. Removal of vaginal cuff is not essential as it neither improves the survival nor reduces the recurrence rate.

Traditionally, laparotomy has been the approach. Currently laparoscopic and robotic surgery are also recommended.

In Stage I, Surgery is the Mainstay of Treatment

Surgical procedures [surgical staging (page 300)]

- **Incision** longitudinal midline or paramedian is of choice for better exposure.
- **Peritoneal washings** (pouring 100 mL of saline) are taken for cytology.
- **Thorough exploration** of liver, diaphragm, omentum, pelvic organs, pelvic and para-aortic lymph nodes, is done.
- Suspicious lesions are biopsied.
- **Not to hold** the uterus by a vulsellum. Instead, traction is given by placing long straight artery forceps on either side of uterine cornu (Fig. 35.6B).
- **Procedure:**
  1. Type 1 hysterectomy (extrafascial): Total abdominal hysterectomy with bilateral salpingo-oophorectomy is done.
  2. **Uterus** is cut open in the operating room—for evaluation of tumor size, cervical extension, and myometrial invasion by gross examination. It may be done by microscopic frozen section.
  3. Patients with stage I G1 tumor postoperative radiation (vaginal brachytherapy or EBRT) may be given when deep myometrial invasion is there.
  4. **High-risk woman: Presence of big tumor** (>2 **cm),** cervical extension, G3 tumor, and myometrial invasion (>1/2 thickness) as determined by frozen section biopsy, indicates pelvic and para-aortic lymphadenectomy.
- **Lymph node sampling** of the following areas is done: (a) Common iliac; (b) External iliac; (c) Internal iliac; (d) Obturator; (e) Para-aortic.
- **Vaginal hysterectomy** may be done selectively (stage I, with well-differentiated tumor) in patients with uterovaginal prolapse or with extreme obesity.
- **Laparoscopic or laparoscopic assisted robotic** hysterectomy (p. 518) with bilateral salpingo-oophorectomy and lymph node sampling are done for staging and treatment of endometrial carcinoma (stage I).

In Stage II, Carcinoma

Management options are:

A. **Radical hysterectomy** bilateral salpingo-oophorectomy with pelvic and para-aortic lymphadenectomy.
B. **Combined radiation and surgery:** Radiation (external and intracavitary) followed 6 weeks by extrafascial total abdominal hysterectomy and bilateral salpingo-oophorectomy.
C. **Initial surgery** simple hysterectomy followed by external and intravaginal radiation.

Radiotherapy

The primary treatment by radiotherapy is indicated in:

- Women found unfit for surgery.
- Women with significant medical comorbidities.
- Surgically inoperable disease.
- Those with high-risk of recurrence.
- Patients with advanced disease for paliation therapy.

  Intracavity brachytherapy with or without external beam pelvic radiation is commonly used.

Contraindications of radiotherapy: Presence of a pelvic mass, pelvic kidney, pyometra, pelvic abscess, previous laparotomies, and/or adhesions with bowel and prior pelvic radiation.

Combined Therapy (Surgery and Radiation)

Combined therapy has shown high degree of success in this disease.

TAH-BSO followed by adjuvant radiotherapy 4–6 weeks after surgery, in a selected case, is done **to prevent locoregional recurrence.**

- **No myometrial invasion stage IA (G1, 2):** Observation only.
- **Myometrial invasion <1/2 thickness (stage IA, G2 disease):** Vaginal vault radiation (5000–6000 cGy) using colpostats afterloading techniques.
- **Myometrial invasion >1/2 thickness (stage IB):** Whole pelvis external beam radiation (4500–5000 cGy) over 5–6 weeks plus vaginal cuff boost.
- **Adnexal spread and/or intraperitoneal disease:** Whole abdominal radiation or chemotherapy (TAP).
- **Radiation therapy:** Adjuvant rediotherapy (brachytherapy and pelvic radiation) reduces locoregional recurrence in cases with high risk endometrial cancer.

Stage III and IV, Endometrial Cancer

In locally advanced disease: Adjuvant chemotherapy followed by pelvic radiation is done. Combination chemotherapy is commonly used. **Drugs comprise:** Doxorubicin paclitaxel (Taxol), adriamycin and cisplatin (TAP).

External pelvic and intracavitary radiation followed by extended hysterectomy 6 weeks later in cases of:

- Highly anaplastic tumor
- Uterine papillary serous carcinoma (UPSC)
- Clear cell carcinoma.

These tumors have got high rate of recurrence both locoregional and systemic.

Chemotherapy

Chemotherapy is used in advanced and recurrent cases or in metastatic lesions.

- **Cytotoxic drugs** are being tried either singly or in combination. **The drugs commonly used are doxorubicin, cisplatin, carboplatin, paclitaxel, and ifosfamide** (Ch. 31, Table 31.7).

Hormonal Therapy

- **Progestogens**—are widely used. Women with presence of steroid hormone receptors [(progesterone receptor (PR) and estrogen receptor (ER)] have significantly high response to progestin therapy.
  Any one of the drugs—17 hydroxyprogesterone caproate (1 g/week IM), medroxyprogesterone acetate (1 g/week IM or 150 mg/day oral) or megesterol acetate (160 mg/day orally) is of use. The drug is to be continued for at least 3 months. If responsive, may be continued for longer period with reduced doses. In cases with early stage disease (stage IG1) with poor surgical risk LNG-IUS may be useful.
- **Selective estrogen receptor modulators (SERMs) and aromatase inhibitors (AI):** Tamoxifen is a nonsteroidal agent with antiestrogenic as well as weakly estrogenic properties. It is used 10 mg twice daily along with progestogen therapy. It blocks the tissue estrogen receptor. It modulates progesterone receptors. It is found very effective when used adjunctively with progesterone (p. 448).

RECURRENT DISEASE

Common sites for recurrence are the vagina and the pelvis. The extrapelvic metastases are seen in the lung, lymph nodes (aortic), liver, brain, and bones. Majority (60%) of recurrences are seen within 2 years of initial therapy.

- Radiation therapy is the choice for isolated recurrence following surgical treatment.
- **Targeted therapy:** Drugs (mTOR inhibitors) including temsirolimus, everolimus and ridaforolimus are found to be effective in cases with recurrence. Combined therapy with everolimus and letrozole is found encouraging.

Follow-up of Patients

Following initial therapy, patient is examined every 4 months for the first 2 years, every 6 months for next 3 years and thereafter, annually (ACOG - 2005). Evaluation of symptoms, thorough clinical examination and X-ray chest (annual) are essential. Other investigations are: Mammography (annual) and CT, MRI when clinically indicated. Regular estimation of serum CA 125 may be helpful in cases with UPSC.

Place of Hormone Replacement Therapy

Its use is limited. In a patient with severe postmenopausal symptoms progestin (medroxyprogesterone acetate, 5–10 mg daily) may be a choice. Nonhormonal therapy (clonidine) can also be used. Urogenital symptoms can be improved using topical estrogen.

Prognosis

Elderly patients, higher stage (FIGO), poorly differentiated tumor, greater degree of myometrial penetration, lymph vascular space invasion are prognostically poor. Aneuploid tumors are prognostically worst. Histologically non-endometrioid tumors are aggressive and carry increased risk of recurrence. The prognostic factors to be considered are tabulated in Tables 24.17 and 24.18.

Fertility Sparing Therapy

Ovarian preservation in a woman with endometrial carcinoma: (a) Young women; (b) Fertility preservation needed; (c) Low grade disease; (d) Early stage disease; (e) Mandatory follow up with a compliant patient.

Fertility sparing therapy without hysterectomy is an option in a carefully selected woman. Myometrial invasion (or adnexal disease) is excluded with imaging studies. Woman with stage I G1 tumor are the candidates. Progestins are used, MPA (oral or IM) or LNG-IUD are the options. Hysterectomy and staging should be done when the lesion fails to regress with hormonal therapy.

TABLE 24.17: Poor prognostic factors in endometrial adenocarcinoma.

- **Age** at diagnosis (older the patient poorer the prognosis).
- **Advanced stage** of the disease.
- **Histologic type** (typical adenocarcinomas—better prognosis, papillary serous, clear cell carcinoma—poor prognosis)
- **Histologic differentiation**
- **Histologic grade:** Grade 3 tumors have 5 times more risk of recurrence and low 5-year survival rate
- **Increased myometrial invasion**
- **Lymphovascular** space invasion
- **Lymph node** metastasis
- **Extension** to cervix
- **Peritoneal cytology**—positive
- **Tumor size** (>2 cm → more lymph node metastasis)
- **Hormone receptor** status (receptor positive tumors have got better prognosis)
- **Ploidy status**—aneuploid tumors have got poor prognosis compared to diploid tumors
- **Oncogene expression** — HER-2/neu, poor prognosis
- **Type II endometrial cancer:** Poor prognosis

TABLE 24.18: 5-year survival rate (FIGO - 1998).

Stage	*Overall survival rate (%)*
IA	90.9%
IB	88.2%
II	71.6%
III	51.4%
IV	8.9%

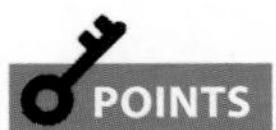

POINTS

- **Carcinoma body** ranks third amongst genital malignancies next to cervix and ovary. In USA, it is the leading site of genital malignancies followed by ovary and cervix. 75% are postmenopausal with the median age of 60. Nulliparity is associated in 30%. **Endometrial cancer** can be estrogen dependent (type-1) and nonestrogen dependent (type II). Prognosis of type I carcinoma is favorable compared to type II. **Women with Lynch syndrome** have 40–60% lifetime risk of endometrial cancer.
- **Use of combined oral contraceptive** is a known protective factor whereas chronic unopposed estrogen stimulation is a known predisposing factor for endometrial carcinoma (Tables 24.14 and 24.16). **Corpus cancer** syndrome encompasses obesity (BMI >30), hypertension and diabetes. Fibroid is associated in 30%. Endometrial hyperplasia precedes carcinoma in 25%. The most common histological type is adenocarcinoma. The pelvic and/or para-aortic glands are involved in about 10% in stage I. **Postmenopausal bleeding** is the predominant feature (75%). In premenopausal women, irregular bleeding is too often related. Once suspected, hysteroscopy and endometrial biopsy or fractional curettage is to be done, not only to diagnose but also to determine the extent of the lesion. The important primary prevention includes restriction of injudicious use of estrogen after menopause in nonhysterectomized women. **Secondary prevention** includes screening of 'high risk' women at least in menopausal period and prophylactic hysterectomy in premalignant lesions of the corpus and in women with Lynch syndrome (HNPCC). **Diagnosis of endometrial carcinoma** includes history, clinical examination, endometrial biopsy and imaging studies. **Mainstay in the treatment** of carcinoma body is total abdominal hysterectomy and bilateral salpingo-oophorectomy with pelvic and para-aortic lymph node sampling. In stage II, radical hysterectomy has to be done. Adjuvant radiation is considered depending on the surgical stage of the disease, myometrial invasion and histologic grade.
- **Primary radiotherapy** is the treatment in surgically risk patients and in advanced stages.
- **Multimodality approach** (chemo and radiation therapy) is used in advanced and recurrent cases or in metastatic lesions.
- **Progestogens are** widely used in well-differentiated carcinoma with adequate estrogen and progesterone receptors. Antiestrogen, tamoxifen is often used along with progestogens to improve the result.
- **Prognosis of endometrial** cancer depends on many factors (Table 24.17) of which depth of myometrial invasion and tumor grade are the most important ones. Younger women with endometrial cancer have a better prognosis when compared with the older women.

GESTATIONAL TROPHOBLASTIC DISEASE

Gestational trophoblastic disease (GTD) is a heterogeneous spectrum of diseases with abnormal trophoblastic proliferation ranging from benign to malignant state. It has varying degree of spread from local invasion to distant metastasis.

Diagnosis of postmolar GTN is made when the hCG level plateaus for 3 or more consecutive weeks or re-elevates. **This may occur in 15–20% following hydatidiform mole.** Some, however, follow abortion, ectopic, and even normal pregnancy.

RISK FACTORS FOR DEVELOPMENT OF GTN

1. Advanced maternal age (>40 years)
2. β-hCG >100,000 IU/L
3. Increased uterine size
4. Bilateral ovarian enlargement (>8 cm)
5. USG—uterine invasion
6. Increased uterine vascularity (USG Doppler)

PERSISTENT GESTATIONAL TROPHOBLASTIC NEOPLASIA (GTN)

Persistent GTN is evidenced by persistence of trophoblastic activity following evacuation of molar pregnancy. **This is clinically diagnosed** when the patient presents with (a) Irregular vaginal bleeding; (b) Subinvolution of the uterus; (c) Persistence of theca lutein cysts; (d) Level of hCG either plateaus or re-elevates after an initial fall. After molar evacuation serum β-hCG becomes normal in about 7–9 weeks.

Postmolar GTN of serious nature may be either invasive mole or choriocarcinoma but **GTN after nonmolar pregnancy is always a choriocarcinoma.**

Classification of GTD and risk factors are discussed in Tables 24.19A and B.

TABLE 24.19A: Classification of GTD (WHO).

Classification
A. Benign trophoblastic lesions
▪ Placental site nodule
▪ Exaggerated placental reaction
B. Hydatidiform moles (HM)
▪ Complete hydatidiform mole
▪ Partial hydatidiform moles
C. Gestational trophoblastic neoplasia
▪ Invasive mole
▪ Choriocarcinoma
▪ Placental site trophoblastic tumor
▪ Epithelioid trophoblastic tumors

TABLE 24.19B: Risk factors of GTD.

Risk factors
▪ **Race:** Asians compared to North Americans or Europeans
▪ **Age:** Extremes of age (<16 and >45)
▪ **Parity:** Increasing parity
▪ **Diet:** Risks of CHM is increased when dietary intake of animal fat, beta-carotene or vitamin A is less
▪ **Genetics:** Autosomal recessive disorder (familial recurrent HM) chromosome 19q
▪ **Risk of recurrence** is increased up to 25% when there is previous 2 or more molar pregnancy

(CHM: complete hydatidiform mole)

Incidence

The incidence of GTN is about 1 in 5,000 pregnancies in oriental countries and 1 in 50,000 in Europe and North America. More than 50% occur after molar pregnancy, about 25% after abortion and/or ectopic pregnancy and a few after normal pregnancy. **Nonmetastatic (locally invasive) lesions develop in 15% and metastatic lesions develop in about 4% of patients after molar evacuation.**

PLACENTAL SITE TROPHOBLASTIC TUMOR

The tumor arises from the trophoblast of the placental bed. Incidence is less than 1% of all patients with GTN. 40–50% of these patients develop metastases. Syncytiotrophoblast cells are generally absent, instead intermediate trophoblast cells are predominant. β-hCG secretion is low but human placental lactogen (hPL) is secreted and this is monitored during the follow up. **The entity is not responsive to chemotherapy. Hysterectomy is the preferred treatment. Serial serum hPL** may be a reliable marker and hPL is useful for immunohistochemical staining to confirm the diagnosis.

Epithelioid trophoblastic tumor (ETT): It is a variant of PSTT (WHO, 2003). Both are relatively chemoresistant and recurrence rate for the both are high (20–30%) despite surgery or chemotherapy.

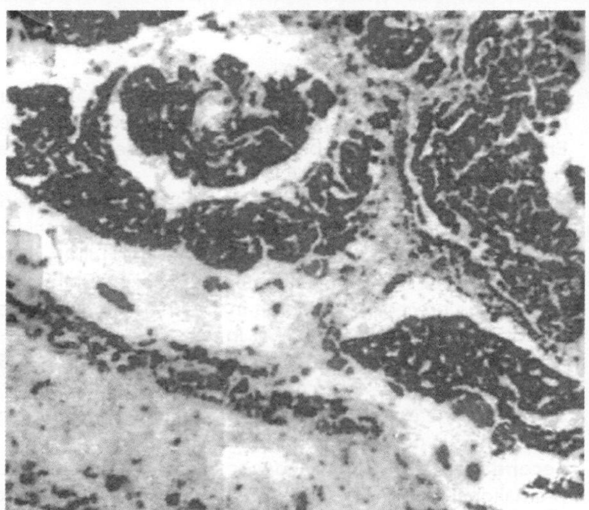

Fig. 24.13: Histological section of invasive mole showing structures of villi with marked trophoblastic proliferation deep in myometrium.

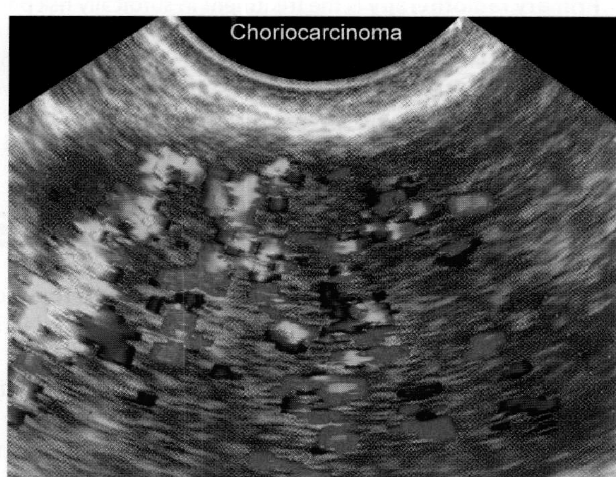

Fig. 24.14: Transvaginal color Doppler scan of choriocarcinoma showing randomly dispersed vessels.

INVASIVE GTN (CHORIOADENOMA DESTRUENS)

Invasive mole comprises about 15% of all GTN.

The prominent features of this type of mole are invasive and destructive potentialities. Invasive mole shows abnormal penetration through the muscle layers of the uterus. The uterine wall may be perforated at multiple areas showing purple, fungating growth with massive intraperitoneal hemorrhage. The neoplasm may invade the pelvic blood vessels and metastasizes to vagina or distant sites as like those in choriocarcinoma.

Diagnosis

- **On laparotomy:** (a) Perforation of the uterus through which purple fungating growth is visible; (b) Hemoperitoneum.
- **Histology:** There is penetration of the uterine wall by the hyperplastic trophoblastic cells which **still retain villus structures. There is no evidence of muscle necrosis** (Fig. 24.13). The materials for uterine curettage are often deceptive as the lesion may be deep inside the myometrium.
- **Persistent high level** of urinary or serum hCG.

CHORIOCARCINOMA

Choriocarcinoma is a highly malignant tumor arising from the chorionic epithelium (Fig. 24.14). It should be remembered that it is not a tumor of the uterus which is secondarily involved.

About 3–5% of all patients with molar pregnancies develop choriocarcinoma. Amongst all patients with choriocarcinoma, around 50% develop following a hydatidiform mole, 30% occur after a miscarriage or an ectopic pregnancy and 20% after an apparently normal pregnancy. **Trophoblastic disease following a normal pregnancy is either choriocarcinoma or PSTT and not a benign or invasive mole.**

Pathology

The primary site is usually anywhere in the uterus. Rarely, it starts in the tube or ovary. Ovarian choriocarcinoma (nongestational) may also be associated with malignant teratoma or dysgerminoma.

Naked Eye Appearances (Fig. 24.15)

The lesion is usually localized nodular type. It looks red, hemorrhagic, and necrotic. At times, the lesion is diffuse involving the entire endometrium. The nodular type may be located deep in the myometrium with overlying

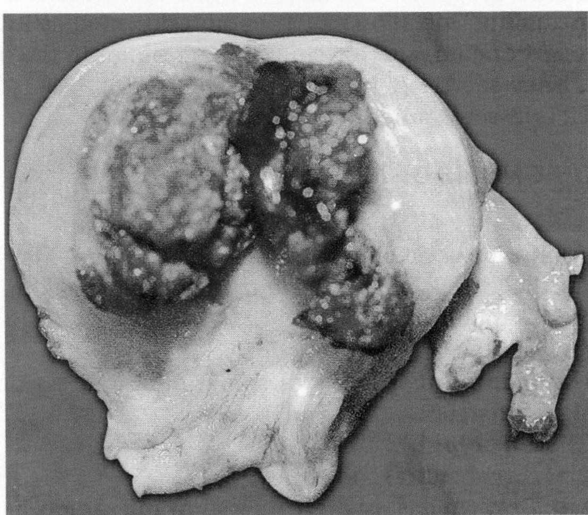

Fig. 24.15: Choriocarcinoma of diffuse type.

endometrium intact. This often gives the false-negative diagnosis on uterine curettage.

Microscopic Appearance (Fig. 24.16)

There are anaplastic sheets or columns of trophoblastic cells invading the uterine musculature. There are **evidences of necrosis and hemorrhage. Villus pattern is completely absent.**

Ovarian Enlargement

Bilateral lutein cysts are present in about 30%. These are due to excessive production of chorionic gonadotropin.

SPREAD OF GTN

Apart from the local spread, vascular erosion takes place early and hence distant metastases occur rapidly. **The common sites of metastases are** lungs (80%), anterior vaginal wall (30%), brain (10%), liver (10%), and others.

CLINICAL FEATURES OF GTN

The clinical features depend on the location of the primary growth and on its secondary deposits.

Patient Profile

There is usually a history of molar pregnancy in recent past. Rarely, its relation with a term pregnancy, abortion or ectopic pregnancy may be established. **GTN after a nonmolar pregnancy is always a choriocarcinoma.**

Symptoms

The following are the usual symptoms:

- Persistent ill health
- Irregular vaginal bleeding, at times brisk
- Continued amenorrhea.

Other symptoms due to metastatic lesions are:

Lung: Cough, breathlessness, hemoptysis
Vaginal: Irregular and at times brisk hemorrhage
Cerebral: Headache, convulsion, paralysis or coma
Liver: Epigastric pain, jaundice.

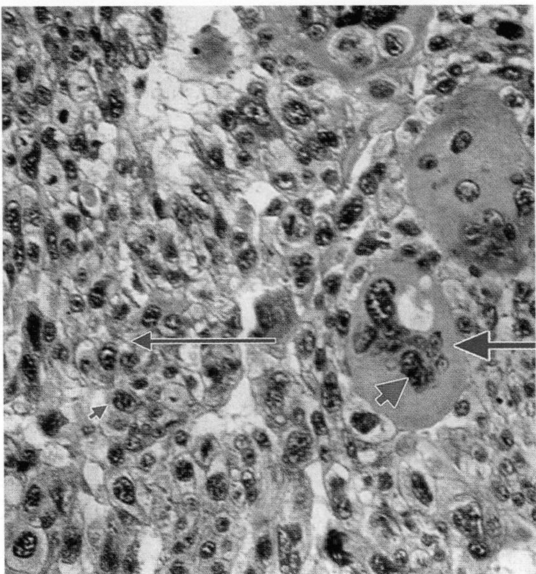

Fig. 24.16: Histologic picture of choriocarcinoma. The cytotrophoblast cells are well-defined with clear cytoplasm (thin arrow). The syncytiotrophoblast cells are arranged in sheets of multinucleated cytoplasm (thick arrow).

Signs

- Patient looks ill
- Pallor of varying degrees.

Physical signs are evident according to the organ involved.

Bimanual examination reveals subinvolution of the uterus. There may be a purplish-red nodule in the lower-third of the anterior vaginal wall (Fig. 24.17). Unilateral or bilateral enlarged ovaries may be palpable through lateral fornices.

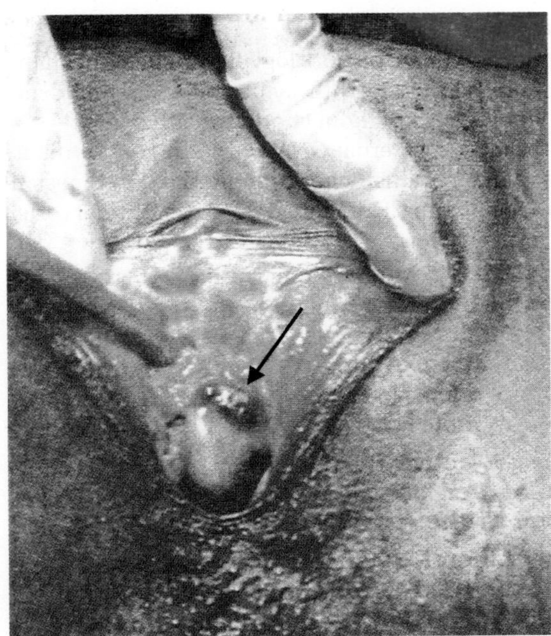

Fig. 24.17: Note the purplish-red metastatic nodule in the lower third of anterior vaginal wall (suburethral). Metastases may occur in vaginal fornices also.

SPECIAL INVESTIGATIONS

The methods extended are not only to establish the diagnosis but also to note the metastatic sites which help in staging.

Metastatic brain lesion is suspected when the ratio of hCG in spinal fluid/in serum is more than 1:60.

DIAGNOSTIC CRITERIA FOR POSTMOLAR GTN (FIGO)

Levels of serum β-hCG are followed up.
- ≥ Four values of plateaued hCG (±10%) over at least 3 weeks time (D:1, 7, 14, 21).
- A rise of hCG of >10% for >3 values over at least 2 weeks time.
- Histologic diagnosis of choriocarcinoma.
- Persistence of hCG beyond 6 months of mole evacuation.

Chest X-ray

X-ray shows 'cannon ball' shadow or 'snow storm' appearance due to numerous tumor emboli (Fig. 24.18). Pleural effusion may be present.

Pelvic Sonography

Sonography helps not only to localize the lesion but to differentiate GTN from a normal pregnancy.

Diagnostic Uterine Curettage

Pretherapy D and C reduces the intrauterine tumor bulk. However, routine D and C for histologic diagnosis is not required. It reveals the characteristic histological pattern. It is emphasized that, the curetted material may not reveal the diagnosis in all the cases, as the lesion may be deep in the myometrium or the uterus may not be the primary site. One should be very careful and alert while doing uterine curettage as brisk hemorrhage may occur for which a lifesaving hysterectomy may have to be done.

Histopathology

Choriocarcinoma, on histology shows sheets of anaplastic trophoblastic tissue with cytotrophoblast and syncytiotrophoblast cells without chorionic villi.

Absence of paternal DNA within the tumor differentiates nongestational choriocarcinoma from gestational choriocarcinoma. Extragonadal germ cell tumors originate from midline loctations such as anterior mediastinum, retroperitoneum, and have no primary tumor in the ovaries. They secrete β–hCG. PSTT secrete HPL (50–100%) and it is lesser in amount (10%) to that of hCG.

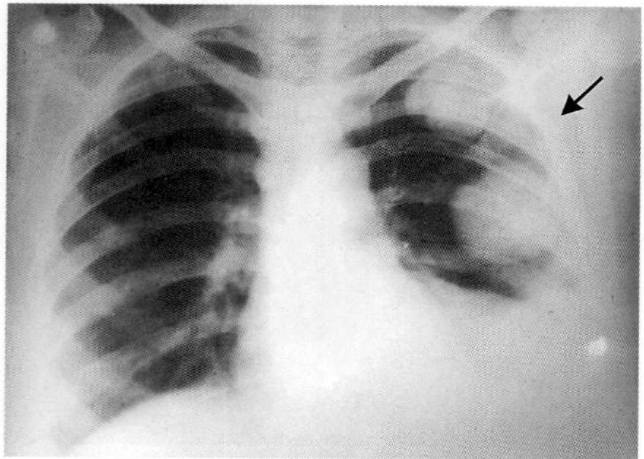

Fig. 24.18: Cannon ball shadow in the left apical and midregion of the lung with pleural effusion in choriocarcinoma.

(*Courtesy:* Eden Hospital, MCH, Kolkata)

DIAGNOSIS OF METASTASES

Vaginal nodules

Excision biopsy or biopsy should not be done. Massive hemorrhage following resection may need packing or selective embolization.

Cerebral

- The ratio of hCG levels in spinal fluid and serum is higher than 60.
- CT scan or MRI.

Liver: CT scan; ultrasonography.

Chest: X-ray (metastasis); CT may show micrometastases which are not visible on a chest radiograph.

Metastases to other sites are uncommon when pelvic examination and chest X-ray are normal.

WHO prognostic scoring system of gestational trophoblastic disease is discussed in Table 24.20.

STAGING

The anatomic staging for gestational trophoblastic tumors (GTT) as described by FIGO is tabulated in Table 24.21.

TABLE 24.20: WHO prognostic scoring system of gestational trophoblastic disease as modified by FIGO (2000).

Parameter	Score			
	0	1	2	4
Age (years)	<40	>40	—	—
Antecedent pregnancy	Mole	Abortion	Term	—
Interval (month)*	<4	4–6	7–12	≥13
Pretreatment hCG (IU/L)	$<10^3$	10^3–$<10^4$	10^4 – $<10^5$	$\geq 10^5$
Largest tumor (cm)	<3	3–4	>5	—
Site of metastases	Lung pelvis	Spleen, kidney	GI tract, liver	Brain
No. of metastases detected	—	1–4	5–8	>8
Prior chemotherapy	—	—	Single drug	Multiple drugs

Total score: <6 is low risk and a total score ≥7 is high risk.
***Interval:** Time between antecedent pregnancy and start of chemotherapy. This scoring is not applicable to PSTT and ETT.

TABLE 24.21: FIGO anatomic staging for GTT.

Stage I	The lesion is confined to the uterus
Stage II	The lesion spreads outside the uterus but is confined to the genital organs
Stage III	The lesion metastasizes to the lungs
Stage IV	The lesion metastasizes to sites such as brain, liver or gastrointestinal tract

Flowchart 24.1: Management of gestational trophoblastic disease (GTD).

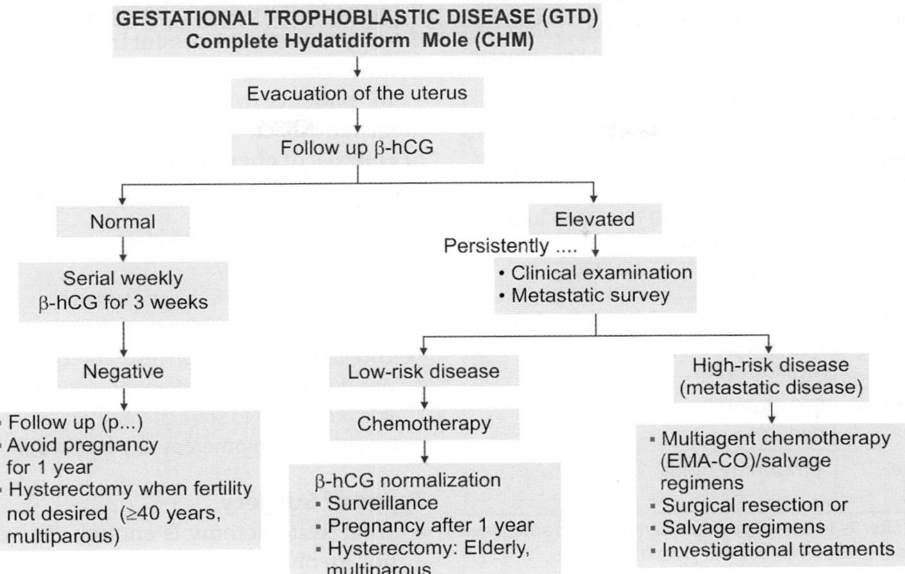

MANAGEMENT OF GTN

- **Preventive**
- **Curative**

Preventive

- **Prophylactic chemotherapy** in 'at risk' women following evacuation of molar pregnancy may be considered. It prevents uterine invasion or metastasis. 'At risk' women are:
  - Age of patient > 40 years.
  - Initial levels of serum hCG ≥ 100,000 IU/mL.
    - hCG level fails to become normal by 7–9 weeks time or there is re-elevation.
    - Histologically diagnosed as infiltrative mole.
  - Evidence of metastases irrespective of the level of hCG.
  - Previous history of a molar pregnancy.
  - Woman who is unreliable for follow up.

Disadvantage of routine chemotherapy is unnecessary exposure of the toxic drugs to all women who may not need it. Majority (80–90%) of women do not develop persistent GTN.

- **Meticulous follow up** following evacuation of hydatidiform mole is essential for at least 6 months to detect early evidence of trophoblastic reactivation. **A single agent chemotherapy is highly effective in nonmetastatic and low-risk metastatic GTN.**
- **Selective hysterectomy** in hydatidiform mole over 35 years. There is 4-fold reduction in the risks of choriocarcinoma.
- In suspected cases, serum hCG is to be determined.

Curative

- **Chemotherapy**
- **Surgery**
- **Radiation**

Chemotherapy

The advent of chemotherapy has revolutionized the treatment of both the nonmetastatic and metastatic lesion of choriocarcinoma. Chemotherapy is now the mainstay in the treatment (Flowchart 24.1).

Whether a single agent (Table 24.22) or multidrug regimen (Tables 24.23 and 24.24) is to be used, depends on the risk factors present. **In general, patients with nonmetastatic (low risk) and good prognosis disease are treated effectively with single agent therapy (methotrexate or actinomycin). The patients with poor prognosis metastatic disease should be treated with combination drug regimen (EMA-CO regimen).**

- **Management of GTN** needs thorough assessment of the extent of the disease. **Chemotherapy regimen is decided** on WHO prognostic scoring.
- In high risk metastatic disease, best results are obtained with EMA-CO protocol (Table 24.24).

Ultra high risk GTN (WHO): Patients in the group are: (a) FIGO high risk group with score of ≥13; (b) Patients with

TABLE 24.22: Single drug regimen in low-risk cases.

Methotrexate	1–1.5 mg/kg	IM/IV	Days 1, 3, 5, and 7
Folinic acid	0.1–0.15 mg/kg	IM	Days 2, 4, 6, and 8

The courses are to be repeated at interval of 7 days.

TABLE 24.23: Mac protocol in low-risk cases.

Methotrexate	1–1.5 mg/kg	IM/IV	Days 1, 3, 5, and 7
Folinic acid	0.1–0.15 mg/kg	IM	Days 2, 4, 6, and 8
Actinomycin D	12 mg/kg	IV	Days 1–5
Cyclophosphamide	3 mg/kg	IV	Days 1–5

The courses are to be repeated at interval of 2 weeks.

TABLE 24.24: EMA-CO protocol in high risk metastatic GTN.

Days	Drug	Dose
Day 1	Etoposide	100 mg/m^2 in 200 mL saline infused over 30 minutes
Day 1	Actinomycin D	0.5 mg IV bolus
	Methotrexate	100 mg/m^2 bolus followed by 200 mg/m^2 IV infusion over 12 hours
Day 2	Etoposide	100 mg/m^2 in 200 mL saline infused over 30 minutes
	Actinomycin D	0.5 mg IV bolus
	Folinic acid	15 mg IM every 12 hours for 4 doses beginning 24 hours after starting methotrexate
Day 8	Cyclophosphamide	600 mg/m^2 IV in saline over 30 minutes
	Vincristine (Oncovin)	1 mg/m^2 IV bolus

The course will restart after 7–14 days, if possible. Generally two additional courses are given after the hCG levels become normal.

metastases in liver, brain or extensive metastasis. These patients tolerate poorly with first line multiagent chemotherapy. This multiagent therapy causes sudden tumor collapse. Many of these patients suffer severe hemorrhage, metabolic acidosis, myelosuppression, septicemia, multiorgan failure and death.

Management: Complications can be avoided by giving initial minimal agents like EP regimen. Etoposide 100 mg/m^2 and cisplatin 20 mg/m^2 on days 1 and 2 are given and repeated weekly for 1–3 weeks. Thereafter the usual full dose regimen EMA-CO is started.

Salvage therapies: Patient failing EMA-CO are mostly salvaged with paclitaxel and etoposide alternating with paclitaxel and cisplatin (TE/TP) or with EP/EMA.

All tests are repeated before each cycle: Quantitative estimation of β-hCG level, complete blood count (CBC), RFT, LFT, thyroid function and imaging studies are to be done. β-hCG levels are high in invasive mole and choriocarcinoma (100–1000,000 mIU/mL), low levels are seen in PSTT, ETT.

Treatment course should not be repeated if:

- WBC <3,000 cu mm
- Polymorphonuclear leukocytes <1500 cu mm
- Platelet counts <100,000 cu mm
- Significant elevation of BUN, SGPT

Continue treatment at 1–3 weekly interval until three consecutive negative weekly hCG titers.

SURVEILLANCE DURING AND AFTER THERAPY OF GTN

Serum hCG value monitoring every week → once negative → every 2 weeks for 3 months → every month for 1 year → every 6–12 months for life or at least 3–5 years.

- **Remission:** 3 consecutive normal weekly hCG values.
- **Response:** >10% decline in hCG during one cycle treatment.
- **Plateau:** ±10% change in hCG during one cycle.
- **Resistance:** 10% rise in hCG during one cycle or plateau for two cycles of chemotherapy.

Place of Hysterectomy

Primary hysterectomy has got a limited place. Chemotherapy alone is successful in curing 85% of patients with nonmetastatic and good prognosis metastatic GTN.

In patients with nonmetastatic or good prognosis metastatic disease, **hysterectomy decreases the number of courses of chemotherapy.**

INDICATIONS OF HYSTERECTOMY

- Lesions confined to the uterus in women aged >35 years, not desirous of fertility.
- Placental site trophoblastic tumor.
- Intractable vaginal bleeding.
- Localized uterine lesion resistant to chemotherapy.
- Accidental uterine perforation during uterine curettage.

It is preferable to start chemotherapy → surgery on day 3 → followed by chemotherapy as per schedule.

Types of Surgery

- Total hysterectomy is enough. The ovaries are usually not involved and if involved, can be effectively cured with postoperative chemotherapy.
- Lung resection (thoracotomy) in pulmonary metastasis in drug resistant cases.
- Craniotomy for control of bleeding.

Radiation

Patients with brain metastases require whole-brain radiation therapy (3000 cGy over 10 days). Intrathecal high dose methotrexate may be administered to prevent hemorrhage and for tumor shrinkage.

Liver Metastasis

Interventional radiology (hepatic artery ligation or embolization) or whole liver radiation (2000 cGy over 10 days) along with chemotherapy may be effective. Hepatic metastasis has a poor prognosis.

Transplacental metastases to the fetus is rare and the prognosis is poor.

Prognosis

The cure rate is almost 100% in low risk and about 70% in high risk metastatic groups.

Recurrences

Overall recurrences are 3% for stage I; 8% for stage II; 4% for stage III and 9% for stage IV. Meantime for recurrence is 6 months. Recurrence rate for PSTT and ETT are about 20–30%.

Prevention of Recurrent Disease

Additional cycle of chemotherapy following normalization of hCG level, should be given as follows: For nonmetastatic disease—one cycle; for good prognosis metastatic disease—two cycles; for poor prognosis metastatic disease—three cycles.

Future Childbirth

There is no adverse effect on the subsequent pregnancy provided the conception occurs after 1 year of completion of chemotherapy. **Pregnancy** should be confirmed by USG early and hCG level is to be measured 6 weeks after delivery to exclude persistent GTN. Incidence of placenta accreta is increased.

Surveillance and follow up is mandatory for all patients at least for 2 years. Serum hCG is measured weekly until it is negative for three consecutive weeks. Thereafter, it is measured monthly for 6 months and 6 monthly thereafter for life.

Increased risk for the development of secondary malignancies like leukemia, colon cancer, and breast cancer has been observed. This is common after treatment with multiple agent chemotherapy. Etoposide is reserved for resistant and high-risk cases only.

Phantom β-hCG: In some patients persistent mildly elevated levels of β-hCG serum persist for a long time. But in reality there is no true β-hCG or no trophoblastic disease is present. This 'phantom' β-hCG is due to heterophile antibodies in the patient's serum that interfere with the β-hCG immune assay and cause a false positive result.

In such a situation patient does not need any active management neither chemotherapy nor hysterectomy. The diagnosis can be confirmed by doing the urine test that will be negative. Heterophile antibodies are not filtered in the urine as these are large glycoprotein molecule.

Quiescent GTN: Following treatment of a HM and choriocarcinoma, persistence of low level (1–300 IU/L) of β-hCG has been observed in few patients for a period of 3 months or longer. There is no evidence of GTN on clinical, radiologic or biochemical study. It is known as quiescent GTN.

This is also considered as premalignant condition as 25% of these cases progress to choriocarcinoma over a period of 6 months to 10 years. Presence of hyperglycosylated hCG (hCG-H) is a marker of invasive cytotrophoblasts. hCG-H can be detected in many cases of quiescent GTD. Majority of these cases do not need any treatment as these are self-resolving. These cases need follow up. Cases with elevated levels of hCG on follow up, need chemotherapy.

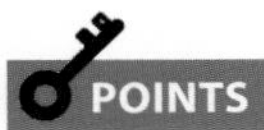

- **Gestational trophoblastic neoplasia** (GTN) encompasses persistent hydatidiform mole, invasive mole, choriocarcinoma and placental site trophoblastic tumor.
- The **incidence of GTN** is about 1 in 5,000 pregnancies in Oriental countries and 1 in 50,000 in Europe and North America. 50% occur after molar pregnancy, 25% after abortion and ectopic and 25% after normal pregnancy. Nonmetastatic lesions develop in 15% and metastatic lesions develop in about 4% of patients after molar evacuation.
- **Trophoblastic cells** normally regress within 3 weeks following delivery. Women treated for GTN should not become pregnant for 6–12 months after the treatment. This helps to assess the level of β-hCG and treatment response. Diagnosis of postmolar GTN is made when the hCG level plateaus for 3 or more consecutive weeks or re-elevates.
- **The invasive mole** is diagnosed on laparotomy and on histology showing hyperplastic trophoblastic cells maintaining villous structures without evidences of muscle necrosis. In choriocarcinoma, the hyperplastic trophoblastic column of cells invades the muscles. There are evidences of hemorrhage and muscle necrosis. The villous pattern is lost.
  The most common site of metastases is lung, followed by anterior vaginal wall, brain and liver.
- **Recurrence rate of GTN** following treatment (hCG level reached normal) is 5% for metastatic good prognosis cases and is 1–2% for nonmetastatic cases (Tables 24.19A and B).
- **hCG monitoring:** All forms of hCG (hCG, core hCG, C- terminal hCG, nicked free beta and the hyperglycosylated) are monitored. To exclude false positive result retest with another assay kit or test for urine hCG may be used.
- **Heterogenicity of β-hCG molecules in GTN** is increased compared to a normal pregnancy. hCG molecules in GTN has higher proportion of nicked β-hCG, β core fragment and free β-hCG. A β-hCG assay for follow up must detect both β-hCG as well as its all the fragments and metabolites. An assay with poor sensitively may fail to detect low levels of β-hCG, leading to incorrect decision and management result. Ultimately there is disease persistence. Patients, following complete remission, have normal pregnancy and live births.
- **Chemotherapy is now the mainstay of treatment (p. 307).**
- **Primary surgery** has got limited place. Hysterectomy is indicated in women aged more than 35 years to improve the efficacy of chemotherapy or to control intractable bleeding. Total hysterectomy is to be done on day 3 of a course of chemotherapy.
- **There is no adverse effect** on subsequent pregnancy, if it occurs after 1 year of chemotherapy. Pregnancy should be confirmed by USG early and serum hCG should be measured 6 weeks after delivery to exclude persistent GTN.
- **Prophylactic chemotherapy** can prevent uterine invasion and metastasis. But it is given selectively.
- **Low-risk GTN cases** (Tables 24.19A and B) are usually treated by single-agent chemotherapy whereas high-risk metastatic cases are treated with multiple-agent chemotherapy. Nonmetastatic and low-risk metastatic GTN cases are completely curable by chemotherapy.
- **Surveillance during and after therapy** of GTN is essential (p. 308).

MALIGNANT TUMORS OF THE OVARY

INCIDENCE

Ovarian malignancy constitutes about 15–20% of genital malignancy. It is the leading cause of cancer death in women next to breast cancer in US and Scandinavian countries. It is much less in Oriental or Latin American and Asian countries including Japan and India. **Approximately, 1 in every 70 newborn females in the United States will live to develop ovarian cancer** and 1 woman in 100 will die of

TABLE 24.25: Variations in incidence, mortality rates and disease burden for ovarian cancer.

Countries	*Incidence (ASR) per 100,000*	*Mortality rate (ASR) per 100,000*
Less developed	5.0	3.1
More developed	9.2	5.0
World average	6.1	3.7

(ASR: age-standardized incidence rates)

the disease. 20% of ovarian neoplasms are malignant. **It is more common amongst nulliparous.** It is the fourth most common cause of cancer deaths in women exceeded only by breast, colon and lung malignancies. Ovarian cancer has the highest mortality of all gynecologic cancers. World wide, there are 2,39,000 new cases and 152,000 deaths from ovarian cancer each year.

EPIDEMIOLOGY AND ETIOLOGICAL FACTORS (TABLE 24.25)

Highest incidence is recorded in the industrialized countries (Sweden, USA, and UK). There is significant reduction in the risk with increasing parity.

- **Nulligravidas** carry a higher risk for ovarian malignancy.
- **Incessant ovulation theory** (Fathalla, 1971) suggests repeated ovulatory trauma to the ovarian epithelial lining is a promoting factor for carcinogenesis. Combined oral contraceptive pills reduce the risk significantly as also repeated pregnancies.
- The role of **ovulation inducing drugs** is yet uncertain. Use of coffee, tobacco, alcohol, and dietary fat has been implicated. Association of ovarian cancer with **talc and asbestos** has also been mentioned. Breastfeeding, tubal ligation, and hysterectomy have been associated with reduction in the risk.

GENETICS AND OVARIAN MALIGNANCY

Hereditary ovarian cancer occurs in two forms:

- **Hereditary breast ovarian cancer (BOC) syndrome** is observed in 80–95% cases of all familial ovarian cancers. *BRCA1* (chromosome 17q21) and *BRCA2* (chromosome 13q12) gene mutations are observed in majority of such cases (serous not mucinous carcinoma). These patients present at an earlier age.
- **Hereditary nonpolyposis colorectal cancer (HNPCC)**—is an autosomal dominant transmission. Women with HNPCC (Lynch II syndrome) have life time risk of about 50% for endometrial cancer and 12% for ovarian cancer. The risks of other cancers like genitourinary in addition to HNPCC are high. It is due to mutations in three DNA mismatch repair genes (MLH1, MSH2, and MSH6).
- A first degree relative: Mother, sister, daughter of an affected individual
- A second degree relative: Maternal or paternal aunt or grandmothers
- **Concept of distal fallopian tube origin (Fig. 24.19)**

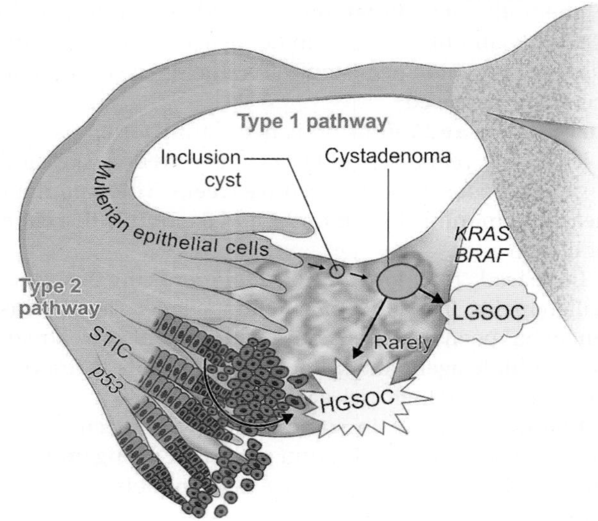

Fig. 24.19: The schematic presentation of distal fallopian tube origin of ovarian carcinoma. The concept of LGSOC and HGSOC with STIC and p53 mutation are shown.

TABLE 24.26: Dualistic pattern of ovarian carcinogenesis.

	Type 1	*Type II*
Carcinogenesis	Incorporation of Müllerian epithelial cells on the ovary causing ovarian endometriosis, cortical inclusion cyst	Incorporation of serous tubal intraepithelial carcinoma (STIC) with exfoliation of cells on the ovarian surface or in the peritoneal cavity
Type of tumor	Borderline tumors; Low-grade serous ovarian cancers (LGSOC), clear cell cancer, mucinous carcinoma	▪ High-grade serous ovarian carcinoma (HGSOC) ▪ Undifferentiated carcinoma
Stage at presentation	Early stage	Advanced stage
Gene mutation	KRAS, BRAF or PTEN, not p-53	P-53 mutations in 100% of cases
Clinical course	Indolent	Highly aggressive from the outset

The two important carcinogenic pathways are shown in Table 24.26.

CATEGORIES OF OVARIAN MALIGNANCY

Categories of ovarian cancer (Table 24.27).

GENERAL CONSIDERATIONS

Malignant epithelial tumors constitute about 90% of all primary ovarian carcinomas. The nonepithelial malignant tumors such as gonadal stromal or germ cell tumors are indeed rare, present special problems in extremes of age and are of pathologist's curiosity. These will be dealt separately. **Thus, in the discussion to follow, only the malignant epithelial tumors will be described.**

TABLE 24.27: Categories of ovarian cancer (PRAT – 2012).

Epithelial (80–85%)	*Germ cell (5%)*	*Sex cord stromal (1%)*	*Metastatic disease (5%)*	*Hereditary (10–15%)*
▪ High-grade serous (70%) ▪ Mucinous (10%) ▪ Endometrioid (10%) ▪ Low-grade serous (5–10%) ▪ Clear cell (5%)	▪ Teratoma (immature) (36%) ▪ Dysgerminoma (33%) ▪ Endometrial sinus tumor (15%) ▪ Embryonal carcinoma (4%) ▪ Choriocarcinoma (2%) ▪ Gonadoblastoma ▪ Mixed germ cell (5%)	▪ Granulosa cell (70%) ▪ Thecoma ▪ Fibroma ▪ Sertoli-Leydig cell ▪ Gynandroblastoma	▪ GI tract 39% ▪ Breast (28%) ▪ Endometrium (20%) ▪ Lymphoma	▪ Hereditary breast and ovarian cancer syndrome ▪ Lynch syndrome

PRIMARY EPITHELIAL

Malignant epithelial tumors include both cystic and solid types. **These are bilateral in about 50%** (Fig. 24.24). Cystic is more common than solid. These may arise de novo as malignant or more commonly, they result from malignant changes of benign cystic tumors.

Endometrioid carcinoma is associated with endometrial carcinoma in 20 % and ovarian endometriosis in 10% cases. In less than 5%, it may arise from the endometrial cyst.

Cystic

Naked eye appearances: The wall of the cystic tumor becomes shaggy. There may be papillary projection at places. Cut section shows solid areas with hemorrhage at places. The papillae become friable, the base becomes broad and indurated. In mucinous type, it is filled up with gelatinous material (Fig. 24.20).

Microscopic picture: The histologic appearance in each type is tabulated in Table 24.28 and shown in Figure 24.21.

Solid (Fig. 24.22)

It attains a moderate size. The external surface is smooth and often lobulated. Subserous blood vessels may be prominent. Cut section shows grayish granular appearance, at times brain-like. There may be irregular cystic spaces due to necrosis.

Microscopic appearance reveals adenocarcinoma or carcinoma without adenomatous pattern.

TABLE 24.28: Epithelial ovarian tumor and histologic appearance.

Tumor types	*Histology*	*Occurrence all ovarian*
Serous cyst carcinoma	Adenocarcinoma	35–40
Mucinous cyst carcinoma	Adenocarcinoma	10–15
Endometrioid or adenoacanthoma	Adenocarcinoma	15–25
Malignant dermoid	Squamous cell carcinoma	Rare
Others: Clear cell adenocarcinoma, malignant Brenner tumor, squamous cell carcinoma, undifferentiated carcinoma.		

FIGO STAGING OF CARCINOMA OVARY (P. 307)

The staging aims at:
- Better choice of adjuvant therapy
- Better assessment of prognosis.

The staging is done following laparotomy (staging laparotomy) and is followed as per FIGO, 2014 (Table 24.29).

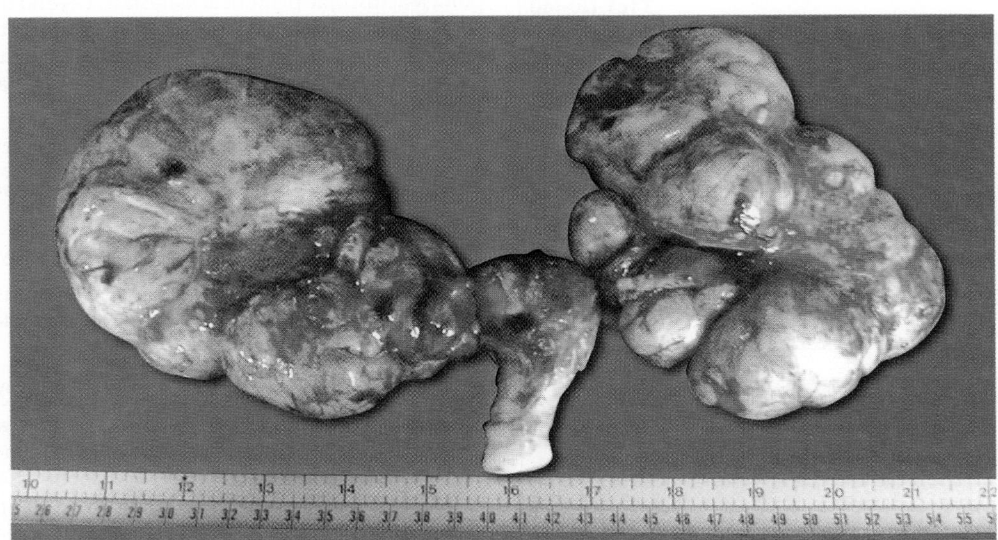

Fig. 24.20: Photograph of a surgical specimen of a huge bilateral mucinous cyst adenocarcinoma. The tumors are lobulated and with areas of hemorrhage and necrosis are seen.

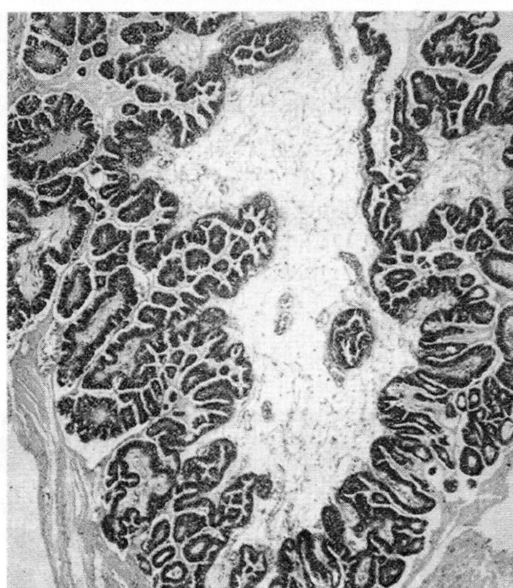

Fig. 24.21: Histologic picture of serous cyst adenocarcinoma. Long papillary outgrowths are seen. There is considerable cellular mitotic activity. This lace-like pattern characterized by slit-like spaces between the papillae is due to extensive coalescence of papillae.

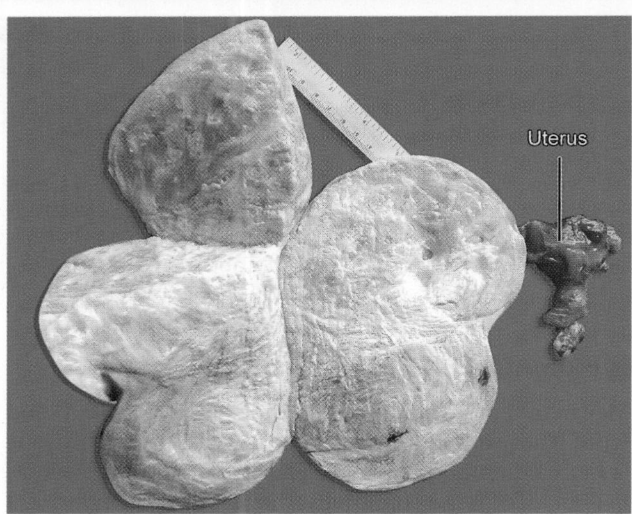

Fig. 24.22: 55-year-old lady presented with pelvic heaviness and AUB. MRI revealed solid ovarian mass. Solid ovarian tumor is cut opened. Histology confirmed ovarian fibroma. The uterus is seen by the side.

TABLE 24.29: FIGO staging of carcinoma of the ovary, tube and peritoneum (2018).

Stage	TNM
Stage I: Tumor confined to ovaries or fallopian tube(s).	**T1-N0-M0**
IA: Tumor limited to 1 ovary (capsule intact) or fallopian tube; no tumor on ovarian or fallopian tube surface; no malignant cells in the ascites or peritoneal washings	**T1a-N0-M0**
IB: Tumor limited to both ovaries (capsules intact) or fallopian tubes; no tumor on ovarian or fallopian tube surface; no malignant cells in the ascites or peritoneal washings	**T1b-N0-M0**
IC: Tumor limited to 1 or both ovaries or fallopian tubes, with any of the following:	
IC1: Surgical spill	**T1c1-N0-M0**
IC2: Capsule ruptured before surgery or tumor on ovarian or fallopian tube surface	**T1c2-N0-M0**
IC3: Malignant cells in the ascites or peritoneal washings	**T1c3-N0-M0**
Stage II: Tumor involves 1 or both ovaries or fallopian tubes with pelvic extension (below pelvic brim) or peritoneal cancer	**T2-N0-M0**
IIA: Extension and/or implants on uterus and/or fallopian tubes and/or ovaries	**T2a-N0-M0**
IIB: Extension to other pelvic intraperitoneal tissues	**T2b-N0-M0**
Stage III: Tumor involves 1 or both ovaries or fallopian tubes, or peritoneal cancer, with cytologically or histologically confirmed spread to the peritoneum outside the pelvis and/or metastasis to the retroperitoneal lymph nodes	**T1/T2-N1-M0**

Contd...

Contd...

Stage	TNM
IIIA1: Positive retroperitoneal lymph nodes only (cytologically or histologically proven):	
IIIA1(i) Metastasis up to 10 mm in greatest dimension	
IIIA1(ii) Metastasis more than 10 mm in greatest dimension	
IIIA2: Microscopic extrapelvic (above the pelvic brim) peritoneal involvement with or without positive retroperitoneal lymph nodes	**T3a2-N0/N1-M0**
IIIB: Macroscopic peritoneal metastasis beyond the pelvis up to 2 cm in greatest dimension, with or without metastasis to the retroperitoneal lymph nodes	**T3b-N0/N1-M0**
IIIC: Macroscopic peritoneal metastasis beyond the pelvis more than 2 cm in greatest dimension, with or without metastasis to the retroperitoneal lymph nodes (includes extension of tumor to capsule of liver and spleen without parenchymal involvement of either organ)	**T3c-N0/N1-M0**
Stage IV: Distant metastasis excluding peritoneal metastases	
Stage IVA: Pleural effusion with positive cytology	
Stage IVB: Parenchymal metastases and metastases to extra-abdominal organs (including inguinal lymph nodes and lymph nodes outside of the abdominal cavity)	**Any T, any N, M1**

Regional lymph nodes (N)	**Distant metastasis (M)**
1. NX: Regional lymph nodes (N) cannot be assessed 2. N0: No regional lymph node metastasis 3. N1: Regional lymph node metastasis	1. MX: Distant metastasis cannot be assessed 2. M0: No distant metastasis 3. M1: Distant metastasis (excluding peritoneal metastasis)

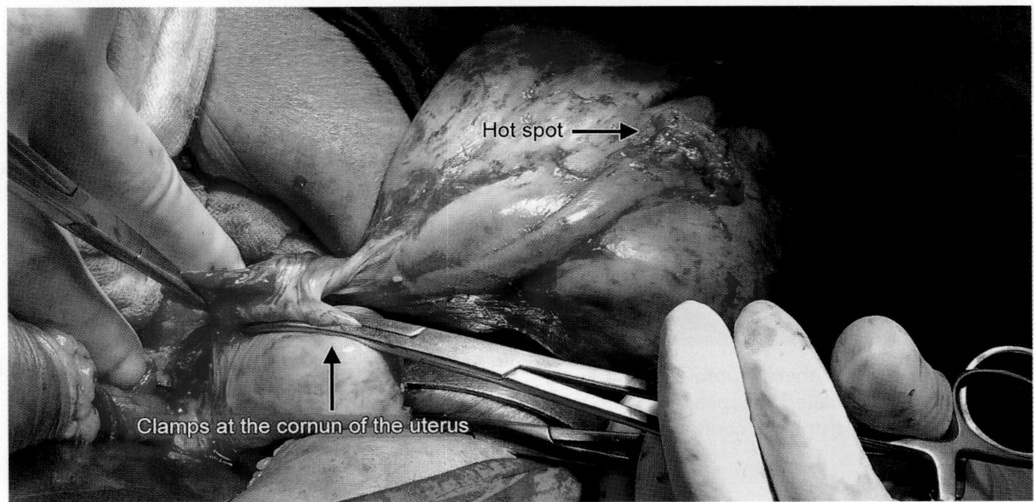

Fig. 24.23: Intraoperative photograph of a huge ovarian serous cyst adenocarcinoma. Note the tube is stretched over the tumor surface. The junction of the peritoneum (arrow) with the fimbrial epithelium [(tubal-peritoneal junction (TPJ)], is the site of carcinogenesis. TPJ is also known as 'hot spot' as that of SCJ for CIN.

SPREAD

Natural path of spread: The tumors spread **along the peritoneal surface** to involve ovarian, parietal and intestinal peritoneal surfaces as well as the undersurface of the diaphragm, particularly on the right side. **The modes of spread are:**

- **Transcelomic (exfoliation of cells)**
- **Lymphatic**
- **Direct**
- **Hematogenous**

Transcelomic

Implantation of malignant cells occurs by:

- Direct exfoliation of cells as in papillary cyst adenocarcinoma.
- Penetration of tumor capsule.
- Rupture of the capsule.

The **exfoliated cells** in the peritoneal fluid flow along the paracolic gutters.

Multiple secondary deposits are formed on the peritoneal surfaces especially in the pouch of Douglas, in the omentum, diaphragm, retroperitoneal nodes, and serous surfaces of the abdominopelvic organs (Fig. 24.23).

Lymphatics

The lymphatic spread is to the draining lymph nodes namely para-aortic and superior gastric nodes. The pelvic nodes may be involved through utero-ovarian, round ligament and peritoneal permeation into the subperitoneal lymphatics (Table 24.30) external iliac, internal iliac, common iliac and inguinal nodes. **The left supraclavicular nodes are enlarged due to** obstruction of the efferent lymphatic channel of the nodes by the tumor emboli, as it enters the thoracic duct just prior to its drainage into the left subclavian vein.

TABLE 24.30: Lymph node involvement in ovarian malignancy (%).

Stage	*Para-aortic (%)*	*Pelvic (%)*
I and II	20	30
III and IV	65	67

Lateral lymphatic spread through the broad ligament to the pelvic nodes may occur. Retrograde lymphatic spread in advanced disease may occur to the inguinal nodes through the round ligament.

Lymphatics of peritoneal surfaces drain through the diaphragm. Other metastatic sites are: Peritoneum, omentum, liver, pleura (effusion) and the diaphragm.

Direct

After the capsule is broken, the spread occurs directly to the adjacent organs such as tubes, broad ligament, intestines, omentum, and uterus.

Hematogenous

The bloodstream metastasis is late and the involved organs are lungs, liver parenchyma, brain, bones, etc.

CLINICOPATHOLOGIC EXPLANATION

Ascites

Ascites is due to obstruction of peritoneal fluid outflow principally through the diaphragm. There is also increased transudation of serum across the peritoneal surfaces. The secretion is not from the tumor bearing peritoneum but from the tumor-free areas.

Liver

The involvement of liver parenchyma is usually blood-borne when the guts are involved.

Contralateral Ovary (Fig. 24.24)

The contralateral ovary is involved in majority of metastatic ovarian malignancy. Even in primary malignancy, the contralateral involvement may be due to retrograde

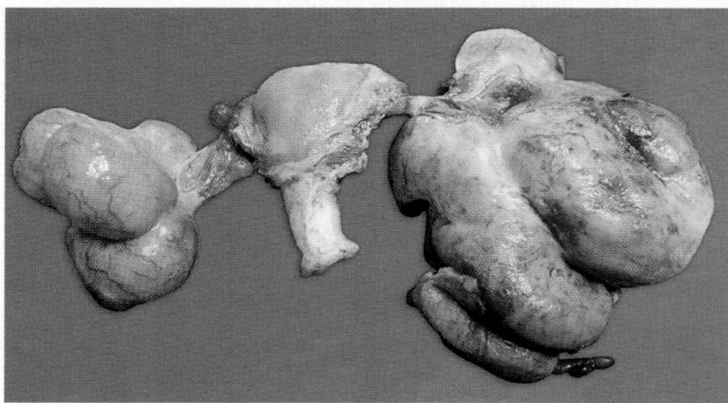

Fig. 24.24: Bilateral malignant epithelial tumors of the ovary. Both the ovaries are enlarged, lobulated in appearance with areas of hemorrhage and necrosis. Histology confirmed mucinous cystadenocarcinoma.

(*Courtesy:* Dr Biswajit Ghosh, Burnpur, WB)

lymphatic spread through para-aortic glands. Direct implantation or multicentric origin may also be a possibility.

Uterus

The body is mostly affected either due to lymphatics or through transtubal spread. The cervical involvement is rare.

Right-sided pleural effusion: More ascitic fluid reaches the right subdiaphragmatic space along the wider right paracolic gutter. This is facilitated by the increased negative suction created by liver during respiration. The fluid so collected can pass freely across the diaphragm. This is because of free communication of submesothelial network of lymphatic capillaries with the corresponding plexuses on the thoracic surface of the diaphragm underlying the pleura on the right side → right pleural effusion. Alternatively, there is more presence of wide pleuroperitoneal sinuses on the right side and hence producing right pleural effusion.

CLINICAL FEATURES

Patient Profile

Although no age is immune to ovarian malignancy, but about 60% of ovarian neoplasms in postmenopausal and about 20% in premenopausal women are malignant. There is increased association of nulliparity and with a family history.

Symptoms

In its **early stage**, ovarian carcinoma is a notoriously silent disease (asymptomatic). The presenting complaints are usually of short duration and insidious in onset. Symptoms are not specific.

- Feeling of abdominal distension and vague discomfort.
- Features of dyspepsia such as flatulence and eructations and pelvic pain.
- Loss of appetite with a sense of bloating after meals.
- In pre-existing tumor:
  - Appearance of dull aching pain and tenderness over one area.
  - Rapid enlargement of the tumor.

Gradually, more pronounced symptoms appear. These are:

- Abdominal swelling which may be rapid.
- Dull abdominal pain.
- Sudden loss of weight.
- Respiratory distress—may be mechanical due to ascites or due to pleural effusion.
- Menstrual abnormality is conspicuously absent except in functioning ovarian tumors (mentioned later in the Ch.).

Signs

The following are the findings in an established case of ovarian malignancy.

- **General examination reveals**
  - Cachexia and pallor of varying degree.
  - Jaundice may be evident in late cases.
  - Left supraclavicular lymph gland (Virchow's) may be enlarged (Fig. 24.25).
  - Edema leg or vulva is characteristic of malignant and not of benign neoplasm.
- **Per abdomen**
  - Liver may be enlarged, firm and nodular.
  - A mass is felt in the hypogastrium; too often it may be bilateral. It has got the following features (Table 21.4, p. 249):
    - Feel—solid or heterogeneous.
    - Mobility—mobile or restricted.
    - Tenderness—usually present.
    - Surfaces—irregular.
    - Margins—well-defined but the lower pole is usually not reached.
    - Percussion—usually dull over the tumor; may be resonant due to overlying intestinal adhesions.

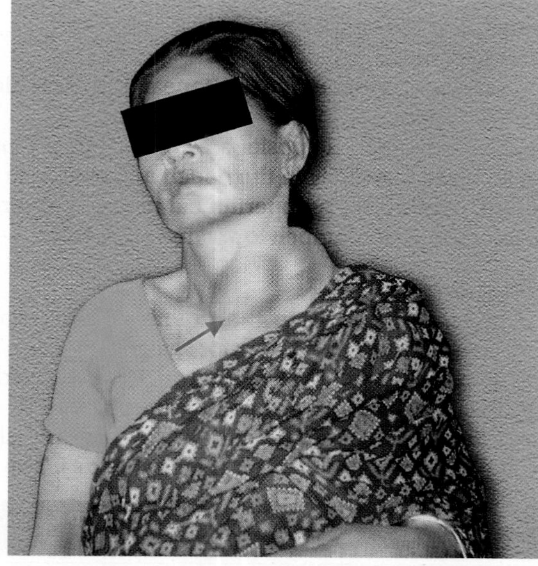

Fig. 24.25: Case of advanced ovarian malignancy with enlarged left supraclavicular glands (Virchow's gland).

(*Courtesy:* Professor S Pati, Dr A Halder, Associate Professor, Department of Gynecology and Obstetrics, NBMCH, Darjeeling)

- **Per vaginam**
  - The uterus may be separated from the mass felt per abdomen.
  - Nodules may be felt through the posterior fornix. If it is more than 1 cm, the diagnosis of malignancy is almost certain.

SPECIAL INVESTIGATIONS

Investigation aims at:

- To confirm malignancy preoperatively
- To identify the extent of lesion
- To detect the primary site.

To Confirm Malignancy

- Cytologic examination for detection of malignant cells is carried out from the fluid collected by abdominal paracentesis or "cul-de-sac" aspiration.
- Tumor marker: In epithelial carcinoma, there is no specific tumor marker. But, elevated CA-125 level >65 U/mL with a pelvic mass may be suggestive. Other biomarkers: HE4, CA-19-9, CA-15-3, OVXI may also be suggestive.

To Identify the Extent of Lesion

- **Straight X-ray** chest to exclude pleural effusion and chest metastasis.
- **Barium enema** to detect any colon or rectal cancer.
- **Cytologic examination** of thoracocentesis fluid.
- **Paracentesis** is done in women with ascites for malignant cell cytology.
- **Ultrasound imaging:** Features suggestive of malignancy are: Multiloculation with thick-walled septa, nodular areas (>6 cm), papillary surface projections or neovascularization (on Doppler study). It can be used to detect involvement of the omentum or contralateral ovary.
- **Computed tomography (CT)** is helpful for retroperitoneal lymph node assessment and detection of metastasis (liver, omentum). It helps in staging of ovarian carcinoma (Fig. 24.26).
- **Magnetic resonance imaging (MRI)** is helpful to determine the nature of ovarian neoplasm and also for the retroperitoneal lymph nodes and detection of metastasis. It can also detect recurrence of the tumor following initial treatment (Fig. 24.27).
- **Positron emission tomography (PET)** can differentiate normal tissues from cancerous tissues. It is more sensitive than CT or MRI (p. 101). CT/PET scans are especially useful for diagnosis of disease recurrence.
- **Intravenous pyelography**.
- Examination under anesthesia.
- Diagnostic uterine curettage.

To Detect the Primary Site

- Barium meal X-ray
- Gastroscopy/colonoscopy
- Mammography.

DIAGNOSIS

- Clinical
- Investigations
- Operative findings
- Histologic confirmation.

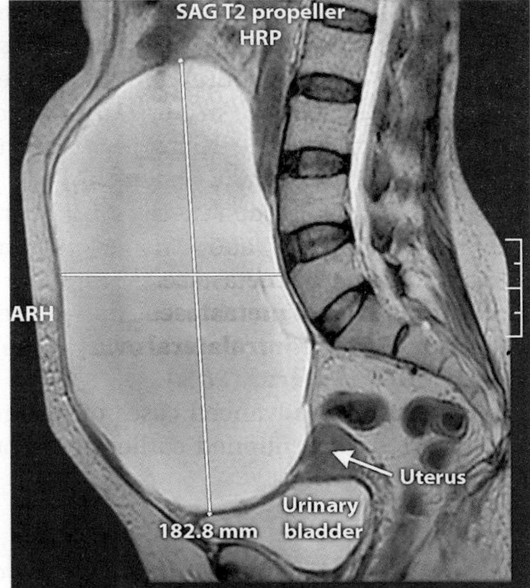

Fig. 24.26: MRI scan of a 47-year-old woman, showing a huge ovarian tumor. Sagittal view of the tumor is seen. Preoperative MRI can detect the anatomic regions that the tumor occupies and presence of any involvement of the surrounding organs and the nodal survey.

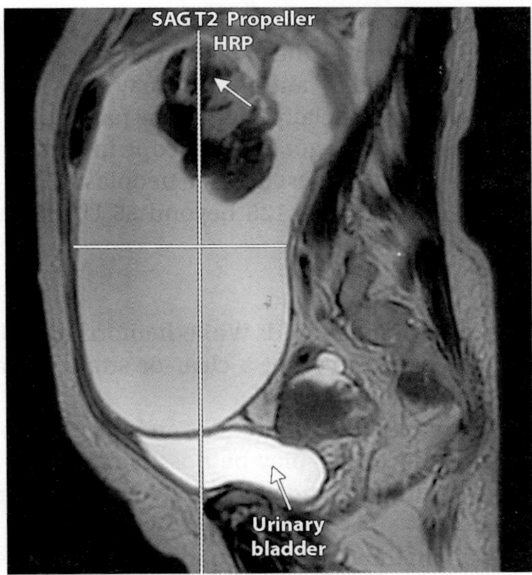

Fig. 24.27: Sagittal view of a MRI image of a 51-year-woman showing a large ovarian tumor. The tumor is heterogeneous in nature. MRI is a nonradioactive imaging modality with excellent soft tissue contrast resolution. It can detect metastatic deposits in liver, peritoneum and retroperitoneal nodes. Tumor showed a solid area in the upper part of the mass (*see* arrow). No lymph nodes are seen to be enlarged.

Clinical

Clinical diagnosis in early stage is very much deceptive because of:

- **No age specificity:** Although more prevalent beyond the age of 45 (40% of ovarian neoplasms are malignant), no age is immune to ovarian cancer. All physicians must be aware of the possible significance of persistent gastrointestinal symptoms in women over the age of 40 with a history of ovarian dysfunction.
- **No specific symptom:** It may remain asymptomatic in about 15% when first diagnosed.

- **Unrelated to duration of symptoms: Even with symptoms** of short duration may have extensive spread, conversely a long-standing tumor may remain benign.
- **Unrelated to the size of the tumor:** A big tumor may remain benign for a long time whereas, a small enlarged ovary may be found malignant.

The cumulative effects of such vagaries explain the fact that at the time of diagnosis, about 70% of patients with epithelial carcinomas have metastases outside the pelvis. **The most common sites of metastases are—peritoneum (85%), omentum (70%), contralateral ovary (70%), liver (35%), lung (25%) and uterus (20%).**

In established and/or advanced cases of malignancy, the clinical features as mentioned earlier are enough to arrive at a diagnosis.

Ancillary Aids

- **Detection of malignant cells** from the ascitic fluid collected by abdominal paracentesis or cul-de-sac aspiration is a positive proof of abdominal malignancies. When combined with presence of a pelvic mass almost confirms ovarian malignancy.
- **Noninvasive methods** such as MRI or CT scan have not yet proved to be much useful in diagnosis. Transvaginal sonography improves the detection rate (p. 100).
- Examination under anesthesia may be useful in doubtful cases, especially in an obese patient.
- Laparoscopy too has got limited scope in confirmation of malignancy. It can just detect a neoplasm.
- Elevation of serum CA 125 beyond 35 U/mL may be suggestive.

Operative Findings

- Nature of peritoneal fluid: While hemorrhagic fluid is very much suggestive but a clear or straw color fluid cannot rule out malignancy.
- Nature of the tumor: Differentiation between a benign and malignant tumor may be possible clinically, with laparotomy findings and with ultrasonographic criteria (p. 249).
- Metastatic nodules on the peritoneal surfaces and omentum.

Histological Diagnosis

All ovarian tumors irrespective of their nature must be subjected to histologic examination. This not only confirms the diagnosis but also identifies the type and grade of malignancy.

MANAGEMENT OF EPITHELIAL OVARIAN CANCER

- **Preventive**
- **Curative**

Preventive

Primary Prevention of Epithelial Ovarian Cancer

Prevention and risk reduction of ovarian cancer is done in three ways: (1) Surveillance; (2) Chemoprevention, (3) Risk reducing surgery.

1. **Surveillance:**
   - Tumor markers screening for ovarian cancer is currently done with serum CA-125, HEP4, OVX1. Multimodal screening (TVS and serum CA-125) and longitudinal biomarker algorithms rather than a predefined cut off value (CA-125 >35 IU/mL) is important.
   - Transvaginal ultrasonography
2. **Chemoprevention: Combined oral contraceptive pills** as a preventive (chemoprevention) measure is recommended to a woman especially belonging to Lynch type II families.
3. **Risk reducing surgery**
   - Opportunistic bilateral salpingectomy
   - Bilateral salpingectomy
   - Risk reducing salpingectomy and delayed oophorectomy in high risk women
   - Opportunistic salpingectomy in general population (family planning)
   - Salpingo-oophorectomy.
4. **Genetic screening for *BRCA1* and *BRCA2*** for women with high risk for ovarian and breast cancer.

The estimated lifetime risks of breast cancer with *BRCA1* and *BRCA2* mutation are 50% and 25% respectively.

Bilateral salpingo-oophorectomy in women following completed child bearing with BRCA mutation can reduce the risk of ovarian cancer significantly. It reduces the risk of breast cancer also.

Guidelines for Management of an Enlarged Ovary

- An ovarian enlargement of 8 cm during childbearing period deserves careful follow up.
- In postmenopausal women, any ovarian enlargement should be assessed by serum CA-125 and transvaginal sonography.
- Cysts that are simple, unilocular, ≤8 cm in diameter with normal serum CA-125—can be managed conservatively. Women should be under follow up with ultrasound scan and serum CA-125 at an interval of 4 months.
- Early laparotomy is indicated in following cases:
  - The ovary enlarges progressively beyond 8 cm while under observation.
  - Any symptomatic ovarian tumor regardless of size.

Secondary Prevention (Screening for Ovarian Cancer)

Natural history of the disease is unknown. There is no preinvasive stage like that of cervical intraepithelial neoplasia. As such, screening aims at detecting early ovarian malignancy in asymptomatic women. Till date no specific method of screening for early detection of epithelial ovarian cancer is available.

Screening procedures

- **Clinical:** Regular and periodic clinical examination of the 'high risk' group is done (Table 24.31). Bimanual pelvic examination in an asymptomatic woman may detect an adnexal mass. However, clinical examination is not very specific.

TABLE 24.31: Women with 'high risk' factors for ovarian cancer.

- **Age** group 40–60 years
- **Familial cancers**: Breast, endometrial, ovarian, colorectal
- **History** of removal of benign ovarian tumor or breast carcinoma
- Women with *BRCA1* and *BRCA2* mutation
- Postmenopausal palpable ovary (volume >8 cm^3)
- Nulliparity
- Early menarche, late menopause
- Relative or absolute infertility
- Dysgenetic gonad
- Fertility drugs use (incessant ovulation)
- Women with BMI >30
- Women workers in asbestos related industries
- Pelvic inflammatory disease

TABLE 24.32: Clinical association of raised serum CA-125.

Cancer	Disease	Others
Ovarian (serous)	Endometriosis	Normal (1%)
Peritoneal, tubal	Peritonitis	Pregnancy
Colon, uterine	Pancreatitis	Mid menstruation
Breast, lung	PID	
Stomach, lung, liver	Leiomyomata	

- **Tumor markers:** CA-125 (Table 24.32) is a glycoprotein, which has been used for screening of epithelial (nonmucinous) cancers of the ovary. Value more than 35 U/mL is suggestive of epithelial ovarian cancer. It is also used for monitoring a patient during chemotherapy and for follow up. But it is not a tumor specific antigen. There are several other conditions, where level of CA-125 is raised.
- **Multimodal screening** (serum CA-125 and TVS) is important. Longitudinal biomarker algorithms rather than a predefined cut off value (>35 IU mL) is more important (UKCTOCS - 2018).

The serum level of CA-125 falls after surgical resection of the tumor or following chemotherapy. Elevated level indicates bulky residual disease or tumor recurrence or resistant clones to chemotherapy. Serum half-life of CA-125 is 20 days.

HE 4 (Human Epididymis 4 protein) is elevated in the serum of woman with serous epithelial ovarian cancer. It is useful in the early stage ovarian cancer. Combination of CA-125 and HE 4 biomarkers study is superior to any other marker in the diagnosis and management of ovarian serous cancers.

Other tumor markers are: Macrophage colony-stimulating factors (M-CSF), OVXI, HER-2/neu, and inhibin.

- **Ultrasound imaging:** Transvaginal color Doppler imaging has been able to differentiate benign from malignant tumors by assessment of its vascular supply and intratumoral blood flow. Increased neoangiogenesis in ovarian malignancy causes central neovascularity. Study of **vascular parameters,** e.g. pulsatility index (PI) <1.0 or resistive index (RI) <0.4 increases the risk of malignancy.

Three-dimensional, contrast enhanced, power Doppler sonography is found to be more diagnostic.
- **Opportunistic bilateral salpingectomy** at the time of surgery for benign adenexal disease or hysterectomy.
- **Risk of malignancy index (RMI): RMI = U × M × CA 125**; U = USG score (one point each for: Multilocular cyst; solid areas; metastasis; ascites; bilateral lesions), M = 3 (postmenopausal women) and CA-125 level in U/mL. The risk of cancer is 75% when the RMI value is > 250.
- **Genetic testing (p. 437).**

PROTECTIVE FACTORS FOR OVARIAN MALIGNANCY

- Combined oral contraceptives
- Pregnancy
- Tubal ligation, hysterectomy
- Breastfeeding
- Low fat and high fiber diet
- DMPA

TREATMENT OF MALIGNANT OVARIAN TUMOR

- **Surgery**
- **Chemotherapy**
- **Radiotherapy**
- **Combined therapy**

Surgical Treatment of Ovarian Cancer

Surgery is the keystone in the primary treatment of ovarian malignancy.

The aims are:
- To stage the disease (staging laparotomy) accurately, thereby allowing better choice of adjuvant therapy and a better assessment of prognosis.
- To perform effective surgical removal.

Surgical Staging for Ovarian Malignancy

- Methods
  - Laparotomy
  - Laparoscopy
  - Laparoscopic assisted robotic sugary
- Procedures
  - **Omentectomy:** From transverse colon
  - **Cytoreduction:** Maximum to reduce the residual disease <1 cm.

Practical Guidelines

- **Liberal vertical incision** to minimize chance of rupture of the tumor and to facilitate better exploration.
- **To note the character of the ascitic fluid**, if any, and to collect sample for cytology. If appreciable fluid is not available, then a sample of peritoneal wash with 100 mL saline in the subdiaphragmatic area and paracolic gutter is to be collected.
- **A systematic (visual and manual) exploration (clock wise)**—palpation of liver, gastrointestinal tract, subdiaphragmatic area, omentum, and para-aortic lymph nodes. This is done in a clockwise fashion starting from the cecum.
- **Pelvic exploration**—nature of the tumor, extent of adhesions, condition of the contralateral ovary, uterus and tubes, and palpation of pelvic lymph nodes.
- **Any metastatic deposit** over the peritoneal surfaces, under surface of the diaphragm should be **biopsied**.

TABLE 24.33: Commonly used regimen for chemotherapy in cases with ovarian epithelial cancer.

Drug	Dose	In fusion time	Cycle	Interval	Toxicity
Carboplatin or	400 mg/m^2 or AUC 5	1 hour	6 cycles	3 weeks	Nephrotoxic, neurotoxic, myelosuppression
Paclitaxel or	175 mg/m^2	3 hour	6 cycles	3 weeks	Neurotoxic, myelosuppression
Docetaxel	75 mg/m^2	1 hour	6 cycles	3 week	Neurotoxic (less), myelosuppression

Pelvic and para-aortic lymph node sampling should be done.

- **In the absence of any metastatic disease**, multiple peritoneal biopsy, scraping from the diaphragm for cytology should be taken. Occult metastasis has been found in about 10–40% of early stage (stage I and II) epithelial ovarian cancer.

Primary Surgery

- **Early stage disease (Stage Ia, G1, G2):**
  - **Young woman** → unilateral oophorectomy (fertility sparing surgery) → routine follow up and monitoring → completion of family → removal of the uterus and the other ovary.
  - **Elderly woman** → hysterectomy and bilateral salpingo-oophorectomy.
  - **In stage Ia, G3 disease and others stage I diseases:** Staging laparotomy → hysterectomy and bilateral salpingo-oophorectomy. Chemotherapy is considered for most patients.
- **Advanced stage disease:** Exploratory laparotomy → **cytoreductive or debulking surgery.** This includes: Total abdominal hysterectomy bilateral salpingo-oophorectomy, complete omentectomy, retroperitoneal lymph node sampling and resection of any metastatic tumor (Figs. 38.64A to C). **Optimum cytoreductive surgery** is aimed to reduce the residual tumor load ≤1–2 cm in diameter. Lesser the residual tumor (optimally debulked) volume (<1 cm), better is the survival.

Maximum cytoreductive surgery may need resection of a segment of bowel, bladder or the lymph nodes. Removal of omental cake by cytoreductive surgery improves the result of subsequent chemotherapy or radiotherapy. Surgery includes resection of large volume diaphragmatic disease. Diaphragmatic stripping, resection of diaphragm full thickness or half thickness, splenectomy, hepatic resection for parenchymal metastatic disease, bowel resection need to be done. Place of retroperitoneal lymphadenectomy is yet to be decided. Appendectomy is done in cases with mucinous ovarian cancer.

ADJUVANT CHEMOTHERAPY

- **In stage Ia (Grade I)** epithelial carcinoma → no adjuvant chemotherapy.
- **In all other stage I disease** → adjuvant chemotherapy with carboplatin and paclitaxel for six cycles.
- **Advanced stage disease.**
  - **Chemotherapy:** Chemotherapy is used widely following surgery to improve the result in terms of survival. Drugs are given for five or six cycles at 3–4 weekly interval (p. 427).
  - **Combination chemotherapy:** Paclitaxel (175 mg/m^2) and carboplatin (400 mg/m^2) are commonly used (Table 24.33).

    Carboplatin is excreted by the kidney. Its effective serum concentration is calculated from Calvert formula. Carboplatin total dose = Desired AUC (area under the curve) × (GFR + 25); AUC value of 5 to 7.5.

  Patients who are hypersensitive to paclitaxel, topotecan 1 mg/m^2 for 1–3 days, every 3 weeks or Gemcitabine 800 mg/m^2, every 3 weeks is given (p. 433
- **Platinum compounds (cisplatin, carboplatin) are the most effective drugs** in terms of tumor response and survival rate. Like alkylating agents they cause cross linkage of DNA strands. **They can be used either singly (Table 24.34) or in combination with paclitaxel (*see* below).**
- **Taxane derivatives** (paclitaxel, docetaxel) are found to be very effective in ovarian cancer (p. 433). Paclitaxel is derived from the bark of the pacific yew tree. Docetaxel is semisynthetic and its side effects are less (peripheral neuropathy). Taxane derivatives prevent cell division by polymerization of microtubules and making them excessively stable. They are found to be effective even in cisplatin resistant ovarian cancer. **Paclitaxel is recommended as the primary treatment of all epithelial ovarian cancer following optimal cytoreductive surgery.**
- **Combination chemotherapy:** Drugs acting in different ways on the cell cycle (p. 433), with different toxicities, are combined. Therefore efficacy is expected to be more and chance of drug resistance is low. **Currently paclitaxel and carboplatin combination chemotherapy is found to have better survival rate in advanced ovarian cancer (Table 24.33).**

Efficacy of **docetaxel** has been found similar to paclitaxel. **Gemcitabine** or **Topotecan** has got similar efficacy (p. 433).

The recommended drugs and doses for chemotherapy of ovarian carcinoma (CAP and CP) are discussed below.

Drugs: Combining paclitaxel, carboplatin either with gemcitabine or pregylated liposomal dexorubicin are used. It is found to be toxic.

- **Maintenance therapy** with agents like pazopanib, oral tyrosine kinase inhibitor (TK1) of VEGFR, PDGFR,

TABLE 24.34: Recommended drugs and doses used as a single agent.

Drug	Dose	Route	Cycle	Interval
Cisplatin	75 mg/m^2	IV	6	4 weeks
Carboplatin	400 mg/m^2	IV	6	4 weeks
Paclitaxel	175 mg/m^2	IV	6	4 weeks
Docetaxel	75 mg/m^2	IV	6	4 weeks

FGFR and poly-ADP (ribose) polymerase (PRAP) inhibitors have been tried (p. 432).

- **Platinum resistence disease** may be treated with: Pegylated liposomal doxorubicin (PRD), topotecan, gemcitabine, etoposide, docetaxel or paclitaxel.
- **Intraperitoneal chemotherapy** is used only for minimal (<2 cm) or microscopic residual disease. The drugs can penetrate only few millimeters. Moreover, serum levels are similar to those seen after IV chemotherapy. Currently both platinum (cisplatin) and taxanes (docetaxel) are used. There is distinct benefit of intraperitoneal cisplatin and docetaxel over their intravenous use.

Primary chemotherapy for advanced ovarian cancer is done either by IV (docetaxel or paclitaxel and carboplatin) or by intraperitoneal chemotherapy to improve the overall survival.

- **Neoadjuvant chemotherapy (NACT) and interval cytoreductive surgery:** Biopsy confirmation is done before chemotherapy.
- **Interval debulking surgery (IDS):** Patients with a advanced stage (stage III and IV) disease, often are at increased risk of primary surgery. 3–4 cycles of NACT followed by IDS and additional chemotherapy are found to improve the survival outcome.

Indications of NACT are:

- Advanced epithelial ovarian cancer (as in imaging studies).
- High risk for surgery.
- Associated comorbid conditions (pleural effusion).
- Predicted (imaging studies) to be suboptimally resected.
  Patient should have histological diagnosis of the tumor (biopsy).
- Following a failed attempt of primary surgery.

Benefits of neoadjuvant chemotherapy are:

- Rapid clinical improvement.
- Subsequent surgery is easier and morbidity is reduced
- Optimum cytoreduction with minimal residual disease may be possible (Flowchart 24.2).
- **Radiotherapy:** There is very little scope of radiotherapy as an adjunct to surgery because of the advent of chemotherapy.
- **Radioactive isotopes (p. 426):** In early cases of ovarian cancer, radioactive phosphorus (^{32}P) is instilled into the peritoneal cavity. The isotopes are taken up by macrophages and the radiation effects are limited to superficial 4–6 mm of peritoneal lining. ^{32}P acts by emitting β-rays. Bowel complications are increased.
- **Hormone therapy:** Tamoxifen, leuprolide acetate (GnRH agonist), aromatase inhibitors are being studied in relapsed cases of ovarian tumor.
- **Immunotherapy:** With the use of *Corynebacterium parvum* and BCG cytokines, interferon or interleukin-2 is under trial. Herceptin, an antibody, when used along with chemotherapy improves the response rate (p. 436). All patients need to be followed up after completion of treatment. Serum level of CA-125 is reviewed. CT evaluation may be needed when there is suspicion of recurrent disease (50–90%).
- **Gene and molecular therapy** (page 437).
- **Fertility sparing surgery (FSS):** Could be done in selected cases when the disease is confined to one ovary (stage IA). Unilateral adnexectomy has got excellent long-term survival. Postoperative chemotherapy may be needed in a few without an adverse effect to these child bearing.

Flowchart 24.2: Management outline for ovarian carcinoma

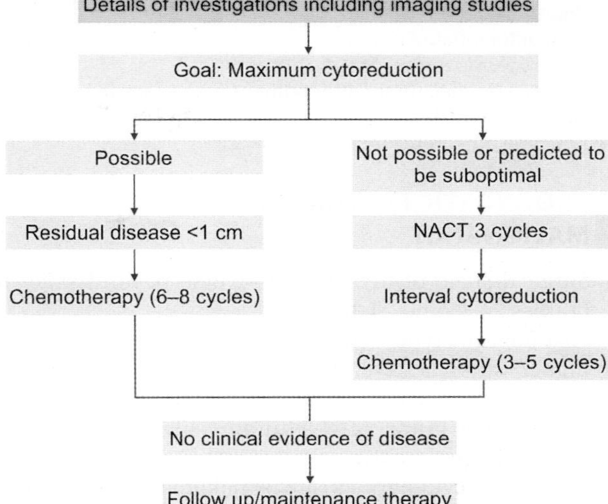

PLACE OF UNILATERAL SALPINGO-OOPHORECTOMY (FSS)

- Tumor confined to one ovary
- Disease stage IA G1
- Capsule intact
- Contralateral ovary clinically normal
- Negative peritoneal washing
- Negative omental biopsy
- Young woman, fertility desired
- Strongly motivated for follow up

Secondary cytoreductive surgery may be done in some selected cases following completion of first line chemotherapy. Selected cases are: (a) Tumor sensitive to platinum based chemotherapy; (b) Prolonged disease free interval; (c) Isolated site recurrence; (d) Absence of ascites; (e) Following initial subopitimal debulking procedure.

REASONS FOR POOR OUTCOME IN OVARIAN CANCER

- Late diagnosis
- No preinvasive stage of the disease
- No effective screening procedure
- No correlation of symptoms with the tumor size
- Extent of tumor spread is often unknown
- Limitations of cytoreductive surgery
- Variable chemosensitivity
- Radiation dose restriction by neighboring organs
- Tumor cells are freely mobile within the peritoneal cavity

A laparoscopy prior to laparotomy is advised. Currently, CT, MRI, and serum CA-125 are being evaluated as an alternative to second look laparotomy. Better survival rate following second look surgery is however questionable.

FAVORABLE PROGNOSTIC FACTORS

- Younger age
- Well differentiated tumor
- Small volume tumor
- Minimal residual tumor after primary cytoreductive surgery
- Absence of ascites
- Cell type other mucinous and clear cell

PROGNOSTIC FACTORS IN OVARIAN MALIGNANCY

- Surgical stage of the disease—worse beyond stage II (Tables 24.35 and 24.36).
- Histological type—endometrioid tumor has got a higher survival rate than serous type because the former tumor is highly well-differentiated.
- Histological grade of the tumor—higher the grade, poorer the prognosis.
- Peritoneal cytology—positive malignant cells, higher the risk.
- Presence of ascites—higher the risk.
- Presence of metastatic disease before cytoreductive surgery—poor the prognosis and shorter the survival.
- Volume of residual tumor after primary surgery—when <5 mm better the prognosis.
- Ploidy status—diploid tumors are prognostically better compared to aneuploid tumors.
- Degree of oncogene expression (p. 431, Ch. 31).

TABLE 24.35: Epithelial ovarian cancer (NIC – 2011C).

Stage	*5-year survival (%)*
Localized (confined to primary site)	92
Regional (regional nodes involved)	72
Distant (metastasis)	27
Unstaged	22

TABLE 24.36: Carcinoma of the ovary 5-year survival rate (FIGO stage).

Stage	*5-year survival rate (%)*
IA	94
IB	92
IC	85
IIA	78
IIB	73
IIIA	59
IIIB	52
IIIC	39
IV	17

PRIMARY PERITONEAL CARCINOMA

Papillary serous carcinoma of the peritoneum is a rare type of primary peritoneal adenocarcinoma (PPA). It constitutes 7–20% of all epithelial ovarian carcinoma.

Criteria for Diagnosis of PPA (GOG – 1993)

- The ovaries are either absent or physiologically normal in size (<4 cm diameter).
- Extraovarian sites are more involved than that of the ovarian surfaces.
- Microscopically, the ovaries are either not involved or exhibit cortical implants <5 mm in depth. There no stromal involvement.
- The histologic and cytologic tumor character is serous type. FIGO staging for ovarian carcinoma is followed. Management is according to ovarian carcinoma grade and staging. Prognosis is similar to that of epithelial ovarian cancer.
- When it is not possible to designate the primary site for ovarian, fallopian tube and peritoneal cancer, it defined as "undesignated".

GERM CELL TUMORS OF THE OVARY

Germ cell tumors constitute about 15–20% of all ovarian neoplasms and they are the second common ovarian tumors. For classification page 241. They have got varying degrees of malignant potentiality. Mature cystic teratoma (dermoid cyst) is the most common germ cell ovarian tumor (95%) and it is benign. Germ cell tumors have the following feature: (1) Occur predominantly in children and young adults. (2) Most are early stage disease, and (3) Usually have good prognosis due to chemoresponsiveness; (4) Fertility sparing surgery may be possible. About 5% of these tumors are malignant. They arise from embryonic germ cells.

IMMATURE TERATOMA

Immature teratomas are derived from the three germ layers — ectoderm, mesoderm and endoderm. These are less common and constitute 35% ovarian teratomas. **It is the most common germ cell malignancies.** It is commonly (50%) seen in women between the ages of 10 and 20 years and rarely seen after menopause. Immature teratomas are almost never bilateral.

Pathology

Varying grades of undifferentiated tissue elements are present. Prognosis depends on the quantity of immature neural tissue elements. The prognosis of immature teratoma depends mainly on the tumor grade and the stage of the disease. Grade 3 tumor has poor prognosis. Serum AFP and LDH levels may be raised. Other tumor markers: CA-125, CA 19-9, CEA are to be done. Mature teratoma carries excellent prognosis.

Treatment

Unilateral oophorectomy with surgical staging is the optimum treatment when the tumor is confined to one ovary. For elderly women hysterectomy and bilateral salpingo-oophorectomy is ideal. **Adjuvant chemotherapy** for patients beyond stage Ia GI is indicated. BEP (*see above*) is preferred, though VAC regimen is also effective.

DYSGERMINOMA

Dysgerminoma is the second most common (33%) malignant germ cell tumor. It arises from undifferentiated form of germ cells. It is often (5%) associated with dysgenetic gonad (Ch. 28). The counterpart of dysgerminoma in male is seminoma. Majority (75%) of the tumors occur before the age of 30 years.

hCG assays are often positive, confusing the diagnosis with pregnancy. It may coexist with pregnancy (20–30%). Dysgerminoma may be associated with choriocarcinoma or endodermal sinus tumor. **Tumor markers** LDH, hCG, lactate dehydrogenase (LDH) may be positive. Karyotyping is needed (presence of Y chromosome) especially when a premenarchal girl presents with a pelvic mass.

Pathology

The shape is usually round or oval and is usually 5–15 cm in diameter; feel is boggy, at times, it is firm rubbery. It may be bilateral (10–20%). Cut section shows pink or yellow color. Microscopic appearance reveals uniform large round cells (monotonous pattern), arranged in cords or clumps with abundant clear cytoplasm. Nuclei are large, irregular, and hyperchromatic with varying degree of mitosis. There is intense infiltration of lymphocytes and plasma cells in the fibrous septum (Fig. 24.28). Lymphocytic infiltration indicates favorable prognosis. In more than 50%, they are potentially malignant.

Clinical features are not specific for the tumor.

Treatment

Majority (75%) of dysgerminomas are confined to one ovary and are stage I at the time of diagnosis.

In a young patient where preservation of fertility is desired, laparotomy for surgical staging should be done. Conservative surgery, unilateral salpingo-oophorectomy may done in early stage I disease. Routine biopsy of normal contralateral ovary should be avoided. The tumor

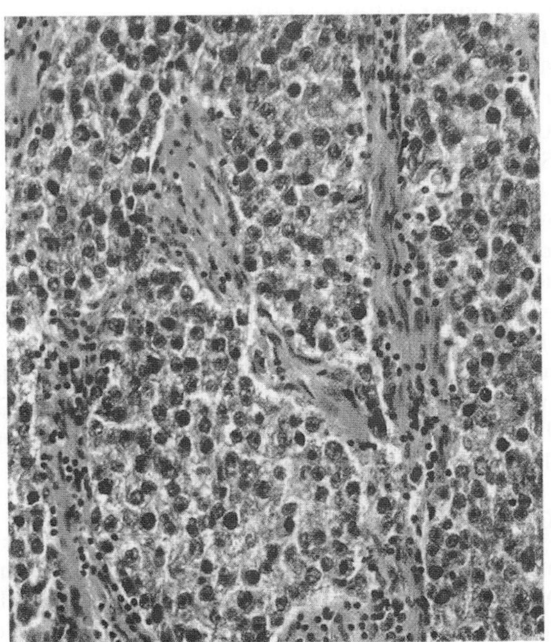

Fig. 24.28: Histologic picture of dysgerminoma cells are mostly uniform (monotonous pattern) in size. The stroma is dense with lymphocytic infiltrate.

TABLE 24.37: Recommended drugs and doses of chemotherapy (BEP, VBP).

Drugs	*Dose*	*Schedule*
Bleomycin (B)	15 units/m^2	Every week
Etoposide (E)	100 mg/m^2	On days 1–3, every 4 weeks
Cisplatin (P)	100 mg/m^2	Every 3 weeks
Vinblastin (V)	12 mg/m^2	Every 3 weeks
Drugs are given IV for 3–4 cycles, combinations used are BEP and VBP		

is sensitive to both chemotherapy and radiotherapy. **Systemic chemotherapy is the treatment of choice, where fertility is to be preserved, even in the presence of metastatic disease.**

Different chemotherapeutic agents are used either singly or in combination (Ch. 31) (Table 24.37). Carboplatin 400 mg/m^2, IV, every 4 weeks, for 6 courses have been used as a single agent therapy where the tumor has been removed completely. BEP (bleomycin, etoposide, and cisplatin), **VBP** (vinblastin, bleomycin, and cisplatin), **VAC** (vincristine, actinomycin, and cyclophosphamide) are the commonly used drugs for the germ cell tumors. The most effective chemotherapeutic regimens used are BEP, VBP and VAC (Table 24.34 and p. 433). Combination chemotherapy has significantly improved the survival rate.

Patient with Y chromosome as detected on karyotyping should have both the ovaries (gonads) removed.

Radiotherapy: Loss of fertility is a problem with radiation therapy. So, radiation therapy is not used in young patients.

Recurrent disease is treated either with combination chemotherapy or radiation therapy. Combination chemotherapy with POMB-ACE (vincristine, bleomycin, methotrexate, cisplatin, etoposide, actinomycin D, and cyclophosphamide) is preferred (p. 433). Radiation therapy is considered for patients who had been treated with combination chemotherapy earlier.

Overall survival following unilateral oophorectomy in early stage (stage Ia) disease 100% and following cisplatin-based combination chemotherapy in advanced disease is 75%.

ENDODERMAL SINUS TUMOR

These tumors arise from the primitive yolk sac.

It is observed mostly between 15 and 20 years of age. **It is the third common (20%) malignant germ cell tumor of the ovary.** Yolk sac tumors are unilateral and are usually solid, more than 10 cm in diameter.

Characteristic histological feature is the presence of cystic spaces lined by flattened epithelium. Within this space a tuft of vascular tissue is often seen. This is called **Schiller-Duval body**. Eosinophilic, hyaline bodies containing alpha fetoprotein and other proteins are also constant microscopic features. Tumor markers are AFP and LDH.

It is highly malignant and spreads to the adjacent structures rapidly. It is usually solid and cut section shows gelatinous or hemorrhagic areas. It is composed of yolk sac endoderm and extraembryonic mesoblasts. Association with dysgerminoma should be kept in mind. Yolk sac tumor patient may present with acute abdomen as these tumors are friable, necrotic and often hemorrhagic serum tumor markers are AFP and LDH.

Treatment

Surgical staging and unilateral salpingo-oophorectomy is generally the treatment of choice. All patients need subsequent chemotherapy. Total hysterectomy and contralateral salpingo-oophorectomy do not improve the prognosis in any way.

Chemotherapy: Routine use of combination chemotherapy has improved the survival significantly. Different combination regimens (VAC, VPB and POMB–ACE) are used (p. 427, 428). Combinations containing platinum-based compounds are associated with better response and survival. Overall 5 year disease specific survival for stage I disease is below 93%.

The tumor produces alpha fetoprotein which is an useful marker (serum level above 20 µg/mL) to monitor regression and detect recurrence.

NONGESTATIONAL OVARIAN CHORIOCARCINOMA

Ovarian choriocarcinoma may be gestational, arising from ovarian pregnancy or metastases from the uterine choriocarcinoma. It may be nongestational arising from one element of a solid teratoma. Pure nongestational choriocarcinoma of the ovary is extremely rare. Most patients present before 20 years of age. Isosexual precocious puberty is common (50%). It consists of both cytotrophoblasts and syncytiotrophoblasts and **secretes gonadotropins (hCG) which is utilized as a marker** in diagnosis and follow up. Nongestational choriocarcinoma is differentiated from gestational choriocarcinoma only by the absence of paternal DNA in the tumor.

Unlike gestational choriocarcinoma, it is not so sensitive to methotrexate. As such, surgery is the primary treatment to be followed by chemotherapy. Combination chemotherapy (MAC, BEP) have been used. Prognosis is poor.

Embryonal carcinoma: Constitutes 4% of all malignant ovarian germ cell tumors. It is seen at a mean age of 15 years. It is a highly aggressive malignant ovarian tumor. The serum tumor markers are AFP, hCG and estrogen. Histology show solid sheets of large polygonal cells with pale eosinophilic cytoplasm with a syncytial pattern.

GONADOBLASTOMA

It is a rare ovarian tumor. It consists of germ cells and gonadal stromal cells. Dysgerminoma is present in 50% of cases. Patients often present with primary amenorrhea, virilism or genital abnormalities. Karyotype is usually 45,X or 46,XX/46,XY. It is bilateral in 30% of cases.

Treatment is surgical removal of the tumor and also the contralateral ovary. Prognosis is excellent.

MIXED GERM CELL TUMORS

Presence of more than one germ cell element (at least two) is considered in this group. Dysgerminoma is the most common (70–80%) tissue element, other is yolk sac tumor. Serum markers for hCG, AFP are to be estimated. Complete surgery followed by chemotherapy (VBP, MAC or VAC) is advised.

Chemotherapy in Germ Cell Tumor

Combination chemotherapy has improved the survival following conservative surgery in advanced malignant germ cell tumors of the ovary. Patients with advanced stage-IA grade I disease need close follow up only. Following combination regimens have been used most commonly. BEP (bleomycin, etoposide, and cisplatin), VBP (vinblastin, bleomycin, and cisplatin) MAC (methotrexate, actinomycin-D, and cyclophosphamide), VAC (vincristine, actinomycin-D, and cyclophosphamide) and POMB-ACE (cisplatin, vincristine, methotrexate, bleomycin, actinomycin-D, cyclophosphamide and etoposide). For details p. 433.

Menstrual function, fertility and other endocrine functions have been found to be normal following use of these drugs.

SEX CORD STROMAL TUMORS

Types

- **Granulosa cell tumors (70%)**
- **Thecomas, fibromas**
- **Sertoli-Leydig cell tumors (androblastoma)**
- **Gynandroblastoma (mixed)**
- **Unclassified.**

Sex cord stromal tumors (SCSTs) constitute 6–10% of all ovarian neoplasms. Peak incidence is over the age of 50. Patients with these tumors often present with features of excess estrogen or androgen. SCSTs are generally confined to one ovary. Majority have slow rate of growth and low malignant potential. **Surgical excision** is the primary treatment. Chemotherapy is less required. **Overall prognosis** of ovarian SCST is excellent. Commonly evaluated **tumor markers** for ovarian SCSTs with malignant potential are inhibin A and B, estrodiol and αFP. They are also known as *'functioning tumors.'*

GRANULOSA CELL TUMORS

Granulosa cell tumors constitute 2% of all ovarian neoplasms. Nearly 70% of all ovarian SCSTs are granulosa cell tumors. Adult form is about 95% and juvenile is 5%. The tumor originates from the 'rests' of primitive granulosa cells unused in folliculogenesis. **It is the most common ovarian stromal tumor.**

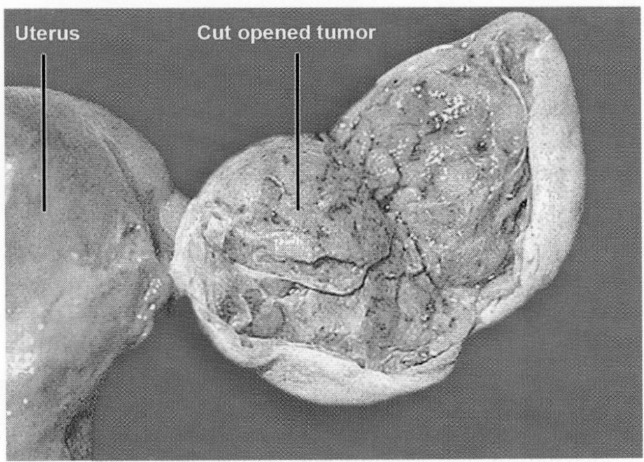

Fig. 24.29: Granulosa cell tumor. Left sided ovary cut opened to show the tumor. Histology confirmed granulosa cell tumor.

It is bilateral only in 2% of cases and is a slow growing tumor. The size varies, so also the consistency—may be solid or cystic. **Cut section** is characteristically yellow or orange (Fig. 24.29) due to its lipid content.

Microscopic Appearance (Fig. 24.30)

The cells are round or polygonal with granular eosinophilic cytoplasm with ill-defined borders. The tumor cell nuclei are variable in size but they are pale, usually grooved or folded and are called **"Coffee bean" nuclei.** Some cells are luteinized containing large polyhedral lipid cells. The cells are arranged in a number of architectural pattern but commonly in folliculoid type. The granulosa cells are arranged in small clusters around a central cavity. These structures are called **Call-Exner bodies and are pathognomonic of granulosa cell tumor.** The juvenile tumor has less number of Call-Exner bodies and less number of "Coffee bean" nuclei compared to the adult

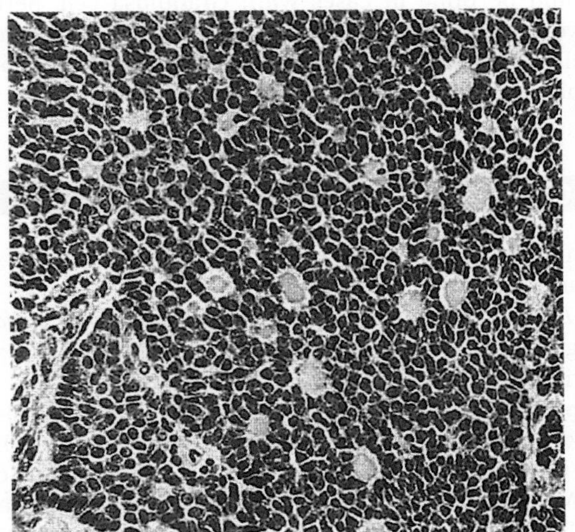

Fig. 24.30: Histologic picture of granulosa cell tumor. Presence of Call-Exner bodies (microfollicular pattern) are diagnostic.

variety. The tumor cells secrete **inhibin (inhibin B)** and it is an useful marker for the disease (see Tumour Markers).

The tumor produces estrogen and AMH. There may be associated endometrial hyperplasia (50%). Unopposed estrogenic stimulation leads to development of endometrial carcinoma in about 5–10% of cases.

Clinical Features

It occurs in all ages, 10% prior to puberty, 40% during child-bearing period, and 50% in postmenopausal women. Apart from the nonspecific features due to tumor mass, it produces **effects caused by hyperestrinism which differs with ages.** These tumors infrequently secrete androgens and may cause virilization.

- **Prior to puberty:** Precocious puberty—commonly iso sexual (p. 40).
- **Childbearing period:** Abnormal uterine bleeding.
- **Postmenopausal:** Bleeding. Associated endometrial hyperplasia or adenocarcinoma is present in 20–30% of cases.

The features of precocious puberty revert back to normal after removal of the tumor. Patient may present with **acute abdomen as** these tumors have the propensity to rupture.

Treatment

Laparotomy and surgical staging is done. Unilateral salpingo-oophorectomy is the optimum treatment for children or women in the reproductive age. Metastatic disease and recurrences have been treated with BEP chemotherapeutic regimens. Overall prognosis is good. Overall 5-year survival rate for stage I disease is about 95%. Life time follow up is essential as recurrence can occur as late as 30 years.

THECOMA-FIBROMA GROUP

Thecoma is predominantly a lesion of postmenopausal age. It may occur as a distinct entity or mixed with granulosa cell tumor. External appearance looks like a fibroma. Cut surface shows islands of yellow tissue separated by gray fibrous septa (Fig. 24.31). Microscopic picture reveals cells like that of cortical stroma with areas of granulosa cells.

Due to excess **estrogen** (tumor marker) production, there is endometrial hyperplasia and often associated with endometrial carcinoma. It is responsible for postmenopausal bleeding. Rarely, it may cause ascites or Meig's syndrome. Often the thecal cells are luteinized. These luteinized thecal cells are either inactive or may produce androgens to induce masculinization.

Treatment

It is surgical removal—total hysterectomy with bilateral salpingo-oophorectomy. In younger age group, conservative surgery may be employed considering the fact that it is mostly benign.

Fibroma in the ovary is usually observed in the postmenopausal women. It is derived from the stromal cells

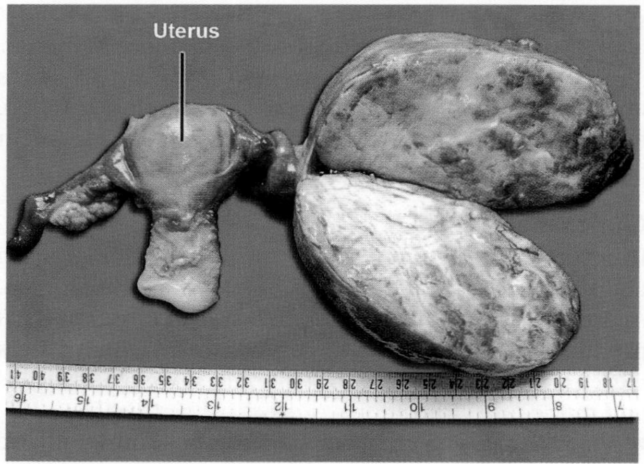

Fig. 24.31: Photograph of a surgical specimen from a 49-year-old woman who suffered abnormal uterine bleeding. The specimen had been halved to show the solid nature of the tumor. Histology revealed thecoma-fibroma.

and are similar to thecomas. Less than 10% are bilateral. Meig's syndrome (ascites, pleural effusion, and ovarian fibroma) is seen in about 1% of cases (p. 241, 545). Excision of fibromas is usually the treatment especially in young women. Fibromas showing increased cellularity and pleomorphic features and mitotic activity may be of low malignant potential. Fibrosarcoma is found in about 1% of cases.

SERTOLI-LEYDIG CELL TUMOR (ANDROBLASTOMA, ARRHENOBLASTOMA)

Sertoli-Leydig cell tumor is very rare and accounts for less than 0.5% of all ovarian tumors and less than 5% of all SCSTs.

They probably arise from the male directed cell rests in the hilum of the ovary, from granulosa cells or from teratomas. The tumor produces predominantly androgens (80%) and, in some cases estrogen 80%. Other tumor markers are: Inhibin and AFP. 80% are stage 1 and most are benign.

The tumors are small, usually unilateral (90%) and solid in consistency. Cut surface shows yellowish tinge with areas of hemorrhage and necrosis. Microscopic picture often resembles to various testicular cells such as Sertoli and Leydig cells. Immunostaining is invaluable to confirm diagnosis.

Clinical Features

The androgens produced by the tumor first lead to **defeminization**—atrophy of the breasts and uterus and amenorrhea followed by **masculinization (50%)**. This is evidenced by male type of distribution of hair, hoarseness of voice, breast atrophy, hirsutism, baldness and clitoral enlargement. Serum testosterone level is elevated.

Treatment is surgical removal of the tumor. The menstruation and fertility may return but the virilizing features fail to regress. Unilateral oophorectomy for younger age group is optimum. For older patients total hysterectomy with bilateral salpingo-oophorectomy is ideal. Adjuvant therapy is needed for poorly differentiated tumor. Combination chemotherapy (VAC or VBP) is needed for recurrent disease. Tumor removal results in rapid resolution of most hormonal effects except deepening of voice and clitoromegaly.

GYNANDROBLASTOMA

This is a very rare type of tumor. It contains both granulosa cell (estrogenic) or Sertoli-Leydig cell (androgenic) types. Usually, it has got a benign course. Surgical removal is the optimum treatment.

Follow-up

All patients of ovarian SCSTs need to be followed up. Stage I disease has got excellent prognosis following surgery. Women with higher stage disease may need adjuvant chemotherapy.

During surgery for ovarian SCSTs, staging laparotomy should be done in cases with: Granulosa cell, Sertoli-Leydig cell, fibrosarcoma, and steroid cell tumors. Well differentiated tumors like fibroma, thecoma, gynandroblastoma may not need staging laparotomy.

METASTATIC TUMORS OF THE OVARY

Metastatic tumors of the ovary constitute about 5% of all ovarian tumors.

The common primary sites from where metastases to the ovaries occur are gastrointestinal tract (pylorus, colon, and rarely small intestine), gallbladder, pancreas, breast, and endometrial carcinoma.

The mode of spread from the primary growth is through retrograde lymphatics or by implantation from metastases within the peritoneal cavity. The malignant cells from the stomach reach the superior gastric group of lymph glands which also receive the lymphatics of the ovaries. Hematogenous spread is also there.

These are usually bilateral, solid with irregular surfaces (Fig. 24.34). Peritoneal metastases are present, so also ascites. The omentum is involved and becomes solid.

Typical: Histologic picture same as that of primary one.

Atypical: The **atypical one is Krukenberg tumor** in which the histological picture differs from that of the primary one.

Metastatic tumors from the GI tract can be associated with sex hormone (estrogen and androgen) production. Patient may present with postmenopausal bleeding.

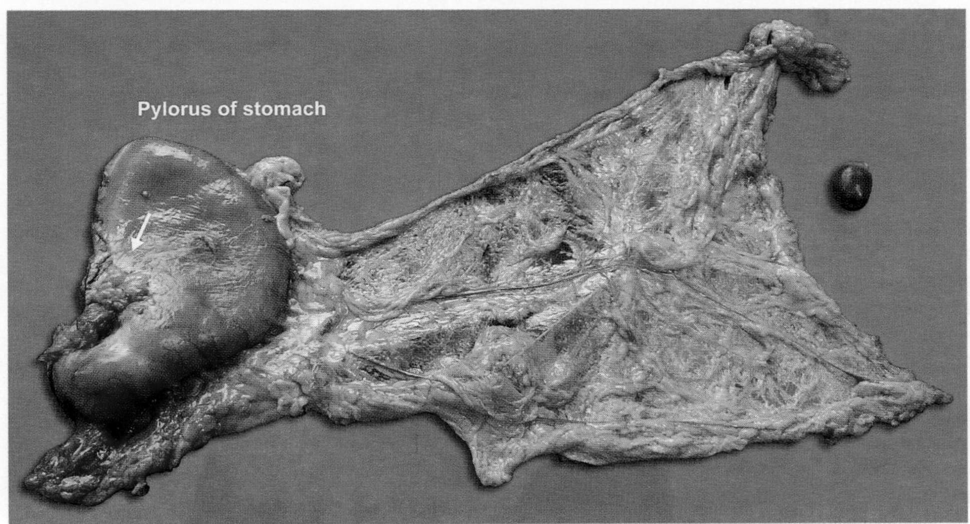

Fig. 24.32: Postoperative photograph of a specimen following partial gastrectomy and omentectomy for carcinoma of the pylorus of the stomach (see arrow).

Case history

Mrs JB 37-year-old lady underwent laparotomy for pelvic abdominal lump with the provisional diagnosis of ovarian tumors. She remained mostly asymptomatic and only late that vague symptoms of upper abdominal discomfort, dyspepsia, fullness and associated pelvic heaviness.
She underwent laparotomy for partial gastrectomy, omentectomy (Fig. 24.32) and total hysterectomy and bilateral salpingo-oophorectomy (Fig. 24.33). Histology confirmed metastatic ovarian tumors (Krukenberg's tumor).

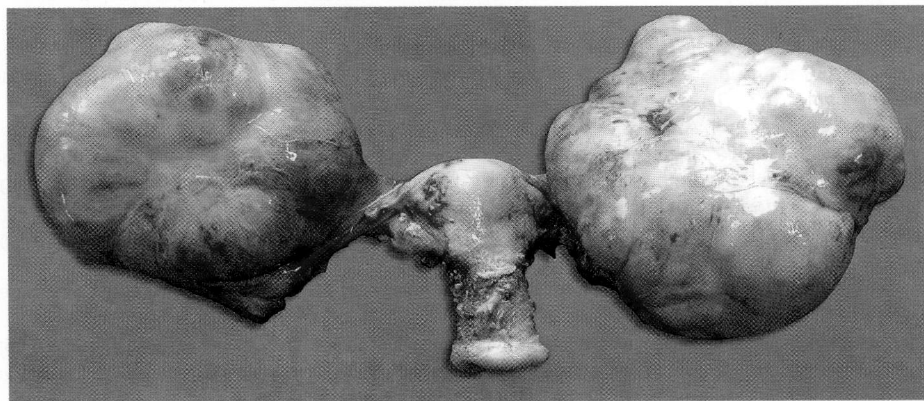

Fig. 24.33: Postoperative photograph of metastatic ovarian tumors following hysterectomy and bilateral salpingo-oophorectomy (Krukenberg's tumor). Primary site of origin was the stomach (the same patient described above). The lesions are usually diagnosed late until the primary disease is advanced. In few cases primary site is not found.

Naked Eye Appearance

The tumor is usually bilateral, solid with smooth surfaces and usually maintaining the shape of the ovary. They typically form rounded or reniform, firm white masses. Sometimes they are bosselated and may attain a big size. There is no tendency of adhesion (i.e. capsule remains intact) (Fig. 24.33).

The cut surfaces usually look yellow or white in color with cystic space at places due to degeneration. Cut surface has waxy consistency.

Histologically, the stroma is highly cellular. The mucin within epithelial cells compresses the nuclei to one pole, producing *'signet ring'* appearance. The scattered **'signet ring' looking cells are characteristic of Krukenberg tumor (Fig. 24.34).**

In most patients with Krukenberg's tumors, the prognosis is poor. Median survival being less than a year. Rarely, no primary site can be identified and the Krukenberg's tumor may be a **primary tumor.**

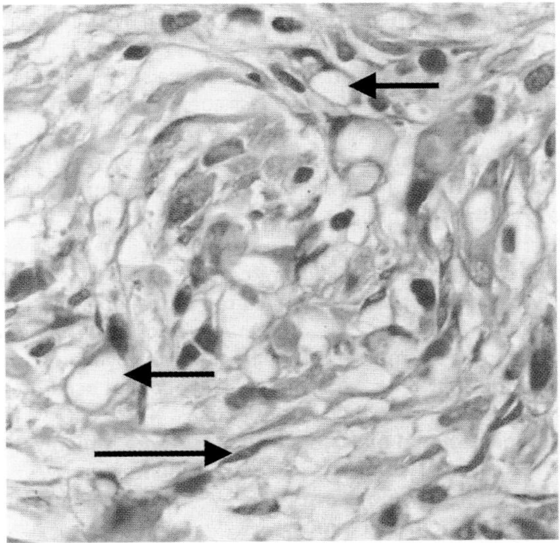

Fig. 24.34: Histologic picture of Krukenberg tumor showing characteristic 'signet ring' appearance. The signet ring cells contain the eccentric nuclei and abundant pale cytoplasm.

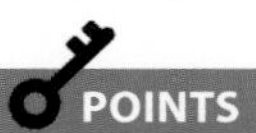

- There is wide geographical variation in the incidence of ovarian malignancy. Incidence is high in Scandinavian countries and US, low in Asian countries (India, Japan). In US about, 1 in every 70 newborn females will line to develop ovarian cancer.
- **The concept of ovarian tumerogenesis** with the distal fallopian tube origin is considered indisputable.
- **Serous cystadenomas** are the most common epithelial tumors. Serous adenocarcinomas have the worst prognosis of epithelial adenocarcinomas.
- About 20% of ovarian neoplasms are malignant. Malignant epithelial tumors constitute about 90% of all primary ovarian carcinomas. The primary mode of spread of epithelial ovarian carcinoma is transcoelomic and it spreads to the visceral and parietal peritoneum, diaphragm and to the retroperitoneal nodes. Most ovarian carcinomas are diagnosed in stages III or IV.
- **Endometrioid carcinoma** is associated with endometrial carcinoma in 20% and ovarian-endometriosis in 10% cases.
- **Patients with familial cancer syndrome** (Lynch type I and II) have a higher risk of developing epithelial ovarian cancer. Mutations of BRCA 1 gene (17 q) and BRCA 2 gene (13 q) have been observed. Inherited ovarian malignancies account for about 10–15% of epithelial ovarian cancers.
- **Incessant ovulation theory** is thought to be factor for carcinogenesis due to repeated ovulatomy trauma.

  The efficacy of screening procedure is not well-documented. However, periodic internal examination supplemented by transvaginal color Doppler sonography to note the ovarian volume, blood flow and estimation of CA-125 in 'high risk' population, can reveal the lesion at the early stage. Gene mutation study for detection of genetic inheritance is not currently recommended.

  Women with high risk factors are: Family history of ovarian, endometrial or breast carcinoma, history of removal of ovarian or breast neoplasm, use of fertility drugs, women with BRCA mutations, nulliparity, and postmenopausal palpable ovary (volume > 8 cm^3) (Table 24.31).
- **Protective factors** for ovarian epithelial adenocarcinomas are: Combined oral contraceptives, pregnancy, tubal ligation, prophylactic salpingectomy, hysterectomy and breastfeeding.
- **Ovarian enlargement less than 8 cm** in diameter in a menstruating women is most commonly functional.
- **Surgery** is the keystone in the primary treatment of ovarian malignancy. The aims are staging of the disease and to perform maximum surgical removal.
- **The ideal definitive surgery** is total hysterectomy with bilateral salpingo-oophorectomy with infracolic omentectomy with pelvic and para-aortic lymph node sampling. In exceptional cases, conservative surgery of unilateral salpingo-oophorectomy is justified.
- **Debulking surgery** with residual tumor nodules <1 cm confers better survival advantage even in advanced stage disease. CT, MRI and PET are effective for detecting residual tumor and the retroperitoneal nodes.
- **Second look surgery** either by laparoscopy or laparotomy is employed either after 12 courses of chemotherapy or after 1 year of primary therapy.

  The 5-year survival rate for patients with borderline epithelial ovarian cancer (grade 0) is close to 100%. For other stages *see* Table 24.35.
- Place of minimally invasive surgical staging of early stage ovarian cancer is accepted. About 15% of women with EOC have early stage disease at diagnosis. MIS for staging and management of early ovarian cancer is safe, feasible and effective when done by a gynecologic oncologist. The outcomes are comparable with that of laparotomy.
- **Chemotherapy** is being widely used following cytoreductive surgery to improve the result in terms of survival.
- **Platinum-based compounds** (cisplatin, carboplatin), either alone or in combination with taxane, prolong the survival rate. Taxane derivatives (paclitaxel, docetaxel) are effective in cisplatin resistant ovarian cancer. Treatment with carboplatin and paclitaxel for 3–6 cycles is desirable for most patients.

  Neoadjuvant chemotherapy is an alternative mode of chemotherapy when preoperative disease assessment is such that optimal cytoreduction is not possible.
- Chemotherapy is given before definitive surgery to debulk cancer. Benefits of this method is that the future surgical intervention is more successful and and is less complicated. Women with advanced ovarian cancer with medical complications are considered for neoadjuvant chemotherapy.
- **The ovarian antigen** CA-125 is useful to monitor the patient during chemotherapy and for follow up.
- **The prognosis of epithelial ovarian carcinoma** depends on many factors. Overexpression of oncogene (HER-2/neu) has been associated with poor prognosis.
- **Germ cell tumors** occur in young women. They are the second most common type of ovarian neoplasm. Most common germ cell tumor is the benign cystic teratoma (dermoid). It is bilateral in 10–15% cases.

  Dysgerminoma is the most common malignant germ cell tumor. It is bilateral in 10% cases. The tumor is highly sensitive to radiation. Multiagent chemotherapy (ectoposide, platinum with or without bleomycin) results in complete remission.
- **Fibroma** is the most common benign solid ovarian tumor.
- **Endodermal sinus tumor** is highly malignant occurring at a median age of 19. Alpha fetoprotein is the tumor marker. Treatment is surgery followed by chemotherapy.
- **Nongestational ovarian choriocarcinoma** is highly malignant. hCG is the tumor marker. It is not responsive to chemotherapy. The treatment is surgery followed by chemotherapy.
- **Multiagent chemotherapy** (BEP, VAC, VBP, CAP) has improved the survival rate as well as childbearing function in patients with malignant germ cell tumors.

Contd...

Contd...

- **Granulosa cell tumor** produces estrogen and may be associated with endometrial hyperplasia or endometrial carcinoma. It occurs 10% prior to puberty and 40% in postmenopausal period. It produces precocious puberty and postmenopausal bleeding. Thecoma is predominantly postmenopausal. There is excess estrogen production.
  Sertoli-Leydig cell tumor (previously called arrhenoblastoma) is very rare. It arises from the male directed cell rests in the hilum of the ovary, from granulosa cells or from teratomas. The tumor produces androgens (80%) and in some cases estrogen.
- **Primary prevention of ovarian cancer:** Current recommendations are to consider: (a) Opportunistic bilateral salpingectomy at the time of surgery for hysterectomy for benign disease or (b) Bilateral salpingo-oophorectomy in women with high risk factors (BRCA mutation), following completed family or (c) Bilateral salpingectomy and delayed oophorectomy.
- **The common primary sites** of metastatic ovarian malignancies are gastrointestinal tract, gallbladder, breast, and endometrial carcinoma. The tumor may be typical or atypical (Krukenberg). The primary sites of Krukenberg are stomach, large bowel and breast. The spread to the ovaries is by retrograde lymphatics. Histologically, it is confirmed by presence of 'signet ring' looking cells.

FALLOPIAN TUBE CARCINOMA

PRIMARY FALLOPIAN TUBE CARCINOMA

Primary carcinoma of the fallopian tube is very rare. The incidence of tubal carcinoma is less than 0.5% of gynecological malignancies.

Predisposing factors: Infertility, nulliparity and family history of ovarian cancer. Similar to ovarian cancer, the association with gene mutations (*BRCA1, BRCA2*), the high risk factors and the protective factors are the same.

Pathology

The site is usually in the ampullary part and the mucosa is commonly affected. The fimbrial end usually gets blocked resulting in hydrosalpinx or hematosalpinx (Fig. 38.57 and 38.58). It is mostly unilateral (80%).

Microscopic appearance: It is mostly adenocarcinoma (papillary serous) 90%.

Spread

Apart from **direct spread**, the **lymphatic** spread to the regional lymph glands (para-aortic) usually occurs. **Blood borne** spread to distant organs can occur in late stages. Transcoelomic spread with exfoliation of cells also occur.

Choriocarcinoma can occur in the fallopian tube following ectopic pregnancy or tubal hydatidiform mole.

Clinical Features

Patient profile: The patients are usually postmenopausal and nulliparous. History of infertility and pelvic infection may be there.

Symptoms

- Vaginal (postmenopausal) bleeding.
- Intermittent profuse watery discharge (hydrops tubae profluens).
- Colicky pain in lower abdomen.

Signs

Bimanual examination reveals a unilateral mass which may be tender. If reduced in size on compression, along with a watery discharge through the cervix, it is very much suspicious.

Diagnosis

- Most often accidentally discovered on laparotomy and histologic examination of the excised tube.
- **Clinical features**—as mentioned earlier.
- Suspected features are:
  - Persistent postmenopausal bleeding with uterine pathology being excluded by curettage.
  - Persistent positive Papanicolaou smear with a negative cervical and endometrial pathology.
  - Serum CA 125 is elevated in most cases (85%).
  - USG: Fluid-filled ovoid mass.
- **Laparoscopy:** In cases of persistent postmenopausal bleeding with a negative uterine pathology.
- **Ultrasound:** A fluid-filled sausage shaped mass separate from the uterus and ovary is seen. Ascites may be present.
- **Other imaging studies:** CT, MRI and PET may be used to differentiate fallopian tube from peritoneal cancer.

Stage

FIGO stage (2018) for fallopian tube cancer is as with the stage for ovarian and peritoneal cancers.

Treatment

Prophylactic surgery in high risk cases needs bilateral salpingo-oophorectomy once child bearing is completed (p. 312).

Actual treatment: Staging laparotomy is similar to ovarian cancer (p. 317). Total hysterectomy with bilateral salpingo-oophorectomy along with omentectomy. This should be followed by **platinum based (carboplatin and paclitaxel) combination chemotherapy** as an adjuvant therapy. In advanced cases, radiotherapy is considered (Ch. 31).

Prognosis

The prognosis is unfavorable mostly due to late diagnosis. The 5-year survival rate ranges between 25 and 40%.

SECONDARY FALLOPIAN TUBE CARCINOMA

This is more common (90%) than the primary. **The common primary sites are** ovary, uterus, breast, and gastrointestinal tract.

The mode of spread from the ovary or uterus is probably by lymphatics rather than a direct one.

SARCOMA UTERUS

Incidence

Sarcoma of the uterus is rare and constitutes about 3% of uterine malignancy.

CLASSIFICATION OF UTERINE SARCOMAS

Pure sarcoma	*Carcinosarcoma (malignant mixed Müllerian tumor)*
A. Homologous ▪ Smooth muscle tumors • Leiomyosarcoma (40%) • Others ▪ Endometrial stromal sarcomas (10–15%) • Low grade • High grade **B. Heterologous** ▪ Rhabdomyosarcoma ▪ Chondrosarcoma ▪ Osteosarcoma, others	**A. Homologous** ▪ Carcinoma + Homologous sarcoma **B. Heterologous** ▪ Carcinoma + heterologous sarcoma ▪ Müllerian adenosarcoma ▪ Lymphoma **C. Müllerian adenosarcoma** **D. Lymphoma**

Leiomyosarcomas are 1–2% of uterine malignancies. **Intravenous leiomyomatosis**—where benign smooth muscle grows into venous channels within the broad ligaments, uterine and iliac veins. Prognosis following surgery is excellent.

Histopathologic diagnostic criteria for uterine leiomyosarcoma depends on the number of mitotic figures (>5 MF/10 HPF), nuclear atypia and presence of coagulative necrosis.

Endometrial stromal tumors arises from endometrial stromal cells. **Endometrial stromal tumors** have chromosomal stromal aberrations observation (6p and 7p). These tumors are less common (10–15%). **Depending on mitotic activity endometrial stromal tumors are of three types:** (1) Endometrial stromal nodule (mostly benign); (2) Endolymphatic stromal myosis (low grade malignancy); (3) Endometrial stromal sarcoma (high grade malignancy).

Undifferentiated sarcoma: These high grade tumors are aggressive (mitosis >10 MF/10 HPF) and have poor prognosis.

Leiomyomatosis peritonealis disseminata—where benign smooth muscle nodules grow over the peritoneal surfaces. It is thought to arise from the metaplasia of subperitoneal mesenchymal stem cells to smooth muscle, fibroblasts, myofibroblasts under the influence of estrogen and progesterone.

Sarcomatous change of fibroid occurs in about 0.1% cases. When it does, the fibroid becomes soft. The cut section shows yellowish appearance with hemorrhage and cystic degeneration. **The whorl appearance is lost (Fig. 24.35).**

Malignant mixed Müllerian tumors (MMMT) of the uterus usually forms a large fleshy mass protruding into the uterine cavity with a broad base. Majority (90%) presents with postmenopausal bleeding.

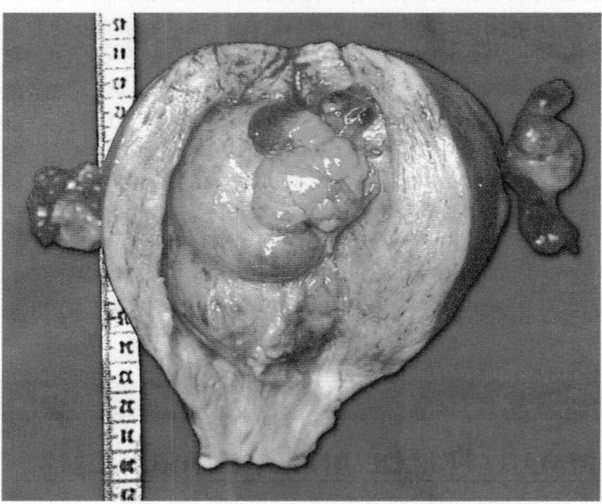

Fig. 24.35: Endometrial stromal sarcoma of uterus.

MICROSCOPIC APPEARANCE

Uterine sarcomas may be pure (single cell type) or mixed (more than one cell type). The tumor is termed *homologous when* the tissue elements are native (smooth muscle) or *heterologous when* tissue elements are not native (cartilage, striated muscle, bones). This is due to the totipotent nature of endometrial stromal cells.

Histologically, three types of cells are seen—spindle, round or combination of the two along with giant cells. **The most common is spindle cell type (Fig. 24.36).**

Malignant mixed Müllerian tumor is evidenced by presence of **both the structures of sarcoma and carcinoma (carcinosarcoma).**

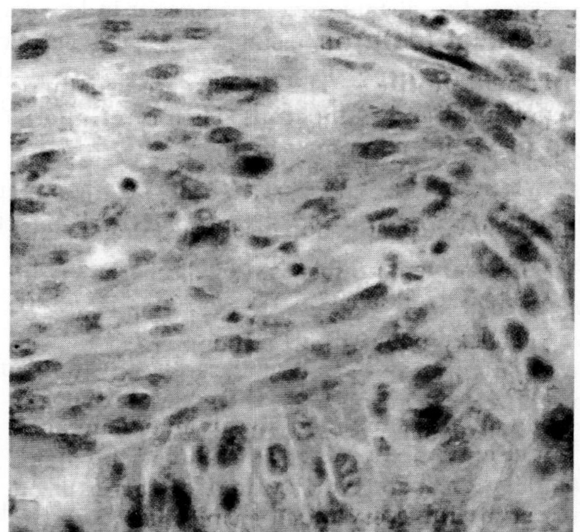

Fig. 24.36: Microscopic picture of leiomyosarcoma showing large spindle-shaped cells with pleomorphic nuclei. There is moderate cellular atypia.

SPREAD

- **Blood borne:** This is the most common mode of spread. The organs involved are liver, lungs, kidneys, brain, bones, etc.
- **Directly** to the adjacent structures.
- **Lymphatic** spread to the regional (pelvic and para-aortic) lymph nodes.

Clinical Features

Patient profile: The age is usually between 40 and 60 years. There may be history of pelvic irradiation either for induction of menopause or malignancy.

Symptoms: There is no specific symptom.

- Irregular premenopausal or postmenopausal vaginal bleeding.
- Abnormal vaginal discharge—offensive, watery foul smelling discharge associated at times with expulsion of fleshy necrotic mass.
- Abdominal pain—due to involvement of the surrounding structures.
- Pyrexia, weakness, and anorexia.
- **Suspected sarcomatous change in a fibroid is evidenced by:**
  - Postmenopausal bleeding
  - Rapid enlargement of fibroid
  - Recurrence following myomectomy or polypectomy.

Pelvic Examination

There is no specific finding. The uterus may be enlarged and irregular. Parametrium may be thickened and indurated.

Speculum examination may reveal a polypoidal mass protruding out through the external os.

DIAGNOSIS

- MRI may be helpful when the uterus is large (Fig. 24.37).
- Diagnosis is made usually following histological examination of the removed uterus.

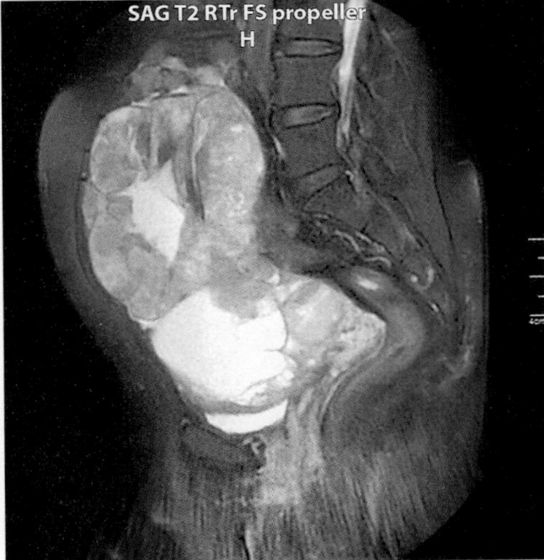

Fig. 24.37: MRI showing a huge pelvic mass (leiomyosarcoma) arising from the uterus with no normal tissue planes for resection.

- Diagnostic uterine curettage and endometrial biopsy may reveal the mucosal form of sarcoma.
- Histologic examination of the removed polyp.
- Serum CA-125 levels may be elevated in cases with carcinosarcoma. CA-125 values may be a useful marker to monitor the disease response.

TREATMENT

- Total hysterectomy with bilateral salpingo-oophorectomy is to be done. This may be followed by adjuvant external pelvic radiation.
- If **the cervix** is also involved, radical hysterectomy should be done.
- **Radiation therapy** (adjuvant) preoperative or postoperative is helpful to decrease the pelvic recurrence in endometrial stromal sarcoma and MMMT.
- **Several chemotherapeutic agents** have been tried in cases with metastatic disease. Doxorubicin, cisplatin gemcitabine, docetaxel and ifosfamide are the drugs used either singly or in combination with varying response.
- Watchful expectancy may be extended in cases of sarcoma detected accidentally from the well-capsulated fibroid following myomectomy.
- Complete resolution has been observed with progestin (provera), letrozole therapy in cases with endometrial stromal tumors.

PROGNOSIS

The prognosis is unsatisfactory. The 5-year survival rate ranges from 10–30%. Sarcoma in fibroid has got a better prognosis.

SARCOMA BOTRYOIDES (EMBRYONAL RHABDOMYOSARCOMA)

Embryonal rhabdomyosarcoma of the cervix is the most common malignant tumor of the vagina in infants and children. It is a highly aggressive tumor. Most are the subtypes of sarcoma botryoides. It is seen almost exclusively in girls below the age of 5 years. In the middle aged women it is seen within the cervix and after menopause within the uterus.

Patients with embryonal rhabdomyosarcomas have improved prognosis. The subtype sarcoma botryoides has the best chance of cure.

Clinical Features

The presenting features are:

- Blood stained watery vaginal discharge.
- Anemia and cachexia.
- Vaginal examination reveals pinkish, "grape-like" polypoidal edematous soft growth arising from the cervix. It may often fill up the whole vagina. It may be pedunculated to protrude outside.

Diagnosis is confirmed by histologic appearances of loose myxomatous stroma, pleomorphic malignant cells with striated rhabdomyoblasts.

Treatment

With the use of multimodality treatment using chemotherapy, surgery and radiation therapy outcome of these patients have improved. Primary chemotherapy followed by conservative surgery to excise the residual tumor have been done. Many patients respond well to primary chemotherapy even without surgery.

Intravenous administration of VAC therapy (vincristine, actinomycin-D, cyclophosphamide) and radiation has been found very much effective. The drugs should be administered every 3 weeks over a period of 6 months. Chemotherapy with local resection of the disease gives better result. Radiation therapy may be needed. The results of multimodality approach are better.

Prognosis

Embryonal rhabdomyosarcomas have the poor prognosis. However, the subtype sarcoma botryoides has been best chance to cure following treatment.

Pseudosarcoma botryoides is a rare, benign vaginal polyp resembling sarcoma botryoides. It is found in vagina of infants and pregnant woman. Large atypical cells may be present but strap cells are absent. Local excision is effective.

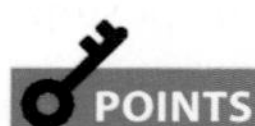

- **Primary carcinoma of the fallopian tube** is rarest (<1%) gynecological malignancy. It is mostly unilateral (80%). Associated hematosalpinx is often present. Classic traid of adnexal mass, intermittent profuse watery discharge (hydrops tubae profluens) and vaginal bleeding is considered pathognomonic for tubal carcinoma. USG/laparoscopy is suggestive and biopsy is confirmatory. Persistent postmenopausal bleeding and/or positive vaginal cytology for adenocarcinoma, in the absence of endometrial carcinoma, the diagnosis of tubal carcinoma should be considered.
- **Total hysterectomy with bilateral salpingo-oophorectomy along with omentectomy is done.** This is followed by platinum based combination chemotherapy as the adjuvant treatment. The prognosis is not good.
  Secondary carcinoma (metastatic) is common (90%), the primary sites are from ovary, uterus, breast or gastrointestinal tract.
- **Uterine sarcoma** comprise less than 5% of uterine malignancies. The most common site of uterine sarcoma is the intramural part.
- **The most common mode of spread** is blood borne. Total hysterectomy with bilateral salpingo-oophorectomy is the surgery. This is followed by multiagent chemotherapy and external pelvic radiation. Mitotic figure is an important prognostic factor for leiomyosarcoma of the uterus. Patients with mitotic rate of less than 5/10 HPF behave as a benign lesion but mitotic rate of more than 10 per 10 HPF are frankly malignant and have got worst prognosis.
- **Sarcoma botryoides** is a special type of mixed mesodermal tumor arising from the cervix. The child, before the age of 8, may be affected. Multimodality approach (multiagent chemotherapy with surgical removal and occasionally radiation) gives better result.

CHAPTER

25 Urinary Problems in Gynecology

CHAPTER OUTLINE

- Anatomy of Vesicourethral Unit
- Urinary Continence
- Genuine Stress Incontinence
- Urge Incontinence
- Overactive Bladder
- Painful Bladder Syndrome
- Voiding Disorder
- Urinary Tract Infections
- Dysuria

ANATOMY OF VESICOURETHRAL UNIT

The bladder and urethra should be considered as a single unit with two major functions—storage of urine and voiding of urine.

Though the two organs are anatomically separate entities but integrated with complex functional interplay.

The descriptive anatomy of the urinary bladder and urethra has been described in Ch. 1. **The anatomic and physiologic peculiarities involved in storage and voiding of urine are to be discussed here.**

BLADDER

The bladder muscles—called detrusor consist of three layers of muscles (Figs. 25.1A and B).

- **Outer longitudinal:** The muscles course downwards from the fundus to bladder neck. At the level of bladder neck, it forms a sling. With this arrangement, it forms an active and dominant role in both storage and voiding.
- **Middle circular:** It is more prominent in the lower part of the bladder.
- **Inner longitudinal:** It courses downwards from the fundus of the bladder and continues in the form of spirals up to the midurethra.

Recent studies, however, suggest that there is frequent interchange of fibers between the bundles and the separate layers are not distinctly defined.

From a functional point of view, the detrusor appears to contract as a single syncytial mass. The detrusor muscles are shown to contain significant amount of acetylcholinesterase.

Trigone: The smooth muscle has got two distinct layers. The deeper one is similar to detrusor. The superficial layer is relatively thin. Traced distally, it fades out in the proximal urethra. It is devoid of acetylcholinesterase but have more cholinergic nerve supply.

Bladder neck: The muscle bundles are largely oblique or longitudinal. They appear to have little or no sphincteric action.

URETHRA

From the functional point of view, the anatomic length of the urethra is divided into three parts.

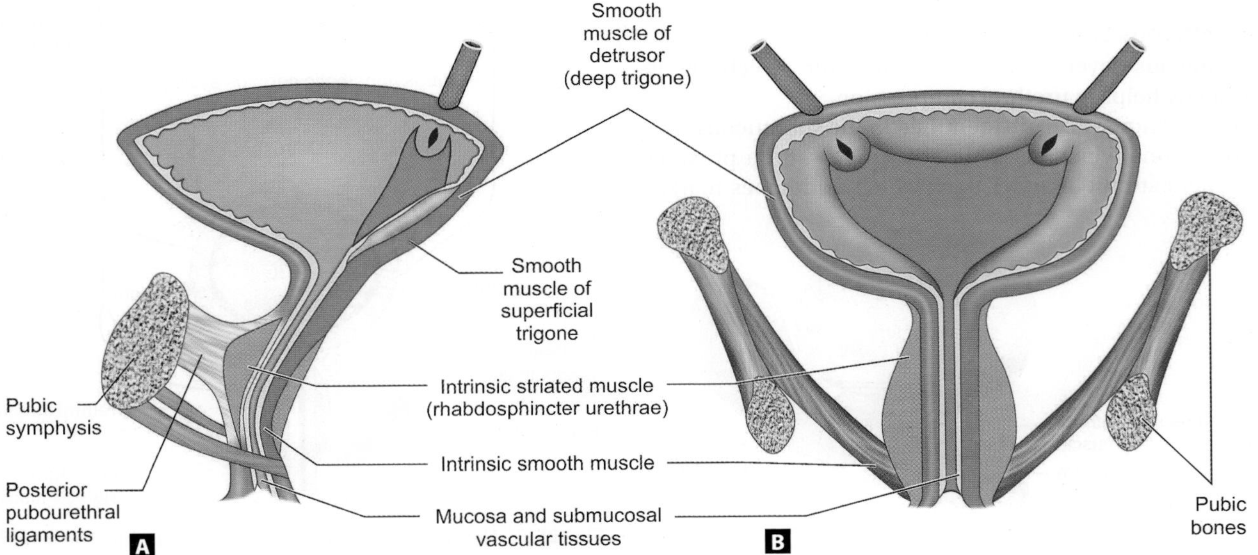

Figs. 25.1A and B: Female bladder and urethra: (A) Sagittal section; (B) Coronal section.

1. **Proximal urethra:** It is weakest part of the urethra. Inner longitudinal muscle of the detrusor fades out in this part of the urethra. It fails to withstand the rise of intravesical or intra-abdominal pressure (IAP).
2. **Midurethra (Figs. 25.1A and B, Fig. 25.2):** This is the strongest part of the urethra. This part has got an additional support by the intrinsic striated muscle (rhabdosphincter urethrae). This muscle encircles the whole urethra and is composed predominantly of skeletal muscle with nerve supply from parasympathetic division of autonomic nerves. This rhabdosphincter is further enforced in the upper part by levator ani muscles (extrinsic muscles) being separated from it by a distinct connective tissue septum. The extrinsic periurethral muscle (levator ani) is supplied by the perineal branch of pudendal nerve. The intrinsic striated muscles (slow twitch fibers) is responsible for **urethral closure at rest**. The extrinsic periurethral striated muscles (first twitch fibers) provide additional **support to urethra on stress.**
3. **Distal urethra:** This part is a passive conduit and is surrounded by collagen tissue. In fact, the entire urethra is rich in elastic and collagen fibers.

Pubourethral ligaments and condensed endopelvic fascia are found to contain smooth muscle fibers. They work together to maintain the normal anatomic support and prevent hypermobility of bladder neck and urethra.

Urethra has got 2 layers of smooth muscle. Outer circular and inner longitudinal. This smooth muscle layers are surrounded by a circular layer of striated muscle.

This striated urogenital sphincter complex includes: (a) Sphincter urethrae; (b) Uretherovaginal sphincter; (c) Compressor urethrae.

These 3 muscles contract simultaneously to constrict the urethrae circumferentially on its entire length. Sphincter urethrae with its slow twitch fibers remains tonically contracted and maintains the continence at rest. The urethero vaginal sphincter having first twitch muscle fibers constrict the urethrae and maintains continence with sudden increased intra abdominal pressure.

Submucous Layer of the Urethra

Submucous layer is the vascular layer which by its plasticity helps in urethral compression.

Two venous plexi are identified in the submucous coat. A distal one which varies little with age and a proximal one beneath the bladder neck which undergoes marked changes with age. In the reproductive period, these vessels give a cavernous appearance to the submucosa which disappears in the postmenopausal period. **This urethral vascular system plays a significant role in the maintenance of resting urethral pressure.**

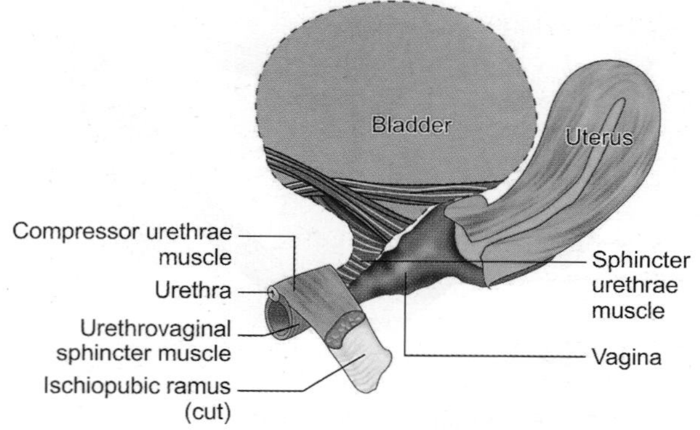

Fig. 25.2: Striated urogenital complex (Rhabdomyosphincter).

Mucous Layer of the Urethra

Mucosa is arranged in longitudinal folds that allow apposition and distension.

SUPPORT TO BLADDER NECK AND URETHRA

Support is maintained by intrinsic and extrinsic factors.

Intrinsic factors: (a) Intrinsic rhabdosphincter urethrae (Figs. 25.1A and B, New Fig. 25.2); (b) Urethral submucosal venous plexus (cavernous plexus); (c) Urethral smooth muscles; (d) Sympathetic activity to maintain urethral tone by α-adrenergic receptors; (e) Estrogen to increase collagen connective tissue.

Extrinsic factors: (a) Contraction of pubococcygeus part of levator ani muscle; (b) Pubourethral ligaments and condensed endopelvic fascia with smooth muscle fibers; (c) Exercise to increase collagen turnover and also to maintain strength of levator ani.

NERVE SUPPLY OF THE VESICOURETHRAL UNIT (FIG. 25.3)

Autonomic

Both the parasympathetic and sympathetic nervous system work with CNS via pontine micturition center (PMC). Parasympathetic nerves originating from S_{2-4} stimulate detrusor contractions through the release of **acetylcholine** (cholinergic nerve fibers). **Parasympathetic division**

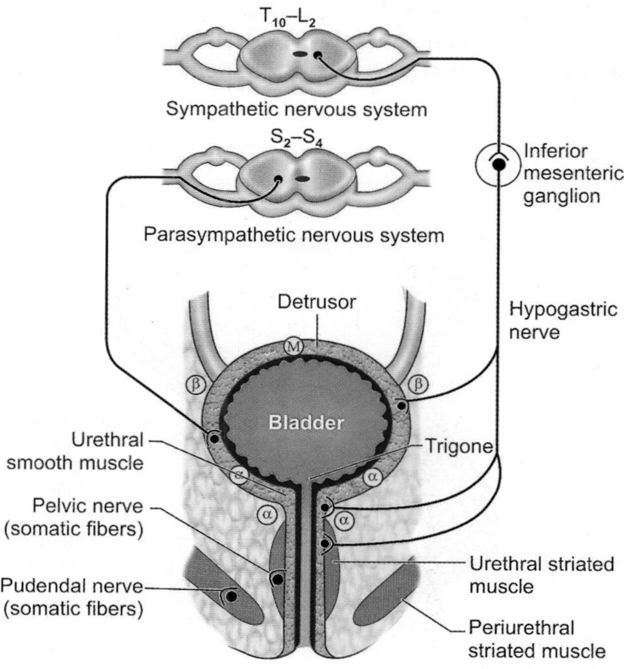

Fig. 25.3: Nerve supply of the vesicourethral unit. The bladder fundus is rich in parasympathetic (muscarinic) receptors (M) and sympathetic β-adrenergic receptors (β). The bladder neck contains higher number of sympathetic α-adrenergic receptors (α).

acts through acetylcholine binding to muscarinic receptors. Preganglionic sympathetic fibers arising from T_{10}–L_2 are also cholinergic but the postganglionic fibers innervating both the bladder and urethra act through the release of **norepinephrine** (adrenergic nerve fibers). Norepinephrine stimulate both α and β adrenergic receptors. **β-adrenergic fibers terminate mainly in the bladder dome. α-adrenergic receptors** are mainly present in the bladder base and urethra. On stimulation α-receptors cause urethral contraction and urine storage and continence. **β-receptors are located mainly on the fundus of the bladder and cause detrusor relaxation**. This helps in storage of urine.

The sympathetic is concerned mainly with the filling and storage phase of micturition. Parasympathetic supply (acetylcholine) is responsible for detrusor contraction and normal voiding. During voiding PMC in the brain inhibits the sympathetic pathway to the urethra. This allows urethra to relax for voiding. Functional brain imaging studies with PET during voiding show activation of cortex, insula and PMC.

Somatic

The somatic supply to the striated muscle of urethra is through the pudendal nerve. The rhabdosphincter is supplied by pelvic splanchnic nerves traveling with the parasympathetic fibers. Extrinsic periurethral striated muscle is supplied by the motor fibers of the pudendal nerves.

PHYSIOLOGY OF MICTURITION

The bladder and urethra should be considered as a single unit with two main functions:

- **Storage of urine**
- **Voiding of urine**

STORAGE PHASE

The urine comes into the bladder drop by drop through the ureteric openings. As the bladder fills, the walls stretch to maintain a constant muscle tone. The bladder usually fills at the rate of 0.5–5 mL/minute from the ureters. The intravesical pressure is raised to remain at almost steady level of about 10 cm of water even with a volume of about 500 mL.

The intravesical pressure is kept lower than that of the urethra by delicately coordinated relaxation of detrusor muscle. **This is possible through number of mechanisms.**

- Proximal urethral musculature acts like a sphincter by maintaining tonic contraction.
- Stretching of the detrusor reflexly contracts the sphincteric muscles of the bladder neck.
- Inhibition of the cholinergic system responsible for detrusor contraction operating from the spinal centers.
- Stimulation of **β-adrenergic receptors results in further relaxation of the detrusor and α-adrenergic dominance leads to contraction of smooth muscles round the bladder neck** (*internal sphincter*).
- *The external sphincter* mechanism consists of periurethral muscle fibers which are of 'slow twitch' variety innervated by the pelvic efferent nerves. The other component of the external sphincter derived from the levator ani, composed of fibers of 'first twitch' variety innervated by the perineal branch of pudendal nerve.
- The external sphincter mechanism contributes the second line guard assisting the first line guard provided by the internal sphincter of the bladder neck.

VOIDING PHASE

When the volume of the bladder reaches about 250 mL, a sensation of bladder filling is perceived. A desire to void is reached, not by increased intravesical pressure but by stimulation of stretch receptors in the bladder wall.

The sensation passes up the spinal roots S_2, S_3 and S_4 **and in untrained bladder** (children), there sets in motion a reflex which automatically contracts the detrusor and results in voiding.

But in the trained adults, this urge can be suppressed especially if the time or place is not convenient. Because in adults, the reflex spinal arc is under control of the hypothalamus and higher areas of the brain (anterior part of the frontal lobes). Cerebral control of micturition is complex but is predominantly controlled by pontine center. Action of detrusor can therefore be voluntarily inhibited (Fig. 25.4).

When the time or the place is convenient, the higher centers via the hypothalamus no longer inhibit the detrusor and the bladder changes from its passive to active role. The detrusor contracts **to raise the intravesical pressure to 30–50 cm of water.** The pressure is further raised to about 100 cm of water by voluntary contraction of the abdominal muscles.

The series of chronologic events to follow in the process of micturition are:

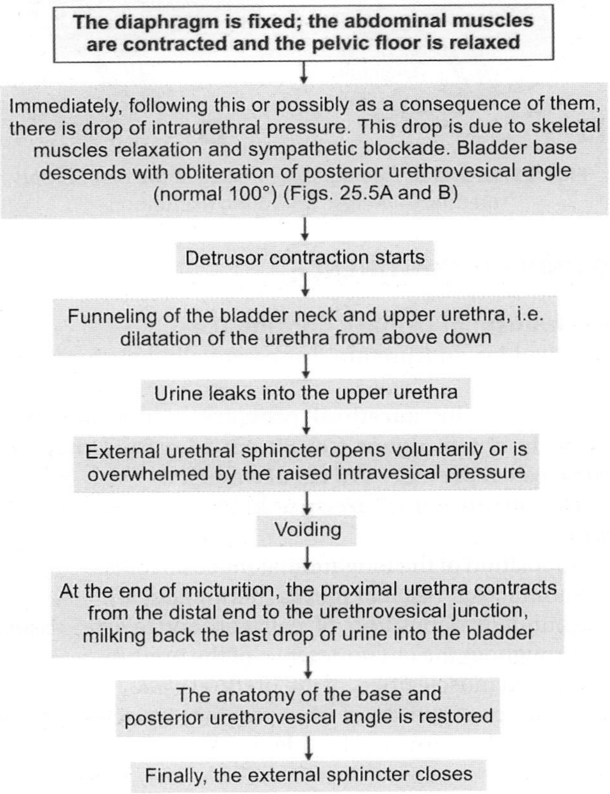

The diaphragm is fixed; the abdominal muscles are contracted and the pelvic floor is relaxed

↓

Immediately, following this or possibly as a consequence of them, there is drop of intraurethral pressure. This drop is due to skeletal muscles relaxation and sympathetic blockade. Bladder base descends with obliteration of posterior urethrovesical angle (normal 100°) (Figs. 25.5A and B)

↓

Detrusor contraction starts

↓

Funneling of the bladder neck and upper urethra, i.e. dilatation of the urethra from above down

↓

Urine leaks into the upper urethra

↓

External urethral sphincter opens voluntarily or is overwhelmed by the raised intravesical pressure

↓

Voiding

↓

At the end of micturition, the proximal urethra contracts from the distal end to the urethrovesical junction, milking back the last drop of urine into the bladder

↓

The anatomy of the base and posterior urethrovesical angle is restored

↓

Finally, the external sphincter closes

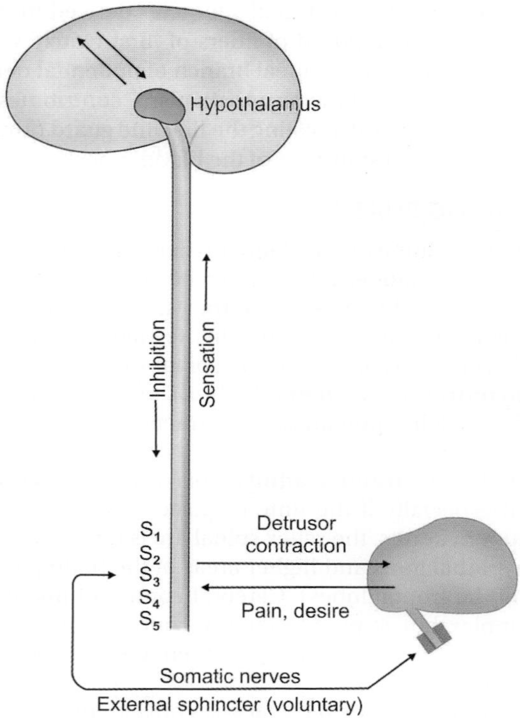

Fig. 25.4: Nervous control of bladder filling and emptying.

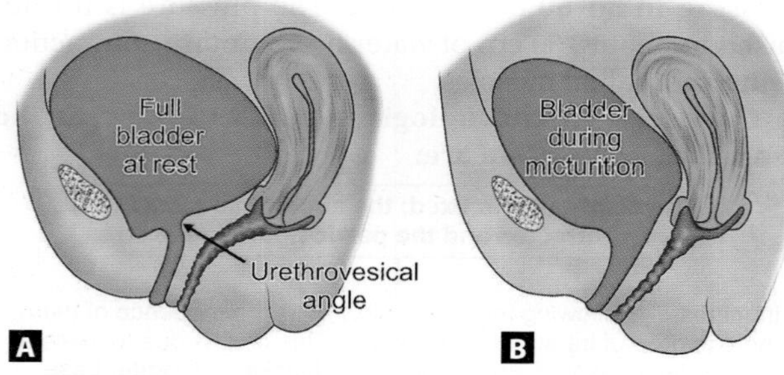

Figs. 25.5A and B: Radiographic tracing of the bladder and urethra. (A) At rest; (B) During micturition.

URINARY CONTINENCE

Mechanism of Urinary Continence

The bladder and urethra are essentially one functional unit.

Normally, **intraurethral pressure at rest and with stress is much higher (20–50 cm of water) than the intravesical pressure (10 cm of water).**

The intraurethral pressure at rest is maintained by the following:

- Apposition of the longitudinal mucosal folds.
- Submucosal vascular plexus (hermetic seal).
- Abundant deposition of collagen and elastic tissues throughout the circumference of the urethra.
- Striated muscle fibers of the urethral wall.
- Tonic contraction of the smooth muscles in the proximal urethra and bladder neck.

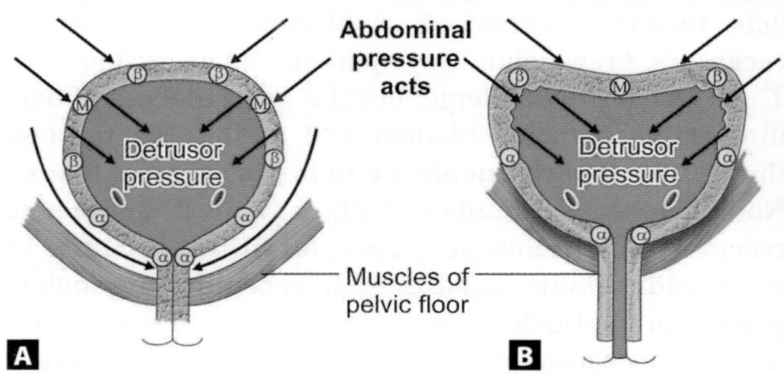

Figs. 25.6A and B: (A) Normally any increase in intra-abdominal pressure (IAP) compresses the upper urethra; (B) If the bladder neck descends, this does not occur.

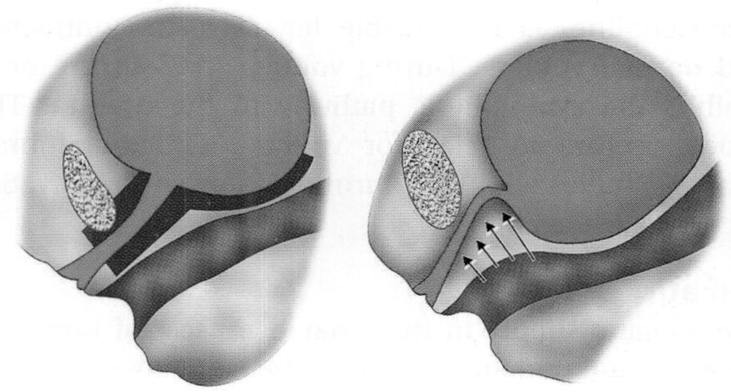

Fig. 25.7: Kinking of the urethra during stress pulling the bladder neck upward and forward.

- Rhabdosphincter in the midurethra and levator ani muscles.
- Part of the intra-abdominal pressure (IAP) is transmitted to the urethra (Figs. 25.6A and B).
- Urethral closing pressure is highest at the mid point of the functional urethra which is above the urogenital diaphragm.

Approximately, one-third of the resting urethral pressure is due to rhabdosphincter effects, one-third to smooth muscle effects and one-third to its vascular plexus.

During stress, with rise of IAP the escape of urine is prevented by the additional factors:

- Centripetal force of IAP transmitted to the proximal urethra which occurs as long as the bladder neck remains above the pelvic diaphragm (Figs. 25.6A and B).
- Reflex contraction of the urethral striated sphincter and periurethral striated musculature during stress.
- Kinking of the urethra (Fig. 25.7) due to:
  - **Hammock-like attachment** of pubocervical fascia with urethra, vagina, and laterally to the arcus tendineus fascia give stability to urethra. During rise in IAP, normally the urethra is compressed against the anterior vaginal wall.
  - **Bladder base rocks** downward and backward.
  - **Bladder neck** is pulled upward and forward behind the symphysis pubis due to preferential better support to the posterior wall of the urethra than to the base of the bladder given by the pubocervical fascia.

URINARY INCONTINENCE

Urinary incontinence is defined as objectively demonstrable involuntary loss of urine so as to cause hygienic and/or social inconvenience for day-to-day activity (Table 25.1).

Pathophysiology of Urinary Incontinence

Basic pathology of incontinence is the rise of intravesical pressure over that of maximum urethral pressure. It may be due to mechanical injury to the supports of the bladder neck following childbirth, trauma (surgery), or due to aging. Overactivity of the detrusor muscles, may also be associated.

Types of Urinary incontinence in women

- **Stress urinary incontinence:** Involuntary loss of urine with effort or physical exertion (e.g. sporting activities) or when sneezing or coughing.
- **Urgency urinary incontinence:** Involuntary loss of urine associated with urgency or sudden, compelling desire to void that is difficult to defer.
- **Mixed urinary incontinence:** Involuntary loss of urine associated with urgency and with physical exertion, sneezing or coughing.
- **Overactive bladder:** Urinary urgency, typically accompanied by frequency and nocturia, with or without urge urinary incontinence, in the absence or urinary tract infection or other obvious pathology.
- **Nocturnal enuresis:** Involuntary loss of urine that occurs during sleep.
- **Functional urinary incontinence:** Involuntary loss of urine that is due to cognitive, functional, or mobility impairments in the presence of an intact lower urinary tract system.
- **Occult stress incontinence:** Stress urinary incontinence that is observed only after the reduction of coexistent pelvic organ prolapse.

Stress Urinary Incontinence (SUI)

SUI is defined as involuntary escape of urine from the external urinary meatus due to sudden rise in IAP. The term, 'urethral sphincter incompetence' seems to be appropriate as it signifies the basic pathology (Table 25.1).

Genuine Stress Incontinence

Definition

Genuine stress incontinence (GSI) is defined, according to the International Continence Society (ICS) as involuntary urethral loss of urine when the intravesical pressure exceeds the maximum urethral pressure **in the absence of detrusor activity**. The diagnosis of GSI should be made following urodynamic assessment only.

TABLE 25.1: Classification of urinary incontinence.

Urethral	*Extraurethral*
▪ Genuine stress incontinence (GSI)	**Acquired**
▪ Urge incontinence	▪ Fistula
▪ Detrusor over activity (DO)	▪ Vesical
▪ Mixed (GSI and DO)	▪ Urethral
▪ Over flow incontinence (acute and chronic)	▪ Ureteral
▪ Functional and transient (infection, pharmacologic, DM)	**Congenital**
	▪ Ectopic ureter
	▪ Epispadias
	▪ Bladder exstrophy

Incidence

The reported incidence in the Western countries is as high as **40% in association with prolapse**. In about 5%, the symptoms may be annoying.

Etiopathogenesis

GSI is strictly an anatomic problem. In the normal continent woman, the bladder neck and the proximal urethra are intra-abdominal and above the pelvic floor in standing position. The urethral pressure exceeds the intravesical pressure.

Urethral sphincter incompetence is principally due to:

- Hypermobility of urethra due to distortion of the normal urethrovesical anatomy.
  - Descent of the bladder neck and proximal urethra which normally lies above the urogenital diaphragm, hinders rise of intraurethral pressure during straining (Fig. 25.6).
- Lowered urethral pressure at rest below the intravesical pressure.

Risk Factors for Stress Urinary Incontinence

- **Developmental weakness** of the supporting structures maintaining the bladder neck and proximal urethra in position. There may be genetic variations in collagen and other connective tissues which normally maintain anatomic and physiologic aspect of the vesicourethral unit.
- **Childbirth trauma:** MRI study revealed damage to the pelvic floor muscles: levator ani, pubovesical muscle and pubocervical fascia. **The injury is more common in gynecoid and least in android pelvis.**
- **Pregnancy:** It is probably functional in nature and related to high level of progesterone. Other factors related to pregnancy and child birth are: difficult vaginal delivery, forceps delivery, or even increased parity.
- **Postmenopausal:** Estrogen deficiency leads to atrophy of the supporting structures.
- **Trauma:** Injury to symphysis pubis due to fracture or following symphysiotomy.
- **Following surgery** like anterior colporrhaphy, local repair of vesicovaginal fistula (VVF) or bladder neck surgery, there may be fibrosis of the urethra and urethral musculature.
- **Age**—increasing age.
- **Obesity (BMI ≥30).**
- **Drugs:** Diuretics.
- **Comorbid conditions:** Diabetes, parkinsonism, and stroke.

Morbid Anatomic Changes

In GSI, the main defects are:

- Intrinsic sphincter dysfunction.
- Bladder base becomes flat and lies in line with the posterior wall of the proximal urethra.
- Descent of the proximal urethra.

TABLE 25.2: Differences in clinical presentation.

Stress incontinence	*Urge incontinence (sensory)*	*Overactive bladder (OAB)*
▪ Leakage of urine coincides with stress ▪ No prior urge to void ▪ Amount—small ▪ Patient—fully aware of it ▪ Micturition—normal	▪ Unable to control the escape of urine, once there is urge to void ▪ Amount—large ▪ Patient—aware of the urge ▪ Urgency and frequency	▪ The incontinence may occur abruptly even without a full bladder or a clinical cause ▪ Amount—large ▪ Patient—not aware of it ▪ Frequency and nocturia

The net effect of these changes is to lower the intraurethral pressure as in early stage of micturition. Thus, even a small rise of intravesical pressure during stress, allows the urine to escape out.

GSI is the ultimate symptom of varying severity due to anatomic urethral hypermobility (80%) and/or intrinsic sphincter deficiency (20%).

Clinical Features

Patient Profile

The patients are usually parous, may be postmenopausal. Often the complaints date back to the last childbirth or some vaginoplastic operation. Sometimes the symptoms may be combined with frequency or urge incontinence. The patient may be obese.

Symptoms

The only symptom is escape of urine with coughing, sneezing or laughing. **The loss of urine has got the following features:**

- Brief and coincides precisely to the period of raised IAP.
- Unassociated with a desire to pass urine.
- Rarely, occurs in supine position or during sleep.
- Patients are fully aware of it.
- The amount of loss is small.

Details of diet, medical history (e.g. diabetes, chronic pulmonary disease, neurological disease), surgical history (spine or genitourinary tract), current medications (sedatives, antipsychotics) must be noted. Because these have direct bearing on urinary incontinence.

Local Examination

Pelvic examination should be done with the full bladder.

- Some degree of **pelvic relaxation** with **cystocele** or cystourethrocele is usually evident.
- **Stress test:** When the patient is asked to cough in (supine and standing position), a few drops of urine are seen escaping from the external urethral meatus.
- **Q-tip test:** The Q-tip test has been tried to predict SUI. A sterile (lubricated with 2% xylocaine jelly) cotton tipped swab is introduced to the level of bladder neck through the urethra. Then the patient is asked to sit and cough (Valsalva). If there is marked upward elevation (>30°) of the cotton tipped swab, **urethra is considered hypermobile**. These patients are benefited with midurethral sling surgery (p. 332).

Differential Diagnosis

Sometimes, there may be clinical confusion with other forms of incontinence such as urge or detrusor instability. The differentiating features are tabulated in Table 25.2.

Special Investigations (Table 25.3)

The investigations aims at:

- To confirm the diagnosis
- To rule out associated pathology.

Midstream urine examination: This should be a routine prior to urodynamic studies to avoid risk of flaring up the infection during invasive procedures. Any woman with a urine dipstick test positive for both leukocytes and nitrites should have a midstream urine specimen for culture and sensitivity. Hematuria, if present, must be thoroughly evaluated with malignant cell cytology, cystourethroscopy and intravenous urography (IVU).

Pad test: An one hour extended pad test is recommended in cases when the clinical stress test is negative.

The patient wears a preweighed sanitary pad, drinks about 500 mL of water and rests for 15 minutes, then performs exercises like walking or climbing stairs for 30 minutes. This is to be followed by provocative exercises such as bending, jumping, coughing, etc. for another 15 minutes. After a period of as hour, the sanitary pad is removed and weighed. **An increase in weight by 1 g is considered as significant loss.**

Frequency volume chart (urinary diary): Patient is asked to record her fluid intake, output, episodes of leakage in relation to time and activity. It should be recorded at least for 3 days. This diary gives an idea about daily urine output, number of voids per day and functional bladder capacity.

Post-void residual urine: The woman is asked to void. A catheter is inserted in the bladder within the next 10 minutes to measure the remaining urine in the bladder. Ultrasonography may be done alternatively. Normally residual urine should be <50 mL. Large amount of residual urine indicates urinary retention (inadequate bladder emptying). Residual volume measurement by ultrasonography is also fairly accurate.

Urodynamic study: If the stress incontinence is the only symptom, there may not be any need for detailed

TABLE 25.3: Diagnosis of genuine stress incontinence (GSI).

▪ **Clinical stress test**—positive ▪ **Pad test**—positive ▪ **Midstream urine analysis**—normal ▪ **Bladder diary** (volume frequency chart) ▪ **Uroflowmetry**—normal ▪ **Cystometry**—normal ▪ **Significant** lowering of urethral closure pressure during strain ▪ **Leak-point pressure** (Valsalva) test—positive ▪ **Cystourethroscopy**—negative finding ▪ **Videocystourethrography (VCU)**—bladder neck funneling ▪ **Transvaginal endosonography**—altered anatomical relationship (descent) of urethrovesical junction and bladder base

urodynamic studies. However, the indications of urodynamic study are—(a) Presence of mixed symptomatology [GSI and overactive bladder (OAB)]; (b) Associated frequency/nocturia/voiding difficulties; (c) Associated neuropathy; or (d) Previous failed surgery.

- ***Uroflowmetry:*** The procedure is simple. The time period of total voiding is recorded by a stop watch and the amount of urine is estimated. **The normal flow rate is 15–25 mL/sec.** If the flow rate drops to less than 10 mL/sec, it indicates atonic bladder or urethral obstruction which can be confirmed by cystometry. The residual urine is to be estimated. Flowmeters can be used to produce a graphic record.

  Low peak flow rate (<15 mL/sec) associated with increased detrusor pressure (> 50 cm H_2O) with prolonged voiding time indicates outflow obstruction. **In stress incontinence**, urinary flow rate is normal with nil or insignificant residual urine.

  If the uroflowmetry is normal, the next step is to submit the patient to cystometry to exclude detrusor instability or urge incontinence.
- ***Cystometry (filling and voiding cystometry):*** **Cystometry** evaluates the change in the bladder during filling and voiding (Table 25.4) to show the pressure volume relationship.

  Principle: Pressure catheters with electronic microtip transducer are used. One pressure catheter is introduced into the bladder. An additional catheter is placed in the bladder to fill it up. Another rectal or vaginal pressure catheter is introduced to measure the IAP. Measurements of total intravesical pressure (P_{ves}), IAP (P_{abd}), and true detrusor pressure (P_{det}) are done. Rectal pressure (P_{abd}) is subtracted from total intravesical pressure (P_{ves}) to obtain true detrusor pressure (P_{det}).

  Technique: Patient sits on the study coach. Normal saline is infused inside the bladder through the filling catheter at the rate of 50–100 mL/min. Continuous recording of fluid volume infused and pressure change is done. Patient may be asked for standing, coughing or heel bouncing, for provocation. During voiding cystometry, filling catheter is removed. Total volume voided, urine flow rate and pressure (P_{abd}, P_{ves} and P_{det}) are recorded. Urge incontinence during filling cystometry indicates detrusor instability. Ambulatory urodynamic studies are thought to be more reliable.

  In GSI, the cystometric evaluation is normal. The values are abnormal in detrusor instability and sensory urge incontinence.

TABLE 25.4: Normal findings in cystometry.

Residual volume	—	0–50 mL
First sensation of urination	—	150–200 mL
Capacity	—	400–600 mL
Intravesical pressure on filling and standing	—	0–15 cm H_2O
Absence of systolic detrusor contraction		
No leakage on coughing		
Able to interrupt the urine flow on command		
Maximum detrusor pressure during voiding	—	<50 cm H_2O
Peak urinary flow rate	—	>15 mL/sec

- **Abnormal cystometry:** (a) Urine leaks on coughing. No rise in detrusor pressure → GSI; (b) Detrusor contractions during filling phase → OAB.
- **Ambulatory monitoring** using microtip pressure transducers (twin channel) is found to increase the detection of OAB. This test is more physiological.
- Use of multichannel pressure recordings plus the video urodynamic system is most accurate.

Urethral pressure profiles

For a continent woman, urethral pressure must be higher than the bladder pressure. Urethral pressure profile test is performed with a special catheter having microtip pressure transducers, which is slowly pulled down from the bladder (filled with 250 mL of normal saline) along the urethra to outside. The transducer measures the intravesical and urethral pressure while it is pulled down. This pressure profile is represented as a curve called **urethral pressure profile**. Maximum urethral closure pressure is obtained by subtracting intravesical pressure from maximum urethral pressure. Unfortunately correlation between urethral pressure and severity of incontinence is poor.

Abnormalities are:

- Functional length of the urethra is decreased usually well below 3 cm.
- Peak urethral pressure decreases both in supine and erect position.
- During strain, there is **significant lowering of the urethral closure pressure compared to intravesical pressure. This is pathognomonic of GSI.**
- **Leak-point pressure test:** It gives an idea about sphincteric strength.

Method: Patient is asked to strain (Valsalva maneuver) when the bladder is filled up to a reasonable volume (200 mL) to increase intravesical pressure. The minimum pressure (cm H_2O) at which leakage is observed is recorded as 'Valsalva (abdominal) leak-point pressure'. If no leakage is observed even at the highest pressure exerted (cm H_2O), it is recorded as 'no leakage'. If reflects maximum urethral closure pressure.

- **Urethral sphincter dysfunction** is common in elderly women. Intrinsic sphincter deficiency (ISD) and urethral hypermobility are often coexistent. ISD is defined when maximum urethral closure pressure is ≤20 cm H_2O. These women are benefited with some obstructive procedures rather than traditional incontinence surgery.

Cystoscopy and urethroscopy—are not done as a routine but can be performed in selected cases. The common indications are (a) Any history of hematuria; (b) Suspected neoplasm; (c) Suspected fistula; (d) History of urgency and frequency to rule out interstitial cystitis and reduced bladder capacity.

Videocystourethrography (VCU), it is not a routine procedure. Special indications are: (a) History of failure of previous surgery and (b) To exclude diverticula and sacculation. Contrast media (35% urografin) is used. Anatomical relationship of bladder neck, urethra, and bladder base are assessed. Similar information can be obtained from transvaginal endosonography. MRI is superior for women with post-void dribble.

Preoperative multichannel urodynamic testing is not necessary before planning primary anti incontinence surgery in women with uncomplicated SUI (ACOG – 2015).

Intravenous urography (IVU) and computed tomography urogram (CTU)—are not a routine procedure. **Indications are:** (a) Patient with hematuria, neuropathic bladder and (b) To rule out congenital anomalies, calculi or fistulae.

Transvaginal endosonography is widely used to assess the anatomy of bladder neck, bladder neck funneling, position and hypermobility. Rectal, perineal, and recently intraurethral probes with three-dimensional images are more informative.

Treatment

- **Preventive**
- **Definitive**

Preventive

Prevention includes avoidance of repeated childbirth trauma and delay in second stage of labor. Management of obesity (normal BMI), diabetes, chronic pulmonary, and neurological diseases are the essential steps in prevention.

Definitive

The treatment aims at:

- Restoration of the function of the muscles of the urethrovesical junction.
- Strengthening the support of the urethra.

- **Conservative**
- **Surgical**

Conservative: To improve the tone of the pelvic floor muscles:

- **Pelvic floor muscle training (supervised):** Basic principle is to strengthen the muscular part of rhabdosphincter and pelvic floor muscle. This will bring back the urethral pressure. Physiotherapy will not, however, strengthen the involuntary muscles of the bladder base and proximal urethra for which surgery is required.

  The pelvic floor muscle training (PFMT) are in the form of drawing up the anus and tightening the vagina for stopping micturition. This squeeze and release is repeated 10 to 15 times with a total of more than 50 contraction. This should be done for several months.
- **Biofeed back therapy:** During PFMT visual, auditory and/or verbal feedback are given to the patient. Vaginal pressure changes are measured with a vaginal probe. Treatment sessions are individualized based on underlying dysfunction. These sessions are found helpful.

  The suitable cases are: GSI of minor degree in cases of recent delivery having poor pelvic muscular tone.
  - Kegel exercises: It is an active pelvic floor muscle training (PFMT) to reduce the problems of urinary incontinence. Patient is taught to contract and hold the levator ani muscles voluntarily for 50–60 times a day. She is asked to do so by squeezing the pelvic floor muscles and the anal sphincter.
  - Use of vaginal devices: Pessaries, bladder neck support prosthesis.
  - Use of vaginal cone with weight ranging from 20–100 g.
  - Electrical stimulation—activation of the pelvic floor muscles by stimulation of pudendal nerves.
  - Diet control in obese patient to reduce weight.
- **Drugs**
  - **Estrogen:** It may be useful in postmenopausal patient (p. 46).
  - **Sympathomimetic drugs (α-adrenergic):** They improve the tone of urethra and bladder neck and thereby symptoms are improved. Imipramine 10–25 mg, orally twice daily is effective. The periurethral levator ani muscles having both the type-I (slow-twitch) and type-II (fast-twitch) fibers are responsible for maintaining continence against sudden increased abdominal pressure.
- **Paraurethral implants:** Implants using Teflon increase the functional length of the urethra. Periurethral injection of GAX collagen (glutaraldehyde cross-linked bovine collagen) is effective in GSI of minor degree. It prevents premature bladder neck opening.

Surgery

- **The principles of surgery are:**
  - Restoration of normal anatomy to maintain bladder neck and proximal urethra as intra-abdominal structures. So that it lies within the abdominal pressure zone (Figs. 25.6A and B).
  - Strengthening the support of bladder neck and proximal urethra. This prevents the funneling of vesicourethral junction in response to raised intravesical pressure.
  - To increase the functional urethral length.
- **The objectives of surgery are:**
  - To elevate the bladder neck so that it lies within the abdominal pressure zone (Figs. 25.6A and B).
  - To support the vesicourethral junction and to prevents its funneling in response to raised intravesical pressure.

Surgery for GSI varies widely. Procedures could be vaginal (plication of the bladder neck) or abdominal (elevation of the bladder neck) or combined (endoscopic bladder neck suspension or sling procedures). *No one single procedure can be ideal for all women. Individualization should be done depending on her age, severity of symptoms and ultimately the experience of the surgeon.* Ideally all patients must be reviewed on the basis of her clinical presentation and urodynamic features.

- **Retropubic cystourethropexy (colposuspension) (Figs. 25.8)**

  Principle of all these operations is to restore the normal anatomy (elevation) of the urethrovesical junction and to prevent the hypermobility of bladder neck. Long-term (5 years) success rate for retropubic cystourethropexy is 80–90%.

  There are several modifications of this operation. This procedure is performed suprapubically (through low abdominal incision) to reach the space of Retzius.

  (a) ***Burch (1961) colposuspension*** is considered the **gold standard** for GSI. The same endopelvic fascia and/or the lateral vaginal fornix is sutured to the ipsilateral iliopectineal ligament [Cooper's ligament, Fig. 25.8(a)]. Vaginal vault mobility is essential. Mild cystocele is corrected with this procedure.

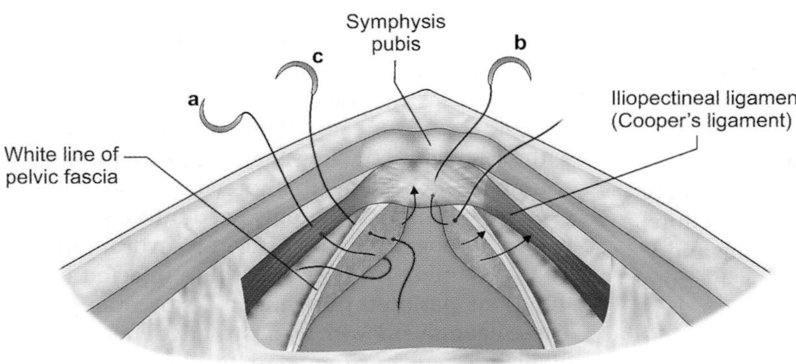

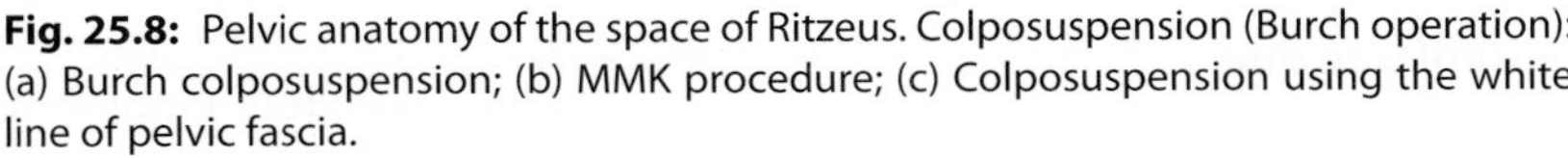

Fig. 25.8: Pelvic anatomy of the space of Ritzeus. Colposuspension (Burch operation): (a) Burch colposuspension; (b) MMK procedure; (c) Colposuspension using the white line of pelvic fascia.

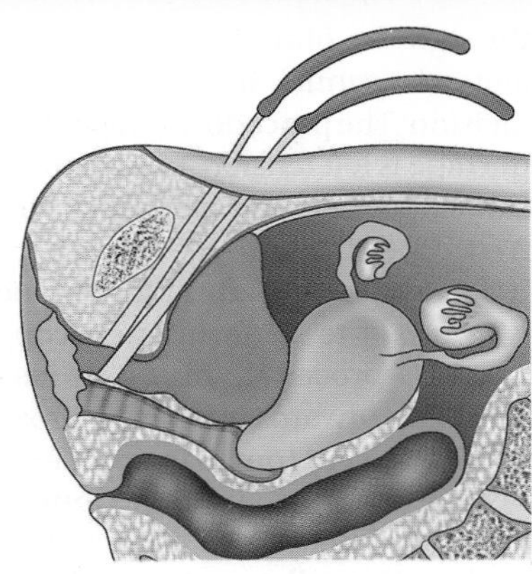

Fig. 25.9: TVT procedure with needles in position. The tape is left tension-free under the urethra.

Complications: Detrusor overactivity, retention of urine, injury to bladder and urethra.

Laparoscopic bladder-neck suspension has been done exactly by the same way as that of an open Burch. Success rate is similar to open method.

- **Retropubic midurethral sling procedures**

  Principles: Normally urethral closure is maintained by the function of three structures: (a) Pubourethral ligaments; (b) Suburethral vaginal hammock and (c) the tone of pubococcygeus muscle.

  Loss of function of these structures results in urinary incontinence. Midurethral sling procedures are designed to provide support to urethra when these anatomical supports are inefficient or lost.

  There are many variations of the procedure. **Principally all involve midurethral placement of a synthetic mesh. The procedures are divided into: (A) Retropubic method**: Tension-free vaginal tape (TVT), and (B) **Transobturator method:** Transobturator tape (TOT).

- **Tension-free vaginal tape (TVT):** It was devised by Petros (1993) and Ulmstem (1996). A Marlex or Goretex tape is passed vaginally in a 'U' shape manner, under the midurethra to the either side with especially designed needles (Fig. 25.9). The needles are passed along the back of the pubic bone to the skin incision one on either side of the midline. Cystoscopy is done at the end of the procedure. Dissection is minimal and the tape is not sutured to any structure (tension-free). This acts by improving the midurethral support. TVT increases urethral coaptation by kinking the urethra during increased IAP. This is less invasive and operative time is short and less hospital stay. Success rate is about 80–90% at 3 years.

  Complications: Urgency, mesh erosion, urinary retention, urge, incontinence, retropubic hematoma, injury to bladder, blood vessels and the intestines. Bladder perforation is a common complication (3–9%).

- **Transobturator tape (TOT) (Figs. 25.10 and 25.11):** It is a minimally invasive procedure designed by Delorme (2001) to support the urethra as a hammock. A 2 cm incision is made in the vagina over the midurethra. A tunnel is created out to the obturator foramen on either side. A multifilament, microporous polypropylene tape is fed through the trocar which passes from the thighfold

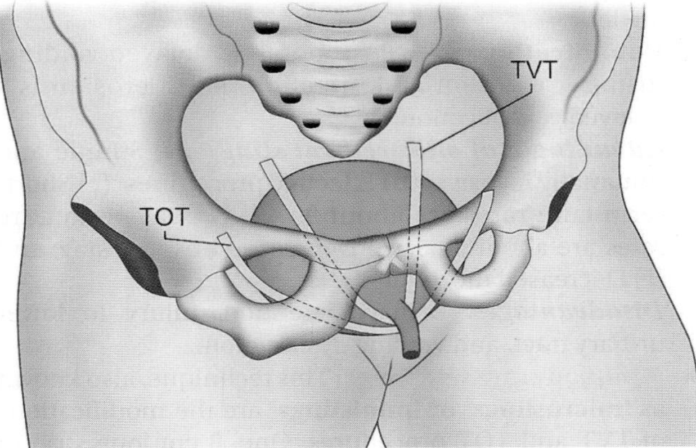

Fig. 25.10: Vaginal tape procedures showing retropubic and transobturator placement (TVT and TOT). The tunnels are seen for each procedure. The tape is left under midurethra without any tension to support it as a hammock.

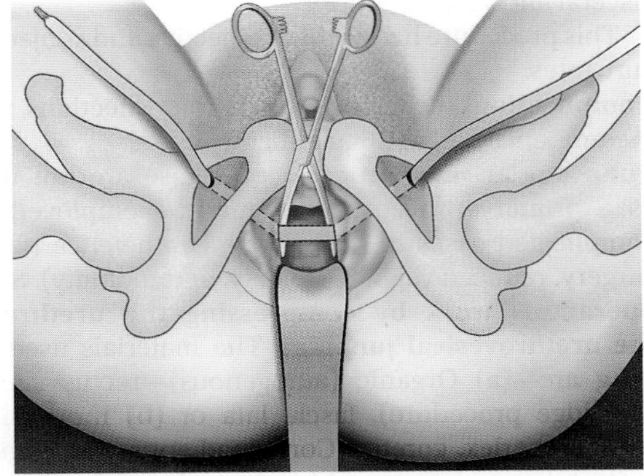

Fig. 25.11: Transobturator tape (TOT) placement. The artery forceps acts as a spacer between the urethra and the mesh. This spacing avoids too much elevation of the urethra and reduces the complication of postoperative retention of urine.

through the obturator foramen from outside to inside along the tunnel. It is finally brought round the vaginal incision. The procedure is repeated on the other side and the tape is left tension-free under the midurethra. It acts similar to a natural hammock supporting the urethra. As it avoids the retropubic space, complications are less. It can be performed under the local anesthetic. There is no need to perform cystoscopy in TOT procedure. The TOT procedure may start inside the vagina and is directed outward (into out approach) or it may be from outside inward (out to in approach).

TOT is day care surgery. **Complications** of bladder injury and that to the obturator neurovascular bundle are less. **Overall success rate (80%), quality of life and satisfaction with these procedures are similar to that of TVT.**

TVT and TOT procedures are recommended as **Grade A**, based on evidence level. Hospital stay, operation time are less.

Complications are: Postoperative delayed voiding, urinary retention and infection. Mesh erosion is a delayed complication.

Advantages of midurethral slings: (a) Simple and minimally invasive; (b) Effective procedures; (c) Short-term cure rates are about 90%; (d) Long-term cure rates are about 80%; (e) Decreased hospital stay; and (f) Decreased morbidity.

Disadvantages: Urinary retention, injury to lower urinary tract, and voiding dysfunction.

- **Minimally invasive slings:** This technique, also known as **'microslings'** or **'minislings'** are the modifications of TVT and TOT procedures. One, 8 cm long strip of polypropylene synthetic mesh is placed across and beneath the midurethra. A small vaginal incision is made beneath the midurethra. The mesh is not passed either through the retropubic space or through the obturator foramen. Thus it avoids the complications of visceral and vascular injury.

  This procedure has got high objective and subjective cure rates.

  Complications: Recurrent urinary tract infections, urge incontinence and voiding difficulty.
- **Pubovaginal sling procedures:** These are not used as a primary procedure but may be employed for complicated cases of sphincter incompetence (failed surgery, reduced vaginal capacity, and mobility). **Sling operations work by compressing the urethra at the urethrovesical junction.** The materials used for sling are—(a) Organic (autogenous)—rectus sheath (Aldridge procedure), fascia lata or (b) Inorganic—silastic, marlex, goretex. Combined approach, vaginal and abdominal (retropubic space) is made. Sling is passed around the bladder neck and is fixed to rectus sheath under **minimal tension to act as a hammock.** Overall success rate is 70%. **Disadvantages are** voiding difficulties, detrusor instability and sling erosion.
- **Intrinsic sphincter deficiency (ISD):** It is commonly seen in women with pelvic trauma, neurologic conditions or scarring of the sphincter. Maximum urethral closure pressure is ≤20 cm of H_2O.

  Treatment of GSI due to ISD are: (a) Periurethral bulking agent (injections); (b) Urethral bladder neck sling procedures; (c) Midurethral synthetic sling; or (d) Use of an artificial urethral device.
- **Urethral bulking agents:** Women having ISD are treated with periurethral bulking agents. Selected women with comorbid conditions that precludes anesthesia are especially suited. Commonly used **bulking agents are** bovine collagen, Teflon, calcium hydroxyapatite or polyacrylamide hydrogel. They are injected transurethrally or periurethrally under cystoscopic guidance. These agents work with an obstructive effect at the level of bladder neck. Compared to surgical procedures, results are for a short period only.
- **Kelly's cystourethroplasty (Howard Kelly, 1914)**
  This is the common surgical procedure employed in GSI with success.

  The technique consists of meticulous exposure of the urethra and the bladder neck vaginally. This is followed by plicating the pubocervical fascia with vertical mattress sutures using 'O' catgut or Vicryl along the proximal urethra and bladder neck. These sutures will strengthen the urethral pressure and assist elevation of the bladder neck.

Advantages are—(a) Simple procedure; (b) Less time is required; (c) Correction of coexistent cystocele; (d) Especially suited for women who are elderly and medically unfit for prolonged surgery.

Disadvantage—Long-term success rate is low (50–60%).

- *Marshall-Marchetti-Krantz (MMK, 1949)*: The principle is to achieve elevation of the urethrovesical junction. Paraurethral and paravesical endopelvic fascia are stitched to the periosteum at the back of the symphysis pubis [Fig. 25.8(b)].

Complications: (a) Hemorrhage during dissection of the space; (b) Urethra and bladder neck injury due to injudicious placement of sutures; (c) Osteitis pubis (MMK procedure); (d) Voiding difficulty; (e) Detrusor instability; (f) Enterocele formation; (g) VVF; (h) Failure and recurrence.

- **Salvage procedures** are suggested where all other procedures have failed hopelessly. Only a small percentage of woman will need this.

  The procedures are:
  - Implantation of artificial sphincter
  - Urinary diversion.

Recommended Surgery for GSI

- **Retropubic**
  - Burch 92% and 80% (curable)
    - Open
    - Laparoscopic
- **Midurethral tape**
  - Tension-free vaginal tape (TVT)
  - Transobturator tape (TOT)
  - Microslings
- **Pubovaginal sling**
  - Autologous
  - Inorganic
- **Endoscopic bladder neck suspension**
- **Intrinsic sphincter deficiency**
- **Bulking agents**
- **Others**
  - Kelly's plication of bladder neck
  - Marshall-Marchetti-Krantz (MMK)
  - Paravaginal repair

URGE INCONTINENCE

Incidence

Urge incontinence due to detrusor overactivity (DO) is the **second common cause of urinary incontinence in an adult female**, the first being the GSI. However, in the elderly group, DO is most common. DO is associated with GSI in about 10–15% of cases when urodynamic studies are done. Overall incidence of DO is 10%. It may be:

- Motor urge incontinence OAB
- Sensory urge incontinence.

Overactive Bladder (Detrusor Overactivity)

Definition

An overactive bladder (OAB) is defined by the International Continence Society as 'one that is shown objectively to contract spontaneously or on provocation during the filling phase while the patient is attempting to inhibit micturition'. Among the elderly women, OAB is the most common cause of urinary incontinence. Overall prevalence is 12–15% in women aged 40 years or more.

Etiology (Table 25.5)

The condition is largely functional and psychosomatic in origin. The patient may be of emotionally labile type or passing through a phase of anxiety, stress. Sometimes, a hypertonic detrusor is even stimulated by bodily movements like getting up from sitting or lying position.

The causative factors are:

- Idiopathic—majority
- Psychosomatic
- Following surgery for incontinence
- Detrusor hyperreflexia (neurogenic)—multiple sclerosis, spinal injuries, early parkinsonism, diabetic neuropathy, cerebrovascular accident, etc.

DO is basically due to acetylcholine induced stimulation of detrusor muscarinic receptors.

Pathophysiology

The pathophysiology is obscure. There may be increased in α-adrenergic activities causing increased detrusor contraction. The identical situation occurs in initiating an event of normal micturition—relaxation of urethral sphincter mechanism followed by contraction of detrusor muscle. Therefore, it is thought that inappropriate detrusor contraction results when there is passage of urine into the proximal urethra due to incompetence of the bladder neck. Incompetent bladder neck → urine in proximal urethra → DO → incontinence. This occurs despite the effort of the individual to inhibit them. Other explanation is change in the detrusor smooth muscle property (due to atherosclerosis or neuropathy) that leads to inappropriate DO. The involuntary contraction occurs at any bladder volumes—either spontaneously or on provocation. There is preceding drop in urethral pressure.

TABLE 25.5: Common causes of urgency, urge incontinence and frequency of micturition.

Gynecological	▪ Genitourinary prolapse ▪ Genuine stress incontinence ▪ Menopause (tissue atrophy due to estrogen deficiency) ▪ Pelvic mass ▪ Pregnancy
Urological	▪ Urinary tract infection ▪ Detrusor overactivity (DO) ▪ Urethral syndrome ▪ Interstitial cystitis
Medical	▪ Diabetes ▪ Neurological lesions (multiple sclerosis, Alzheimer's disease) ▪ Diuretic therapy
Others	▪ Psychological and idiopathic

Symptoms

There is involuntary loss of urine without any prior urge to urinate. **Most common symptoms are urgency, frequency (> 8 times/day), nocturia (> once/night) and bed wetting**. It should be remembered that the entity is too often associated with GSI (Table 25.6).

Special Investigations

- **Maintenance of urinary diary** (frequency volume chart) for 4 days.
- **Detailed neurological examination** is made to exclude neurological disorders (stroke, multiple sclerosis). Cranial nerves are examined.
- **Midstream examination** of urine for culture and sensitivity test.
- **Uroflowmetry:** In idiopathic group, the flow rate is high and the voiding time is short.
- **Cystometry:**
  - Urge to pass urine is provoked at a much lower bladder filling of 100–175 mL of water.
  - True detrusor pressure increases by more than 15 cm of water during bladder filling with 200 mL of fluid.
- **Cystourethroscopy:** This is to exclude the associated local pathology. The findings are normal or coarse trabeculation and diverticulae of bladder may be seen. Bladder capacity is reduced.
- **VCU** may reveal bladder trabeculation, diverticulae and vesicoureteric reflux.

Treatment

General measures

- Psychosomatic problems should be treated by psychotherapy.
- Other medical problems (neurological, diabetes) should be properly attended.

Behavioral therapy

- To limit the intake of fluid to 1 liter/day
- To reduce tea and coffee
- Drugs—diuretics may be stopped if possible
- Bladder retraining.

When combined with stress incontinence, OAB, bladder is to be treated first before proceeding to surgical correction for stress incontinence.

Failed surgical treatment of stress incontinence is to be evaluated for the presence of unstable bladder.

TABLE 25.6: Clinical presentation and diagnosis of GSI and urge incontinence (sensory and motor).

	Genuine stress incontinence (GSI)	Urge incontinence (sensory)	Overactive bladder (OAB)
Definition	Involuntary escape of urine when intravesical pressure exceeds maximum urethral pressure in the absence of detrusor activity	Involuntary leakage of urine accompanied by or immediately preceeded by urgency	Leakage of urine due to sudden, spontaneous, detrusor contraction (detrusor instability), without any clinical cause
Clinical presentation			
▪ **Stress prior to leakage**	Always present	Nil	Nil (urodynamic diagnosis)
▪ **Urge prior to leakage**	Nil	Present	Present except in neurologic disease
▪ **Awareness**	Present	Present	Not present
▪ **Control of loss**	Can control	Can control with adequate encouragement	Cannot control despite strong encouragement
▪ **Amount**	Small	Large	Large
Midstream urine examination	Not informative	Evidences of infection	Usually non-informative
Uroflowmetry	Normal	Normal	High in idiopathic group
Cystometry	During strain, there is significant lowering of the urethral pressure. (urethral pressure profile)	Normal	Urge to pass urine is provoked at much lower bladder filling Detrusor pressure is increased during filling
Cystourethroscopy	Normal	Offending factor present (Table 25.7)	Diminished bladder capacity
Lateral cystourethrography	Funneling of the proximal urethra	Normal	Normal

Bladder retraining: This is useful in idiopathic group. This can be achieved by bladder drill, biofeedback or hypnotherapy.

In bladder drill, the patient is instructed to void by the clock at progressively increasing intervals over a 6-week time period. The initial response is quite good but the failure rate is high. Simultaneous antimuscarinic drug therapy improves the result. The drill is, however, not useful where neurologic disease is responsible for unstable bladder.

Drug therapy

Aims are to—(a) Inhibit bladder contractility; (b) Increase bladder neck and urethral resistance.

The drugs (Table 25.7) have mostly got anticholinergic properties, thereby minimizes detrusor irritability. When administered along with bladder retraining, there is improvement of results. Antimuscarinic drugs are tried along with behavioral training.

In addition, the peri or postmenopausal women are often helped by estrogen therapy. It has shown to raise the sensory threshold.

Intravesical therapy

Capsaicin is a neurotoxin and is obtained from red chillies. Intravesical use of capsaicin in 30% alcohol improve symptoms in patients with neurogenic DO (multiple sclerosis).

TABLE 25.7: Drugs used in overactive bladder.

Nature	Drugs with dosage	Specially used to relieve	Common side effects	Contraindications
Anticholinergic, Antimuscarinic Musculotropic relaxants	Oxybutynin chloride 5 mg PO thrice daily/ transdermal patch 3.9 mg twice/week	▪ Frequency ▪ Urgency	Dry mouth and skin, constipation, blurred vision	▪ Glaucoma ▪ Myasthenia gravis ▪ Intestinal obstruction ▪ Ulcerative colitis ▪ Urinary retention
Antimuscarinic (detrusor selective)	Tolterodine 1–2 mg, PO, BID	▪ Frequency ▪ Urgency	— Do —	
Antimuscarinic (M-3 selective)	Solifenacin 5–10 mg, PO daily	▪ Frequency ▪ Urgency	— Do — Flatulence, chest pain	
M-3 selective antimuscarinic	Darifenacin 7.5–15 mg PO daily	Frequency Urgency	— Do —	
β-3 adrenergic agonist	Mirabegron 25–50 mg. PO daily	Frequency	Tachycardia, UTI	Uncontrolled hypertension
Antimuscarinic	Trospium 40–60 mg PO daily	Nocturnal enuresis	Dyspnea, chest pain, asthenia	Renal and hepatic dysfunction

Other agents used are: Onabotulinum toxin A is a neurotoxin found to effective in intractable DO. It is injected into the bladder wall via cystoscopy.

Surgery

In intractable cases not relieved by drugs or bladder irritability due to neurologic disease, surgery may be of help. Pelvic floor electrical stimulation can improve the symptoms. Direct sacral neuromodulation (S3) and peripheral neuromodulation through peripheral tibial nerve stimulation (PTN) to sacral nerve plexus could be done. It improves symptoms and quality of life. Augmentation cystoplasty (to increase bladder capacity) or urinary diversion (ideal conduit) are the alternatives.

Mixed incontinence of stress and urge may be present. Urodynamic studies are indicated in such a case. In such a situation, symptoms are prioritized. Treatment is initiated towards the predominant symptoms. Conservative management should be tried first. Antimuscarinic drugs are tried. However, in many women (50–60%), urge symptoms are improved after midurethral sling procedure (p.342).

PAINFUL BLADDER SYNDROME

Painful bladder syndrome (PBS) is a chronic inflammatory condition resulting in painful voiding. According to the International Continence Society (2002), **PBS is defined** as the presence of suprapubic pain related to bladder filling associated with other symptoms like frequency, in the absence of urinary tract infection or other pathology. Therefore urgency and pain are the two important diagnostic criteria of PBS. Painful bladder syndrome is more prevalent in women than in men. **Interstitial cystitis**, is considered within the spectrum of PBS.

Pathophysiology is not known. The probable causes are allergy, autoimmune, infective, toxins or leaky urothelium secondary to poor glycosaminoglycan layer.

Symptoms

The clinical presentation varies widely. Symptoms include urgency, frequency, pelvic and lower urinary tract pain, dyspareunia and urinary incontinence.

Diagnosis

PBS is a diagnosis of exclusion. On cystoscopy bladder frequently appears normal. On distension, petechial hemorrhages with oozing of blood from the surface is often seen. The differential diagnosis includes cystitis, trigonitis, tuberculosis, overactive bladder (OAB), bladder stones, or cancer, diverticula, and urogenital atrophy due to estrogen deficiency.

Treatment

As the diagnosis of PBS is difficult, treatment is directed to control the symptoms mainly.

Usually multiple interventions are done. Behavioral therapy, pelvic floor physical therapy, medications including hormones and bladder instillation are the treatment options.

- **Diet:** Alcohol, spices, citrus and caffeinated drinks are avoided as they are found to increase bladder inflammation and pain.
- **Drugs:** Urinary tract analgesics like hyoscyamine, phenyl salicylate may reduce urethral irritation. Pentosan Polysulfate, (100 mg thrice a day) decreases urothelial permeability. It helps to repair the glycosaminoglycan layer of the bladder epithelium.
- **Surgery:** Bladder instillation therapy—with agents like steroids, sodium bicarbonate, botulinum toxin and dimethyl sulfoxide (DMSO), heparin has been found to be helpful. They need to be repeated weekly for a minimum of 6 weeks.
- **Other treatments:** Tricyclic antidepressants, antihistamines, transcutaneous electrical nerve stimulation (TENS) antihistamines and acupuncture have been tried as neuromodulation.

OVERFLOW INCONTINENCE

This occurs as a result of prolonged and neglected retention. Its mechanism is probably the overdistension of the bladder pulls open the internal sphincter. There may be compensatory detrusor hypertrophy.

The causes of overflow incontinence are the same as retention of urine which will be mentioned later in the Chapter.

Urodynamic Findings

Uroflowmetry reveals low flow rate and significant residual urine.

Cystometry reveals large capacity of the bladder and no rise of detrusor pressure during voiding.

Treatment

Surgical treatment of obstruction, if any, has to be done.

In cases of non-obstructive group, continuous catheter drainage is required. Intermittent clamping of the catheter is to be done prior to its removal. Following removal of the catheter, the residual urine has to be measured. It should not be more than 100 mL, preferably 50 mL. If more than 100 mL, the continuous drainage is reinstituted.

VOIDING DISORDER

Definition

Difficulty in emptying the bladder is due to dysfunction of effective detrusor contraction and/or urethral sphincter mechanism. Anuria must be excluded. Voiding difficulties may lead to **retention of urine** either **acute** *(inability to void more than 12 hours without catheterization)* or **chronic** *(inability to empty the bladder more than 50% of its volume).*

Retention of Urine

Causes

- **Postoperative:** The most common cause of retention in gynecology. This may occur following any operation on the vagina or perineum.

TABLE 25.8: Gynecological pathology causing retention of urine.

Period of life	*Associated disorders*	*Provisional diagnosis*
Postmenarchal	**Primary amenorrhea**	**Cryptomenorrhea**
Childbearing period	Short period of secondary amenorrhea	Retroverted gravid uterus
	Menorrhagia	Uterine fibroid impacted in pouch of Douglas
	No menstrual abnormality	Impacted ovarian tumor, cervical or broad ligament fibroid
	Irregular bleeding with pain	Pelvic hematocele
	Irregular bleeding with fever	Pelvic abscess)

The factors operating are:
- Obstructive due to postoperative edema in the neighborhood of the stitch line.
- Reflex spasm of bladder sphincters specially following anterior colporrhaphy.
- Reflex spasm of the levators following perineorrhaphy.
- Postoperative vaginal packing so often given following vaginal plastic operations.

Following radical operation:
- Denervation of the nerve supply of the bladder which travels from $S_{2,3,4}$ in the parametrium. This especially happens in Wertheim's operation, where extensive dissection of the parametrium is carried out.

- **Obstructive conditions intrinsic to the urethra**
  - Cicatricial stenosis following operations for repair of a urethrovaginal fistula or caruncle.
  - Urethral angulation in cases with big cystocele.
  - Bladder neck obstruction in postmenopausal women.
  - After sling operation for stress incontinence.
  - Cancer of the urethra, bladder neck, vulva, paraurethral cyst and tumor.
- **Bladder detrusor may fail to contract**
  - *Diseases*—multiple sclerosis (detrusor-sphincter dyssynergia), Parkinson's disease, neuropathy.
  - *Drugs*—epidural anesthesia antidepressant, ganglion blockers.
  - *Psychogenic*—hysteria, fear, modesty or shyness.
- **Spasm of external sphincter**
  - Nervousness and embarrassment or unaccustomed position.
  - Perineal injuries due to operation.
  - Urethritis.
- **Gynecological causes (Table 25.8):** A pelvic tumor or a mass in the pelvis may produce retention of urine. The diagnosis is usually made by giving attention to associated symptoms.

Retention is caused by the tumor interfering with the opening of internal sphincter of the urethra.

Investigations

Should be designed on the basis of etiology. Neurological examination should done as a routine.

Management

The treatment aims at:
- To relieve the symptom
- To treat the primary cause, when present.

Acute retention: Catheterization is to be done by using an autoclaved soft rubber catheter. Due aseptic precautions are to be taken as described in Ch. 9. If the patient fails to pass urine normally again after 8 hours, a self-retaining catheter is to be introduced for continuous drainage for at least 24–48 hours.

Chronic retention: In cases of chronic retention with marked overdistension of the bladder, it is better to put a self-retaining catheter.

URINARY TRACT INFECTIONS

About 20% of all women have urinary tract infections (UTI) during their lifetime. Moreover, in cases of asymptomatic bacteriuria, the infection remains in the urinary tract for a long period of time.

Prevalence

The prevalence of UTI up to 11 years is about 1% for boys and 3% for girls. In older girls, there is 10-fold increase in incidence as compared to boys. The incidence of asymptomatic bacteriuria in female is about 4%. In pregnancy, it rises to 10%.

- **Factors for increased UTI in females:**
  - Short urethra (4 cm)
  - Close proximity of the external urethral meatus to the areas (vulva and lower-third of vagina) contaminated heavily with bacteria
  - Sexual intercourse
  - Catheterization.
- **Aggravating factors during pregnancy are:**

Stasis of urine in bladder → multiplication of bacteria → influx of the infected urine into the ureters and renal pelves due to laxity of the vesicoureteral sphincters due to edema.

Organisms: The most common organism is *Escherichia coli* which is present in about 80–90% cases. Others are *Pseudomonas, Klebsiella, Proteus, Enterococci, Staphylococcus,* etc.

Predisposing Factors

- **The lower urethra is colonized** with bacteria early in life but the bacteria are nonpathogenic. The protective effect of estrogen is also lacking.
- **Sexual intercourse** increases the ascent of the organisms from the lower urethra into the bladder.
- **Full bladder:** Provided bladder is kept empty completely and regularly, there is least chance of UTI.

- **Catheterization:** This is probably the most common cause of introducing the organisms from the lower urethra into the bladder whatever meticulous aseptic technique being taken.
- **Hypoestrogenic state** as in postmenopausal women—when defense of the bladder and urethral mucosa is diminished.
- **Immunocompromising disorders** like diabetes mellitus, human immunodeficiency virus (HIV).

Routes of Infection

- **Ascending**
- **Hematogenous**
- **Lymphatic**

Ascending—is the most common route of infection. The organisms from the anorectal region, lower vagina and vulva gain access to the urethra and thence to the bladder and kidneys.

Hematogenous—spread involving the kidneys is from the intestine or septic tonsils or other septic foci.

Lymphatic—spread is either from the adjacent ascending colon or genital organs (cervicitis). The kidneys may be affected from the bladder through periureteral lymphatics.

Clinical Presentations

Asymptomatic Bacteriuria

The term asymptomatic bacteriuria is used when a bacterial count of the same species over 10^5/mL in midstream specimen of urine on two occasions is detected without symptom of urinary infection. Counts less than 10^5/mL indicate contamination of urine from the urethra or external genitalia. Nearly 30% of women with asymptomatic bacteriuria develop symptoms of UTI at a later date, if left untreated.

The entity is found related with high incidence of urinary tract abnormality—congenital or acquired. The woman runs a greater risk of developing chronic renal lesion later in life.

Lower Urinary Tract Infection

Urethritis: The symptoms include dysuria, frequency and urgency of micturition. Pain is typically scalding during the act of micturition. Urethra is tender on palpation. Often, pus may be squeezed out from the urethra.

Apart from clean catch midstream urine for culture, the expressed pus should be submitted for Gram stain for intracellular diplococci suggestive of gonorrhea and culture for trichomonas *Chlamydia* and *Neisseria gonorrheae*. Urethritis, chlamydia, *Trichomonas vaginalis* and *N. gonorrhoeae* are the common cause of urethritis. Nucleic acid amplification tests (NAATs) of urine help the detection.

Urethral syndrome: It is a chronic nonspecific form of urethritis probably due to urethral hypersensitivity. Infection should be excluded. The symptoms include dysuria, frequency, nocturia and urgency of micturition. Urethroscopy reveals reddened, chronically inflamed urethral mucosa and spasm of the bladder neck. Benzodiazepines, Amitriptyline. Antibiotics (doxycycline) and estrogen replacement therapy give short-term relief. Progressive urethral dilatation has been the treatment of choice. Cryosurgery has been found to be effective to relief the symptoms.

Cystitis: Cystitis is the most common of the urinary tract infections.

Symptoms include dysuria, frequency and urgency of micturition and pain. It produces painful micturition especially at the end of the act. There may be suprapubic tenderness and may have constitutional upset.

Investigations: Midstream clean catch urine for microscopic examination, culture and drug sensitivity is to be done in every case.

Microscopic examination usually reveals plenty of pus cells and occasional red blood cells. The culture will detect the organism within 24 hours and it usually exceeds 10^5/mL of urine.

Sterile pyuria (negative culture in presence of plenty of pus cells) alerts the possibility of tubercular infection. In suspected tuberculosis, at least three early morning urine specimens have to be collected and cultured.

The presence of red blood cells in the absence of pus cells or negative culture suggests pathology other than infection.

Apart from midstream urine, other methods of collection of urine are—suprapubic needle aspiration and urethral catheterization.

Pyelitis: Symptoms include acute aching pain over the loins and fever with chills and rigor. There is frequency of micturition and dysuria. There may be anorexia, nausea or vomiting.

The patient looks ill with dry tongue. The pulse rate is proportionate with temperature. There is varying degrees of loin tenderness.

Investigations

Midstream urine examination reveals plenty of pus cells and red blood corpuscles. Culture will detect the organism.

Blood examination shows leukocytosis; urea and creatinine level may be raised.

In chronic or recurrent UTI, more extended investigative protocols such as intravenous pyelography (IVP) and cystoscopy is indicated.

Prevention

The following guidelines are prescribed in an attempt **to prevent infection to lower urinary tract.**

- **To maintain proper perineal hygiene**. This consists of cleansing the vulvar region at least daily, wiping the rectum away from the urethra.
- **Prophylaxis of the coital infection:** To void urine immediately following coitus. A single dose of nitrofurantoin 50 mg following coital act is an effective means of prophylaxis. This is helpful in women who have history of postcoital exacerbation of infection.
- **Catheter infection:** Whatever aseptic measures are taken, use of catheter favors introduction of infection. Catheter should preferably be avoided.

- **Bacteriological monitoring** of urine should be done, periodically and after removal, when an indwelling catheter is used for a long time.
- **Plenty of fluid intake** should be encouraged.

Protective mechanisms against UTI have been described in Table 25.8.

Management Principles

- To isolate the organism and drug sensitivity, if time permits prior to antimicrobial therapy.
- To administer effective drug for an adequate length of time (7–10 days).
- To prevent reinfection.
- **General measures:** Plenty of water to drink (3–4 liters a day) for proper hydration.
- **Antimicrobial agents:** Appropriate antibiotic to be started for an adequate length of time (7–10 days).

One negative culture two weeks after the course of therapy is considered cure.

- **Prevention of reinfection:** Presence of any organic pathology is to be treated. Outflow tract obstruction, if present, may have to be dilated.

In reinfection, the appropriate drug is to be continued for at least 2 weeks. This is to be followed by nitrofurantoin 50 mg or norfloxacin 400 mg daily for 4–6 months.

URETHRAL DIVERTICULUM

It is the outpouching of the urethral mucosa into the vaginal tissues. It is observed in 1% to 5% of the women. **Causes are:** (a) Congenital; (b) Acute; (c) Chronic inflammatory and (d) traumatic. Infection and obstruction of periurethral glands resulting in formation of retention cysts. Repeated infections and ultimate rupture into the lumen of urethra is the cause.

The outpouching remains and give rise to the diverticulum. *E. coli* or gonococcus is the common cause. **Symptoms and signs:** (3Ds). (a) Post void Dribbling; (b) Dysuria and (c) Dyspareunia. Occasionally hematuria may be there.
Diagnosis: (a) Pelvic examination: A tender cystic mass in the mid or distal urethra; (b) Urethroscopy is helpful; (c) MRI axial image can help the detection; (d) Double balloon triple lumen catheter is also helpful to the diagnosis.
Treatment: (a) If asymptomatic—no treatment is needed; (b) Mild symptoms—may be treated with antibiotics; (c) Surgical management (diverticulectomy)—dissection of the diverticulum is done to make it free. The diverticular neck is excised by sharp dissection. The urethral wall is repaired with interrupted 4-0 polyglycolic suture. The vaginal incision is closed.
Complications: Urethrovaginal fistula (5–8%), development of SUI, recurrence of diverticulum and stricture of urethra (5%). Malignant change is rare.

DYSURIA

Definition

Dysuria or difficulty in passing urine is a common symptom in gynecology. The difficulty may be painful—or merely mechanical.

Causes

Mechanical Factors

- All the factors leading to retention of urine are usually preceded by dysuria.
- Uterine prolapse with big cystocele.

Factors for painful micturition:

- **Causes in the bladder:** The bladder lesions include—cystitis due to infection with *E. coli* or tuberculosis, stone, radiation drug induced (cyclophosphamide), eosinophilic or due to papilloma or carcinoma.

  Cystitis or other lesions in the bladder cause painful micturition specially at the end of the act.
- **Causes in the urethra:** Here, the pain is scalding during the act. Urethral lesions responsible are—urethritis due to specific or nonspecific organisms, tender caruncle, prolapse of urethral mucosa, kraurosis, urethral carcinoma, etc.
- **Trauma** during catheterization, operation or due to trauma of the external urethral meatus during coitus 'honeymoon cystitis'.
- **Postoperative** causes of dysuria may be due to:
  - Cystitis or urethritis
  - Precipitated by catheterization
  - Trauma around the bladder neck and urethra.

Frequency of Urination

Table 25.5.

URETHRAL CARUNCLE (Fig. 25.12)

DEFINITION

It is a benign lesion of the urethra, clinically characterized by a pedunculated, reddish-appearance mass protruding out of the external urethral meatus.

PATHOGENESIS

It is presumably infective in origin and usually confined to postmenopausal women. It is usually single and arises from the posterior wall of the urethra.

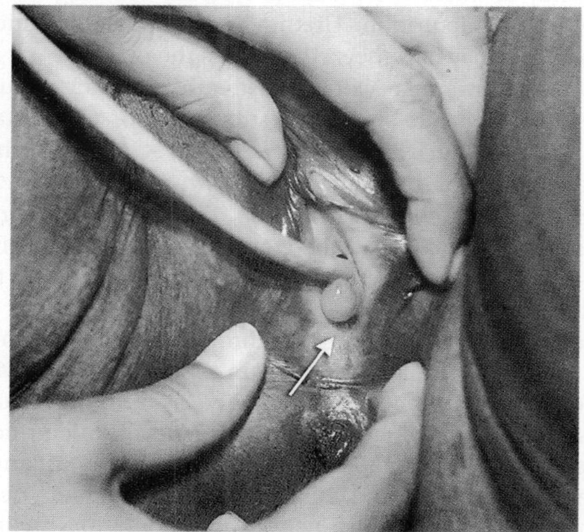

Fig. 25.12: Urethral caruncle (arrow).

Naked eye: The size is small, usually not exceeding 0.5 cm. It looks reddish (Fig. 25.12).

Microscopic appearance: It consists of vascularized granulation tissue covered by transitional or stratified squamous epithelium. **Three types are described**—granulomatous, angiomatous and papillomatous depending upon the histologic appearance.

CLINICAL FEATURES

The patients are usually postmenopausal.

Symptoms:

- Irregular bleeding per vaginam
- Urinary complaints such as painful micturition, frequency or even retention
- Dyspareunia.

Signs: A small angry red-looking, pea-shaped mass protruding out of the external urethral meatus. It may be tender or bleeds to touch.

Differential diagnosis: The lesion is often confused with prolapse of the urethral mucosa and urethral malignancy.

TREATMENT

Excision biopsy is the definitive surgery. The raw area may be sutured or cauterized. Continuous bladder drainage is required for a few days.

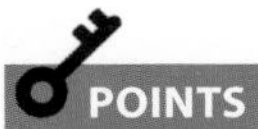

POINTS

- **The sympathetic supply** to the bladder is concerned mainly with the filling and storage of urine. The parasympathetic is important for normal voiding.
- **Parasympathetic nervous system** (acetylcholine receptor) activate detrusor contraction. Sympathetic system in bladder (β-receptor) causes relaxation and in the urethra (α-receptor) causes contraction.
- **Urethral sphincters** for continence are: (a) Intrinsic rhabdosphincter urethrae (containing 'slow twitch fibers'); (b) Extrinsic sphincter of levator ani (containing both 'slow and fast twitch' fibers).
- **Intrinsic urethral sphincter** maintains urethral closure at rest, whereas extrinsic sphincter maintain urethral closure during stress (cough, sneeze).
- **Normally urethral closure pressure** is maintained effectively. Any rise in intra-abdominal pressure (IAP) transmitted equally to the bladder and the proximal urethra. This mechanism maintains the pressure gradient (Figs. 25.6A and B).
- **Approximately**, one-third of the resting urethral pressure is due to rhabdosphincter effects, one-third to smooth muscle effects and one-third to submucous vascular plexus of the urethra.
- **The intravesical pressure** is about 10 cm of water and is much lower than the urethral pressure (20–50 cm of water).
- Normally **first sensation of urination** is felt at 150–200 mL of bladder volume and functional bladder capacity is 400–600 mL.
- **Continence** is a state of balance between urethral closure pressure versus detrusor contraction pressure.
- **Urinary incontinence** is either urethral or extraurethral in origin (Table 25.1).
- **Nearly 30% of women** suffer from some degree of urinary incontinence during their life time.
- **Genuine stress incontinence (GSI)** is defined as involuntary urethral loss of urine when intravesical pressure exceeds the maximum urethral pressure in the absence of the detrusor activity.
- **GSI** is due to anatomic hypermobility of bladder-neck and urethra (80%) and also due to urethral intrinsic sphincteric incompetence (20%).
- **GSI** is often confused with urge incontinence (sensory) and detrusor instability (motor) (Tables 25.2 and 25.6). During strain, there is significant lowering of the urethral closure pressure. This is pathognomonic of GSI.
- **Thorough urodynamic investigations** are essential in certain conditions to get maximum benefit of treatment. However, it is not recommended as a routine neither it is to be done before any conservative treatment.
- **Patient with urodynamic features** of both GSI and overactive bladder (OAB), OAB is to be treated prior to continence surgery.
- **UTI** must be treated before any urodynamic investigation. A urine dipstick test is done for all women with UI. Women with urine tests positive for both leukocytes and nitrites should have a midstream urine specimen for culture and sensitivity.
- **IVU**, cystourethroscopy or videocystourethrography should not be performed as a routine investigation.
- **USG** (transvaginal, perineal or intraurethral) is becoming more informative in assessing a patient with urinary symptoms.
- **Cystometry** confirms the diagnosis of DO but GSI is a diagnosis of exclusion.
- **Vaginal delivery** causes damage to anatomical supports of the bladder neck, urethra and the pelvic floor nerves. It is an important cause for genitourinary prolapse and GSI.
- **Individualization** of a patient for a particular type of incontinence surgery is essential. Important deciding factors are: (a) severity of symptoms; (b) patient's age; (c) associated complications and (d) experience of the surgeon.
- **The objectives of** the surgical treatment are to elevate the bladder neck along with proximal urethra and to support the vesicourethral junction to prevent funneling during stress. Surgical treatment of GSI vary depending on an individual patient.
- **Approximate success rate (5 years)** for individual procedure is: Cystourethroplasty 50–60%; cystourethropexy (MMK) 80–90%, Burch 85–90%, endoscopic bladder neck suspension 50%.
- **In TVT procedure** a macroporous tape made of polypropylene is placed U-shaped under the midurethra, lying tension-free. Overall cure rate of this procedure is 84–90%. Injury to the bladder (during trocar insertion), hemorrhage in the retropubic space, tape rejection or erosion are the complications.
- **TOT** is a simple procedure where a polypropylene macroporous tape is placed under the midurethra. The tape passes through the obturator foramen either from outside in (TOT) or from inside-out (TVT-O). It maintains the natural suspension of the urethra. As it avoids the retropubic space, the complications are less. It can be done under local anesthetic. Success rate is similar to that of TVT.

Contd...

Contd...

- **Minimally invasive slings** (micro/minislings) are done by placing one 8 cm long strip of prolyproylene synthetic mesh across and beneath the midurethra. The procedure is a modification of TVT or TOT but the tape is passed neither through the retropubic space nor through the obturator foramen. It avoids the complications of visceral and vascular injury. It is highly effective.
- **Recommended surgical procedures** for GSI as based on evidence are as mentioned in.
- **Detrusor overactivity (DO)** is defined as an unstable bladder, objectively to contract spontaneously or on provocation during the filling phase while the patient is attempting to inhibit it. It is the second common cause of urinary incontinence in adult female, the first being GSI. It is the most common cause in elderly women. The diagnosis is based on urodynamic assessment.
- **Intrinsic urethral sphincter dysfunction** is best treated by periurethral collagen injection, a sling procedure or by an artificial sphincter.
- **The etiology of overactive bladder (OAB)** is largely functional and psychosomatic in origin. True detrusor pressure increases by more than 15 cm of water during bladder filling even with 100–175 mL of fluid.
- **Overactive bladder (OAB)** is a symptomatic diagnosis whereas detrusor overactivity is a diagnosis confirmed on cystometry. OAB has got spontaneous remissions and exacerbations.
- **Bladder retraining**, behavioral therapy and anticholinergic drugs are effective to control symptoms of OAB on majority of patients. Dosage of anticholinergic drugs need to be increased gradually to a level as to produce side effects (Table 25.7). Anticholinergic agents decrease detrusor activity.
- **Oxybutynin** should be the first choice for women with OAB or mixed UI if bladder training is ineffective. When oxybutynin is not tolerated, darifenacin, solifenacin, tolterodine, trospium or transdermal formulation of oxybutynin is considered.
- **PBS** is a chronic inflammatory condition associated with urgency and painful voiding. It is a diagnosis of exclusion. Urinary tract infection must be ruled out. It is associated with altered epithelial permeability, mast cell activation and upregulation of sensory afferent nerves. Treatment is directed to control the symptoms. Diet and drugs (to control inflammation), surgery and neuromodulation therapy are the options.
- **Sensory urge incontinence** is usually associated with infection or foreign body. The treatment is by appropriate antibiotic therapy and hormone replacement therapy (HRT) in postmenopausal women.
- **Important causes of urgency**, urge incontinence and frequency of micturition are gynecological, urological or medical disorders (Table 25.5).
- **There is increased risk of UTI** in females than in males. The most common organism is *Escherichia coli*.
- **Recurrent UTI** need to be investigated with cystoscopy and intravenous urography. In a chronic case, following an appropriate drug therapy for 2 weeks, nitrofurantoin 50 mg or norfloxacin 400 mg daily bed time for 3–4 months is to be continued.
- **Urethral syndrome** is a chronic form of painful micturition due to urethral hypersensitivity in the absence of UTI.
- **Negative culture** in presence of plenty of pus cells alerts to the possibility of tubercular infection.
- **The presence of red blood cells** in the absence of pus cells or negative culture suggests pathology other than infection.
- **Apart from midstream urine**, other methods of collection of urine are suprapubic needle aspiration and urethral catheterization.
- **Voiding disorders** are defined as difficulty in emptying bladder due to dysfunction of effective detrusor contraction and/or sphincter mechanism.
- **Low peak flow rate (<15 mL/sec)** associated with increased detrusor pressure (>50 cm H_2O), with prolonged voiding time indicates outflow obstruction.
- **Retention of urine** may be acute (inability to void over 12 hours without catheterization) or chronic (inability to empty bladder more than 50% of its volume). Desire to void is felt at a bladder volume of 150–200 mL and functional bladder capacity is 400–500 mL.
- **Common causes of retention of urine** in gynecology are postoperative, retroverted gravid uterus, impacted uterine fibroid or ovarian tumor in the pouch of Douglas (POD), cervical fibroid or cryptomenorrhea.
- **Investigations and management** for retention of urine should be designed according to the etiology.
- **Urethral caruncle** is a benign lesion arising from posterior wall of the urethra. It is commonly seen in postmenopausal women. Histologically, it may be granulomatous, angiomatous or papillomatous in type. Excision biopsy is the definitive surgery.

CHAPTER

26 Genitourinary Fistula

CHAPTER OUTLINE

- Genitourinary Fistula
- Vesicovaginal Fistula
- Urethrovaginal Fistula
- Ureteric Injury in Gynecologic Surgery
- Rectovaginal Fistula

GENITOURINARY FISTULA

DEFINITION

A fistula is an abnormal communication between two or more epithelial surfaces. **Genitourinary fistula** is an abnormal communication between the urinary and genital tract **either acquired or congenital (rare)** with involuntary escape of urine into the vagina.

The incidence is estimated to be approximately 0.2–1% among gynecological admissions in referral hospitals of the developing countries. The incidence is; however, going down in India with progressive improvement in maternal and child health care.

Fistula May be

Congenital (rare): It is due to abnormal fusion of ureteric bud and the Müllerian duct with the urogenital sinus or due to abnormal development of the urorectal septum.

Acquired: Abnormal communication that develops between the bladder, urethra or ureter and genital tract.

Genitourinary fistulae have further been classified depending upon: (a) Distance of fistula's distal edge from the external urinary meatus; (b) Size of the fistula (c) Extent of fibrosis at the fistulae margin; (d) Vaginal length; (e) Special factors like postradiation, failed repair, etc. (Table 26.1).

VESICOVAGINAL FISTULA (VVF)

DEFINITION

There is communication between the bladder, the vagina and the urine escapes into the vagina causing true incontinence (Fig. 26.2). **This is the most common type of genitourinary fistula.**

TABLE 26.1: Types of vesicovaginal fistula (VVF) based on complexity (Elkin, 1999).

Fistula	Simple	Complicated
Size	Up to 3 cm	>3 cm
Location	High vaginal	Midvaginal
Bladder involvement	Supratrigonal	Trigonal area
Pelvic malignancy	Absent	Present
Prior radiation	Absent	Present
Vaginal length	Normal	Shortened
*The complicated group has poor result.		

FOLLOWING ARE THE TYPES OF FISTULA (ACQUIRED) (FIG. 26.1)

Bladder
- Vesicovaginal (most common)
- Vesicourethrovaginal
- Vesicouterine
- Vesicocervical

Urethra
- Urethrovaginal

Ureter
- Ureterovaginal
- Ureterouterine
- Ureterocervical
- Vesicoureterovaginal

CAUSES

- **Obstetrical**
- **Gynecological**

Obstetrical

In the developing countries, the most common cause is obstetrical and constitutes about 80–90% of cases, as opposed to only 5–15% in the developed countries. The fistula may be due to ischemia or following trauma. In India obstetric fistula is on the decline.

Ischemic: It results from prolonged compression effect on the bladder base between the head and symphysis pubis

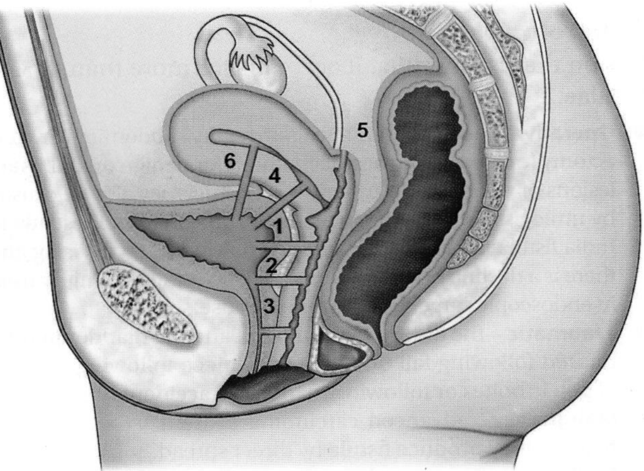

Fig. 26.1: Types of genitourinary fistula: (1) Vesicovaginal; (2) Vesicourethrovaginal; (3) Urethrovaginal; (4) Vesicocervical; (5) Ureterovaginal; (6) Vesicouterine.

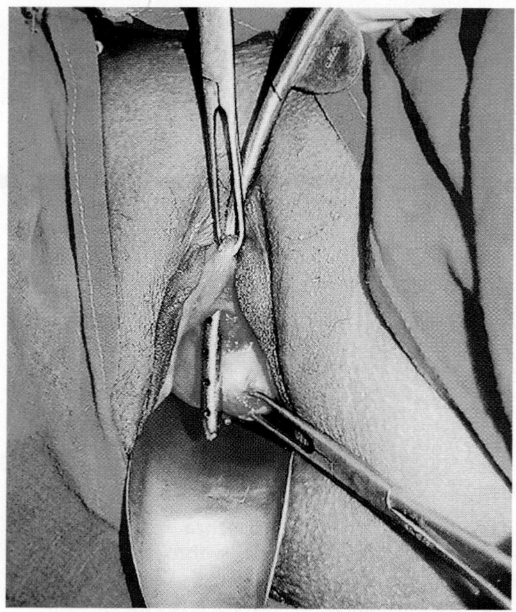

Fig. 26.2: Midvaginal obstetric fistula (VVF). It was of moderate size to allow a metal catheter which is clearly visible.

(*Courtesy:* Dr P Mukherjee, Professor and Head, Department of Gynecology and Obstetrics, Medical College, Kolkata)

in **obstructed labor** → ischemic necrosis → infection → sloughing → fistula. **Thus, it takes few days (3–5) following delivery to produce such type of fistula.**

Traumatic: This may be caused by:

- **Instrumental vaginal delivery** such as **destructive operations** or **forceps** especially with Kielland. The injury may also be inflicted by the **bony spicule** of the fetal skull in **craniotomy operation.**
- **Abdominal operations** such as hysterectomy for ruptured uterus or cesarean section especially a repeat one or for cesarean hysterectomy. The injury may be direct or ischemic following a part of the bladder wall being caught in the suture.

This type of direct traumatic fistula usually follows soon after delivery.

Gynecological

It is on the rise in India. It accounts for more than 80% of fistulae.

- **Operative injury**—anterior colporrhaphy, abdominal hysterectomy (open or laparoscopic method) for benign or malignant lesions or removal of Gartner's cyst. Fistula may also be caused by urologists, colorectal and general surgeon also. Presently in India fistula following injury during pelvic surgery is rising and there is a decline in obstetric causes. Electrothermal injury used in endoscopic surgery, is a common cause.
- **Traumatic**—the anterior vaginal wall and the bladder may be injured following fall on a pointed object, following fracture of pelvic bones or following road traffic accidents.
- **Malignancy**—advanced carcinoma of the cervix, vagina or bladder may produce fistula by direct spread.
- **Radiation**—there may be ischemic necrosis by endarteritis obliterans due to radiation effect, when the carcinoma cervix is treated by radiation. It takes usually long time (1–2 years) to produce such fistula.
- **Infective**—chronic granulomatous lesions such as vaginal tuberculosis, lymphogranuloma venereum, schistosomiasis or actinomycosis may produce fistula.

Thus, the fistula tract may be lined by fibrous, granulation tissue, infective extension or malignant cells.

Other causes are: Infection (lymphogranuloma venereum), sexual assault.

TYPES

Fistula may be classified as—(i) Simple (healthy tissues with good access) or (ii) **Complicated** (tissue loss, fibrosis, difficult access, associated with RVF) (Table 26.1).

Depending upon the site of the fistula, it may be:

Juxtacervical (close to the cervix): The communication is between the supratrigonal region of the bladder and the vagina (vault fistula).

Midvaginal: The communication is between the base (trigone) of the bladder and vagina.

Juxtaurethral: The communication is between the neck of the bladder and vagina (may involve the upper urethra as well).

Subsymphysial: Circumferential loss of tissue in the region of bladder neck and urethra. The fistula margin is fixed to the bone.

CLINICAL FEATURES

Patient Profile

In the developing countries, obstetrical fistula being common, the patients are usually young primiparous with history of difficult labor or instrumental delivery in recent past. In others, it is related with the relevant events (recent pelvic surgery, open or laparoscopic).

Symptoms

- **Continuous escape of urine per vaginam** (true incontinence) is the classic symptom. The patient has got no urge to pass urine. However, if the fistula is small, the escape of urine occurs in certain positions and the patient can also pass urine normally. Such history has got a positive correlation with the related events mentioned in the etiology.

  Leakage of urine following **direct surgical injury** occurs from the first postoperative day whereas in **obstetric fistulae** symptoms may take 7–14 days to appear urethral fistulae that are situated high up, often presents with features of stress incontinence.

  VVF may present from days to weeks **after laparoscopic surgery** (hysterectomy).

  Women with vesicocervical or vesicouterine fistulae may hold urine at the level of the uterine isthmus and may remain continent. But they complain of cyclical hematuria at the time of menstruation (menouria). Sometimes women may complain of intermittent leakage of urine.

  Information of prior surgeries, pelvic malignancy, radiation therapy, prior failed surgery should be mentioned.
- There is associated pruritus vulvae.

Signs

Vulvar inspection

- Escape of ammonia smelling watery discharge per vaginam is characteristic.
- Evidences of sodden and excoriation of the vulvar skin.
- Varying degrees of perineal tear may be present.

Internal examination: If the fistula is big enough, its position, size and tissues at the margins are to be noted.

At times, there may be varying degrees of vaginal atresia so as to make the fistula inaccessible.

Speculum examination: A Sims' speculum in Sims' position gives a good view of the anterior vaginal wall when the vagina becomes ballooned up by air because of negative suction.

- The size, site and number of fistula.
- Often, the bladder mucosa may be visibly prolapsed through a big fistula (Fig. 26.2).
- A tiny fistula is evidenced by a puckered area of vaginal mucosa.

Associated clinical features that may be present in cases of such fistula are:

- Secondary amenorrhea of hypothalamic origin (menstruation resumes following successful repair).
- Complete perineal tear or rectovaginal fistula.
- Foot-drop due to prolonged compression of the sacral nerve roots by the fetal head during labor (rare).

Confirmation of Diagnosis

The diagnosis is most often made from the typical history and local examination. But, sometimes confusion arises in a case of tiny fistula for which additional methods are to be employed (Table 26.2). **The confused clinical conditions are** stress incontinence, ureterovaginal and urethrovaginal fistula.

To confirm the diagnosis, followings are helpful:

- Examination under anesthesia (EUA) is needed for better evaluation.
- The patient is placed in Sims' or knee chest position and while examining the anterior vaginal wall, bubbles of air are seen through the small tiny fistula when the woman coughs.
- **Dye test:** A speculum is introduced and the anterior vaginal wall is swabbed dry. When the methylene blue solution is introduced into the bladder by a catheter, the dye will be seen coming out through the opening.
- **A metal catheter passed** through the external urethral meatus into the bladder when comes out through the fistula not only confirms the VVF but ensures patency of the urethra (Fig. 26.2).
- **Three-swab (tampon) test:** The three-swab test not only confirms the VVF but also differentiates it from ureterovaginal and urethrovaginal fistula (Table 26.3).

TABLE 26.2: Summary in clinical diagnosis.

Big fistula	▪ Visible fistula tract ▪ Obvious escape of urine
Tiny fistula	▪ Dye test ▪ In knee-chest position escape of bubbles of air when the patient coughs ▪ Three-swab test
Confusion in diagnosis	▪ Cystoscopy

TABLE 26.3: Three-swab (tampon) test.

Observation	*Inference*
Upper most swab soaked with urine but unstained with dye. The lower two fistula swabs remain dry	Ureterovaginal fistula
Upper and lower swabs remain dry but the middle swab stained with dye	Vesicovaginal fistula
The upper two swabs remain dry but the lower swab stained with dye	Urethrovaginal fistula

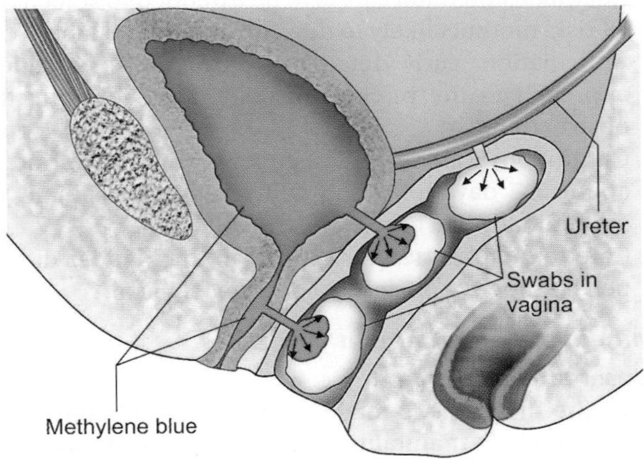

Fig. 26.3: Three-swab (tampon) test using methylene blue.

Procedure of Three-Swab Test (Table 26.3 and Fig. 26.3)

Three cotton swabs are placed in the vagina—one at the vault, one at the middle and one just above the introitus. The methylene blue or indigo carmine is instilled into the bladder through a rubber catheter and the patient is asked to walk for about 5 minutes. She is then asked to lie down and the swabs are removed for inspection (Fig. 26.3).

INVESTIGATIONS

Imaging studies

- **Intravenous urography (IVU) or intravenous contrast enhanced CT scanning:** For the diagnosis of ureterovaginal fistula. It is associated in 10% of cases with VVF.
- **Retrograde pyelography:** For the diagnosis of exact site of ureterovaginal fistula.
- **Voiding cystourethrography** (VCUG) can detect leakage in the vagina.
- **Sinography** (fistulography) for intestinogenital fistula.
- **Hysterosalpingography** (lateral view) for diagnosis of vesicouterine fistula when there is history of hematuria (Youssef's syndrome).
- **Ultrasound, computed tomography (CT) and magnetic resonance imaging (MRI)** are done for evaluation of complex fistulae. Where involvement of ureter or intestines are there.
- **Endoscopy studies:** Cystourethroscopy is done in selective cases. The added information are: Exact level, number and location of the fistula and its relationship to ureteric orifices and bladder neck.
- **Examination under anesthesia** is helpful for identification of small fistulae. A metallic probe may be used for exploration (Fig. 26.2).

TREATMENT OF VVF

- **Preventive**
- **Operative**

Preventive

Obstetric fistula in the developing world can be prevented with safe motherhood initiative **(WHO - 1987)**. Women with obstetric VVF is considered as a maternal 'near-miss'. Gynecological fistula—can be prevented with better anticipation and improved surgical skill.

The Following Guidelines are Prescribed

- Adequate antenatal care is to be extended to screen out 'at risk' mothers likely to develop obstructed labor.
- Anticipation, early detection (partograph) and ideal approach in the method of delivery in relieving the obstruction.
- Continuous bladder drainage for a variable period of about 5–7 days following delivery either vaginally or abdominally in a case of obstructed labor.
- Care to be taken to avoid injury to the bladder during pelvic surgery—obstetrical or gynecological.

Immediate Management

Conservative treatment

Once the diagnosis is made, continuous catheterization for 4–8 weeks is maintained. This may help spontaneous closure of small size (2 mm to 2 cm diameter) fistula tract in about 50–60% cases. Unobstructed outflow tract helps epithelialization, provided the tissue damage is minimum. The management of most genitourinary fistula needs a team approach both by the gynecologists, nursing staff and the urologists. **These socially ostracized women need realistic counseling. Otherwise treatment failure may cause further devastation.**

Operative

Local repair of the fistula is done.

Principles of Surgery

- A correct preoperative assessment and preparation
- Timely repair
- Repair should be tension free
- Presence of healthy vascular tissue at the fistula margin
- Postoperative bladder drainage.

Preoperative Assessment

- Fistula status: Assessment is done as regards the site, size, number, mobility and extent of fibrosis at the margins of the fistula.
- Urethral involvement is assessed by introducing a metal catheter through external urethral meatus into the bladder.
- To ascertain the position of the ureteric openings in relation to a big fistula, cystoscopy is indicated.
- **To exclude associated rectovaginal fistula or complete perineal tear**.
- Complete hemogram and urea, creatinine (renal function) estimation are done.

Preoperative Preparations

- **Improvement of the general condition** is essential prior to surgery.
- **Local infection** in the vulva should be treated by application of silicone barrier cream with antibiotics.
- **Urinary infection**, if any, should be corrected beforehand. Preoperative collection is best to be done through ureteric catheterization. Urine collected through vaginal speculum will not serve the purpose because of contamination. It is advised to start urinary antibiotics at least 3–5 days prior to surgery.

Definitive Surgery

Time of repair

The ideal time of surgery is usually after 6 weeks to 3 months following delivery. By this time, the general condition improves and local tissues are likely to be free from infection. Further delay is likely to produce more fibrosis and unnecessary prolongs the misery of the patient. Surgical repair of an uncomplicated (without infection) fistula may be done early without routine waiting for 6 weeks.

Advantages of vaginal route repair are: Less blood loss, less morbidity, short hospital stay. Ureteral stents may be placed when needed.

Surgical fistula if recognized within 24 hours, immediate repair may be done provided it is small. Otherwise it should be repaired after 10–12 weeks. Radiation fistulae should be repaired after 12 months.

Route of repair

It mostly depends upon the access to the fistula site and the tissue mobility of the vagina. Either the **abdominal or vaginal route** may be approached according to the choice and expertize of the surgeon (Table 26.4).

Suture materials

Polyglactin (Vicryl) 2–0 suture material is preferred for both the bladder and vagina. Polydioxanone (PDS) 4–0 on a 13 mm round bodied needle is used for the ureter. 3–0 PDS on a 30 mm round bodied needle is used for bowel surgery.

Local repair by flap splitting method is the preferred surgery (Figs. 26.4A to E).

Principles of Surgery (Boxes 26.1 and 26.2)

- Perfect asepsis and good exposure of the fistula.
- Excision (minimal) of the scar tissue round the margins.
- Mobilization of the bladder wall from the vagina.
- Suturing the bladder wall **without tension** in two layers.

First layer is with polyglactin (Vicryl) 2–0 suture (p. 547) on a 30 mm needle is preferred. Interrupted stitches (3 mm apart) excluding the bladder mucosa are done.

TABLE 26.4: Other routes of repair of bladder fistula.

- **Transperitoneal**—vesicouterine fistula; ureteric fistula
- **Transvesical**—high and fixed fistulae (extraperitoneal) at the vault: Inaccessible by vaginal route
- **Transperitoneal or transvesical** approach are done in selective cases. Indications are:
  - Fistula located high up and vagina is narrow
  - Fistula is close to ureteric openings
  - Previous failed repair
  - Fistula is large or complex
  - When an interpositional graft is needed.

Second layer is with interrupted sutures using the same suture material taking the muscle and fascial layer of the bladder wall, burying the first suture line.

- Apposition of the vaginal wall by interrupted sutures using same suture material No. 'O' (Figs. 26.4A to E).
- Closure must be water-tight and is tested by dye instillation into the bladder at the end of the operation.
- To maintain continuous bladder drainage by an indwelling catheter for 10–14 days (Box 26.3).

Saucerization (Paring and Suturing)

This operation was originally devised by **James Marion Sims (1852) of USA**. He used to repair (Fig. 38.2) the fistula in **Sims' position** (p. 85) exposing the fistula with **Sims' speculum** and after paring the margins, **sutured the fistula with silver wire**. Saucerization is the closure of a small fistula using interrupted stitches without dissection of bladder from the vagina. This may be employed in a very small fistula using Vicryl (2-0).

Latzko technique is used to repair a VVF that develops following total hysterectomy operation. Principle of this operation is to produce **partial colpocleisis (obliteration of the vagina around the fistula)**. This procedure is suitable for a fistula which is small and high in the vagina.

Box 26.1: Principal steps.

- Vaginal mucosa is dissected off the bladder wall around the fistula site.
- The fistula tract is excised.
- Bladder mucosal edges are approximated with interrupted sutures (2–0 Vicryl).
- Two additional suture layers are used to appose the muscle and fascia.
- Vaginal mucosa is closed by interrupted sutures using same suture material. Continuous bladder drainage by indwelling catheter is maintained for 10–14 days.

Box 26.2: Modifications of vaginal operations (Table 26.4).

- **Ureteric openings close to the margins:** To introduce ureteric catheter prior to repair to prevent inclusion of the ureteric opening in suture.
- **Involvement of the bladder neck:** Suprapubic or vaginal cystostomy prior hand as temporary urinary diversion to keep the repair area free from getting wet.
- **Associated with other pathology CPT or rectovaginal fistula (RVF):** To repair the VVF first followed by repair of the CPT or RVF in the same sitting.

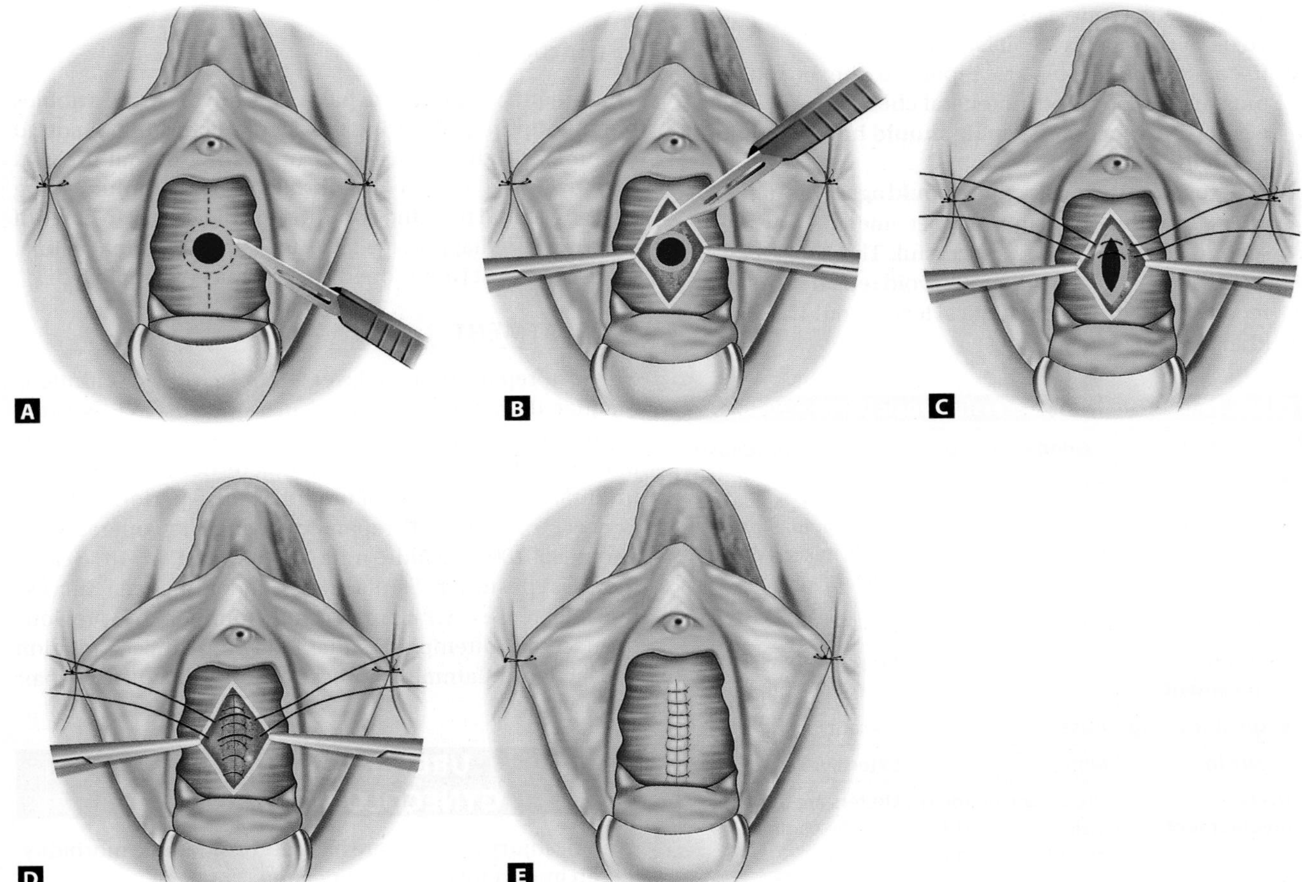

Figs. 26.4A to E: Principal steps of repair of old VVF by flap method: (A) Line of incision; (B) Separation of the vaginal wall from the bladder, to excise the fibrous tissues around the margin of fistula; (C) Closure of the bladder opening by interrupted sutures taking bites through the muscle wall excluding the bladder mucosa; (D) Reinforcing interrupted sutures taking superficial muscle and bladder fascia; (E) Look of the suture line after final repair.

Box 26.3: Special postoperative care.

- Urinary antiseptics either given at random or appropriate to the sensitivity report.
- Continuous blood drainage for about 10–14 days.
- The patient is advised to pass urine frequently (say 1 hourly) following removal of catheter. The interval is gradually increased.
- Nursing care for fluid balance, urine output and to detect any catheter block.

Use of Graft (Interpositional Flaps)

Repair of a big fistula may need interposition of tissue grafts to fill space and with new blood supply. Different tissues may be used.

Martius graft

Bulbocavernous muscle and labial fat pedicle graft is used for big bladder neck fistula.

Other tissues used are: Gracillis muscle, omental pedicle graft (transperitoneal approach) or peritoneal flap.

Laparoscopic repair of genitourinary fistula currently being done in selected cases.

Advice during discharge

- To pass urine more frequently.
- To avoid intercourse for at least 3 months.
- To defer pregnancy for at least 1 year.
- If conception occurs, to report to the hospital and must have mandatory antenatal check-up and hospital delivery. **A successful repair should have an abdominal delivery.**

  If repair fails, local repair should again be attempted after 3 months. The fistula may become smaller when the second attempt may be successful. The best chance of cure is at the first operation. To avoid repeated failures of repair skilled urological surgical team should be involved (Table 26.5).

TABLE 26.5: Criteria for successful repair (WHO – 2006).

Criteria	*Good prognosis*	*Uncertain prognosis*
No. of fistula	Single	Multiple
Site	Vesicovaginal fistula (VVF)	Rectovaginal fistula (RVF), mixed (VVF and RVF)
Size	<4 cm	>4 cm
Urethral involvement	Absent	Present
Vaginal scarring	Absent	Present
Tissue loss	Minimal	Extensive
Ureter involvement	Ureters are draining inside the bladder, not into the vagina	Ureters are draining into the vagina
Circumferential defect (urethra separated from the bladder)	Absent	Present

Principles in the Management of Gynecological VVF

- **Detected during operation:** To repair immediately in two layers.
- **Detected in the postoperative period:** To put an indwelling catheter for about 10–14 days. If fails, repair is to be done after 3 months.
- **Malignant or postradiation fistula:** Any of the following may relief the symptoms—(a) Ileal bladder; (b) Anterior exenteration; (c) Colpocleisis.
- **Infective fistula:** Eradication of the specific infection be done first followed by local repair.

URETHROVAGINAL FISTULA

CAUSES

- Part or whole of the urethra is involved along with bladder. The causes are the same as those of VVF.
- Small isolated urethrovaginal fistula is caused by:
  - Injury inflicted during anterior colporrhaphy, urethroplasty, suspension or sling operation for stress incontinence.
  - Residual fistula left behind following repair of vesicourethrovaginal fistula.

DIAGNOSIS

The patient has got urge to pass urine but the urine dribbles out into the vagina during the act of micturition. A sound or a metal catheter passed through the external urethral meatus when comes out through the communicating urethrovaginal opening confirms the diagnosis. In cases of confusion in diagnosis with VVF or ureterovaginal fistula, three-swab test (mentioned earlier) may be employed.

TREATMENT

Surgical repair in two layers followed by continuous bladder drainage as outlined in repair of VVF is satisfactory. Prior suprapubic or vaginal cystostomy ensures better success. In cases of complete destruction of the urethra, reconstruction of urethra is to be performed.

Success rate of VVF repair following first operation is about 80–100%. Failure rate is 10% and in 10% cases there is posterior fistula stress incontinence. Success rate decreases with increasing number of previous unsuccessful attempts. Fistulas following cancer, radiation and active inflammatory diseases are difficult to repair successfully.

URETERIC INJURY IN GYNECOLOGIC SURGERY

Ureteric injury through rare has got considerable morbidity. It is an important cause for litigation.

CAUSES

- **Acquired**
- **Congenital**

Acquired

This is common and usually follows trauma during pelvic surgery. Although commonly associated with difficult surgery like abdominal hysterectomy in cervical fibroid, broad ligament fibroid, endometriosis, ovarian malignancy or radical hysterectomy, it may be injured even in apparently simple hysterectomy—abdominal or vaginal (rare). Use of thermal energy during laparascopic hysterectomy may cause ureteric injury.

Congenital

The aberrant ureter may open into the vault of vagina, uterus or into urethra.

INJURY TO THE URETER DURING GYNECOLOGICAL SURGERY

Because of close anatomical association between ureter and genital organs, ureteric injury is not uncommon during gynecological surgery. Overall incidence is 0.5–1% of all pelvic operations. About 75% of ureteral injury result from gynecological operations and 75% of them occur following abdominal gynecological procedures.

Important anatomical locations where ureteric injury is more common.

- At the level of infundibulopelvic ligament—where ureter runs parallel to ovarian vessels at the same place. Ureter forms the posterior boundary of ovarian fossa. Any inflammatory or malignant processes will involve the ureter.
- Deep in the pelvis, below the level of ischial spine, where ureter lies lateral to the peritoneum of uterosacral ligament.
- At the level of internal cervical os, 1.5 cm lateral to the cervix where uterine artery crosses the ureter from above.
- Over the anterior vaginal fornix, within the ureteric tunnel of cardinal ligament (tunnel of Wertheim) where it turns anteriorly and medially to enter the bladder.
- Where it traverses through the musculature of bladder (intravesical part).
- Any congenital malformation (duplex ureter) makes it more vulnerable to injury at any of these sites.

Nature of Ureteral Injury

Severity of ureteric injury may be any of the following types:

- Simple kinking or angulation—causing obstruction.
- Ischemic injury resulting from trauma to ureteric sheath endangering its blood supply.
- Ligature incorporation.
- Crushing injury by clamps followed by necrosis.
- Transection—either partial or complete.
- Segmental resection either accidental or planned.
- Thermal injury during minimally invasive surgical procedure when diathermy (monopolar or bipolar) or laser energy is used (p. 514).
- Injury by staplers during laparoscopic surgery.

Gynecological Operations and Ureteric Injury

Risk of injury is more where pelvic anatomy is distorted due to presence of any pelvic pathology. Common pathological conditions are:

- Cervical fibroid or low corporeal fibroid
- Broad ligament tumor
- Pelvic endometriosis
- Gynecological malignancy
- Pelvic hematoma
- Tubo-ovarian mass, pelvic adhesions
- Reapplication of a clamp to the pedicle of uterine artery following its initial slip
- Presacral neuronectomy (endoscopic)
- Ovarian remnant—when needs removal
- Radical hysterectomy
- Vaginal hysterectomy (rare)
- Colposuspension
- Laparoscopically assisted vaginal hysterectomy (LAVH).

DIAGNOSIS

Signs and symptoms are subtle and often overlooked. Fever, flank pain, hematuria, abdominal distension, urine leakage (vaginally), peritonitis, ileus and retroperitoneal urinoma should raise the suspicion.

a. *Escape of urine through vagina* following the operative procedure is suspicious.
b. The patient has got *urge to pass urine and can pass urine normally.*
c. *Three-swab test* differentiates it from VVF (Table 26.3).
d. *Intravenous indigo carmine test*—if the urine in the vagina is unstained following three-swab test, indigo carmine is injected intravenously. If urine becomes blue (generally within 4–5 minutes) the diagnosis of ureterovaginal fistula is established.
e. *Cystoscopy*—should be performed to determine the side of ureterovaginal fistula. There is no spurt of urine from the ureteric orifice of the affected side.
f. When a *ureteric catheter* is passed under cystoscopic guidance, obstruction is met when the catheter tip reaches the site of injury.
g. *Excretory urography (IVU)* confirms the side and site of fistula. The tract of ureterovaginal fistula is also outlined.
h. *Renal ultrasound* is a noninvasive method. Hydronephrosis and retroperitoneal urinomas when seen, are helpful to the diagnosis (ureteral ligation).
i. *Computed tomography (CT)* showing contrast extravasation is the most consistent to the diagnosis.

Preoperative detection of ureteral laceration can be made by seeing the leakage of dye at the site, following intravenous injection of indigo carmine. When the ureter is ligated or kinked, gradually increasing ureteric dilatation will be noticed, instead of dye leakage.

MANAGEMENT OF URETERIC INJURY

- **Preventive**
- **Operative**

Preventive Measures

A thorough knowledge of pelvic anatomy is essential. Where there is any doubt, the following measures may be of help, if taken either during preoperative or intraoperative period.

- **Intravenous urography** (preoperative)—is helpful in certain situation (e.g. pelvic tumors), to ascertain the course of the ureters. Any congenital abnormality is also revealed.
- **Placement of ureteral catheters** (preoperative or intraoperative) to facilitate detection and dissection of ureters. Unfortunately in a fibrotic pelvic condition (endometriosis) palpation may be difficult.
- **Direct visualization and/or palpation of ureters** throughout its pelvic course wherever possible.
- **Uriglow**—ureteric catheters within built incorporated light source for better localization has been tried.
- **Adequate exposure of pelvic organs** is a must. Inadequate incision leads to inadequate exposure and dissection. This may lead to blind clamping or suturing.
- **Meticulous care during dissection** not to damage the sheath of ureter so that longitudinal vessels are not destroyed.
- **To follow the important axiom of surgery**—any important structure at risk of inadvertent injury must be carefully dissected and adequately exposed.
- **To avoid blind clamping** of blood vessels.

Operative

Management of ureteric injury depends on the following factors—(a) Time of detection: Intraoperative or postoperative; (b) Type and severity of injury; (c) Anatomical level; (d) Mobility of the ureter and bladder; (e) Pathology leading to ureter injury; (f) Patient's general condition and prognosis.

PRINCIPLES OF URETERIC REPAIR

- Not to damage the ureteric sheath and its blood supply during dissection
- Ureteric mobilization and tension-free anastomosis
- Watertight closure with PDS 4–0 on a 13 mm needle is used
- Sent with a ureteric catheter
- Passive drain at the anastomotic site to prevent urine accumulation.

Management of Injury when Recognized During Operation

Ureteral sheath denudation: No intervention, rarely ureteral stenting (double J or Pig tail), if a long segment is involved.

Ureteral kinking (due to closely placed sutures): Immediate removal of suture.

Ureteral ligation: Deligation immediately → assessment of viability by blood flow and ureteral peristalsis. Ureteral stenting may be needed if any doubt.

Ureteral crushing (clamp injury): Remove the clamp → check the viability → ureteral stenting → extraperitoneal drainage at the site is placed.

URETERIC TRANSECTION

Partial

Primary repair over ureteral stent.

Complete

(i) In the middle-third → end-to-end anastomosis over an ureteral stent (ureteroureterostomy) following adequate mobilization of both the segments. Otherwise (complicated) ureteroileal interposition is done; (ii) In the lower-third → ureteroneocystostomy with psoas hitch over an ureteral stent.

Thermal injury resection and management according to the length of transection.

Ureteric implantation into the bladder (ureteroneocystostomy) must be done without any tension. High mobilization of bladder is needed and bladder dome is sutured to the psoas muscle on that side (**psoas hitch**). To prevent vesicoureteric reflux, ureter is implanted through submucosal tunnel in the posterior wall of the bladder.

Bladder flap procedure (modified Boari-Ockerblad) is an alternative when the ureter is short or the injury is at the level of pelvic brim (Fig. 26.5). An obliquely placed bladder flap is outlined. The flap is rolled into a tube and the ureter is reimplanted in the submucosal tunnel without tension.

Alternatively, **ureteroileoneocystostomy** would be done.

Thermal Injury

Depending upon the severity it may need resection and management according to transection.

Complications Following Repair of Ureteric Injury

(a) Stricture; (b) Infection; (c) Ureteric obstruction; (d) Reflux of urine; (e) Stent or Boari flap complications.

RECTOVAGINAL FISTULA

DEFINITION

Abnormal communication between the rectum and vagina with involuntary escape of flatus and/or feces into the vagina is called rectovaginal fistula (RVF) (Fig. 26.6).

Causes

- Acquired
- Congenital

Acquired

Obstetrical

- **Incomplete healing or unrepaired recent CPT** is the most common cause of RVF.
- Instrumental injury inflicted during destructive operation or operative vaginal delivery.
- **Obstructed labor:** The rectum is protected by peritoneum of pouch of Douglas in its upper-third, by

the perineal body in the lower-third and by the curved sacrum in the middle-third. However, if the sacrum is flat, during obstructed labor the compression effect produces pressure necrosis → infection → sloughing → fistula. It is rare these days.

Gynecological

- Following incomplete healing of repair of old CPT (most common).
- **Trauma** inflicted inadvertently and remains unrecognized in operations like—perineorrhaphy, repair of enterocele, vaginal tubectomy, posterior colpotomy to drain the pelvic abscess, reconstruction of vagina, etc.
- Fall on a sharp pointed object.
- Malignancy of the vagina (common), cervix or bowel.
- Pelvic radiation therapy.
- Lymphogranuloma venereum or tuberculosis of the vagina.
- Diverticulitis of the sigmoid colon → abscess → bursts into the vagina.
- Inflammatory bowel disease: Crohn's disease involving the anal canal or lower rectum.

Congenital

The anal canal may open into the vestibule or in the vagina.

DIAGNOSIS

- Involuntary escape of flatus and/or feces into the vagina. If the fistula is small, there is incontinence of flatus and loose stool only but not of hard stool.
- Rectovaginal examination reveals the site and size of the fistula.
- Confirmation may be **done by a probe passing** through the vagina into the rectum. If necessary, methylene blue dye is introduced into the rectum which is seen escaping out through the fistula into the vagina. Examination under anesthesia may be conducted to facilitate clinical diagnosis (Fig. 26.6).
- Barium enema or, CT scanning proctoscopy, colonoscopy may be needed when malignancy or inflammatory bowel diseases are suspected.

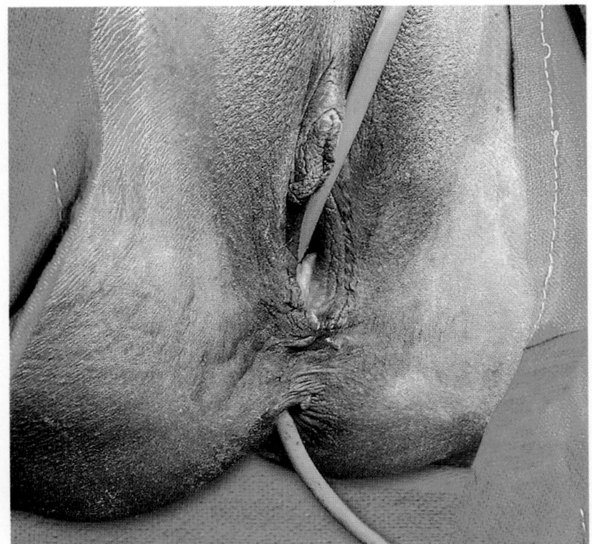

Fig. 26.6: Rectovaginal fistula (RVF) following traumatic forceps delivery. It was of moderate size so as to pass a rubber catheter through the vagina and it is clearly seen to come out through the anus.

INVESTIGATIONS

- Barium enema
- Barium meal and follow through may be needed to confirm the site of intestinal fistula

Sigmoidoscopy and proctoscopy are helpful for the diagnosis of inflammatory bowel disease or for taking biopsy of fistula edge.

TREATMENT

- **Preventive**
- **Conservative**
- **Definitive**

Preventive

Preventive aspects include good intranatal care, identification of CPT and its effective repair. Consciousness about the possible injury of the rectum in gynecologic surgery mentioned and its effective and appropriate surgery minimize the incidence of fistula.

Conservative

Small size fistula may be followed up conservatively for spontaneous healing.

Definitive Surgery Includes

- Transvaginal approach is commonly done.
- Transvaginal fistulotomy and purse string method of repair is also done
- Situated low down—to make it a complete perineal tear and repair it as that of CPT.
- Situated in the middle-third—repair by flap method.

Repair by flap method: Repair is commonly done transvaginally. The scar-margin is excised. Vaginal wall separated from the underlying rectal wall. This wide tissue mobilization helps repair without any tension. Repair is done in layers. Suture material used is polydioxanone (PDS) 3-0 on a 30 mm needle. Pre- and postoperative bowel management are similar to that in repair of CPT.

- Treatment of RVF depends on the size, site and the underlying cause. Small size fistula following obstetric injury may be followed up conservatively for spontaneous healing.
- Situated high up—preliminary colostomy → local repair after 3 weeks → closure of colostomy after 3 weeks.
- The preoperative preparations of one stage vaginal repair are like those mentioned in repair of CPT.

Success rate of repair depends upon the underlying cause and method of repair. Success of repair following obstetric injury vary from 80–100%. Fistulas due to cancer, radiation or active inflammatory diseases are difficult to treat successfully.

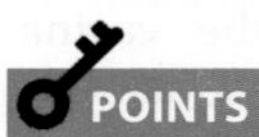

- **The incidence of genitourinary fistula** ranges between 0.2–1% among gynecological admissions of the developing countries. Vesicovaginal fistula is the common one.
- **The majority** (80–90%) is obstetrical following ischemia due to obstructed labor. In the developed countries, the fistula is mostly gynecological (80%).
- **The fistula is best revealed** in Sims' position using Sims' speculum (Sims' triad). In tiny fistula, diagnosis is made by **three swab test** (Table 26.3). The test also differentiates it from ureterovaginal fistula. Investigations are needed to diagnose it exactly.
- **Fistula** may be congenital (rare) or acquired. Acquired fistulas are classified depending upon number of factors (Table 26.1).
- **Route of repair** of VVF depends on many factors (p. 352). Transperitoneal or transvesical approach are done in selective case (Table 26.4). Vaginal route approach is preferred.

  Local repair by flap splitting method between 3 months following delivery is the preferred surgery. Continuous bladder drainage for 10–14 days following surgery should be a must. Special postoperative care is essential for success. If repair fails, local repair should be attempted after 3 months. In traumatic fistula, especially gynecological, the repair should be done immediately during primary surgery. However, if detected in the postoperative period, the continuous bladder drainage is to be kept for about 10–14 days failing which repair is to be done after 3 months. There are some favorable factors for successful repair.
- **Ureterovaginal fistula** is common following difficult abdominal hysterectomy for cervical or broad ligament fibroid, endometriosis, ovarian malignancy or radical hysterectomy (p. 354). It may also occur following vaginal hysterectomy or otherwise, in a case of simple hysterectomy. There are some anatomical locations as well as pelvic pathologies where ureteric injury is more likely (p. 355). Nature of ureteric injury may vary from kinking to complete transection. **Three swab test** differentiates it from a tiny VVF. Further investigations are needed to confirm the diagnosis and also to know the side and site of injury. End-to-end anastomosis during surgery or ureteroneocystostomy is the preferred surgery in late cases.
- **Rectovaginal fistula** is common following incomplete healing or unrepaired recent complete perineal tear. Other causes of RVF are obstetric, gynecological or congenital (p. 357).
- **Diagnosis** (p. 357) is important as regard the site and size of fistula.
- **Definitive surgery** for RVF may be as that of a repair of a CPT or by flap method or repair with prior colostomy (p. 357).
- Ureter can be distinguished from the pelvic vessels by (a) observing the peristalsis after stimulation with a surgical instruments and by (b) noting the longitudinal blood vessels.
- To minimize ureteric injury during a difficult surgery following precautions should be followed: (a) dissection should be careful with identification of the anatomy; (b) to operate from known anatomic areas into the unknown and (c) rarely in cases with obscure anatomy dissection may be retroperitoneal to start with.

CHAPTER

27 Genital Tract Injuries and Anorectal Dysfunctions

CHAPTER OUTLINE

- Introduction
- Complete Perineal Tear
- Coital Injuries
- Rape Victims
- Direct Trauma
- Foreign Bodies
- Functional Anorectal Dysfunctions
- Anal Incontinence

INTRODUCTION

The genital tract and the adjacent pelvic organs are subjected to strain of vaginal delivery either spontaneous or assisted. Many patients may have full recovery from the injuries but a substantial number may produce permanent legacies which lead to major gynecological problems. The following are some of such major obstetric legacies (Table 27.1).

All are dealt in appropriate chapters, only the severe form of perineal injuries, i.e. old complete perineal tear will be dealt within this chapter. **It is thus appropriately considered that obstetrics is a branch of preventive medicine.**

COMPLETE PERINEAL TEAR

DEFINITION

Tear of the perineal body involving the sphincter ani externus with or without involvement of the anorectal mucosa is called **complete perineal tear (CPT)**. It is called old when passed beyond an arbitrary period of 3 months following the injury (Fig. 27.1).

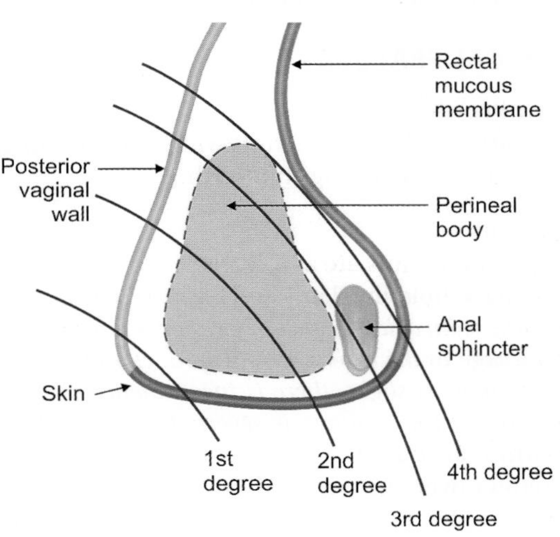

Fig. 27.1: Diagrammatic representation showing different degrees of perineal tear (from author's "Dutta's Textbook of Obstetrics).

ETIOLOGY

- **Obstetrical**
- **Gynecological**

TABLE 27.1: Obstetric legacies leading to major gynecological problems.

Pelvic organ prolapse (Ch. 16)
Perineal injuries including complete perineal tear
Genitourinary and rectovaginal fistula (Ch. 26)
Anal incontinence (AI)
Anal fissure
Tender perineal and vaginal scar
Backache
Eversion cervix with cervicitis (p. 221)
Ill health and chronic debilitating state

CLASSIFICATION OF OBSTETRIC (RCOG) ANAL SPHINCTER INJURY

First degree	Injury to perineal skin only
Second degree	Injury to perineum involving perineal muscles but not the anal sphincter
Third degree	Injury to perineum involving anal sphincter complex ▪ 3a: <50% of EAS thickness torn ▪ 3b: >50% of EAS thickness torn ▪ 3c: Both EAS and IAS torn
Fourth degree	Injury to perineum involving anal sphincter complex (EAS and IAS) and anal epithelium

(RCOG: Royal College of Obstetrician and Gynecologist; EAS: external anal sphincter; IAS: internal anal sphincter)

Obstetrical

Perineal injury (3° and 4°) results from **over stretching** or **sudden stretching** of the perineum during childbirth. It is more common when the perineum is **inelastic**.

RISK FACTORS FOR THIRD DEGREE TEARS (RCOG – 2007)

- Primigravida
- Big baby (>3 kg)
- Face to pubis delivery
- Midline episiotomy
- Forceps delivery
- Outlet contraction with narrow pubic arch
- Shoulder dystocia
- Precipitate labor
- Scar in the perineum
- Prolonged second stage

Gynecological

Direct injury on the perineum by fall may lead to trauma on the perineum to the extent of CPT.

CLINICAL FEATURES

Patient Profile

Patients are usually primiparous with a history suggestive of inadequate care during childbirth.

Symptoms

The chief complaints are as follows:

- Inability to hold the flatus and feces. *While incontinence of flatus is invariable, that of feces depends on the extent of damage of the external anal sphincter* (Table 27.2). *If the damage is slight, there is incontinence of only loose stool but if the damage is severe, there is incontinence of hard stool as well.*
- Soreness over the perianal region is due to constant irritation by the stool. It is often surprising that, the condition may remain asymptomatic for many years and only discovered accidentally during pelvic examination. **Overactivity of the levator ani muscle makes the patient continent with the stool; the incontinence of flatus being ignored.**

Signs

Inspection of the perineum reveals:

- There is absence of perineum. Vaginal and rectal mucous membranes are found to be continuous, only separated by a bridge of fibrous tissue (**rectal mucosa is reddish and the vaginal one is pinkish in color) (Fig. 27.2)**.
- Visible dimple on the skin on either side of the fused mucosa may be present. These represent the retracted torn ends of the sphincter ani externus which have got subcutaneous attachment.

Radial wrinkling of the skin is present only on the posterior aspect of the anal opening.

TABLE 27.2: Structures torn in CPT.

- Posterior perineal skin or/and vaginal wall
- Perineal muscles
- Perineal body
- Anal sphincter complex
- Varying degrees of anorectal mucous membrane

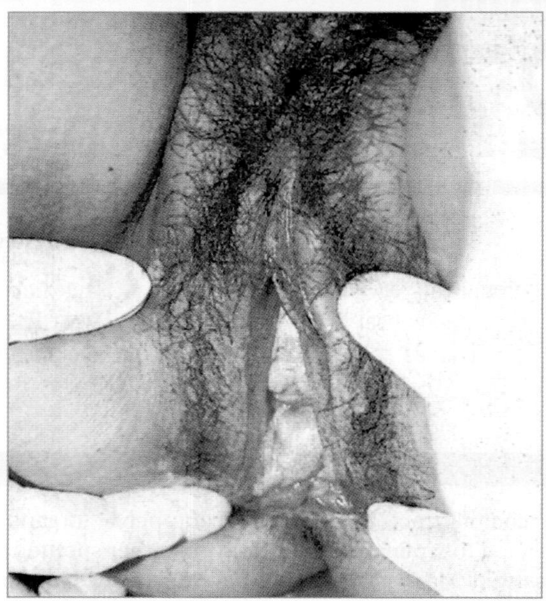

Fig. 27.2: Old complete perineal tear. Note the absence of perineum and the pinkish vaginal mucosa is continuous with reddish rectal mucosa.

Palpation: There is absence of the sphincteric grip evidenced when a finger is introduced into the rectum. The anal canal is separated from the vagina only by a septum (c.f. urinary incontinence)

It is surprising that in spite of deficit of the perineum, there is no prolapse. This is because of overactivity of the levator ani muscle. If prolapse is found along with CPT, it is more likely pre-existing.

Diagnosis: Endoanal imaging (Fig. 27.3): Endoanal or transvaginal ultrasound (EAS or TVS) can diagnose the defect in both the internal anal sphincter (IAS) and external anal sphincter (EAS). EAS can image the puborectalis muscle and perineal body also. **Perineal body thickness more than 12 mm is sufficient to maintain anal continence.**

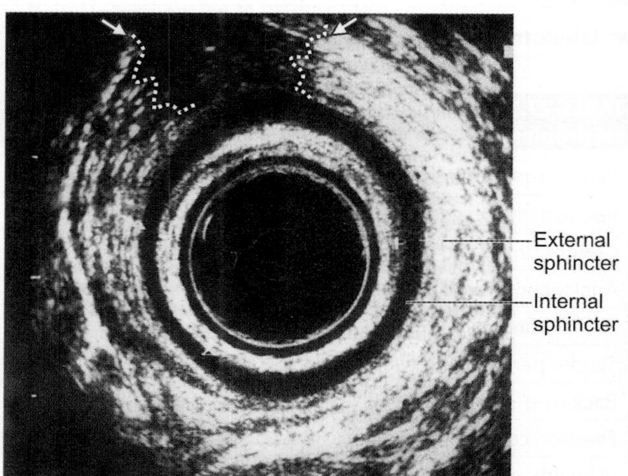

Fig. 27.3: Endoanal ultrasound image showing a defect in both the external and internal sphincters anteriorly (*see* arrows).

MRI imaging is good to detect the morphology of EAS. It is not commonly used. **Electromyography** detects the electrical activity of the muscles.

DIFFERENTIAL DIAGNOSIS

A rectovaginal fistula situated low down may at times be confused with CPT. This is especially in cases where overlying skin remains intact. **Rectovaginal fistula causes more inconvenience to the patient than CPT.**

TREATMENT

See from Author's "Dutta's Textbook of Obstetrics" Ch. 29.

- **Preventive**
- **Operative**

Preventive

Proper conduct in the second stage of labor taking due care of the perineum when it is likely to be damaged is the effective step to prevent undue lacerations (Table 27.3).

The prevention of the perineal injuries in normal delivery includes:

- More attention should be paid not to the perineum but to the controlled delivery of the head.
- Delivery by early extension is to be avoided.
- Slow delivery of the head during forceps delivery maintaning the correct direction of pull
- To deliver the head in between contractions.
- To perform timely episiotomy (when indicated).
- To take care during delivery of the shoulders as the wider bisacromial diameter (12 cm) emerges out of the introitus.

Operative

The definitive surgery is repair of the **anal sphincter complex (sphincteroplasty) with restoration of the perineal body (perineorrhaphy)**.

This should preferably be done between 2 and 3 months following the injury. **The best time of repair is, however, within 24 hours of the injury, if detected immediately following delivery**.

By 2 months time, the local infection subsides, general condition of the patient improves and the baby can be kept at home. If kept more, there is more fibrosis on the margins and unnecessary prolonged inconvenience to the patient. **Repair without such delay is generally advocated.**

Preoperative Investigations

There is no special preoperative investigation except the stool should be examined for evidence of intestinal infestations like hookworm, *Ascaris* or *Entamoeba histolytica*, which are common in the tropical countries. Their presence needs eradication prior to surgery.

TABLE 27.3: Prophylaxis to perineal injuries during delivery.

- Delivery of the head by early extension is to be avoided
- Controlled delivery of the flexed head in between uterine contractions
- Timely and judicious mediolateral episiotomy especially in primigravidae, occipitoposterior, face, breech or forceps delivery

Preoperative Preparations

- The patient should admitted at least 3 days prior to surgery.
- The patient should have low residual diet consisting of milk, bread, lime-whey for 2 days prior to surgery.
- Intestinal antiseptics are prescribed starting from 2 days prior to surgery. Any one of the drugs may be given—neomycin 250 mg thrice daily, erythromycin 500 mg thrice daily, metronidazole 400 mg thrice daily.
- Enema and bowel wash are given daily, for 2 days prior to operation. The idea is to clear the lower bowel. Enema should not be given in the morning of the operation.

Principles of Surgery (Warren Flap Method)

- An inverted V-shaped incision is made on the posterior vaginal mucosa (Fig. 27.4A).
- Mobilization of the rectal wall from the overlying vaginal wall.
- Mobilization of the torn ends of the sphincter ani externus.
- Suturing of the rectal wall in two layers.
- Approximation of the torn ends of the sphincters by interrupted sutures.
- Apposition of the musculofascial structures of the perineal body by 2–3 interrupted sutures.
- Apposition of the vaginal wall and skin of the perineum by interrupted sutures.

Steps of Operation (Figs. 27.4A to G)

Preliminaries: As in anterior colporrhaphy.

Actual steps

Mobilization of the rectum and anal sphincter

- Two Allis tissue forceps are placed on either side of the fused rectovaginal mucosa and are retracted laterally by the assistant.
- An inverted V-shaped incision is made over the fused mucosa extending from one end to the other (Fig. 27.4A).
- Two Allis forceps are placed on either side on the lower end of the labium minus.
- Incision over the fused mucosa is extended upwards from each end up to the lower end of the labium minus.
- The posterior vaginal wall is dissected off from the rectum and the rectum is well-mobilized (Fig. 27.4B).
- Two more Allis forceps are placed beyond the skin dimple on either side. Incision is made from each end of the fused mucosa downwards over the skin dimple (site of torn end of the sphincter ani externus).
- The incision lines now look almost to the letter 'H'.
- Torn end of the anal sphincter of each side is held by Allis forceps and is well-mobilized (Fig. 27.4D).

  Repair: Prior to repair, the scar tissue on the rectal margins is to be excised.
- The rectal wall is sutured by interrupted sutures using polydioxanone (PDS) 3-0 on 30 mm needle starting from the apex. The knots are placed inside the lumen (Fig. 27.4B).

Contd...

Contd...

- The pararectal fascia is approximated over the first layer by interrupted sutures using the same suture materials (Fig. 27.4C).
- **Anal sphincteroplasty:** *Repair is done by two methods:* (1) **End-to-end technique is commonly done**; and (2) **Overlapping method is done in a case with old tear.** However, these is no superiority of one method over the other. The torn ends of the sphincter ani externus are approximated in front of the repaired rectum by a sutures using PDS No. '2-0'. This is enforced by one or two interrupted sutures (Figs. 27.4D and E). Results of repair of EAS either by an overlapping or an end-to-end approximation method, are the same.
- Redundant portion of the vaginal mucosa is excised.
- Two or three interrupted sutures are placed through the fibromuscular tissues of the perineal body using Vicryl No. 'O' (Fig. 27.4F).
- The rest of the steps are like that of perineorrhaphy.

Special Postoperative Care

- Nonresidual diet is given from 3rd day onwards; the full diet is given on 6th day.
- Bowel should not be moved for about 4–5 days.
- Lactulose 10 mL twice daily beginning on the 2nd day and increasing the dose up to 30 mL on the 3rd day is a satisfactory regimen to soften the stool.
- If the patient fails to pass stool and is having discomfort, compound enema (olive oil or liquid paraffin, glycerine and normal saline, each 4 oz) may be given by a rubber catheter.
- Antibiotics (cefuroxime 1.5 and metronidazole 500 mg—IV) are used to cover the perioperative period.
- Intestinal antiseptics should be continued for about 5 days (*see* above).

Advice on Discharge

- Stool is kept soft using a laxative at bed time.
- Contraceptive practice to postpone pregnancy.
- To review the woman after 6 weeks of repair.
- To have antenatal check-up when she is pregnant and a mandatory hospital delivery. **In future vaginal delivery, liberal mediolateral episiotomy may be done.**
- Women who are symptomatic or have abnormal endoanal ultrasonography (USG) and/or manometry after repair should be **delivered by elective cesarean section.**

Complications of Repair Operations

- Complete dehiscence
- Incomplete dehiscence leading to rectovaginal fistula
- Difficulty in defecation because of too much tightening of the sphincter
- Dyspareunia
- Persistence of incontinence of flatus or feces. Endoanal USG or anorectal manometry is to be done to detect any residual defects (20–30%).

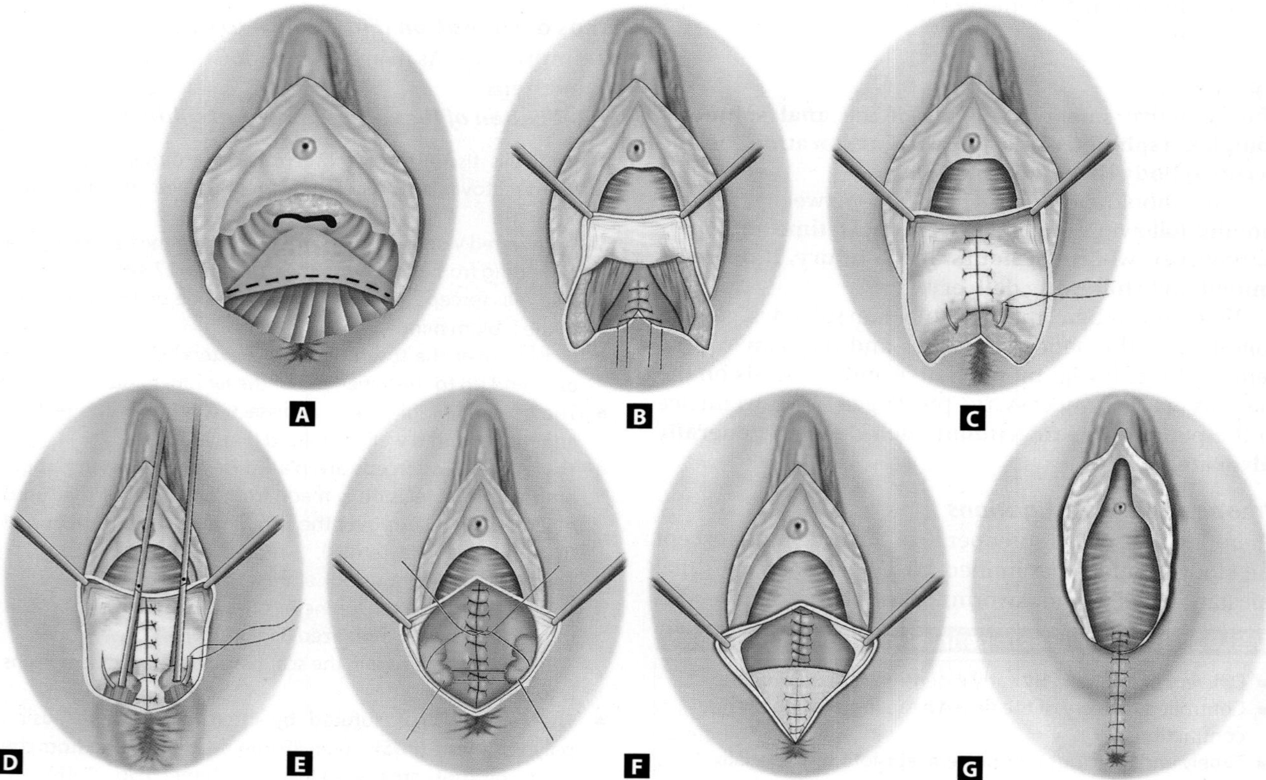

Figs. 27.4A to G: Principal steps of repair of complete perineal tear.

COITAL INJURIES

The following are the nature of coital injuries:

- Minor hemorrhage due to tearing of the hymen or bruising of the vagina or urethra may occur at defloration. No treatment is usually required.
- Severe hemorrhage may occur, if the tear spreads to involve the vestibule or the region of the clitoris. Lacerations of the anterior vaginal wall may occur usually following rape.
- Very rarely, rupture of the vault of the vagina may occur to expose the peritoneal cavity. This usually occurs in—(a) rape, (b) very young girls, (c) postmenopausal atrophy and (d) following vaginal/abdominal hysterectomy. Bowels and omentum may prolapse through the ruptured vault and cause shock and peritonitis.

MANAGEMENT

Small tears need no treatment; only pressure application is enough. Larger lacerations have to be repaired. If the vault has ruptured, it is preferable to perform laparotomy or laparoscopy and repair the vault and to tackle any associated pathology.

RAPE VICTIMS

Rape is a sexual assault. It is a legal term. It refers to any penetration of a body orifice with threat of force or actual force and nonconsent. Sexual violence is defined as any sexual act performed by one person on another without consent. Worldwide 7.2% women experienced nonpartner sexual violence. It is lower in Asia compared to North America and Africa.

The victims may be of any age groups—premenarchal, childbearing or even postmenopausal. The very young, mentally and physically handicapped and the very old are the common victims.

FORENSIC CONSIDERATIONS

- Rape is a legal diagnosis. The medical evidences and examinations are of value only to the court.
- Referral may be through police, hospital, doctor or by self-referral.
- Due consent is to be taken from the victim and the examination is made early and in the presence of a third party or chaperone. Confidentiality is to be maintained.
- Detailed statement from the victim, examination findings are recorded. Collected materials are labeled properly and should be submitted for expert examination.
- Sperm are detected in the vagina up to 7–9 days and motile sperm up to 8 hours. It should be borne in mind while interpretating the findings that about 10% adult males are azoospermic or oligospermic. It is also observed that in one-third, sperm are not ejaculated in the vagina and millions are vasectomized and that many rape victims douche before reporting for examination.

MANAGEMENT

Management aims at:

- Examination with clinical and evidential protocols.
- To treat any local injury
- To perform appropriate tests
- To prevent infection and sexually transmitted diseases (STDs)
- To prevent pregnancy (emergency contraception)
- Medicolegal procedure
- To provide emotional support to the victim.

MEDICOLEGAL PROCEDURES AND DOCUMENTATION

- To document history in detail.
- To examine her thoroughly (genital/nongenital) and to note the injuries.
- To collect the clothings, hair samples by combing pubic hair and finger nail scrapings, vaginal secretions for DNA typing.
- To collect samples for sperm, acid phosphatase from the affected site (vagina, rectum, and pharynx). Photographs of injuries are taken for forensic evidence.
- To send specimens to forensic authorities with record.

Local Injuries

The injuries may be in the form of bruises, lacerations around the neck, buttocks or vulva. Extensive lacerations in the area of hymen, vagina, urethra, even the vaginal vault may be there. There may be major injuries especially in young virgins or premenarchal girls. The injuries should be repaired under general anesthesia. In premenarchal girls, to increase the vaginal defense, small dose of estrogen is given orally daily for 2 weeks (0.01 mg ethinyl estradiol).

To Prevent Infections and STIs

Infection may be genital as well as extragenital (pharynx). **Rape victim runs the risk of infection with gonorrhea, syphilis, *Chlamydia*, *Trichomonas*, HIV, Hepatitis B and others (Ch. 11).** Blood for serological test for syphilis (RPR) and cervical and urethral smear for *Gonococcus* are to be collected for bacteriological study (NAATs). Cultures of cervical mucus should also be done for microbiological study.

Since about 6 weeks must elapse after exposure before the serology becomes positive, a positive test at the first visit indicates that the victim has already been exposed. If negative, surveillance blood testing for HIV, syphilis are repeated at 6 weeks, 3 months and 6 months when initial tests results are negative.

Drugs commonly used for the prevention of STIs are given in the Table 27.4.

TABLE 27.4: Drugs used for prevention of infection and STIs.

▪ Ceftriaxone 250 mg IM is given—single dose for gonorrhoea Plus
▪ Azithromycin, 1 g PO—for *Chlamydia*.

To Prevent Pregnancy

Due care is to be taken to prevent pregnancy. **This is, however, not applicable** in premenarchal girls, in women protected by pills or intrauterine device (IUD) or permanent sterilization. If the patient is at risk of pregnancy, emergency contraception is advised (p. 412).

Medicolegal Procedures

Details of history and examination especially the injuries are documented. All clothings and undergarments are collected and labeled properly. Smears of vaginal secretions are made to document the presence of sperm, acid phosphatase and for deoxyribonucleic acid (DNA) typing. Collected swabs are refrigerated until they are processed. Pubic hair combings is done to obtain pubic hair of the assaulter. Finger nail scrapings are obtained for DNA typing of the perpetrator.

To Provide Emotional Support

To treat the psychic trauma (rape trauma syndrome), which usually lasts for a variable period—sympathetic handling, counseling, and assurance is done.

The acute phase lasts for hours to days. The victim may present with features of fear, depression, guilt, sleeplessness and eating disorders.

The late phase or the reorganization phase consists of nightmares, flash backs or phobias. It may last for months to years. The victim is allowed to express her feelings, anxieties and fears. She should be reassured as far as possible. Other healthcare personnel may be involved to counsel her if needed. Follow-up visit should be planned within 4–6 weeks before she is discharged.

Follow-up

The follow-up should be arranged in 1–4 weeks. The protocols to be maintained are:

- Serological test for syphilis, human immunodeficiency virus (HIV)
- Test of cure by culture for gonorrhea
- Urine test for pregnancy, if suspected
- Reassurance and support.

DIRECT TRAUMA

Accident, as falling astride on any sharp or pointed object, is not uncommon especially in young girls. It may produce bruising of the vulva or at times give rise to vulvar hematoma (Fig. 27.5).

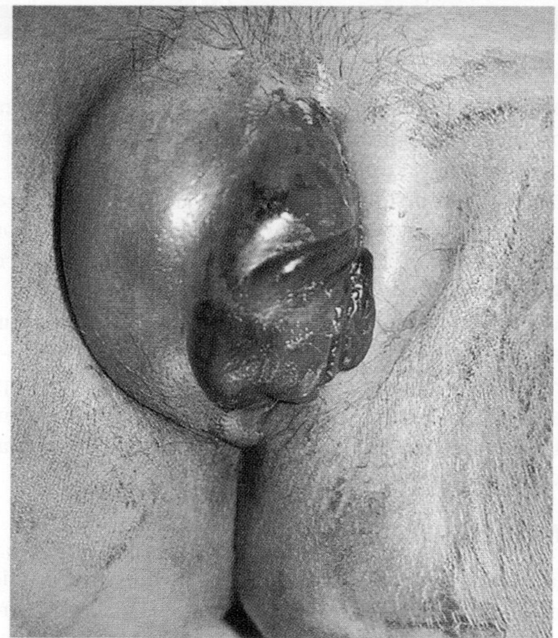

Fig. 27.5: A 17-year-old girl suffered extensive vulvar hematoma following a fall on a chair.

Major accident may involve fracture of pelvic bones causing injuries to pelvic viscera like bladder or rectum apart from vagina. There may be supralevator hematoma.

Even, falling on a sharp object may produce the above puncture or perforate the vaginal wall with injury of the surrounding viscera.

MANAGEMENT

Assessment of the general condition and the nature and extent of the injuries inflicted should be done first. Small vulvar hematoma, if not spreading may be left alone but if it is a big one or spreading, along with resuscitative measures, the hematoma is to be tackled under general anesthesia.

This includes scooping of the blood clots after giving an incision, secure hemostasis and obliteration of the dead space by interrupted mattress sutures.

In supralevator hematoma or in cases of suspected gut injuries, laparotomy is indicated and appropriate measures taken.

FOREIGN BODIES

Various types of foreign bodies may be placed either in the vagina or uterus and retained for a prolonged period often unnoticed by the patient. The articles so placed are either introduced by the patient or at times by a physician. Such articles are of varying nature, only few of them are mentioned below.

In the vagina

- Coins, toys, small stones either introduced out of curiosity by children or perversion in adults
- Forgotten menstrual tampon or diaphragm, cervical cap or condom used as contraceptives
- Articles introduced to procure abortion
- Packs, swabs or dressings
- Forgotten pessary.

In the uterus

- Retained intrauterine contraceptive device (IUCD) for a long time
- Old gauze packs
- Articles inserted for procuring abortion.

EFFECTS

The effects depend upon the nature of the foreign body, duration of its existence and amount of tissue damage.

Any material left inside invites infection. This especially happens in rubber goods, foreign bodies, swabs or gauze packs. There is foul smelling discharge.

Retained and forgotten pessary may cause vaginitis, sloughing and ulceration. It may produce vesicovaginal fistula and may be a precursor of vaginal carcinoma. Prolonged retention of IUD may cause menorrhagia, irregular bleeding and if left even in postmenopausal period, may produce pyometra or postmenopausal bleeding.

MANAGEMENT

Once diagnosed, the foreign body is to be removed. In children, it may not be easy and it is better to expose the vagina under general anesthesia using aural or nasal speculum.

FUNCTIONAL ANORECTAL DYSFUNCTIONS

Functional anorectal dysfunctions include:
(a) Functional fecal incontinence; (b) Functional anorectal pain and (c) Functional defecation disorders. However, organic disease has to be excluded in all such cases.

ANAL INCONTINENCE

Anal incontinence (AI) is defined as the involuntary loss of flatus, liquid or solid stool through the anus, that causes a social or hygienic problem impairing the quality of one's life significantly. Over all prevalence of A1 varies between 2 and 28%.

The important **mechanism for anal continence and normal defecation procedures are**:

- Competent anal sphincter complex (both IAS and EAS). EAS is composed of striated muscle supplied by a somatic nerve. It is under voluntary control. **EAS** is **responsible for anal canal's squeeze pressure**. IAS is composed of smooth muscle and supplied by autonomic nerves. **IAS maintains the resting pressure**.
- Puborectalis part of the levator ani muscle (puborectal sling), maintains the anorectal angle (Figs. 27.6A and B).
- Normal anorectal sensation when stool enters rectum, reflexly induces contraction of the EAS (squeeze muscle). This reflex phenomenon of contraction of the EAS and relaxation of the IAS is known as **rectoanal inhibitory reflex (RAIR)**.

  The process of **"sampling"** refers to the recognition of anal epithelium to rectal contents (gas, liquid or solid).
- Intact pudendal nerve innervation is essential.
- Optimum rectal capacity, compliance and distensibility acts as a storage of stool. Once, the process of "sampling" is initiated IAS relaxes and the EAS contracts.

CAUSES OF ANAL INCONTINENCE

- ***Age:*** Increasing age
- Obesity
- ***Obstetric trauma:*** Anal sphincter injury
- Forceps delivery
- High parity
- Operative procedures (perineorrhaphy)
- Pelvic organ prolapse
- Anal fistula and anal surgery
- Chronic obstructive pulmonary disease (COPD)
- Spinal cord injury
- Diarrhoea
- Irritable bowel syndrome (IBS)
- Crohn's disease
- Psychosis
- Congenital anomalies (neurogenic)

Anorectal manometry can detect the IAS resting pressure and EAS squeeze pressure. Decreased pressure readings suggest sphincter dysfunction, myopathy or neuropathy.

Treatment of anal incontinence depends upon the individual patient's etiology and severity of anal incontinence.

Medical management

- Biofeedback therapy may be effective for some women to increase neuromuscular tone.
- Pelvic floor muscle training exercises (Kegel's exercise) combined with biofeedback are beneficial.
- **Drugs:** Loperamide, slows down intestinal transit time, reduces stool volume and also increases the resting tone. It is useful. Other drugs are: Diphenoxylate and amitriptyline.

Surgical management

- Sphincteroplasty (p. 361)
- Other surgical procedures (p. 362).

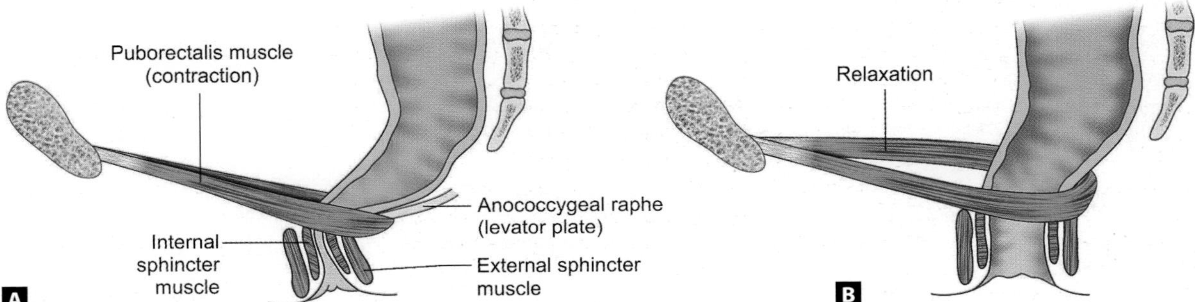

Figs. 27.6A and B: Anorectal canal, anal sphincters and puborectalis muscle. (A) Anal continence is maintained due to the angulation at the anorectal junction (nearly 90°) created by the puborectalis muscle; (B) Relaxation of puborectalis muscle during defecation. The rectal canal is opened up and the angulation is lost.

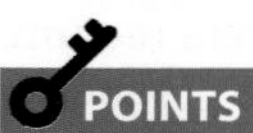

- **Obstetric legacies** leading to gross gynecological problems include—genital prolapse, perineal injuries, fistula, backache, chronic cervicitis and ill health. Gross injury to the perineum is mostly due to mismanaged second stage of labor.
- **In complete perineal tear**, there is absence of perineum and the vaginal and rectal mucous membranes are found to be continuous.
- **The definitive surgery** is anal sphincteroplasty and perineorrhaphy. The best time is within 24 hours of injury and in late cases after 2 months. Bowel preparations are to be done prior to surgery.
- **Postoperative management** and advice on discharge are important for success of repair (p. 362).
- **Minor hemorrhage** due to tearing of the hymen is the most common coital injury. Severe injury results from rape in very young girls or postmenopausal atrophy.
- **Rape** is a legal diagnosis. Due consent is to be taken from the victim and the examination is made in presence of a third party or chaperone. **Management of rape victims aims at**—treatment of the local injuries, prevention of infection and STD, prevention of pregnancy, medicolegal procedures and emotional support to the victim (p. 364). Emergency contraception is advised if the victim is at risk of pregnancy (Ch 30).
- **Direct injury** to the vulva may at times produces hematoma which requires resuscitation and exploration under general anesthesia. **Foreign bodies**— placed in the vagina for a prolonged period are pessary and diaphragm or cervical cap used as contraceptives. IUD may be forgotten and retained for a prolonged period in the uterus. Once diagnosed, the foreign bodies are to be removed.
- **Uterine injury** in gynecologic surgery is relatively uncommon compared to pregnant uterus. Interference is indicated in deteriorating general condition, suspected gut injury and with the features of developing peritonitis. In infective or malignant condition, laparotomy is seriously to be thought of.
- **Functional fecal incontinence** is defined as recurrent uncontrolled passage of fetal material for more than 3 months in an individual with anatomically normal defecatory muscles that function abnormally.
- **Anal incontinence (AI)** is defined as the involuntary loss flatus, liquid or solid stool through the anus.
- **EAS sphincter** is responsible for anal squeeze pressure whereas **IAS** maintains the resting pressure.
- **Causes of AI** are many (p. 359), but obstetric trauma and increasing age are the important ones.
- **Management** of AI may be medical (p. 361) or anal sphincteroplasty or other surgical procedures.

CHAPTER 28 Disorders of Sexual Development

CHAPTER OUTLINE

DEFINITION

Disorders of sexual development (DSD) may be defined as the presence of both male and female external and/or internal genital organs in the same individual causing confusion in the diagnosis of true sex. The incidence is about 2 per 1,000.

EMBRYOLOGICAL CONSIDERATIONS

The development of the gonads and genitalia has been described in Chapter 3. Only its schematic representation is depicted in Flowchart 28.1.

DETERMINATION OF SEX

In determining the sex, the following factors are to be considered—**(1)** Genetic sex; **(2)** Chromosomal sex; **(3)** External and internal anatomic sex; **(4)** Gonadal sex; **(5)** Hormonal sex; **(6)** Psychologic sex; **(7)** Sex of rearing.

In the newborn, the diagnosis of the apparent sex is determined by the appearance of the external genital organs. In the adolescence, however, in addition to the appearance of external genitalia, sex of rearing, psychogenic sex and the appearance of secondary sex characters should be taken into consideration.

Flowchart 28.1: Schematic representation of development of gonads.

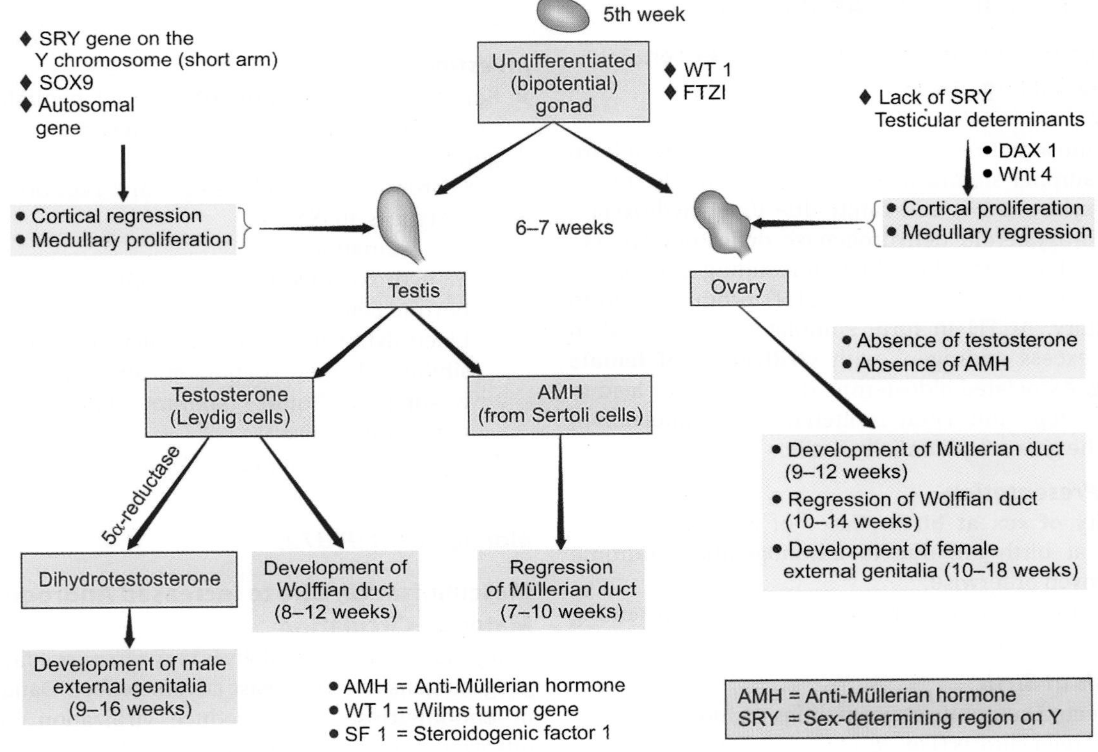

Ultimately disorders of sexual development are the conditions due to abnormal development or differentiation of chromosomal, gonadal or genital organs. These are discussed under the following categories.

NOMENCLATURE

- An association of female gonads with male external genitalia (female pseudohermaphrodite).
- An association of male gonads with female external genitalia (male pseudohermaphrodite).
- An individual possessing both ovaries and testes with ambiguity of genital organs (true hermaphrodite).
- Gonadal dysgenesis—abnormal gonads.
- Embryonic testicular regression.

Classification of DSD (Hughes, 2008)

A. Sex chromosome DSD (45X, 46X/46XY, 46XX/46XY, 47 XXY)
B. 46 XY DSD [disorders of (gonadal) testicular development and/or function]
- Gonadal dysgenesis (complete or partial)
- Ovotesticular DSD
- Disorders of androgen action

C. 46 XX DSD (disorders of ovarian development and/or function):
- Dysgenesis
- Androgen excess

D. Others: Müllerian agenesis/hypoplasia
- Syndromic associations (cloacal anomalies)

46, XX DISORDERS OF SEXUAL DEVELOPMENT

FEMALE PSEUDOHERMAPHRODITISM

Adrenogenital Syndrome (Congenital Adrenal Hyperplasia) (Fig. 28.1)

Etiology

It is an autosomal recessive disorder. It is due to inborn error of adrenal steroid metabolism, commonly due to 21-hydroxylase (95%) and rarely due to 11-hydroxylase or 3β-hydroxysteroid dehydrogenase deficiency (p. 63). There is lack of cortisol production resulting in excess of adrenocorticotropic hormone (ACTH) production from the pituitary. ACTH in turn, stimulates the adrenal to produce excess androgens with **virilization of female offspring**. Associated aldosterone deficiency may lead to excess salt depletion. There is often history of affection of sibling. The girls are potentially fertile.

Clinical Presentation

Ambiguity of sex at birth: Cases of ambiguity of sex detected at birth are due to adrenogenital syndrome unless proved otherwise.

Hirsutism and amenorrhea may be the presenting features around puberty in milder form.

Diagnosis at Birth

The suspected anatomic abnormalities include:
- An enlarged clitoris (Fig. 28.1).
- Presence of penile urethra or hypospadius.

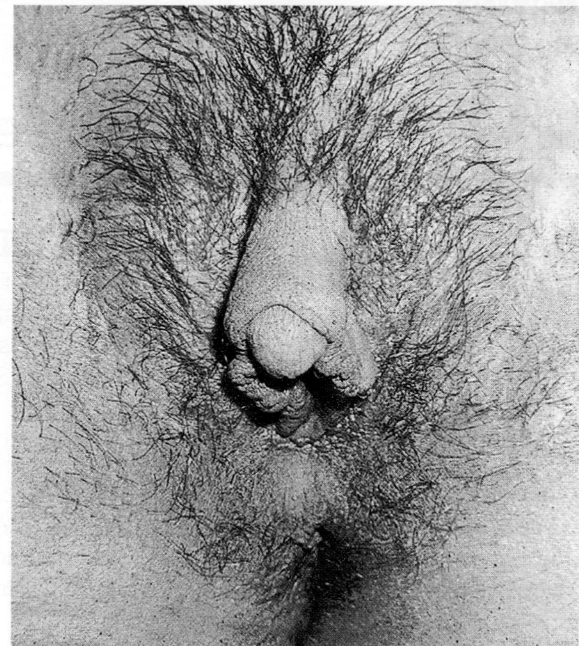

Fig. 28.1: Enlarged clitoris, fused labia minora in adrenogenital syndrome.
(*Courtesy*: Prof BN Chakravorty, IRM, Kolkata)

- Associated metabolic abnormality—salt wasting (hyponatremia, hyperkalemia) and hypotension may be present.
- Fusion of the labia minora.
- The presence of any one or more of the above features necessitates further investigations for confirmation of an early diagnosis.

Investigations

- Sonographic evaluation of internal genitalia shows presence of uterus, fallopian tubes and vagina. The gonads are ovaries.
- Sex chromatin study reveals positive Barr body.
- Karyotype is 46, XX.
- Serum estimation
  - 17-hydroxyprogesterone (17-OHP) is elevated to beyond 800 ng/dL.
  - Electrolyte values are estimated to check the possibility of their depletion and producing "salt wasting syndrome" (sodium and chloride—low, potassium—raised).
- Urinary excretion of pregnanetriol and 17 ketosteroids are markedly elevated.

Management (P. 372)

Masculinization Due to Increased Androgen in Maternal Circulation

Drug-induced androgenicity is very rare nowadays. Newer progestogens have got least adverse effect. Danazol used in endometriosis may produce virilization in female offsprings, if continued during inadvertent pregnancy. Rarely, the androgen source may be adrenal tumor, androgen secreting tumor, Sertoli-Leydig cell tumor or Cushing's syndrome of the mother.

There may be confusion in diagnosis of sex at birth. The history of intake of androgenic drug is often present. The source of excess androgen can be detected by appropriate investigations. To rule out adrenogenital syndrome, serum 17-hydroxyprogesterone is to be measured. **This is not elevated in any of the conditions mentioned.**

45, XO SEX CHROMOSOME DSD

GONADAL DYSGENESIS (45, XO DSD)

The term is employed for patients with female habitus in whom the gonads are imperfectly developed.

This may be due to nondisjunction of maternal chromosome leading to 45, XO (> 50%) or a mosaic pattern (46, XX/45, XO). The germ cells either fail to develop or fail to reach the gonads. The gonads are represented by white streaks without any germ cell.

TURNER'S SYNDROME (HENRY TURNER, 1938)

The cases usually present as primary amenorrhea with delayed secondary sexual characters.

The syndrome is characterized by short stature (height <150 cm), webbing of the neck, cubitus valgus, broad shield chest, low hair line on the neck, micrognathia, high arched palate, skin nevi, autoimmune disorders (thyroditis), lymphedema, short fourth metatarsals, and poor development of secondary sexual characters. They are mentally retarded and often associated with coarctation of aorta (Figs. 28.2A to C). Renal anomalies (horseshoe kidneys) and multiglandular autoimmune disorders are common. 45X is the most common chromosomal abnormality and 99% of fetuses are aborted.

Vagina, uterus and fallopian tubes are present. The uterus is small but is responsive to exogenous estrogen. Gonads are 'streaks' (fibrous tissue) without any follicle nor any potentiality to produce hormone (chromosomally incompetent ovarian failure). Associated autoimmune disorders like Hashimoto's thyroiditis, Addison's disease, hypothyroidism, diabetes are common.

Investigations

Confirmation of the clinical diagnosis is by the following:

- Sex chromatin study is negative
- Karyotype is 45, XO
- Serum E_2 is very low
- Serum follicle-stimulating hormone (FSH) and luteinizing hormone (LH) are elevated
- Autoantibodies may be present (Ch. 29).

Thus, there is hypergonadotrophic hypogonadism state.

Mosaic variety: In mosaic variety, the classic features of Turner are absent. The individual is of normal height. Ovaries are 'streaks' with few follicles. Occasionally, menstruation can occur for few cycles until the follicles are exhausted. Pregnancy has also been recorded.

- Sex chromatin is doubtful.
- Karyotype is 46, XX/45, XO.

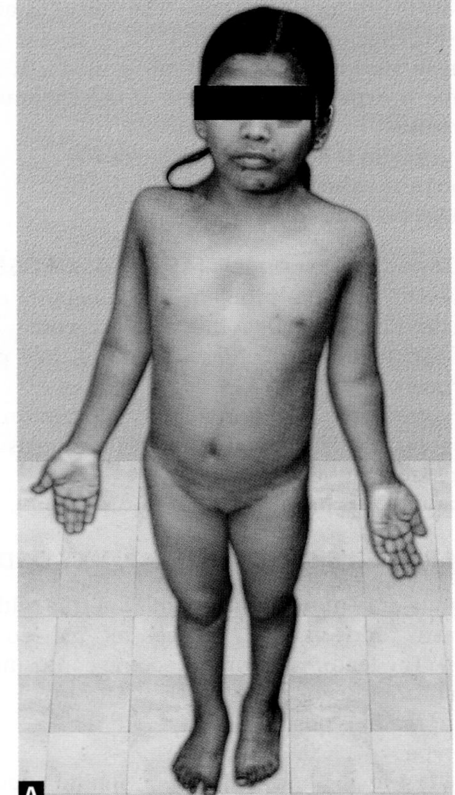

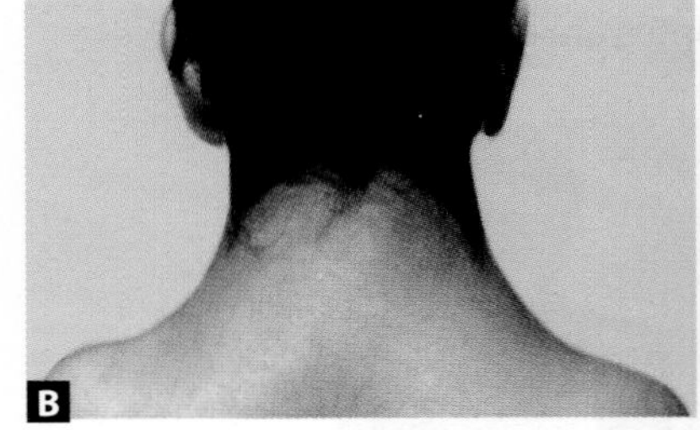

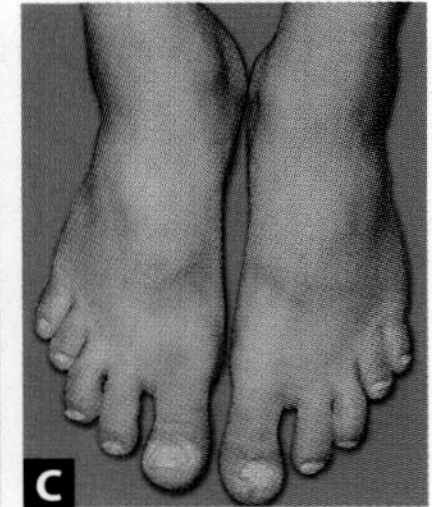

Figs. 28.2A to C: Turner's syndrome: (A) 17-year-old girl with Turner's syndrome (45, X). Characteristic somatic abnormalities seen are: Short stature (130 cm), shield chest, widely apart nipples, cubitus valgus, short neck and absent secondary sex characters; (B) The same girl with webbing of the neck and low hair line; (C) Deformity of the metatarsal bones in Turner's syndrome.

Management

P. 372.

Structural Abnormality of X Chromosome

Deletion of genetic material from short arm of 'X' chromosome leads to somatic features of Turner's syndrome (short stature). Loss of the long arm near the centromere leads to primary amenorrhea.

Pure Gonadal Dysgenesis or Gonadal Agenesis

The patients usually present as primary amenorrhea with delayed development of secondary sexual characters. **The stature is average.**

The vagina, uterus and tubes are present although infantile. Gonads are bilateral 'streaks' without any potentiality to produce hormones. The uterus is, however, sensitive to exogenous estrogen.

As these patients have got no gonads, a female phenotype is expected regardless of the chromosomal complement.

- Sex chromatin is doubtful
- Karyotype is either 46, XX or 46, XY
- FSH levels are raised.

Mixed Gonadal Dysgenesis (45, X/46, XY DSD)

Some present with the problem of ambiguous external genitalia at birth. Usually, the patients come around puberty for features of masculinization or primary amenorrhea.

There are features of partial masculinization of the external genitalia. The gonad of one side is testis and on the other side a 'streak'.

The karyotype is usually 45, XO/46, XY.

KLINEFELTER'S SYNDROME (47, XXY DSD)

The patients are eunuchoid in build, infertile with small penis, testis and varying degrees of gynecomastias (Fig. 28.3). The features at times become confusing when first seen in adolescence (Fig. 28.4).

- Sex chromatin is positive.
- Karyotype is 47, XXY or 48, XXXY.
- Genitalia—small and infantile. Genital ducts are Wolffian.
- Serum gonadotropins are elevated

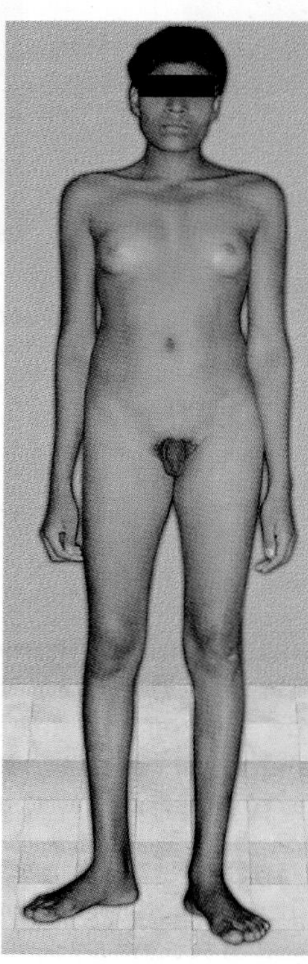

Fig. 28.3: A case of Klinefelter's syndrome having gynecomastias. (*Courtesy*: Dr B Ghosh, Burnpur)

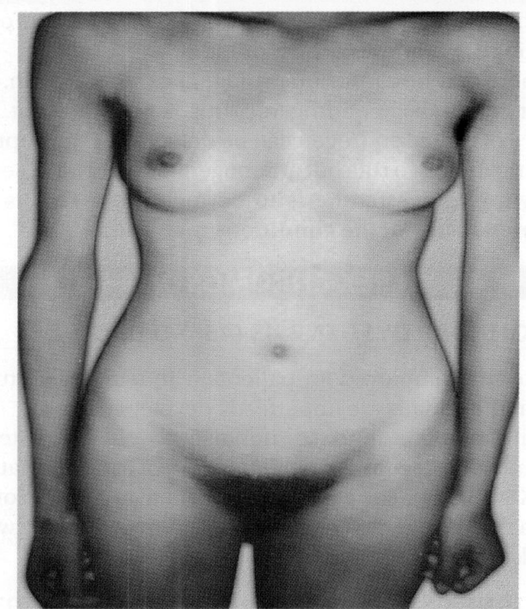

Fig. 28.4: A case of sex reversal 47, XXY female Klinefelter. (*Courtesy*: Prof BN Chakravorty, IRM, Kolkata)

- Testes are small and firm
- Infertility is due to oligo-azoospermia
- Serum testosterone: Low
- Often suffer psychological abnormalities, diabetes and breast cancer
- Fertility is possible with ICSI
- Most common cause of testicular failure.

Cases of sex reversal 47, XXY female Klinefelter have been recorded (Fig. 28.4). Breasts are well-developed and secondary sexual characters are of female (Fig. 28.4).

46, XY DISORDER OF SEXUAL DEVELOPMENT

ANDROGEN INSENSITIVITY SYNDROME (TESTICULAR FEMINIZATION)

The condition is inherited as a X-linked recessive gene. It includes a variety of phenotypical males depending upon the degree of androgen receptor (AR) response to androgens. The ultimate phenotype depends on whether the ARs are absent, present but functionally abnormal or normal but decreased in number. Based on these AIS may be:

A. Complete variety
B. Incomplete variety: Presentations may be:
   - Infertile men with bifid scrotum
   - Infertile men with under masculinization
   - Infertile men with azoospermia or severe oligospermia

- The cases are rarely diagnosed prior to puberty.
- Usually presents with primary amenorrhea and or infertility.
- They are phenotypically and psychologically female.
- Breast development is adequate (Fig. 28.5).
- The nipples are small with pale areola.

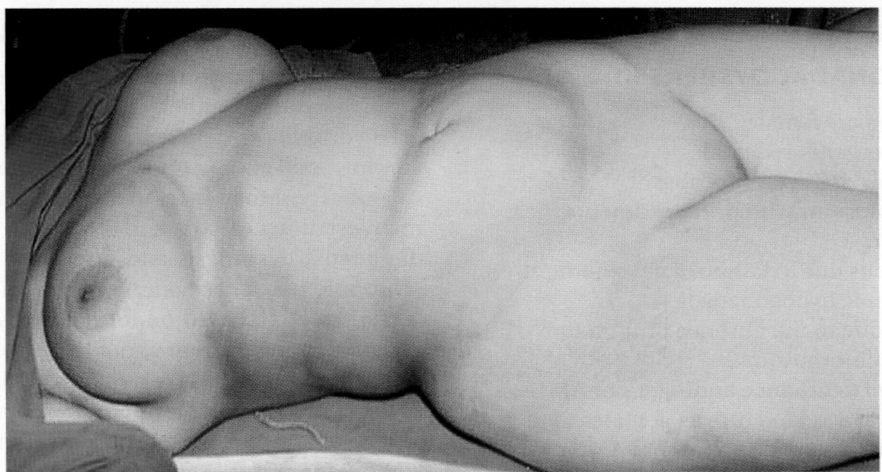

Fig. 28.5: A case of androgen insensitivity syndrome. Breasts are well-developed, pubic hair absent. (*Courtesy*: Prof BN Chakravorty, IRM, Kolkata).

- There is eunuchoidal tendency (long arms, with big hands, and feet).
- Absent or sparse axillary and pubic hair (Fig. 28.5).
- External genitalia looks like female.
- Vagina is short and blind (Fig. 28.6). The upper two-thirds of vagina, uterus and tubes are absent due to the effect of anti-Müllerian hormone (AMH). The gonads (Sertoli cells) secrete AMH.
- They have tissue receptor defect for normal androgens function. This leads to the development of female phenotype.
- The enzyme 5α-reductase (type 2) deficiency (autosomal recessive disorder) results in failure conversion of testosterone to dihydrotestosterone (DHT). This causes impaired virilization of the male external genitalia in fetal life.
- Defects in androgen receptor gene located on the X chromosome.
- Either there is lack of androgen cytosol receptor or the receptor is mutated (defective).
- At puberty the conversion of testosterone to estrogen stimulates breast growth.
- Gonads (testes) are either placed in the labia, or inguinal canal or intra-abdominal (Figs. 28.6 and 28.7).

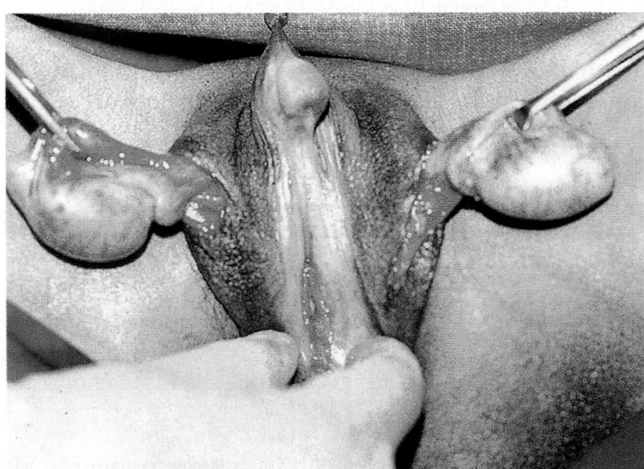

Fig. 28.6: Bilateral labial gonads (testes) and short blind vagina in testicular feminization.
(*Courtesy*: Prof BN Chakravorty, IRM, Kolkata)

Investigations

- Sex chromatin is negative
- **Karyotype is 46, XY**
- Serum testosterone is within average for normal males
- Serum E_2 level is high than normal for males
- Serum LH level is normal or slightly elevated
- Confirmation of diagnosis is by gonadal biopsy.

Gonadal biopsy

- Seminiferous tubules are small and hyalinized
- Spermatogenesis is absent
- Leydig and Sertoli cells are normal.

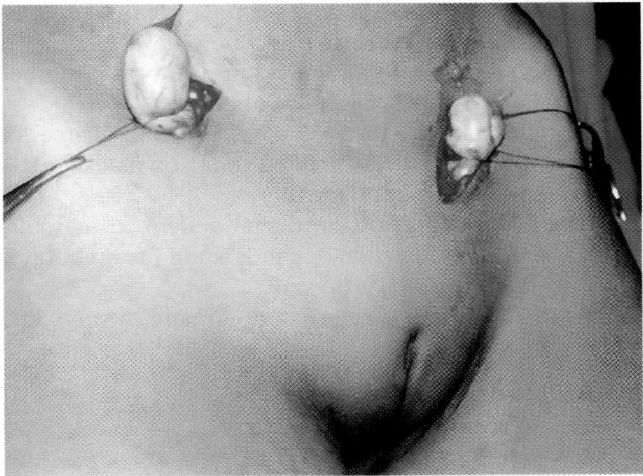

Fig. 28.7: Testicular feminization—bilateral inguinal gonads.
(*Courtesy*: Prof BN Chakravorty, IRM, Kolkata)

Management (p. 372)

46, XY DSD (SWYER SYNDROME)

COMPLETE GONADAL DYSGENESIS

- External genitalia are female.
- Internal genital organs are female.
- Secondary sexual characters are absent.
- The individual presents with primary amenorrhea.
- Karyotype 46, XY.
- Gonads are fibrous due to failure of development.
- Hypergonadotropic hypogonadism
- Testis is absent due to the absence or mutation of SRY or TDF on the Y chromosome.
- Streak gonads fail to produce androgens or AMH.
- These patients are reared up as females and have normal Müllerian system due to absent AMH.
- Patients with Y chromosome need gonadectomy as the risks of gonadal tumor are high (GCT).
- Estrogen and progestin therapy is given for development of breast and secondary sexual characters.
- **Pregnancy is possible with IVF and donor oocytes.**

Testicular regression syndrome: In this condition, testes are normal in development but regressed later on. It may be unilateral or bilateral. External genitalia is normal male.

TRUE HERMAPHRODITISM

OVOTESTICULAR DISORDERS (46, XY DSD)

The condition is common among Bantu tribes in Southern part of Africa.

The entity is due to chromosomal defect and genetic cause.

Types

Both the testicular and ovarian tissues are present in an individual in different combinations.

- Ovotestis on each side (most common)
- Testis on one side (right), ovary on the other (left) side
- Testis or ovary on one side and ovotestis on the other.

It is probable that fertilization by a sperm carrying one 'X' chromosome, which contains some male determining material from 'Y' gives rise to this condition.

- The common presentation is ambiguity of external genitalia and under masculinization.
- The internal structures depend on the degree of differentiation of the associated gonad on that side.
- Most have a vagina and the uterus
- The differentiation of the ductal system to masculinization or feminization depends upon the amount of testosterone or AMH is present.
- About 75% develop gynecomastia and nearly 50% menstruate.

Investigations

- Sex chromatin is usually positive.
- Karyotype is usually 46, XX (70%), rest are 46, XY and rarely mosaic XX/XY.
- Confirmation of diagnosis is by gonadal biopsy.

DIAGNOSIS OF DSD

At birth: Most cases of ambiguous genitalia detected at birth are due to either congenital adrenal hyperplasia (21-hydroxylase deficiency) or to androgenic drugs administered to the mother in early pregnancy.

At puberty: Most cases presented at puberty are late manifestations of congenital adrenal hyperplasia, those of gonadal dysgenesis and rarely androgen insensitivity syndrome (testicular feminization). Diagnosis and sex of rearing need to based on further investigations. Till then assignment of gender should be postponed. In these conditions, the child is reared up as girl and she is brought to the clinician either for poor development of secondary sexual characters or for primary amenorrhea with or without hirsutism.

DIAGNOSIS OF AMBIGUOUS GENITALIA

It is a major diagnostic problem. Multidisciplinary team approach by endocrinologist, geneticist, neonatologist, psychiatrist and urologist is needed. Newborn metabolic and electrolyte status should be assessed. Severe hyperkalemia, hyponatremia and hypoglycemia (CAH) may be life-threatening.

Thorough physical examination to note:

- Life-threatening conditions with features of vomiting, dehydration, diarrhea or shock must be excluded (adrenal failure).
- Height and secondary sexual characters.
- Presence of vagina or urogenital sinus.
- Length of phallus: In a normal newborn clitoris measures <1 cm and penis is <2.5 cm, in length.
- Urethral meatus: Opening into perineal area or into urogenital sinus or hypospadias is noted.
- Labioscrotal folds: Degree of fusion is noted.
- Location of gonads: Gonads may be felt in the inguinal or in the labial region or may be in the abdomen.

A normal looking girl with primary amenorrhea who have normal breast development but no uterus may be either a case of Mayer-Rokitansky-Küster-Hauser (MRKH) syndrome or testicular feminization syndrome. The diagnostic features are given in Table 28.1.

The couple is counseled for the need of appropriate determination of gender and sex of rearing.

The diagnostic features are described in the Table 28.2.

MANAGEMENT OF DSD

BASIC GUIDELINES

Gender assignment rests on—(a) Projected appearance of genitalia after puberty; (b) Penile length, and (c) Prospect of future fertility.

- It is always better to diagnose the correct nature of DSD at birth or as early as possible. This is essential not only to correct the underlying disorders promptly but also to

TALBE 28.1: Differentiation between androgen insensitivity syndrome (AIS) and Müllerian agenesis (MRKH).

Characters	*Androgen insensitivity syndrome*	*Müllerian agenesis (MRKH syndrome)*
Sexual hair (pubic and axillary)	Absent or sparce	Normal female
Primary amenorrhea	Present	Present
Vagina	Short and blind	Absent
Clitoris	Enlarged	Normal as in female
Gonads: ▪ **Structure** ▪ **Location**	▪ Testes ▪ Inguinal, labial or abdominal	▪ Ovary ▪ Abdominal
Breasts	Developed	Developed
Serum testosterone level	Slightly elevated	Normal as in female
Müllerian system (uterus)	Absent	Absent or rudimentary
Wolffian system	Absent	Absent
Karyotype	46, XY	46, XX
Associated anomalies	Rare	Skeletal 12% and urological (renal) 47%

avoid the adverse psychological effect on the child and the family.

- If the diagnosis remains uncertain or the corrective surgery is deferred for the future, the baby should be reared up as female.

1. **Management of Adrenogenital Syndrome:** Hydrocortisone 10–20 mg/m^2 body surface area per day is given to suppress the excess ACTH secretion. Mineralocorticoid (fluorocortisone) is also given in cases with 21-hydroxylase deficiency. Cases with salt loss must be replaced carefully. Thereafter, a long-term therapy with corticosteroid is essential to suppress the adrenocortical hyperfunction.

   Once the neonate is stable, surgery to reduce the enlarged clitoris (reduction clitoroplasty) may be done. Reconstructive surgery includes clitoroplasty and vaginoplasty. **Timing of surgery is debated. However, it is recommended to perform vaginoplasty with the onset of puberty.** The reproductive potentiality remains unaffected, if treated early. **Prenatal diagnosis** is possible with chorion villus sampling at early weeks (9–12 weeks) of pregnancy using DNA probes. 17-OHP level in the amniotic fluid (amniocentesis) is elevated. Prenatal therapy with dexamethasone or termination of pregnancy is the option.

2. **In cases of Gonadal Dysgenesis**, karyotyping should be done. **The presence of 'Y' chromatin necessitates**

TABLE 28.2: Entity, clinical presentation, diagnosis and possible reproductive outcome of an individual with DSD.

Characters (DSD)	*Clinical presentation*	*Diagnostic criteria*	*Reproductive outcome*
Adrenogenital syndrome 46 XX DSD (androgen excess)	▪ Ambiguity of sex at birth	▪ Sonographic evaluation of internal genital organs ▪ Karyotype 46, XX ▪ Serum 17 hydroxyprogesterone ↑ ▪ Urinary pregnanetriol ↑ >5 µg/100 mL	Pregnancy possible
Gonadal dysgenesis ▪ Turner's syndrome sex chromosome DSD	▪ Primary amenorrhea ▪ Poor secondary sexual characters ▪ Short stature ▪ Webbing of neck ▪ Cubitus valgus ▪ Genitalia underdeveloped	▪ Karyotype 45, XO ▪ Bilateral 'streak' gonads ▪ Serum: E_2 ↓ and FSH ↑	Pregnancy with donor oocyte
▪ Mosaic Turner sex chromosome DSD	▪ Primary/secondary amenorrhea ▪ Average height ▪ Poor secondary sexual characters ▪ Genitalia underdeveloped	▪ Karyotype 45, XO/46, XX ▪ Bilateral 'streak' gonads	Pregnancy possible
Pure gonadal dysgenesis 46 XX or 46 XY DSD	▪ Primary amenorrhea ▪ Delayed secondary sexual characters ▪ Average height ▪ Genitalia underdeveloped	▪ Karyotype—46, XX or 46, XY ▪ Bilateral 'streak' gonads	Rare
Mixed gonadal dysgenesis 45 X/46 XY DSD	▪ At birth: Ambiguous sex ▪ At puberty: • Virilism with amenorrhea • External genitalia—partial masculinization • Internal genitalia may have unilateral Müllerian development	▪ Karyotype —45 XO/46 XY ▪ Gonads—testis on one side and on the other side a 'streak'	Depends on anatomic sex

Contd...

Contd...

Characters (DSD)	Clinical presentation	Diagnostic criteria	Reproductive outcome
Androgen insensitivity syndrome (46 XY DSD)	▪ Primary amenorrhea ▪ Infertility ▪ Phenotypically female ▪ Breast development—good ▪ External genitalia—female	▪ Axillary and pubic hair scanty or absent ▪ Short, blind vagina ▪ Gonads—labial, inguinal or abdominal ▪ Karyotype—46, XY ▪ Gonads are testes	Incomplete variety: Possible
Sex chromosome DSD (Klinefelter's syndrome)	▪ Eunuchoid ▪ Infertility (azoospermia) ▪ Gynecomastia	▪ External genitalia—male ▪ Genital ducts—Wolffian ▪ Gonads—testes (small) ▪ Sex chromatin—positive ▪ Karyotype—47, XXY	May be possible with ICSI
Complete gonadal dysgenesis (Swyer syndrome) 46 XY DSD	▪ Amenorrhea ▪ Secondary sex characters absent ▪ External genitalia female	▪ Karyotype 46 XY ▪ Gonadal–fibrous tissues ▪ Internal genitalia female	Rare with IVF and donor oocytes

removal of the gonads as there is chance of dysgerminoma, seminoma or gonadoblastoma in such gonads. Substitution therapy using cyclic estrogen and progestogen will help to develop secondary sexual characters.

Turner's syndrome (gonadal dysgenesis)

- Exogenous growth hormone (GH) can increase the height.
- Low dose estrogen (conjugated estrogen 0.625 mg) orally daily for 25 days with progestin (medroxyprogesterone acetate 5 mg daily) for last 10 days is started after 13 years of age.

3. **In cases of Androgen Insensitivity Syndrome**, the individual may be reared up as a girl. The ectopic gonads (testes) are to be removed (Figs. 28.6 and 28.7) as the risks of gonadal malignancy [gonadoblastoma or dysgerminoma are high (20–30%)]. **Vaginoplasty is done after the growth is completed (16–18 years) with development of secondary sexual characters.** After gonadectomy, long-term estrogen replacement therapy should be prescribed for its effect on vaginal epithelium, osteoporosis and cardiovascular system (p. 374).

   Conversion as a male need surgical and medical management. Size of the phallus and feasibility of constructing a penile urethra need consideration. Use of the testosterone before puberty enlarges the phallus in cases with 5α reductase deficiency. In the incomplete variety of AIS, pregnancy may be possible with IUI or IVF-ICSI though sperm counts are very low.
4. **In rare variety of true hermaphrodite**, the change of sex depends on sex of rearing, psychologic and the anatomic sex. The genitalia inconsistent with sex assignment should be surgically removed or modified. In general, it is possible to change the external genitalia from male to female but less from female to male. Management depends upon the phenotype. The gonads are to be removed to be followed by substitution therapy.

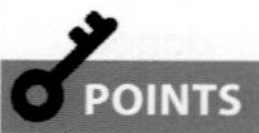

POINTS

- **The incidence** of disorders of sexual development **(DSD)** is about 2 per 1,000.
- **Female pseudohermaphroditism (46 XX DSD)** is the association of female gonads with male external genitalia.
- **Male pseudohermaphroditism (46 XY DSD)** is the association of male gonads with female external genitalia.
- **True hermaphrodite (ovotesticular DSD)** is an individual possessing both ovaries and testes with ambiguity of genital organs.
- **46, XX (female pseudohermaphroditism)** is due to congenital adrenal hyperplasia (most common) or due to increased androgen in maternal circulation.
- **Ambiguity of sex at birth** is due to adrenogenital syndrome unless proved otherwise. The entity is confirmed by elevated serum 17 hydroxyprogesterone and urinary pregnanetriol with karyotype 46, XX. Prenatal diagnosis can be made by CVS or amniocentesis using DNA probe.
- **MRKH (Mayer-Rokitansky-Küster-Hauser) syndrome** is the second common cause of primary amenorrhea.
- **Disorders of gonadal development** include—gonadal dysgenesis, gonadal agenesis and mixed gonadal dysgenesis.
  Turner's syndrome (sex chromosome DSD) is the most common variety of gonadal dysgenesis. It is the most common cause of primary amenorrhea. The individual is short (<60"), absence of secondary sexual characters with webbing of the neck and having 'streak' gonads. Karyotype is 45, XO with low serum E_2 and elevated serum FSH. There may be mosaic Turner with karyotype—46, XX/45, XO.
- In pure gonadal dysgenesis, the karyotype is either 46, XX or 46, XY. In mixed gonadal dysgenesis, the karyotype is usually 45, XO or 46, XY.
- About one-third of women with **gonadal dysgenesis** have major cardiovascular or renal abnormalities. Individuals with gonadal dysgenesis should have karyotyping done to determine the presence of Y chromosome.

Contd...

Contd...

- **Testicular feminization (46, XY DSD)** is rarely diagnosed prior to puberty. The patient is phenotypically female with short blind vagina and gonads (testes) are in the labia or inguinal canal or intra-abdominal. Sex chromatin is negative. Karyotype is 46, **XY**. Confirmation is by gonadal biopsy (structures of testis). Gonadal estrogen secretion induces normal pubertal feminization and breast development.
- **Androgen insensitivity (46, XY DSD)** syndrome may be partial or complete. Phenotypical expression depends upon the degree of function of androgen receptors.
  In Klinefelter's syndrome (sex chromosome DSD), the sex chromatin is positive and the karyotype is 47, XXY or 48, XXXY. Serum gonadotropin is elevated.
- **In true hermaphrodite (46, XX DSD)**, ovotestis is the most common presentation. Sex chromatin is positive. Karyotype is usually 46, XX or 46, XY. Confirmation is by gonadal biopsy.
- **A normal looking girl** with primary amenorrhea, who has normal breast development but absent uterus, may be either a case of MRKH syndrome or androgen insensitivity syndrome (Table 28.1).
- **Gonadal dysgenesis (sex chromosome DSD)** and uterovaginal anomalies are the common causes of primary amenorrhea.
- **Management of DSD**
  - **Congenital adrenogenital syndrome (46, XX DSD)** should be treated by hydrocortisone or dexamethasone. Apart from reduction clitoroplasty, the corrective surgery should be deferred till puberty.
  - **Cases of gonadal dysgenesis (sex chromosome DSD)** should be treated by substitution therapy with estrogen and progestogen. In presence of 'Y' chromosome, gonadectomy should be done to prevent malignancy.
  - **In 46, XY (AI)**, gonadectomy is to be done after the development of secondary sexual characters (puberty) to be followed by estrogen supplementation therapy.
  - **In true hermaphrodite 46, XY DSD (ovotesticular)**, the genitalia inconsistent with sex assignment should be surgically removed or modified.

CHAPTER

29 Amenorrhea

CHAPTER OUTLINE

DEFINITION

Amenorrhea literally means absence of menstruation. It is a symptom and not a disease. Overall prevalence of pathologic amenorrhea is about 3–4%.

There are at least five basic factors *involved in the onset and continuation of normal menstruation. These are (Fig. 29.1):*

- Normal female chromosomal pattern (46,XX)
- Coordinated hypothalamo-pituitary-ovarian (HPO) axis
- Anatomical presence and patency of the outflow tract

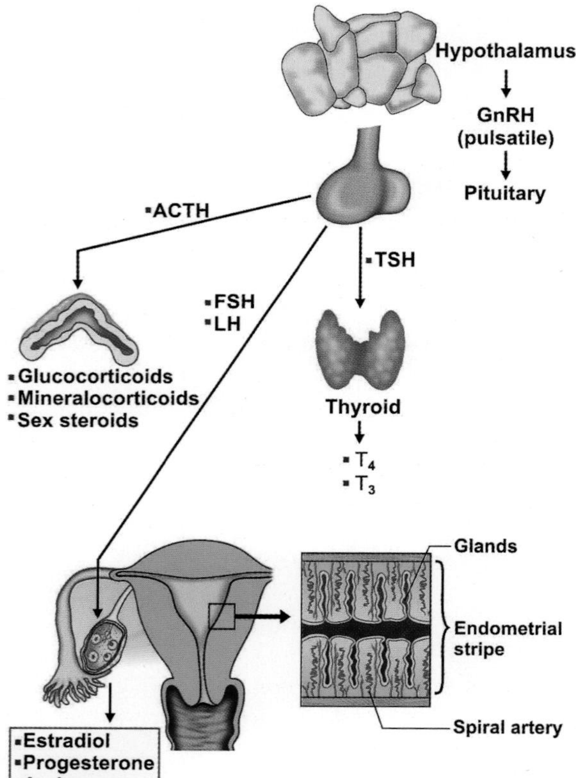

Fig. 29.1: Schematic representation of the coordinated function of hypothalamic–pituitary–ovarian and endometrial axis. Support of thyroid at adrenal glands are essential. Development of ovarian follicles and the endometrium results in menstruation.

- Responsive endometrium
- Active support of thyroid and adrenal glands.

CLINICAL TYPES

For descriptive purposes, the following types are conveniently described (Flowchart 29.1). This will help the clinicians to sort out the clinicopathological entity.

Physiological

Before Puberty

The pituitary gonadotropins are not adequate enough to stimulate the ovarian follicles for effective steroidogenesis → estrogen levels are not sufficient enough to cause bleeding from the endometrium.

During Pregnancy

Large amount of estrogens and chorionic gonadotropins secreted from the trophoblasts suppress the pituitary gonadotropins → no maturation of the ovarian follicles.

During Lactation

High level of prolactin → inhibits ovarian response to follicle-stimulating hormone (FSH) → no follicular growth → hypoestrogenic state → no menstruation. If the patient does not breastfeed her baby, the menstruation returns by 6th week following delivery in about 40% and by 12th week in 80% of cases. If the patient breastfeeds her baby,

Flowchart 29.1: Clinical types of amenorrhea.

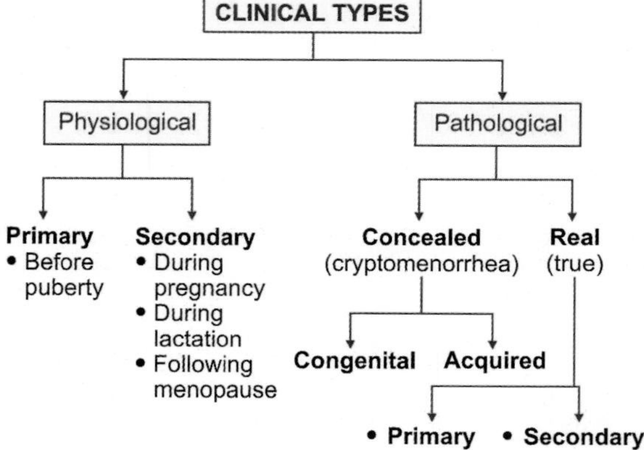

the menstruation may be suspended in about 70% until the baby stops breastfeeding.

Following Menopause

No more responsive follicles are available in the ovaries for the gonadotropins to act. As a result, there is cessation of estrogen production from the ovaries with elevation of pituitary gonadotropins.

Pathological

Cryptomenorrhea

In cryptomenorrhea, there is periodic shedding of the endometrium and bleeding but the menstrual blood fails to come out from the genital tract due to obstruction in the passage.

Causes

- **Congenital**
- **Acquired**

Congenital

- Imperforate hymen
- Transverse vaginal septum
- Atresia of upper-third of vagina and cervix.

Morbid pathological changes, clinical features and treatment of the congenital etiology have been described in Chapter 4.

Acquired

- Stenosis of the cervix following amputation, deep cauterization and conization.
- Secondary vaginal atresia following neglected and difficult vaginal delivery.

Pathology

There is only accumulation of blood in the uterine cavity resulting in hematometra. In neglected cases, the blood may enter the tubes whose fimbrial ends get blocked resulting in distension of the tubes by blood → hematosalpinx. May result in endometriosis (c.f. retrograde menstruation).

Clinical features

The patients with history of any of the etiological factors mentioned earlier, complain of:

- Amenorrhea dated back from the events
- Periodic pain lower abdomen.

Pelvic examination reveals the offending lesion either in the vagina or cervix. The uterus is symmetrically enlarged.

Treatment

Simple dilatation of the cervix so as to drain the collected blood is enough. In cases of secondary atresia of the vagina, reconstructive surgery is to be performed, to maintain the patency.

SUMMARY OF CRYPTOMENORRHEA

Cryptomenorrhea is a condition where the menstrual blood fails to come out from the genital tract due to obstruction in the passage.

Causes

The most common cause is congenital due to imperforate hymen. The acquired cause is rare due to cervical stenosis following amputation, conization or deep cauterization.

Pathophysiology

If the site of obstruction is low down in the vagina, the accumulated blood results in hematocolpos → hematometra → hematosalpinx. If the obstruction is at the cervix, it will produce hematometra → hematosalpinx. **Hematocolpos produces marked elongation of the urethra → retention of urine.**

Clinical features

The patient aged about 13–15 (congenital type) complains of periodic pain lower abdomen. Hematocolpos is usually associated with urinary problems to the extent of retention of urine. Abdominal examination reveals an uniform globular mass in the hypogastrium. Vulvar inspection reveals the bulging hymen. Rectal examination confirms the fullness of the vagina and uterine mass.

Management

- Cruciate incision of the hymen and drainage of blood (Fig. 4.3).
- Dilatation of the cervix in stenosis.

PRIMARY AMENORRHEA

DEFINITION

A young girl who has not yet menstruated by her 16 years of age is having primary amenorrhea rather than delayed menarche. The normal upper age limit for menarche is 15 years.

In view of lower mean age of menarche, currently a cut off value at **14 years** (in the absence of secondary sexual characters) and **16 years** (regardless of the presence of secondary sexual characters) is being considered.

Etiopathogenesis

The **causes of primary amenorrhea are** grouped as follows:

- **Hypergonadotropic hypogonadism (43%)**
  - *Primary ovarian failure* (p. 389).
  - *Resistant ovarian syndrome* (p. 389).
  - *Galactosemia*: Due to premature ovarian failure (p. 389).
  - *Enzyme deficiency (17-α-hydroxylase deficiency)*—characterized by ↓ cortisol and ↑ adrenocorticotropic hormone (ACTH), ↑ mineralocorticoids production, ↑ progesterone (>3 ng/mL). There is hypertension with hypernatremia and hypokalemia. The individual may be 46,XX or 46,XY with primary amenorrhea and no secondary sexual characters.
  - *Others*—gonadotropin receptor mutations—rarely FSH and/or LH levels are high as the respective receptor may be absent or mutated.
- **Developmental defect of genital tract (30%)**
  - Müllerian agenesis/dysgenesis
  - Imperforate hymen (Fig. 4.3).
  - Transverse vaginal septum (TVS)
  - Atresia upper-third of vagina and cervix (Fig. 4.6)
  - Complete absence of vagina (Fig. 29.2)
  - Absence of uterus in Mayer-Rokitansky-Küster-Hauser (MRKH) syndrome (Fig. 29.3 and Table 28.1).
- **Hypogonadotropic hypogonadism (27%)**
  - *Delayed puberty (constitutional)*—delayed gonadotropin-releasing hormone (GnRH) pulse reactivation.

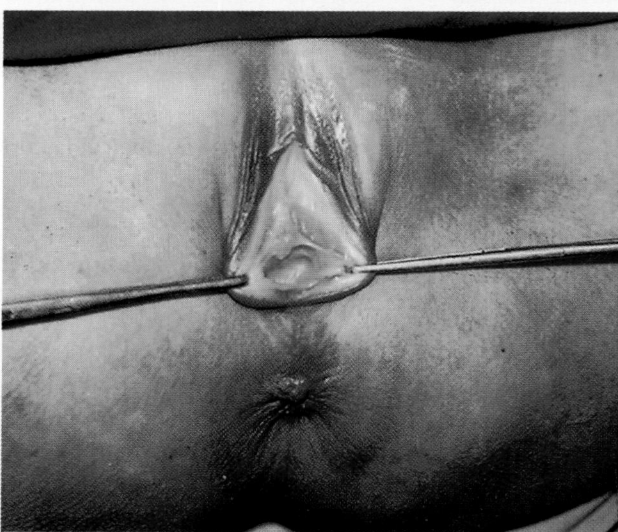

Fig. 29.2: Complete absence of vagina.
(*Courtesy:* Prof KM Gun)

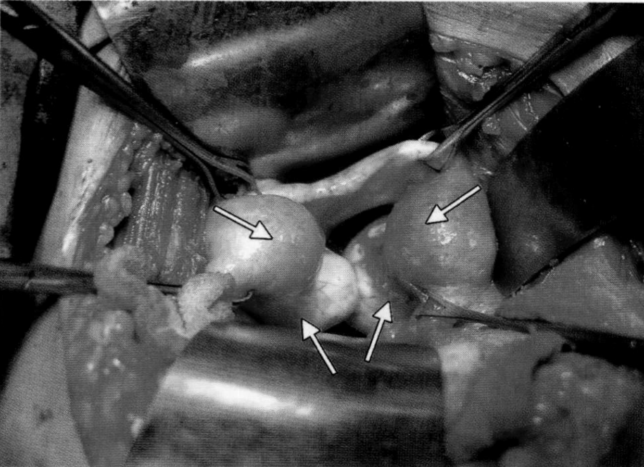

Fig. 29.3: Müllerian agenesis with small uterine knobs one on either side (down arrow). Normal ovaries are seen (up arrows). Cervix and vagina were absent in this case.
(*Courtesy:* Dr PK Biswas, Professor, Department of Obstetrics and Gynecology, CNMCH, Kolkata)

- *Hypothalamic and pituitary dysfunction*—gonadotropin deficiency due to stress, weight loss, excessive exercise, anorexia nervosa, chronic disease (tuberculosis).
- *Kallmann's syndrome*—inadequate GnRH pulse secretion—reduced FSH and luteinizing hormone (LH) (p. 390).
- *Central nervous system tumors*—craniopharyngioma → reduced GnRH secretion → reduced FSH and LH.

■ **Abnormal chromosomal pattern**
- Turner's syndrome (45,X) (Figs. 28.2A and B)
- Various mosaic states 45,X/46,XX
- Pure gonadal dysgenesis (46,XX or 46,XY)—phenotypically female with streak gonads. Stature is average with some secondary sexual characters
- Androgen insensitivity syndrome (testicular feminization syndrome) 46,XY (Fig. 28.5)
- Partial deletions of the X chromosome (46,XX).

When part of one X chromosome is missing—deletion of long arm of X chromosome (Xq^-) leads to streak gonads and amenorrhea but no somatic abnormalities. Deletion of short arm of X chromosome (Xp^-) usually leads to somatic features similar to Turner's syndrome.

■ **Dysfunction of thyroid and adrenal cortex**
- Adrenogenital syndrome (Figs. 28.1 and 33.1).
- Cretinism.

■ **Metabolic disorders**
- Juvenile diabetes.

■ **Systemic illness**
- Malnutrition, anemia
- Weight loss
- Tuberculosis.

■ **Unresponsive endometrium**
- *Congenital:* Uterine synechiae (tubercular).

INVESTIGATIONS (FLOWCHART 29.2)

The basic disorders responsible for primary amenorrhea almost always have some specific clinical manifestations. The diagnosis and management of cryptomenorrhea of congenital variety has already been described in Ch. 4. **Only the true primary amenorrhea is dealt with here.**

When to start investigations?

The following guidelines may be of help:
- No period by 16 years of age in the presence of normal secondary sexual characters.
- No period by the age of 14 in the absence of growth or development of secondary sexual characters.

However, the formula may not be applicable in all cases. A patient may come with typical features suggestive of Turner and there is no point to defer the investigation or a patient of 14 with absence of vagina should not be told to come after 2 years for investigation. Even in primary amenorrhea, the possibility of pregnancy should be kept in mind, as pregnancy can occur even prior to menarche.

The investigation protocols can be grouped as:

History

Certain types of primary amenorrhea are of heredofamilial in nature. Delayed menarche or androgen insensitivity syndrome often runs in family, the later one is often found in multiple siblings of the same family and their maternal aunts.

Medical diseases: Genital tuberculosis or diabetes though rare, may be responsible for primary amenorrhea. Such type of amenorrhea is usually associated with hypogonadism.

Other features: Abnormal loss or gain in weight within short span of time is suggestive of some metabolic disorders.

Clinical Examination

With few exceptions, the physical signs (height, weight, arm span) are so apparent that the clinical diagnosis of etiological factors of primary amenorrhea does not seem to be difficult. The diagnosis of some common causes based on clinical examinations are tabulated in Table 29.1.

Flowchart 29.2: Evaluation of patent with primary amenorrhea.

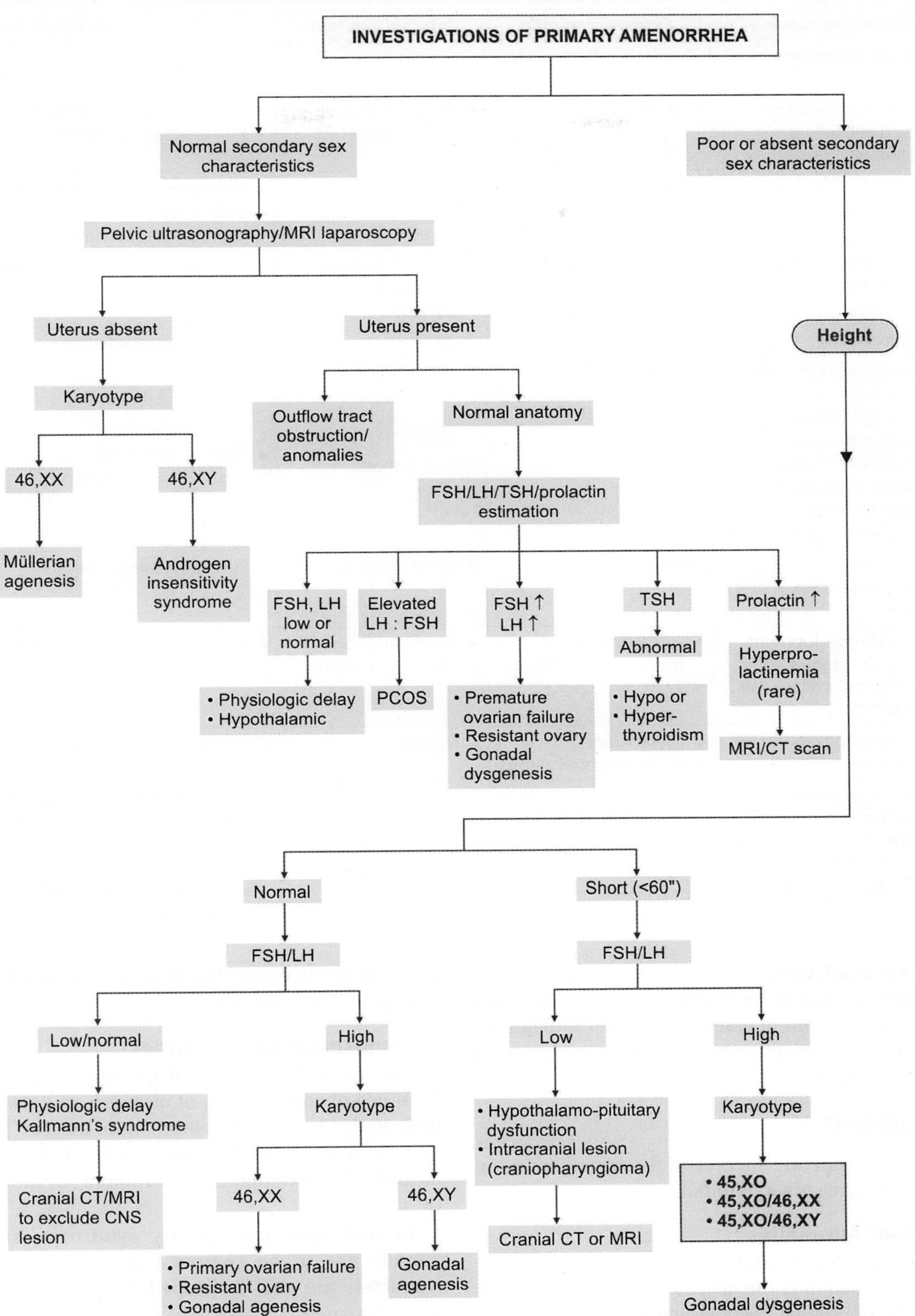

(FSH: follicle-stimulating hormone; LH: luteinizing hormone; TSH: thyroid-stimulating hormone; PCOS: polycystic ovary syndrome; CNS: central nervous system; MRI: magnetic resonance imaging, CT: computed tomography)

TABLE 29.1: Diagnosis of primary amenorrhea based on clinical examination.

Physical appearance	External genitalia	Internal genitalia	Probable diagnosis
Secondary sex characters Stature			
▪ Normal breast development ▪ Normal sexual hair ▪ Average stature	▪ Normal	▪ Absence of vagina ▪ Absent uterus	▪ Müllerian agenesis (Mayer-Rokitansky-Küster-Hauser syndrome)
—do—	—do—	▪ Normal	▪ Unresponsive endometrium—receptor defect (rare) ▪ Uterine synechiae (rare)
▪ Poor breast development ▪ Scanty pubic hair ▪ Average stature	▪ Underdeveloped	▪ Underdeveloped (vaginal rugosity absent)	▪ Hypogonadotropic hypogonadism
▪ Tall and lanky	—do—	—do—	▪ Primary ovarian failure
▪ Poor secondary sex characters ▪ Stature—short ▪ Webbing of the neck and cubitus valgus present ▪ Congenital malformations of cardiac, renal or great vessels (coarctation of aorta) ▪ Phenotypically female	—do—	—do— 'Streak' gonads	▪ Turner's syndrome
▪ Average height ▪ Delayed secondary sex characters	Normal	Bilateral 'streak' gonads	▪ Pure gonadal dysgenesis
▪ Normal breast development without areolar pigmentation ▪ Scanty pubic and axillary hair ▪ Average stature	▪ Labial or inguinal gonads (Figs. 27.6 and 27.7)	▪ Short blind vagina ▪ Absence of uterus	▪ Androgen insensitivity syndrome
▪ Normal phenotypically female ▪ Average stature	▪ Labial fusion ▪ Enlargement of clitoris	▪ Normal	▪ Adrenogenital syndrome (late onset)
▪ Features of (hypogonadotropic hypogonadism) • Short stature • Mental retardation • Obesity, retintis pigmentosa	▪ Underdeveloped	▪ Underdeveloped	▪ Cretinism due to hypothyroidism ▪ Hypothalamopituitary dysfunction (rare) • Kallmann's syndrome • Prader-Labhart-Willi syndrome • Laurence-Moon-Bardet–Biedl syndrome (rare)

Special Investigations

The investigation should be restricted for corroboration of clinical diagnosis and in cases where clinical diagnosis remains disputed. The appropriate investigation protocol is tabulated in Tables 29.2 and 29.3.

MANAGEMENT

The scope of therapeutic success in the management of primary amenorrhea is very limited.

Development Anomalies

Complete agenesis of vagina

Vaginal reconstruction is the accepted form of treatment. The principle of vaginal reconstruction is to create an avascular space between the bladder and rectum. The patency is to be maintained by a mold and graft. **The commonly used materials for graft** are skin or amniotic membranes. The result are quite satisfactory so far as the coital act is concerned. **The ideal time of operation** is prior to or soon after marriage.

Chromosomal Abnormalities

In Turner or other types of gonadal dysgenesis, short-term use of combination of estrogen and progestogen is indicated at least for development of breasts (p. 374). **The gonads of XY gonadal dysgenesis should be removed** for its increased development of seminoma or dysgerminoma (p. 374).

In androgen insensitivity syndrome, the ectopic gonads are to be removed after the secondary sex characters are well-developed, because they may turn to malignancy. Substitution therapy after gonadectomy is indicated to maintain the secondary sex characters. Hormone replacement therapy (HRT) with conjugated equine estrogen (Premarin 0.625 mg daily) is adequate (p. 374).

TABLE 29.2: Special investigations in a case of primary amenorrhea to corroborate clinical diagnosis.

Probable diagnosis	*Investigations*	*Findings*	*Management*
Müllerian agenesis (Mayer-Rokitansky-Küster-Hauser syndrome)	▪ Ultrasonography ▪ MRI ▪ Laparoscopy ▪ Karyotype ▪ Intravenous pyelogram (IVP) ▪ Urinary tract abnormalities (30%)	▪ Uterus—absent ▪ Tubes—present ▪ Ovaries—normal ▪ 46,XX	Endocrinologically normal. They can have children following reconstructive surgery or using surrogacy. Uterine transplantation is the alternative for fertility improvement
Unresponsive endometrium	▪ *Progesterone challenge test ▪ Hysterosalpingography (HSG)/hysteroscopy ▪ Hormonal studies (FSH/E_2)	▪ Negative ▪ Normal uterine cavity ▪ Normal/high	Mutation in estrogen receptor (ERα) gene. Exogenous estrogen induce minimal changes with high doses. Pregnancy may be possible, other option is surrogacy
Uterine synechiae	▪ Progesterone challenge test ▪ HSG ▪ Hysteroscopy/saline infusion sonography	▪ Negative ▪ Honeycomb appearance ▪ Direct visualization	Endocrinologically normal. Hysteroscopic adhesiolysis is the preferred treatment. Successful pregnancy is possible
Tubercular (p. 113)	▪ Blood—erythrocyte sedimentation rate (ESR) ▪ X-ray chest ▪ Mantoux test ▪ Endometrial biopsy	▪ Raised ▪ May have positive finding ▪ Positive (usually) ▪ Positive lesion may be detected	Antitubercular drug therapy. Pregnancy is possible
Hypogonadotropic-hypogonadism	▪ Progesterone challenge test ▪ Serum gonadotropins ▪ Serum estradiol	▪ Negative ▪ Low <5 mIU/mL ▪ Low (<20 pg/mL)	Often respond with GnRH stimulation with increase in FSH and LH levels. Basic defect in CNS—hypothalamus (KAL gene defect)
Primary ovarian failure (p. 389) (hypergonadotropic-hypogonadism)	▪ Karyotype ▪ Serum estradiol ▪ Serum gonadotropins ▪ Ovarian biopsy (ovaries—small/streak), ovarian biopsy is not essential for diagnosis	▪ 46,XX ▪ Low (<20 pg/mL) ▪ Elevated >40 mIU/mL ▪ (a) A follicular (common), (b) follicular or (c) autoimmune (lymphocytic infiltration) type. Follicles are present in resistant ovarian syndrome	May have pregnancy with egg donation as long as the uterus is normal
Turner (p. 369)	▪ Laparoscopy ▪ Serum gonadotropins ▪ Karyotype	▪ 'Streak' gonads ▪ High ▪ 45,XO or 45,XO/46,XX	Mosaic individual may have follicles that develop with gonadotropin stimulation. Rarely ovulation and pregnancy can occur
Androgen insensitivity syndrome (p. 370)	▪ Laparoscopy ▪ Serum testosterone ▪ Karyotype ▪ Gonadal biopsy	▪ Uterus—absent; tubes—absent ▪ Equal to normal males ▪ 46,XY ▪ Testicular structure	Flow chart 29.2
Adrenogenital syndrome	▪ Karyotype ▪ Serum 17-hydroxyprogesterone ▪ Urinary pregnanetriol	▪ 46,XX ▪ Elevated (>8 ng/mL) ▪ Elevated	Flow chart 29.2
Thyroid dysfunction (hypo)	▪ Serum thyroid-stimulating hormone (TSH) ▪ T_3, T_4	▪ Elevated ▪ Lowered	Flow chart 29.2
Hypergonadotropic Hypogonadism	▪ Karyotype ▪ CT scan or MRI	46,XX CNS, H-P-O axis lesion to rule out	Ovulation induction with GnRH

*The test is performed by tablet medroxyprogesterone 10 mg daily or micronized progesterone 200 mg daily for 10 days or administrating progesterone in oil suspension 75 mg IM. Withdrawal bleeding usually occurs within 10 days, if the test is positive

TABLE 29.3: Types of amenorrhea.

Type of hypogonadism	Serum levels of LH/FSH	Estrogen levels	Pathology
Hypergonadotropic	High (FSH >30 mL/IU/mL)	Low	Ovary
Hypogonadotropic	Low (FSH <5 mL IU/mL)	Low	CNS: Hypothalamic-pituitary
Eugonadotropic	Normal	Normal	Varied

Hypothalamo-pituitary-ovarian (HPO) Axis Defect

Patients with delayed puberty, following exclusion of other causes, should be counseled and reassured. Otherwise puberty may be induced using oral estrogen and progestin therapy when there is severe delay.

Gross defects in the form of adiposogenital dystrophy or pituitary dwarfism are not amenable to any form of therapy. In mild disorders, it is possible to induce ovulation and menstruation either by treatment with gonadotropins or with GnRH analogs. Individuals with isolated gonadotropin deficiency (Kallmann's syndrome) can be treated for induction of menstruation or ovulation. Pulsatile administration of GnRH is used for induction of ovulation. Estrogen and progestin therapy is given for menstruation.

Hypothalamic-pituitary tumors (craniopharyngioma, prolactinoma) may need therapy, surgical excision or radiotherapy. Team approach involving a gynecologist, an endocrinologist, a neurosurgeon, and a radiotherapist is ideal.

Thyroid and Adrenal Dysfunction

Gross thyroid hypoplasia (cretinism) does not respond to thyroid replacement therapy. However, mild hypothyroidism may have good result with replacement therapy. Adrenogenital syndrome with enlarged clitoris should be treated by surgical removal of clitoris (clitoroplasty) as early as possible to avoid psychological problems. Corticosteroid therapy should be continued for a prolonged period.

Corticosteroid replacement therapy is given for 17-α-hydroxylase deficiency state.

Prolactinomas need to be treated with dopamine agonists (p. 391).

Metabolic and Nutritional

Diabetes and tuberculosis are to be treated by antidiabetic and antitubercular drug respectively. Correction of anemia and improvement of nutrition status may resume menstruation. Correction of malabsorption, weight loss, stress, and chronic diseases are to be done when indicated.

Unresponsive Endometrium

Uterine synechiae of tubercular origin should be treated by antitubercular drugs supplemented by adhesiolysis and intrauterine contraceptive device (IUCD) insertion. Hysteroscopic (p. 520) release of adhesions using scissors or electrocautery can be done. To prevent recurrence of adhesion formation, high dose estrogen and progestin therapy is given monthly for withdrawal bleeding. There is no known treatment as yet for congenital unresponsive endometrium (receptor defect).

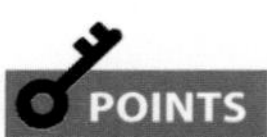

POINTS

- **Amenorrhea** is physiological before puberty, during pregnancy and lactation and following menopause.
- **Most common cause** of amenorrhea in a woman of reproductive age is pregnancy.
- **Regular menstruation** indicates cyclical ovarian function in response to intact hypothalamo-pituitary-ovarian (HPO) axis. On the other hand amenorrhea and oligomenorrhea indicates ovarian, endometrial and/or hypothalamo-pituitary-ovarian (HPO) axis dysfunction.
- The **most common cause of secondary amenorrhea** (pathological) is hypothalamic dysfunction.
- **Most common cause of cryptomenorrhea** is imperforate hymen. The symptoms include periodic lower abdominal pain and occasional retention of urine. The treatment is cruciate incision of the hymen and drainage of blood.
- **More common causes of primary amenorrhea** are gonadal failure, abnormal chromosomal pattern, developmental defect of genital tract and disturbed function of the hypothalamo-pituitary-ovarian axis.
  As such **detailed history, clinical examination** and **specific investigations** most often clinch the diagnosis of primary amenorrhea (Tables 29.1 and 29.2).
- **Women with primary amenorrhea** due to hypogonadotropic hypogonadism, should have CT scan to rule out CNS lesion. Karyotyping is not needed.
- **Individuals with gonadal dysgenesis** and X chromosomal abnormality are less than 150 cm in height.
- **The scope of therapeutic success** in the management of primary amenorrhea is very limited.
- **XY gonads** should be removed for its increased risk of malignancy. Substitution estrogen therapy should be prescribed for the development and maintenance of secondary sex characters.
- **Amenorrheic patients** may belong to any of the four groups: (a) Hypergonadotropic hypogonadism; (b) Hypogonadotropic hypogonadism; (c) Hyperprolactinemia; or (d) Normogonadotropic anovulation.
- **Hypothalamic hypogonadism** is associated with reduced FSH and LH. There is no follicular growth and estradiol production.
- **Other common causes of primary amemorrhea are**: (a) Hypergonadotropic hypogonadism; (b) Chromosomal abnormality; (c) Developmental defect of Müllerian system (MRKH syndrome); (d) Hypogonadotropic hypogonadism; (e) Dysfunction of thyroid; and adrenal gland; (f) Systemic illness, malnutrition and juvenile diabetes.
- **Women with Müllerian abnormalities** have associated renal abnormalities in about one-third of cases.
- *Conditions where breast development is absent and uterus is present (estrogen deficient state): (a) Gonadal failure (45, XO, dysgenesis), 17α hydroxylase deficiency; (b) Hypothalamic failure: Neurotransmitter defect, Kallmann syndrome, craniophanyngioma; (c) Pituitary failure: Isolated gonadotropin deficiency (thalassemia major).*
- *Conditions where breast development present but uterus absent: Testicular feminization*
- *Conditions where breast development absent and uterus absent: 17α hydroxylase deficiency with 46,XY karyotype (male). These individuals have: Hypernatremia, hypokalemia, decreased cortisol, elevated ACTH, raised mineralocorticoid levels, hypertension, raised serum progesterone >3 ng/mL. Treatment: Cortisol administration in addition to sex steroids.*

SECONDARY AMENORRHEA

DEFINITION

It is the absence of menstruation for 6 months or more in a woman in whom normal menstruation has been established.

The physiological causes and cryptomenorrhea has been described earlier in this chapter. Only the true secondary amenorrhea will be discussed here.

ETIOLOGY

The causes of **true** secondary amenorrhea with the possible mechanism are outlined in Table 29.4. However, amenorrhea in a women with reproductive age should be considered as pregnancy unless proved otherwise.

COMMON CAUSES

Details have been discussed in Tables 29.4 and 29.5.

TABLE 29.4: Etiopathogenesis of secondary amenorrhea.

Etiology	*Mechanism*
Uterine factors ▪ Tubercular endometritis ▪ Postradiation ▪ Synechiae ▪ Surgical removal	 ▪ Destruction of the endometrium or inhibition of ovarian function by tubercular toxin ▪ Destruction of the endometrium ▪ Intrauterine adhesions → amenorrhea ▪ Ablation of endometrium by laser, resectoscope (p. 522)
Ovarian factors ▪ Polycystic ovarian syndrome ▪ Premature ovarian failure ▪ Resistant ovarian syndrome (Savage's syndrome) ▪ Chemotherapy (Alkalyting agents)	 ▪ Tonically elevated LH → increased androgen production from the theca (PCOS) cells and stroma of the ovaries → decrease SHBG → increased unbound estrogens and androgens → pituitary sensitivity to GnRH is increased → preferential increased production of LH, decreased production of FSH due to inhibin. Disturbed adrenal function is also implicated in androgen excess. A state of hyperandrogenism produces amenorrhea by its antiestrogenic action ▪ Absence of follicle or accelerated rate of depletion of follicles in the ovaries ▪ Follicles are present but are resistant to gonadotropins (defect in FSH receptor)
Hyperestrogenic state ▪ Persistent follicles in metropathia ▪ Feminizing tumor of the ovary (granulosa cell tumor)	 ▪ The estrogen level remains high and there is no fluctuation ▪ As such, so long as endometrial support is not lost, amenorrhea continues
Androgen excess **Masculinizing tumor of the ovary** (Sertoli-Leydig cell tumor)	▪ Androgen excess opposes the effect of estrogen on the endometrium (p. 386)
Hypoestrogenic state ▪ Oophorectomy ▪ Pelvic radiation	 ▪ Removal of the site of production of estrogens ▪ Makes the ovaries unresponsive to gonadotropins
Pituitary factors ▪ Adenoma (prolactinoma) ▪ Cushing's disease ▪ Acromegaly ▪ Sheehan's syndrome ▪ Simmond's disease (unrelated to pregnancy)	 ▪ Microadenoma usually associated with hyperprolactinemia. It either inhibits ovarian steroidogenesis directly or inhibits pituitary gonadotropin release . ▪ There is partial or complete destruction of the pituitary by ischemia caused by venous thrombosis following severe postpartum hemorrhage and shock. The principal hormones affected are growth hormone, gonadotropins, TSH, adrenocorticotropins, and prolactin
Hypothalamic factors ▪ Psychogenic shock, stress, anorexia nervosa, strenuous exercise, pseudocyesis, etc.	 ▪ Inhibit the release of GnRH or affect dopamine metabolism. There is low level of estrogen and LH but FSH level remains normal (*see* below)
▪ Congenital malformation ▪ Trauma: Accidents, surgery or radiotherapy ▪ Infection: Tubercular or sarcoid granulomas ▪ Tumors: Craniopharyngioma, meningioma	Lead to hypogonadotropic hypogonadism. There may be hyperprolactinemia due to altered dopamine inhibition. Tumors of the hypothalamus or pituitary need surgical excision or radiotherapy. Management needs a team approach including a neurosurgeon, a radiotherapist and an endocrinologist
Adrenal factors ▪ Adrenal tumor or hyperplasia ▪ Cushing's syndrome	 ▪ Androgen excess opposes the effect of estrogen on the endometrium —do—

Contd...

Contd...

Etiology	*Mechanism*
Thyroid factors ▪ Hypothyroid state	 ▪ Raised TSH and hyperprolactinemia by direct action of TRH on the galactophore cells in the pituitary
General disease ▪ Malnutrition, tuberculosis, chronic nephritis, diabetes, etc.	 ▪ Probably affecting the hypothalamo-pituitary-ovarian axis
Iatrogenic ▪ Contraceptive pills (post pill amenorrhea) ▪ Psychotrophic drugs: Phenothiazine derivatives ▪ Antihypertensive drugs: Reserpine or dopamine antagonists	 ▪ Suppression of GnRH release ▪ Dopamine receptor blocking agents raise the prolactin level ▪ Dopamine depleting agents raise the prolactin level

(LH: luteinizing hormone; PCOS: polycystic ovary syndrome; SHBG: sex hormone-binding globulin; GnRH: gonadotropin-releasing hormone; FSH: follicle-stimulating hormone; TSH: thyroid-stimulating hormone)

TABLE 29.5: Common causes of secondary amenorrhea.

Hypothalamus	*Pituitary*	*Ovary*	*Uterine*	*Systemic*
▪ ***Stress*** ▪ ***Postpill*** ▪ ***Weight:*** Either too much loss or too much gain ▪ ***Drugs:*** Psychotropic and antihypertensive drugs	▪ Adenoma ▪ Sheehan's	▪ Polycystic ovary syndrome (PCOS) ▪ Premature ovarian failure	▪ Synechiae (Spontaneous or induced)	▪ Malnutrition ▪ Hypothyroid state ▪ Diabetes

CLINICAL FEATURES AND DIAGNOSIS OF SECONDARY AMENORRHEA

UTERINE FACTORS

TUBERCULAR ENDOMETRITIS

The family history or past history of tuberculosis in the patient herself may or may not be present. Physical and pelvic examination may not be informative. The diagnosis is often accidentally made following diagnostic curettage or at laparotomy or laparoscopy.

UTERINE SYNECHIAE (SYN: ASHERMAN'S SYNDROME)

There is formation of adhesions following post-abortal and puerperal curettage and also following diagnostic curettage in dysfunctional uterine bleeding. Rarely, it follows tubercular endometritis. Menstrual abnormalities include hypomenorrhea, oligomenorrhea or amenorrhea. Progesterone challenge test is negative. Hysterosalpingography shows honeycomb appearance (Fig. 38.76). Transvaginal sonography or saline infusion sonography is helpful to the diagnosis. But definitive diagnosis is made by hysteroscopy. Hysteroscopy reveals the extent of adhesions directly. It has got its therapeutic value also (p. 521).

OVARIAN FACTORS

POLYCYSTIC OVARIAN SYNDROME (PCOS)

Polycystic ovarian syndrome was originally described in 1935 by Stein and Leventhal as a syndrome manifested by amenorrhea, hirsutism, and obesity associated with enlarged polycystic ovaries.

It is the **most common endocrine disorder** in a woman of reproductive age.

Etiology

This heterogeneous disorder is characterized by excessive androgen production by the ovaries mainly. **PCOS is a multifactorial and polygenic condition.** Dysregulation of the CYP 11a gene, upregulation of enzymes in androgen biosynthetic pathology have been suggested. Insulin receptor gene on chromosome 19p13.2 are also involved.

Diagnosis *is based upon the presence of any two of the following three criteria* [American Society for Reproductive Medicine (ASRM)/European Society of Human Reproduction and Embryology (ESHRE), 2018].

- Oligo and/or anovulation.
- Hyperandrogenism (clinical and/or biochemical).
- Polycystic ovaries.

Other etiologies [congenital adrenal hyperplasia (CAH)], thyroid dysfunction, hyperprolactinemia, Cushing syndrome) are to be excluded. The incidence varies between 0.5–4%, more common amongst infertile women. It is prevalent in young reproductive age group (20–30%). Polycystic ovary may be seen in about 20% of normal women. Hyperandrogenism is considered the key feature for the syndrome. Not all women with isolated polycystic appearing ovary (PAO) have PCOS. With other insults of genetic, environmental (weight gain and psychological stress), may develop PCOS.

Pathology

Typically, the ovaries are enlarged. Ovarian volume is increased ≥10 cm^3. Stroma is increased. The capsule is

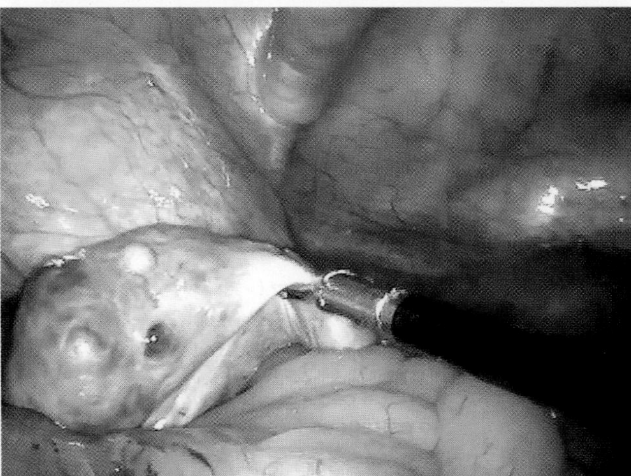

Fig. 29.4: Laparoscopic view of polycystic changes (PCOS) of the ovary. Multiple small peripheral cysts are seen on the ovarian surface.

thickened and pearly white in color. Presence of multiple (≥12) follicular cysts measuring about 2–9 mm in diameter are crowded around the cortex (Fig. 29.4).

Histology

There is thickening of tunica albuginea. The cysts are the follicles at varying stages of maturation and atresia. There is theca cell hypertrophy (stromal hyperthecosis). Patient may present with features of diabetes mellitus (insulin resistance).

Clinical Features

The patient complains of increasing obesity (abdominal—50%), menstrual abnormalities (70%) in the form of oligomenorrhea, amenorrhea or dysfunctional uterine bleeding (DUB) and infertility. Presence of hirsutism and acne (Fig. 29.5) are the important features (70%). Virilism is rare.

Acanthosis nigricans is characterized by specific skin changes due to insulin resistance. The skin is thickened and pigmented (gray brown). Commonly affected sites are nape of the neck, inner thighs, groin and axilla (Fig. 29.6).

HAIR-AN syndrome in patients with PCOS is characterized by **h**yperandrogenism, **i**nsulin **r**esistance and **a**canthosis **n**igricans.

Internal examination reveals bilateral enlarged cystic ovaries which may not be revealed due to obesity.

Investigations

- **Sonography:** Transvaginal sonography (8 MHz) is especially useful in obese patient (BMI ≥ 25/23). Ovaries are enlarged in volume (≥10 cm^3). Increased number (≥20) of peripherally arranged follicles per ovary (2–9 mm) are seen (Fig. 29.7).
- **Serum values:**
  - LH level is elevated and/or the ratio LH: FSH is >3:1.
  - Raised level of estradiol and estrone—the estrone level is markedly elevated.
  - SHBG level is reduced.

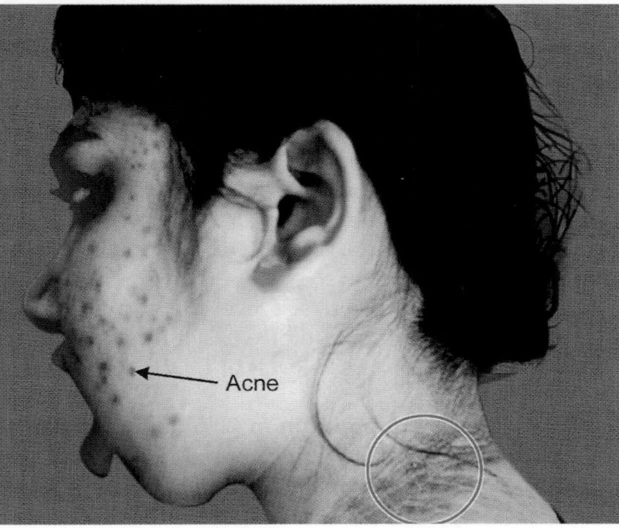

Fig. 29.5: Hirsutism, acne, acanthosis nigricans in PCOS (red circle).

(*Courtesy*: Prof BN Chakravorty, IRM, Kolkata)

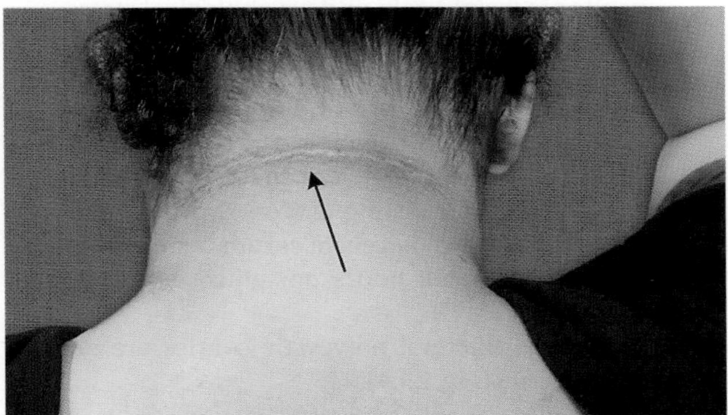

Fig. 29.6: Acanthosis nigricans in PCOS.

(*Courtesy:* Prof BN Chakravorty, IRM, Kolkata)

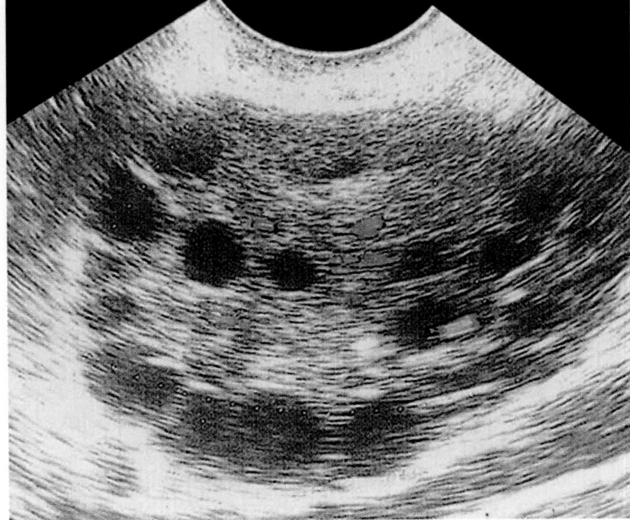

Fig. 29.7: Color Doppler (TV) scan showing numerous small cysts with increased ovarian stroma and vascularity—typical of PCOS.

- Hyperandrogenism—mainly from the ovary but less from the adrenals. Androstenedione is raised (3–5 ng/mL).
- Raised serum testosterone (>1.5 ng/mL) and dehydroepiandrosterone sulfate (DHEAS) levels.
- Elevated LH or raised LH/FSH ratio is there. But it is neither specific nor diagnostic of PCOS.
- Women with hirsutim have raised levels of dihydrotestosterone (DHT) with the presence of the enzyme 5α-reductase.
- These women have raised levels of 3α-androstenediol glucoronide (3α-diol-G). Nonhirsute women with PCOS have raised levels of T, *DHEAS or but not 3α-diol-G)*
- Raised levels of prolactin in 20% due to increased pulsatility of GnRH.
- *More of serine phosphorylation instead of tyrosine phosphorylation is observed in the insulin receptor.*
- 31% women with PCOS have impaired OGT and 7.5% diabetes.
- Genetic predisposition of PCOS is clear. There are several susceptible genes. Two major environmental insults are weight gain and psychological stress.
- Elevated insulin levels stimulate adipocyte production of adipokines. There is release of many inflammatory mediators and other factors like IL-6, TNFα and leptin and decrease in adiponectin.
- **Insulin resistance (IR):** Raised fasting insulin levels >25 μIU/mL and fasting glucose/insulin ratio <4.5 suggests IR (50%). Levels of serum insulin response >300 μIU/mL at 2 hours postglucose (75 g) load, suggests severe IR.

- **Laparoscopy:** Bilateral polycystic ovaries are characteristic of PCOS (Fig. 29.4).

Pathophysiology

Exact pathophysiology of PCOS is not clearly understood. It may be discussed under the following heads (Fig. 29.8):

- Hypothalamic-pituitary compartment abnormality
- Androgen excess and hirsutism
- Anovulation
- Obesity and insulin resistance
- Long-term consequences.

Hypothalamic-pituitary Compartment in PCOS

- Increased pulse frequency of GnRH leads to increased pulse frequency of LH. **Leptin** (a peptide, secreted by fat cells and by the ovarian follicle), insulin resistance and hyperandrogenemia are responsible for this.
- GnRH is preferential to LH rather than FSH (Fig. 29.8).
- Increased pulse frequency and amplitude of LH results in tonically elevated level of LH (Fig. 29.9).
- FSH level is not increased. This is mainly due to the negative feedback effect of chronically elevated estrogen and the follicular inhibin.
- Increased free estradiol due to reduced sex hormone binding globulin (SHBG) bears positive feedback relationship to LH.
- The LH : FSH ratio is increased.

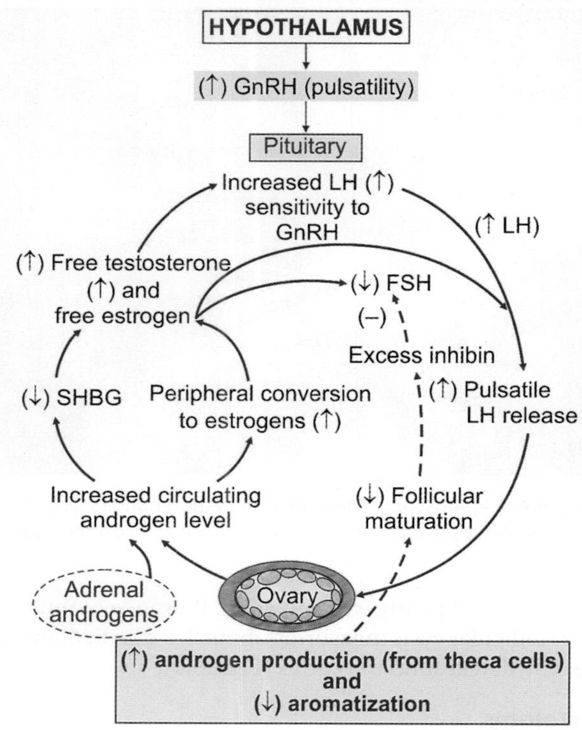

Fig. 29.8: Hypothalamic-pituitary compartment in PCOS.

Hypothalamus → increased pulse frequency of GnRH → pituitary sensitivity to GnRH↑ → increased pulse frequency of LH (*preferential*) compared to FSH → LH (↑) : FSH (↓)

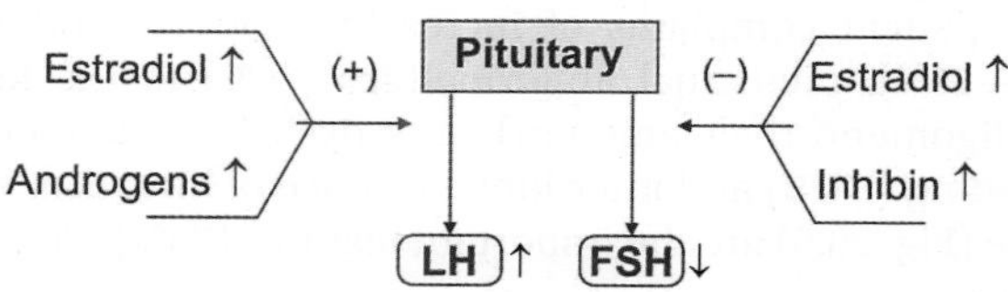

Fig. 29.9: Increased pulse frequency of LH in the pathogenesis of PCOS.

Androgen Excess

Abnormal regulation of the androgen forming enzyme (P450 C17) is thought to be the main cause for **excess production of androgens from the ovaries** and adrenals. The principal sources of androgens are: (a) Ovary; (b) Adrenal; (c) Systemic metabolic alteration.

- **Ovary** produces excess androgens due to: (a) Stimulation of theca cells by high LH; (b) P450 C17 enzyme hyperfunction; (c) Defective aromatization of androgens to estrogen; (d) Stimulation of theca cells by IGF-1 (insulin growth factor-1) (Fig. 29.10).
- **Adrenals** are stimulated to produce excess androgens by: (a) Stress; (b) P450 C17 enzyme hyperfunction; (c) Associated high prolactin level (20%).
- **Systemic metabolic alteration**
  - **Hyperinsulinemia** causes: (a) Stimulation of theca cells to produce more androgens; (b) Insulin results in more free IGF-1. By autocrine action, IGF-1

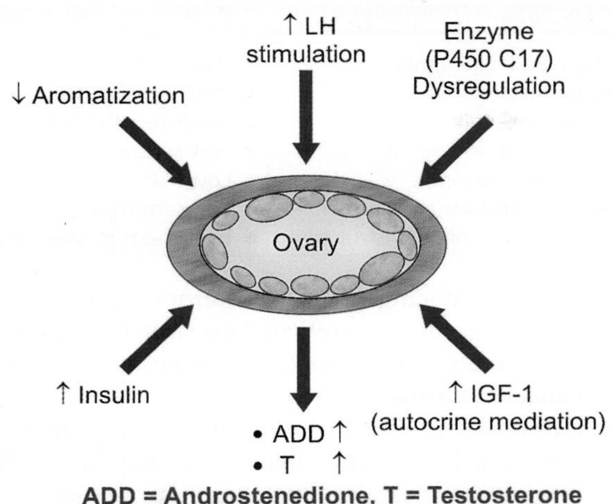

Fig. 29.10: Ovary as a source of excess androgens in the pathogenesis of PCOS.

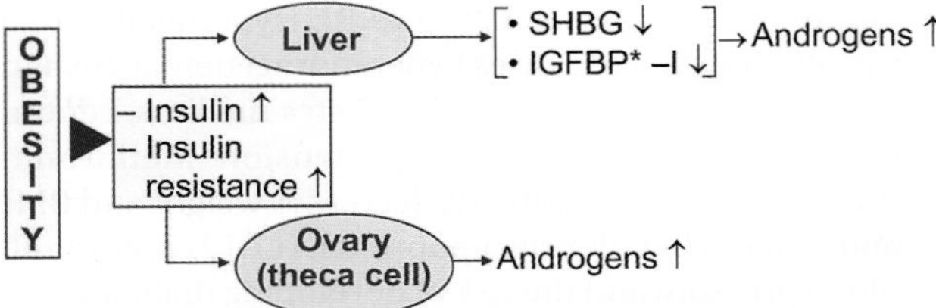

Fig. 29.11: Hyperinsulinemia in the pathogenesis of PCOS.

stimulates theca cells to produce more androgens; (c) Insulin inhibits hepatic synthesis of SHBG, resulting in more free level of androgens (Fig. 29.11). **Features suggestive of insulin resistance are:** BMI >25 kg/m^2, acanthosis nigricans and waist to hip ratio >0.85.

- **Hyperprolactinemia:** In about 20% cases, there may be mild elevation of prolactin level due to increased pulsitivity of GnRH or due to dopamine deficiency or both. The prolactin further stimulates adrenal androgen production.

Whatever may be the etiology, the endocrinologic effects of PCOS produce a vicious cycle of events as shown in the Figure 29.8.

Anovulation

Because of **low FSH level**, follicular growth is arrested at different phases of maturation (2–10 mm diameter). The net effect is diminished estradiol and increased inhibin production. **Due to elevated LH**, there is hypertrophy of theca cells and more androgens are produced either from theca cells or stroma (Fig. 29.12).

There is defective FSH induced aromatization of androgens to estrogens.

Follicular microenvironment is therefore more androgenic rather than estrogenic.

Unless there is estrogenic follicular microenvironment, follicular growth, maturation, and ovulation cannot occur. There is huge number of atretic follicles that contribute

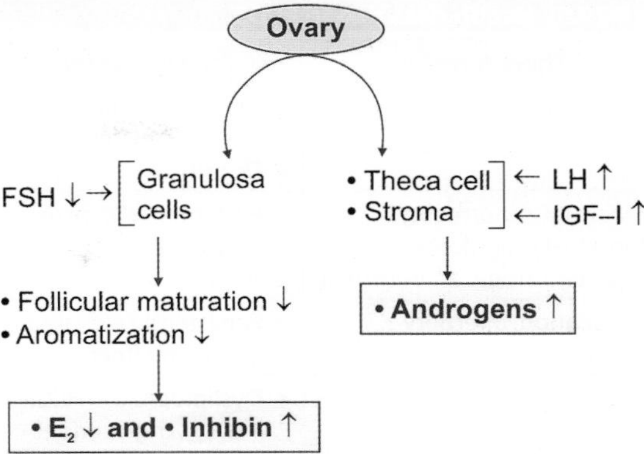

Fig. 29.12: Anovulation in the pathogenesis of PCOS.

to increased ovarian stroma (hyperthecosis). LH level is tonically elevated without any surge. LH surge is essential for ovulation to occur.

Obesity and Insulin Resistance

Obesity (central) is recognized as an important contributory factor. Apart from excess production of androgens, obesity is also associated with reduced SHBG. It also induces insulin resistance and hyperinsulinemia which in turn increases the gonadal androgen production. PCOS is thought to have a dominant mode of inheritance as about 50% of first degree relatives have PCOS.

Etiology of insulin resistance is unknown. Mutations of the insulin receptor gene in the peripheral target tissues (muscle and adipose tissue) and reduced tyrosine autophosphorylation of the insulin receptor, is currently thought to be an important cause. Increased central body fat leads to android obesity.

Long-term Consequences (Table 29.6)

Long-term consequences in a patient suffering from PCOS includes: The **excess androgens** (mainly androstenedione) either from the ovaries (mainly) or adrenals are peripherally aromatized to estrone (E_1). There is concomitant **diminished SHBG. Cumulative excess unbound E_2 and estrone results in a tonic hyperestrogenic state** (Fig. 29.13). There is endometrial hyperplasia.

Investigations in a Case of PCOS

- Ultrasonography (transvaginal preferred).
- Reassessment of BMI, BP (blood pressure), waist circumference
- Serum levels of FSH, LH, TSH, total testosterone, prolactin, DHEAS, 17 OHP
- 2 hours oral glucose tolerance test (GTT)
- Lipid profile.

Management: Polycystic Ovarian Syndrome

Management of PCOS needs individualization of the patient. It depends on her presenting symptoms, like menstrual disorder, subfertility, obesity, hirsutism or combined symptoms. Patient counseling is important.

TABLE 29.6: Health risks due to PCOS

Short-term	***Long-term***
▪ Obesity	▪ Diabetes mellitus (10%) (insulin resistance) ▪ Obesity
▪ Menstrual abnormality: Menstrual irregularity—oligomenorrhea, amenorrhea	▪ Endometrial cancer ▪ Ovarian cancer
▪ Anovulation, infertility	▪ Persistently elevated estrogen effect
▪ Miscarriage	▪ Dyslipidemia: ↓HDL, ↑LDL, ↑triglycerides
▪ Abnormal lipid profile	▪ Hypertension
▪ Androgen excess: • Acne • Hirsutism • Alopecia	▪ Cardiovascular disease ▪ Coronary artery disease ▪ Hyperhomocysteinemia ▪ Inflammatory adipocytokines
▪ Insulin resistance: • Glucose intolerance	▪ Obstructive sleep apnea (obesity)
• Acanthosis nigricans	▪ Increased mortality

(HDL: high-density lipoprotein; LDL: low-density lipoprotein)

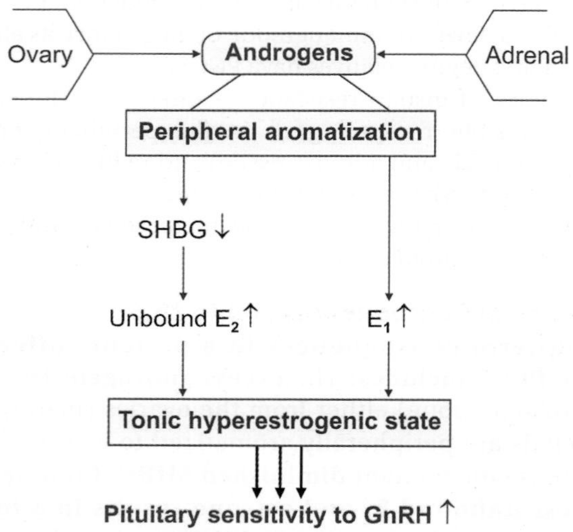

Fig. 29.13: hyperestrogenic state as a consequence of PCOS.

Treatment is primarily targeted to correct the biochemical abnormalities (Table 29.7).

Weight reduction in obese patients is the first line of treatment. Body mass index (BMI) <25 improves menstrual disorders, infertility, impaired glucose intolerance (insulin resistance), hyperandrogenemia (hirsutism, acne), and obesity. Weight reduction (2–5%) improves the metabolic syndrome and reproductive function (read below). **Exercise** is found beneficial.

Fertility not Desired

- **Management of hyperandrogenemia (p. 484)**
  - **Combined oral contraceptive pills** are effective. Progestin suppresses LH and estrogen improves SHBG, reducing free testosterone level. Newer progestins (desogestrel) are best suited (Table 30.4). COCs reduces the risks of endometrial and ovarian cancer to normal.
  - **Hirsutism** is due to anovulation, high androgen and insulin levels, decreased hepatic SHBG production and also due to genetic sensitivity of hair follicles to androgens. Correction of metabolic syndrome (Table 29.8), improves it. **Antiandrogens** (cyproterone acetate, spironolactone, flutamide) may be used (p. 451).
- **Metabolic syndrome (Table 29.8):** Hyperinsulinemia (insulin resistance) causes hyperandrogenemia. Insulin resistance is associated with diabetes mellitus, central obesity, dyslipidemia and hypertension. Metformin, increases insulin sensitivity, decreases weight and BMI and reduces low-density lipoprotein (LDL) cholesterol, blood pressure and the risk of developing diabetes.
- **Hyperinsulinemia** contributes hyperandrogenemia in women with PCOS. Hyperinsulinemia increases the risk of dyslipidemia, cardiovascular disease, and diabetes mellitus. Insulin resistance is the principal abnormality to cause metabolic syndrome (Table 29.8).

Metformin (p. 201) is used as an oral insulin sensitizing agent (*see* below).

Endometrial hyperplasia causes abnormal uterine bleeding. Chronic anovulation, hyperestrogenemia, obesity, and hyperinsulinemia cause endometrial hyperplasia even endometrial cancer. Endometrial biopsy may have to be done.

Combined oral contraceptives (COCs) is the treatment of choice to prevent endometrial hyperplasia and abnormal bleeding and endometrial cancer.

TABLE 29.7: Biochemical abnormalities associated with PCOS.

▪ Hyperandrogenemia ▪ Hyperinsulinemia ▪ Hyperlipidemia ▪ High serum estrogens (estradiol, estrone) ▪ Androgenic ovarian follicular microenvironment (anovulation)	▪ Hyperprolactinemia ▪ Insulin resistance ▪ Hypersecretion of LH ▪ Low serum SHBG ▪ Low FSH ▪ Low serum progesterone ▪ hyperhomocysteinemia

Treatment for Subfertility

Chronic anovulation is the common cause of infertility. Improvement of metabolic syndrome is essential.

Ovulation induction is usually achieved by clomiphene citrate or letrozole following correction of other biochemical abnormalities (Table 29.7). In unresponsive cases, pure FSH

TABLE 29.8: Metabolic syndrome (diagnostic criteria).

1. Triglyceride levels ≥150 mg/dL
2. HDL-cholesterol <50 mg/dL
3. Blood pressure ≥130/85 mm Hg
4. Fasting glucose ≥110 mg/dL
5. Waist circumference >78 cm
Presence of three abnormal findings out of the five

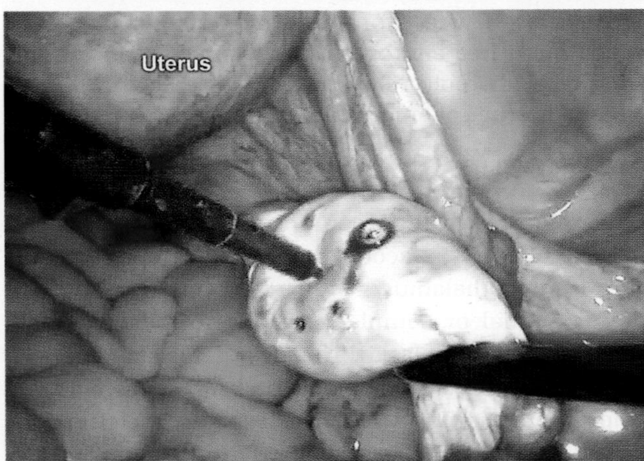

Fig. 29.14: Laparoscopic ovarian drilling using diathermy.

or human menopausal gonadotropin (HMG) along with human chorionic gonadotropin (hCG) may be administered backed up with monitoring facilities (Ch. 17).

Insulin sensitizers: Women with PCOS and hyperinsulinemia with BMI >25 kg/m^2, ovulate satisfactorily when clomiphene is combined with metformin.

Metformin improves metabolic syndrome by reducing all the parameters: weight, BMI (hyperinsulinemia, hyperandrogenism), BP and lipid abnormalities. 500 mg thrice daily is found to correct the biochemical abnormalities. Pioglitazone and rosiglitazone are also being used in cases, resistant to metformin (Ch. 17).

Surgery (Fig. 29.14): Laparoscopic ovarian drilling (LOD) is done for cases found resistant to medical therapy (p. 500). Ovarian surface cysts are punctured up to a depth of 2–4 mm. The cysts are vaporized using monopolar cutting current (20–30 W). 4–6 punctures are made in each ovary. It has replaced the conventional wedge resection of the ovaries. Pregnancy rates following ovarian diathermy are higher. **Bariatric surgery** may be indicated in some PCOS women who are morbidly obese.

Treatment in Women with PCOS

Obesity and metabolic syndrome	• Exercise, diet • Change in lifestyle • Metformin
Subfertility	• Ovulation induction: Letrozole, ± Metformin, ± Gonadotropins
AUB	• Progestins, COCs
Body hair	• Antiandrogens • COCs

(AUB: abnormal uterine bleeding; COCs: combined oral contraceptives)

PREMATURE OVARIAN INSUFFICIENCY

Premature ovarian insufficiency (POI) (failure) is defined when ovarian failure occurs **before the age of 40**. It occurs in about 1% of the female population. During intrauterine life either there is failure of germ cell migration or there may be normal germ cell migration but an accelerated rate of germ cell depletion (apoptosis) due to various reasons (later). This results in either no follicle or only few follicles left behind in the ovary by the time they reach puberty.

Causes of Premature Ovarian Failure (POF)

- **Genetic:** (a) Turner's syndrome (45,XO), (45,X/46,XX); (b) Gonadal dysgenesis 46, XX, 46, XY; (c) Trisomy 18 and 13; (d) X-chromosome deletion, translocation.
- **Autoimmune:** (a) Autoantibodies: antinuclear antibodies (ANA), lupus anticoagulant; (b) Polyglandular autoimmune syndrome (antibodies against thyroid, parathyroid, adrenal, islet cells of pancreas).
- **Infections:** Mumps, tuberculosis.
- **Iatrogenic:** Radiation therapy, chemotherapy (cyclophosphamide), surgery (hysterectomy, bilateral ovarian cystectomy).
- **Metabolic:** Galactosemia, 17α-hydroxylase deficiency. In galactosemia, the enzyme galactose-1-phosphate uridyl transferase is absent. Follicles are destroyed to the toxic effects of galactose.
- **Environmental:** Smoking, pesticides.
- **FSH receptor** absent or postreceptor defect (Savage's syndrome).
- **Idiopathic.**
- **POF/POI:** Often POI is a transient state before the actual onset of POF. Occasionally, women with POI, may ovulate and conceive. Histologically, the ovaries of a woman with POI may show either sclerotic changes as seen a postmenopausal ovary or may have primordial follicles (30%). Ovaries may look like normal ovaries. This condition is an autoimmune state or gonadotropin receptor defect also known as gonadotropin resistant ovary syndrome.

Diagnosis/Investigations

- History of amenorrhea in less than 35 years of age.
- Serum gonadotropin level (FSH >40 mIU/mL) two values at interval of 4 weeks, are high.
- Serum E_2 level is low (<20 pg/mL).
- Karyotype abnormality (*see* above).
- Organ specific humoral antibody (antithyroid most common).
- Ovarian biopsy (afollicular, follicular, and autoimmune variety) **is not essential to the diagnosis**. In autoimmune variety, there is perifollicular lymphocyte infiltration. In **resistant *ovarian syndrome***, follicles are present. FSH receptor is either absent or defective.
- Patient presents with amenorrhea—primary (25%) or secondary (75%). Features of hypoestrogenic state like hot flashes, vaginal dryness, dyspareunia and psychological symptoms are there.
- The possibility of autoimmune disorders should be considered below the age of 35. For this, antithyroid antibodies, rheumatoid factor and antinuclear antibodies should be measured.
- In younger patients (age below 30) karyotype is to be done to rule out chromosomal abnormality.
- Management (p. 395).

MASCULINIZING OVARIAN TUMOR

There are features of gradual defeminization followed by appearance of masculinizing features such as hoarseness of voice, hirsutism, and enlargement of clitoris. Abdominal and pelvic examinations reveal an adnexal tumor; the exact nature is confirmed by biopsy. Serum testosterone level is elevated to >2 ng/mL while DHEAS level is normal.

HYPOTHALAMIC (FACTORS) AMENORRHEA

Hypothalamic dysfunction is one of the major causes of true secondary amenorrhea. There is often history suggestive of **stress, exercise, rapid gain or loss of weight**.

WEIGHT RELATED AMENORRHEA

Female athletes, runners, ballet dancers are under constant stress and performing strenuous exercise. They have high level of corticotropin releasing hormone (CRH). The levels of ACTH, cortisol and endogenous opioids are high. Stress and exercise increase the levels of opioid peptides [β endorphin (β EP)], catechol-estrogens, and CRH. All these inhibit GnRH release. Leptin levels are low. Low leptin levels stimulate neuropeptide Y (↑NPY) which stimulates hunger and alter GnRH pulsatility. CRH directly inhibits GnRH secretion via raised endogenous opioids. They are more likely to develop amenorrhea due to **decrease in GnRH pulse frequency.** According to body weight hypothesis, body weight should be above critical level to achieve menarche and regular menstruation. To achieve menarche, body fat should reach 17% of the body weight and for regularity of menstruation body fat should be maintained at least at 22%. The ratio of body fat to total body weight is more important. Leptin, a hormone produced by adipocytes, links between body composition and H-P-O axis. Reduction of body fat by about one-third will result in menstrual abnormality. Weight loss leads to hypothalamic dysfunction leading to failure of normal GnRH release, thyroid dysfunction and release of growth hormone. Menstruation becomes irregular when the BMI is <19 kg/m^2.

These subjects are hypoestrogenic and have got elevated prolactin and cortisol level. Leptin level is found low.

ANOREXIA NERVOSA

It is a state of self-imposed starvation. This is a psychosexual problem where the patient suffers from the illusion of excessive body fat and distorted body image. Patient denies food and is markedly under weight. Amenorrhea is the rule. Constipation is common. Release of GnRH is affected. **FSH and LH levels are low, cortisol level is high**. This may be a life-threatening disorder.

OBESITY

Obese women so often suffer from irregular menstrual bleeding. Excess number of fat cells in obese women, convert peripheral androgens to estrogen (aromatization). There is also low level of sex-hormone binding globulin, which helps free androgens to be converted to estrone. Obesity with polycystic ovarian disease can cause oligomenorrhea or amenorrhea.

KALLMANN'S SYNDROME

Embryologically GnRH neurones develop in the ectodermal olfactory placode before they migrate finally to the hypothalamus. GnRH neurones are absent due to partial or complete agenesis of olfactory bulb (olfactogenital dysplasia). This disorder is characterized by hypogonadotropic hypogonadism, anosmia and color blindness. The woman presents with cleft palate, unilateral renal agenesis, epilepsy, and neurosensory hearing loss. There may be associated cleft lip and palate. Patients present with primary amenorrhea. These women have hypogonadism, increased wingspan to height ratio. Mode of inheritance is due to a variety of genetic mutations in the KAL-I gene (X-linked) or as an autosomal dominant or recessive fashion. Menstruation can be induced with combined estrogen and progestin therapy. Induction of ovulation is successful with exogenous gonadotropins.

Isolated gonadotropin deficiency is a rare pituitary disease. Women present with amenorrhea and do not respond to GnRH. They almost always have an associated disorder like thalassemia major with iron deposition in the pituitary/retina. Occasionally, it is associated with prepubertal hypothyroidism, mumps or encephalitis.

PSEUDOCYASIS

Woman presents with secondary amenorrhea and symptoms of pregnancy. Endocrine studies revealed alterations with LH pulse frequency and elevated levels of androgen. Raised levels of prolactin with or without galactorrhea have also been observed.

Functional hypothalamic amenorrhea (FHA):

- FHA is defined as the development of secondary amenorrhea in the absence of any drug intake, strenuous exercise, environmental stress, weight loss and without any pathology in the uterus, ovary or in the pituitary. The women with FHA have an abnormal cyclic variation of GnRH pulsatility. This is mostly due to abnormality in CNS neurotransmitters following increased opioid activity. These women have reduced GnRH pulse frequency and normal pulse amplitude. There is reduced secretion of LH and also reduced secretion of FSH, PRL and TSH. However, these women have normal pituitary response GnRH.
- Hypothalamic dysfunction: The condition when GnRH is produced to facilitate gonadotropin stimulation to the ovaries producing E_2 (≥30 pg/mL), sufficient for proliferation of endometrium. This disorder is known as hypothalamic pituitary "dysfunction". However, when the E_2 levels fall 40 pg/mL, (arbitrary value), it is considered as hypothalamic pituitary failure.

PITUITARY FACTORS

ADENOMA

In adenoma either micro or macro, there is usually associated inappropriate lactation (galactorrhea), secondary amenorrhea, and infertility. There may be headache with disturbed vision.

Serum prolactin level is raised beyond 100 ng/mL. X-ray sella turcica may reveal space occupying lesion. CT or MRI scan is more informative.

Hyperprolactinemia and Amenorrhea

Prolactin inhibits GnRH pulse secretion through elevated levels of dopamine (p. 56). Gonadotropin levels are suppressed. Hyperprolactinemia inhibits ovarian steroidogenesis. It is responsible for secondary amenorrhea in about 30% of women. **There is anovulation and hypogonodotropic hypogonadism**.

Pituitary Adenoma (Prolactinoma)

Prolactin is a protein hormone having 199 amino acids with a molecular weight of 23,000 daltons. Prolactin has got various forms, called as "little" or (monomer), "big" (dimer) or "big big" (multimeric) prolactin (glycosylated form) respectively. Little prolactin (90%) has got more biological activity. Prolactin is synthesized and released primarily by the lactotrophs located in the anterior pituitary gland. **Extrapituitary sites of PRL production include** decidua, endometrium, lungs, etc. Prolactin secretion from the anterior pituitary is under the inhibitory control of dopamine. Dopamine is produced in the arcuate nucleus of the hypothalamus and is released in the portal hypophyseal vessels. Hyperprolactinemia is commonly due to pituitary adenomas (microadenoma or macroadenoma). There are other various causes of hyperprolactinemia. *Normal plasma level of prolactin is 1–20 ng/mL.*

Causes of Hyperprolactinemia

Physiological

- Stress and exercise (raised endogenous opioids)
- Pregnancy
- Stimulation of nipples
- Sleep
- Idiopathic

Hypothalamus and Pituitary

- Craniopharyngioma
- Sarcoidosis
- Tuberculosis
- Meningiomas
- Primary hypothyroidism
- Multiple endocrine disorder (Cushing's syndrome, acromegaly)
- Pituitary adenomas (prolactinomas)
- Resection of pituitary stalk.

Neurogenic

- Chest wall lesions
- Empty sella syndrome
- Spinal cord lesions

Drugs

- Alprazolam
- Ranitidine
- Isoniazid
- Sertalin
- Cimetidine
- Cisapride
- Fluoxetine
- Combined oral contraceptives
- Depo-Provera
- Monoamine oxidase (MAO)
- Valproic acid
- Danazol

(↓) Decreased hypothalamic prolactin-inhibiting factor (PIF):

- Phenothiazines
- Metoclopramide
- Methyldopa
- Reserpine
- Antidepressants
- Estrogens

- Atenolol

Others

- Renal failure — (↓) Decreased prolactin (PRL) clearance

(↑) Increased PRL production:

- Cirrhosis of liver
- PCOS
- Idiopathic

Diagnosis of Pituitary Adenomas

Prolactin level is more than 100 ng/mL is often associated with prolactinoma. Most of the adenomas are microadenoma (diameter less than 1 cm). "Coned down" and lateral views of the sella turcica by CT/MRI can detect gross abnormalities, calcification of tumor. Microadenomas rarely progress to macroadenomas. CT is helpful for macroadenomas. MRI with better resolution is superior to CT. It has no radiation risk.

Visual field examination is essential to detect any compression effect on the optic nerves.

Treatment: p. 395.

SHEEHAN'S SYNDROME

There is history of severe postpartum hemorrhage, shock or severe infection. Depending upon the degree of anterior pituitary necrosis, the features vary. **The common manifestations are** failing lactation, loss of pubic and axillary hair, lethargy, hypotension, secondary amenorrhea, and atrophy of the breasts and genitalia. Gonadotropin level is low, so also T_3, T_4, and cortisol. The hormones affected in order of frequency are growth hormone (GH), prolactin, gonadotropins (FSH and LH), TSH, and ACTH. Hyponatremia may be present (30%). The syndrome may develop slowly over 8–10 years time.

Management

Replacement therapy with appropriate hormones including corticosteroid and thyroid are needed. Fertility can be achieved in these women with hMG and hCG. Clomiphene is ineffective.

Eugonadotropic amenorrhea:

- Polycystic ovarian syndrome
- Thyroid disorders
- Hyperprolactinemia
- Ovarian tumors (hormone producing)
- Congenital adrenal hyperplasia
- Androgen insensitivity syndrome.

ADRENAL FACTORS

ADRENAL TUMOR OR HYPERPLASIA

There is secondary amenorrhea, infertility, acne, and features of defeminization followed by virilization (hoarseness of voice, hirsutism, and enlargement of clitoris). In both the conditions there is excess production of androgens. Serum level of DHEAS correlate well with daily urinary 17-KS excretion. **Rise of serum DHEAS and urinary 17-ketosteroid levels are suppressed with dexamethasone 2 mg daily for 2 days in adrenal hyperplasia but not in tumor**. For confirmation of the diagnosis of tumor, intravenous pyelogram (IVP), MRI, CT scan or sonography is helpful.

Level of serum testosterone >200 ng/dL is suggestive of an ovarian androgen secreting tumor. Whereas level of (DHEAS) >800 μg/dL is suggestive of an adrenal tumor. Urinary 17-ketosteroid excretion is high in a case with adrenal tumor. Ovarian neoplasm could be diagnosed with ultrasonographic examination (endovaginal or abdominal).

Late onset congenital adrenal hyperplasia (CAH) is due to enzyme defect (21-hydroxylase, 11β-hydrolase or 3β-hydroxysteroid dehydrogenase) and leads to excess androgen production. But there is relative decrease in cortisol production. 21-hydroxylase deficiency is most common (90%). It is an autosomal recessive disorder.

Serum (morning sample) level of 17-hydroxy-progesterone [17-OHP(I)] >800 ng/dL is diagnostic of 21-hydroxylase deficiency. Level of serum 17-OHP <200 ng/dL virtually rules out the diagnosis of CAH. There is significant rise in 17-OHP level following ACTH stimulation test.

CUSHING'S SYNDROME

Cushing first described the syndrome in 1932. Androgens are formed as intermediate products in the synthesis of cortisol. The elevated cortisol level found in Cushing's syndrome encompasses two distinct pathologic entities.

- Cushing disease (ACTH dependent)
- Adrenal tumor (ACTH independent).

In Cushing disease, there is excess production of ACTH from the anterior pituitary or from ectopic sites. Basophil adenoma (microadenoma) is present in about 75% of cases. The increased ACTH causes hyperstimulation of adrenal cortex leading to its hyperplasia which in turn leads to excess production of cortisol and androgens.

ACTH independent causes (adrenal adenoma or cancer) may be iatrogenic (high dose corticosteroid therapy) or adrenal tumor.

The cause of adrenal mischief is cortisol secreting adenoma which produces excess cortisol. The androgen production is usually less but may be markedly elevated in presence of adrenal carcinoma.

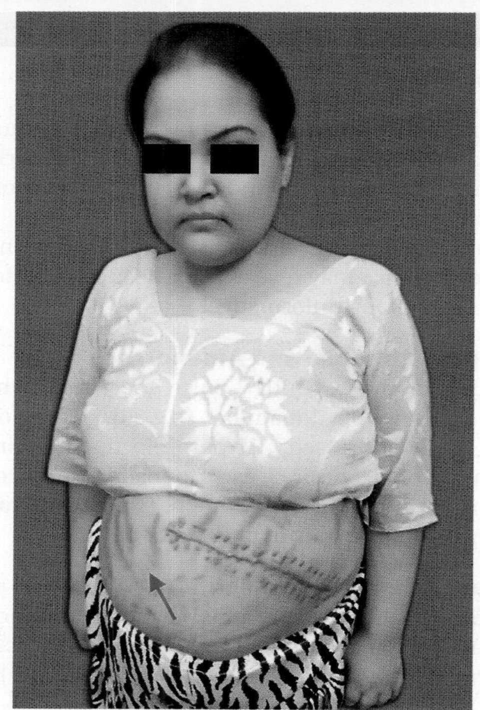

Fig. 29.15: 19-year-old girl, BMI 36, presented with frontal balding, amenorrhea, central obesity and purple abdominal striae (arrow). Investigations including CECT confirmed the diagnosis Cushing's syndrome (non-ACTH dependent) due to adrenal adenoma (left). Abdominal scar of operation seen.

Symptoms include weakness, oligomenorrhea, amenorrhea, acne, and hirsutism. Virilism is rare. **Signs include**, moon facies, centripetal obesity, and abdominal striae (Fig. 29.15) muscle wasting and weakness.

The syndrome is often associated with hypertension, osteoporosis and insulin dependent diabetes.

The screening test consists of dexamethasone supression test (1 mg) ingested at 11 pm and serum cortisol obtained at 8 am the following day. **Level less than 5 μg/100 mL essentially rules out the Cushing's syndrome**. Value of 24 hour urinary free cortisol >250 μg is diagnostic of Cushing's syndrome. Serum ACTH is elevated in Cushing disease but not in adrenal tumor. CT or MRI can detect adrenal tumor.

THYROID DYSFUNCTION

Both hypo- and hyperthyroid states may produce secondary amenorrhea and anovulation, the former is common. Serum TSH is raised, while T3 and T4 values are lowered in hypothyroid state. In subclinical hypothyroid state, while serum TSH is elevated but T4 is normal. **Serum prolactin may be raised** even beyond 20 ng/mL in hypothyroid state. This is due to increased sensitivity of prolactin secreting cells of anterior pituitary to TRH. Elevated prolactin causes rise in central levels of dopamine. Dopamine alters GnRH pulse secretion.

POSTPILL AMENORRHEA

It is observed in less than 1% of the women following the use of combined oral contraceptive pills. The association is more coincidental rather than causal. Fertility rate is normal following discontinuation of the drug. Spontaneous resumption of menstruation occurs in majority of cases after a varying period. Otherwise such amenorrhea should be investigated as in other cases of secondary amenorrhea.

GENERAL DISEASE

Malnutrition, tuberculosis both pulmonary and pelvic, diabetes, and chronic nephritis are all implicated. Their diagnostic criteria vary accordingly. Straight X-ray chest in pulmonary tuberculosis, blood sugar in diabetes, urine analysis, and blood urea in chronic nephritis are helpful to substantiate the diagnosis.

INVESTIGATIONS OF SECONDARY AMENORRHEA

Investigations aims at:

- To diagnose or confirm the etiological factor.
- To guide the management protocol either to restore menstruation and/or fertility.

It should be emphasized that **pregnancy must be excluded** prior hand irrespective of the status of the women—married, unmarried, widow, divorced or separated.

With the etiological factors in mind, one should proceed for investigations (Flowchart 29.3).

DETAILED HISTORY

Enquiry should be made about:

- Mode of onset—whether sudden or gradual preceded by hypomenorrhea or oligomenorrhea.
- Sudden change in environment, emotional stress, psychogenic shock, or eating disorder (anorexia nervosa).
- Sudden change in weight—loss or gain.
- Intake of psychotropic or antihypertensive drugs like reserpine or methyldopa. Intake of oral 'pills' or its recent withdrawal. History of radiotherapy and chemotherapy or surgery.
- Appearance of abnormal manifestations either coinciding or preceeding the amenorrhea, such as:
  - Acne, hirsutism (excessive growth of hair in normal and abnormal sites in female) or change in voice.
  - Inappropriate lactation (galactorrhea)—abnormal secretion of milk unrelated to pregnancy and lactation.
  - Headache or visual disturbances.
  - Hot flashes and vaginal dryness.
- Obstetric history—overzealous curettage leading to synechiae.
  - Cesarean section may be extended to hysterectomy of which the patient may be unaware.
  - Severe postpartum hemorrhage, or shock or infection.
  - Postpartum or postabortal uterine curettage.
  - Prolonged lactation—the patient may be amenorrheic since childbirth or she may have one or two periods, followed by amenorrhea.
- Medical history of tuberculosis (pulmonary or extrapulmonary), diabetes, chronic nephritis or overt hypothyroid state should be enquired.
- Family history—premature menopause often runs in the family (mother or sisters).

GENERAL EXAMINATION

The following features are to be noted:

- Nutritional status
- BP
- Cold calmy skin (thyroid)
- Extreme emaciation or marked obesity (BMI)
- Presence of acne or hirsutism or Acanthosis
- Discharge of milk from the breasts.

Abdominal Examination

- Presence of striae associated with obesity may be related to Cushing disease.
- A mass in the lower abdomen.

Pelvic Examination

- Enlargement of clitoris.
- Adnexal mass suggestive of tubercular tubo-ovarian mass or ovarian tumor.

With the above methods, either a probable diagnosis is made or no abnormality is detected to account for amenorrhea. **The latter group is much more common and these are investigated as outlined below.**

Even though there is no inappropriate galactorrhea, serum prolactin, TSH estimations, and X-ray sella turcica are mandatory. **If these are normal, the following protocols are followed:**

Step I

Progesterone challenge test is employed. **If withdrawal bleeding occurs, it proves**—(a) The intact hypothalamopituitary ovarian axis; (b) There is adequate endogenous estrogens (serum E_2 level more than 40 pg/mL) to promote progesterone receptors in the endometrium; (c) Anatomically patent outflow tract; (d) Endometrium is responsive.

Estimation of serum testosterone, prolactin TSH, oral GTT, and fasting lipid profile should be done in a case of PCOS.

If withdrawal bleeding fails to occur, it signifies—(i) lack of progesterone receptors in the endometrium or (ii) diseased endometrium. To differentiate between the two, one is to proceed to step II.

Step II

Estrogen-progesterone challenge test—ethinyl estradiol 0.02 mg or conjugated equine estrogen 1.25 mg is to be taken daily for 25 days. Medroxyprogesterone acetate 10 mg daily is added from day 15–25. Alternately, one course

Flowchart 29.3: Evaluation of a patient with secondary amenorrhea.

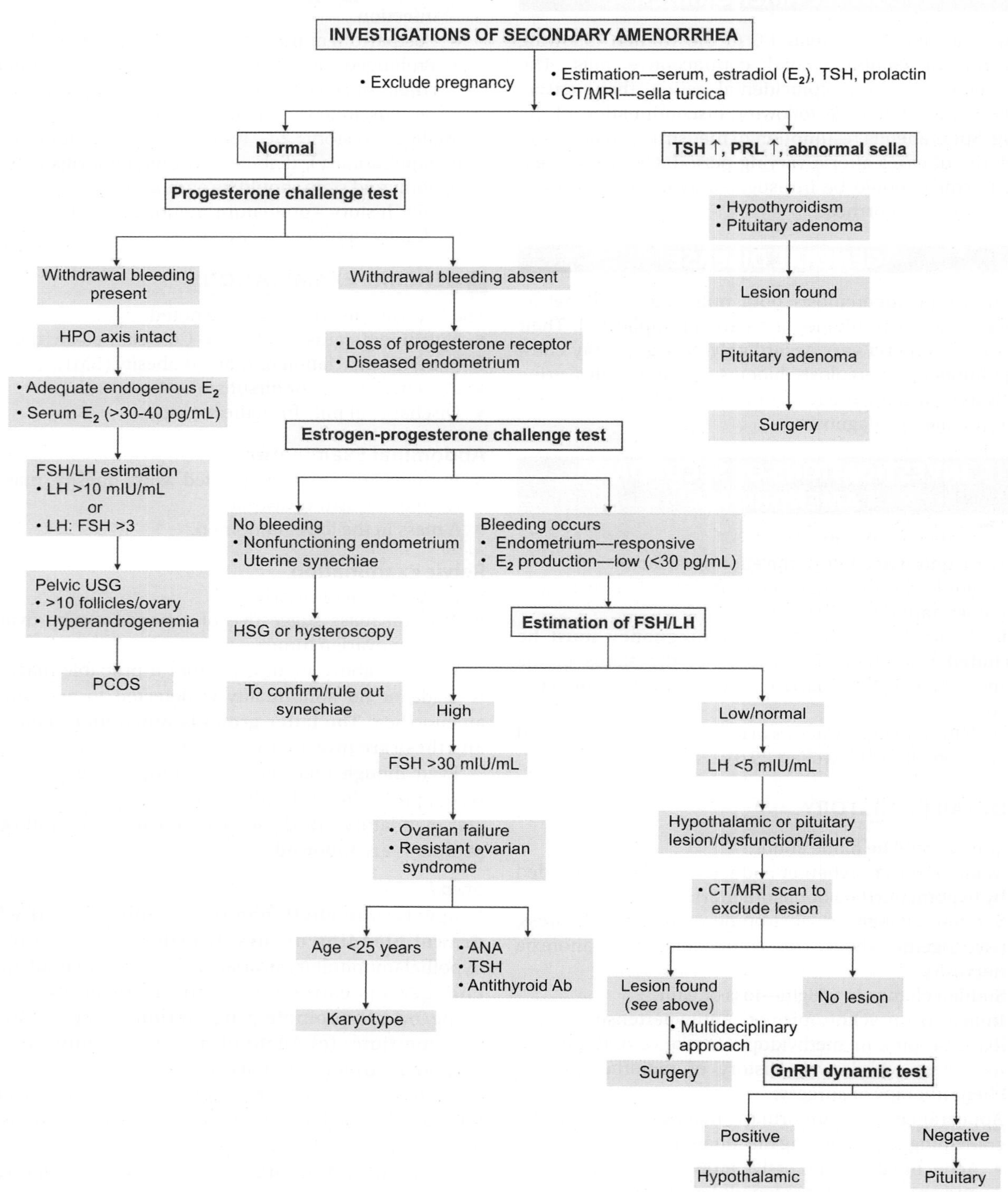

(TSH: thyroid-stimulating hormone; CT: computed tomography; MRI: magnetic resonance imaging; PRL: prolactin; FSH: follicle-stimulating hormone; LH: luteinizing hormone; USG: ultrasonography; PCOS: polycystic ovary syndrome; HSG: hysterosalpingography; GnRH: gonadotropin-releasing hormone)

of oral contraceptive pill is given and to observe whether withdrawal bleeding occurs or not.

If there is no bleeding, it signifies local endometrial lesion such as uterine synechiae. This is to be confirmed by **HSG or hysteroscopy**.

If withdrawal bleeding occurs, it indicates the presence of responsive endometrium but the endogenous estrogen production is inadequate. As such, to determine whether the underlying defect lies in the ovary or in the pituitary, one is to proceed to step III.

Step III

Estimation of serum gonadotropins is to be done. If the level of serum **FSH is more** than 40 mIU/mL, the case is one of premature ovarian failure or resistant ovarian syndrome. Ovarian biopsy is not recommended to confirm the diagnosis or to differentiate the two entities.

If, however, the level of FSH is either normal or low, it signifies pituitary dysfunction. Whether the disturbed pituitary function is primary or secondary to hypothalamus, one should proceed to step IV.

Step IV

GnRH dynamic test: If with GnRH administration, there is rise of pituitary gonadotropins, it is probably a case of hypothalamic dysfunction. In cases of primary pituitary disorder, there will be no rise of gonadotropins. The result is however inconclusive.

If possible, pituitary tumor have to be excluded by X-ray sella turcica, CT or MRI, scan even though the prolactin level is normal.

MANAGEMENT OF SECONDARY AMENORRHEA

NO ABNORMALITY DETECTED

- The patient is not anxious about amenorrhea and or fertility. No treatment is required. Only assurance is given and too often, menstruation resumes within 6 months to a year.
- **The patient is anxious for amenorrhea** but **not for fertility**.
  - With normal endogenous estrogen: Oral combined steroidal contraceptives are prescribed and to be continued for at least three cycles.
  - With low endogenous estrogen: Ethinyl estradiol 0.02 mg or CEE 1.25 mg daily is to be taken for 25 days. Medroxyprogesterone acetate 10 mg daily is added from day 16–25.
- **The patient desires for fertility**—couple needs evaluation (Ch. 17).

  Husband's semen analysis in primary infertility and the tubal factor of the women are to be evaluated prior to induction of ovulation either using clomiphene, letrozole or gonadotropins (details in Ch. 17).

CASES WITH DETECTABLE CAUSE

- **Anxiety and stress**—may be corrected by assurance and psychotherapy.
- **Systemic illness and malnutrition**: To improve the health status and appropriate therapy for systemic illness.
- **Exercise induced** amenorrhea is cured with limitation of activity and appropriate diet.

HYPERPROLACTINEMIA, INAPPROPRIATE GALACTORRHEA

Treatment—medical: Bromocriptine (lysergic acid derivative) is a dopamine agonist is effective. Common side effects are: Giddiness, nausea, vomiting, headache, constipation, and orthostatic hypotension. **Cabergoline** is a long acting selective dopamine agonist. It has less side effects, greater potency and longer duration of action. It is given 0.25 mg or 0.5 mg once or twice weekly. **Bromocriptine:** Dose may be gradually increased to reduce the adverse effects. There is shrinkage of the tumor with therapy. Prolactin levels usually decrease within 2–3 weeks of treatment. Menses, ovulation, and fertility return when prolactin level returns to normal. Pregnancy following treatment is high. Most women need induction of ovulation. **Cabergoline can be continued safely in pregnancy when required as it is not teratogenic. Surgery** is considered when there is failure of medical therapy. **Transnasal—transsphenoidal microsurgical resection (adenectomy) is done. Complications of surgery are**: Meningitis, diabetes insipidus, leakage of cerebrospinal fluid (CSF) and recurrence. Radiation therapy is not commonly preferred. Radiation therapy is used for large macroadenomas and for cases with large residual tumor after surgery.

Risk: Panhypopituitarism may develop following radiation therapy. Damage to the optic nerves may occur.

PREMATURE OVARIAN FAILURE

- To prevent or to minimize postmenopausal health hazards, HRT should be judiciously employed.
- In proved cases of autoimmune disorders, corticosteroids may be of help.
- Fertility potentiality is far and remote. However, induction of ovulation may be hopefully tried in presence of follicle. This may be achieved by administration of sequential estrogen and progesterone or by use of GnRH agonist, followed by administration of gonadotropins for ovulation induction.
- Spontaneous recovery and pregnancy have been reported in an occasional case of premature ovarian failure.
- IVF with donor's oocyte with total replacement of hormones can increase the chance of pregnancy.
- In the presence of 'Y' chromosome, gonadectomy is to be done to avoid malignancy.

ADRENAL DISORDERS

Treatment of Cushing's disease: Pituitary tumor is treated by transsphenoidal microsurgical resection or by external beam radiation. Excess cortisol due to adrenal tumor is cured by simple adrenalectomy. Many patients need medical therapy either before or after surgery to maintain normal cortisol level. Metyrapone (adrenocorticolytic drug) may be used to produce medical adrenalectomy. Enzyme inhibitors like aminoglutethimide or metyrapone has been used to block excess cortisol production. Ketoconazole inhibits adrenal steroid biosynthesis. It is also used for long-term benefit.

Adult onset adrenal hyperplasia: Dexamethasone replacement therapy is given. A dose of 0.25–0.5 mg may be adequate. Periodic serum cortisol level is to be checked and is maintained at >2 μg/dL and serum 17-OHP should be between 400 and 1200 ng/dL.

HYPOTHYROID STATE

It should be treated by thyroxine 1.6 μg/kg of body weight per day may be started.

HYPERANDROGENIC STATE

Suppression of hyperandrogenism can be achieved using oral contraceptives, glucocorticoids or antiandrogen preparations.

UTERINE SYNECHIAE

Hysteroscopic adhesiolysis followed by insertion of IUD is effective. Addition of oral contraceptive pills for three months may help in regeneration of the endometrium. Successful pregnancy and live birth rate is about 70–80% following treatment. There may be recurrence in about 30% of cases.

OVARIAN TUMOR

Appropriate surgery is done (p. 495).

ANOREXIA NERVOSA

It needs multidisciplinary team approach. Behavioral therapy, psychiatric consultation are helpful. Hospitalization may be needed in severe cases.

RESULTS

The following conclusions are made about the fate of the patients having amenorrhea.

In primary amenorrhea, more investigations are often done to find out the cause with minimal effect. In fact, in most of the cases where menstruation occurs are the young girls whose menarche is delayed in onset.

In secondary amenorrhea, with comparative fewer investigations, the result is satisfactory. But the percentage of cures falls steeply as the duration of amenorrhea lengthens. However, with or without treatment, spontaneous resumption of menstruation occurs in about 60% cases of secondary amenorrhea of more than one year's duration.

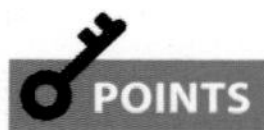

- **Common causes of secondary amenorrhea** are hypothalamic dysfunction, PCOS, stress, premature ovarian failure, and hypothyroid state (Table 29.5). **PCOS is the most common endocrine disorder in women (20–25%).**
- **Majority of women with PCOS** have android obesity (BMI >25), elevated levels of biologically active LH. About 40% of women with PCOS have hyperinsulinemia and impaired glucose tolerance and androgen excess.
- **PCOS is a heterogeneous condition.** Presence of two out of the three following criteria is essential to define PCOS (ESHRE/ASRM): (a) Oligo- and/or anovulation; (b) Hyperandrogenism (clinical or biochemical); (c) Polycystic ovaries.
- **In polycystic ovarian syndrome (PCOS)**, there is excess androgen production by the ovaries. Typically, the ovaries are enlarged, capsule is thickened with multiple cysts along with hypertrophy of theca cells (stromal hyperthecosis).
- **Management of PCOS** needs patient individualization. Weight reduction is an important step. Correction of hyperandrogenemia, hyperprolactinemia, hyperinsulinemia and elevated LH levels are the others. Metformin ameliorates the biochemical abnormalities. Ovulation induction has higher success when clomiphene is combined with metformin (insulin sensitizing agent). In refractory cases, laparoscopic ovarian drilling or laser vaporization of multiple cysts of the ovaries is better than wedge resection.
- **About 50% of women with PCOS** have insulin resistance and impaired glucose tolerance. Metabolic syndrome is improved by metformin. Hyperandrogenism is managed by COCs or by other drugs.
- **Long-term risk of PCOS patients**, if left untreated includes, diabetes mellitus (metabolic syndrome), dyslipidemia, hypertension and endometrial carcinoma, obstructive sleep apnea.
- **Common causes of uterine synechiae** are tubercular endometritis, overzealous postabortal or puerperal curettage.
- **Level of serum FSH** can differentiate hypogonadotropic hypogonadism from estrogen deficiency due to ovarian failure.
- **Serum FSH level >40 mIU/mL**, establishes the diagnosis of ovarian failure or hypergonadotropic hypogonadism.
- When uterine bleeding fails to occur after progestin therapy, level of endogenous estradiol is below 40 pg/mL.
- **When withdrawal bleeding occurs** following progestin challenge test, it suggests: (a) Intact hypothalamo-pituitary-ovarian axis; (b) Serum E_2 level is more than 40 pg/mL; (c) Outflow tract is present and is patent anatomically; (d) Endometrium is responsive.
- **The triad for diagnosis** of premature ovarian failure include amenorrhea, raised gonadotropins and low serum estradiol. Karyotype should be done for younger (<30 years) age group. Serum antibodies are positive in autoimmune variety. Ovarian biopsy is not essential to the diagnosis.
- **Serum level** (morning sample) of 17-OHP when >8 ng/mL establishes the diagnosis of late onset congenital adrenal hyperplasia.
- **Abnormal secretion of GnRH results** in amenorrhea is about 30% of women. Stress-induced amenorrhea is due to increased level of opioids (β-endorphin) in CNS, causing interference of GnRH release. Increased leptin level is associated with hypothalamic amenorrhea.
- **Hypothalamic dysfunction** (severe weight loss, stress, exercise) results in decreased GnRH secretion. There is decreased gonadotropin secretion and ovulation resulting in hypoestrogenic state.
- **Weight loss** when 15% below the ideal body weight can cause amenorrhea due to hypothalamic dysfunction.

Contd...

Contd...

- **Exercise induced amenorrhea** is also due to reduced GnRH pulse secretion, resulting in decreased LH pulses.
- **Hyperprolactinemia** is associated with anovulation, amenorrhea or galactorrhea. Causes of hyperprolactinemia are many. Most common cause of mildly raised prolactin level is stress. Majority of women with hyperprolactinemia, amenorrhea and galactorrhea will have prolactinoma. Most microadenomas (<1 cm in diameter) do not enlarge with time. Bromocriptine shrinks 80–90% of macroadenomas. Most common side effects of bromocriptine therapy are nausea, vomiting, and orthostatic hypotension. Cabergoline is more effective and is better tolerated.
- **MRI** is the best diagnostic modality for pituitary adenomas or empty sella syndrome.
- **Hyperprolactinemia** is present in 15% of all anovulatory women. Nearly 60% of all women with galactorrhea have hyperprolactinemia. Nearly 90% of women with galactorrhea and amenorrhea have hyperprolactinemia. About 5% of women with hyperprolactinemia have hypothyroidism.
- **Bromocriptine** treatment returns prolactin level to normal in 90%, induces ovulation in 80% and cures galactorrhea in 60% of cases.
- **Combined oral contraceptives** do not stimulate the growth of prolactin secreting microadenomas.
- **Pregnancy induced by bromocriptine** is not associated with an increased risk of congenital malformation or multiple pregnancy.
- **Surgical treatment** of prolactinomas is done when there is failure of medical treatment but long-term recurrence rate is about 20%.
- **In masculinizing ovarian tumor**, serum testosterone is elevated to >2 ng/mL while DHEAS is normal. Elevated DHEAS reflects adrenal androgen excess. Serum levels of DHEAS correlate well with daily urinary 17-KS excretion.
- **In Sheehan's syndrome**, there is failing lactation, loss of pubic and axillary hair, secondary amenorrhea and atrophy of the breasts. Hormones affected in order of frequency are GH, FSH, LH, TSH, and ACTH.
- **In Cushing disease**, there is excess production of ACTH leading to excess secretion of cortisol and androgen production. The symptoms of Cushing syndrome include weakness, amenorrhea, acne and hirsutism; signs include moon facies, centripetal obesity, and abdominal striae.
- **The diagnosis** of a case of secondary amenorrhea is difficult to make out from the clinical examination (Flowchart 29.3). Pregnancy must be excluded prior hand. Even though, there is no galactorrhea, serum prolactin, TSH estimation, and X-ray sella turcica are mandatory as the first step of investigation. When no abnormality is detected and the patient is not anxious about amenorrhea and or fertility, no treatment is required.
- **In primary amenorrhea**, more investigations are often done to find out the cause with minimal effect. In secondary amenorrhea, with comparative fewer investigations, the result is satisfactory.
- **Drugs associated** with hyperprolactinemia are: (a) Antidepressants (alprazolam, fluoxetine); (b) Antihypertensives (atenolol, methyldopa); (c) H_2 receptor blockers (ranitidine, cemetidine); (d) Hormones (COCs, MPA); (e) Phenothiazines and others (domperidone).

CHAPTER

30 Contraception

CHAPTER OUTLINE

INTRODUCTION

Rapid population growth (96% in developing countries) is a critical issue worldwide. Family planning methods save women's lives preventing unintended pregnancies. **Slower population growth conserves resources, improves health and living standards.**

Benefits of fertility control are interrelated. **Benefits are** improved quality of life, better health, less physical and emotional stress of life, better education, job, and economic opportunities. Benefits are enjoyed by the couple, the children, other family members, the community and the country.

Contraception and fertility control are not synonymous. Fertility control includes both fertility inhibition (contraception) and fertility stimulation. While the fertility stimulation is related to the problem of the infertile couples, **the term contraception includes all measures, temporary or permanent, designed to prevent pregnancy due to the coital act.**

Ideal contraceptive methods should be highly (100%) effective, acceptable, safe, reversible, cheap, having non-contraceptive benefits, simple to use and requiring minimal motivation, maintenance and supervision.

METHODS OF CONTRACEPTIONS

The various methods of contraception are schematically depicted here (Flowchart 30.1 and Table 30.1).

Flowchart 30.1: Contraceptive methods.

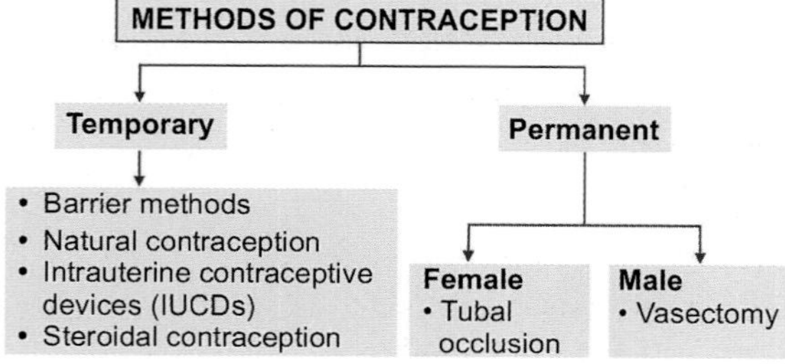

Contraceptive effectiveness chart (WHO, 2007)	*Pregnancy/ 100 WY*
Most effective methods: Implants (p. 411), IUDs (p. 496), sterilization (male and female) (p. 414)	0.1–0.2
Very effective methods: Injectables, LAM COCs, POPs, patch, vaginal rings	0.3–9
Effective methods: Male condom, diaphragm, female condom, fertility awareness methods	2–20
Least effective methods: Spermicides	10–30
No WHO Category: Withdrawal, no method	4–85

TEMPORARY METHODS

Temporary methods are commonly used to postpone or to space births. However, these methods are also frequently being used by the couples (Table 30.2) even though they desire no more children.

INTRAUTERINE CONTRACEPTIVE DEVICES

The intrauterine contraceptive devices (IUCDs) have been used worldwide. It is a safe, effective and reversible method of contraception. The efficacy of IUCDs are comparable with surgical sterilization.

There has been a significant improvement in its design and content. The idea is to obtain maximum efficacy without increasing the adverse effects. **The device is classified as open**, when it has got no circumscribed aperture of more than 5 mm so that a loop of intestine or omentum cannot enter and become strangulated if, accidentally, the device perforates through the uterus into the peritoneal cavity. Cu-T, Cu-7, multiload are examples of open devices. **The device may be medicated (bioactive)** by incorporating a metal copper, in devices like Cu-T 380A, Multiload-375 (Figs. 30.1A to C) or it may be hormonally active (LNG-IUS).

TABLE 30.1: Methods of contraception used by women of reproductive age (15–49) in different countries.

Country	Methods used (Percent)								
	Sterilization		COC	IUCD	Barrier	Implant/ Injectable	Others	Any method	Unmet need
	F	M							
India (2007–2008)	35.8	1.1	3.6	1.8	5.5	-	15	54.8	20.5
Banglasesh (2011)	5	1.2	27.2	0.7	5.5	12.3	10	61.2	13.5
UK (2008–2009)	8	21	28	10	27	3	12	84	—
US (2011–2013)	15.5	5.5	16.0	LARCS 7.2 (IUDs + implant)	9.4	4.4	4.1	61.7	—

(COC: combined oral contraceptive; IUCD: intrauterine contraceptive devices)

TABLE 30.2: Failure rate of contraceptive methods in first 12 months of use.

Methods	Pregnancy rate per 100 Women years (approx.)	
	Typical use	Perfect use
No method	85	
Natural (calendar, temperature, mucus)	25	3
Withdrawal	27	4
Lactational amenorrhea		2
Condom (male)	15	2
Condom (female)	21	5
Diaphragm	16	6
IUCD:		
Cu T 380A	0.8	0.6
LNG-IUS	0.1	0.1
Combined oral pill	8	0.1
Progestin-only pill	9	0.3
Patch	9	0.3
DMPA and NET injectables	6	0.2
Norplant	0.5	0.5
Implanon	0.01	0.01
Vasectomy	0.5	0.1
Tubectomy	0.5	0.15
Failure rate is less when methods are used correctly and consistently		

(IUCD: intrauterine contraceptive devices; CU-T: copper-T; LNG: levonorgestrel; DMPA: depot medroxyprogesterone acetate; NET: norethisterone)

Types of IUCDs: The copper T-380A is commonly used. The amount of copper that comes out of the device on daily basis amounts to less than that ingested in the normal diet.

Hormone-containing IUDs either releasing progesterone (progestasert) or levonorgestrel (LNG-IUS) has also been introduced. Nowadays, the following medicated IUDs are in use:

- Cu-T 380A
- Multiload 375
- LNG-IUS
- Skyla

Description of the Devices (Figs. 30.1A to C)

Cu-T 380A: It is a medicated device containing copper. It carries 380 mm^2 of copper in total. The vertical stem is wrapped with 314 mm^2 of fine copper and each arm has a 33 mm^2 copper bracelet. The sum of these is 380 mm^2 **(Fig. 30.1A)**. Two strings extend from the base of the stem. The stem of the device is made of polyethylene frame. These two threads are used for detection and removal of the device. In spite of copper being radiopaque, additional barium sulfate is incorporated in the device. The device is replaced **every 10 years**. However, this Cu-T 380A device has been used to prevent pregnancy for 20 years. Women desiring for continued contraception, the existing device can be removed at the end of the schedule time and a new device can be inserted during the same time. Apart from the use of Cu-T as a contraceptive, it is used following synecolysis to prevent recurrent adhesion formation. **Devices containing less than 300 mm^2 of copper have higher failure rate.**

Multiload Cu-375: The device is available in a sterilized sealed packet with an applicator. There is no introducer and no plunger. It has 375 mm^2 surface area of copper wire wound around its vertical stem. **Replacement is every 5 years** (Fig. 30.1B).

Levonorgestrel-intrauterine system (LNG-IUS) (Fig. 30.1C): This is a T-shaped device, with polydimethylsiloxane membrane around the stem which acts as a steroid reservoir. Total amount of levonorgestrel is 52 mg and is released at the rate 20 μg/day. **This device is to be replaced every 7 years though approved for 5 years.** Its efficacy is comparable to sterilization operation. It has many noncontraceptive benefits also (p. 404).

Skyla: It is a newer device with 13.5 μg LNG-releasing per day.

This IU device with a smaller body than Mirena has been approved for up to 3 years.

Mode of Action

Mechanism of antifertility effect of all the IUDs is not yet clear. They act predominantly in the uterine cavity and do not inhibit ovulation. Probable factors are:

- **Biochemical and histological changes in the endometrium:** There is a nonspecific inflammatory reaction along with biochemical changes in the endometrium. This accumulates throughout the uterine lumen, cervical canal and the fallopian tubes. This affects the function and viability of the gametes. Thus, it prevents fertilization, reduces chance of zygote formation and implantation. Lysosomal disintegration from the macrophages attached to the device liberates

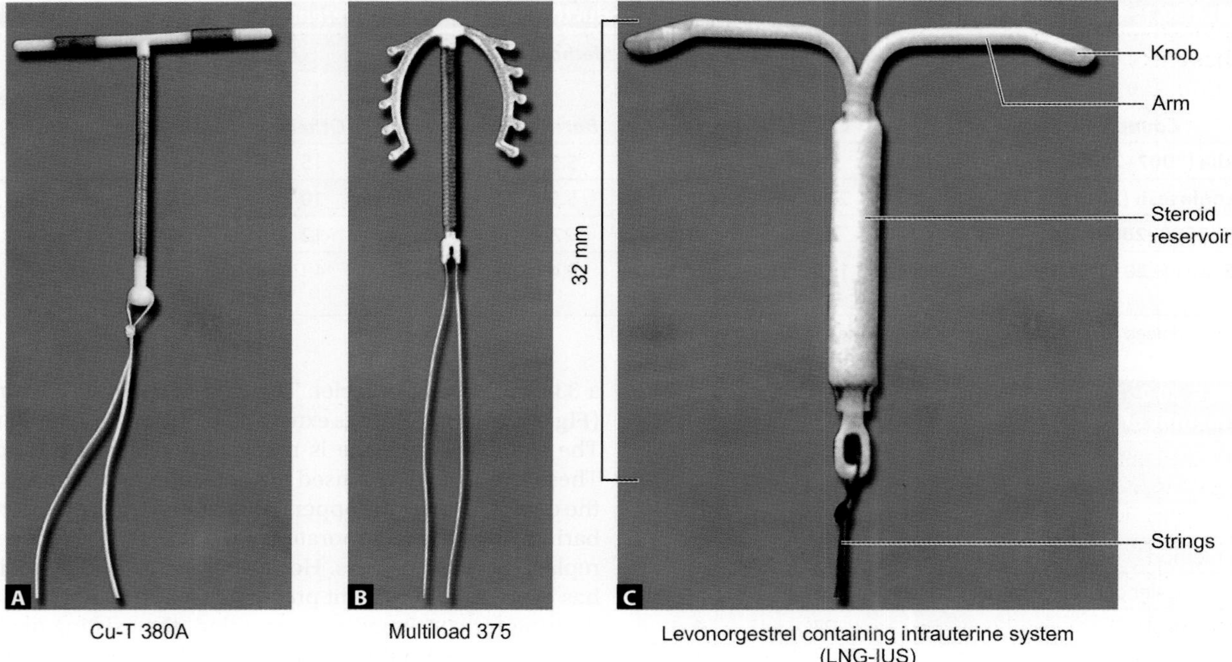

Figs. 30.1A to D: Commonly used intrauterine devices.

prostaglandins, which are toxic to spermatozoa. Macrophages cause phagocytosis of spermatozoa.

- **Endometrial inflammatory response** decreases sperm transport and impedes the ability of sperm to fertilize the ovum.
- **Copper devices:** Ionized copper has got an additional local antifertility effect by **preventing blastocyst implantation through enzymatic interference**. Copper initiates the release of cytokines which are cytotoxic. Serum copper level is not increased. The copper ion impedes sperm transport and viability in the cervical mucus. These actions of IUD, prevent sperm to reach the tubes. So there is no fertilization.
- **Levonorgestrel-IUS (Mirena):** It induces strong and uniform suppression of endometrium. Cervical mucus becomes very thick and scantly. It impedes sperm motility and access to the upper genital tract. Anovulation and insufficient luteal phase activity has also been mentioned. It decreases tubal motility. Serum progesterone level is not increased.

Contraindications for Insertion of IUCD

- Pregnancy or suspected pregnancy.
- Undiagnosed genital tract bleeding.
- Acute pelvic infection current or within 3 months.
- Distortion of the shape of the uterine cavity as in fibroid or congenital uterine malformation.
- Severe dysmenorrhea.
- Known or suspected uterine or cervical neoplasia.
- Postpartum or postabortal endometritis in last 3 months or infected abortion.
- Sexually transmitted infections (STIs): Current or within 3 months.
- Trophoblastic disease.
- Significant immunosuppression.

Contd...

Contd...

Additionally for Cu-T are:

- Wilson disease.
- Copper allergy.

For **LNG-IUS** are:

- Hepatic tumor or hepatocellular disease (active).
- Current breast cancer.
- Severe arterial disease.

Time of Insertion

- **Interval** (when the insertion is made in the interconceptional period beyond 6 weeks following childbirth or abortion): **It is preferable to insert 2–3 days after the period is over**. But it can be inserted any time during the cycle, provided she is not pregnant. It can be safely inserted even during menstrual phase which has certain advantages (open cervical canal, distended uterine cavity, less cramp). However, during **lactational amenorrhea**, it can be inserted at any time.
- **Postabortal:** Immediately following termination of pregnancy by suction evacuation or D and E, or following spontaneous abortion, the device may be inserted. The additional advantage of preventing uterine synechia can help in motivation for insertion.
- **Cu-T 380A** can be used as an emergency contraception up to 5 days following unprotected coitus (p. 412)

Immediate Postpartum:

- **Post-placental** within 10 minutes after expulsion of placenta following vaginal delivery.
- **Intracesarean** insertion during cesarean delivery, after removal of the placenta and before closure of the uterine incision.
- **Within 48 hours after delivery** before the patient is discharged from the hospital.
- **Extended postpartum/interval any time after 6 weeks.**

- **Advantages are:** (a) Safe and highly effective; (b) immediate action; (c) Long-term protection; (d) Special benefit to women having limited access or no access to postpartum care; (e) Immediate return to fertility after removal; (f) No need of frequent visits and no further cost; (g) High continuation rates and user satisfaction. However, the expulsion rate is high.

Methods of Insertion (Figs. 30.2 to 30.5)

- **Cu-T 200**
- **Cu-T 380A**

Preliminaries

(1) History-taking and examinations (general and pelvic) to exclude any contraindication of insertion. (2) Patient is informed about the various problems, the device is shown to her and consent is obtained. (3) **The insertion is done in the outpatient department**, taking aseptic precautions without sedation or anesthesia. To reduce cramping pain ibuprofen [Nonsteroidal anti-inflammatory drug (NSAID)] may be given (200–400 mg) 30 minutes before insertion. (4) **Placement of the device inside the inserter**—the device is taken out from the sealed packet. The thread, the vertical stem and then the horizontal stem folded to the vertical stem are introduced through the distal end of the inserter. The device is now ready for introduction. **"No touch" insertion method is preferred** (*see* below).

Actual steps

(1) The patient empties her bladder and is placed in lithotomy position. Uterine size and position are ascertained by pelvic examination. (2) Posterior vaginal speculum is introduced and the vagina and cervix are cleansed by antiseptic lotion. (3) The anterior lip of the cervix is grasped by Allis forceps. A sound is passed through the cervical canal to note the position of the uterus and the length of the uterine cavity. The appropriate length of the inserter is adjusted depending on the length of the uterine cavity. (4) The inserter with the device placed inside is then introduced through the cervical canal right up to the fundus and after positioning it by the guard, the inserter is withdrawn keeping the plunger in position. **Thus, the device is**

Contd...

Contd...

not pushed out of the tube but held in place by the plunger while the inserter is withdrawn (withdrawal technique in Figure 30.2). (5) The excess of the nylon thread beyond 2–3 cm from the external os is cut. Then the Allis forceps and the posterior vaginal speculum are taken off. **'No-touch' insertion technique** includes: (i) Loading the IUD in the inserter without opening the sterile package. The loaded inserter is now taken out of the package without touching the distal end. (ii) Not to touch the vaginal wall and the speculum while introducing the loaded IUD inserter through the cervical canal.

- **Multiload Cu-375:** The applicator with the device is just to be taken out of the sealed packet in a 'no-touch' method and **the same is pushed through the cervical canal up to the fundus of the uterus**. The applicator is then withdrawn (Fig. 30.3).
- **LNG-IUS:** The details of insertion are to be followed as in the instruction package (Fig. 30.4).

Principal steps

The initial steps are the same as in Cu-T 380A.

Sterile package is opened up. The arms of the device should be kept horizontal. The slider is pushed up, to draw the IUCD within the insertion tube.

- The uterocervical length is measured by the uterine sound.
- The flange on the inserter tube is positioned from the IUCD tip according to this uterocervical length.
- The inserter tube with the device is gently inserted within the uterus, until the flange is at 1.5–2 cm from the external os.
- The arms of the device are then released by pulling the slider back to the raised white line on the handle. To hold this position for about 20–30 seconds to allow the arms to open fully.
- The inserter is then gently guided into the uterine cavity until its flange touches the cervix (Fig. 30.5).
- The device is released by holding the inserter firmly in position and pulling the slider back all the way.
- The threads are released automatically. The inserter is then removed slowly.
- The threads are then trimmed preserving 3 cm length outside the cervix (same as in Cu-T 380A)

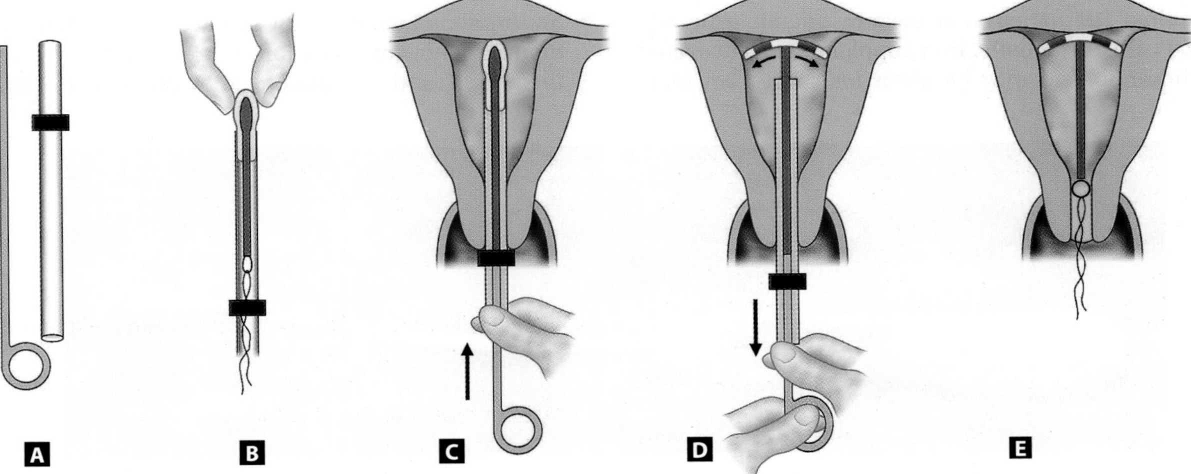

Figs. 30.2A to E: Withdrawal technique of insertion of Cu-T.

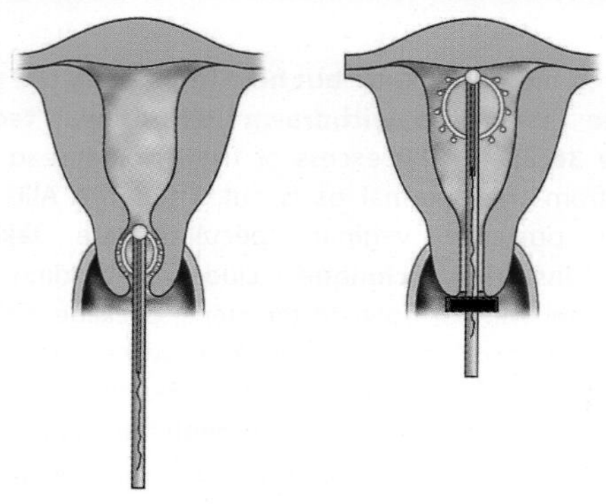

Fig. 30.3: Technique of insertion of multiload IUCDs.

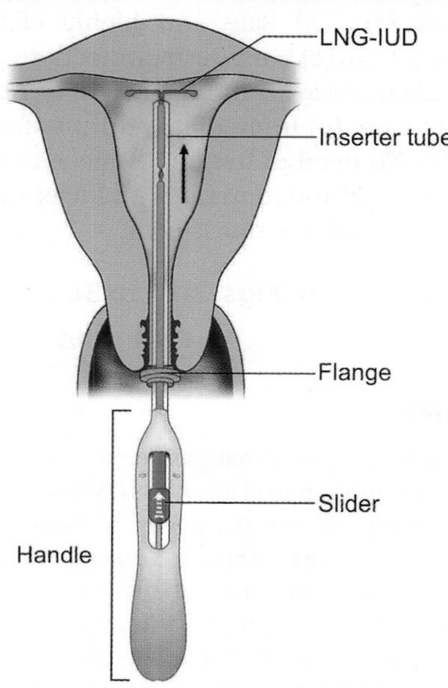

Fig. 30.4: Insertion method of LNG-IUS.

Instructions to the Patient

The possible symptoms of pain and slight vaginal bleeding should be explained. The patient should be advised to feel the thread periodically by the finger. The patient is checked after 1 month and then annually.

Complications

Immediate

- **Cramp-like pain:** It is transient but, at times, severe and usually lasts for half to 1 hour. It is relieved by analgesic (ibuprofen) taking before insertion or antispasmodic drugs.
- **Syncopal attack:** Pain and syncopal attack are more often found in nulliparous or when the device is large enough to distend the uterine cavity.
- **Partial or complete perforation:** It is due to faulty technique of insertion but liable to be met within lactational period when the uterus remains small and soft.

Remote

- **Pain:** The pain is more or less proportionate to the degree of myometrial distension. A proper size of the device may minimize the pain.
- **Abnormal menstrual bleeding:** The excessive bleeding involves increased menstrual blood loss, prolongation of duration of period and intermenstrual bleeding. The patient may become anemic especially who is already anemic. Iron supplement is advocated. Tranexamic acid may be given for short-term relief. **Menstrual loss is much less with the use of third-generation IUDs** (p. 404).

  Women using LNG-IUS have less (60%) blood loss. Nearly 50% of women develop amenorrhea and 25% have oligomenorrhea after 24 months of use.
- **Pelvic inflammatory disease (PID):** The risk of developing PID with the use of current devices, is not increased. Infections with gonorrhea, chlamydia and rarely with actinomyces are seen. Women with symptomatic infection, the IUCD is removed and antibiotic therapy is given. Women with existing infection like purulent vaginal discharge, adnexal tenderness or cervical motion tenderness, laboratory testing should be done and IUCD insertion is delayed. Newer IUDs reduce the risk (p. 404). It is the procedure not the device or the thread, is the risk of infection.

  Pain, abnormal uterine bleeding (AUB) and PID are the main factors related to its discontinuation (10–15%).
- **Spontaneous expulsion:** Usually occurs within a few months following insertion, more commonly during the period, at times, unnoticed by the patient. Failure

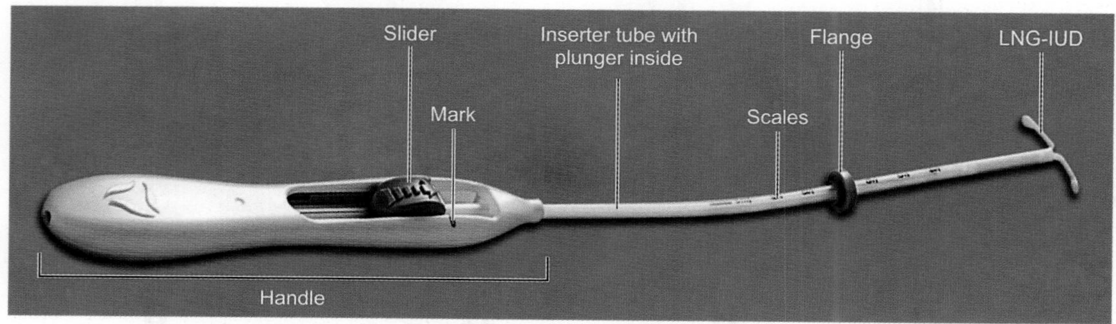

Fig. 30.5: LNG-IUS insertion device. Different parts of the device are shown.

to palpate the thread which could be felt before, is an urgent ground to report to the physician. **The expulsion rate is about 5%.** The rate is, however, more following postabortal or puerperal insertions. The expulsion rate is markedly reduced in the successive years. Another device of appropriate size may be reintroduced and this is likely to be retained. **The newer IUDs have got less expulsion rate.**

- **Perforation of the uterus:** It is rare and the incidence is about 1 in 1,000 insertions. Most perforations occur at the time of insertion but the migration may also occur following initial partial perforation with subsequent myometrial contraction. **It is, however, less common when the device is introduced by the withdrawal technique.**

Diagnosis of uterine perforation: Nonvisibility of the threads through the external os and the appearance of pelvic symptoms after a long asymptomatic period are suspicious. **Negative findings on exploration** of the uterine cavity by a probe is suggestive. **Ultrasonography** can detect the IUD in abdominal cavity and is better than radiography. **Plain X-ray**, anteroposterior and lateral view, following introduction of a radiopaque probe (uterine sound) into the uterine cavity, is conclusive. The device is found away from the opaque shadow placed in the uterine cavity, if it has perforated the uterine wall (Fig. 30.6).

Management

Lippes Loop

As it is an open device made of inert material, it will cause no harm if left in the peritoneal cavity. Adhesions and intestinal injury are unlikely. But for psychological reason or otherwise, **it is better to remove it by laparoscopy or by laparotomy.**

Copper Device

A copper-bearing device induces an intense local inflammatory reaction with adhesions with the surrounding structures. Thus, as soon as the diagnosis is made, it is to be removed by laparoscopy or laparotomy.

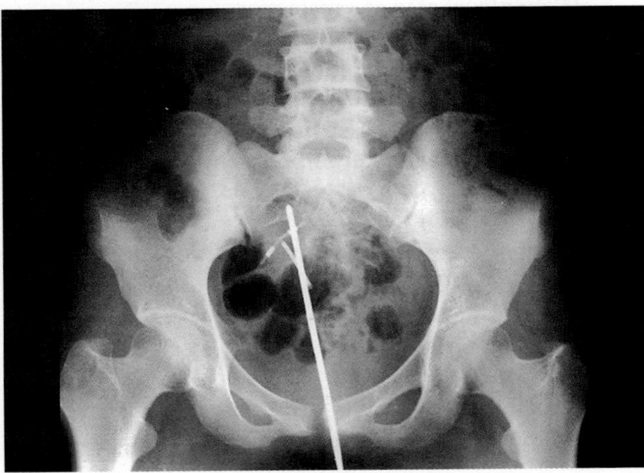

Fig. 30.6: Plain X-ray of the pelvis with a uterine sound placed inside the uterine cavity—the displaced intrauterine contraceptive device (IUCD) seems inside the uterine cavity with anteroposterior (AP) view. Lateral view is needed for confirmation.

(*Courtesy*: Dr Swati Shirodkar, HOD, Department of Obstetrics and Gynecology, MGM Medical College, Aurangabad)

Pregnancy

The pregnancy rate with the device in situ is rare. Lowest pregnancy rates are observed with Cu-T 380A (0.8–HWY) and LNG-IUS (0.2–HWY). When pregnancy occurs with a device in situ, there is risk of ectopic pregnancy (0.02%). IUD can thus prevent a uterine but not an ectopic pregnancy. IUCDs do not increase the viral shedding or reduce the antiretroviral therapy efficacy (ACOG, 2012). Third generation of IUDs like Cu-T 380A and LNG-IUS give some amount of protection against an ectopic pregnancy.

Management of a pregnant woman with device in situ: **If the thread is visible** through the cervix it is best to remove the device. This will minimize complications like miscarriage, preterm labor, sepsis, placenta previa, abruption, cesarean delivery, low birth weight baby, including malformations. **However, if the thread is not visible,** it is better to counsel the patient about the risks involved in continuing pregnancy. Pelvic ultrasound must be carried out to locate the pregnancy. When the pregnancy is undesired, manual vacuum aspiration can be done to remove the pregnancy and the device. The device is expected to be expelled spontaneously with the delivery of the placenta.

Indications for Removal of IUDs

- Persistent excessive regular or irregular uterine bleeding
- Flaring-up of salpingitis
- Perforation of the uterus
- IUD has come out of place (partial expulsion)
- Pregnancy occurring with the device in situ
- Woman desirous of a baby
- Missing thread
- One year after menopause
- When effective lifespan of the device is over.

IUD removal is simple and can be done at any time. It is done by pulling the strings gently and slowly with forceps.

Missing Threads

The thread may not be visible through the cervical os due to—(a) Thread coiled inside; (b) Thread torn through; (c) Device expelled outside unnoticed by the patient; (d) Device perforated the uterine wall and is lying in the peritoneal cavity, and (e) Device pulled up by the growing uterus in pregnancy.

Methods of Identification

Pregnancy is to be excluded first:

- **Ultrasonography** can detect the IUD either within the uterine cavity or in the peritoneal cavity (if perforated). It is preferred to radiography (Fig. 30.7).
- **Hysteroscopy** can be used for direct visualization of the uterine cavity and it could be removed simultaneously (Fig. 30.8).
- **Sounding** the uterine cavity by a probe (Fig. 30.8).

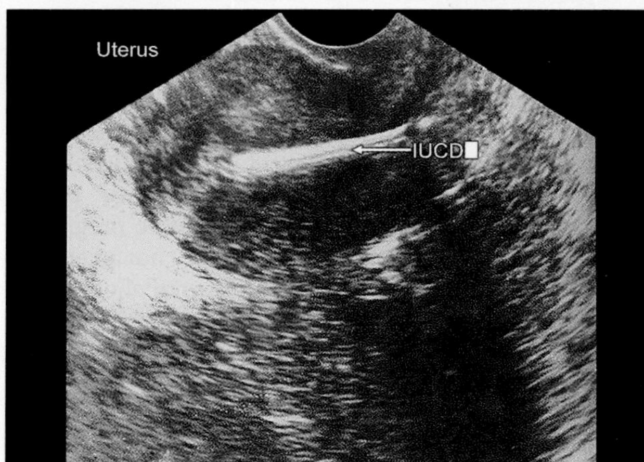

Fig. 30.7: Ultrasonogram showing the Cu-T inside the uterine cavity. Thread was missing in this case.

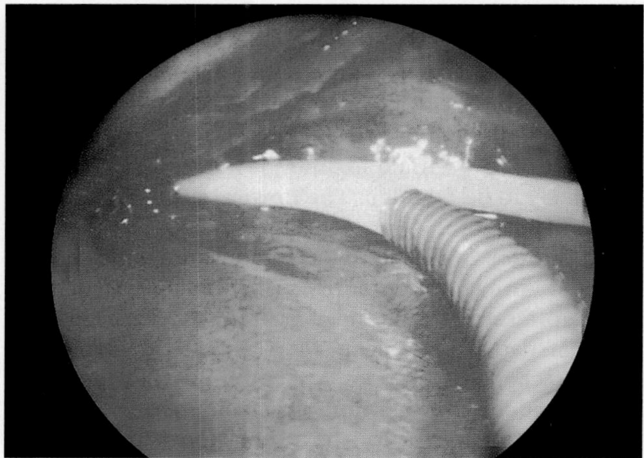

Fig. 30.8: Hysteroscopic view of IUCD in uterine cavity. The threads are coiled inside.

- If negative, **plain X-ray** after introducing radiopaque probe (uterine sound) into the uterine cavity. This will not only reveal the presence or absence of the device but also its existence outside the uterine cavity (Fig. 30.6).

Removal

- **Device inside the uterine cavity:** It can be removed by any of the following methods mentioned here.
  - Especially designed blunt hook.
  - Hysteroscopically under direct vision (Fig. 30.8)
  - Uterine curette
  - Artery forceps.
- **Outside the uterus but inside the abdominal cavity:** (a) Laparoscopy; (b) Laparotomy (rarely).

Advantages of Third Generation of IUDs

Cu-T 380A, multiload-375 and levonorgestrel-IUS.

- Higher efficacy with lowest pregnancy rate (less than one per 100 women every year).
- Used as LARC with longer duration of action (5–10 years).
- Low expulsion rate and fewer indications for medical removal (Table 30.3).

TABLE 30.3: Safety and advantages of IUD (Cu devices and hormone-releasing IUDs).

Advantages
▪ Inexpensive: Cu-T distributed free of cost through government channel
▪ Simplicity in techniques of insertion and most cost effective of all methods
▪ Prolonged contraceptive protection after insertion (5–10 years) and suitable for the rural population of developing countries
▪ Systemic side effects are nil. Suitable for hypertensives, breastfeeding women and epileptics
▪ Reversibility to fertility is prompt after removal
Failure rate—0.1–2/HWY

- Risk of ectopic pregnancy is significantly reduced (Cu-T 380A and LNG-IUS: 0.02 HWY).
- Risk of PID is reduced, anemia is improved.
- **Noncontraceptive benefits, especially with LNG-IUD:**
  - **Significant reduction** in menstrual blood loss, menorrhagia, dysmenorrhea, and premenstrual tension syndrome (PMS).
  - It can be used **in the treatment of** endometrial hyperplasia, adenomyosis, endometriosis, and uterine leiomyomas.
- **Safety and advantages of LNG-IUS**
  - Use is associated with reduction in the risk endometrial and cervical carcinoma.
  - LNG-IUS—can be used as a fertility sparing treatment of early stage endometrial carcinoma.
  - Safe and as effective as an alternative to sterilization method.
  - Higher level of user satisfaction.
  - It can be used **as an alternative to** hysterectomy for menorrhagia, dysfunctional uterine bleeding (DUB).
  - It provides excellent benefits of **hormone replacement therapy** (HRT) when used over the transition years of reproduction to perimenopause (fibroplant, p. 423).

Disadvantages of Third Generation of IUDs

- Expensive (LNG-IUS).
- LNG-IUS is not available through government channel in India currently.
- Amenorrhea (5%).
- Malpositioning with long duration of use may cause pregnancy (failure) or expulsion.

Summary of IUD

Intrauterine contraceptive device is a safe and widely acceptable reversible method of contraception for spacing of births. Amongst many, either a copper impregnated device like Cu-T, multiload or a hormone-releasing device like LNG-IUS is commonly used. **Its mode of action:** It produces nonspecific biochemical and histological changes in the endometrium and ionized copper has got spermolytic and gametotoxic effects. LNG-IUS induces uniform suppression of endometrium and produces very scanty cervical mucus. Both copper and LNG-IUS can be offered to young or nulliparous women. Symptomatic women with IUCDs should be treated with antibiotics—regiment (CDC, 2015) till she is symptom free. Otherwise the device should be removed. The device can be introduced in the interval period or following abortion or following childbirth. The introduction is an outdoor procedure and can be done even by a trained paramedical personnel without anesthesia. The technique employed is 'withdrawal' in Cu-T. **The immediate complications** include cramp-like pains or even syncopal attacks. **The delayed complications** include pelvic pain, menstrual irregularities, expulsion of the IUD or even perforation of the uterus. Complications are much less with third generation of IUDs. **The indications of its removal are** missing threads, persistent pelvic pain, menorrhagia, pregnancy, displacement of the device and flaring up of pelvic infection. Multiload 375 is replaced after 5 years, Cu-T 380A after 10 years and LNG-IUS after 5 years. **The failure rate is** about 0.5–2 per HWY. **Devices less than 300 mm^3 of copper have higher failure role.** Copper device can also be used as postcoital contraception and following synaecholysis.

POINTS

- **Modes of antifertility effects of IUCDs are:** (a) Nonspecific inflammatory reaction along with biochemical (gametotoxic) changes in the endometrium; (b) Copper devices release ionized copper that prevents blastocyst implantation; (c) LNG-IUS—suppresses endometrium, as it makes cervical mucus scanty (p. 399).
- **The introduction of IUCDs** (Cu-T, multiload) is an OPD procedure without anesthesia taking full aseptic precautions. **'No touch' insertion** technique is preferred (p.401).
- **Intrauterine contraceptive devices (IUCDs):** (a) This is an effective method of contraception with failure rate of 0.5–2 HWY; (b) It is also the most effective method of emergency contraception; (c) It can be used by nulliparous women; (d) IUCDs containing <300 mm^2 copper have higher failure rate; (e) Irregular and heavy bleeding may be the side effects and the reason for removal; (f) Third generation IUCDs have higher efficacy and reduced side effects; (g) Risks of ectopic pregnancy is also reduced (p. 402).
- **The contraindications** of insertion of IUD are: PID, suspected pregnancy, DUB or suspicious cervix. The failure (pregnancy) rate is about 0.5–2 HWY. There is risk of ectopic pregnancy 1–2%. Third generation IUDs have minimal side effects and lowest pregnancy rate (p. 402).
- **Immediate complications of IUDs** include pain, syncopal attack, and uterine perforation. **Remote complications** include—pain, abnormal uterine bleeding, pelvic infection, spontaneous expulsion or even perforation of the uterus (p. 402).
- **Indications of removal of IUD are**—excessive uterine bleeding, flaring up of pelvic infection, uterine perforation, pregnancy, missing thread, and patient desirous of a baby (p. 403).
- **There are many reasons for missing threads** (p. 403) and management depends on whether it is within the uterine cavity or within the peritoneal cavity.
- **Apart from contraception**, the IUD is used as an emergency contraception and following synaecholysis.
- The **replacement time** for Cu-T 200B is 4 years, multiload 250—3 years, Cu-T 380A—10 years, multiload 375—5 years and LNG-IUS is 5 years.
- **LNG-IUS** has got many noncontraceptive **health benefits**. It is a very safe and effective method for prolonged use.

STEROIDAL CONTRACEPTIONS

Enovid (norethynodrel 10 mg and mestranol 0.15 mg) was used in the first contraceptive field trial in Puerto Rico in 1956 by Pincus and his colleagues. Currently, 30 μg dose of estrogen has been reduced to 20 μg or even 10 μg to minimize the side effects of estrogen without reducing the efficacy. Types of steroidal contraceptives have been discussed in Flowchart 30.2.

COMBINED ORAL CONTRACEPTIVES (PILLS)

The combined oral steroidal contraceptives is the most effective reversible method of contraception. In the combination pill, **the commonly used progestins are either levonorgestrel, or norethisterone, or desogestrel and the estrogens are principally confined to either ethinylestradiol or mestranol** (3-methyl ether of ethinylestradiol). Currently, 'lipid friendly' is **third-generation progestins,** namely desogestrel, gestodene, norgestimate are available. Some of the preparations available in the market are mentioned in Table 30.4. Only Mala-N is distributed through government channel free of cost (Fig. 30.9).

Fourth generation: Drospirenone which is an analog of spironolactone is used as progestin. It has antiandrogenic and antimineralocorticoid action. It causes retention of K^+ (hyperkalemia). So drospirenone should not be used in patients with renal, adrenal or hepatic dysfunction.

Mode of Action

The probable mechanisms of contraception are:

- **Inhibition of ovulation:** Both the hormones synergistically act on the hypothalamopituitary (HP) axis. Estrogen suppresses GnRH, follicle-stimulating hormone (FSH) and prevents follicular growth and progestins suppress luteinizing hormone (LH) and prevent ovulation. The release of gonadotropin-releasing hormones (GnRH) from the hypothalamus is prevented through a negative feedback mechanism. There is thus no peak (pulsatile) release of FSH and LH from the anterior pituitary. So follicular growth is either not

Flowchart 30.2: Types of steroidal contraceptives.

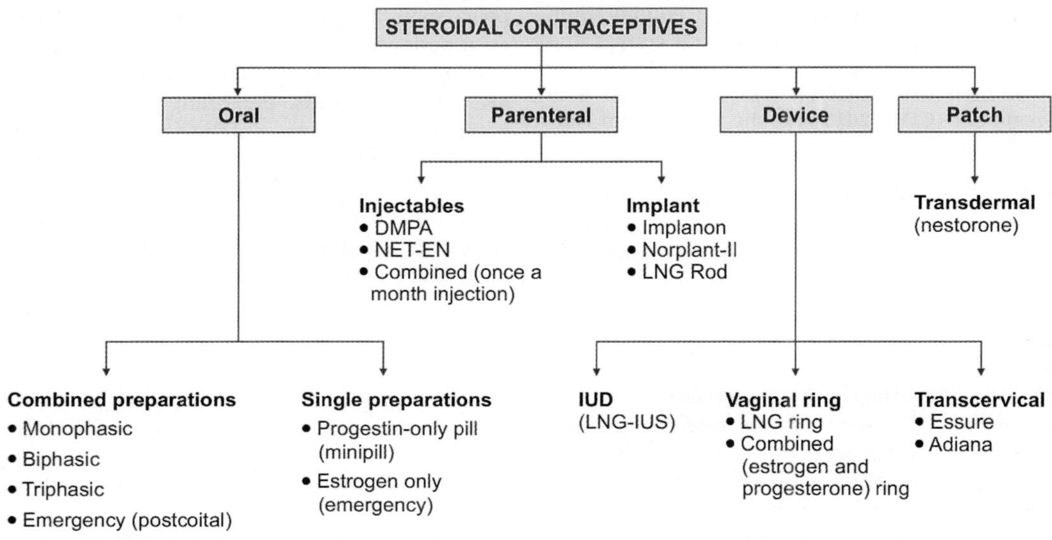

(DMPA: depot medroxyprogesterone acetate; NET-EN: norethisterone enanthate; LNG: levonorgestrel; LNG-IUS: levonorgestrel-intrauterine system; IUD: intrauterine devices)

TABLE 30.4: Some of the oral contraceptives and their composition.

	Composition		
Commercial names	***Progestins (mg)***	***Estrogen (μg)***	***No. of tablets***
1. **Mala-N (Government of India)**	Levonorgestrel (0.15)	Ethinyl estradiol (30)	21 + 7 iron tablets
2. **Mala-D**	Levonorgestrel (0.15)	—do—	21 + 7 iron tablets
3. **Loette (Wyeth)**	Desogestrel (0.15)	Ethinyl estradiol (20)	21
4. **Yasmin (Schering)**	Drospirenone 3 mg (p. 405)	Ethinyl estradiol (30)	21

Depending on the amount of ethinyl estradiol (E) and the types of progestin (P) used, pills are defined as: **1st generation**—with E 50 μg or more; **2nd generation**—with E 20–35 μg and P as levonorgestrel or norgestimate; **3rd generation**—with E 20–30 μg and P as desogestrel or gestodene; **4th generation**—E as third generation, with P as drospirenone, dienogest or nomegestrol. Low dose pills have E less than 50 μg.

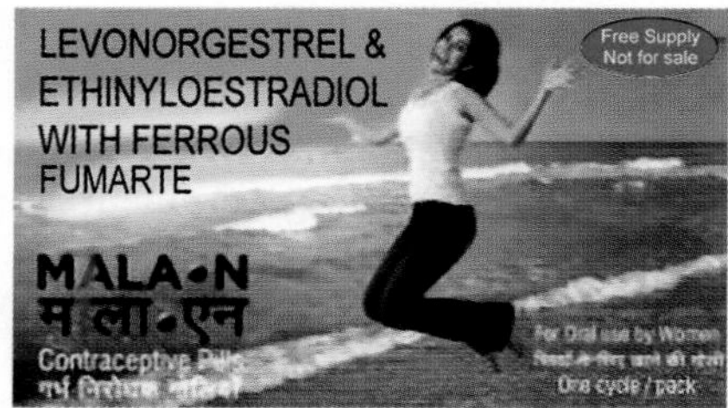

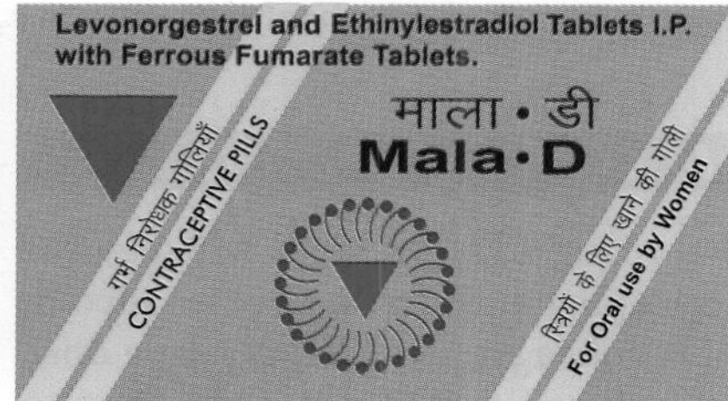

Fig. 30.9: Some commonly used oral contraceptives.

initiated or if initiated, recruitment does not occur. There is no ovulation.

- **Producing static endometrial hypoplasia:** There is stromal edema, decidual reaction and regression of the glands making endometrium nonreceptive to the embryo.
- **Alteration of the character of the cervical mucus** (thick, viscid, and scanty) so as to prevent sperm penetration.
- **Probably interferes** with tubal motility and alters tubal transport. Thus, even though accidental breakthrough ovulation occurs, the other mechanisms prevent conception.

Estrogen inhibits FSH rise and prevents follicular growth. It is also useful for better cycle control and to prevent breakthrough bleeding.

Progestin: Anovulatory effect is primarily by inhibiting LH surge. **It is also helpful to counteract the adverse effects of estrogen on the endometrium** (endometrial hyperplasia and heavy withdrawal bleeding). It is also responsible for changes in the cervical mucus (vide supra).

Selection of the Patient

History and general examination should be thorough, taking special care to screen cases for contraindications (headache, migraine). Examination of the breasts for any nodules, weight, and blood pressure are to be noted.

Pelvic examination to exclude cervical pathology, is mandatory. Pregnancy must be excluded.

Cervical cytology to exclude abnormal cells, is to be done. Thus, any woman of reproductive age group without any systemic disease and contraindications listed, is a suitable candidate for combined pill therapy. Growth and development of the pubertal and sexually active girls are not affected by the use of 'pill.'

How to Prescribe a Pill?

(Patient instruction): New users should normally start their pill packet **on day one of their cycle**. One tablet is to be taken daily preferably at bed time for consecutive 21 days. It is continued for 21 days and then has a 7 days break, with this routine, there is contraceptive protection from the first pill. Next pack should be started on the eighth day, irrespective of bleeding (same day of the week, the pill finished). **Thus, a simple regime of "3 weeks on and 1 week off" is to be followed**. Packing of 28 tablets, there should be no break between packs. Seven of the pills are dummies and contain either iron or vitamin preparations. However, a woman can start the pill up to day 5 of the bleeding. In that case, she is advised to use a condom for the next 7 days. The pill should be started on the day after abortion. Following childbirth in nonlactating woman, it is started after 3 weeks, and in lactating woman, it is to be withheld for 6 months (*see* later in the Ch.).

Follow-up: The patient should be followed up based on her symptoms. The patient above the age 35 should be checked more frequently.

Missed pills: Normally, there is return of pituitary and ovarian follicular activity during the pill-free interval (PFI) of 7 days. Breakthrough ovulation may occur in about 20% cases during the time. Lengthening of PFI due to omissions, malabsorption, or vomiting either at the start or at the end of a packet, increases the risk of breakthrough ovulation and, therefore, pregnancy.

Management

When a woman forgets to take **one pill** (late up to 24 hours), she should take the missed pill at once and continue the rest as schedule. There is nothing to worry.

When she **misses two pills or more** she should take 2 pills on each of the next 2 days and then continue the rest as scheduled. Extra precaution has to be taken for next 7 days either by using a condom or by avoiding sex. Alternatively, a new pack can be started and a barrier method to be used additionally for a week. If she misses any of the **7 inactive pills** (in a 28-day pack only) she should throw away the missed pills. She should take the remaining pills one a day and start the new pack as usual. Failure of withdrawal bleeding during the pill free interval, pregnancy should be excluded with medical tests. COCs are not teratogenic when taken accidentally in early pregnancy.

Drug Interactions

Effectiveness of some drugs (aspirin, oral anticoagulants, oral hypoglycemics, lamotrigine) are decreased and that for some other drugs (beta blockers, corticosteroids, diazepam, aminophylline) are increased by oral contraceptives.

MEDICAL ELIGIBILITY CRITERIA FOR CONTRACEPTIVE USE (WHO/FRM/FPP)		
COMBINED ORAL CONTRACEPTIVES (COCs)		
Indications of COCs	***Contraindications of COCs***	
No restriction of use (WHO Category–1)	**Relative (WHO Category–2 and 3)**	**Absolute (WHO Category–4)**
▪ Age: Menarche to 40 years ▪ Postabortion ▪ Anemia (iron deficiency, malaria) ▪ HIV or AIDS (additional to condom use) ▪ GTN following normal hCG level ▪ History of ectopic pregnancy ▪ Endometriosis, uterine fibroid, ovarian or endometrial cancer ▪ Dysmenorrhea, DUB ▪ Pelvic inflammatory disease ▪ Epilepsy ▪ Thyroid disease ▪ Varicose veins ▪ Tuberculosis ▪ Benign breast disease	**A. WHO Category–2 (advantages outweigh the risks)** ▪ Age ≥40 years ▪ Smoker <35 years ▪ History of jaundice ▪ Mild hypertension ▪ Gallbladder disease ▪ Diabetes ▪ Sickle cell disease ▪ Headache ▪ Cancer cervix or CIN **B. WHO Category–3 (risks outweigh the advantages)** ▪ Unexplained vaginal bleeding ▪ Hyperlipidemia ▪ Liver tumors (benign) ▪ Breastfeeding (postpartum 6 weeks to 6 months) ▪ Heavy smoker (>20 cigarettes/day) ▪ Past breast cancer	**A. Circulatory diseases (past or present)** ▪ Arterial or venous thrombosis ▪ Severe hypertension ▪ History of stroke ▪ Heart disease: Valvular, ischemic ▪ Diabetes with vascular complications ▪ Migraine with focal neurologic symptoms **B. Diseases of the liver** ▪ Active liver disease, jaundice ▪ Liver adenoma, carcinoma **C. Others** ▪ Pregnancy ▪ Breastfeeding (postpartum 6 weeks) ▪ Major surgery or prolonged immobilization ▪ Estrogen-dependent neoplasms, e.g. breast cancer

(GTN: gestational trophoblastic neoplasia; CIN: cervical intraepithelial neoplasia; HIV: human immunodeficiency virus; AIDS: acquired immunodeficiency syndrome; hCG: human chorionic gonadotropin; DUB: dysfunctional uterine bleeding)

Additional Contraception

To ensure 100% efficacy, additional mechanical contraceptives (usually condom) are to be used in the following circumstances:

- **When broad-spectrum antibiotics like** ampicillin, ciprofloxacin, tetracycline, doxycycline are used—as they impair the absorption of ethinyl estradiol.
- **When enzyme-inducing drugs are used,** e.g. (a) Barbiturates; (b) All antiepileptic drugs except sodium valproate and clonazepam; (c) Rifampicin; (d) Ketoconazole; (e) Griseofulvin; (f) Protease inhibitor (ritonavir); and (g) Nevirapine—under such circumstances, high dose preparations (ethinyl estradiol of 50 μg or more) are to be used to counter-balance the increased liver metabolism.

Indications for Withdrawal

While the majority tolerates the combined pill, in some susceptible individuals, gross adverse symptoms develop which necessitate its withdrawal. The indications for withdrawal of the pill are—(a) Severe migraine; (b) Visual or speech disturbances; (c) Sudden chest pain; (d) Unexplained fainting attack or acute vertigo; (e) Severe cramps and pains in legs; (f) Excessive weight gain; (g) Severe depression; (h) Prior to surgery (it should be withheld for at least 6 weeks to minimize postoperative vascular complications), and (i) Patient wanting pregnancy.

Continuous and Extended Use of COCs

Extended continues regimens: Contain 84 days of active pills followed by 7 days of hormone free interval (HFI). Withdrawal bleeding is only four times a year. Any monophasic pill may be used in this manner. Failure rate is also less.

Return of fertility: The suppressive effects on H-P-O axis disappear quickly following stoppage of low dose COCs. Normal endocrine function returns. Ovulation returns within 3 months of withdrawal of the drug in 90% cases. Women who conceive inadvertently while taking COCs, there is no risks of fetal congenital malformations.

Withdrawal bleeding: It is bleeding that is seen during the hormone free interval, whereas bleeding that occurs during the time when active pills are being taken is called breakthrogh bleeding. **Breakthrough bleeding** is due to insufficient estrogen to support the endometrium.

How Long can the Pill be Continued?

Potential benefits of pills are greater when compared to risks, in a well-selected individual. A woman who does not smoke and has no other risk factor for cardiovascular disease, may continue the pill (with careful monitoring) until the age of 50 years. This offers the dual advantages of effective contraception and HRT. However, for spacing of births, use of 3 to 5 years is considered enough and safe.

General and Metabolic Effects of COCs

The combined preparations containing estrogen and progestin have got a wide range of metabolic activities which affect almost all the systems of the body. The changes are almost similar to those of pregnancy and almost completely revert back to normal after the drug is withdrawn. **The effects are related either to the estrogen (OGN) or to the progestin (PGN) or to both (OGN + PGN) of the compounds.**

Health Benefits of Combined Oral Contraceptives (COCs)

- **Contraceptive benefits:** (a) Protection against unwanted pregnancy (failure rate—0.1 per 100 women years); (b) Convenient to use; (c) Not intercourse related; (d) Reversibility; and (e) Improving maternal and child health care.
- **Noncontraceptive health benefits:** *Improvement of menstrual abnormalities*—(1) Regulation of menstrual cycle (Table 30.5); (2) Reduction of dysmenorrhea (40%); (3) Reduction of menorrhagia (50%); (4) Reduction of PMS; (5) Reduction of Mittelschmerz syndrome; (6) Protection against iron-deficiency anemia. **Protection against health disorders**—(7) PID (thick cervical mucus); (8) Ectopic pregnancy; (9) Endometriosis; (10) Fibroid uterus; (11) Hirsutism and acne; (12) Functional ovarian cysts; (13) Benign breast disease; (14) Osteopenia and postmenopausal osteoporotic fractures; (15) Autoimmune disorders of thyroid; (16) Rheumatoid arthritis; (17) Increases bone mineral density. **Prevention of malignancies**—(18) Endometrial cancer (50%); (19) Epithelial ovarian cancer (50%); (20) Colorectal cancer (40%).

Adverse Effects of COCs

Minor Complications

The minor complications or ailments are:

- **Nausea, vomiting, headache (OGN) and leg cramps (PGN):** These are transient and often subside following continuous use for 2–3 cycles.
- **Mastalgia (OGN + PGN):** Heaviness or even tenderness in the breast is often transient.
- **Weight gain (PGN):** Though progestins have got an anabolic effect due to its chemical relation to testosterone, use of low-dose COCs does not cause any increase in weight.
- **Chloasma (OGN) and acne (PGN):** These are annoying for cosmetic reasons. Low-dose oral contraceptives improves acne as levonorgestrel preparations are less androgenic.

TABLE 30.5: Combined oral contraceptives (COCs).

Health benefits of COCs
▪ Highly effective ▪ Good cycle control ▪ Well-tolerated in majority ▪ Additional health benefits are many (*see* above) ▪ Low-dose pill with 'lipid friendly' progestins further reduces the risk ▪ Extended regimens are available ▪ Return of fertility rate is prompt *Failure rate—0.1 (HWY)*

- **Menstrual abnormalities:** ***Breakthrough bleeding (BTB):*** It is commonly due to subthreshold blood level of hormones. Other causes of breakthrough bleeding in pill takers are: (a) Disturbance of drug absorption—diarrhea, vomiting; (b) Use of enzyme, inducing drugs (mentioned earlier), missing pills, use of low dose pills; (c) Pregnancy complications (miscarriage); (d) Diseases—cervical ectopy or carcinoma. Usually, it settles after 3–4 cycles when there is no other specific cause for BTB. Exogenous estrogen (conjugated estrogen 1.25 mg or estradiol 2 mg) given daily for 7 days can control the bleeding. Doubling up the active pills for 2–3 days, or until bleeding stops, is helpful. A pill containing higher dose of estrogen, with different progestin could be helpful. BTB is not associated with any increased failure rate. **Hypomenorrhea (PGN):** It is of little significance although disturbing to the patient. It is due to the local endometrial changes. **Menorrhagia (OGN):** It is usually pre-existing and use of compounds with progestin preponderance is helpful. **Amenorrhea (OGN or PGN):** Postpill amenorrhea of more than 6 months duration occurs in less than 1% cases. The association is casual not causal. It is usually more in women with pre-existing functional menstrual disorders. Spontaneous resumption of menstruation occurs in 6 months for majority of cases. A refractory case (≥6 months) should be investigated as a case of secondary amenorrhea.
- **Libido:** Libido may be diminished **(PGN)** probably due to dryness of the vagina. More often, it may either remain static or, at times, may even increase due to loss of fear of pregnancy.
- **Leukorrhea:** It may be due to excessive cervical mucus secretion **(OGN)** or due to increased preponderance of monilial infection **(OGN + PGN)**.

Major Complications

The major complications are:

- **Depression:** Low-dose estrogen preparations are not associated with depression.
- **Hypertension (OGN):** Current low dose COCs rarely cause significant hypertension. Pre-existing hypertension is likely to be aggravated. Changes are seen only in systolic but not in diastolic blood pressure. The effect on blood pressure is thought to involve the renin-angiotensin system. There is marked increase in plasma angiotensinogen. The changes, however, reverse back to normal 3–6 months after stoppage of pill.
- **Vascular complications (OGN):** (a) **Venous thromboembolism (VTE):** The overall risk is to the extent of 3–4 times more than the non-users. Pre-existing hypertension, diabetes, obesity thrombophilias (inherited or acquired) and elderly patient (over 35, especially with smoking habits) are some of the important risk factors. Ethinyl estradiol used with a dose of 20 µg in the pill markedly reduce the incidence. Current studies estimate the annual number of nonfatal VTE per 100,000 users as: no COC use = 5, second-generation COC = 15, COC-containing desogestrel and gestodene = 30, pregnancy = 60. The absolute risk is very small compared to pregnancy. The most important risk factor is genetic thrombophilia (factor V Leiden mutation). This is rare in Asians (0.4%) compared to Caucasian (5%). (b) **Arterial thrombosis: The high-risk factors for myocardial infarction and stroke (ischemic and hemorrhagic) are hypertension, smoking habit, age over 35 and diabetes.** Women with multiple risk factors for cardiovascular disease generally should not use COCs.
- **Cholestatic jaundice:** Susceptibility is increased in women with previous history of idiopathic recurrent jaundice in pregnancy or hepatitis.
- **Neoplastic risks and the benefits:** Combined oral contraceptives (COCs) **reduce the risk of epithelial ovarian (50% ↓) and endometrial (50% ↓) carcinoma**. This protective effect persists for 10–15 years even after stopping the method following a use of 6 months to 1 year.
  There is reduction in **colorectal carcinoma (20%)**.
  Breast cancer: COCs use increases the risk of breast cancer by 25% and the risk disappears after cessation of use. The absolute risk is low.
  Cervical cancer: COC increase the risk of cancer cervix with increasing duration of use. Adenocarcinoma of the cervix is more compared to squamous cell. However, pill users should have regular HPV-DNA and **cervical cytology screening. No increased risk of hepatocellular adenomas** have been found with low dose preparations. It gives protection against benign cystic breast disease and cystic ovaries.
- **Death:** Risk of death for a woman using COCs is about 1.5/100,000. It is significantly low.

General and Metabolic Effects

Carbohydrate (PGN): Progestins impair glucose tolerance promoting insulin resistance and hyperglycemia. This was observed in preparations containing 150 µg or more levonorgestrel. Low-dose COCs have no effect on insulin, HbA1C, and fasting glucose levels. **Protein (OGN):** Estrogen has got some stimulatory effect on the hepatic secretion of many proteins. The level of sex hormone-binding globulin (SHBG) is increased. **Lipid (OGN):** Plasma lipids and lipoproteins are increased. Total cholesterol and triglycerides are increased. Low dose estrogen increases high-density lipoprotein (HDL) cholesterol and decreases low-density lipoprotein (LDL) cholesterol thereby exerts its protective effect against atherosclerosis. Progestins, however, decrease HDL cholesterol and increase LDL cholesterol thereby promote heart disease. Preparations with more selective, lipid friendly, and third generation progestins namely desogestrel, gestodene or norgestimate, HDL level is somewhat elevated. However, most changes are within the normal range and not clinically relevant. **Vitamins and minerals:** Vitamin B_6, B_{12}, folic acid, calcium, manganese, zinc, and ascorbic acid levels are decreased while vitamins A and K levels are increased.

Effects on Organs

- **Hypothalamopituitary axis:** Both FSH and LH levels remain low as found in early proliferative phase and remain throughout the cycle at such static low level.

- **Ovary:** Ovarian function remains quiescent with occasional evidence of breakthrough ovulation. There is evidence of fibrosis, progressive wastage of unripe ova with advancing age without evidence of corpus luteum. The endogenous hormones remain static at a low level.
- **Endometrium (PGN):** Stromal edema, decidual reaction and glandular exhaustion out of depletion of glycogen are more or less constant findings.
- **Cervix (PGN + OGN):** Increased glandular hyperplasia and downgrowth of the endocervical epithelium beyond the squamocolumnar junction gives the appearance of an ectopy. Relative risk of cervical cancer with COC use is 1.1. It may be due to the persistent exposure of the pill users to HPV infection or due to their more sexual activity.
- **Uterus (OGN):** Uterus may be slightly enlarged. Low-dose COCs do not usually increase the size of a pre-existing fibroid. COCs can reduce the amount of menstrual bleeding.
- **Vagina (PGN):** Cytohormonal study reflects the picture of early luteal phase.
- **Other organs:** (a) **Liver:** The liver functions are depressed; (b) **Gastrointestinal tract (GIT):** There is increased incidence of mesenteric vein thrombosis; (c) **Urinary:** There is increased incidence of urinary tract infection but is probably related to increase in sexual activity.

Effects on Reproduction

- **Risk to fetus:** When COC is taken during early pregnancy inadvertently there is no greater risk of significant congenital anomaly. Risk of congenital abnormality in general is 2–3%.
- **Lactation (OGN + PGN):** Lactation is probably affected by a reduction in the milk production and also by alteration of the quality of the milk (reduction of protein and fat content). Moreover, significant amount of the steroids are ingested by the infant, the effects are as yet unknown. Mini-pill is a better alternative for the breastfeeders.

Types of Oral Contraceptive Formulations

In multiphasic preparation, minimum doses are provided for contraceptive effect in the early part of the cycle and slightly higher doses later in the cycle to prevent breakthrough bleeding. It is an attempt to minimize undesirable side effects of lipid metabolism.

1. a. Monophasic (fixed dose): Combined pills (COCs)
   b. Multiphasic (different dose combinations) with different tablet color): It may be biphasic, triphasic or four phasic.
2. OC formulations and regimens: Most covers 28 days (4 weeks). Many combinations are—21 days (3 weeks) followed by 7 days hormone-free interval (HFI).

Most products contain spacer pills (iron) in the HFI. Bleeding usually occurs during the HFI (or 3–4 days). Some preparation contains active tablets for 24 days and HFI is 4 days. They are more effective than 21 days pill.

CENTCHROMAN (CHHAYA/SAHELI)

Female: *Ormeloxifene* is a research product of Central Drug Research Institute (CDRI) of Lucknow, India. It is a nonsteroidal compound with potent antiestrogenic and weak-estrogenic properties. It is taken orally (30 mg) twice a week for first 3 months then once a week. It works primarily by preventing implantation of fertilized ovum. It creates asynchrony between developing zygote and the endometrium causing implantation failure. It does not inhibit ovulation.

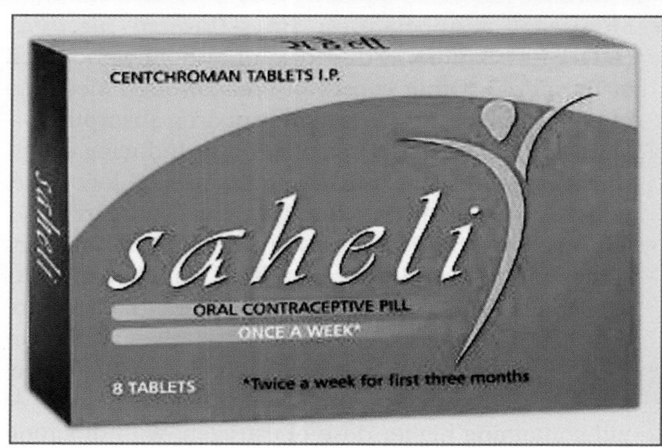

Side effects are a few. It is avoided in polycystic ovarian disease, cervical cell hyperplasia, with liver (jaundice) and kidney diseases, and in tuberculosis. There may be a tendency of oligomenorrhea. The failure rate is about 1–4 per 100 women years of use. Failure rate is less with increased doses. It is devoid of any significant adverse metabolic and hormonal effect. This may also be used as safely by the lactating women and an emergency contraceptive. It is highly safe, effective and a reversible method. It has no teratogenic effect and return of fertility is immediate. It is sold against prescription only and not over the counter.

Noncontraceptive use: Because of its potent antiestrogenic activity, centchroman is being currently tried in the management of DUB, endometrial hyperplasia, endometriosis and breast cancer. It is used as HRT, because of its weak estrogenic property.

PROGESTOGEN-ONLY CONTRACEPTIONS

Progestogen-only contraception includes:

- **Oral:** POPs
- **Parenterals:** DMPA, NET-EN, implants (Implanon)
- **LNG-IUS** (p. 399).

Progestin-only Pill (POP/Minipill)

Progestin-only pill is devoid of any estrogen compound. It contains very low dose of a progestin in any one of the following forms—levonorgestrel 75 µg, norethisterone 350 µg, desogestrel 75 µg, lynestrenol 500 µg or norgestrel 30 µg. **It has to be taken daily from the first day of the cycle.**

Mechanism of action: It works mainly by making cervical mucus thick and viscous, thereby prevents sperm penetration. Endometrium becomes atrophic, so blastocyst implantation is also hindered. In about 2% of cases, ovulation is inhibited and 50% women ovulate normally.

How to prescribe a minipill?: The first pill has to be taken on the first day of the cycle and then continuously. It has to be taken regularly and at the same time of the day. There must be no break between the packs. **Delay in intake** for more than 3 hours, the woman should have the missed pill immediately and the next one as scheduled. Extra precaution has to be taken for next 2 days.

Advantages: (a) Side effects attributed to estrogen in the combined pill are totally eliminated; (b) No adverse effect on lactation and hence can be suitably prescribed in lactating women and as such it is often called 'Lactation Pill';

(c) Easy to take as there is no 'On and Off' regime; (d) It may be prescribed in patient having (medical disorders) hypertension, fibroid, diabetes, epilepsy, smoking, and history of thromboembolism, HIV positive women; (e) Reduces the risk of PID and endometrial cancer.

Disadvantages: (a) There may be acne, mastalgia, headache, breakthrough bleeding, or at times amenorrhea in about 20–30% cases; (b) All the side effects, attributed to progestins may be evident; (c) Simple cysts of the ovary may be seen, but they do not require any surgery; (d) Failure rate is about 0.3–2 per 100 women years of use. Failure is more in young compared to women over 40. Women using drugs that induce liver microsomal enzymes to alter a metabolism (mentioned above) should avoid this method of contraception.

Contraindications: (a) Pregnancy; (b) Unexplained vaginal bleeding; (c) Recent breast cancer; (d) Arterial disease; (e) Thromboembolic disease; (f) Women taking antiseizure drugs.

Injectable Progestins

The preparations commonly used are depomedroxy-progesterone acetate (DMPA) and norethisterone enanthate (NET-EN). Both are administered intramuscularly (deltoid or gluteus muscle) within 5 days of the cycle. The injection should be deep, Z-tract technique and the site not to be massaged. DMPA in a dose of 150 mg every three months (WHO, 4 months) or 300 mg every six months; NET-EN in a dose of 200 mg given at two monthly intervals.

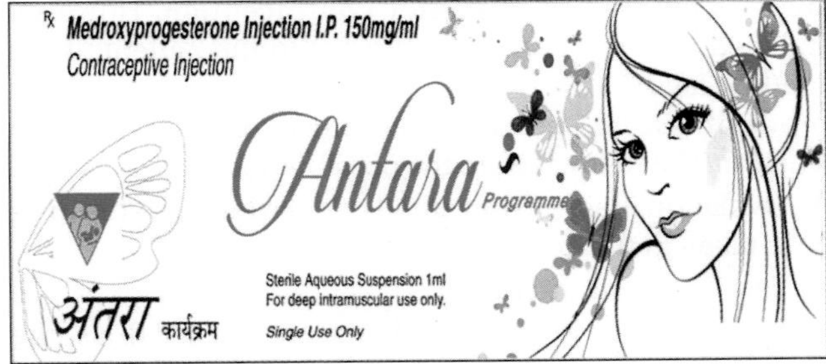

Depo-SubQ provera 104 (Uniject) contains 104 mg of DMPA. It is given subcutaneously over the anterior thigh or abdomen at every 90 days. It suppresses ovulation for 3 months as it is absorbed more slowly.

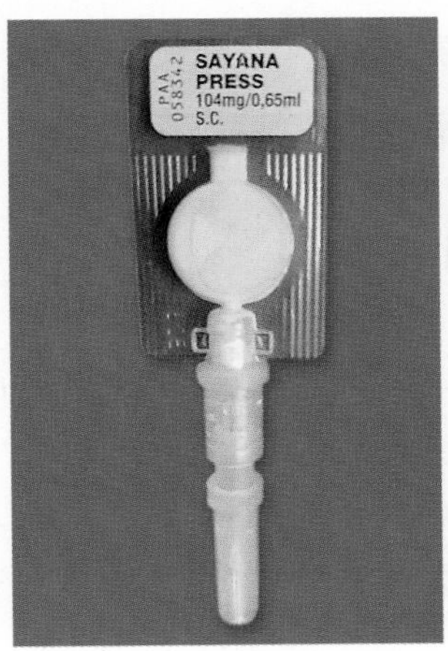

Medroxyprogesterone acetate (SAYANA PRESS): Inj. 104 mg/ 0.65 mL. It is available as a prefilled single dose injector. The injector needs to be activated by pushing the needle shield firmly towards the port, before use. The medicine appears white and uniform. The suspension is to be shaken vigorously just before use. It is given by SC injection into the anterior thigh or abdomen every 3 months (12–14 weeks). It is administered by a healthcare professional or by the woman herself.

Mechanism of action: (a) Inhibition of ovulation—by suppressing the midcycle LH peak; (b) Cervical mucus becomes thick and viscid thereby prevents sperm penetration; (c) Endometrium is atrophic preventing blastocyst implantation.

Advantages: (a) It eliminates regular medication as imposed by oral pill; (b) It can be used safely during lactation. It probably increases the milk secretion without altering its composition; (c) No estrogen-related side effects; (d) Menstrual symptoms, e.g. menorrhagia, dysmenorrhea are reduced; (e) Protective against endometrial cancer; (f) Can be used as an interim contraception before vasectomy becomes effective; (g) Reduction in PID, endometriosis, ectopic pregnancy and ovarian cancer. **The noncontraceptive benefits** are DMPA reduces the risk of—salpingitis, endometrial cancer, iron deficiency anemia, sickle cell problems, and endometriosis.

Disadvantages: **Failure rate** for DMPA—(0–0.3) (HWY). There is chance of irregular bleeding and occasional phase of amenorrhea. Return of fertility after their discontinuation is **usually delayed** for several months (6–12 months). However, with NET-EN the return of fertility is quicker. Loss of bone mineral density (reversible) has been observed with long-term use of depot provera. It is suitable for adolescents and the perimenopausal women. However, most bone lost is restored within 5 years of stoppage. Overweight, insulin-resistant women may develop diabetes. **Other side effects are** depression, weight gain, and headache.

Contraindications: Women with high-risk factors for osteoporosis, breast cancer, and the others are same as in POP (*see* above).

Implant

Nexplanon is a progestin-only delivery system containing 3 ketodesogestrel **(etonogestrel)**. It is a long-term (up to 3 years) reversible contraception (Fig. 30.10). It consists of a single closed capsule (made of ethylene vinyl acetate copolymer 40 mm × 2 mm) and contains 68 mg of etonogestrel (ENG). It releases the hormone about 60 μg, gradually reduced to 30 μg per day **over 3 years.** Implanon does not cause decrease in bone mineral density.

Mechanism of action: It inhibits ovulation in 90% of the cycles for the first year. It has got its supplementary effect on endometrium (atrophy) and cervical mucus (thick) as well.

Insertion: The capsule is inserted subdermally, in the inner aspect of the nondominant arm, 6–8 cm above the elbow fold. It is inserted between biceps and triceps muscles. Preloaded sterile applicator is available. No incision is required. Removal is done by making a 2 mm incision at the tip of the implant and pushing the rod until it pops out. It is done under local anesthetic. It is ideally inserted within D-5 of a menstrual cycle, immediately after abortion and 3 weeks after postpartum.

Removal: Implanon should be removed within 3 years of insertion. Loss of contraceptive action is immediate.

Advantages are the same as with DMPA. Others are (a) Highly effective for long-term use and rapidly reversible; (b) Suited for women who have completed their family

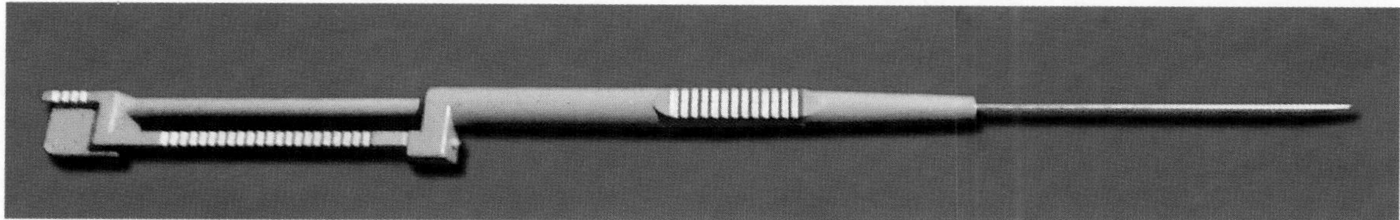

Fig. 30.10: Single implant rod—Implanon.

but do not desire permanent sterilization. **Efficacy of Nexplanon** is extremely high with Pearl indices of 0.01. This safe and effective method is considered as 'reversible sterilization'. **Drawbacks** are frequent irregular menstrual bleeding, spotting and amenorrhea are common. Difficulty in removal is felt occasionally. Nexplanon can be imaged (X-ray, USG, MRI); if not palpable during removal. **Contraindications** are similar to POP (p. 411).

Norplant-II (Jadelle)

Two rods of 4 cm long with diameter of 2.5 mm is used. Each rod contains 75 mg of levonorgestrel. It releases 50 µg of levonorgestrel per day. Contraceptive efficacy is similar to combined pills. Failure rate is 0.06 per 100 women years. It is used for 3 years. The rods are easier to insert and remove.

Long-acting reversible contraception (LARC) needs only one time motivation for long-term use. There is no risk of user error once it is placed in the body. LARCs are highly effective and immediately reversible with rapid return of fertility after its removal. Contraindications of LARCs are very few. It is recommended for the lactating women. It can be used in the postpartum or postabortal period. It has high continuation rate and user satisfaction. It is offered as first line contraception (ACOG, 2009). The common LARC methods are: Copper-T 380A, LNG-IUS, Implants [Nexplanon (p. 411)]

EMERGENCY CONTRACEPTION (SYN: POSTCOITAL CONTRACEPTION)

- **Hormones**
- **Antiprogesterone**
- **IUD**
- **Others**

Indications of emergency contraception: Unprotected intercourse, condom rupture, missed pill, delay in taking POP for more than 3 hours, sexual assault or rape and first time intercourse, as known to be always unplanned. Risk of pregnancy following a single act of unprotected coitus around the time of ovulation, is 8%.

Hormones (Table 30.6)

Morning-after pill: This is not true contraception, but has rightly been called interception, preventing conception in case of accidental unprotected exposure around the time of ovulation. Drugs commonly used are ethinyl estradiol 2.5 mg. The drug is taken orally twice daily for 5 days, beginning soon after the exposure but not later than 72 hours.

Levonorgestrel (E. pills) 0.75 mg, two doses given at 12 hours interval, is very successful and without any side effects. The two tablets (1.50 mg) can be taken as a single dose also (Fig. 30.11). The first dose should be taken within 72 hours may be taken up to 120 hours.

No fetal adverse effect has been observed when there is failure of emergency contraception. However, induced abortion should be offered to the patient, if the method fails.

TABLE 30.6: Emergency contraceptives.

Drug	*Dose*	*Pregnancy rate (%)*
Levonorgestrel (POP)	150 mg (single dose) Or 0.75 mg stat and after 12 hours	0–1
Copper IUDs (gold standard)	Insertion within 5 days	0–1
Ulipristal acetate (SPRM)	30 mg PO within 120 hour	0–1
Ethinyl estradiol 50 µg + Norgestrel 0.25 mg (COC) (Yuzpe method)	2 tab stat and 2 after 12 hours	0–2
Mifepristone RU 486 (PA)	100 mg single dose	0–0.6

(POP: progestin-only pill; IUDs: intrauterine devices; SPRM: selective progesterone receptor modulator; COC: combined oral contraceptives; PO: per oral)

Mode of action: The exact mechanism of action remains unclear. The following are the possibilities:

- Ovulation is either prevented or delayed when the drug is taken in the beginning of the cycle.
- Fertilization is interfered.
- Implantation is prevented (except E. pills) as the endometrium is rendered unfavorable.
- Interferes with the function of corpus luteum or may cause luteolysis.

Drawbacks: Nausea and vomiting are much more intense with estrogen use. Antiemetic (meclizine) should be prescribed.

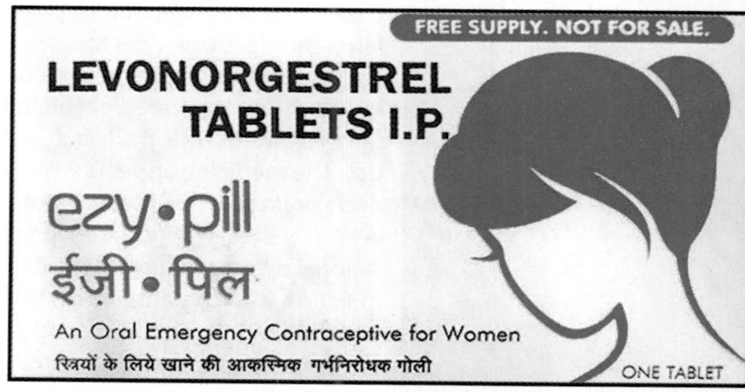

Fig. 30.11: Levonorgestrel (LNG) pill.

Copper IUD

Introduction of a copper IUD within a maximum period of 5 days can prevent conception following accidental unprotected exposure. This prevents implantation. Failure rate is about 0–1%. It is the gold standard method to be offered to all women for EC.

Advantage: It can be kept in place for 10 years if desired as a regular method of contraception.

Postcoital contraception is only employed as an emergency measure and is not effective if used as a regular method of contraception.

Yuzpe method (Combined hormonal regimen) is equally effective. Two tablets of Ovral (0.25 mg levonorgestrel and 50 μg ethinyl estradiol) should be taken as early as possible after coitus (<72 hours) and two more tablets are to be taken 12 hours later.

Oral antiemetic (10 mg metoclopramide) may be taken 1 hour before each dose to reduce the problem of nausea and vomiting.

Antiprogesterone

Antiprogesterone (RU 486-mifepristone) binds competitively to progesterone receptors and nullifies the effect of endogenous progesterone.

Dose: A single dose of 100 mg is to be taken within 5 days of intercourse. Implantation is prevented due to its antiprogesterone effect. Pregnancy rate is 0–0.6%.

Ulipristal acetate as an EC is superior to levonor-gestrel. It is a progesterone receptor modulator. A single dose 30 mg, to be taken orally as soon as possible or within 120 hours of coitus. It acts by suppressing follicular and endometrial growth. It delays ovulation and inhibits implantation. It should neither be prescribed in women with severe hepatic dysfunction nor with severe asthma.

SUMMARY OF ORAL CONTRACEPTIVES

- **Combined pills (COCs)**
- **Triphasic pill**
- **Emergency (postcoital) contraception**
- **Minipill**

- **Conventional combined preparations:** The widely used oral contraceptives consist of tablets containing estrogen and progestin compounds. It is the most effective and reversible method of contraception. Each tablet usually contains 30 mg of ethinyl estradiol and 1 mg of norethisterone or 0.3 mg norgestrel. **It has got trigger action**—(a) inhibition of ovulation, (b) production of static endometrial hypoplasia, and (c) alteration of the character of the cervical mucus. **Its use is absolutely contraindicated in cases** with circulatory diseases, liver diseases, severe migraine, and estrogen-dependent tumor. The pill should be started from the day one of a cycle and continued as '3 weeks on and 1 week off' regime. Periodic check-up is essential, especially when prescribed in women above the age of 35. **The pill should be withdrawn** if complications arise such as severe migraine, chest pain, visual disturbances, etc.

  The beneficial effects are relief of dysmenorrhea, premenstrual tension, endometriosis, acne, hirsutism, and lesser chance of ectopic and PID. It gives protection against ovarian and endometrial carcinomas.

  The minor side effects are nausea, vomiting, breakthrough bleeding, mastalgia, leg cramp, weight gain, hypomenorrhea or amenorrhea. The major complications are rare and include depression, hypertension and thromboembolic manifestations. The failure rate is about 0.1 per HWY.
- **Triphasic pill:** It has got lesser amount of steroids than the conventional monophasic tablets. There is lesser effect on lipid metabolism.
- **Emergency:** Following rape or accidental exposure, either levonorgestrel, 0.75 mg two doses at 12 hours interval or two tablets of the COC preparations are to be taken soon after coitus and two more tablets after 12 hours are quite effective in preventing conception. The first dose should be taken within 72 hours.
- **Minipill:** The pill contains low doses of progestin— norgestrel 30 mg, levonorgestrel 75 μg or desogestrel 75 μg. It should be taken daily and can be safely prescribed during lactation. It is best suited where estrogen is contraindicated.

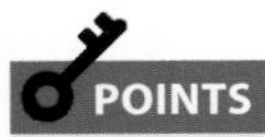

KEY POINTS

- **Medical eligibility criteria** (WHO) for the use of any method of contraception is **categorized as: (1)** No restriction for use of the method; **(2)** Advantages of using the method generally outweigh the theoretical or proven risks; **(3)** Theoretical or proven risks usually outweigh the advantages of using the method; **(4)** Health risks are unacceptable if the contraceptive method is used.
- **Combined oral contraceptives (COCs)** are very reliable apart from their many other **health benefits** (p. 408).
- **Mechanism of action of COCs are:** (a) Inhibition of ovulation by suppression of FSH and LH; (b) Making endometrium nonreceptive for implantation (endometrial hypoplasia); (c) Making cervical mucus thick, viscid and scanty; (d) Probably alters tubal motility.
- **Absolute contraindications** of oral pills (p. 407), major side effects (p. 408) and indications of withdrawal of pills (p. 509) have been discussed.
- The **newer low-dose pills** with more specific and 'lipid friendly' progestins reduce the health risk further.
- **Drospirenone** containing COC is useful in treating PMS, PMDD. It should not be used in women with renal, adrenal or hepatic dysfunction.
- **A woman who does not smoke** and has no other risk factor for cardiovascular disease, may continue the pill (with careful monitoring) until the age of 50.
- **Combined oral contraceptives:** (a) Contain estrogen and progestin compounds; (b) Third-generation progesterone may increase the risk of VTE; (c) Current users of COCs have an increased risk of breast cancer (RR 1.24); (d) With perfect use, failure rate is 0.1 per 100 WY; (e) It is contraindicated in women with arterial or venous disease.
- **Progestogen-only contraceptions:** (a) Does not inhibit ovulation completely; (b) Irregular vaginal bleeding is often associated and it may be the reason for discontinuation; (c) LNG-IUS may cause amenorrhea due to endometrial atrophy. DMPA use in adolescents and perimenopausal women should be after consideration of other methods. Importantly, most bone mass loss during DMPA use is restored within 5 years after its discontinuation; (d) DMPA does not increase the risk of cardiovascular disease but is associated with decreased BMD.

Contd...

Contd...

- **Low-dose progestin pill (minipill)** is advantageous in lactating women, as it has got no adverse effect on breast milk. It can be used as a suitable alternative where estrogen is contraindicated (p. 408).
- **Overall safety of DMPA** is clearly greater than COC. **Norplant and Implanon** are safe and effective for long-term use. Both are considered as 'reversible sterilization'.
- **Emergency contraception** includes hormones, IUD and antiprogesterone (RU 486). Within 72 hours, hormonal preparations are effective; within 5 days, IUD is effective and Ru 486 should be taken within day 27 of cycle irrespective of the day and number of intercourse (p. 412).
- **Centchroman** in a nonsteroidal antiestrogenic compound used as once a week contraceptive pill. It acts by preventing the implantation of the fertilized ovum. It has many benefits (p. 410).

STERILIZATION

Permanent sterilization may be done either for the male or female. Sterilization is a highly effective and safe method. In contrast to other methods, which are reversible or temporary, sterilization should be considered permanent. If a women who have tubal sterilization, wish to conceive, IVF is method can be used otherwise tubal reconstructive surgery is the alternative. For male anastomosis of vas deferens could be done. **The operation done on male is vasectomy and that on the female is tubal occlusion, or tubectomy**.

COUPLE COUNSELING

Couple must be counseled adequately before any permanent procedure is undertaken. Individual procedure must be discussed in terms of benefits, risks, side effects, failure rate, and reversibility.

Surgery

Advantages of vasectomy over tubectomy: (a) Can be done in the clinic under local anesthesia; (b) No entry to peritoneal cavity; (c) Less time needed (20 minutes); (d) Complications are less; (e) No hospital admission or stay; (f) Highly effective; (g) Minimum side effects; (h) Low cost; and (i) Simple to perform.

MALE STERILIZATION

Vasectomy (Fig. 30.12)

It is a permanent sterilization operation done in the male where a segment of vas deferens of both the sides are resected and the cut ends are ligated.

Advantages: (a) The operative technique is simple and can be performed by one with minimal training; (b) The operation can be done as an outdoor procedure or in a mass camp even in remote villages; (c) Complications—immediate or late are fewer; (d) Failure rate is minimal—0.15% and there is a fair chance of success of reversal anastomosis operation (70–80%); (e) The overall cost is minimal in terms of equipment, hospital stay and doctor's training.

Drawbacks: (a) Additional contraceptive protection is needed for about 2–3 months following operations, i.e. till the semen becomes free of sperm; (b) Frigidity or impotency when occurs is mostly psychological.

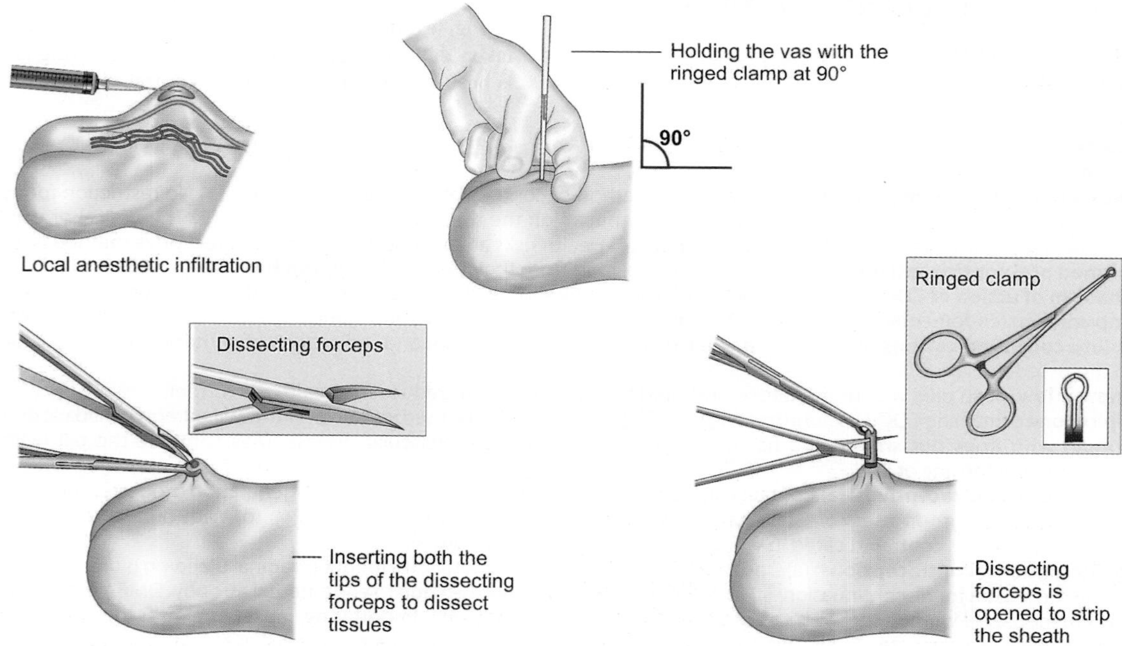

Fig. 30.12: Method of no-scalpel vasectomy (NSV) operation.

Selection of candidates: Sexually active and psychologically adjusted husband having the desired number of children is an ideal one.

No-scalpel Vasectomy

No-scalpel vasectomy (NSV) is commonly done at present in India. It was popularized by Dr Li Shun Qiang of China in 1991.

Technique

Written consent of the person is taken following counseling. The operation is done as an outdoor procedure or in the camp. The local area is shaved and cleaned with povidone-iodine lotion. Full surgical asepsis has to be maintained during operation. Procedure is done under local anesthetic.

The vasa is palpated with three fingers of the left hand; index and thumb in front and the middle behind. This is done at the level midway between the top of the testis and the base of the penis. The vasa is grasped with a ringed clump applied perpendicularly on the skin overlying the vasa. The skin is punctured with the sharp pointed end of the medial blade of dissecting forceps. The puncture point is enlarged by spreading the tissues (dartos muscle and spermatic fascia) inserting both the tips of the dissecting forceps. The vasa is elevated with the dissecting forceps and in hold with the ringed clamp. At least 1 cm of length of vasa is made free and mobilized. The vasa is ligated at two places 1 cm apart by No. '00' chromic catgut and the segment of the vasa in between the ligatures is resected out. Division of the vasa should be accompanied by fascial interposition or diathermy. This reduces the failure rate. Hemostasis is secured. No skin suturing is needed. Wound dressing is done and a small pressure bandage is applied. The same procedure is repeated on the other side. A scrotal suspensory bandage is worn. The patient is allowed to go home after half an hour. Histological examination of the excised segment of the vasa should be done for confirmation if the surgeon is in any doubt.

Advices

Antibiotic (Injection Penidure LA 6 IM) is administered as a routine and an analgesic is prescribed. Heavy work or cycling is restricted for about 2 weeks, while usual activities can be resumed forthwith. For check-up, the patient should report back after 1 week, or earlier, if complication arises. **Additional contraceptive should be used for 3–4 months.**

NSV takes less time, helps faster recovery due to less tissue injury. Complications are significantly less. However, it needs training on the part of the surgeon.

Precaution

The man does not become sterile soon after the operation as the semen is stored in the distal part of the vasa channels for a varying period of about 3 months. It requires about 20 ejaculations to empty the stored semen. Semen should be examined either by one test after 16 weeks or by two tests at 12 and 16 weeks after vasectomy and if the two consecutive semen analyses show absence of spermatozoa, the man is declared as sterile. Till then, additional contraceptive (condom or DMPA to wife) should be advised.

Complications

Complications of NSV are significantly less.

- **Immediate:** (a) Wound sepsis which may lead to scrotal cellulitis or abscess; (b) Scrotal hematoma.
- **Remote:** (a) Frigidity or impotency: It is mostly psychological in origin; (b) Sperm granuloma is due to inflammatory reaction to sperm leakage. This can be prevented by cauterization or fulguration of the cut ends; (c) Chronic intrascrotal pain and discomfort (post-vasectomy syndrome) may be due to scar tissue formation, or tubular distension of the epididymis; (d) There is no increase in testicular cancer or heart disease. Risk of prostate cancer is considered to have no causal association; (e) Spontaneous recanalization (1 in 2,000) is rare.

Other Methods to Block the Vasa

- **Electrocoagulation** may be used to encourage scar tissue formation.
- **Fascial interposition** following ligation, excision, and cautery. This is done to prevent recanalization.

FEMALE STERILIZATION

Occlusion of the fallopian tubes in some form is the underlying principle to achieve female sterilization. It is the most popular method of terminal contraception all over the world.

Indications

1. **Family planning purposes:** This is the principal indication in most of the developing countries.
2. **Socioeconomic:** An individual is adopted to accept the method after having the desired number of children.
3. **Medicosurgical indications (female partner):** (a) Medical diseases such as heart disease, diabetes, chronic renal disease, hypertension are likely to worsen, if repeated pregnancies occur; (b) During third time repeat cesarean section or following repair of prolapse to avoid complications.
4. **Risk-reducing salpingectomy:** As a preventive measure against serous ovarian and peritoneal cancer.

Time of Operation

1. **During puerperium (puerperal):** If the patient is otherwise healthy, the operation can be done 24–48 hours following delivery. Its chief advantage is technical simplicity. Hospital stay and rest at home following delivery are enough to help the patient to recover simultaneously from the two events, i.e. delivery and operation.
2. **Interval:** The operation is done beyond 3 months following delivery or abortion. **The ideal time of operation is following the menstrual period in the proliferative phase**
3. **Concurrent with medical termination of pregnancy (MTP) and at the time of cesarean section:** Sterilization is performed along with termination of pregnancy. This is mostly done, especially in the urban centers.
4. **Concurrent with cesarean delivery** with prior consent.

Methods of Female Sterilization

Occlusion by resection of a segment of both the fallopian tubes (commonly called tubectomy) is the widely accepted procedure. Currently, occlusion of the tubes with rings or clips or electrocoagulation using a laparoscope is gaining popularity. Hysterectomy during the childbearing period has got an incidental sterilization effect but should not be done for sterilization purpose.

Tubectomy

It is an operation where resection of a segment of both the fallopian tubes is done to achieve permanent sterilization. The approach may be:

- **Abdominal**
- **Vaginal**

Abdominal

- **Conventional**
- **Minilaparotomy**

Conventional (Laparotomy)

Steps

- **Anesthesia:** The operation can be done under general or spinal or local anesthesia. **In mass camp, local anesthesia is preferable.** In case of local anesthesia, premedication with injection morphine 15 mg or injection pethidine 100 mg with phenergan 50 mg IM is to be administered at least 30–45 minutes prior to surgery. The incisional area is infiltrated with 1% lignocaine.
- **Incision: In puerperal cases**, where the uterus is felt per abdomen, the incision is made two fingers breadth (1") below the fundal height and in interval cases, the incision is made 2 fingers' breadth above the symphysis pubis. The incision may be either midline or paramedian or transverse. The abdomen is opened by the usual procedure.
- **Delivery of the tube:** The index finger is introduced through the incision. The finger is passed across the posterior surface of the uterus and then to the posterior leaf of the broad ligament from where the tube is hooked out. **The tube is identified by** the fimbrial end and mesosalpinx containing utero-ovarian anastomotic vessels.

Techniques (Figs. 30.13A to F)

- **Pomeroy's:** A loop is made by holding the tube by an Allis forceps in such a way that the major part of the loop consists mainly of isthmus and part of the ampullary part of the tube (at the junction of proximal and middle third). Through an avascular area in the mesosalpinx, a needle threaded with No. '0' chromic catgut is passed and both the limbs of the loop are firmly tied together. About 1–1.5 cm of the segment of the loop distal to the ligature is excised. The tube is so excised as to leave behind about 1.5 cm of intact tube adjacent to uterus. **Segment of the loop removed is to be inspected to be sure that the wall has not been partially resected and to send it for histology.** The same procedure is repeated on the other side. Because of the absorption of the absorbable ligature, the cut ends become independently sealed off and are separated after a few weeks. **Advantages:** It is easy, safe, and very effective in spite of the simplicity of the technique. The failure rate is 0.1–0.5%. The cut ends become independently sealed off and retract widely from each other (Fig. 30.13C).

Contd...

Contd...

- **Uchida technique:** A saline solution is injected subserosally in the midportion of the tube to create a bleb. The serous coat is incised along the antimesenteric border to expose the muscular tube. The tube is ligated with No. '0' chromic catgut on either side and about 3–5 cm of the tube is resected off. The ligated proximal stump is allowed to retract beneath the serous coat. The serous coat is closed with a fine suture in such a way that the proximal stump is buried but the distal stump is open to the peritoneal cavity. No failure in this method has been observed so far.
- **Irving method:** The tube is ligated on either side and mid-portion of the tube (between the ties) is excised. The free medial end of the tube is then turned back and buried into the posterior uterine wall creating a myometrial tunnel (Fig. 30.13D).
- **Madlener technique (Fig. 30.13E):** It is the easiest method. The loop of the tube is crushed with an artery forceps. The crushed area is tied with black silk. **The loop is not excised**. The failure rate is very high to the extent of 7% and hence, it is abandoned in preference to the Pomeroy's technique.
- **Kroener** method of fimbriectomy is not a common procedure (Fig. 30.13F).

The abdomen is closed in layers. Antibiotics are given routinely in the postoperative period. The abdominal stitches are removed on the 5th day and the patient is discharged. However, if the patient has satisfactory postoperative progress, she may be discharged after 48 hours. The stitches may be removed in the outpatient department.

Minilaparotomy (MINI-LAP)

When the tubectomy is done through a small abdominal incision along with some device, the procedure is called mini-lap. It has been popularized by Uchida of Japan ever since 1961.

Steps

(1) **Anesthesia:** Always under local anesthesia: (2) **Plan of incision:** As described in conventional method but the incision should be $1/2"–3/4"$; (3) Especially designed retractor may be introduced after the abdomen is opened; (4) Uterus is elevated or pushed to one side or the other by the elevator that has already been introduced transvaginally into the uterine cavity. This helps manipulation of the tube in bringing it close to the incisional area, when it is seized by artery forceps; (5) The appropriate technique of tubectomy is performed on one side and then repeated on the other side; (6) The peritoneum is closed by purse string suture.

Once conversant with the technique, it can be performed with satisfaction to the patient. It also benefits the organization (turn over of the patient per bed is more than that in the conventional method). The patient is usually discharged within 24–48 hours.

Vaginal ligation: Tubectomy through the vaginal route may be done along with vaginal plastic operation or in isolation. When done in isolation, **the approach to the tube is through posterior colpotomy.** Surgeon needs additional skill of vaginal surgery. Interval cases (uterus <12 weeks) are most suited. It is done under general or spinal anesthesia. It takes longer time. Laparotomy may sometimes be needed due to difficulties.

Complications: Hemorrhage, broad ligament hematoma, and rarely rectal injury. Dyspareunia may be a late complication.

Advantage: Short hospital stay is convenient in obese women. Its limitation and relative merits and demerits are given in Table 30.7.

Laparoscopic Sterilization

Laparoscopy is the commonly employed method of endoscopic sterilization (Fig. 30.14). It is gradually becoming more popular—especially, in the camps (Fig. 30.15). The procedure is mostly done under local anesthesia. The operation is done in the interval period, concurrent with vaginal termination of pregnancy or 6 weeks following delivery. It should not be done within 6 weeks of delivery.

The procedure can be done either with single or double puncture technique. The tubes are occluded either by a **silastic ring** (silicone rubber with 5% barium sulfate) devised by **Fallope** or by **Filshie clip** is made of titanium lined with silicone rubber. Only 4 mm of the tube is destroyed. Failure rate is 0.1%. **Hulka-Clemens Spring clip** is also used. **Electrosurgical methods:** Desicates the tissue by heating. Unipolar or bipolar method of tubal coagulation is used. Bipolar cautery is safer than unipolar one but it has higher failure rates (2.1%). Laser photocoagulation is not popular because of high recanalization rate.

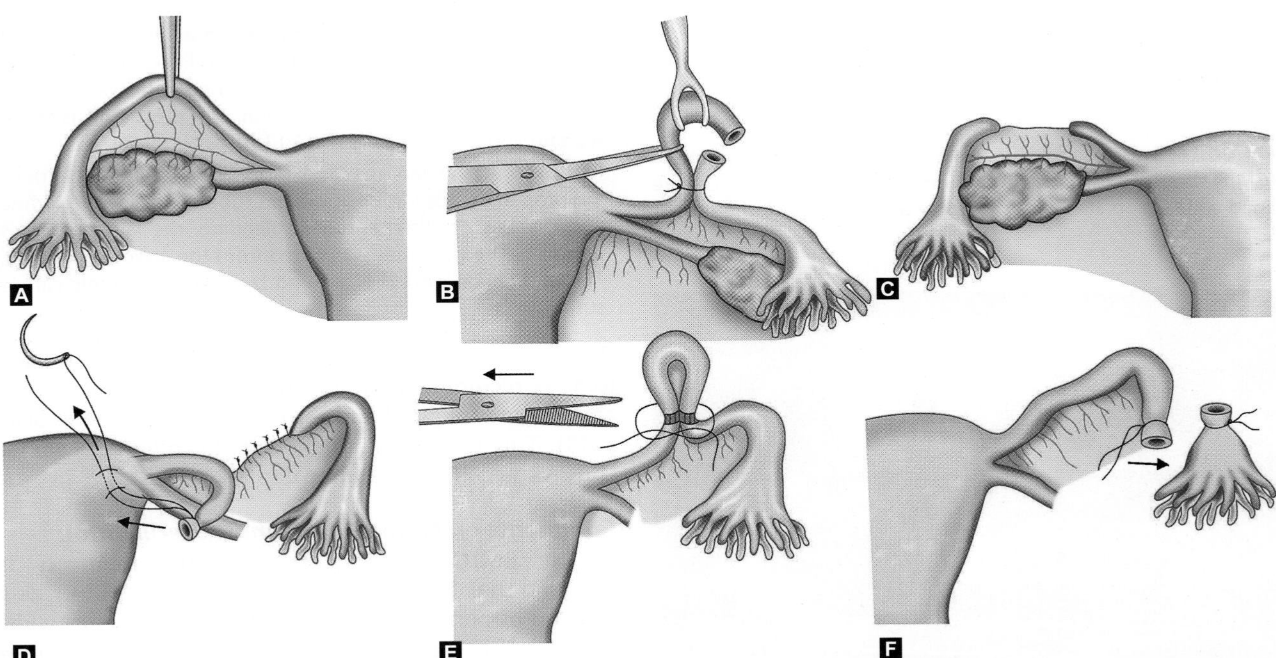

Figs. 30.13A to F: Steps of tubectomy by Pomeroy's method: (A) A segment of the fallopian tube is lifted up; (B) The loop is ligated with chromic catgut and is cut (about 1.5 cm); (C) End result of the operation—note wide separation; (D) **Irving procedure:** The medial cut end is buried in the myometrium posteriorly and the distal cut end is buried in the mesosalpinx; (E) **Madlener procedure**; (F) **Kroener procedure:** The ampullary end of the tube is ligated and resected.

TABLE 30.7: Mini-lap vis-a-vis laparoscopic sterilization.

Features	*Mini-lap*	*Laparoscopic sterilization*
Principle	Resection of portion of the tube	Using bipolar cautery sialistic band (Fallopering) or Filshie clip
Personnel	Any medical personnel with surgical skill	Should only be performed by persons with special training
Selection of time	Any time—puerperium, interval, with MTP	Should not be done within 6 weeks of delivery or with enlarged uterus
Contraindication	Practically none. Can be done in conditions contraindicated for laparoscopy	Lung lesions, organic heart diseases, intra-abdominal adhesions, extreme obesity
Complication life-threatening	Minimal but usually not	Minimal but at times fatal
Hospital stay	3–5 days	3–4 hours
Failure rate	0.1–0.3%	0.2–0.6%
Reversibility	Difficult due to adhesions and reduced remnant tubal length	Easier and effective. Only 4 mm of the tube is destroyed with the Filshie clip

(MTP: medical termination of pregnancy)

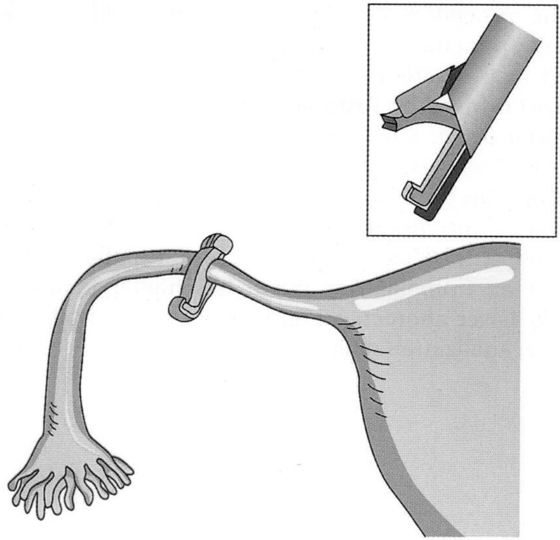

Fig. 30.14: Laparoscopic tubal sterilization by Filshie clip. Filshie (GM Filshie) clip is made of titanium and the inner surfaces are lined with silicon. It is easier to apply and damage to the tube is less.

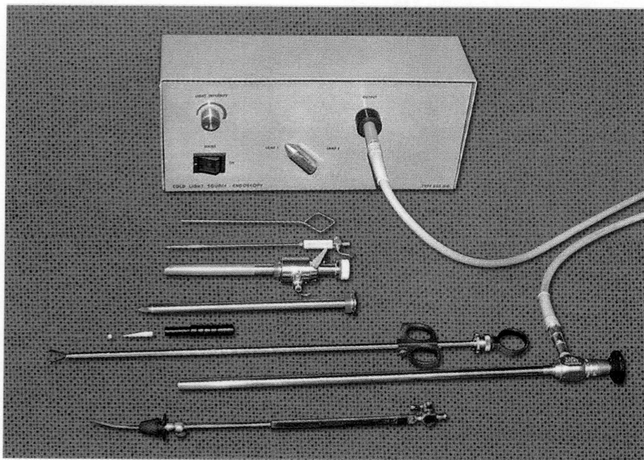

Fig. 30.15: Laparoscopic instruments for tubal sterilization.

Principal Steps (Single Puncture Technique)

Premedication: Pethidine hydrochloride 75–100 mg with phenergan 25 mg and atropine sulfate 0.65 mg are given intramuscularly about half an hour prior to operation.

Local anesthesia: Taking usual aseptic precautions about 10 mL of 1% lignocaine hydrochloride is to be infiltrated at the puncture site (just below the umbilicus) down up to the peritoneum.

Position of the patient: The patient is placed in lithotomy position. The operating table is tilted to approximately <15° of Trendelenburg position. Usual aseptic precaution is taken as in abdominal and vaginal operations. The bladder should be fully emptied by a metal catheter. Pelvic examination is done methodically. A uterine manipulator is introduced through the cervical canal for manipulation for visualization of tubes and uterus at a later step.

Contd...

Contd...

Producing pneumoperitoneum: A small skin incision (1.25 cm) is made just below the umbilicus. The Veress needle is introduced through the incision with 45° angulation into the peritoneal cavity. The abdomen is inflated with about 2 liters of gas (carbon dioxide or nitrous oxide or room air or oxygen). Choice of gas depends upon the method of sterilization.

Introduction of the trocar and laparoscope with ring-loaed applicator: Two silastic rings are loaded one after the other on the applicator with the help of a loader and pusher. The trocar with cannula is introduced through the incision previously made with a twisting movement. The trocar is removed and the laparoscope together with ring applicator is inserted through the cannula (Fig. 30.14).

The ring loaded applicator approaches one side of the tube and grasps **at the junction of the proximal and middle third of the tube.** A loop of the tube (2.5 cm) is lifted up, drawn into the cylinder of the applicator and the ring is slipped into the base of the loop under direct vision. The procedure is to be repeated on the other side (Fig. 30.14).

Removal of the laparoscope: After viewing that the rings are properly placed in position, the tubal loops looking white and there is no intraperitoneal bleeding, the laparoscope is removed. The gas or air is deflated from the abdominal cavity. The abdominal wound is sutured by a single chromic catgut suture.

Risk reducing salpingectomy: Bilateral total salpingectomy is recommended as it reduces the risk of ovarian cancer (endometroid and serous types) up to 34% (SGO, 2013). This is especially beneficial for high-risk women (BRCA 1 or BRCA 2 mutation).

Comments on Methods of Female Sterilization

In the LMIC, mini-lap remains the mainstay in the National Family Planning Program (NFPP) as a method of permanent sterilization. It is safe, has wider applicability, is less expensive and has got a less failure rate compared to laparoscopic sterilization. However, for a quick turnover in an organized mass camp, laparoscopic sterilization offers a promising success (Table 30.8).

Hazards of Tubal Sterilization

Immediate: These are related to general anesthesia and to the particular method used in sterilization. The related complications have already been discussed (Tables 30.7 and 30.8).

Remote: (a) Specific for the approach; (b) Related to the sterilization.

- The remote complications specific for the approach of the operation, abdominal or vaginal have already been described.
- The complications related to sterilization can be grouped into: (a) **General complications:** These include occasional obesity, psychological upset; (b) **Gynecological:** (i) Chronic pelvic pain, (ii) Congestive dysmenorrhea, (iii) Menstrual abnormalities in the form of menorrhagia, hypomenorrhea or irregular periods. Pelvic pain, menorrhagia along with cystic ovaries **constitute a**

TABLE 30.8: Female sterilization.

	Abdominal approach	*Vaginal approach*
Surgeon	Can be performed by any one conversant with surgery	Can be done only by a surgeon conversant with vaginal plastic operation
Time of operation	Can be done at any time, puerperal or interval	Interval period is most suited. May be done in other times, provided the uterus is smaller than 12 weeks
Contraindication	Practically—nil, uterus <12 weeks size	Associated TO mass, uterus—>12 weeks
Anesthesia	Can be done under local anesthesia	General or spinal anesthesia is usually needed
Complication during operation	Easy to tackle	Difficult at times and laparotomy may be necessary
Duration of operation	Shorter time	Longer time
Complications: *Immediate*	Few Wound infection, peritonitis—rare	Few Hemorrhage, revealed or broad ligament hematoma, injury to the rectum
Late	Incisional hernia, failure rate—less	Dyspareunia, failure rate—more
Hospital stay	Longer—5–6 days Shorter with mini-lap (24–48 hours)	Shorter—24–48 hours

post-ligation syndrome. It may be vascular in origin. However, the incidence can be minimized, if the blood vessels adjacent to the mesosalpinx are not unduly disturbed; (iv) Alteration in libido.

Failure Rate

The overall failure rate in tubal sterilization is about 0.7%, **the Pomeroy's technique being the lowest 0.1–0.5%**, in contrast to the Madlener's, being 1.5–7%. The failure rate is increased when it is done during hysterotomy or during cesarean section. Failure rates of laparoscopic sterilization depend upon the individual method (electrocoagulation—unipolar 0.75%, bipolar 2.1%, Fallope ring 1.7%, Filshie clip 0.1%). Failure may be due to **fistula formation or due to spontaneous reanastomosis**.

Mortality following tubal sterilization is estimated to be 72 per 100,000 for all methods. Laparoscopic procedures carried the mortality rate of 5–10 per 100,000 compared to 7 per 100,000 for puerperal ligations.

Reversibility

Informed consent must be obtained after **adequate counseling**. Couple must understand the permanency of the procedure, its occasional failure rate, the risks and side effects, and its alternatives. Unfortunately, regret is not uncommon. Microsurgical techniques give excellent result for tubal reanastomosis. Pregnancy rates after reversal are high (80%) following use of clips and rings. Reversal of vasectomy with restoration of vasa patency is possible up to 90% of cases. But pregnancy rate is low (50%).

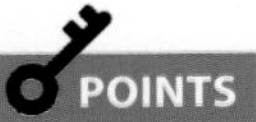

- **Sterilization** is the permanent method of surgical contraception. In male, it is vasectomy and that in female, it is tubectomy.
- **No scalpel vasectomy (NSV)** is commonly done in India.
- **Tubectomy** could be done by abdominal (common) or by vaginal route. Abdominally, it is done by conventional laparotomy or by minilaparotomy procedure (p. 416). Pomeroy's method is commonly done.
- **A man is not sterilized** immediately after vasectomy. As such, additional condom should be advised for at least 3 months (p. 415).
- **No scalpel vasectomy (NVS)** is done under local anesthetic making a tiny puncture over the stretched skin of the vasa (p. 415). It has fewer complications. Both the NSV and scalpel vasectomy (SV) are safe.
- **Globally, tubal sterilization** is the most common method (20%) of contraception followed by IUDs (15%), oral contraceptives (8%) and condoms (5%).
- **Counseling for sterilization** should be done with all information (p. 422).
- **Female sterilization** operation can be done during puerperium (puerperal), in interval period or concurrent with MTP or cesarean delivery (p. 415). Hysteroscopic methods of sterilization include insertion of quinacrine pellet and **essure (microcoil)**.
- **Reversal of sterilization** is not always successful. This should be counseled to the couple before sterilization operation.
- Apart from **conventional or mini-lap** abdominal method, **laparoscopic sterilization** is very popular and effective.
- **Contraceptive prescription** should be on an **individual basis**. In an individual, the method may vary according to her phase of reproductive life. **Teenage girls, older women** and **sex workers** should also be protected (p. 422).

BARRIER METHODS

These methods prevent sperm deposition in the vagina or prevent sperm penetration through the cervical canal. The objective is achieved by mechanical devices or by chemical means which produce sperm immobilization, or by combined means. The following are used (***see* the box below**).

Types of Barrier Methods

- **Mechanical**
  Male: Condom
  Female: Condom, diaphragm, cervical cap
- **Chemical** (vaginal contraceptives)
  Creams: Delfen (nonoxynol-9, 12.5%)
  Jelly: Koromex, Volpar paste
  Foam tablets: Aerosol foams, T or Contab, Sponge (today)
- **Combination**
  Combined use of mechanical and chemical methods

CONDOM (MALE)

Condoms are made of polyurethane or latex. Polyurethane condoms are thinner and suitable to those who are sensitive to latex rubber. It is the most widely practiced method used by the male. In India, one particular brand (latex) is widely marketed as 'Nirodh'. The efficacy of condoms can be augmented by improving the quality of the products and by adding spermicidal agents during its use. **Protection against sexually transmitted disease (STD) is an additional advantage**. Occasionally, the partner may be allergic to latex.

The method is suitable for couples who want to space their families and who have contraindications to the use of oral contraceptive or IUD. These are also suitable to those who have infrequent sexual intercourse.

FEMALE CONDOM (FEMIDOM) (FIG. 30.16A)

It is a pouch made of polyurethane which lines the vagina and also the external genitalia. It is 17 cm in length with one flexible polyurethane ring at each end. Inner ring at the closed end is smaller compared to the outer ring. Inner ring is inserted at the apex of the vagina and the outer ring remains outside. It gives protection against STIs cytomegalovirus (CMV) [HIV, hepatitis B virus (HBV)] and pelvic inflammatory disease. It is expensive. Multiple uses can be made with washing, drying, and with lubrication. Failure rate is about 5–21/HWY.

Use of Condom

(a) As an elective contraceptive method; (b) As an interim form of contraception during pill use, following vasectomy operation (*see* later) and if an IUD is thought lost until a new IUD can be fitted; (c) During the treatment of trichomonal vaginitis of the wife, the husband should use it during the course of treatment irrespective of contraceptive practice; (d) Immunological infertility—male partner to use for 3 months. For other noncontraceptive benefits (Table 30.9).

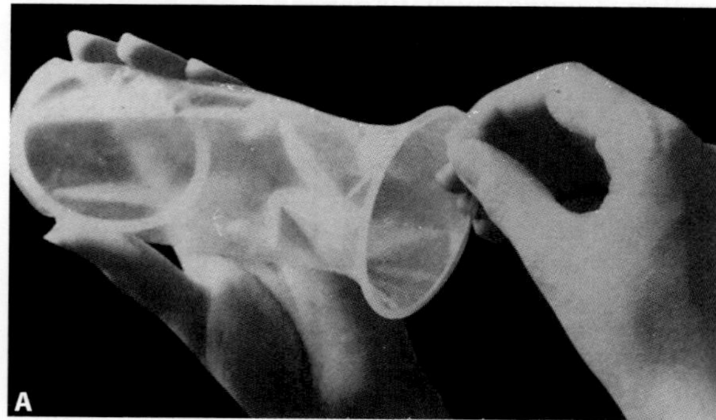
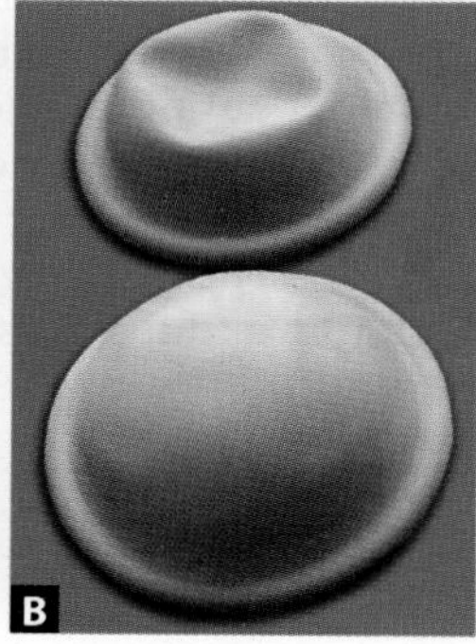
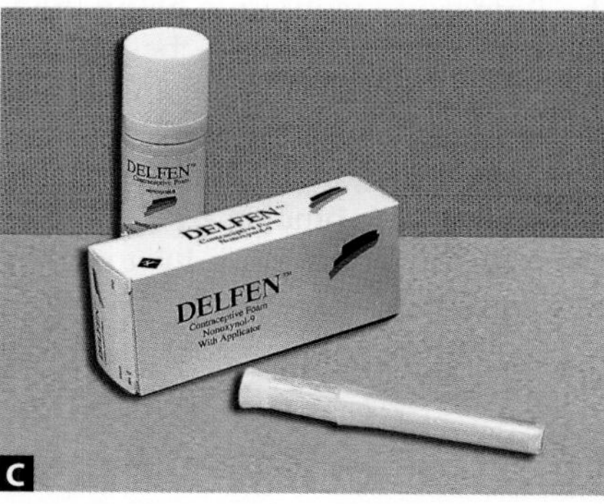

Figs. 30.16A to C: (A) Female condom; (B) Commonly used conventional contraceptive (diaphragm); (C) Vaginal contraceptive (nonoxynol-9, 12.5%).

TABLE 30.9: Condom.

Advantages		*Disadvantages*
▪ Cheaper with no contraindications	NIRODH Lubricated condoms	▪ May accidentally break or slip off during coitus
▪ No side effects		▪ Inadequate sexual pleasure
▪ Easy to carry, simple to use and disposable		▪ Allergic reaction (latex)
▪ Protection against sexually transmitted diseases, e.g. gonorrhea, chlamydia, HPV and HIV		▪ To discard after one coital act.
▪ Protection against pelvic inflammatory diseases		
▪ Reduces the incidence of tubal infertility and ectopic pregnancy		
▪ Protection against cervical cell abnormalities		
▪ Useful where the coital act is infrequent and irregular		
Precautions: (a) To use a fresh condom for every act of coitus; (b) To cover the penis with condom prior to genital contact; (c) Create a reservoir at the tip; (d) To withdraw while the penis is still erect; (e) To grasp the base of the condom during withdrawal.		

Failure rate—15 (HWY). (HPV: human papilloma virus; HIV: human immunodeficiency virus)

TABLE 30.10: Diaphragm.

Advantages	*Disadvantages*
▪ Cheap ▪ Can be used repeatedly for a long time ▪ Reduces PID/STIs to some extent ▪ Protects against cervical precancer and cancer	▪ Requires help of a doctor or paramedical person to measure the size required ▪ Risk of vaginal irritation, abrasion and urinary tract infection are there ▪ Not suitable for women with uterine prolapse.

Failure rate—16 (HWY)
(PID: pelvic inflammatory disease; STIs: sexually transmitted diseases)

DIAPHRAGM (TABLE 30.10 AND FIG. 30.16B)

It is an intravaginal device made of latex with flexible metal or spring ring at the margin. Its diameter varies from 5 cm to 10 cm. It requires a medical or paramedical personnel to measure the size of the device. The largest size should be used without any discomfort or undue pressure. Caya (FDA approved) is a single dose diaphragm that does not require fitting by a medical person. **Failure rate:** Typical use 13–17%; perfect use 4–8%. Diaphragm and cervical cap may also reduce the risk of cervical cancer. Diaphragm should completely cover the cervix. As it cannot effectively prevent ascent of the sperms alongside the margin of the device, additional chemical spermicidal agent should be placed on the superior surface of the device during insertion, so that it remains in contact with the cervix. **The device is introduced up to 3 hours before intercourse and is to be kept for at least 8 hours after the last coital act.** Ill-fitting and accidental displacement during intercourse increase the failure rate.

VAGINAL CONTRACEPTIVES (FIG. 30.16C)

Spermicides

Spermicides are available as vaginal foams, gels, creams, tablets, and suppositories. Usually, they contain **surfactants like nonoxynol-9, octoxynol or benzalkonium chloride. The cream or jelly** is introduced high in the vagina with the help of the applicator soon before coitus. The duration of maximum effectiveness is usually not more than one hour. **Foam tablets** (1–2) are to be introduced high in the vagina at least 5 minutes prior to intercourse. In isolation, it is not effective (18–29 HWY), but enhances the efficacy of condom or diaphragm when used along with it. There may be occasional local allergic manifestations either in the vagina or vulva.

Spermicide-Microbicide combination supports the natural defense maintaining the acidic pH and acts as antimicrobial also. They are controlled by the female. These agents are protective against STIs including HIV. The agents containing surfactant, destroy the sperm membrane and also the outer envelops of the virus and bacteria.

Vaginal Contraceptive Sponge (Today)

It is made of polyurethane impregnated with 1 g of nonoxynol-9 as a spermicide. Nonoxynol-9 acts as a surfactant which either immobilizes or kills sperm. **It releases spermicide during coitus, absorbs ejaculate and blocks the entrance to the cervical canal. The sponge should not be removed for 6 hours after intercourse. Its failure rate (HWY) is about—parous women: 32–20, nulliparous 16–9.** Currently, it is observed that nonoxynol-9 is not effective in preventing cervical gonorrhea, chlamydia or HIV infection. Moreover, it produces lesions in the genital tract when used frequently. Those lesions are associated with increased risk of HIV transmission.

FERTILITY AWARENESS METHOD (TABLE 30.11)

Fertility awareness method requires partner's cooperation. The woman should know the fertile time of her menstrual cycle.

Rhythm Method

This is the only method approved by the Roman Catholic Church. **The method is based on identification of the fertile period of a cycle and to abstain from sexual intercourse during that period.** This requires partner's cooperation. The methods to determine the approximate time of ovulation and the fertile period include—(a) Recording of previous menstrual cycles (**calendar rhythm**); (b) Noting the basal body temperature chart (**temperature rhythm**); (c) Noting excessive mucoid vaginal discharge (**mucus rhythm**). **The users of the calendar method** obtain the period of abstinence from calculations based on the previous twelve menstrual cycle records. **The first unsafe day is obtained** by subtracting 20 days from the length of the shortest cycle and **last unsafe day** by deducting 10 days from the longest cycle. **Users of temperature rhythm** require abstinence until the third day of the rise of temperature. **Users of mucus rhythm** require abstinence on all days of noticeable mucus and for 3 days thereafter.

Coitus Interruptus (Withdrawal) (Table 30.12)

It is the oldest and probably the most widely accepted contraceptive method used by man. **It necessitates withdrawal of penis shortly before ejaculation.** It requires sufficient self-control by the man so that withdrawal of penis precede ejaculation.

TABLE 30.11: Fertility awareness methods (rhythm method).

Advantages	*Disadvantages*
▪ No cost ▪ Lack of side effects ▪ The period of abstinence is determined by calculating the length of the woman's previous menstrual cycles. Three assumptions are considered: (a) Human ovum can be fertilized for about 24 hours after ovulation; (b) Sperm can fertilize 3–5 day after coitus; (c) Ovulation usually occurs 12–16 days before the onset of menstruation	▪ Difficult to calculate the safe period reliably ▪ Needs several months training to use these methods ▪ Compulsory abstinence from sexual act during certain periods ▪ Not applicable during lactational amenorrhea or when the periods are irregular

Failure rate—20–30 (HWY)

TABLE 30.12: Coitus Interruptus.

Advantages	Disadvantages
▪ No appliance is required ▪ No cost	▪ Requires sufficient self-control by the man ▪ The woman may develop anxiety neurosis, vaginismus or pelvic congestion ▪ Chance of pregnancy is more: • Precoital secretion may contain sperm • Accidental chance of sperm

Failure rate—20 (HWY)

Breastfeeding, Lactational Amenorrhea (LAM)

Prolonged and exclusive (6 months) breastfeeding offer a natural protection against pregnancy. The criteria for successful of LAM are: Continuous amenorrhea and exclusive breastfeeding up to 6 months. Night nursing is highly protective. This is more effective in women who are **amenorrheic than those who are menstruating**. The risk of pregnancy to a woman who is exclusively breastfeeding for 6 months and amenorrheic is **less than 2% in the first 6 months**. Otherwise, the **failure rate** is high (1–10%). Thus during breastfeeding, additional contraceptive support should be given by condom, IUCD or injectable steroids where available, to provide complete contraception.

When the woman is **exclusively breastfeeding**, a contraceptive method should be used in the **3rd postpartum month and with partial or no breastfeeding, she should use it in the 3rd postpartum week**.

Fertility awareness based methods are: (a) **Natural contraception** (rhythm method, coitus interruptus, and LAM); (b) **Barrier method** (condoms, diaphragm, and spermicides).

CONTRACEPTIVE COUNSELING AND PRESCRIPTION

Pregnancy carries an overall maternal mortality around 400 per 100,000 total births in the developing countries (India 167/100,000 LB) and the same in the developed countries is less than 10. Whereas annual number of deaths per 100,000 exposed to pill is 1.3 and with that of IUDs is 1. The same from tubal sterilization is 1.2 and vasectomy is 0.1. The risks of death from automobile driving is 1 in 6,000 per year. Contraception usually carries less risk compared to pregnancy. **Importantly, benefits of contraceptive use outweigh the risks of pregnancy.**

No single universally acceptable method has yet been discovered. The individual should have the liberty to choose any of the currently available well-tested method, which may even vary at each phase in her reproductive life. If one compares the risks and benefits of any contraceptive, it is observed that more deaths occur as a result of unplanned pregnancies than from the hazards of any modern contraceptive method (excluding 'pill' users over 35 who smoke).

Important factors for the selection of any contraceptive method for an individual are—relative safety, effectiveness, side effects, and willingness to use the method correctly and consistently. The other factors to consider are the frequency of coitus, the need of lactation and prevention of STIs. Acceptability is probably the most critical factor in the effectiveness of a contraceptive method. Couple (client) should be helped to make an informed choice. A clear account of the risks and the benefits for an individual method is given. Regular follow-up and compliance with the instructions are to be ensured. It is also essential that an informed (verbal) consent is obtained and recorded.

STERILIZATION COUNSELING

It includes a discussion of the following issues: (a) Desire of the individual partner (male/female); (b) Procedure selection; (c) Failure rate; (d) Risks and side effects; (e) Issue of reversibility. Reversal is more likely to be successful after laparoscopic clips compared to laparotomy procedures. However, the risks of ectopic pregnancy is there; and (f) Options for alternative long active (equally effective) reversible methods (implants, Cu-T 380A) should be given.

PRESCRIPTION

Conventional contraceptives can be safely prescribed during the entire reproductive period as elective choice or as an alternative to 'pill' or IUD if they are contraindicated or unacceptable to the couple. As such only the advice regarding the use of 'pill' or IUD during different phases of reproductive life is discussed.

Adolescent Girls

Low-dose combined pills are most effective for the sexually active adolescents. It is the contraceptive of choice. However, **DMPA or norplant** may be an alternative when accepted. There is no concern about their future reproductive endocrinologic function or the epiphyseal closure in postmenarchal girls.

Newly Married Couple

A highly effective and acceptable contraceptive like DMPA, or POPs, could be prescribed. IUD may not be prescribed. As such COCs are recommended provided there is no contraindication. Apart from effective contraception 'COCs' have got many noncontraceptive benefits as well (p. 408).

Spacing of Births

▪ **Postabortal** ▪ **Postpartum** ▪ **Interval**

Postabortal

The contraceptive practice should be started soon following the abortion process is completed. DMPA, POPs or COCs could be a choice. IUD is an alternative.

Postpartum

▪ **Nonlactating** ▪ **Lactating**

Nonlactating

Contraceptive practice should be started after 3 weeks. 'POP' is good; IUD is an equally effective alternative. Injectable DMPA could be used as it is devoid of any estrogen-related side effects. Implanon (etonogestrel) may be prescribed.

Lactating

In fully lactating women (5-6 feeds and spending about 60 minutes in 24 hours), the contraceptive practice may be safely withheld for 10 weeks postpartum. For doubtful adverse effects of steroids on lactation and on the babies through the ingested milk, **'pill' is better withheld. Minipill (POP) or injectable steroid (DMPA)** is ideal. Alternatively, IUD can be inserted.

Interval

Below the age of 35 years, she can have her choice to either 'pill' or IUD following adequate counseling. In women above the age of 35, especially who are smokers, IUD should be inserted in preference to 'pill'. Injectables (DMPA) or implant (Implanon) is the other alternative.

To stop future pregnancies: The decision to advise permanent sterilization should be judiciously given, especially to the under-privileged women in the face of high perinatal and infant mortality rate. The cases are to be individualized. However, a two-child formula is usually recommended and as such, a couple having two children who have been fully immunized can have permanent sterilization (husband or wife). If the couple is not motivated to undergo the sterilization operation, any of the temporary methods is to be prescribed till the end of the reproductive period of the wife. Women who have completed their family but do not desire for permanent sterilization, may use IUD (CU-T 380A) or implant if accepted.

Older Women

Contraception should be prescribed to avoid unplanned pregnancy. Low dose pills can be continued till menopause (with monitoring) in the low-risk group. Progestin-only pill, injectable progestin (DMPA), LNG-IUS are the other alternatives. Barrier methods and vaginal spermicides can be used either as a primary or back-up method. Usually, fertility is reduced after 40 years of age.

Women at risk of STIs need dual protection against pregnancy and STIs. They should use condom with spermicides or use another contraceptive (DMPA, COC, or POP), method in conjunction with condom.

Women using enzyme inducers are advised to take COCs having more than usual dosage or other method of contraception (DMPA, IUDs). **Emergency contraception (postcoital contraception)** when required as emergency, POP, IUD or other methods can be used (p. 412).

ONGOING TRIALS AND SELECTIVE AVAILABILITY

The following are used on trial basis or are available in selected countries:

- **Combined injectable contraceptives (CICs):** Both estrogen and progestin are combined in these monthly injectables. Preparations available are: DMPA 25 mg with estradiol cypionate 5 mg (Cyclofem) and NET-EN 50 mg with estradiol valerate 5 mg (Mesigyna). It is given within first 5 days of menstruation. Next injection should be on the same date of each month (4-week schedule). Fertility return is quick.

  Drawbacks: (a) Irregular or prolonged menstrual bleeding; (b) Not suitable for nursing mothers. It is has been currently withdrawn from the market.
- **Transdermal patch: Patch** contains 0.75 μg ethynyl estradiol and 6 mg norelgestromin. When used as a cream to the skin provides effective contraception. Patch delivers 150 μg norelgestromin (progestin) and 20 μg ethinylestradiol daily. It has an area of 20 cm^2 (4.5 × 4.5 cm). The patch is used weekly for 3 weeks and one week off for withdrawal bleeding. It is well-tolerated, safe and effective.

  Drawbacks: Patch detachment, skin reaction and high failure in overweight women (>90 kg). It is applied over the buttocks, upper and outer arm, or lower abdomen but not over the breasts. Failure rate is 1.2 per 100 women years. Patch failure rate is high in woman weighing ≥90 kg. Patch may increase the risk of VTE.
- **Vaginal ring:** Containing levonorgestrel covered by silastic tubing has been introduced. They are 5 and 6 cm in diameter. The vaginal ring delivers levonorgestrel (20 μg/day) to maintain a constant blood level like norplant. The rings are replaced by 90 days. Pregnancy rate is 3 per 100 women. This method is under woman's control.
- **Combined ring (Nuva ring):** Soft, flexible transparent ethylene vinyl ring releases ethinyl estradiol (15 μg) and etonogestrel (metabolite of desogestrel) 120 μg daily over a period of 21 days. The ring is inserted on the first day of menses and is worn for 3 weeks. The ring must be reinserted within the next 3 hours, if removed for any reason, vaginal route use avoids GI absorption, first pass liver metabolism and has lowest systemic estrogenic side effects. It is then removed and after 1 week (after the withdrawal bleed) a new ring is inserted. It acts by inhibiting ovulation. Pearl index is 0.65 and cycle control is good. The ring (54 mm diameter and 4 mm thick) is inserted within 5 days of menses. Side effects are, headache, leukorrhea, vaginitis, and expulsion.
- **Fibroplant (LNG):** Similar to Mirena, a smaller version of levonorgestrel system is currently being tested. Its small size is suitable for the perimenopausal women in whom the uterus shrinks. It releases LNG at the rate of 14 μg/day. It is also used as an HRT for postmenopausal women.
- **Uniplant:** It is a single rod implant, containing 55 mg of nomegestrol (newer progestin) with a release rate of 100 μg per day. It provides contraception for one year.
- **Biodegradable implants** are under study. **Capronor** (single capsule) releases levonorgestrel from the polymer E-caprolactone at a rate 10 times faster than from silastic. The longer capsule contains 26 mg of levonorgestrel and inhibits ovulation in about 50% of cycles. Contraceptive efficacy is comparable to norplant. The capsule begins to disappear after 12 months.
- **Injectable contraceptive (biodegradable)** in the form of microspheres using copolymer (lactide-glycolide) have been studied. Hormone currently used in the microsphere (0.06–0.1 mm diameter) is either norethindrone acetate or norethindrone combined with ethinyl estradiol. Injection is given over the gluteal muscle. Unlike implant, microspheres cannot be removed once injected.
- **Luteinizing hormone-releasing hormone (LHRH)** agonist (buserelin) and antagonist (cetrorelix) acts by preventing the pituitary response to the endogenous GnRH. They have the potential to arrest follicular growth and endometrial development. Unwanted side effects (loss of libido and hot flushes) are avoided using add-back therapy. Long-term effects are not known as yet.
- **Newer IUDs—a frameless IUD (GyneFix)** is made of six copper beads (330 mm^2 of Cu) on a monofilament polypropylene thread. The upper and lower beads are

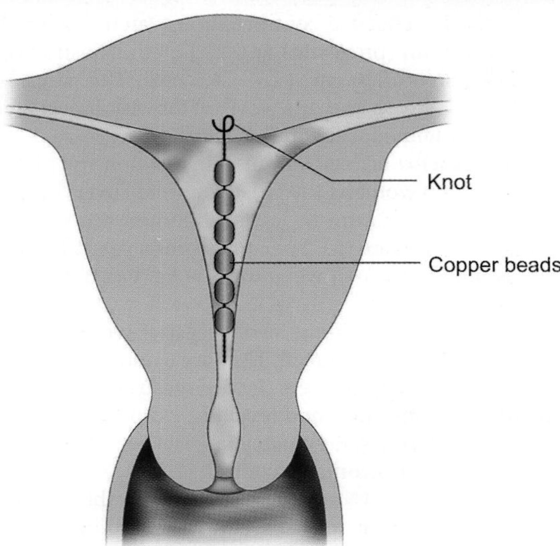

Fig. 30.17: Frameless intrauterine devices (IUD) (GyneFix).

crimped onto the thread. The thread is knotted at one end which is embedded into the fundal myometrium to a depth of 1 cm. This anchors the device at the fundus. **The advantages** of the device (Fig. 30.17) over the framed ones are significantly reduced risk of expulsion, dysmenorrhea, bleeding, and infection. Threadless (Butterfly) IUD is also found promising to reduce the risk of side effects (infection). It can be removed with a hook when required. This device is especially suited for nulligravid women.

TRANSCERVICAL STERILIZATION

- **Quinacrine pellet,** 252 mg is inserted on two occasions one month apart into the uterine cavity transcervically through a hysteroscope during the proliferative phase. It is repeated in the next cycle. It acts as a sclerosing agent. Pregnancy rate is 2–3 per 100 woman years. WHO does not recommend it due to its carcinogenic concern.
- **Adiana** has been withdrawn from the market.
- **Essure** is a 4 cm long, 2 mm diameter, microcoil (spring-like device) made of nickel-titanium steel alloy coil within which lie polyethylene terephthalate fibers (Fig. 30.18). **It is inserted into each fallopian tube transcervically using a hysteroscope.** The tube is blocked permanently when scar tissue grows into the device. To ensure proper placement and total occlusion of essure a hysterosalpingogram is done three months after. Its success rate is similar to surgical sterilization (<1%). **For the first 3 months, the woman needs to use a temporary contraceptive method** in addition, till the scar tissue is formed.

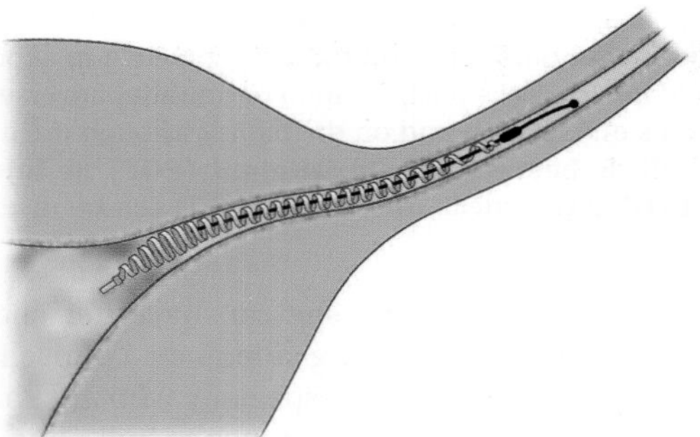

Fig. 30.18: Essure device within the intramural portion of the fallopian tube. It is inserted using a hysteroscope.

- **Ovion eclipse** is under trial. Compared to Essure, it is short in length by 2 cm.
- **Ovabloc (third generation)** causes immediate tubal occlusion. Silicon matrix is instilled into the fallopian tube that becomes solid immediately. Tubal blockage is to be verified by HSG after 3 months. Success rate is nearly 100%.

MALE CONTRACEPTION METHODS

Testosterone or a combination of testosterone and progestin (monthly injection or implant) is found to suppress sperm production. Testosterone undecanoate is used and found successful.

- **GnRH analog** produce a decline in sperm density, sperm mobility, and a decrease in testosterone level. The marked loss of libido makes it unacceptable. Add-back therapy (testosterone) is used to overcome the side effects.
- **Gossypol:** It has been discovered in China; an extract from cotton seed. It acts directly on the seminiferous tubules inhibiting spermatogenesis. The side effects are fatigue, decreased libido, and delayed recovery of sperm count. The serious side effects are hypokalemic paralysis and cardiac arrhythmias.

Intra vas device (IVD): Two plugs are implanted in each vas to block sperm transport through the vasa deferens. Plugs could be removed to make it a reversible procedure. Its contraceptive effectiveness is being studied.

KEY POINTS

- **Barrier methods** of contraception include condom, diaphragm and vaginal contraceptives (chemicals and sponge today).
- **Natural contraception includes**—rhythm method, coitus interruptus, and breastfeeding (p. 421).
- **Conventional contraceptive methods** include use of condom, vaginal diaphragm, spermicidals, and rhythm method.
- **Fertility awareness methods** (periodic abstinence) are mostly dependent upon the compliance of use.
- **Barrier methods** have high failure rate unless used correctly and consistently.
- These must be fitted by a health professional.
- Male condoms can reduce the risk of STIs including HIV.
- **Spermicide and microbicide** are used as combined agents. In isolation, these should not be used (p. 421).
- Lactational amenorrhea is an effective method of contraception. Failure rate is 2 per 100 WY.
- **Contraceptive counseling and prescription**—should consider the relative safety, effectiveness, and side effects of the method. It is important that the method is used correctly and consistently (p. 422).
- **It is hard to predict** contraceptive trends in the immediate future as the results of contraceptive research are still unclear about the risks and benefits.

CHAPTER 31 Basic Principles of Radiation Therapy, Chemotherapy, Immunotherapy and Gene Therapy in Gynecology

CHAPTER OUTLINE

INTRODUCTION

Radiotherapy and chemotherapy are the important modalities of therapy for human cancers apart from surgery. They may have a curative role (e.g. radiotherapy in carcinoma cervix and chemotherapy in gestational trophoblastic neoplasia) when used as a primary therapy. **Multidisciplinary approach** is needed for the treatment of some malignancies to improve the outcome. Radiotherapy and/or chemotherapy should be considered even for palliation of incurable symptoms. The basic principles of radiotherapy and chemotherapy in relation to gynecologic malignancies have been discussed in the Chapter. Current understanding in immunotherapy and gene therapy have also been highlighted.

RADIATION THERAPY

RADIOBIOLOGY OF NORMAL TISSUES

The effects of radiation on tissues are generally of two types: (1) Loss of mature functional cells by apoptosis (programmed cell death). This usually occurs within 24 hours of radiation. (2) Loss of cellular reproductive capacity. The severity depends upon the total dose of radiation, length of time over which radiotherapy is delivered and the radiosensitivity of the particular cell types. Usually lost cells are replaced by proliferation of surviving stem cells or progenitor cells.

Ionizing radiation used for therapy may be: (a) Electromagnetic radiation; (b) Particulate radiation.

Electromagnetic Radiation

This consists of quanta of energy and wavelength (photon radiation). They are of two types—X-rays and gamma rays. These electromagnetic waves travels in discrete bundles called 'photons'.

- **Gamma rays** are produced spontaneously as a result of decay of the **atomic nucleus** of some radioactive isotopes. ^{60}Cobalt or ^{192}Iridium is a source of γ-rays.
- **X-rays** are produced **outside the atomic nucleus**. When fast-moving electrons approach the fields around the nuclei of atoms of a target material (tungsten), they are deflected from their path. The energy thus emitted in the form of electromagnetic radiation (photons) is X-rays. Machines such as betatron (circular fashion) and linear accelerator (linear fashion) can accelerate electrons with high kinetic energy. Therefore, X-rays generated by these machines are very high in energy.
- **X-rays and gamma rays** are collectively called photons. When photons interact with matter (tissue), three effects are observed: **(1) Photoelectric effect**; **(2) Compton scattering**; and **(3) Pair production**. In human radiation therapy, **compton scattering** is the major interaction of photons with tissue (Fig. 31.1). X-rays and gamma rays have shorter wavelength and high frequency. They have high kinetic energy. X-rays and gamma rays possess considerable power of tissue penetration depending on the photon energy and the density of the matter through which they pass. The photon energy produced from radioactive cobalt is 1.2 million electron volts (MeV). External photon beam radiation is usually derived from a linear accelerator (p. 427).

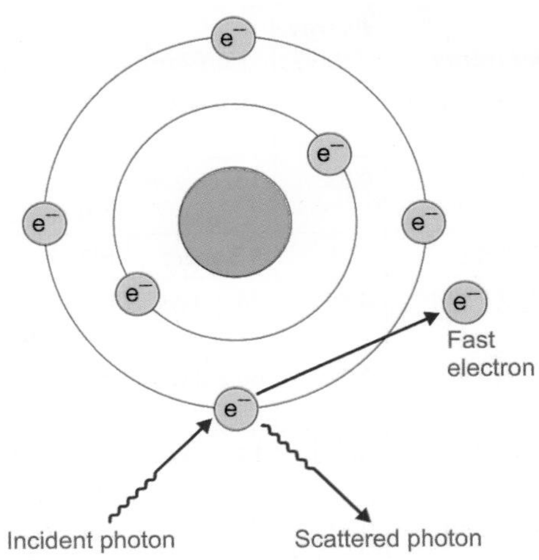

Fig. 31.1: Compton scattering effect.

Principles of Radiation Physics and Radiobiology

- In the treatment of gynecologic malignancy the most common source of radiation is electromagnetic (photon) radiation. Photons are generally referred to as X-rays or gamma rays.
- **Radioactive nuclei particles** give off alpha and beta particles and gamma rays.
- **Radium 226, Cesium 137, Gold 198, Iodine 125, Cobalt 60, Iridium 192** are used as radioactive sources for therapeutic purpose (Table 31.1).
- **Radioactive substances** are encapsulated to absorb alpha and beta particles leaving gamma rays to attain therapeutic purpose.
- **Oxygen enhancement ratio (OER):** The ratio of radiation dose required for a given level of cell killing under hypoxic condition compared with the dose needed in air.
- **Inverse square law:** Dose of radiation at a particular point varies inversely proportional to the square of the distance from the source of radiation.
- **Fractional cell kill:** Each radiation dose kills a constant fraction of the tumor cells.
- **Radiation dose rate:** Large radiation doses per fraction cause the largest number of tumor cell kills; at the same time the large doses may cause maximum damage on normal tissues. Ultimately this is the cause of many early and late complications.
- **Radiation resistance:** Tumor cells are mostly sensitive to the effects of radiation. This results in tumor regression or tumor repopulation during or after radiation treatment. Radiation resistance associated with (a) rapid cell repair of radiation damage; (b) Active concentration of chemical radio-protectors; or (c) Cellular hypoxia.
- **Cell cycle dependency of cell kill:** Actively proliferating tumor cells are most after often killed by radiation therapy. Ionizing radiation has its greatest cell kill effect during the mitotic phase (M phase) and to some extent in the late G-1 phase and in early deoxyribonucleic acid (DNA) synthesis phase.
- **Radiosensitivity:** p. 428

TABLE 31.1: Radioactive isotopes used in gynecological malignancies.

Element isotope	Energy (MeV)	Half-life	Clinical use
Cesium 137 (^{137}Cs)	0.662	30 years	LDR intracavitary, interstitial
Radium 226 (^{226}Ra)	0.83	1626 years	LDR intracavitary, interstitial
Cobalt 60 (^{60}Co)	1.25	5.3 years	HDR intracavitary
Iridium 192 (^{192}Ir)	0.38	74.2 days	Interstitial implant and intracavitary
Iodine 125 (^{125}I)	0.028	60.2 days	Interstitial implant (permanent)
Phosphorus 32 (^{32}P)	None	14.3 days	Intracavitary (permanent)
Gold 198 (^{198}Au)	0.412	2.7 days	Interstitial (permanent)

Particulate Radiation

This consists of atomic subparticles such as electrons, protons, and neutrons. Only electrons (β-rays) are used in radiotherapy.

TECHNIQUES OF RADIATION THERAPY

Brachytherapy

It gives a very high dose of radiation where the source of radiation is placed within, or close to the tumor. The application may be: (a) Intracavitary; (b) Interstitial; or (c) Surface (skin). Damage to normal tissues is less as there is rapid falloff of radiation around the source (inverse square law).

Intracavitary: The devices for brachytherapy consist of hollow stem (intrauterine tandem), which is placed within the uterine cavity (Fig. 31.2). Specially designed devices used for vaginal placements are called vaginal ovoids or colpostats.

Interstitial: The form of brachytherapy consists of placement of radioactive sources (needles, wires or seeds) within the tissues. Commonly used sources are Iridium 192 (^{192}Ir), Cesium 137 (^{137}Cs), and Cobalt 60 (^{60}Co). Small volume of tumor, as in early cases of vaginal carcinoma, can be treated with the method. Normal tissues are spared from radiation injury.

Intraperitoneal: Intraperitoneal instillation (^{32}P) is another mode of local therapy.

After loading technique: It is a modern development of brachytherapy to prevent radiation complications to the personnel. A mock insertion of applicators is performed and X-ray is taken to note their exact position. After loading technique may be manual or by remote control. Later on, live radioactive sources are introduced by remote control in identical manner. Remote after loading system uses selectron (^{137}Cs) or high-dose selectron (^{60}Co). Remote

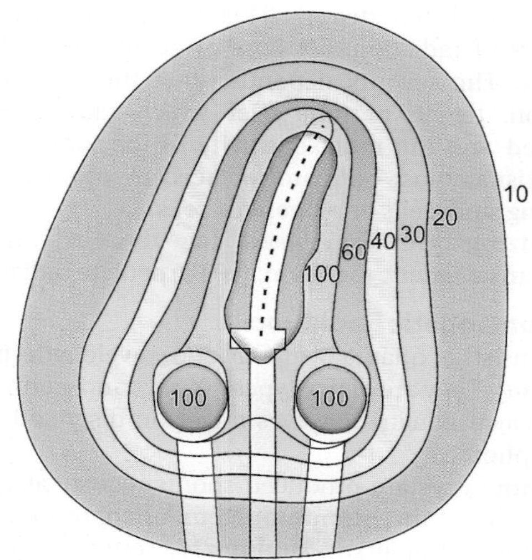

Fig. 31.2: Isodose distribution curve with intracavitary irradiation.

control systems allow complete protection of staff from radiation exposure.

Brachytherapy can be either low dose rate (LDR) or a high dose rate (HDR) system. LDR require hospital admission and deliver dose at about 50–100 cGy/hour. HDR systems are commonly done as outpatient basis. The dose rate delivered is at 100 cGy/minute.

Advantages: Localized high radiation dose to a small tumor volume with high local control. Radiation dose in the surrounding normal tissues is less as there is sharp fall off according to inverse square law (*see* above).

Disadvantages: (a) Large tumors are usually unsuitable unless used following external beam radiation therapy (EBRT) and/or chemotherapy; (b) Risks of exposure to medical and nursing personnel due to gamma rays.

External Beam Radiotherapy

External beam radiotherapy (EBRT) or teletherapy is the treatment with beams of ionizing radiation produced from a source external to the patient. Superficial tumors may be treated with X-rays of low energy in the range of 80–300 KV. Deep-seated tumors are usually treated using megavoltage photons.

Cobalt 60 is the common teletherapy source for EBRT, the other one is Cesium 137. External radiation therapy is used to treat large volumes (tumor, lymph nodes, parametrium) of tumor (p. 294). It is designed to deliver a uniform radiation dose to the tumor volume without 'hot' (excess dose) or 'cold' (under dose) spots. Accurate tumor localization and volume measurement are essential. Greater the tumor volume, higher the radiation dose required.

Instillation of Radioisotopes into the Peritoneal or Pleural Cavity

Radioactive isotopes of either gold or phosphorus, linked to carrier colloids, are commonly used in ovarian cancer. This can give radiation only to a depth of 4–8 mm. Radioactive chromic phosphate (^{32}P) emits pure β-rays and has got longer half-life (14.3 days) and deeper penetration (8 mm) power compared to radio gold (^{198}Au). Small volume of tumor in the peritoneal or pleural cavity is treated with solution of radioisotopes.

Palliative radiotherapy is aimed to achieve quick symptom control. It may have little or no impact on the survival outcome of the patient. Lowest dose of therapy is preferred so that normal tissue damage is avoided.

MEASUREMENT OF RADIATION

Radiation absorption dose (Gray) is the unit used to measure the amount of energy absorbed per unit mass of tissue. **One gray (Gy) is equivalent to 1 Joule/kg which is equivalent to 100 rads. Currently, the term centigray (cGy) is used. One cGy is equivalent to one rad.** Amount of radiation the patient receives is calculated by **dosimetry**. Homogeneous irradiation of tissues is desirable (Fig. 31.2). Primary tumor should receive high dose. Brachytherapy and teletherapy should be combined to provide adequate irradiation to the primary tumor as well as the pelvic lymph nodes and the parametrium (Fig. 31.3).

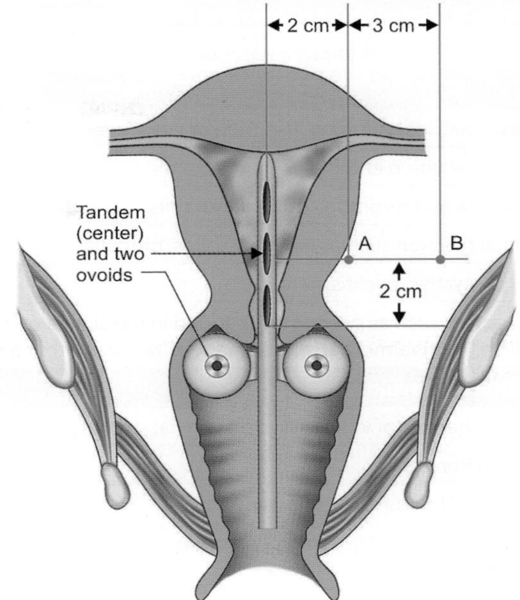

Fig. 31.3: Tandem (center) and two ovoids placement for carcinoma cervix (Manchester technique). Points A and B are the reference points (p. 294).

Biological Effects of Radiation (Radiobiology)

Radiation has got two modes of action:

1. **Direct action:** Where the radiation is absorbed, it causes damage to DNA directly. This is the predominant mechanism of action of particulate radiation (neutrons).
2. **Indirect action:** Where the radiation interact with other substances (H_2O) in the cell to produce free radicals (OH^-) which in turn damages the DNA.

Radiation, depending on the dose and time of exposure may cause (a) gene mutation; (b) abnormal cell mitosis; and (c) derangement of reproductive ability of the cell—'progeria'.

Compton effect produces fast electrons by dislodging orbital electrons of tissues, through which they pass. This fast electron ionizes molecules along its path. There is production of free hydrogen atoms, free hydroxyl radicals, and H_2O_2. These ionized molecules react with proteins, enzymes, and nucleic acids resulting in structural and functional alteration of a cell.

The target for radiation injury is DNA. Ultimately, there is limited cell mitosis and mitotic cell death. There is cytoplasmic vacuolation and fragmentation. Ionizing radiation also produces damage to nuclear and plasma membranes.

This **effect of ionizing radiation** is common for both the normal and neoplastic tissues, encountered in the radiation path. Radiation complications are mainly due to interaction with the normal tissues (Table 31.2). **When the radiation effect to a cell is sublethal, cellular DNA may undergo repair and the cell survives. Lethal effect kills the cell.**

TABLE 31.2: Radiation reactions and their management.

Radiation reactions	*Management*
Early	
Anorexia, nausea, vomiting, lassitude or even fever	▪ Antiemetics (p. 425) ▪ Antihistaminics
Diarrhea (radiation enteritis)	Intravenous fluid therapy to correct electrolyte imbalance
Leukopenia and thrombocytopenia, anemia	Hematinics, blood transfusion, G–CSF, erythropoietin (EPO) (Table 31.13)
Intestinal reaction such as enteritis, colitis, proctitis	Antispasmodics, analgesics, antidiarrheal agents
Urinary—cystitis, pyelitis, hematuria	Urinary antiseptics and analgesics
Skin reaction such as peeling often found in moist area of the vulva. This is almost absent in megavoltage radiotherapy	▪ To keep the area dry ▪ Application of 1% aqueous gentian violet
Late (due to vasculitis and fibrosis)	
Atrophic changes of vulvar skin and vaginal stricture	Markedly minimized with megavoltage therapy
Radiation fibrosis	Often confused with recurrence of growth
Pathological fracture due to osteoporosis	Usual treatment for fracture. There is no problem in union
Intestine—stricture, bleeding per rectum, perforation, obstruction	Appropriate therapy
Malabsorption syndrome with megaloblastic anemia	Administration of folic acid
Proctosigmoiditis	Steroid enemas, antidiarrheal agents
Fistula	
Vesicovaginal *or* rectovaginal	Difficult to treat locally
Usually occurs 1–2 years following primary therapy	Colpocleisis may be an alternative
Ovary	Radiation damage, menopausal symptoms

Radiation Dose

According to the **'inverse square law'** there is reduction of radiation at a distance from the source in brachytherapy. This protects the normal tissues (isodose distribution curve, Fig. 31.2).

A planning computer calculates the field sizes, the dose from each field and the angles of the treatment machine. High energy machines spare the skin and deliver more radiation below the skin surface. Linear accelerators which deliver X-rays of 4–8 MeV are used currently. Treatment is carried out in a especially protected room. During the treatment time, the patient should be alone and he/she is supervised using a television camera. Safety precautions of radiation are maintained.

Radiocurability is the elimination of tumor at the primary or metastatic site due to a direct effect of radiation.

Radiosensitivity means the response of the tumor to irradiation. Radiosensitivity is measured in terms of loss of cellular proliferative capacity due to the damage to DNA. Accumulation of sublethal injury following repeat radiation leads to ultimate DNA damage and cell death. Radiosensitivity varies with the type of cancer.

a. **Highly sensitive:** Dysgerminoma, embryonal cancer, small cell cancer and lymphoma.
b. **Moderately sensitive:** Squamous cell cancer, adenocarcinoma.
c. **Poorly sensitive:** Melanoma, glioma

Radiosensitivity depends on several factors.

- **Tissue hypoxia:** Higher the hypoxic fraction of cells, the less (2–3 times) is the radiation response. Hypoxic cells are more resistant to radiation compared to toxic cells.
- **Proportion of mitotic (clonogenic) cells:** Clonogenic cells are more radiosensitive.
- **Cell cycle:** Mitotic cells (M phase) and G2 cells are more radiosensitive compared to late S-phase cells (Fig. 31.4).
- **Tumor specificity:** Certain tumors (dysgerminomas) are more radiosensitive than the others.
- **Tumor volume:** Smaller the tumor volume → lesser the hypoxic cells → less the radiation dose better the radiation response.

Lesser the photon wavelength more is the penetrating power and energy of ionizing radiation. Supervoltage and megavoltage radiation (^{60}Co, ^{137}Cs, ^{226}Ra, betatron, linear accelerator) have the following advantages over the orthovoltage one. They have higher energy of radiation, less skin injury, less lateral scattering, and more tissue penetration at a greater depth. They are suitable for the deep seated tumors (e.g. carcinomas of the cervix and endometrium).

Fractionation is the division of a total dose of external beam radiotherapy into small (daily) doses. Thus it spares normal tissue damage preferentially. External beam radiotherapy is usually fractionated and is given once daily for five times a week. A dose of 180–220 cGy per fraction is used. This is based on the ability of the cells to accumulate and repair the sublethal injury. Tumor tissue takes longer time to recover from radiation damage compared to normal tissue. Fractionation allows **normal tissue** (intestinal mucosa, bone marrow) to repair sublethal injury (sparing effect). On the other hand irradiation results in accumulation of sublethal damage and ultimate loss of reproductive capacity in **tumor tissue**.

Radiation dose prescription should include the total dose, number of fractions with dose and time for each fraction (e.g. 40 Gy in 20 fractions given five times weekly can be completed in 4 weeks at 2 Gy per fraction).

ADVANCES IN RADIATION THERAPY

High linear energy transfer: X-rays and γ-rays are less effective against hypoxic cells compared to oxygenated cells. **Fast neutrons** or negative π mesons (pions) or protons are very effective against the hypoxic cells. **Fast neutron** beam for radiotherapy are generated by the cyclotron and the D-T generator. The neutron is emitted with an energy of 14–16 MeV.

Negative π mesons (pions) with energies between 40 and 70 MeV have a depth range in tissue of about 6–13 cm. It has high biologic effectiveness and a low dependence on oxygen.

RADIOPOTENTIATORS AND HYPOXIC CELL SENSITIZERS

Compared to well-oxygenated cells, hypoxic cells require about three times the radiation dose, to obtain the same proportion of cell kill. Hypoxic cell can be sensitized to ionizing radiation to improve the **oxygen enhancement ratio (OER)** by different chemical compounds.

Number of **chemotherapeutic agents** have been found to potentiate the radiation effect and also to sensitize the hypoxic cells (Table 31.3). Exact mechanism is not well-understood. Use of hyperbaric oxygen to increase radiosensitivity is of doubtful benefit. Moreover this technique is cumbersome.

Intraoperative radiation of large fraction of 1500–2500 cGy are delivered directly to the area selected. Periaortic node irradiation (biopsy proven) at the time of staging laparotomy is possible.

Hyperthermia is found helpful as an active anti-neoplastic agent and a significant radiosensitizer.

NEW TECHNOLOGY FOR RADIATION THERAPY

Three-dimensional Conformal Radiation Therapy (3D CRT)

3D CRT uses imaging modalities (CT, MRI, and PET scanning). Beam placement using a CT simulation is used. 3D conformal radiotherapy (3D CRT) can shape the beam to conform to the target. **Computerized dosimetry is currently used.** This can help to arrange the beams to maximize dose to the tumor and minimize dose to normal tissues (Table 31.4).

Intensity Modulated Radiation Therapy (IMRT)

IMRT uses the power of computers to shape and perform thousands of iterations of planning to maximize the tumor dose and to minimize normal tissue dose. Both 3D CRT and IMRT use small collimator "leaves" to shape the beam finely. These "leaves" are mobile and can vary the beam intensity. It allows irregular shapes (tumor) to be treated and has the benefit of reduced radiation to normal tissues (bowel, bladder).

Tomotherapy and cone-beam CT may allow more precise localization of beam and verification of dose delivered.

Stereotactic Radiotherapy and Gamma Knife Radiation

The are similar to IMRT and 3D CRT to allow precise high dose delivery of external radiation. Stereoatactic radiation uses a modification of linear accelerator.

Treatment Field for Carcinoma Cervix

Superior border—between L_4 and L_5 to include the common iliac nodes. **Inferior border**—2 cm below the inferior margin of obturator foramen to include the obturator nodes. **Lateral borders**—1.5–2 cm lateral to the margins of the pelvic brim.

Lead compensators are used in the path of external beam radiation to prevent overdose to the central portion of the pelvis, which has received high dosage from brachytherapy.

TABLE 31.3: Radiopotentiators, hypoxic cell sensitizers.

Chemotherapeutic agents
▪ Cisplatin ▪ Paclitaxel ▪ Gemcitabine ▪ Doxorubicin
Others
▪ Metronidazole ▪ Tumor necrosis factor (TNF) ▪ Interferon ▪ Acyclovir

TABLE 31.4: Tissue tolerance of radiation dose (normal).

Organ/tissue	*Dose tolerance (Gy)*
Cervix	>120
Vaginal mucosa	70–75
Urinary bladder	60–70
Rectum	60–70
Small bowel	45–50
Liver	25–35
Kidney	20–23
Ovary	Young women (< 40 yrs): 4Gy-sterilized 30% Older women (> 40 yrs): 4Gy-sterilized 100%

Radiotherapy in Epithelial Ovarian Carcinoma

Chemotherapy has replaced radiotherapy both for the management of early and advanced disease. **However, it may be used in the following cases who fail to respond with chemotherapy: (a) Metastatic deposits over the peritoneal surfaces; (b) Lymph node metastasis; (c) Palliation for painful recurrences in the pelvis or bone.**

Moving strip technique is used to irradiate whole of abdomen. Presence of residual disease following debulking procedures in a case of ovarian carcinoma is treated with this technique. Whole abdomen is divided into contiguous strips of 2.5 cm wide area. Each strip is irradiated from front and back over 2 days and the field is gradually moved up. Cobalt 60 machine is generally used and a total tumor dose of 2600–2800 cGy is delivered. Pelvic boost of 2000–3000 cGy is given additionally. Kidneys and right lobe of liver are shielded with lead to reduce the dose to these organs. **Bulky residual disease (>2 cm) is not suitable for radiotherapy.**

Use of radiotherapy for individual organ malignancy—see respective Chapters.

Radiation reactions and their management—*see* Table 31.2. **Contraindications of radiotherapy**—p. 292.

CHEMOTHERAPY

GENERAL CONSIDERATIONS

Use of cytotoxic chemotherapy has got the following objectives:

- **Complete remission of the tumor**
- **Partial remission (30%) with improvement of median survival**
- **To prevent recurrence of the tumor**
- **To alleviate the symptoms, so as to improve the quality of life (palliation).**

Effective chemotherapy is designed to kill selectively the malignant cells without producing serious irreversible harm to normal cells. The substances as yet available, damage both cancerous and normal tissues but in contradistinction to normal tissues, cancerous tissues cannot recover from the insult.

CELL KINETICS

Cell cycle time denotes the amount of time needed by a proliferating cell to progress through the cell cycle and produce a new daughter cell. Cell cycle times vary widely (12–217 hours) but are relatively constant for a specific tumor type.

Normal cells have the inherent capacity to multiply. There is also constant and balanced cell loss. Normal cells may be classified as:

- **Proliferating cells** (bone marrow, intestinal mucosa)—undergo constant cell division.
- **Quiescent cells** (liver)—can proliferate under special conditions (injury), otherwise they are in quiescent phase.
- **Static cells** (neurons)—rarely proliferate.

Cancer cells undergo uncontrolled and excessive proliferation compared to cell loss. Speed of cell division is the same compared to a normal cell.

Doubling time of human tumor is defined as the time taken by a tumor mass to double its size. Doubling time varies depending upon the specific type of the tumor. Tumor growth depends on growth fraction and cell death. **Growth fraction** is the number of cells in the tumor mass that are actively involved in the phase of cell division.

Gompertzian growth states that when a tumor volume increases in size, its mass doubling time becomes progressively longer.

Cell Cycle

There are four phases of cell cycle. These are G_1, S, G_2, and M (Fig. 31.4). The duration of the cycle from M phase to M phase is called **generation time**. Tumor cells do not have faster generation time. Normal tissues have huge number of cells in the G_0 phase (out of cycle), in contrast to tumor cells, where more cells are in the active phase of cell division.

Cell cycle concept is very important for cancer chemotherapy. Dividing tumor cells are most sensitive to cytotoxic agents whereas cells in the G_0 are relatively insensitive (Fig. 31.4).

Varieties of Malignancy

The credibility of the use of cancerolytic drugs depends upon the fact that in all malignancies, dissemination occurs at some stage of the disease and local treatment may not suffice. Proper understanding of cell cycle has evolved legitimate synergistic combinations of drugs with better cancer killing potentialities and less side effects (Fig. 31.5).

Broadly speaking, chemotherapeutic drugs are of two varieties depending on the basis of their cell cycle specificity (Fig. 31.4):

- Cell cycle specific agents which act on proliferating cells only (Table 31.5).
- Cell cycle nonspecific agents which destroy both resting and cycling cells (Table 31.5).

It is observed that antitumor agents kill a constant fraction of cells (rather than a constant number) with each course of therapy. This is called log kill hypothesis. Intermittent courses of therapy are found useful to destroy more tumor cells.

Principles

- Rapidly growing tumors are more amenable than slow growing tumors.
- A constant fraction of neoplastic cells are killed with each dose of cytotoxic drug.
- Effect of drugs depends on: Tumor mass, sensitivity and growth rate of tumor cells
- High dose intermittent course of chemotherapy may result in high cell kill and optimal destruction of the tumor (dose intensity).

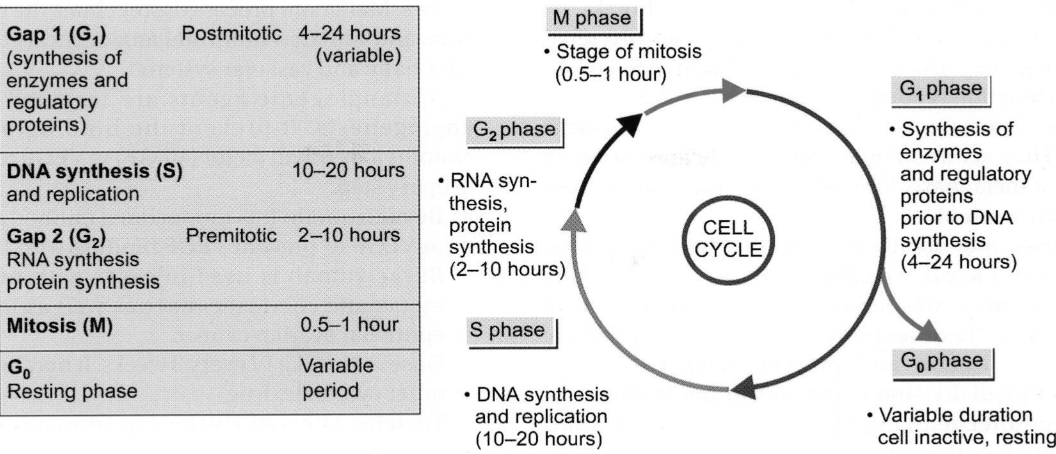

Gap 1 (G_1) (synthesis of enzymes and regulatory proteins)	Postmitotic	4–24 hours (variable)
DNA synthesis (S) and replication		10–20 hours
Gap 2 (G_2) RNA synthesis protein synthesis	Premitotic	2–10 hours
Mitosis (M)		0.5–1 hour
G_0 Resting phase		Variable period

Fig. 31.4: The cell cycle and cell generation time.

TABLE 31.5: Drug activity in the cell cycle.

Cell cycle	Nonspecific	Cyclophosphamide
Cell cycle	Specific	
	On G_1	Actinomycin, Doxorubicin
	On S phase	Methotrexate, 5 FU, Doxorubicin, Gemcitabine, Topotecan
	On G_2	Bleomycin, Etoposide, Cisplatin, Carboplatin
	On M phase	Vinblastine, Vincristine, Taxanes
	G_0	Nitrosoureas (BCNU, CCNU)

- Combination agent chemotherapy is superior to single agent.
- Drug dose is adjusted according to the tolerance of the patient. Before starting any chemotherapy, pretreatment evaluation should be done (p. 425).

Single Agent versus Combination Agents

- Combined chemotherapeutic agents attack different phases of cell cycle (synergistic effect), so reduces the tumor volume effectively.
- Use of combination (cell cycle specific and cell cycle nonspecific) chemotherapy enhances tumor cell kill compared to single drug therapy.
- Because of toxicity, drug dose and duration of therapy cannot be increased when single agent chemotherapy is used.
- Emergence of drug resistance is more with single agent therapy.

MECHANISMS OF DRUG RESISTANCE

- Increased repair of DNA
- Decrease in cellular drug uptake
- Increased level of target enzyme to make the cell immune to the drug
- Increase in drug degradation
- Spontaneous tumor cell mutations

CLASSIFICATION OF CYTOTOXIC DRUGS

Classification is based principally on structural similarity and mechanism of action:

- **Alkylating agents:** These drugs transfer their alkyl radical to nucleic acids (DNA). **They prevent cell division by cross-linking the DNA strands. They produce single and double stranded DNA break.** Cyclophosphamide inhibits DNA synthesis in addition. *These are cell cycle nonspecific agents (CCNS).*
  Examples: Cyclophosphamide (endoxan), ifosfamide.
- **Platinum (PTL)** analogs—form PTL-DNA adducts that interrupt the DNA synthesis. It is given by IV or IP for epithelial ovarian carcinomas.
  Side effects: Vomiting, nausea, hypomagnesemia, nephrotoxicity (needs copious hydration), ototoxicity peripheral neuropathy.
  Carboplatin dose is calculated on glomerular filtration rate (GFR) or creatinine clearance.
  Toxicities: Myelosuppression, thrombocytopenia, anemia, alopecia, hepatotoxicity and neurotoxicity.
- **Platinum agents:** Cisplatin, carboplatin, oxaliplatin.
- **Antimetabolites** act by inhibiting essential metabolic processes that are required for synthesis of purines, pyrimidines, and nucleic acids.
  Examples:
  - *Methotrexate:* Folic acid antagonist, prevents reduction of folic acid to folinic acid by inhibiting the enzyme dihydrofolate reductase.
  - *5-fluorouracil:* Pyrimidine analog, blocks thymidine synthesis and prevents DNA replication.
  - *6-mercaptopurine:* Purine derivatives—competitive attachment to enzymatic catalytic site.
  - *Gemcitabine* (2', 2'-fluorodeoxy cytabidine) is an antimetabolite. It binds to DNA to form a wrong base pair and stops DNA synthesis. It is used against ovarian, breast, and cervica l carcinoma.
- **Antibiotics:** *These are cell cycle nonspecific agents.* They prevent DNA replication, causes single and double stranded DNA break, e.g. actinomycin D, bleomycin, doxorubicin, mitomycin C, adriamycin.

- **Bleomycin:** Cause single strand DNA breaks by hydroxyl radical formation. It is given IV and excreted by the kidney. Dose reduction may be needed when renal function is compromised (see carboplation).

■ **Plant derivatives and taxanes:** *These are cell cycle specific agents.* They act as spindle poison and cause arrest of mitosis at metaphase. Vincristine and vinblastine (from plant ***Vinca rosea***).
- **Taxanes** are obtained from the bark of pacific yew tree (***Taxus brevifolia***). Important members of this group are paclitaxel (taxol) and docetaxol (synthetic). **Taxanes** promote microtubule assembly and stabilization and prevent depolymerization. **Thus by cell division is arrested at the M phase.**
- **Camptothecin analogs** (topotecan and irinotecan) inhibit topoisomerase-1, thereby causes single stranded DNA break.
- **Vinca alkaloids (plant derivatives):** Vinca alkaloids (vinorelbine, vincristine)—bind to the β-tubulin subunits of the mitotic spindles. This prevents microtubule (polymerization) during mitosis. *These drugs affect the M phases of the cell cycle. It increases cell radiosensitivity.*

■ **Topoisomerase inhibitors:** Functions of topoisomerase (TOPO) enzymes are to unwind and rewind DNA to help DNA replication. Inhibitors to TOPO isomerase interefere with this function and block DNA synthesis. There are two categories of inhibitors. Camptothecins (Topotecan) inhibit TOPO I and podophyllotoxin (Etoposide) inhibit TOPO II.

■ **Poly-ADP-ribose polymerase (PARP) inhibitors:** Olaparib is a PARP inhibitor. It is used in cases (known to be *BRCA1* and *BRCA2* mutation carriers) with ovarian cancer resistant to platinum drugs.

Targeted agents: Tyrosine kinase inhibitors (TKI): Sunitinib, Pazopanib are used to target the VEGF angiogenesis pathway.

For further details see author's Manual of Obstetrics and Gynecology for the postgraduates.

■ **Doxorubicin and the liposomal formulation** inhibit the enzymes needed for RNA synthesis, and DNA transcription, replication.

It also inhibits topoisomerase II. It is given by IV injection. Extravasation causes soft tissue and skin necrosis and ulceration. It is metabolized by the liver.

Toxicities: Myelosuppression, alopecia, cardiac failure (CCF) and cardiomyopathy. **Liposomal doxorubicin** has a esynthetic lipid like membrane around the molecule. This promotes tumor uptake of the drug and also reduces the risk of cardiotoxicity. It is given IV; dose: 40–50 mg/m^2 every 4 weeks.

Cardiomyopathy is less common. Others: Skin toxicity, especially palmar plantar erythrodysesthesia (PPE) is more common. Before therapy, patient need to be evaluated for liver and cardiac function tests.

■ **Antiangiogenesis agents:** Angiogenesis is a process of new blood vessel formation. The blood vessels are remodeled for transport of oxygen and nutrient to tissues. Malignant process dysregulates the normal balance and initiates abnormal angiogenesis through the lymphatic and vascular system.

Antiangiogenic agents are targeted to inhibit angiogenesis. It prevent the binding of vascular endothelial growth factor (VEGF) to VEGF receptor as a primary step.
- **Bevacizumab:** It is monoclonal antibody that binds to VEGF to prevent VEGF binding with its receptor. Bevacizumab is used in cases with recurrent or metastatic cervical cancer as well as in recurrent epithelial ovarian cancer.

  Dose: 15 mg/kg IV every 3 weeks. It may be given with other cytotoxic drug.

  Toxicity: Minimal; rise in blood pressure may lead to hypertensive crisis, intestinal perforation has been reported.

■ **Mammalian target of rapamycin inhibitors:** Mammalian target of rapamycin (mTOR) is a protein kinase. It regulates membrane trafficking, transcription, translation and maintain cytoskeleton. mTOR increases production of VEGR.

Rapamycin inhibits mTOR. Temsirolimus, everolimus are currently being studied in gynecological cancers.

Hormones: The drugs induce regression of a hormone responsive tumor and also increase anabolic processes.

Progesterone preparations, e.g. hydroxyprogesterone caproate, medroxyprogesterone acetate, megestrol acetate.

Antiestrogen—tamoxifen acts by competitive receptor binding—thus helpful in estrogen dependent tumors.

■ **Toxicity: The toxic reactions depend on the type of drug used. The toxic reactions are tabulated in Table 31.7.**

Routes of Administration

■ **Oral:** Alkylating drugs (PARP inhibitors) are mainly used orally. The intermittent therapy allows recovery of normal cells.

■ **Parenteral:** Administration (intravenous—commonly, intra-arterial) at interval of 1–4 weeks allows bone marrow to recover.

■ **Intraperitoneal (IP):** Systemic administration is more effective. Drug penetration will be only 3–6 cells deep.

Objectives of chemotherapy: (a) As a primary treatment of cancer; (b) As an adjunct to radiation therapy; (c) As a neoadjuvant therapy, used for advanced disease following which additional treatment is planned; (d) By direct instillation (intraperitoneal chemotherapy).

Means to assess the response of chemotherapy: (a) Clinical and physical examination; (b) Assessing by imaging studies, e.g. CT or MRI; (c) Serial measurement of specific tumor markers (i.e. CA-125 for epithelial ovarian cancer, β-hCG for GTN); (d) Detection of hypermetabolic state by PET or PET-CT (Table 31.6).

Pretreatment Evaluation

Chemotherapeutic agents are highly toxic to the erythropoietic system, bone marrow in particular. The drugs are

TABLE 31:6: Response evaluation criteria in solid tumors (RECIST).

Criterion	Features
Complete response (CR)	Disappearance of all target lesions
Partial response (PR)	30% decrease in the sum of greatest diameters of target lesions
Progressive disease (PD)	20% increase in the sum of greatest diameters of target lesions
Stable disease (SD)	Small changes that do not meet the above criteria

mostly metabolized in the liver and are excreted through the kidneys. The patients are also immunocompromised and as such, any source of infection is to be treated.

Pretreatment evaluation of all the important organ function is of paramount importance.

- **Hematological**—complete hemogram and platelet count (>100,000)
- **Serum**—electrolytes
- **Renal functions**—serum urea, uric acid, creatinine, and creatinine clearance (especially when cisplatin is used)
- **Liver functions**—serum proteins, liver enzymes, bilirubin
- **Cardiac function**—baseline ECG, echocardiography to assess ventricular ejection fraction when cardiotoxic drug (doxorubicin) is used
- **Pulmonary function**—when bleomycin is used
- **Throat swab, urine**—for culture and sensitivity.

Calculation of Dose

The dose of a chemotherapeutic agent is usually calculated as square meter of body surface area. It provides a better measure of potential toxicity than body weight. **The surface area closely reflects cardiac output and blood flow.** There is minimal change of surface area during entire course of therapy compared to body weight. Nomogram is used for calculating body surface area of adults.

Uses of Drugs

Commonly used chemotherapy agents, type of neoplasm their average dosage, route of therapy, toxicity, and precautions are mentioned in Tables 31.7 to 31.9. It should be noted that this schedule is flexible and treatment must be individualized according to patient.

It is imperative that all cases undergoing chemotherapy should be monitored (Tables 31.10). **Minor complications like nausea, vomiting, alopecia, glossitis should not preclude full treatment protocol.** The benefits are to be weighed against toxic effects.

Use of Antiemetics

Nausea and vomiting are the most common side effects. It is due to stimulation of chemoreceptor trigger zone (CTZ) which secretes neurotransmitters (serotonin, dopamine, and histamine) to activate the vomiting center (Table 31.12).

Ondansetron (5 HT_3 receptor antagonist), dexamethasone and metoclopramide are commonly used.

TABLE 31.7: Commonly used chemotherapeutic agents, use, toxicity, and precautions.

Drugs	*Dosage and route of therapy*	*Type of neoplasm*	*Toxicity (important)*	*Precaution*
▪ **Alkylating agent** • Cyclophosphamide (Endoxan)	750–1,000 mg/m^2 of body surface/IV. Single dose every 3 weeks 50–110 mg/m^2 by mouth (PO)	▪ Carcinoma • Ovary • Endometrium • Cervix • Fallopian tube	Bone marrow depression (BMD), alopecia, cystitis	Adequate fluid intake
• Ifosfamide (Ifex)	7–10 g/m^2 IV over 3–5 days, to be repeated every 3–4 weeks	▪ **Carcinoma** and **sarcoma** of • Ovary • Cervix • Endometrium	BMD, alopecia, cystitis	Uro-protectant (mesna)
• Cisplatin (Cis-diamine dichloroplatinum) • Carboplatin	50–75 mg/m^2 IV every 1–3 weeks—usually 4–6 such 300–400 mg/m^2 IV. Repeat every 3–4 weeks for 6 courses	• Ovary • Endometirum • Cervix	Nephrotoxicity, neurotoxicity, myelosuppression, thrombocytopenia	Adequate pre-hydration, monitor renal function
• Oxaliplatin	59–130 mg/m^2 IV over 2 hours, every 3 weeks	• Ovary	Myelosuppression, peripheral neuropathy	Contraindicated in hepatic and renal dysfunction
▪ **Antimetabolites** • Methotrexate	10–30 mg/day PO × 5 days 240 mg/m^2 IV with leucovorin rescue	▪ Choriocarcinoma ▪ Carcinoma • Ovary • Cervix	BMD, megaloblastic anemia, stomatitis, vomiting, alopecia, hepatic/pulmonary fibrosis	Adequate renal function and urine output to maintain
• 5-Fluorouracil (5-Fu)	10–15 mg/kg/day IV × 5 days. Repeat after 3–4 weeks. 10–15 mg/kg IV weekly, maximum up to 1 gram	▪ Carcinoma • Ovary • Endometrium	Bone mineral density, diarrhea, stomatitis, alopecia	Dose reduction with compromised renal, hepatic or bone marrow function

Contd...

Contd...

Drugs	Dosage and route of therapy	Type of neoplasm	Toxicity (important)	Precaution
• Gemcitabine	800–1000 mg/m^2 IV weekly every 3 weeks	▪ Carcinoma • Breast • Ovary • Leiomyosarcoma of uterus	Myelosuppression	None
▪ **Antibiotics** • Actinomycin D	0.5 mg/m^2/IV/weekly, repeat 3–4 weeks or 0.5 mg/m^2/IV daily × 5 days 15 µg/kg/day IV or 0.5 mg/day for 5 days	▪ Embryonal rhabdomyosarcoma, choriocarcinoma, ovarian germ cell tumors	BMD, stomatitis, hyperpigmentation in areas of irradiation	Dose adjustment in liver disease and decrease bone marrow function
• Mitomycin C	8 mg/m^2/IV every 3 weeks	▪ Cancer cervix	Neutropenia, thrombocytopenia, oral ulceration	Prevention of extravasation
• Doxorubicin (Adriamycin)	50 mg/m^2/IV weekly. Repeat every 3–4 weeks	▪ Adenocarcinoma ▪ Endometrium ▪ Ovary ▪ Vagina ▪ Tube ▪ Uterine sarcoma	BMD, alopecia, cardiac toxicity, myopathy, stomatitis	Avoid insignificant heart disease, ECG monitoring
▪ **Antiangiogenic agents** • Bevacizumab	15 mg/kg IV every 3 weeks	▪ Metastatic or recurrent: Ovarian and cervical cancer	Rise in BP	Hypertension
▪ **Targeted agents** • PARP inhibitors • Olaparib	400 mg PO twice day	▪ Ovarian cancer resistant to platinum drugs (*BRCA1* and *BRCA2* mutation carriers)	Fatigue	Poor health
• Bleomycin	10–12 mg/m^2/IV/IM weekly	▪ Squamous cell cancer of skin, vulva, cervix ▪ Choriocarcinoma, germ cell and sex cord stromal tumors of ovary	**Skin:** Hyperpigmentation, ulceration, alopecia. **Pulmonary:** Pneumonitis, fibrosis, dyspnea	Avoid in renal or pulmonary disease
▪ **Plant derived** • Vincristine (Oncovin)	0.4–1.4 mg/m^2 IV weekly	▪ Uterine sarcoma ▪ Ovarian germ cell tumor	Paresthesia, weakness, loss of reflexes, foot drop, BMD, reticulocytopenia, alopecia, hoarseness, anemia	Avoid extravasation, dose adjustment with liver disease
• Vinblastine (Velban)	5–6 mg/m^2 IV every 1–2 weeks	▪ Choriocarcinoma	BMD, neutropenia, alopecia, peripheral neuropathy depression, weakness	Avoid extravasation, dose adjustment with liver disease
• Etoposide (Epipodophyllotoxin)	100 mg/m^2 IV on days — 1,3 and 5 repeat every 3–4 weeks	▪ GTN ▪ Germ cell tumors	Leukopenia, thrombocytopenia, alopecia, headache, fever	Dose reduction up to 50% to prevent toxicity
▪ **Taxanes** • Paclitaxel (taxol) • Docetaxel	135–250 mg/m^2 IV over 3 hours every 3–4 weeks; 60–100 mg/m^2 IV over 1 hour every 3–4 weeks	▪ Carcinoma ▪ Ovary ▪ Endometrium ▪ Cervix ▪ Ovarian carcinoma	BMD, dyspnea, hypotension, cardiotoxicity, alopecia, stomatitis myelosuppression, mucositis	Cardiac monitoring, premedication with steroids
▪ **Camptothecin analogs** • Topotecan	1.5 mg/m^2 IV/day for 5 days; 4 mg/m^2 IV on D-1, D-8 every 3 weeks	▪ Ovary ▪ Cervix	BMD, alopecia, fever malaise	To guard against neutropenia

TABLE 31.8: Other chemotherapeutic agents: Use, toxicity and precautions.

▪ **Hormones** **Progestogens** • 17α-Hydroxyprogesterone caproate (1 g IM twice a week for 1 year) • Medroxyprogesterone acetate (Depo-Provera) (400–800 mg orally/IM weekly for 1 year) • Megestrol acetate (Megace) (40–120 mg tablet oral/day for 1 year) – **Type of carcinoma:** Endometrium – **Toxicity:** Hepatic dysfunction, alopecia – **Precaution:** Monitor liver function	▪ **Antiestrogen** • Tamoxifen (10–20 mg twice daily orally) – **Type of carcinoma:** Breast (ER +ve), endometrium – **Toxicity:** Hot flashes, pruritus vulvae, vaginal bleeding • Leuprolide (Lupron) (1 mg daily SC) – **Type of carcinoma:** Endometrium – **Toxicity:** Antiestrogen effects – **Precaution:** Add back therapy

TABLE 31.9: Formalities maintained in systemic chemotherapy.

- Drugs used in combination should not be mixed together
- The infusion set should be flushed with normal saline between the administration of each drug
- To avoid sclerosis of the vein, the drugs should be washed through with normal saline
- Extravasation should be avoided (Table 31.11)
- Antiemetics should be given before start of therapy
- Fertility sparing therapy (surgery, chemotherapy and radiotherapy) is considered for a woman desiring fertility preservation. See Ca cervix (p. 284) Ca ovary (p. 309) Ca endometrium (p. 297)

TABLE 31.10: Toxic effects of the cytotoxic drugs and their management.

Tissue or organ affected	*Toxic effects and drugs*	*Management*
Gastrointestinal	Nausea, vomiting, oral ulceration, stomatitis, necrotizing enterocolitis, diarrhea **Drugs:** Cisplatin, methotrexate, paclitaxel, docetaxel, etoposide	Antiemetics used for emetogenic chemotherapy ▪ Dexamethasone 20 mg IV ▪ Ondansetron 8 mg IV every 4 hours 2–3 doses ▪ Metoclopramide 80–120 mg IV every 3–4 hours
Hair roots	Alopecia **Drugs:** Paclitaxel, cyclophosphamide	Generally reversible
Hematological (bone-marrow)	Anemia, granulocytopenia, thrombocytopenia. The danger level being: Hb percent <8 g percent, leukocyte count <3,000/mm^3 and platelet count <20,000/mm^3 **Drugs:** Paclitaxel, etoposide, carboplatin	Blood transfusion, platelet transfusion, drug dose may be modified. Granulocyte colony-stimulating factor (G-CSF) and granulocyte macrophage colony-stimulating factor (GM-CSF) have been used (250 μg/m^2, subcutaneously) for myelostimulation
Skin	Dermatitis, pigmentation (bleomycin), extravasation (Table 31.11), skin necrosis **Drugs:** Sctinomycin D, doxorubicin	For extravasation and skin necrosis—removal of intravenous line, local infiltration of corticosteroids, ice pack therapy
Cardiac	Cardiomyopathy, cardiac failure, arrhythmias, endocardial fibrosis **Drugs:** Doxorubicin, cyclophosphamide), toxic myocarditis (paclitaxel)	Discontinuation of drug, drug and dose modification, consult cardiologist
Liver	Hepatitis, elevated transaminases, and bilirubin **Drugs:** Methotrexate	Discontinuation of drug, drug and dose modification
Lungs	Fibrosis (bleomycin, alkylating agents doxorubicin)	Pulmonary function tests, to stop therapy, steroids may be helpful
Nervous system	Neurotoxicity, ototoxicity, peripheral neuropathy **Drugs:** Cisplatin, ifosfamide	Vitamin B complex, pyridoxine therapy, drug and dose modification
Urinary system	Renal failure, azotemia (cisplatin), hemorrhagic cystitis (cyclophosphamide, ifosfamide), red urine **Drugs:** Doxorubicin	Prehydration and mannitol-induced diuresis before therapy, avoid simultaneous use of nephrotoxic drugs (aminoglycosides). **Mesna** is used for hemorrhagic cystitis due to cyclophosphamide or ifosfamide
Immune system	Suppression of cellular and humoral immunity, loss of host defense mechanism	Usually reversible
Metabolic	Hyperkalemia, hyperuricemia, hypocalcemia—due to rapid tumor lysis. Hyponatremia— due to inappropriate ADH secretion	Estimation of serum electrolytes and appropriate correction

Contd...

Contd...

Tissue or organ affected	Toxic effects and drugs	Management
Surgical wound	Delayed healing	—
Gonads	Infertility, amenorrhea, premature ovarian failure	Patient counseling
Embryo	Teratogenic effect, congenital malformations	Patient counseling, to assess risk and benefit
Second malignancies	Due to mutagenic effect—leukemia **Drugs:** Melphalan	—

TABLE 31.11: Chemotherapeutic drugs and tissue injury following extravasation.

Name	Tissue injuries	Drugs
Vesicants	Skin ulceration, tissue necrosis and sloughing	Doxorubicin, actinomycin D, paclitaxel
Exfoliants	Skin exfoliation	Cisplatin, topotecan, docetaxel
Irritants	Skin irritation	Carboplatin, etoposide
Inflammants	Inflammation of the skin	Methotrexate
Neutral drugs	–	Bleomycin, cyclophosphamide, gemcitabine, ifosfamide

TABLE 31.12: Antiemetic drugs used during chemotherapy.

Drugs 5 HT_3 (SRA)	Dose	Tim
Ondansetron	Oral: 24 mg IV: 8 mg	Before therapy
Granisetron	Oral: 2 mg IV: 1 mg	Before chemotherapy
Dexamethasone (Decadron)	Oral: 12 mg Oral: 8 mg	Before chemotherapy Daily: Days 2–4

(5 HT_3: 5-hydroxytryptamine-3; SRA: Serotonin receptor antagonists

Targeted therapies are aimed to increase the efficacy and decrease the toxicity of anticancer therapy. Three therapies target the pathway of angiogenesis, cell cycle and apoptosis in tumor cells. Several broad categories of targeted therapies exist. These are bevacizumab, pazopanib, and temsirolimus. **Monoclonal antibodies** are commonly used. However, these therapies cannot replace the cytotoxic drugs and are used in combinations.

Growth Factor Therapy

To minimize the hematologic toxicity (myelosuppression, acute granulocytopenia, thrombocytopenia) of the chemotherapy, these molecules are used (Table 31.13). These are mostly from the cytokines family (p. 429).

TABLE 31.13: Use of growth factors in the management of cancers.

Cytokines	Functions
▪ **Granulocyte-macrophage colony stimulating factor (GM-CSF)**	▪ Stimulates hematopoiesis ▪ Activates granulocytes and macrophages
▪ **Granulocyte-colony stimulating factor (G-CSF) (filgrastim, pegfilgrastim)**	Activates granulocytes
▪ **Erythropoietin (epoetin alfa, darbepoetin alfa)**	Stimulates erythroid growth and development

IMMUNOTHERAPY

The following considerations have led to the idea that host immune response can prevent tumor growth:

- Immune suppressed patients are more likely to develop malignant disease.
- Therapy with monoclonal antibodies is found to destroy tumor cells, which is due to antibody dependent cellular cytotoxicity.
- Natural killer (NK) cells (lymphoid cells) and lymphokine-activated killer (LAK) cells together with IL-2, TNF, IFN can cause tumor cell destruction (adoptive immunotherapy).
- Cytotoxic T cells lyse infected cells or signal B cells to produce antibody.

CYTOKINES AND CANCER THERAPY

Cytokines are polypeptides secreted by different immune cells like, monocytes, macrophages, T cells, and tumor cells. Cytokines are pleiotropic. Their functions include regulation of cell immune activity (interferons, interleukins), hematopoiesis [granulocyte colony stimulating factor (G-CSF) and granulocyte macrophase colony stimulating factor (GM-CSF)], and cytotoxic activity (interleukins and tumor necrosis factor). ***The overall cytotoxic mechanism are:*** *(a) stimulation of NK cells and macrophages, (b) antiangiogenic effects and (c) inhibition of expression of oncogenes (HER-2/neu). They also increase the sensitivity of tumor cells to cytotoxic drugs.*

PRINCIPLES OF IMMUNOTHERAPY

- Tumor mass must be reduced to a minimum (<10^8 cells) by radical surgery, chemotherapy or radiation before immunotherapy.
- Immunotherapy approach should be a combined one.
- Any single agent therapy is often ineffective.
- Immunotherapy is more effective against tumors that are highly antigenic.

MODULATION OF IMMUNE SYSTEM (BIOLOGICAL RESPONSE MODIFIERS)

Approaches to augment the immune response to human tumor include:

- Active immunotherapy (to induce host immune response).
  - Biological immunostimulants—administration of *Bacillurs Calmette-Guérin* (BCG) and *Corynebacterium parvum*. HPV vaccine (nonavalent) for the prevention of vulvar, vaginal or cervical cancers.
  - Chemical immunostimulants—levamisole, cimetidine.

- Cytokines, interferons (IFN), interleukins (IL-2), chemokines, tumor necrosis factor (TNFα).
- Chemotherapeutic drugs—cisplatin, doxorubicin.

■ Passive immunotherapy (immunologically active substances are directly transferred to the host).

- Cytokines: Interferon, TNF
- LAK cells: Together with IL-2
- Monoclonal antibodies
- Activated macrophages: Interferon.

Immunotherapy has its limitations. Immune response enhancement leading to rejection of tumor can occur when the following conditions are fulfilled:

- Biological response modifiers are in direct contact with tumors
- Tumor bulk is minimal
- Blood supply is good
- Monoclonal antibodies to be conjugated with agents (chemotherapy drugs, toxins, interferon) for precise delivery to tumor cells.

GENETICS AND GYNECOLOGIC MALIGNANCY

Familial cancer of the breast, ovary, colon, endometrium, and other sites have been observed in the female members of affected families. Well-defined cancer family syndromes with autosomal dominant inheritance pattern have been described (p. 310). *When life-time risk of ovarian cancer in the population as a whole is 1.4%, it is about 5% when one first degree relative is affected and it rises to 7% when two or more first degree relatives are affected.*

Genetic basis of ovarian and breast malignancy have been explained (p. 310). Malignant change is seen with point mutations, gene amplification, chromosomal aberration or translocation. **Three types of genes (oncogenes, tumor suppressor genes, and DNA mismatch repair genes)** are involved with malignant change. Point mutation, deletion and insertion are the important changes observed in malignancy.

■ **Oncogenes are** dominant whereas **tumor suppressor genes (*p53*)** are recessive in function at cellular level. Oncogene activate cell proliferation to malignant behavior whereas tumor suppressor genes (*BRCA1*) restrain cell growth. However, majority of ovarian cancers are not associated with familial predisposition. Familial cancer account for less than 10% of all cases of ovarian cancer and have an early age of onset.

Early detection of cancer may be possible by detecting mutated copies of a gene products (*p53*, HER-2/neu K-RAS), using polymerase or ligase chain reaction. Several oncogene products (HER-2/neu, K-ras, C-myc, p21), tumor suppressor gene products (*p53*, P16, PRB) are currently being investigated as independent **prognostic markers.**

Apoptosis means programmed cell death. There may be intentional induction of cell death. Mature cells die to give way to more differentiated and specialized cells. If a cell becomes immortal, cancer can result. Apoptosis of cells is blocked by mutation in genes (BCL-2 or TP53). These mutated cells are suddenly free to continue replication and propagating their mutations. This genetic mutability is an early step of developing cancers.

Oncogenes regulate cell growth in a positive fashion. Oncogenes include transforming genes of viruses and normal cellular genes that are activated by mutations to promote cell growth to a partly malignant behavior. It needs one mutational events for its gain of function (dominant).

Selected oncogenes and associated tumors are Ha-ras-bladder cancer; Neu-erb-B2—breast, ovary and gastric cancer.

■ **Tumor suppressor gene** (antioncogene): Suppresses cellular growth, proliferation and malignant phenotype. It needs two mutational events (point mutation, deletions) for its loss of function (recessive).

Study for detection of gene mutation is mainly restricted to research purpose only.

Common tumor suppressor genes and their chromosome location are:

RB1 (13q), *p53* (17p), *BRCA1* (17q), *BRCA2* (13q), *WT1* (11q).

Loss of cell apoptosis due to gene mutation may lead to cancer.

■ **Mismatch repair genes (total six)** work in concert to repair DNA damage that occur in the course of a normal cell division or that result from exogenous or endogenous mutagenic agents. Germ line mutations in mismatch repair genes is responsible for many hereditary cancers (colorectal, endometrial, and uroepithelial). Common mismatch repair genes are MLH-1, MSH-2, MSH-6.

Telomerase: Reactivation of telomerase activity to restore telomere sequences is absent in a normal cell. Cells having significant telomerase activity become immortal and turn into cancer cells.

Gene therapy: The effects of **oncogene function** can be transformed by two approaches. One attempt is to remove the oncogene product or to block its function. Alternatively, one can use antisense oligonucleotides in an attempt to block the production of oncogene by preventing the transcription of chromosomal DNA to RNA. Antisense oligonucleotide can be administered systemically. Cytokine gene transfer to tumor cells stimulates a systemic immune response and destroy tumor cells. Cells are engineered to produce cytokines including interleukines 2,4,5, and 6, TNF and others. Clinical trials are in progress in patients with squamous cell carcinoma, ovarian epithelial cell carcinoma with this technology.

In cervical carcinoma, recurrent loss of heterozygosity (LOH) is identified. Active immunotherapy is effective.

Ovarian cancer: Point mutations of the *p53* (17P) gene are the most frequent genetic alteration. Loss of heterozygosity (LOH) on chromosome 17q has been noted.

Cytokines provide stimulatory signals important for T cell activation. Such cytokine milieu can be enhanced by local injection at the tumor site to promote the acquisition of cellular immunity. Tumor cells are genetically engineered to produce molecule of interest (IL-2, 4, 5, 6, MF-CSF, TNF) and are used as vaccines. Trials are in progress with this technology to prevent squamous cell cancer, colon cancer, ovarian epithelial cancer, and lung cancer.

TUMOR MARKERS

A tumor marker is a substance that is selectively produced by the neoplastic tissue. It is then released into the blood where from it can be detected.

Ideal tumor marker should fulfil the following criteria:

- *It should be produced only by the tumor cells.*
- *It should be specific.*
- *Its measurement either in the blood or urine should be sensitive enough to detect microscopic or subclinical disease.*

Uses of Tumor markers

- Assessment of risk of an individual without the disease so as to use it for **screening purpose**.
- Screening an individual to **detect** a cancer earlier before the appearance of clinical presentation.
- Tumor marker to **establish the tissue of origin** and to **differentiate the condition as benign or malignant.**
- **Assessment of prognosis** of a patient—risk of recurrence, metastasis.
- Ability of a marker to predict the **sensitivity or resistance to specific therapy**.
- **Monitoring the patient** during the course of therapy as regard the response to therapy.
- Tumor marker should represent the tumor volume correctly.

Tumor marker is useful in screening, diagnosis and management of a case and for follow-up. However, the detection of tumor marker is seldom made before the cell population becomes 10^{10}.

A list of tumor markers is given in Table 31.14.

TABLE 31.14: Commonly used gynecological tumor markers.

Marker	*Tissue of origin of cancer*
Human chorionic gonadotropin (hCG)	Trophoblastic and some germ cell tumor (dysgerminoma, embryonal carcinoma)
Alpha fetoprotein (AFP)	Germ cell tumor (yolk sac, immature teratoma tumor), dysgerminoma and others: Gastric, lung cancers
CA-125	Ovarian epithelial tumors (benign and malignant), endometrial carcinoma, endometriosis, PID, fibroid, salpingitis. Pancreatitis, normal women, non-ovarian cancers: Breast, pancreas, stomach, liver.
HE 4	Serous epithelial ovarian cancer, urologic cancer, lung cancer, endometrial cancer
Carcinoembryonic antigen (CEA)	Ovarian (serous, endometrioid), cervical carcinoma (squamous cell), endometrial cancer, colon and pancreatic cancers
Tumor associated glycoprotein-72 (TAG-72)	Epithelial ovarian tumor (EOT)
Macrophage colony stimulating factor (M-CSF)	Epithelial ovarian tumor (EOT)
Squamous cell carcinoma antigen (SCC)	Carcinoma cervix, vulvar and vaginal squamous cell carcinoma
Lactate dehydrogenase (LDH)	Ovarian germ cell tumors (dysgerminoma)
CA 15–3, OVX 1, OVX 2 HER-2/neu (oncogene product) HE 4	Ovarian epithelial carcinoma
Galactosyltransferase associated with tumor (GAT)	To differentiate ovarian cancer from endometriosis
Estrogen Progesterone Testosterone	Gonadal stromal tumors
Inhibin, anti-Müllerian hormone (AMH)	Granulosa cell tumor, mucinous and endometrioid cancers
Cell free DNA	Epithelial ovarian carcinoma (EOC)
Glycodelin	Serous ovarian cancer
CYFRA 21-1	Endometrial cancer, ovarian and cervical cancer

KEY POINTS

- ***Electromagnetic radiation** is a form of energy that has no mass or charge. It travels with the speed of light. For therapeutic purpose, radium, and cesium are commonly used.*
- **Effect of radiation** at a point varies inversely as the square of the distance from the source (inverse square law).
- **Brachytherapy** is the common form of radiation therapy especially when the tumor volume is small. After-loading technique is the modern development. Teletherapy is used to deliver to homogeneous radiation dose to a large volume of tumor.

Contd...

Contd...

- ***Rad** is the absorbed dose. Recently, the unit Gray (Joule/kg) is used. One centigray (cGy) is equivalent to one rad.*
- **Biological effects of radiation** are due to fast electron, that ionizes molecules to produce free radicals. Target for radiation injury is DNA. Tumor tissue recovers from radiation damage more slowly compared to normal tissue. Each delivered radiation dose kills a constant fraction of human cells. Oxygen can cause radiation-induced DNA damage permanent.
- **Radiocurability** of a tumor depends upon the biological behavior of the cells. It is not identical to radiosensitivity which depends several factors (p. 425).
- **There may be localized or systemic radiation reactions** for which appropriate therapy is needed. Early reaction is curable but the late reactions produce severe morbidity. Radiation reaction commonly affects GI tract, bone marrow, and bladder (p. 435).
- **The cell replication** cycle consists of M (mitosis), G_1 (RNA and protein synthesis), S (DNA synthesis) and G_2 (RNA and protein synthesis) phases. Cells, not in the replication cycle, are in G_0 phase (p. 431). Diving tumor cells (M phase) are most sensitive to cytotoxic agents. Radiation acts on cells primarily in M phase.
- **Large tumors** have smaller growth fractions and longer mass doubling time. Cytotoxic agents act on various phases of the cell cycle. They primarily affect rapidly proliferating cells. Rapidly growing tumors are more curable to treatment. Drugs commonly used are alkylating agents, antimetabolites, antibiotics, plant alkaloids, and hormones. Toxic effects varies from slight to more severe one, even to the extent of death (p. 433 and 434).
- ***Cisplatin** is more nephrotoxic and myelosuppressive compared to carboplatin. Doxorubicin is cardiotoxic. Bleomycin is associated with pulmonary toxicity. Vincristine and cisplatin cause peripheral neurotoxicity. Alopecia can occur with any chemotherapy. Taxol (paclitaxel and docetaxel) is a powerful antineoplastic agent that disrupts microtubule function (polymerization) (p. 433).*
- **Antiangiogenic agents** TOPO inhibitors (p. 488), mTOR inhibitors and the PARP inhibitors are being used to increase the tumor cell kill.
- **Combination therapy** is preferred. It gives a synergistic effect by acting at different cell sites and reduces the development of drug resistance (p. 433).
- **Multiple chemotherapeutic agents** have been used to kill cancer cells. They have also been used to sensitize cells to radiation. Chemoradiation improves outcome especially with squamous cell cancers.
- **Pretreatment evaluation** and proper monitoring during therapy are mandatory to prevent or minimize the toxicity (p. 432). Growth factors or granulocyte colony-stimulating factor are used to prevent hemorrhagic toxicity of chemotherapy.
- **Immunotherapy** in malignancy—is being explored recently. Cytokines (polypeptides) have antitumor and immune stimulating effects. Augmentation of immune system is achieved by active (interferon, IL-2) and passive (LAK cells) immunotherapy.
- ***Tumor markers** indicate the presence and also the site of tumor origin. It is useful in screening, diagnosis, and management of cases and also for follow up. Gynecological tumor markers in common use are—hCG in trophoblastic tumor, AFP in germ cell tumor, cancer antigen (CA)-125 in ovarian epithelial tumor and SCC in carcinoma cervix. HER-2/neu, an oncogene product is used for epithelial ovarian cancer (p. 438).*
- **Familial cancer** (breast, ovary, colon, endometrial) is explained on the basis of genes (oncogene, tumor suppressor gene, and mutator gene). Point mutation, deletion and insertion are the important changes. Gene therapy to the tissues at risk by insertion of normal copies of genes is a way forward.

CHAPTER

32 Hormones in Gynecological Practice

CHAPTER OUTLINE

NOMENCLATURES

- **Hormones**
- **Factors**
- **Analogs**
- **Agonists**
- **Antagonists**

- **Hormones:** Hormone is a substance that is produced in a special tissue and released into the bloodstream. Hormones travel to **distant cells** to have its desired effects.
- **Factors:** Factors are substances that modulate cell function and proliferation by acting upon the cell membrane receptors. They act locally (unlike the hormones) by autocrine and paracrine mechanism.
- **Analogs:** An analog is a synthetic substance with a structure mostly similar to a natural one but different from it in certain component. It may have agonist and/or antagonist function at the cellular level. Gonadotropin-releasing hormone (GnRH) analog acts as an agonist (upregulation) initially but on chronic therapy, it antagonizes (downregulation) the pituitary GnRH receptors.
- **Agonists:** Agonist is a substance that has increased affinity for cell receptors and it stimulates the cellular physiological response.
- **Antagonists:** An antagonist tends to nullify the action of another substance binding on its receptor without eliciting a biological response. There is a blockage of receptor response. Tamoxifen blocks estrogen receptor whereas mifepristone blocks progesterone receptors.

Because of relative lack of receptor specificity, an antagonist for one class of hormone can have an antagonistic effect on another class of hormone.

Antagonists may have adverse effects apart from the intended use.

CELLULAR FUNCTION

A cell function is modulated by any of the *three ways*:

1. **Endocrine** when a hormone in circulation (blood or lymph) regulates the function of a cell at a distant site.
2. **Paracrine** function is when a regulating substance diffuses from one cell to a contiguous cell (intercellular) and modulates the cell function. Insulin-like growth factor-II (IGF-II) is produced by the theca cells of ovary. It stimulates granulosa cell proliferation when it diffuses to it.
3. **Autocrine** function is explained when a regulating substance produced by a cell act upon the receptor on the same cell. It modulates the function of the same cell (intracellular). IGF-II is said to have autocrine function when it is produced by and acts on luteinized granulosa cells.

HYPOTHALAMIC HORMONES

GnRH

It is used for activation of hypothalamo-pituitary-gonadal function (p. 54).

- **Diagnostic**
- **Therapeutic**

- **Diagnostic:** The GnRH stimulation test is used to differentiate an amenorrhea of pituitary from hypothalamic in origin (p. 395).

An intravenous (IV) dose of GnRH 50–100 μg is given to stimulate pituitary. The maximal response is observed at 15–30 minutes for luteinizing hormone (LH) and 30–60 minutes for follicle-stimulating hormone (FSH). **The absence of response usually denotes pituitary fault.** However, the result may not be unequivocal and as such, requires cautious interpretation.

- **Therapeutic:** The pulsatile nature of hypothalamic GnRH in the control of gonadotropin secretion affords a physiological basis for the **activation of pituitary gonadal axis.**
  - ***Induction of ovulation:*** **It is suitable in cases with** idiopathic **hypogonadotropic hypogonadism** who have failed to respond with clomiphene. Pulsatile administration of GnRH (2.5–20 μg/pulse) at a constant interval (60–90 minutes) induces ovulation effectively. GnRH therapy results follicular growth and development similar to a normal cycle. In hypothalamic causes of anovulation, GnRH is most effective. For IV route, portable minipump is used. For subcutaneous route high dose (20 μg) is needed. **The main advantages of pulsatile administration are** lower incidence of hyperstimulation syndrome

and multiple pregnancy when compared to human menopausal gonadotropins (hMG).

Other uses through activation of pituitary-gonadal axis:

- **Delayed puberty**—to activate the pituitary-gonadal axis (p. 43)
- **Functional hypothalamic amenorrhea** to stimulate hypothalamic-pituitary-ovarian (HPO) axis for ovarian follicular development
- **Cryptorchidism**
- **Hypogonadotropic hypogonadism (p. 377)**.

GnRH Analogs

GnRH analogs (agonists and antagonists) have been synthesized by substitution of amino acids at different positions of GnRH molecule. This is done to overcome the short half-life, as well as to alter the functions of GnRH. **GnRH agonists have longer half lives (3–8 hours) and greater potencies (15–200 times).**

GnRH Agonist

This is produced when there is substitution of amino acids at 6 and 10 positions (Fig. 7.2, p. 54). This makes GnRH more stable with increased receptor affinity.

Mode of Action

Initially, there is stimulation of anterior pituitary resulting in increased secretion of FSH and LH **(upregulation)**. This is called **flare effect**. After 1–3 weeks, there is profound suppression of secretion **(downregulation)** due to loss of pituitary GnRH receptor sensitivity. This leads to a fall in pituitary gonadotropic hormones—LH and FSH, consequently the gonadal secretion (hypogonadotropic hypogonadal state). **The net effect is production of medical hypophysectomy**.

Mode of Administration

It can be used by intranasal and subcutaneous route and the biodegradable implants last for a month (Table 32.1).

Use of GnRH Agonists

- **Controlled ovarian stimulation in IVF:** Suppression of endogenous pituitary gonadotropin secretion by downregulation with GnRH analogs followed by administration of hMG or FSH allows good quality stimulation with superovulation. The problems of suboptimal response and premature luteinization due to endogenous LH surge are thus avoided. This will allow significantly higher number of oocyte retrieval and significant improvement in pregnancy rate. It is preferable to support the luteal phase with hCG.

  Protocol: *Two types of protocols are commonly used with probably of equal efficacy (p. 207).*

  a. Long protocol: The GnRH analogs are given from 21st day of previous cycle to desensitize the pituitary [LH level < 5 mIU/mL and estradiol (E_2) <30 pg/mL or when ultrasonogram (USG) fails to detect follicle] before the hMG or FSH is given. **The benefits include** less need of cycle monitoring, high pregnancy, and livebirth rates.

  b. Short protocol: The hMG or FSH is given soon after administration of GnRH agonists on day 2 and before the pituitary is desensitized. **The advantages of short protocol** are the economy and convenience, using for a short period of time.
- **Induction of ovulation with higher baseline LH in polycystic ovarian syndrome (PCOS):** In refractory cases of ovulation induction, especially in patient with polycystic ovaries (PCO), when the endogenous LH level is high, GnRH analogs offer a good success with long protocol regimen. It is used in the in vitro fertilization (IVF) cycles (p. 207).
- **Endometriosis:** By producing medical hypophysectomy and thereby, a hypoestrogenic state, it produces atrophy of the ectopic endometrium. **GnRH agonists are very effective in relieving the pain and reducing adhesion formation.**
- **Leiomyoma:** By producing hypoestrogenic state, they will produce shrinkage of the tumor by about 60% after 3–6 months treatment. But the size comes back to previous state after the drug is withdrawn. The drug cannot replace surgery. Blood loss during operation is less but surgical dissection may be difficult due to softening of the myoma. **GnRH antagonist** (depot cetrorelix) preoperative treatment has faster response (14 days) and is equally effective (p. 232).
- **Precocious puberty (p. 40):** In only constitutional variety, to inhibit the premature activation of hypothalamo-pituitary-gonadal axis, the analogs are safe and highly effective.

  Dose: 100 μg intranasally twice daily for 6 months or until the chronological ages are matched (Ch. 5).
- **Hirsutism:** In the idiopathic group, by suppressing the pituitary-gonadal axis, the excess hair growth can be arrested with the use of GnRH analogs.

  Dose: Nafarelin 100 μg per day subcutaneously will decrease the serum level of total and free testosterone and there is clinical improvement of hirsutism.
- **Dysfunctional uterine bleeding (DUB):** During the time, the patient waiting for operation or during the period to improve the anemic state (p. 159).
- **Premenstrual syndrome (PMS)/premenstrual dysphoric disorder (PMDD) (p. 150):** It is used for diagnostic as well as therapeutic purpose.

  For diagnostic purpose, a depot preparation is administered for 3 months. Leuprorelin acetate,

TABLE 32.1: Common preparations (GnRH agonists) available with their dose and route of administration.

Preparation	*Dose*	*Route*
Buserelin (Suprefact)	300–600 μg daily 200–500 μg daily	Intranasal, subcutaneous
Nafarelin	400–800 μg daily	Intranasal
Goserelin (Zoladex)	3.6 mg every 28 days	Subcutaneous implant
Leuprorelin (acetate)	3.75 mg every 28 days	Subcutaneous or intramuscular (IM)
Triptorelin (Decapeptyl)	3 mg every 28 days	Intramuscular

11.25 mg is given every 3 months for maximum 6 months. Relief of symptoms confirm the diagnosis (p. 150).

Symptoms due to hypoestrogenism is a problem. Add-back therapy may be needed (*see* below).

- **Advanced breast carcinoma** in premenopausal women (Estrogen dependent).
- **Contraception:** Used for ovulation inhibition and suppression of spermatogenesis (female and male) (Ch. 30).

  Used in male: (i) GnRH analogs produce a decline in sperm density, sperm mobility and testosterone level. The marked loss of libido makes it unacceptable. Currently, use of GnRH antagonist along with testosterone (add-back therapy) is found to overcome the problem. (ii) Prostatic cancer (hormone dependent).

  Used in female: GnRH analogs act by preventing the pituitary response to endogenous GnRH. Buserelin is given intranasally (Table 32.1). **Add-back therapy** is effective to prevent the hypoestrogenic symptoms (*see* below).
- **Endometrial resection/ablation:** Prior to endometrial resection, GnRH analogs are used to suppress the endometrial growth (p. 522).

Clinical use of GnRH and GnRH Agonists

- Induction of ovulation
- Controlled ovarian stimulation in IVF
- Delayed puberty
- Functional hypothalamic amenorrhea
- Hypogonadotropic hypogonadism
- Cryptochidism
- Endometriosis
- Polycystic ovarian syndrome
- Leiomyomas
- Precocious puberty
- Hirsutism
- AUB
- PMS/PMDD
- Breast Carcinoma
- Prior to endometrial resection (TCRE)
- Ovulation inhibition
- Suppression of spermatogenesis
- Contraception
- Prostatic cancer

GnRH Antagonist

It is synthesized by modification of amino acids at positions 1, 2, 3, 6 and 10 (Ganirelix, Cetrorelix). Minimum effective dose to prevent premature LH surge is 0.25 mg SC. Elagolix ,an oral GnRH antagonoist , is used for the control pain in endometriosis. ***The important properties of GnRH agonist and antagonist are given in Table 32.2.***

Hazards of GnRH Analogs

Side effects are predominantly due to hypogonadotropic and hypoestrogenic state. The important **side effects are** hot flashes, vaginal dryness, dyspareunia, headache, and depression (menopause-like symptoms, Ch. 6). Acne, muscle pain, back pain, dry skin are also noted. There is decrease in both, the trabecular (lumbar spine) and cortical (femoral neck) bone mineral density (osteoporosis) when used for more than 6 months. They do not produce significant changes in lipid metabolism. For long-term use, GnRH analogs have been used with low-dose estrogen and progestin (**add-back therapy**) to minimize the side effects. **Add-back therapy** consists

TABLE 32.2: Important properties of GnRH agonist and antagonist.

GnRH agonist	*GnRH antagonist*
Suppression of endogenous LH surge	Suppression of endogenous LH surge
Initial flare effect	Immediate suppression of gonadotropins
Duration of treatment —long	Short
Estrogen deficiency symptoms—present	Absent, well tolerated
Need of gonadotropin stimulation—dose and duration—more	Less
Pituitary function recovery—slow	Quick recovery following therapy
Risk of OHSS—present	Less OHSS (p. 444)
Expensive	Less expensive

of low-dose combined estrogen (conjugated estrogen 0.625 mg) and progestin (medroxyprogesterone 2.5 mg) therapy regimens daily. **Add-back therapy prevents bone loss and other side effects.**

GONADOTROPINS

The use of gonadotropins in clinical use lies on the principle that gonadotropic hormones act on the ovaries to induce ovulation. **The gonadotropins, used widely today, are derived from urine obtained from postmenopausal women.** Human gonadotropin can also be obtained from extract of cadaveric pituitary glands. Human pituitary gonadotropin (hPG) is predominantly FSH. It is not easily available.

The most commonly used commercial preparation is hMG. One ampoule of hMG (pergonal) contains LH activity of 75 IU and FSH activity of 75 IU. Purified FSH (Metrodin-75 IU/ampoule) is available with minimum LH. Highly purified preparation of human FSH can be administered subcutaneously. Recombinant FSH (Gonal F or Recagon) is now available. It is administered by subcutaneous route.

hCG is known to have a biological action like LH surge and is available in ampoules with 1000–5000 IU. **It is obtained from urine of pregnant women.** Recombinant gonadotropins (FSH, LH, and hCG) are used for ovarian stimulation according to the need of individual woman and to optimize oocyte quality and cycle fecundity.

Limitations

- It is expensive.
- It should only be used with back-up facilities for monitoring the response by basal body temperature (BBT), cervical mucus study, supplemented by serial serum estradiol estimation, and sonographic measurement of follicular enlargement (Ch. 17).

As such, its use is limited only in women with adequate ovarian reserve (p. 444).

Indications

- Anovulatory infertility where other factors (tubal, uterine, male) have been excluded.
- Induction of superovulation in assisted reproduction (p. 207).
- hCG is administered for luteal phase support especially when GnRH agonist is used.
- Treatment of male infertility (hypogonadotropic hypogonadism) (p. 201).
- Treatment of cryptorchidism.
- Hypogonadotropic hypogonadism (WHO Group-I, p. 212) with or without amenorrhea.
- Failed clomiphene induction especially in patients with PCOS.
- Unexplained infertility.

Contraindications

- High level of endogenous FSH, indicating ovarian failure (p. 287 and 294)
- Overt thyroid or adrenal dysfunction
- Pituitary tumor
- Indeterminate uterine bleeding.

Treatment Protocol

The drug dose schedule should be individualized to get the best result. As a rule, a higher dose is required in cases of secondary amenorrhea due to pituitary failure and a smaller dose may be required in ovulatory failure or corpus luteal insufficiency.

Women with hypogonadotropic hypogonadism should be treated with hMG (FSH and LH). Treatment with hMG begins following spontaneous menses or induced withdrawal bleeding. A daily dose of 1–2 ampoules of hMG is given intramuscularly for at least 5 days and continued thereafter, with the same dose or an increasing dose with cervical mucus study, E_2 estimation and sonographic (transvaginal) folliculometry at interval of 2–3 days or earlier until the preovulatory follicular diameter measures 18–20 mm (p. 207 and 208). The hMG is then discontinued and after 24 hours, hCG is given intramuscularly for ovulation. The dose of hCG is 5,000 IU for induction of ovulation. The patient is advised to have sexual intercourse on a number of occasions over the next 36–72 hours progesterone support.

In some cases, for adequate ovarian follicular growth, high doses of FSH (4–6 ampoules per day) may be needed.

High responders are those women who have exaggerated response in follicular development. The diagnostic features are enlarged ovaries with large number of follicles, elevated serum estradiol (>3,000 pg/mL).

Management Options

- **Coasting**
  - To continue GnRH agonist.
  - No gonadotropin stimulation.
  - To give hCG once estradiol level is within the normal range (*see* above).
- **Oocyte retrieval and fertilization**—freezing all embryos and no transfer to avoid ovarian hyperstimulation syndrome (OHSS).
- **To delay** embryo transfer until the symptoms subside.
- **To cancel** the treatment cycle.

These women have good prognosis in subsequent cycles.

Poor responders are those women who develop fewer follicle (<3) and have serum estradiol <500 pg/mL in spite of high doses of gonadotropins.

Management Options

- To use higher doses of gonadotropin stimulation.
- To decrease the doses of GnRH agonist.
- To use GnRH antagonist instead of long-acting agonist.

These women have relatively poor prognosis.

Results of Gonadotropin Uses

Cumulative pregnancy rate is about 90% after 6 cycles treatment. Spontaneous miscarriage rate is high (20%). Risk of ectopic pregnancy is high. Multiple pregnancy rate is between 10 and 30%. Majority are twins. There is no increased incidence of congenital malformation of the fetus.

- **Ovarian reserve** means the quantity as well as quality of follicles present in the ovary. The total number of oocytes declines with the age of a woman since her birth. **Inhibin B** secreted by the competent follicles, exerts negative feedback on pituitary FSH secretion (p. 62). With the progressive fall in **follicle number** as with age, inhibin B level is reduced. There is rise in FSH level even in the early follicular phase.
- **Detection of diminished ovarian reserve (DOR): Tests for detection of DOR** can indentify the women who are likely to have poor response with gonadotropin and lower pregnancy rate:
  - Levels of cycle D_3 serum FSH >10–15 IU/L.
  - Levels of D_3 serum estradiol >60–80 pg/mL.
  - *Clomiphene citrate challenge test:* Levels of D_3 serum FSH and estradiol are measured. The women is given clomiphene citrate (100 mg daily from D_5–D_9). Serum levels of FSH is measured again on D_{10} and elevated values of serum FSH (more than 2 SD of the mean) are obtained.
  - Levels of serum anti-Müllerian hormone (AMH)—low (0.2–0.7 ng/mL).
  - Levels of basal serum inhibin B—low (<40 pg/mL). However, it is not a reliable measure.
  - **Antral follicle count (AFC):** Total number of antral follicles (measuring 2–10 mm) in both the ovaries using transvaginal sonography (TVS) is proportional to the number of primordial follicles present in the ovaries. So, a low AFC indicates poor ovarian reserve. A woman in her reproductive age, usually have 20–150 growing follicles in the ovaries at any time. A count of <10 predicts poor reserve.

- **Ovarian volume measurement (OVM)**: Ovarian volume decreases with progressive follicular loss. Poor ovarian reserve indicates poor outcome with IVF. Women need counseling for alternatives like donor oocyte or adoption.

Hazards of ovulation induction (p. 210)

Ovarian Hyperstimulation Syndrome

The OHSS is characterized by multiple follicular development and ovarian enlargement following hCG stimulation. *It occurs mostly with the conception cycle.* The clinical features appear about 3-6 days after the ovulating dose of hCG is administered. It is an iatrogenic and potentially a life-threatening complication of superovulation.

Risk Factors for OHSS

Young age <30 years, PCOS, serum E_2 >2,500 pg/mL, rapidly rising serum E_2 levels (>75% rise from previous day), ovarian 'necklace sign' on USG (multiple small follicles) (Fig. 32.1) hCG administration, and multiple pregnancy.

Pathophysiology

This is poorly understood. Increased capillary permeability leads to leakage of fluid from the peritoneal and ovarian surfaces. Variety of chemical mediators like cytokines, vascular epidermal growth factor (VEGF), prorenin, renin, and nitric oxide (NO) system are thought to be stimulated with hCG administration.

Prevention

Complete prevention may not be possible but severity can be reduced (Table 32.3). The important steps to be taken are:

- Use of GnRH antagonists for pituitary downregulation.
- Low starting dose of gonadotropins in high-risk women.
- Metformin cotreatment during gonadotropin stimulation in women with PCOS.
- Close monitoring of the superovulation cycles using TVS and serum estradiol estimation (p. 207).

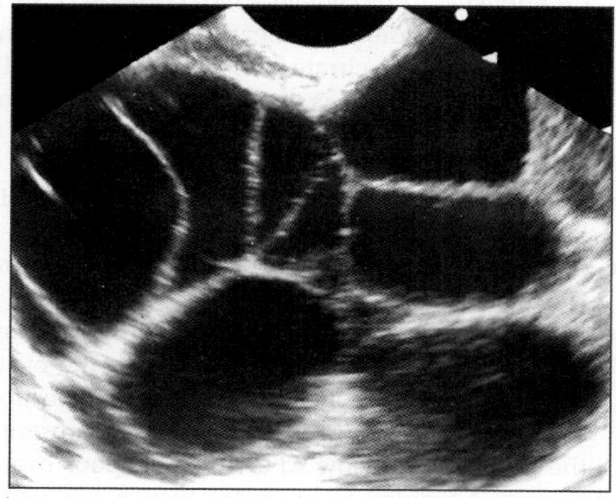

Fig. 32.1: Ultrasonographic view of ovarian hyperstimulation syndrome (OHSS). Enlargement of the ovary with multiple follicles.

TABLE 32.3: Classification of OHSS.

Severity	*Clinical features*
Mild (10–20%)	▪ Abdominal bloating, mild pain ▪ Ovarian size <5 cm
Moderate (5–10%)	▪ Nausea, vomiting, diarrhea ▪ Ultrasonographic (USG) evidence of ascites ▪ Ovarian size: 8–12 cm ▪ Normal laboratory values
Severe (1–2%)	▪ Clinical ascites, sometimes hydrothorax ▪ Acute respiratory distress syndrome (ARDS) ▪ Hemoconcentration (hematocrit > 45%, WBC count >15,000/mL) ▪ Oliguria with raised serum creatinine ▪ Hyponatremia, hyperkalemia ▪ Liver dysfunction ▪ Anasarca ▪ Ovarian size >12 cm
Critical (rare)	▪ Tense ascites, severe end organ dysfunction ▪ Hematocrit >55% ▪ WBC count >25,000/mL ▪ Oliguria with serum creatinine >1.6 mg/dL ▪ Renal failure ▪ Thromboembolic complications ▪ Ovarian size >12 cm

- To withhold ovulatory dose of hCG in susceptible cases and to cancel the cycle or to delay the dose of hCG injection (coasting).
- Follicular aspiration after hCG administration and cryopreservation of oocytes or embryos for future use may reduce the severity of symptoms (coasting and cryopreservation).
- **Dopamine agoinst:** Cabergoline is found to be effective as it inhibits the action of VEGF.
- Aspiration of immature oocytes and in vitro maturation (IVM) are done. Subsequently intracytoplasmic sperm injection (ICSI) is performed on IVM oocytes and embryos are transferred to the hormonally prepared uterus.
- Progesterone should be used for luteal phase support (p. 208) instead of hCG.

Management

Management of OHSS is mainly supportive. Moderate and severe cases are to be admitted.

- To monitor complete hemogram, liver function tests (LFTs), renal function tests (RFTs), electrolytes, coagulation profile, electrocardiography (ECG), and urine output.
- Chest X-ray (shielding the pelvis), monitoring of O_2 saturation is needed when there is respiratory compromise.
- TVS is to be done to assess ovarian volume and ascites.
- Oral fluid is continued to prevent hemoconcentration and to maintain renal perfusion. Normal saline 150 mL/hour IV is given when hematocrit is >45%.
- To relieve respiratory distress, abdominal paracentesis may be done under USG guidance.

- Human albumin (50 mL of 25%) may be administered to correct hypovolemia. It may be repeated.
- Pain is controlled with paracetamol or pethidine.
- Intensive care management (ICM) is needed for specific complications like renal failure.
- Surgery is rarely indicated.

ANTIGONADOTROPINS

Commonly used drugs

- **Danazol**
- **Gestrinone**

Danazol

Danazol is an isoxazole derivative of 17-alpha ethinyl testosterone. It has got both androgenic and anabolic properties. **It is strictly antigonadotropin but acts as an androgen agonist** (Table 32.4).

Mode of Action

The mechanism of action is complex and includes the following:

- Acting on the hypothalamo-pituitary-gonadal axis → depression of frequency of GnRH pulses → suppression of pituitary FSH and LH surge. There is, however, no change in the basal gonadotropin level. Due to this reason the word 'pseudomenopause' seems misnomer; while the estrogen level is reduced but **unlike menopause, the gonadotropins remain static in base levels.**
- Reduces the liver synthesis of sex hormone-binding globulin (SHBG) and as such, free testosterone is increased which in turn has got direct action on endometrial atrophy.
- Acts directly on the ovaries, inhibiting the enzymes responsible for steroidogenesis. Estrogen level is low.
- Binds with steroid receptors on the endometrium and also in the ectopic endometrial sites.
- It causes endometrial atrophy.
- Immunologic effects of danazol include decrease in serum immunoglobulins (Igs), interleukin-1 (Il-1) and tumor necrosis factor (TNF) production. This effect helps in the regression of endometriosis.

The net result is production of an hypoestrogenic and hyperandrogenic and anabolic state.

Precautions

It should be commenced in the early follicular phase of the menstrual cycle. **Barrier method of contraception** should be used to avoid being administered during early pregnancy following accidental ovulation. There is a chance of virilization of the female offspring. **It is contraindicated in liver disease.**

Dose

Depending upon the indication and response, the dose varies from 200–800 mg daily orally. It is used less commonly.

Lower doses of 100 mg/day is also used. Duration of therapy is usually 4–6 months. Improvement following treatment is about 90%. Recurrence rate is 15–30% within 2 years of therapy. Therapeutic effectiveness of danazol with GnRH agonist appear to be the same.

Side Effects (Table 32.5)

The side effects are mostly related to hypoestrogenic and androgenic activity. However, most of these effects revert back to normal soon following stoppage of the therapy. It is recommended that the patient should discontinue the treatment, if they develop hirsutism or hoarseness of voice.

TABLE 32.4: Indications of danazol.

▪ Endometriosis	▪ Precocious puberty
▪ DUB (menorrhagia)	▪ PMS/PMDD (p. 150)
▪ Symptomatic fibroid	▪ Benign fibrocystic disease of the breasts (breast pain)
▪ Prior to hysteroscopic endometrial ablation, to make the endometrium thin	

(DUB: dysfunctional uterine bleeding; PMS: premenstrual syndrome; PMDD: premenstrual dysphoric disorder)

Gestrinone

Gestrinone is a derivative of 19-norethisterone. It is an androgen-agonist and progesterone agonist-antagonist. It markedly reduces SHBG levels and thus increases the free testosterone. It reduces the secretion of FSH and LH. It has a much longer half-life and the dose required to produce equivalent results, is much smaller than danazol.

Dose

2.5 mg twice weekly starting on first day of cycle with second dose 3 days later, repeated on same two days preferably at same time each week.

Side Effects

This are the same to those of danazol but usually less marked.

TABLE 32.5: Side effects of danazol.

Hypoestrogenic	*Androgenic*		*Metabolic and others*
▪ Diminished breast size	▪ Acne	▪ Oily skin	▪ Elevation of LDL, total cholesterol
▪ Decreased libido	▪ Edema	▪ Weight gain	▪ Reduction of HDL
▪ Atrophic vaginitis	▪ Hirsutism		▪ Decrease in TBG and total thyroxine level
▪ Hot flashes, sweats	▪ Deepening of voice (irreversible)		▪ Weakness, GI disturbances

(LDL: low-density lipoprotein; HDL: high-density lipoprotein; TBG: thyroxine-binding globulin; GI: gastrointestinal)

GONADAL HORMONES

There are three gonadal steroid hormones. These are estrogen, progesterone, and androgen.

MECHANISM OF ACTION

Steroid sex hormones are well-absorbed through the skin and the gut. While most are subjected to extensive hepatic metabolic inactivation, there is some enterohepatic recirculation especially of estrogens. This circulation may be interrupted by diarrhea to cause loss of efficacy. The sex hormones are transported in the blood non-specifically by albumin and specifically by SHBG.

Steroid hormone receptors are complex proteins inside the target cell. The steroid penetrates the cell membrane and mediates action via receptors within the nucleus in the cytoplasm (Fig. 7.6).

ESTROGENS

Natural estrogens are 18-carbon atom steroids. Estradiol is the most active natural estrogen in human uses. Clinical and metabolic effects of estrogens and their grades of potency are different (Table 32.6).

Preparations Available

- **Natural**
- **Synthetic**

Natural

(a) It is available in the form of water soluble conjugated estrogen as Premarin [conjugated equine estrogen (CEE)]. It is obtained from the urine of pregnant mares. It is available as tablets 0.3 mg, 0.625 mg, and 1.25 mg and as injection of 20 mg ampoules for IM or IV injection. (b) Estradiol valerate used for priming the endometrium in donor oocyte program (Ch. 17).

Synthetic

- **Oral**
- **Injectable**
- **Cream/gel**
- **Pessary**
- **Implant**
- **Patch**

Oral: This is the best route for synthetic preparations.

- Ethinyl estradiol (Lynoral): 0.01 mg and 0.05 mg daily is commonly used
- Estradiol valerate: 1–2 mg

TABLE 32.6: Clinical and metabolic effects of estrogens and their grades of potency in comparison to 17β-estradiol.

	Suppression effect		*Increase in serum level*	
Types of estrogen	**Hot flashes**	**FSH**	**HDL**	**SHBG**
17β-estradiol	100	100	100	100
Conjugated equine estrogen (CEE)	120	110	150	300
Estriol	30	20		
Ethinyl estradiol	12,000	12,000	40,000	50,000

(FSH: follicle-stimulating hormone; HDL: high-density lipoprotein; SHBG: sex hormone-binding globulin)

- CEE: 0.3 or 0.625 mg
- Estriol succinate (Evalon): 1–2 mg.

Injectable: (a) Estradiol ester as progynon depot (Schering): 10 mg ampoule; (b) Estradiol benzoate or dipropionate: 1 mg and 5 mg ampoule.

Cream: (a) Vaginal cream–dienestrol (0.1 mg/g), estriol (1 mg/g); (b) Percutaneous cream delivers 3 mg of estradiol in each daily 5 g applicator of cream.

Gel: 17β-estradiol gel, 1 mg to be applied once daily over the skin of the lower trunk.

Pessary: Dienestrol or estradiol acetate pessary (inserted for 90 days).

Implants: Subcutaneous implants of 50 mg and 100 mg of 17β-estradiol effect lasts for 6 months.

Transdermal patch: It contains 17β-estradiol releasing about 0.05–0.1 mg of estradiol in 24 hours. Patch should be applied below the waist line and changed twice a week.

Therapy

- **Replacement therapy**
- **Pharmacotherapy**

Replacement Therapy

Ovarian hypofunction: Estrogen daily × 21 days followed by norethisterone or medroxyprogesterone 5 mg × last 10 days (p. 373).

Menopausal symptoms:

- Cyclic or continuous therapy in the form of estradiol or conjugated estrogens
- Postmenopausal hormone replacement therapy (HRT) in a symptomatic women (p. 50)
  - To reduce vasomotor symptoms
  - To prevent osteoporosis
  - To prevent cardiovascular disease.

It is administered either cyclic or continuous. Progestogen should be added to reduce endometrial carcinoma. However, in hysterectomized individuals, progestogen is not added. **It is especially indicated** in premature ovarian failure (POF), gonadal dysgenesis and in surgical menopause (details in Ch. 6).

- Genitourinary symptoms of menopause is observed when serum estradiol level is <35 pg/mL.
- **Common symptoms are:**
  - **Vaginal dryness**, burning and irritation
  - **Sexual difficulty** due to lack of lubrication, causing pain
  - **Urinary symptoms:** Urgency, dysuria and recurrent UTI. Treatment options are: To use local estrogens in the form of vaginal cream, tablet, ring or oral tablets. Commonly used estrogens are: Conjugated estrogens or 17 β-estradiol.

Pharmacotherapy

The estrogen is most commonly used along with progestogen and as such, the use of the combined therapy is discussed later on. **The indications of only the estrogen therapy are mentioned here.**

Oral contraception

While the combined estrogen and progestogen preparations are widely used throughout the globe, estrogen in isolation is only used as postcoital contraception (details in Ch. 30).

Vaginitis

Senile or atrophic vaginitis—either vaginal cream or oral estrogens may be equally effective (Ch. 6).

Vulvovaginitis

Vulvovaginitis in childhood, foreign body in the vagina or sexual assault—low dose of oral estrogen or vaginal cream helps in increasing the vaginal defense and hastens recovery (p. 457).

Intersex state

In Turner's syndrome (45, XO) or **gonadal dysgenesis (46, XY)**, estrogen therapy is helpful for the growth and development of the secondary sexual characters (Ch. 28).

In **androgen insensitivity syndrome (46, XY)**, after gonadectomy supplementary estrogen therapy is indicated to prevent regression of the breast development, osteoporosis and cardiovascular complications (Ch. 28).

The estrogen is used cyclically as ethinyl estradiol 0.01 mg twice daily for 25 days. However, in prolonged use, progestogen in the form of medroxyprogesterone acetate 10 mg daily is added from day 16–25, to minimize the adverse effects of estrogen. Alternatively, a combined oral 'pill' may be prescribed.

Dysfunctional uterine bleeding

The estrogen in pharmacological doses causes rapid growth of endometrium. As such, acute bleeding can be stopped by oral conjugated estrogen in a dose of 10 mg a day. The bleeding usually stops within 24 hours. Alternatively, 25 mg may be given intravenously every 4 hours for 3 doses (p. 159).

Delayed puberty

If the breast development fails to start even at the age of 14, 10 μg of estrogen daily may be of help. In cases of irregular bleeding or when the breast development is well-advanced, progestogens may be added (Ch. 5).

Cervical mucus hostility

To improve the quality of the cervical mucus in infertility, low dose of estrogen (ethinyl estradiol 0.01 mg) may be given cyclically, from day 1–14.

An Adjunct with Clomiphene Therapy

In cases of hypoestrogenic state with hypomenorrhea, small dose of estrogen is of help to improve the quality of the cervical mucus.

Genuine stress incontinence (GSI) in postmenopausal women to improve the tone of collagen tissue.

Comments

Oral route with preparations of ethinyl estradiol is widely used because of its efficacy, low cost, and minimal intolerance. Vaginal cream used in atrophic vaginitis has got its local and systemic effects.

Intramuscular (IM) administration of progynon depot 10 mg at interval of one month is helpful as a prophylaxis against postmenopausal symptoms, following hysterectomy with bilateral salpingo-oophorectomy in premenopausal women.

Adverse Effects

Minor ailments are:

- Nausea, vomiting
- Breast tenderness
- Breakthrough bleeding
- Weight gain

Major effects include: Increased incidence of endometrial carcinoma, thromboembolism, cerebral thrombosis, and hemorrhage.

To minimize breakthrough bleeding and prevent endometrial carcinomas and vascular complications, progestogens should be combined with estrogen therapy. **Contraindications** of use are important (Table 32.7).

ANTIESTROGEN

- **Clomiphene**
- **Aromatase inhibitors**
- **Tamoxifen**

Clomiphene

Clomiphene citrate is a nonsteroid triphenylethylene compound with a structure similar to that of stilbestrol. The commercially available form is a mixture of two isomers, enclomiphene—a potent antiestrogen and zuclomiphene—a weak antiestrogen.

Mode of Action

In the hypothalamus, clomiphene citrate binds to estrogen receptors, occupies the nuclear site for a long time (weeks). The negative feedback of endogenous estrogen is thus prevented. The frequency of pulsatile GnRH secretion is thereby increased which in turn results in rise of pulse frequency of both LH and FSH. Antiestrogenic effects are observed at the level of cervix and endometrium.

During therapy with clomiphene citrate (CC), there is rise in serum levels of LH and FSH and also the levels of serum E_2.

Indications

- Anovulatory infertility where other factors have been excluded.
- Induction of ovulation—the ideal case is one of normogonadotropic-normoprolactinemic disorders of ovulation.
- Assisted reproductive techniques in producing superovulation.
- Male infertility with defective spermatogenesis due to hypogonadotropic hypogonadism.

TABLE 32.7: Contraindications of estrogen therapy (p. 57).

- Undiagnosed genital bleeding
- History of venous thromboembolism
- Active liver disease
- Severe hypertension
- Organic heart disease
- Estrogen dependent neoplasia (breast)

Mode of Administration

Adjuvant drugs: Adjuvant drugs are used when there is failure with clomiphene therapy (Ch. 17).

Contraindications

- Patients who are hypogonadotropic and hypoestrogenic.
- Presence of cystic ovaries.

Side Effects

These include visual disturbances, headache, hot flashes, breast tenderness, abdominal discomfort, loss of hair, rashes, ovarian enlargement and multiple pregnancy. Hyperstimulation syndrome (p. 444) is less likely.

Results

While successful induction can be achieved by 90%, pregnancy rate is about 50%. The **reduced pregnancy rate may be due to its** antiestrogenic effect on endometrium cervical mucus and the oocyte. There may be the presence of other factors for infertility including luteal phase defect (LPD) and luteinized unruptured follicle (LUF) (p. 197). Chance of multiple pregnancy ranges 0–5%.

Aromatase Inhibitors

It inhibits the **enzyme aromatase** in the granulosa cells of ovarian follicles (p. 61 and 62). It suppresses estrogen (E_2) synthesis. It increases the level of FSH. Intra-ovarian androgen levels are also increased. This enhances sensitivity to FSH. No differences in adverse effect or congenital anomalies when compared to CC. Letrozole in combination with gonadotropins may be used in poor responders for IVF.

Letrozole, 2.5 mg given from D3 to D7 increases the release of gonadotropins from the pituitary and stimulates development of ovarian follicle. It suppresses ovarian estradiol secretion and reduces estrogen induced negative feedback. As a result, levels of FSH rises. Intraovarian androgens are increased which increase FSH sensitivity. As opposed to clomiphene, it has no peripheral antiestrogenic effects on the endometrium and the cervical mucus. Half-life of letrozole is 45 hours. Letrozole is used either as a firstline therapy (alternative to clomiphene) or in clomiphene-resistant women (p. 203) with anovulatory infertility. Pregnancy rates are comparable or better than that of clomiphene. Multiple pregnancy rates are low (monofollicular development).

Anastrozole, another aromatase inhibitor is found to be effective in reducing the growth of pelvic endometriosis and in pain relief.

Aromatase inhibitors are primarily used for the treatment of breast cancer in postmenopausal women.

Tamoxifen (SERMs)

Tamoxifen [selective estrogen receptor modulators (SERMs)], is similar to clomiphene both structurally and functionally. It has got both **estrogen antagonist and agonist effects.**

- It is a competitive inhibitor to estrogen at the receptor site. **Antiestrogenic** function of raloxifene is more selective in **uterus and breasts**.
- It decreases antithrombin III and increases the SHBG level (agonist action). Venous thromboembolism (VTE) is increased.
- It can be used for induction of ovulation in doses of 20 mg per day for 5 days, in cases of intolerance to clomiphene.
- It is widely used for the treatment of benign breast diseases.
- In postmenopausal breast carcinoma, it is given in doses of 10 mg twice daily for 2 years as an adjuvant therapy. It is effective both in estrogen receptor positive and negative cases.
- In recurrent endometrial carcinoma, it inhibits the binding of estradiol to the estrogen receptor. Tamoxifen increases the progesterone receptors. A dose of 20–40 mg per day has been used. Low grade tumors and hormone receptor positive tumors have got better response.
- Raloxifene (p. 50) therapy (60 mg a day) is effective in regression of endometriosis.
- Bazedoxifene (BZA) is a SERM. It is used in combination with CEE to improve the vasomotor symptoms and prevents postmenstrual bone loss. Combination of CEE (0.45 mg) PLUS BZA (20 mg) do not cause change in breast density and endometrial thickness.

Side Effects

Hot flashes, vaginal dryness, risks of thromboembolism and risks of endometrial carcinoma on prolonged use.

PROGESTERONE

Progesterone is a natural hormone (C-21 steroid) produced mainly by the theca lutein cells of the corpus luteum (p. 71). It is also secreted by the adrenal cortex in small amount. During pregnancy, placenta is the main source. Progesterone produces secretory changes in an estrogen primed endometrium. Natural progesterones are rapidly metabolized and inactivated when administered by the oral route and as such, it is to be used parenterally. During the last few decades, a number of compounds were synthesized having the properties of progesterone and could be given in tablet form. **These are called progestational agents, gestagens, progestogens** or **progestins**. Classification of progestogens and their grades of progestational activity are given in Tables 32.8 and 32.9.

Uses

- **Diagnostic**
- **Therapeutic**

Diagnostic

Progesterone challenge test: In the investigation of pathological amenorrhea, this test is employed. If withdrawal bleeding occurs, it proves (a) **Intact HPO axis;**

TABLE 32.8: Classifications of progestogens.

	Progesterone derivative	*Progesterone content*
I.	**Progesterone**	Natural progesterone
II.	**Pregnane progestogens** They do not alter carbohydrate metabolism	17 α-hydroxyprogesterone caproate Medroxyprogesterone acetate Chlormadinone acetate Cyproterone acetate
III.	**Norpregnane progestogens**	▪ Nomegestrol acetate ▪ Gestonorone caproate
IV.	**Stereoisomer of progesterone: Retroprogesterone** They do not inhibit ovulation	▪ Dydrogesterone
V.	**19 norprogesterone derivatives** (norpregnanes)	▪ Demegestone ▪ Promegestone ▪ Nestorone ▪ Trimegestone
VI.	**Alkyl derivatives of 19 nortestosterone**	
	A. *Estrone steroids* They alter carbohydrate metabolism slightly. Metabolically, they are converted into norethisterone	▪ Norethisterone ▪ Norethisterone acetate ▪ Norethynodrel ▪ Ethynodiol diacetate ▪ Lynestrenol ▪ Norgestrel
	B. *Gonane steroids* They have excellent contraceptive efficacy and cycle control. Side effects are less. They are more potent than the estrone steroids	▪ Levonorgestrel ▪ Desogestrel ▪ Etonogestrel (3-keto-desogestrel) ▪ Gestodene ▪ Norgestimate ▪ Norelgestromin ▪ Dienogest
VII.	**Spironolactone derivatives**	Drospirenone
VIII.	**Unsaturated 19 nor-steroid**	Gestrinone

(b) There is adequate **endogenous estrogen** (>40 pg/mL); (c) The **endometrium is responsive**; and (d) The **uterovaginal canal** is patent. The individual is likely to respond to ovulation induction drugs (p. 395).

Dose

Medroxyprogesterone acetate 10 mg daily for 5 days is given orally.

Limitations of the test

Some women may bleed with fluctuating levels of estrogen as in hypothalamic amenorrhea or in early stages of POF. Secondly women with high androgen levels (PCOS and CAH) may have atrophic endometrium and may fail to bleed.

TABLE 32.9: Metabolic effects of progestogens and their grades of progestational activity.

	Progestogens	Progestational activity	Androgenic activity	Anti-androgenic activity	Levels of SHBG ↓
1.	**Progesterone**	1	–	+	–
2.	**Cyproterone acetate**	4	–	+++	–
3.	**Medroxyprogesterone**	4	+	–	+
4.	**Norethisterone**	4	+	–	–
5.	**Norgestimate**	4	+	–	–
6.	**Drospirenone**	4	–	+	–
7.	**Dienogest**	4	–	+	–
8.	**Nomegestrol**	5	–	+	–
9.	**Levonorgestrel**	6	++	–	++
10.	**Desogestrel**	8	+	–	–
11.	**Gestodene**	9	+	–	+
12.	**Nestorone**	10	–	–	–
13.	**Trimegestone**	10	–	+	?

Progestational activity is graded 1–10; considering progesterone as 1, 10 being the most potent
SHBG = sex hormone-binding globulin;
(–) = no effect
(+) = effect
(++) = strong effect
(+++) = very strong effect

Therapeutic Indications

Contraception

Combined preparations of estrogen and progestogen are widely used as contraceptive pill (Ch. 30). Uses of only progestogens as contraception are:

- Minipill (oral) (p. 410)
- Levonorgestrel: Emergency contraception (p. 411).
- Depot medroxyprogesterone acetate (DMPA) (injectable)
- Norethisterone enanthate: NET-EN (injectable)
- Implant (implanon subdermally) (p. 411)
- Vaginal ring containing levonorgestrel (p. 423)
- Levonorgestrel-intrauterine system (LNG-IUS)—containing L-norgestrel (p. 398).

Dysfunctional uterine bleeding

Progestogen administration will cause secretory changes in the endometrium. Thus, it is very active in cases of anovulatory than in an ovulatory DUB. The therapy is ideal in puberty, adolescent and those approaching menopause.

To stop bleeding, norethisterone or norethisterone acetate 5 mg thrice daily is quite effective. To regulate the cycle, the same preparation is used from D_5–D_{25} or from D_{15}–D_{25} of cycle.

Mode of Action

Progesterone decreases synthesis of estrogen receptors in the endometrium.

- It converts estradiol to less potent estrone through enzymatic action.
- It inhibits mitotic activity of the endometrial cells.
- It induces the enzyme estradiol dehydrogenase—which degrades estradiol in the endometrium.
- Over all progesterone acts as an antiestrogen on the endometrium.

Endometriosis

The use of progestogens induces a hyperprogestogenic-hypoestrogenic state. Progestogens cause decidualization of endometrial tissue. There will be atrophy of the glands, fibrosis and atrophy of the ectopic endometrial tissues. Progestins also reduce the nerve fiber density and nerve growth factor expression in endometriotic lesions.

The drugs commonly used are medroxyprogesterone acetate or dydrogesterone or derivatives of 19-norethisterone.

Dose

Norethisterone 5 mg or medroxyprogesterone 10 mg twice or thrice daily and continued for 6–9 months. The patient remains amenorrheic.

Alternatively, IM injection of medroxyprogesterone acetate 100 mg every 2 weeks for 4 doses and then 200 mg every month for 4 doses will produce amenorrhea. This is suitable in cases of older women who have completed family.

Dysmenorrhea

Dydrogesterone 5 mg starting from day 5 for 20 days, relieves dysmenorrhea probably by inhibiting uterine contractions. The ovulation is not suppressed. Use of LNG-IUD and progestin implant (implanon) is found to be effective in cases with pelvic endometriosis or adenomyosis.

Luteal phase defect (LPD) (p. 203)

In a proven case, daily IM injection of 12.5 mg progesterone in oil, beginning 2–3 days after the ovulation until menstruation occurs or if conception has taken place, until 10–12 weeks of gestation. Micronized progesterone 100 mg thrice daily can be administered either vaginally or orally. Vaginal suppositories 25 mg twice daily starting 2–3 days after the BBT rise is equally effective.

Endometrial hyperplasia and endometrial carcinoma

Its role in endometrial carcinoma depends on the number of steroid receptors on the tumor. **Well-differentiated grade I endometrial carcinoma has got the highest number of receptors**. These cases are suitable for progestogen therapy. Recurrent endometrial carcinoma having good steroid receptor status is also suitable.

Dose

17α-hydroxyprogesterone caproate 1,000 mg IM daily for 1 week, weekly for 3 months and thereafter at interval of 2 weeks for 1 year. Alternatively, medroxyprogesterone acetate 400 mg IM weekly for 3 months and then every 2 weeks for 1 year.

TABLE 32.10: Side effect of progestogens.

▪ Nausea—subsides gradually	
▪ Leg cramps	
▪ Mastalgia	
▪ Weight gain due to salt and water retention	
▪ Acne	due to androgenic progestins
▪ Scanty periods	
▪ Loss of libido	
▪ Virilism	
▪ Headaches—migraines should be excluded	
▪ Depression and mood changes—may be due to low level of pyridoxine as progestins alter the tryptophan metabolism	
▪ Lipid profile—increase in LDL and decrease in HDL level	

Premenstrual syndrome (PMS) (p. 150)

Controversy exists with the hypothesis that progesterone deficiency may be the cause. So, progestogens have been tried to relieve the symptoms. Dydrogesterone 5 mg twice daily from day 5 for 20 days in each cycle for 3–6 cycles may be tried.

Luteal support

It is usually given on the day after oocyte retrieval for ART (p. 208). Progesterone is used in any of these forms.

- Vaginal suppository 200 mg twice daily
- Micronized progesterone orally 200 mg twice daily. It is usually continued for about 14 days (p. 208).
- Progesterone in oil 50 mg IM daily

Postponement of menstruation

In order to post-pone the menstruation, norethisterone preparation 5 mg tablet thrice daily is to be taken at least 3 days prior to the expected date of menstruation. This should be continued till such time when the patient wishes to have her period. The period usually starts after 48–72 hours. **This should not be taken casually, as it may disturb the menstrual pattern**. There is no contraceptive protection during the period of intake of medicine.

Hormone replacement therapy (HRT)

Progestins are combined with estrogen as an HRT for postmenopausal woman whose uterus is present. This prevents endometrial hyperplasia. They can be used cyclically for last 12–14 days of the cycle or continuously with estrogen (p. 50).

Side Effects

Progestogens side effects are as mentioned in Table 32.10.

COMBINED PREPARATIONS (ESTROGEN AND PROGESTOGEN)

- **Diagnostic**
- **Therapeutic**

Diagnostic

The combined preparations may be used as estrogen-progesterone challenge test in amenorrhea to exclude uterine pathology. **If bleeding fails to occur, it suggests uterine synechiae.**

Therapeutic

- Contraception—the most common and widely use of combined preparations is in the field of fertility control (details in Ch. 30)
- DUB (p. 159)
- Endometriosis (p. 252)
- Dysmenorrhea (p. 149)
- Postponement of period
- Premenstrual symptoms (PMS) (p. 150)
- Idiopathic hirsutism—cyclic therapy of combined preparations containing 50 μg of ethinyl estradiol together with new progestin is more effective (p. 484)
- HRT (p. 50).

ANTIPROGESTERONE

Mifepristone (RU 486)

It is a competitive antagonist of progesterone and glucocorticoid receptors. It is a derivative of 19-nortestosterone. It binds competitively to progesterone receptors and nullifies the effect of endogenous progesterone. As a result, there is an increased release of prostaglandins from the endometrium, resulting in menstrual bleeding or termination of early pregnancy.

Three important biochemical characters of RU 486 are **high affinity for progesterone receptors, long half-life and active metabolites**.

Uses

Therapeutic abortion: It is an effective abortifacient up to 7 weeks. Combination of prostaglandins as vaginal pessary 48 hours after RU 486, increases its efficacy.

Dose

Tablet 200 mg to 600 mg (1 tablet = 200 mg) orally, followed immediatly or up to 72 hours later by misoprostol 400 μg (PGE_1) oral or 800 μg vaginal pessary, sublingual or buccal. Success rate is 95–100%.

Emergency contraception: A single dose of 10 mg is to be taken on 27th day of the cycle irrespective of the day and number of intercourse. Efficiency is 95–100%.

Induction of labor: Mifepristone has been used for cervical ripening. It is given orally.

Uterine fibroids: Mifepristone therapy (5–50 mg daily) for 12 weeks is given. Shrinkage of leiomyomas volume occurs by about 50%. It reduces the symptoms (pain relief) also.

Endometriosis: A dose of 50 mg/day for 6 months is found to reduce pelvic pain and the extent of spread.

Ectopic pregnancy: Injection of mifepristone into the ectopic pregnancy (unruptured sac) is used as a medical management.

Cushing's syndrome: As it blocks the glucocorticoid receptors.

Side Effects

Minor side effects are nausea, vomiting, headache and cramp. There is risk of ongoing pregnancy (failure of medical induction of abortion) in about 1% of cases. Evacuation of the uterus should be done for such a failure. **Other side effects are:** Vasomotor symptoms (40%), endometrial hyperplasia (due to unopposed estrogen effect). Asoprisnil, a SPRM is found to avoid estrogen deficiency symptoms.

Contraindications

- Age >35 years
- Heavy smoker
- Adrenal insufficiency
- Corticosteroid therapy.

ANDROGENS

In a female, androgen (testosterone) sources are adrenal cortex (25%), ovaries (25%), and in adipose tissues from peripheral conversion (50%). Most of the androgens are metabolized in the liver and are excreted as 17-ketosteroid. About **80%** of circulating testosterone is bound to **SHBG**, **19%** to **albumin** and **remaining 1% is free**. In adult female, blood testosterone level is around 20–80 ng/dL. Testosterone is converted to dihydrotestosterone within the target cell by the action of 5α-reductase and then combines with the specific receptors and is transported to the nucleus.

Androgens are partly anabolic and effect sebum formation and are implicated in acne during adolescence. Testosterone, particularly, influences the growth of hair on face and body.

Therapeutic Aspect

Androgens are not active by oral route. Methyltestosterone is used as sublingual tablets to bypass the enterohepatic circulation. **Its use in clinical practice is now a rarity.**

It may be used in cases of frigidity and premenstrual syndrome either orally or as an implant. In postmenopausal or perimenopausal woman, androgens are combined with estrogen to improve libido.

Its use in male infertility has been discussed in Ch. 17. Testosterone derivatives like danazol (isoxazole derivative of 17α-ethinyl testosterone), gestrinone (19-nortestosterone derivative) are used in different clinical situations (p. 259).

Antiandrogens

- **Cyproterone acetate**
- **Spironolactone**
- **Flutamide**
- **Finasteride**
- **Cyproterone Acetate:** It is an antiandrogenic progestogen [17-hydroxyprogesterone (17-OHP)]. **It inhibits gonadotropin secretion and also acts as a competetive androgen receptor antagonist.**

It decreases 5α-reductase activity and reduces LH secretion. It induces hepatic enzymes and increases the metabolic clearance of plasma androgens. It also acts as a potent progestogen having agonist effects on progesterone receptors.

Uses: It is used in the idiopathic hirsutism or hyperandrogenic state (p. 486).

Dose: Cyproterone acetate, 2 mg is most frequently used in combination with ethinyl estradiol.

Available preparation (COCs) containing cyproterone acetate, 2 mg and ethinyl estradiol, 35 μg may be given from day 5 for 21 days.

Treatment: It is to be continued for at least 6 months.

Side effects: Weight gain, loss of libido, mastalgia.

- **Spironolactone: It is an androgen receptor antagonist. It is an antialdosterone diuretic. It also inhibits androgen biosynthesis from ovary and adrenal.**
  - Inhibits 5α-reductase activity
  - It competes with androgen at the receptor sites.

  Dose: The dose varies from 25–150 mg per day. This may produce hyponatremia and hyperkalemia for which initial monitoring of serum potassium and creatinine is necessary at doses above 100 mg per day.

  Important side effects: Menstrual irregularity (DUB), fatigue, diuresis, electrolyte imbalance (hyperkalemia and hyponatremia), gynecomastia and hepatotoxicity.
- **Flutamide:** It is a **nonsteroidal androgen receptor antagonist.** It blocks the androgen receptor sites. Dose of 250 mg daily for 6 months is optimum.

  Important side effects are dry skin, decreased libido and hepatotoxicity.
- **Finasteride**: It inhibits 5α-reductase activity. A dose of 5 mg daily is effective for hirsutism without any side effects.
- **Ketoconazole** inhibits the enzyme (cytochrome P 450) for androgen synthesis in both adrenal and gonads. A dose of 200 mg daily PO is adequate to reduce the level of androgens.
- **Dexamethasone side effects:** Hepatitis and for other antiandrogens.

ADRENOCORTICAL HORMONES

- **Diagnostic**
- **Therapeutic**

DIAGNOSTIC

Dexamethasone suppression test

Principle

A base level plasma cortisol is estimated at 8 a.m. Dexamethasone 1 mg orally is given at 11 p.m.

Plasma cortisol level is estimated in the following morning at 8 am.

In normal individual, the cortisol levels are suppressed below 1.8 μg/dL, but in Cushing's syndrome, the cortisol levels fall but do not go below 10 μg/100 mL.

THERAPEUTIC

Dexamethasone is used mostly in hyperandrogenic state.

- **Hirsutism:** Dexamethasone 0.25–0.75 mg tablet daily at bedtime effectively suppresses adrenocorticotropic hormone (ACTH). It is used for at least a period of 6–12 months. It should be withheld in obese patient.
- **Adrenal hyperplasia:** Dexamethasone 0.5–0.75 mg in divided doses.
- **Polycystic ovary:** Along with combined estrogen and progestogen preparations (oral pill), dexamethasone 0.25–0.5 mg is given at bed time.
- **As an adjuvant therapy** with clomiphene citrate in induction of ovulation with elevated LH.
- **Pubertal menorrhagia** due to idiopathic thrombocytopenic purpura.
- **Hydrotubation** along with antibiotics, in cases of partial tubal obstruction due to adhesions or following tubal anastomosis.
- **Intraperitoneal instillation** may be done to minimize adhesions during pelvic surgery, especially tubal microsurgery.
- **Local antipruritic cream.**

THYROID HORMONE

Hypothyroidism is often associated with menorrhagia or oligomenorrhea, abnormal uterine bleeding (AUB), and amenorrhea. Sometimes it is associated with recurrent miscarriage and subfertility. After the diagnosis is established by radioimmunoassay (RIA) of thyroid-stimulating hormone (TSH), T4, free thyroxine (FT4), FT4 index, and T3, substitution therapy with eltroxin is given orally as per the need (p. 201).

- **Women with hyperthyroidism** commonly present with anovulation, anovulatory DUB. Woman needs to be treated with antithyroid drugs (propylthiouracil or carbimazole).
- **Hypothyroidism** associated with hyperprolactinemia and excess dopamine disrupts the normal pulsality of GnRH secretion. Ultimately it affects the normal cyclic of gonadotropin secretion and prevents ovulation.

A summary of hormones in gynecology is given in Flowchart 32.1.

Flowchart 32.1: Hormones in gynecology.

USES OF HORMONES IN GYNECOLOGY

Diagnostic
- GnRH stimulation test
- ACTH stimulation test
- TRH stimulation test
- Progesterone challenge test
- Estrogen and progesterone challenge test
- Dexamethasone suppression test

Fertility control

Stimulation (induction of ovulation)

Assisted reproduction
Combination of:
- GnRH
- GnRH analogs
- Gonadotropins
- Letrozole
- Clomiphene
- hCG

Dysovulatory infertility:
- Letrozole
- Clomiphene
- Gonadotropins
- Dexamethasone
- Thyroxine
- Metformin
- Dopamine agonist

Inhibition
- Estrogen
- Combined estrogen + progesterone
- Progesterone

Pharmacotherapeutics
- GnRH, GnRH analogs
- Gonadotropins
- Antigonadotropins
  - Danazol
  - Estrogens
  - Progesterone
  - Androgens
- Estrogens
- Antiestrogens
  - Clomiphene
  - Tamoxifen
  - Aromatase inhibitors
  - Selective estrogen receptor modulators (SERMs)
- Progesterone
- Antiprogesterone
  - RU 486 (mifepristone)
  - Estrogens
  - SERMs

  Androgens
  Antiandrogens
  - Cyproterone acetate
  - Spironolactone
  - Flutamide
  - Finasteride
- Adrenocortical hormones
- Thyroid hormones

(GnRH: gonadotropin-releasing hormone; ACTH: adrenocorticotropic hormone; TRH: thyrotropin-releasing hormone; hCG: human chorionic gonadotropin; SERM: selective estrogen receptor modulators)

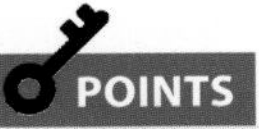

- **GnRH stimulation** is used to differentiate an amenorrhea of pituitary from hypothalamic in origin. The absence of response usually denotes pituitary fault.
- **For induction of ovulation**, GnRH is effective in cases of idiopathic hypogonadotropic hypogonadism.
- **GnRH analogs** (agonists and antagonists) have been synthesized by substitution of amino acids at different position of GnRH molecule (p. 441). GnRH antagonists has got some advantages over GnRH agonist (Table 32.2).
- **The GnRH analogs** stop the normal pattern of GnRH secretion leading to loss of pituitary GnRH receptors and thereby down regulation. This leads to fall in pituitary gonadotropins and consequently the gonadal secretion. The net effect is of medical hypophysectomy.
- **GnRH analogs** are used for superovulation in IVF program and in therapeutic considerations to all conditions related to high estrogen level such as precocious puberty, endometriosis, fibroid, DUB, breast carcinoma and the alike. In achieving superovulation, either a long protocol or a short protocol regimen is followed under proper monitoring.
- **Gonadotropic hormones** act on the ovaries to induce ovulation. Both FSH and LH (Pergonal) or pure FSH (Metronidazole) are available and are obtained from the urine of postmenopausal women. hCG is obtained from the urine of pregnant women.
  Gonadotropins are expensive and require close monitoring not only for induction of ovulation but also to prevent hyperstimulation syndrome. The induction of ovulation with gonadotropins is indicated in hypogonadotropic hypogonadism with or without amenorrhea and in failed clomiphene, in patients with PCOS.
  There is increased incidence of multiple pregnancy (20–30%) and hyperstimulation syndrome (1–20%).
- **Ovarian hyperstimulation syndrome** (OHSS) usually appears about 3–6 days after the ovulating dose of hCG.
  Increased vascular permeability due to VEGF and activation of NO system, leads to leakage of fluid from peritoneal and ovarian surfaces. OHSS may be mild (10–20%), moderate (5–10%) or severe (1–2%) (p. 444).
  In severe cases, correction of hypovolemia, electrolyte imbalance, metabolic acidosis and blood coagulopathy have to be done. Intensive care monitoring may be needed for a few (p. 444).

Contd...

Contd...

- **Ovarian reserve** means the quantity as well as quality of the follicles present in the ovary. There are tests to determine the ovarian reserve. Poor ovarian reserve indicates poor outcome following stimulation of ovulation (p. 443).
- **Danazol** is strictly an antigonadotropin but acts as an androgen agonist. Its use is wide like that of GnRH analogs. It should be started in the early follicular phase and barrier methods of contraception should be used.
  The side effects of danazol are due to hypoestrogenic, androgenic and metabolic changes (Table 32.4). The drug should be discontinued, if the patient develops hirsutism or hoarseness of voice.
- **Gestrinone** is an androgen agonist and progesterone agonist-antagonist. The dose is 2.5 mg twice or thrice a week. Side effects are like those of danazol but less marked.
- **The sex hormones** are transported in the blood nonspecifically by albumin and specifically by SHBG.
  Cell nucleus is the principle site of action of the steroids as opposed to the cell membranes of gonadotropins.
  Estrogens are used as hormone replacement therapy (HRT) in postmenopausal women even in otherwise symptom-free cases to prevent osteoporosis and cardiovascular disease.
- **Estrogens are graded** depending upon their suppression effect on hot flashes, FSH levels, and increase in the serum levels of HDL, SHBG and corticosteroid-binding globulin (CBG). Ethinyl estradiol is more potent compared to conjugated equine estrogen (CEE).
- **Clomiphene** is antiestrogenic. In the hypothalamus, it binds to the estrogen receptors preventing the negative feedback effect of endogenous estrogens to GnRH resulting in more synthesis of gonadotropins.
- **Tamoxifen** is also an antiestrogen and is widely used in benign breast disease. Raloxifen is a more selective antiestrogen.
- **Letrozole** is a specific aromatase inhibitor. It inhibits the enzyme aromatase to suppress synthesis of estrogen. It enhances the secretion of pituitary FSH for the growth and development of follicles. It is used for induction of ovulation in women with anovulatory infertility.
- **Progestogens** are classified according to their structural derivatives and progestogen content (Table 32.7). They are also classified according to their metabolic effects and also with the grades of progestational activity (Table 32.8).
- **Progestogens** are used as diagnostic test to evaluate the cause of amenorrhea. In presence of withdrawal bleeding, it signifies intact hypothalamo-pituitary-ovarian axis and there is endogenous estrogen production.
- **Combined estrogen and progestogen** preparations are commonly used as oral contraceptives.
- **RU 486** is antiprogesterone and is effective in termination of early pregnancy.
- **Mifepristone** reduces the size of myomas by 50% and also reduces other symptoms. It can reduce the pelvic pain in a case with endometriosis.
- **Contraindication of estrogen** use are: Undiagnosed vaginal bleeding, venous thromboembolism, estrogen dependent neoplasia (breast) (Table 32.5).
- **The source of androgens in female** are adrenal, ovary and peripheral adipose tissues. The blood level of testosterone in female is less than 1 ng/mL. Virilization is usually associated with testosterone level >2 ng/mL.
- **Cyproterone, spironolactone, flutamide** and **finasteride** are antiandrogens. These are used in idiopathic hirsutism and hyperandrogenic state (p. 486).
- **Dexamethasone suppression test** is of help to differentiate Cushing's syndrome (adrenal tumor) from Cushing's disease (increased pituitary secretion of ACTH); level of plasma cortisol $\leq$5 μg/dL largely excludes Cushing's syndrome.

CHAPTER

33 Gynecological Problems from Birth to Adolescence

CHAPTER OUTLINE

INTRODUCTION

Pediatric and adolescent gynecology encompasses gynecological diseases of children from birth to adolescence. Care needs to include children's physiology, psychology and the developmental issues. It covers a spectrum of gynecological problems including congenital anomalies, problems due to infection (vulvovaginitis), precocious development, menstrual abnormalities and neoplasm. To prevent the problems of teenage pregnancy and sexually transmitted infections, contraceptive counseling has a place. Children are mostly accompanied by the parents for the problems.

For descriptive purpose, the entire span from birth to adolescence is arbitrarily divided into three phases. Each phase has got distinct problems of its own.

1. Neonates, toddlers and infants <5 years
2. Premenarcheal 5–11 years
3. Perimenarcheal to adolescence 12–18 years.

Common clinical problems in different periods have been described in Table 33.1.

Gynecologists need specific communication skill considering the psychological and developmental milestones of the girl child and the adolescent.

GYNECOLOGICAL EXAMINATION IN A CHILD

This includes history, and brief examination of breasts and external genitalia. Inspection of vulva, vagina, cervix and if necessary a rectal examination may needed. During examination, a parent should be present. An infant may be examined at her mother's lap, knee chest or in the frog leg position. Lithotomy is generally used for girls of 4–5 years of age or older. Once optimally positioned, the introitus, hymen and lower vagina are inspected. Each labium may be pulled laterally using the thumb and the forefingers. Vaginoscopy may be done using hysteroscope or cystoscope with illumination. A minor girl or child must have the consent of a parent whereas a girl of 18 may consent herself. In certain situations, the girl may need examination under anesthesia (EUA).

"Child friendly" pictures, objects, or distracting conversation may ease fear and allow smooth examination.

NEONATES, TODDLERS AND INFANTS

Clitoral Enlargement

Causes

Not infrequently, female babies are born with slightly enlarged clitoris. There is usually no evidence of

TABLE 33.1: Common clinical problems in different periods.

Period	*Common problems*	
<5 years (neonates, toddlers and infants)	▪ Diagnosis of sex at birth (clitoral enlargement) ▪ Genital crisis ▪ Labial adhesions ▪ Imperforate hymen ▪ Hydro or mucocolpos	▪ Ectopic anus ▪ Nipple discharge
5–11 years (premenarcheal)	▪ Vulvovaginitis in childhood ▪ Abnormal vaginal discharge ▪ Vaginal bleeding ▪ Precocious puberty (p. 40)	▪ Trauma to the genital tract (Ch. 27) ▪ White lesion of the vulva (Ch. 18) ▪ Neoplasm (Ch. 24)
12–18 years (perimenarcheal to adolescence)	▪ Menstrual abnormalities (p. 40) ▪ Delayed puberty (p. 43) ▪ Hirsutism (p. 459) ▪ Neoplasm (Ch. 24) ▪ Primary amenorrhea (Ch. 29) ▪ Leukorrhea (p. 459)	▪ Congenital anomalies of the vagina (vaginal anomalies and uterine anomalies) (p. 35). ▪ Disorders of sexual development (Ch. 28) ▪ Miscellaneous problems

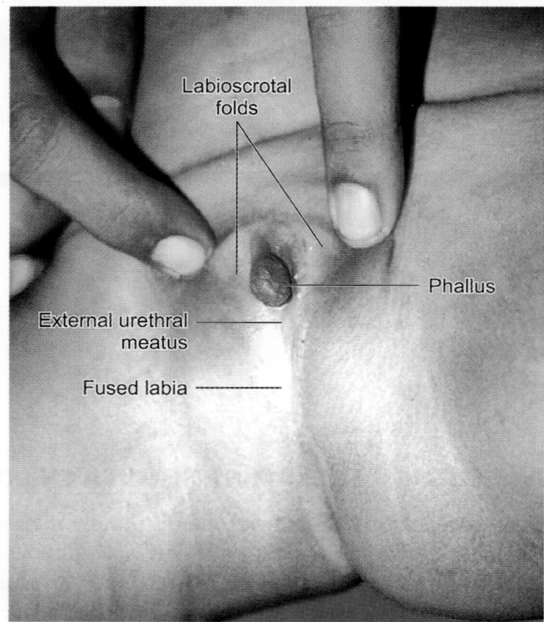

Fig. 33.1: Newborn baby with enlarged phallus due to adrenogenital syndrome causing confusing in the diagnosis of sex.

intrauterine androgen stimulation of the child. Careful history taking reveals development of some degree of masculinizing features of the mother during pregnancy, probably due to increased adrenocortical activity (Fig. 33.1).

Rarely, the enlargement may be due to a disorder of sexual development, adrenogenital syndrome (46,XX DSD). This may cause confusion in the determination of sex at birth (Ch. 28, Fig. 28.1).

Management

In the idiopathic group, no treatment is required. However, an apparently female child with enlarged phallus and impalpable gonads requires at least estimation of serum 17-OHP, urinary 17 ketosteroid and chromosomal analysis to rule out congenital adrenal hyperplasia (p. 368) (Fig. 33.1).

Bleeding per Vaginam

It usually occurs within 10 days following birth; mostly blood stained but, at times, frank bleeding. This is due to decline in level of estrogen, which is unable to support the endometrium, resulting in withdrawal bleeding. There is no cause for concern. Vaginal bleeding may rarely be due to McCune-Albright syndrome with (premature menarche, polyostotic fibrous dysplasia).

Enlarged Breasts

It is due to effect of maternal estrogen and progesterone, there may be some development of duct and alveolar system of the breasts. Withdrawal of hormonal suppression of prolactin leads to discharge from the nipple called 'witch's milk'. No treatment is required; only assurance is enough.

Neonatal Leukorrhea

This is due to excessive secretion of cervical mucus from the hypertrophied cervical glands under the influence of estrogen.

Labial Adhesion (Adhesive Vulvitis)

It is the condition when the labia minora have adhered together.

Causes: Commonly, it is due to mild infection of the vulva which is favored by lack of local defense due to absence of estrogen. There is denudation of the surface epithelium of the labia minora → adhesions.

The adhesions of the labia minora start from behind forward leaving a small opening at the foremost tip through which urine escapes out.

Rarely, it may be a manifestation of minor form of masculinization following maternal intake of androgen during pregnancy.

Diagnosis: The condition usually appears within 2–3 years of birth. The mother usually, anxious about the entity, brings to the notice of the physician for not visualizing the vaginal opening. The adhesions may cause difficulty in micturition or periodic attacks of urinary tract infection. There may be inflammation of the vestibule and vagina.

Examination reveals adhesions of labia minora obliterating the vaginal opening and, at times, even the external urethral meatus (Fig. 33.2A). A thin vertical line in midplane is pathognomonic for this adhesive vulvitis. Confusion arises with:

- Imperforate hymen
- Agenesis of vagina
- Intersex.

In *imperforate hymen* and *agenesis of vagina*, the labia minora and external urethral meatus are clearly visible. In *intersexuality*, there is usually associated clitoral enlargement (p. 368).

Treatment: Separation of the adhesions using fingers or by a probe (introitoplasty) is almost always effective (Figs. 33.2A and B). The raw area is treated with topical application of estrogen or any other antibiotic ointment to prevent reagglutination. Good perineal hygiene should be maintained. Surgical separation for fused labia (introitoplasty) is rarely needed.

Mucocolpos or Hydrocolpos

Pathophysiology: Usually, there is an imperforate hymen or a transverse vaginal septum just above the hymen. Due to excess estrogen stimulation acquired in utero from the mother, there is increased secretion of mucus or watery discharge from the cervical and uterine glands. If a large quantity of fluid is collected in the vagina, it produces hydro- or mucocolpos. It may rarely be big enough to produce an abdominal swelling.

This is rarely met beyond 1 year of age because the uterine and vaginal transudation is not produced in sufficient quantity beyond that age.

Later on, the candidate may be the subject of hematocolpos → hematometra →may cause endometriosis at a later age (Management, p. 33).

Ovarian Enlargement

After the withdrawal of maternal estrogen, there is transient elevation of gonadotropins in neonates. This influence of elevated gonadotropins can stimulate to produce ovarian follicular cysts. These usually regress spontaneously. As such, the cysts need no surgery unless complicated.

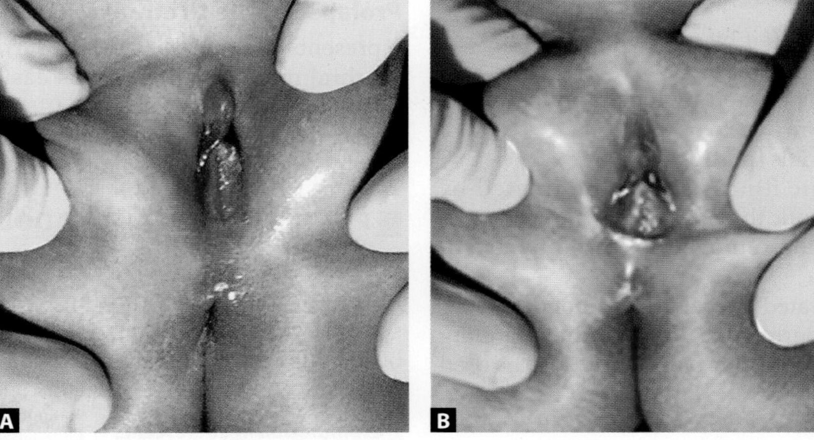

Figs. 33.2A and B: (A) Labial adhesions in a 1½-year-old girl; (B) Separation of adhesions by fingers. Local application of estrogen ointment is helpful.

Ectopic Anus

The anal canal may open either in the vestibule or in the vagina. The details have been described in Chapter 4.

PREMENARCHEAL

Vulvovaginitis

The premenarcheal girls are specially vulnerable to vaginal infection: Lack or very low level of circulatory estrogen → lack of stratification of vaginal epithelium → lack of glycogen and absence of Doderlein's bacillus → no acid formation → vaginal pH remains high, around 7 → infection.

Causes of Vulvovaginitis in Premenarcheal Girls

- Poor vulvar and perineal hygiene
- Poorly estrogenized vulvovaginal epithelium
- Close proximity of the openings of vagina, urethra and the anus
- Lack of protective labial fat pad and pubic hair
- Vaginal infections are associated with vulvovaginitis
- Infections: Nongonococcal—*chlamydia, Candida, Trichomonas, Gardnerella, E. Coli* and gonococcal
- Foreign body
- Threadworm infestation (*Enterobius vermicularis*)
- Systemic ill health/infections
- Skin disorders: Lichen sclerosus, psoriasis, eczema
- Chemical irritants, allergies (soap, bubble bath)
- Sexual abuse

Symptoms

- Vaginal discharge: Purulent or blood-stained in the presence of foreign body.
- Pruritus or soreness in external genitalia.
- Painful urination.
- Vaginal bleeding.

Signs

Vulva becomes edematous and red or even ulcerated. Vaginal inspection using aural speculum reveals congested epithelium with pent-up discharge. The offending foreign body may be detected. The examination may be done under anesthesia. It should be remembered that the vaginal epithelium in young girls looks red. Rectal examination is often helpful to detect the foreign body.

Investigations

- Examination under anesthesia
- **Vaginoscopy** is needed to visualize the upper vagina for bleeding, foreign body or neoplasm. Specially designed speculum (Huffman Graves) is inserted into the vagina. For better visualization, water cystoscope (to wash away secretions, debris or blood) or laparoscope (8 mm) may be used.

  Bacteriological examination of the discharge either by Gram stain or hanging drop preparation or culture, to identify the causative organism (p. 134).
- Smear from the anal area for detection of pin or threadworm.
- Stool examination may reveal the threadworm.
- Blood examination for estimation of sugar in suspected cases of juvenile diabetes.
- Urine for protein, sugar and culture study and NAAT.

Treatment

As the cause remains obscure in majority, the principles to be followed are as follows:

- **Vulvar hygiene:** Proper wiping (front to back) will reduce rectal flora to invade the vulvovaginal area.
  - Sitz baths are very helpful in relieving symptoms (baking soda in water).
  - Avoiding chemical irritants—soaps, shampoos, etc.
  - To keep the local area dry.
  - To wear cotton undergarments.

Medication

- To reduce the overgrowth of pathogenic bacteria, amoxicillin 20–40 mg/kg/day in 3 divided doses is effective.
- In refractory cases, estrogen locally as cream twice daily for 3 weeks is effective to improve the vaginal defense and to promote healing.

Specific therapy

- Trichomoniasis is treated by metronidazole (100 mg thrice daily for 10 days).
- Monilial infection is treated by local application of clotrimazole 1% cream.
- For gonococcal vaginitis (p. 121).
- Associated systemic illness should be treated by intramuscular antibiotic therapy.
- Foreign body is to be removed followed by use of estrogen therapy.
- Helminthes is eradicated by oral use of albendazole.
- Allergic or contact dermatitis: To avoid the offending agents. Topical hydrocortisone ointment (2%) to be used twice daily.

Leukorrhea (p. 459)

As the puberty approaches, there may be excessive white discharge per vaginam. It is nonoffensive and nonirritant. It is due to excessive production of mucus from the cervical glands and increased transudation from the vaginal epithelium.

Neoplasm

The neoplastic conditions encountered during this period are usually ovarian in origin and rarely from the cervix and vagina. The ovarian neoplasms are malignant in about 25%. Germ cell tumors are common (70%). Granulosa cell tumor is estrogen-producing tumor and may cause precocious puberty. Mixed germ cell tumor is highly malignant and dysgerminoma is intermediary in position, provided the capsule remains intact. The benign tumors are cystic teratoma (30%) and epithelial tumors (Ch. 21).

Sarcoma Botryoides or Endodermal Sinus Tumors of the Vagina

It should be remembered that the entity is most often present prior to 6 years of age (p. 330). Vaginoscopy may need to be done. Both are aggressive cancers and need prompt diagnosis.

Vaginal Bleeding

Common causes of vaginal bleeding in premenarcheal girls

- Foreign body in the vagina
- Trauma
- Infection (vulvovaginitis)
- Leech bite
- Prolapse of the urethral mucosa
- Neoplastic conditions (mentioned earlier)
- Sexual abuse
- Precocious puberty
- Isolated menarche
- McCune-Albright syndrome
- Shigella vaginitis.

Leech Bite

This is more prevalent in tropics where pond bath is quite common. The bleeding may, at times, be brisk and requires varying amount of blood transfusion. Bleeding usually stops spontaneously but may, at times, require hemostatic suture.

Prolapse of the Urethral Mucosa

It presents as a vascular swelling surrounding the external urethral meatus which bleeds easily. Prolapse may be partial or complete (entire 360° urethra). Treatment is conservative. Local application of estrogen cream is found helpful. Surgery is needed rarely when necrosis is present.

POSTMENARCHEAL TO ADOLESCENCE

Adolescence

The period of life beginning with the appearance of secondary sexual characters and terminating with cessation of somatic growth is described as adolescence.

Indications of gynecologic examination in adolescents
▪ Vaginal bleeding ▪ Delayed puberty ▪ Persistent vaginal discharge ▪ Primary amenorrhea and cyclic pain (imperforate hymen, vaginal septum or agenesis) ▪ Suspicion of genital tract neoplasia

Common problems in adolescents
▪ Menstrual disorders ▪ Delayed puberty (p. 43) ▪ Hirsutism ▪ Leukorrhea ▪ Neoplasm ▪ Disorders of sexual development (DSD) ▪ Teenage pregnancy ▪ Sexual abuse

Menstrual Disorders

The neurohormonal mechanism essential for maintenance of normal menstruation takes some time (usually 2–3 years) to come to a normal balance. Till then, various types of menstrual abnormalities may occur, causing concern to the young girls or their parents (p. 43).

Common causes of vaginal bleeding in premenarcheal girls	*Other causes of abnormal vaginal bleeding*
▪ **Hypothalamic-Pituitary-Ovarian (HPO) axis dys-function** • Dysfunctional uterine bleeding (DUB • Stress • Obesity ▪ **Endocrinopathies** • Thyroid dysfunction • Polycystic ovarian syndrome (PCOS) • Prolactinoma • Congenital adrenal hyperplasia	▪ **Inflammatory** • Vulvovaginitis • Endometritis • Pelvic inflammatory disease PID. ▪ **Traumatic** • Foreign body • Sexual abuse • Drug effects ▪ **Others** • Pregnancy (abortion problems) • Bleeding disorders [idiopathic thrombocytopenic purpura (ITP) • Local—polyps and neoplasms.

Management

Improvement of general health and assurance are enough in majority. It is expected that after a certain period of time, the menstrual cycles become normal with the onset of regular ovulation.

Delayed Manifestations of the Disorders of Sexual Development (DSD)

While majority of cases of intersex are diagnosed at birth, there are cases where the diagnosis is only revealed after puberty. These are:

- Mild degrees of CAH (p. 368) with late mani-festations of postpubertal hyperandrogenism
- Gonadal dysgenesis (p. 372)
- Androgen insensitivity syndrome (p. 372).

Hirsutism

Hirsutism is one of the manifestations of hyperandrogenism and often causes problems to the young girls. One should not forget to elicit iatrogenic cause of hirsutism following intake of androgenic steroids, corticosteroid or synthetic progestogens. The causes and management of hirsutism are discussed on page 481.

Physiologic Vaginal Discharge (Leukorrhea)

Diagnostic criteria:

- Gray-white or yellowish in color
- Nonpurulent
- Thick in nature, seen to be 'pasted' to undergarments
- Irritations and erythema may be present
- Subsides of its own and needs assurance
- Symptomatic children need sitz bath and frequent changing of underwear
- Microscopic examination of the discharge—show sheets of vaginal epithelial cells.

Excessive vaginal secretion in this period may be due to:

- Relative hyperoestrogenic phase
- Malnutrition and ill health
- Congenital ectopy (erosion)
- Sexual excitement or masturbation
- Vaginal adenosis (rare).

Vaginal adenosis: It is present in about 30–50% of the teenagers who had diethylstilbestrol (DES) exposure in utero. This is a benign condition. In these girls, the junction between the Müllerian ducts and the sinovaginal bulb may not be sharply demarcated. As the Müllerian elements invade the sinovaginal bulb, remnants may remain as areas of adenosis in adult vagina. The columnar epithelium of the endocervix extends onto the ectocervix and also variable part of the vaginal fornices. There is thus copious vaginal secretion from the columnar epithelium. The pathology regresses spontaneously in due course of time. Rarely, it may progress to clear cell carcinoma.

Congenital ectopy: Congenital ectopy producing copious discharge should be cauterized. In others, assurance and improvement of general condition cure the state.

Infective discharge during the period may be due to:

- Nonspecific infection following unhygienic use of menstrual pads or foreign body in the vagina.
- Specific infections such as *Trichomonas vaginalis* or Monilial infection.
- New growths from the vagina or cervix.

The investigations and management have been mentioned earlier in this Chapter.

Neoplasm

Ovarian—functional cysts which are rare in premenarcheal period are quite common during this period. They are usually 6–8 cm in diameters and usually regress within 3–6 months. These are usually follicular cysts.

Most common neoplastic cyst during this period is cystic teratoma (dermoid cyst). The others, though rare, are benign epithelial tumors, sex cord stromal tumors (granulosa cell tumors), germ cell tumors: dysgerminoma, mixed germ cell tumor or androblastoma. **Germ cell tumors constitute 50–75% of all ovarian neoplasms in this age group (p. 320).**

The patients usually come late with symptoms. Common symptoms are lump in the lower abdomen (Table 33.2), acute pain abdomen or, at times, with retention of urine.

Pain from and ovarian cyst may be due to: (a) Stretching or expansion of the ovarian cortex; (b) Rupture of an cyst to cause hemorrhage in the peritoneal cavity; (c) Torsion of the cyst.

About 75–85% of ovarian neoplasms in premenarcheal girls are benign. **Ovarian torsion** may occur as the supporting ovarian ligaments are long. Torsion may occur without a ovarian mass. The ovary is swollen and enlarged after the torsion as the lymphatic drainage is blocked. Many cases of ovarian torsion had normal vascular flow on ultrasound Doppler study. Torsion is more common in the right side as the sigmoid colon is on the left which prevents the left ovary from twisting. Right sided torsion needs to be differentiated from appendicitis.

Diagnosis

The diagnosis is made by abdominal, bimanual vaginal or rectal examination. Ultrasound is an invaluable tool in the diagnosis of ovarian mass. CT, MRI may be needed in few cases of pelvic mass with uncertain diagnosis. Preoperative work-up needs tumor markers estimation (serum CA 125, α fetoprotein, hCG, inhibin, LDH, CEA and testosterone) in these adolescent girls.

Treatment

A suspected functional cyst (6–8 cm) may be observed for 3–6 months. Unilocular functional cysts usually resolve spontaneously. **Surgical therapy is needed** in cases where there are symptoms, masses that fail to resolve or masses with solid or multilocular appearance on ultrasound

TABLE 33.2: Common causes of lump in lower abdomen.

Age	Causes
<5 years	▪ Hydro or mucocolpos, neonatal ovarian cyst
5–11 years	▪ Retention of urine due to vulvovaginitis ▪ Pelvic neoplasm, ovarian cyst
12–18 years	▪ Pregnancy ▪ Retention of urine ▪ Ovarian tumor ▪ Hematometra ▪ Encysted peritonitis

(Flowchart 33.1). Complications may arise as in adult: torsion, hemorrhage, or rupture.

Laparoscopy is usually done when an adnexal mass appears to be benign. However, prompt **laparotomy should be done when there are evidences of malignancy**.

The surgery is usually conservative (detorsion ovariotomy or ovarian cystectomy) considering her future fertility and endocrine functions. Detorsion of the ovary should be done regardless of its appearance. Most will regain function and vascularity (Fig. 21.15). The edema subsides gradually. Risk of embolism from a thrombosed ovarian vein is rare. Adolescent groups usually have borderline epithelial or germ cell tumors. In such a situation, the affected ovary is removed and a formal staging is done (fertility sparing surgery). Unilateral salpingo-oophorectomy is justified for most young girls with stage-I (Stage IA or IB), Grade 1 or 2 disease. During surgery opposite ovary should be carefully examined. Biopsy of the other healthy normal looking ovary is not recommended.

Germ cell tumors are highly responsive to chemotherapy (p. 322). However, if the capsule is ruptured, radical surgery, i.e. total hysterectomy with bilateral salpingo-oophorectomy is to be done followed by radiotherapy or chemotherapy.

A problem may arise when an apparently cystic epithelial benign ovarian tumor is removed, which ultimately proves histologically malignant. In such cases, in consultation with an oncologist, chemotherapy followed by relaparotomy and removal of uterus with contralateral tube and ovary may be done. This should be followed by chemotherapy.

Alternatively, the patient may be treated with chemotherapy alone with follow-up.

Uterus: Sarcoma botryoides (p. 330).

Vagina: Clear cell adenocarcinoma of the vagina.

Sexually Transmitted Infections

Sexually transmitted infections (STIs) are increasing among the adolescents. Lack of sex education, absence of contraceptive use is the cause. The younger the age of first intercourse, the higher the risk for STIs. *Chlamydia* infection, though most common, other infections are human papillomavirus (HPV) (p. 269), human immunodeficiency virus (HIV) (p. 127), gonorrhea (p. 121), hepatitis B, syphilis (p. 123) and others (Ch. 12). Impact on health due to STI complications include—cervical metaplasia, pelvic inflammatory disease (PID) and its consequences (p. 106).

Major problems faced with the management of adolescent STIs are denial of history and symptoms. Fear and social embarrassment cause delay or, at times, incomplete treatment.

Treatment

Sex education among the adolescent girls, practice of safer sex and maintenance of perineal hygiene are essential.

Flowchart 33.1: Management of ovarian enlargement.

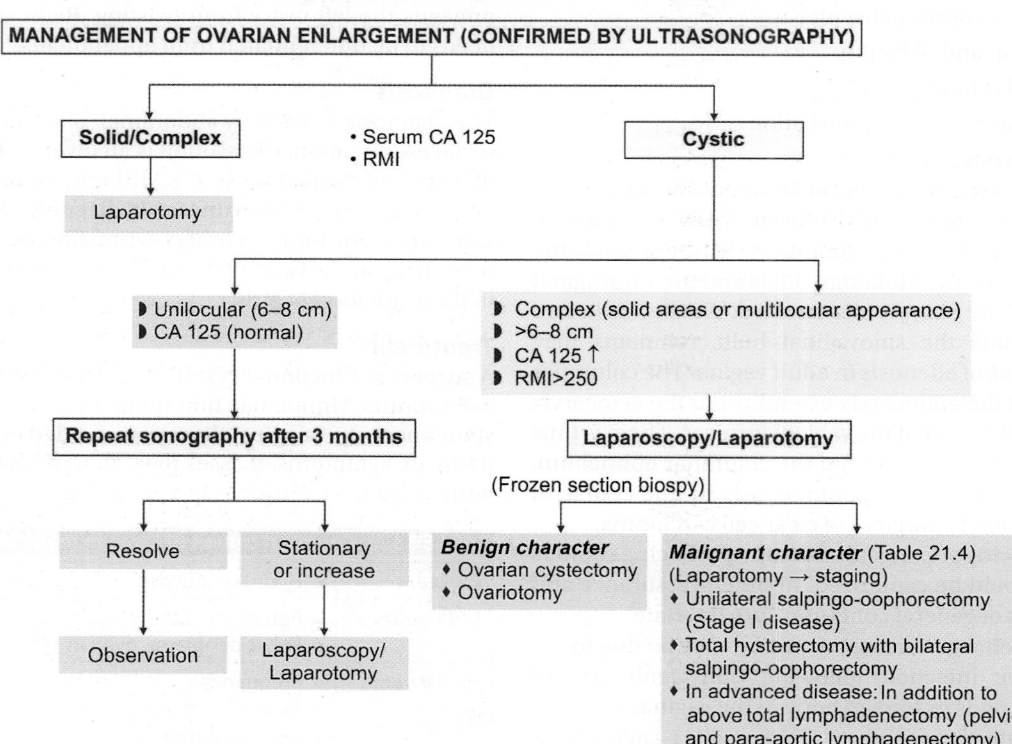

(RMI: risk of malignancy index; CA: cancer antigen)

HPV vaccination is offered. Proper use of condoms protects STIs. **Treatment of STIs** among the adolescents is the same that for the adults (p. 122).

Miscellaneous Problems

Acne

This is of concern due to cosmetic reason. The cause is due to excess androgen secretion by the ovaries (PCOS) and the adrenals. Therapy is aimed to lower the androgen levels. Drugs commonly prescribed are: (a) **Combined oral contraceptives (COCs)**; (b) **Antiandrogens (spironolactone)**; or (c) **5α-reductase inhibitors (finastride)**. Dermatologist may be consulted. Topical retinoids (tazarotene) [creams/gels are effective. Benzoyl peroxide (BPO) and antibiotic erythromycin or clindamycin] combined agent are used for acne. It may pass off spontaneously.

Obesity

Obesity is best assessed by calculating body mass index (BMI). BMI is expressed as weight (kg) divided by the height squared (m^2). Ideal BMI should be between 20 and 24. BMI 25 or more is called over weight, Whereas BMI 30 or more is considered obese (Table 33.3). Obesity increases the risk of insulin resistance, cardiovascular (e.g. hypertension), dyslipidemia, and metabolic (e.g. diabetes) diseases.

Usually, it is due to overeating and constitutional. Rarely, it may be due to hypofunction of pituitary or manifestation of PCOS Cushing's syndrome even at a younger age.

Girls with PCOS are likely to be obese. They are diagnosed by elevated BMI and waist-hip ratio. Obese women may present with a central distribution of body fat with **"apple-shaped"** body pattern (Figs. 33.3 and 33.4). Otherwise, there may be excess fat deposition in the hips and buttocks with **"pear-shaped"** body pattern. They often suffer from metabolic syndrome in their adult life. **Choice of treatment** for these girls are weight reduction, exercise, with or without insulin sensitizing agents (metformin).

There is a strong relationship between morbidity, mortality and increased BMI (>25 kg/m^2). Associated morbidities in an adult are hypertension, diabetes mellitus, dyslipidemia, heart diseases, stroke, arthritis, sleep apnea and increased operative morbidity and mortality. Gynecologic morbidities are: Menstrual abnormalities, endometrial hyperplasia, endometrial cancer, breast cancer and ovarian cancer.

TABLE 33.3: Classification of obesity.

BMI	*Weight*
18.5–24.9	Normal
25.0–29.9	Overweight
>30.0	Obesity
30–34.9	Class I
35–39.9	Class II
>40	Class III

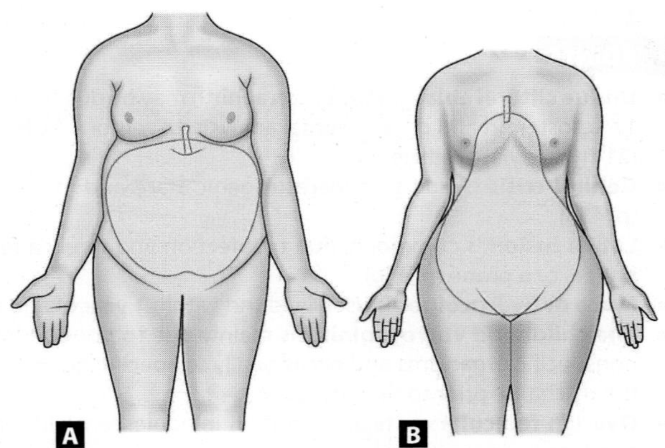

Figs. 33.3A and B: (A) Android; (B) Gynoid obesity pattern.

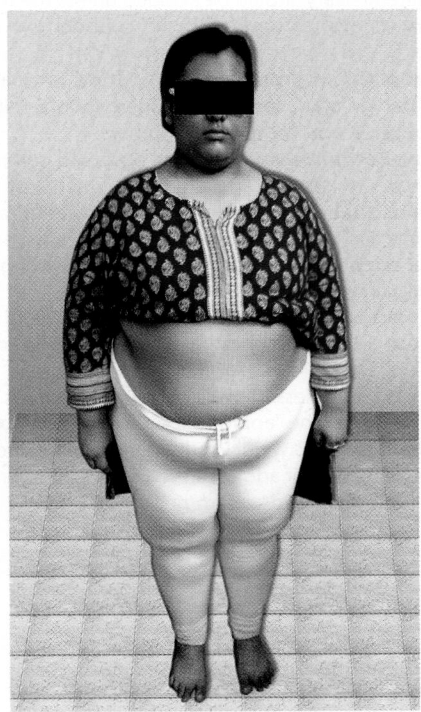

Fig. 33.4: A 17-year-old obese girl with elevated BMI (BMI: 33) and raised waist-hip ratio. She presented with secondary amenorrhea due to PCOS. Central distribution of body fat (android pattern) is seen. This pattern of obesity predicts insulin resistance.

Abnormal Height

Apart from constitutional as found in premenarcheal period, abnormal tallness is due to:

- **Hypersecretion** of the growth hormone from the anterior pituitary. This may be due to pituitary eosinophilic adenoma resulting in gigantism. The treatment is excision of the pituitary adenoma. If the features are well-established, it is, however irreversible.
- **Primary ovarian failure:** There 'is lack' of endogenous estrogen → delayed closure of the epiphysis of long bones. There is associated unopposed action of the growth hormone from the anterior pituitary resulting in linear growth of the long bones (p. 395).

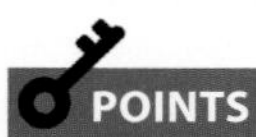

POINTS

- **Undue clitoral enlargement** seen at birth may be due to disorders of sexual development. It requires at least estimation of 17-OHP, 17 ketosteroid and chromosomal analysis. Levels of 17-OHP >800 ng/dL are virtually diagnostic of congenital adrenal hyperplasia (21-hydroxylase deficiency).
- **Genital crisis** is due to hyperestrogenic state and includes bleeding per vaginam, enlarged breasts and neonatal leukorrhea (p. 455).
- **Labial fusion** is commonly due to infection and rarely a feature of intersexuality. Separation of the adhesions is effective using fingers or a probe (p. 456).
- **Muco or hydrocolpos** is usually found within 1 year of age and results from imperforate hymen.
- **The childhood vulvovaginitis** is mainly due to poor perineal hygiene. Vulvovaginitis in premenarcheal period is mostly due to nonspecific organisms and occasionally to specific gonococcal infection. Bacteriological examination should be carried out from the discharge prior to therapy.
- **Ovarian follicular cysts** are common in adolescent girls and are usually self-limiting. An ovarian enlargement more than 5 cm needs to be investigated.
- **Ovarian neoplasm** constitute about 1% of all neoplasms in premenarcheal girls. Tumors are usually unilateral. Biopsy of the contralateral ovary should be avoided unless the tumor is dysgerminoma or immature teratoma.
- **Surgery** for ovarian tumors should consider two important issues: (1) Removal of the neoplasm and (2) Preservation of future fertility.
- **The neoplasm in premenarcheal period** is usually ovarian and, in about 25%, it is malignant. The common type is germ cell tumor (benign cystic teratoma, dysgerminoma, mixed germ cell tumor). The others are granulosa cell tumor or epithelial tumors. The benign tumors are epithelial tumors.
- **Sarcoma botryoides** is most often observed before the age of 8 years (p. 330).
- In a tall girl—to achieve arrest of bone growth, estrogen therapy for 3–6 months may be effective.
- **The menstrual disorders** in adolescent period are usually self-limiting and the hormones should not be used injudiciously. Assurance and improvement of health are enough in majority.
- **Vaginal adenosis** is present in about 30–50% of girls with history of DES exposure and is a benign lesion. Rarely, it progresses to clear cell carcinoma.
- **Most common ovarian neoplasm** in adolescence is benign cystic teratoma (p. 243).
- **STIs** are increasing among the adolescents. Sex education, HPV vaccination, use of condoms and treatment of STIs are essential (p. 461).
- **Obesity** is best assessed by calculating body mass index (BMI) (p. 461) and waist-hip ratio and both are elevated. Body pattern of an obese girl may be "apple-shaped" or "pear-shaped" depending upon the deposition of fat (Fig. 33.3).
- **Treatment** includes weight reduction, exercise and/or insulin sensitizing agents.
- **Acne** is a problem of adolescent girls. It is commonly due to excess androgens (PCOS). Therapy may be systemic (antiandrogens) and/or topical retinoids cream/gel.

CHAPTER

34 Special Topics

CHAPTER OUTLINE

ABNORMAL VAGINAL DISCHARGE

INTRODUCTION

Abnormal vaginal discharge is a frequent complaint of women seen in the gynecologic clinic. The discharge may be an excess of normal or it may pathological. It may be blood-stained or contaminated with urine or stool, all of which are however excluded from the discussion made below.

Characteristics of normal vaginal fluid: *It is watery, white in color, nonodorous with pH around 4.0. Microscopically, it contains squamous epithelial cells and a few bacteria. Lactobacilli (Doderlein bacilli, page 5), few gram-negative bacteria and anaerobes are present without any white or red blood cells.*

Causes of abnormal discharge are schematically presented in Flowchart 34.1, Tables 34.1 and 34.2.

LEUKORRHEA

Definition

Leukorrhea is strictly defined as an excessive normal vaginal discharge.

The term leukorrhea should fulfill the following criteria:

- The excess secretion is evident from persistent vulvar moistness or staining of the undergarments (brownish-yellow on drying) or need to wear a vulvar pad.
- It is nonpurulent and nonoffensive.
- It is nonirritant and never causes pruritus.

Physiologic excess: The normal secretion is expected to increase in conditions when the estrogen levels become high. Such conditions are:

- **During puberty:** Increased levels of endogenous estrogen lead to marked overgrowth of the endocervical epithelium which may encroach onto the ectocervix producing congenital ectopy (erosion) → increased secretion.
- **During menstrual cycle:**
  - **Around ovulation:** Peak rise of estrogen → increase in secretory activity of the cervical glands.
  - **Premenstrual** pelvic congestion and increased mucus secretion from the hypertrophied endometrial glands.
- **Pregnancy:** There is hyperestrinism with increased vascularity. This leads to increased vaginal transudate and cervical gland secretion.

Flowchart 34.1: Causes of abnormal vaginal discharge.

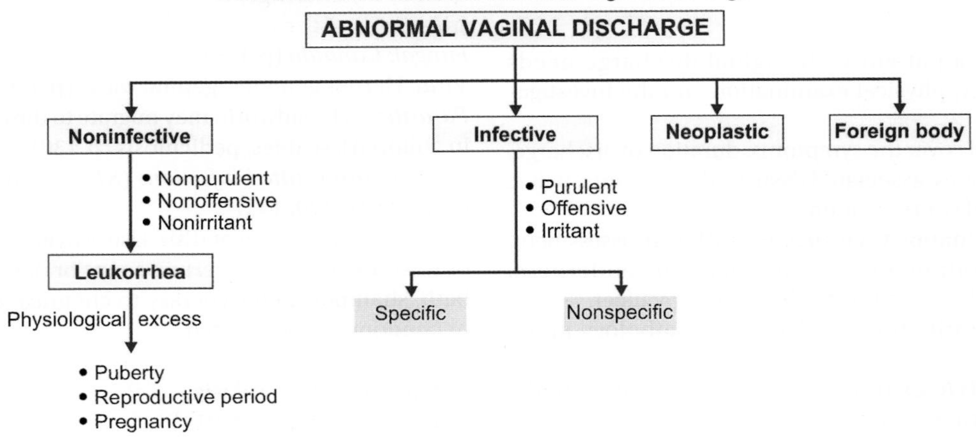

TABLE 34.1: Life table of abnormal vaginal discharge.

Period of life	*Associated symptoms*	*Probable diagnosis*
Early neonatal	Nil	Leukorrhea
Period up to premenarcheal	■ Nil ■ Offensive ■ Vulvar itching	■ Ill health ■ Foreign body ■ Threadworm
Puberty	Nil	Leukorrhea
Reproductive period ***Nonpregnant*** Related to menstrual cycle	Nil	Leukorrhea
Pill users	■ Nil ■ Pruritus	■ Leukorrhea ■ Moniliasis
Any time	■ Nil ■ Pruritus ■ Offensive	■ Ill health ■ Infective vaginitis ■ Neoplasm ■ Foreign body
During **antibiotic therapy**	Pruritus	Moniliasis
Diabetes	Pruritus	Moniliasis
Pregnancy	■ Nil ■ Pruritus	■ Leukorrhea ■ Vaginitis (moniliasis)
Postmeno-pausal	■ Nil ■ Pruritus/diabetic ■ Offensive	■ Senile vaginitis ■ Moniliasis ■ Pyometra ■ Neoplasm

- **During sexual excitement,** when there is abundant secretion from the Bartholin's glands.

Cervical cause: Noninfective cervical lesion may produce excessive secretion, which pours out at the vulva. Such lesions are—cervical ectopy, chronic cervicitis, mucous polyp and ectropion (cervical glands are exposed to the vagina).

Vaginal cause: Increased vaginal transudation occurs in conditions associated with increased pelvic congestion. The conditions are uterine prolapse, acquired retroverted uterus, chronic pelvic inflammation, 'pill' use and vaginal adenosis. Ill health is one of the important causes of excessive discharge. It produces excess exfoliation of the superficial cells.

Diagnosis

Evaluation of a patient with vaginal discharge needs detailed history, physical examination and the investigations.

History should cover the symptoms, duration of discharge, any prior episodes, associated dysuria, dyspareunia, pelvic pain and use of contraception.

Physical examination to cover: General health assessment, abdominal examination for any mass or tenderness, Inspection of the vulva for the discharge any ulcer.

Speculum examination: To detect any pathology in the cervix, vagina.

Bimanual pelvic examination: For any foreign body, adnexal tenderness or mass.

Investigations to be organized for the discharge are: Microbiological study (p. 89) Pap smear, urine for RE and CS and tests for PCR/NAAT for the pathogens (p. 89).

Treatment

The following are the guidelines:

- Improvement of general health.
- Cervical factors require surgical treatment like electrocautery, cryosurgery or trachelorrhaphy.
- Pelvic lesions producing vaginal leukorrhea require appropriate therapy for the pathology.
- Pill users may have to stop 'pill' temporarily, if the symptom is very much annoying.
- Above all, local hygiene has to be maintained meticulously.
- Treatment for specific infection.

PRURITUS VULVAE

About 10% of patients attending the gynecologic clinic complain of vulvar itching.

Definition

Pruritus means sense of itching. When it is confined to the vulva, it is called pruritus vulvae. It should not be confused with pain.

Mechanisms of Itching

The possible mechanisms of the repetitive '**itch-scratch**' cycle are mediated through the following:

- Special sensory innervation of the area.
- Underlying vascular instability (greatly influenced by emotion) results in production of histamine-like substance → induction of itching.
- Aggravation at night because of:
  - Absence of distraction of mind
  - Tired central nervous system
  - Local warmth and lack of aeration.

Etiology

Vaginal discharge: The most common cause of pruritus vulvae is vaginal discharges either due to *Trichomonas vaginalis* or *Candida albicans* or both (p. 135).

Local skin lesions: The lesions may be either localized or generalized. Such lesions include—psoriasis, seborrheic dermatitis, intertrigo, etc.

Infections of the vulva

Fungal: Candida (p. 135).

Viral: Herpes genitalis, genital warts (p. 126).

Parasitic—Threadworm may migrate to the area (especially in children), scabies, pediculosis (p. 130).

Sexually transmitted infections (STIs): Gonorrhea, trichomoniasis (p. 120, 133)

Allergy or contact dermatitis: Use of nylon under-garments or washing those with certain soaps or detergents, bubble bath, shampoos, idiosyncrasy to chemical contraceptives or condom is often related.

Non-neoplastic epithelial disorders of the vulva (p. 213)

- Squamous hyperplasia.
- Lichen sclerosus (p. 214).

TABLE 34.2: Common causes of vaginitis and abnormal vaginal discharge.

	Cause	Nature
Infective	■ Trichomonas vaginitis (p. 134) ■ Monilial vaginitis (p. 135) ■ Bacterial vaginosis (p. 125) ■ Cervicitis	■ Frothy yellow discharge ■ Curdy white in flakes, pruritic ■ Gray-white, fishy odor and nonpruritic ■ Mucoid discharge
Atrophic	Postmenopausal	■ Discharge is not prominent ■ Irritation is prominent
Foreign body	■ Forgotten pessary, tampon ■ Mechanical irritation	Offensive, copious, purulent, often blood stained
Chemical	■ Douches, latex condoms, deodorants ■ Chemical irritation contact dermatitis or allergy	Soreness is pronounced than the discharge
Excretions	Contamination with urine or feces producing secondary vaginitis	Offensive discharge with pruritus
Neoplasms	Fibroid polyp or genital malignancy	Serosanguinous, often offensive

Neoplastic epithelial disorders

- Vulvar intraepithelial neoplasia (VIN) (p. 266).
- Paget's disease (p. 267).
- Invasive carcinoma of the vulva (p. 279).

Pruritus vulvae due to some systemic diseases

- **Medical disorders:** Glycosuria (diabetes mellitus) causes local changes in the skin (raw beef color) and pruritus. It favors the growth of *Candida*. Others: Thyroid disorders, chronic liver disease, autoimmune disorders.
- **Dermatological causes:** Contact dermatitis, drug allergy.
- **Deficiency state:** Deficiencies of iron, folic acid, vitamin B_{12} and vitamin A are all implicated.
- **Psychosomatic causes:** When no cause is detected, psychic factor is to be excluded. Mental anxiety or sexual frustration may be responsible for scratching.

Investigations

It should be borne in mind that pruritus vulvae is a manifestation of some underlying pathology either located at the site or elsewhere in the body. **The investigations should include**:

Detailed history regarding: Age of onset, intensity of itching, duration, associated vaginal discharge, contraceptive practice, relation with psychologic upset or neurosis, allergy to nylon, soap or particular detergents.

General examination: Thorough systemic examination is needed. Examination for diabetes mellitus, liver, and thyroid disorders, hematological diseases are to be made.

Local examination: The extent of the lesion is to be noted.

Special investigations:

- Microscopic examination of the vaginal discharge or vulvar scraping to detect *Candida* or *Trichomonas vaginalis.*
- Urine for sugar, protein and pus cells.
- Blood—complete blood count, postprandial glucose. Detailed hematological work-up (polycythemia, leukemia), thyroid profile, liver function, and renal function tests are carried out.
- Stool—ova, parasites, and cysts are to be looked for.
- In long-standing cases (more than one year) especially with vulvar epithelial disorders, biopsy either random or colposcopic directed, is to be taken to note the type of skin changes and exclude malignancy.

Treatment

General principles

- Appropriate local hygiene is to be taken care of.
- To use loose fitting undergarments preferably made of cotton to keep the area aerated.
- To prevent the vicious cycle of '**itch-scratch**'.
  Local application of antibiotics or clobetasol propionate 0.05% (p. 215) ointment may be helpful. If the skin is atrophic, estrogen or testosterone cream may be helpful.
- **To treat the specific etiological factor** causing pruritus by appropriate therapy—local or systemic.

Surgery: Surgery may be needed when biopsy confirms features of neoplasia (VIN or invasion).

PELVIC PAIN

Pain is an unpleasant sensory and emotional experience associated with actual or potential tissue damage. Pain is a protective mechanism. Pelvic pain is a common symptom in gynecology. It may be present in **acute form** or **in chronic form**. It should be remembered that the pain is just a symptom of an underlying disorder. **Sensation of pain is found to depend on many factors in an individual, e.g. subjective feel, emotional status, genetic factors, experience, gender, pain threshold, anxiety and expectations. Women have a lower pain threshold and tolerance.**

NEUROPHYSIOLOGY OF PAIN

Pain may be (a) somatic (somatic nervous system) or (b) viscera (autonomic nervous system).

Impulse generated due to depolarization of a peri-pheral nerve ending (transduction) → transmission of the nerve impulse → modulation (control of impulse transmission to neurons by neurotransmitters) → perception of pain.

Unlike somatic structures, which are well-represented in the cerebral cortex in terms of localization, visceral structures are poorly localized in the cerebral cortex. Thus,

TABLE 34.3: Localization of referred pain.

Organs	*Site of referred pain*
Body of uterus	Hypogastrium, anterior and medial aspect of thighs
Fallopian tubes and ovaries	Above the mid-inguinal point
Cervix	Upper sacral region
Uterosacral ligament	Lower sacral region

the pain arising from the pelvic organs is often localized not to the organ but referred to the skin area supplied by the same spinal nerve (Table 34.3). Various neuromodulators (prostaglandins, endorphins) and neurotransmitters (norepinephrine, serotonin) are involved to modify the pain sensation in the brain. Visceral pain may be due to distension, stretching, hypoxia, necrosis, chemical irritants or inflammation of the viscera. Pelvic pain may be splanchnic or referred. One finger 'trigger point' tenderness is suggestive of nerve entrapment (ilioinguinal). Similarly 'ovarian point' tenderness suggests pelvic congestion syndrome (p. 150).

ACUTE PELVIC PAIN

Acute pain is of short duration and generally the symptoms are proportionate to the extent of tissue damage. In chronic pelvic pain, the onset is insidious and the degree of pain is not proportionate to the extent of structural tissue damage.

Most often, the basic mechanism of acute pain is due to irritation of the peritoneum by either blood or infection. The causes of acute pelvic pain are given in Table 34.4.

Diagnosis

A meticulous history-taking and examinations—systemic, abdominal and pelvic, most often clinch the diagnosis.

General physical examination: It includes facial expression, pallor, temperature, pulse, and BP recording.

Abdominal examination: Inspection (previous scars), palpation in all the quadrants for distension, tenderness, wall rigidity, ascites, auscultation (bowel sounds) are done. Pelvic examination including rectal examination for pelvic and colorectal pathology is done.

Guidelines in clinical diagnosis:

- Pain of gynecologic origin usually starts in the lower abdomen and then spreads to the entire abdomen.
- Pain preceded by amenorrhea is usually obstetrically related—**disturbed ectopic pregnancy should be kept in mind.**
- Anorexia, nausea and vomiting are usually correlated well with gastrointestinal mischief.
- Frequency of micturition, dysuria with or without fever point to the diagnosis of urinary tract infection.
- Fever with chills and rigor is most often associated with acute pelvic inflammatory disease (PID).
- Pain with syncopal attacks with collapse suggests intraperitoneal hemorrhage.
- Abdominopelvic lump along with more or less stable vital signs points towards complicated pelvic tumor.

TABLE 34.4: Causes of acute pelvic pain.

Mechanism	*Clinical conditions*
Hemoperitoneum—peritoneal irritation	▪ Disturbed tubal pregnancy ▪ Ruptured chocolate cyst ▪ Ruptured corpus luteum or follicular cyst
Infection—peritoneal irritation	Acute PID, tubo-ovarian abscess
Chemical irritation	Following HSG
Uterine cramp	Abortion, dysmenorrhea
Vascular complication with neurologic involvement	Axial rotation of ovarian tumor pedicle
Visceral distension	▪ Intracystic hemorrhage ▪ Hyperstimulation syndrome ▪ Hematometra or pyometra
Nongynecological	▪ Appendicitis ▪ UTI, pyelonephritis, renal calculus ▪ Intestinal obstruction ▪ Rectus sheath hematoma ▪ Mesenteric lymph adenitis ▪ Pancreatitis ▪ Musculoskeletal pain

(PID: pelvic inflammatory disease; HSG: hysterosalpingography; UTI: urinary tract infection)

- **Localized pain** on anterior abdominal wall is often due to nerve entrapment or musculofascial pain. It is differentiated from intra-abdominal pain by **Cornett sign**. Pain usually decreases on asking the patient to rise and sit.

Musculofacial pain (Table 34.5): Pudendal neuralgia (S2, S3, S4): Causes a sharp, severe and shooting pain over the area of perineum through its three branches (perineal, inferior rectal and dorsal nerve of the clitotris) (Table 34.5).

Pain may get worse by sitting.

Investigations

Basic investigations to substantiate the clinical diagnosis as when indicated include:

- **Blood:** Complete blood count (CBC) is done. An increase in white cell count especially with a shift to left may indicate infection. Decreased hemoglobin level with low hematocrit value indicates hypovolemia.

TABLE 34.5: Site and tissue origin of pelvic pain (with innervations).

Site(s) of pain	*Muscle with innervations*
▪ Pelvic floor, anus, perineum, lower vagina	Pyriformis (S2-S4, L1-L2)
▪ Pelvic floor, vagina, rectum	Pubococcygeus (S3, S4)
▪ Pelvic floor, buttock, anterior thigh	Obturator (L2, L3, L4)
▪ Lower abdomen, anterior vulva, urethra, clitoris	Iliopsoas (L1-L2)
▪ Ovaries	T9–T10, sympathetics: aortic and superior mesenteric plexus

- **Midstream urine for microscopic examination and culture** is to be done to diagnose urinary tract infection (UTI). Presence of pus cells, bacteria and red blood cells suggests UTI.
- **Urine for immunological test of pregnancy**: A positive test needs to be followed with serial β and human chorionic gonadotropin (hCG) measurement, transvaginal sonography (TVS) to rule out ectopic pregnancy.
  With these protocols, diagnosis is established in majority and for those remaining undiagnosed cases, the following are to be employed.
- **Transvaginal or transabdominal sonography** is useful for adnexal pathology, like torsion, ectopic pregnancy or any uterine mass (fibroid). Three-dimensional (3D) sonography with color Doppler is more informative.
- **X-ray abdomen** (upright, supine and lateral decubitus film) is to be done to diagnose—intestinal obstruction or perforation. Perforation of air-filled viscus is evident by presence of free air under the diaphragm. Free fluid suggests ruptured cyst. Calculus can be evident from X-ray.
- **Computed tomography (CT):** It can detect pelvic, gastrointestinal (GI), and urinary tract (calculi) pathologies. Contrast enhanced computed tomography (CECT) and multidetector CT (MDCT) is more informative.
- **Magnetic resonance imaging (MRI):** It is an important tool when initial sonography is nondiagnostic, especially in an obese patient.
- **Laparoscopy** is helpful to visualize the pelvic pathology. Surprisingly, laparoscopic examination confirms the provisional clinical diagnosis in only 25% of the cases. In acute PID, aspiration of the tubal exudate is to be done for microbial study.

Management

The patients are most often critically ill. Intensive resuscitative or supportive measures are to be taken. The definitive treatment of some of the common events are formulated in Table 34.6.

TABLE 34.6: Management options for acute pelvic pain.

Definite diagnosis	***Immediate laparotomy*** ▪ Hemoperitoneum ▪ Rupture tubo-ovarian abscess ▪ Twisted ovarian cyst (p. 247) ▪ Tubal ectopic rupture
	Institution of medical therapy ▪ Urinary tract infection (p. 344) ▪ Pelvic inflammatory disease (p. 106) ▪ Gastroenteritis ▪ Hyperstimulation syndrome (p. 444)
Doubtful diagnosis	▪ To be subjected to diagnostic sonography or CT or MRI or laparoscopy ▪ Observation

CHRONIC PELVIC PAIN

Chronic pelvic pain (CPP): It is defined as the noncyclic pain (nonmenstrual) of 6 months duration or more localized to the pelvis, anterior abdominal wall below the pelvis or lower back, severe enough to cause functional disability that require medical or surgical treatment.

CPP is a common problem (10%) seen in the gynecologic outpatient. Approximately 20–30% of laparoscopies and 10% of all hysterectomies are done due to CPP.

Diagnosis

While it is comparatively easy to diagnose the cyclic chronic pelvic pain, it is difficult at times to pinpoint the diagnosis of acyclic (Table 34.7) and the nongynecologic group. However, meticulous history-taking and thorough clinical examinations—abdominal and vaginal with the possibility in mind, are often enough to clinch the diagnosis.

In confused state, without any detectable pelvic pathology to account for CPP, **the following guidelines are of help to arrive at the diagnosis.**

- **Nerve entrapment pain** is localized to a particular point of the lower abdominal wall. This may be due to entrapment of ilioinguinal, iliohypogastric or genitofemoral nerve. This pain is often differentiated by **Cornett sign** (p. 471). Local infiltration of bupivacaine 0.25% and relief of pain is a confirmatory test. It is therapeutic also. Surgical exploration and excision of the nerve is also recommended.
- **Trigger point (TRP):** It is the hyperirritable area within a muscle to cause chronic pain. This pain is due to neuromuscular end plate dysfunction with sustained acetylcholine release to cause sarcomere shortening and making the muscle band taut. TRPs may be there in the muscle of the abdominal wall; pelvic floor and pelvic girdle to cause CCP.

TABLE 34.7: Common gynecologic causes of chronic pelvic pain.

Cyclic	*Acyclic*
▪ **Intermenstrual pain** (Mittelschmerz) ▪ **Dysmenorrhea** • Spasmodic • Congestive ▪ **Premenstrual syndrome** ▪ **Pelvic congestion syndrome** ▪ **Endometriosis** ▪ **Adenomyosis** ▪ **Ovarian remnant syndrome** ▪ **Uterine fibroids** ▪ **IUCD**	▪ **Endometriosis, adenomyosis** ▪ **Pelvic inflammatory disease (PID)** ▪ **Tubo-ovarian abscess** ▪ **Uterine displacement** • Retroversion • Prolapse ▪ Uterine fibroid ▪ Ovarian cyst • Functional • Neoplastic ▪ Pelvic adhesions disease secondary to PID, endometriosis or postsurgical ▪ Intrauterine device (IUD) ▪ Trapped or residual ovarian syndrome (p. 469) ▪ Idiopathic • Pelvic varicosities • Psychosomatic

Treatment: It is inactivation of the TRP and to release the taut muscle band. Analgesics, muscle relaxants, biofeedback or electrical stimulation is helpful.

- **Pessary test:** In mobile retroverted uterus or slight degree of uterine descent, a pessary test may be employed. The pessary is inserted and kept for 3 months. If the symptoms are relieved, the diagnosis is certain and surgical correction is advisable.
- **Combined oral contraceptive pills:** Cases with functional ovarian cyst producing CPP are given cyclic oral contraceptive (OC) for 3 months. The functional cyst is likely to regress with the relief of symptoms. The same therapeutic test can be employed to relieve the midmenstrual pain or primary dysmenorrhea by making the cycle anovular.
- **Transcutaneous electric nerve stimulation (TENS)** is helpful in cases by inhibiting the transmission of nerve impulse via unmyelinated fibers.
- **Cognitive and behavioral therapy (CBT)** to be given to patients as it has benefits.
- **Pain mapping** is useful especially in assessment of adhesions.
- **Patient having IUD** and pelvic pain should be cautiously interpreted. **The possibility of PID or ectopic pregnancy should be kept in mind.**
- **Nongynecological disorders** as cause of CPP should be kept in mind (Table 34.8). These are mostly related with disorders of bowel (spastic colon, irritable bowel syndrome). Spasm or rigidity of muscles especially those of vertebral column suggests orthopedic, neurologic or rheumatic lesion.
- **CPP without any organic lesion:** The women are usually parous and perimenopausal. These cases may be attributed to pelvic congestion, or may be due to psychosomatic disturbances.
- **Pelvic congestion syndrome** (Taylor syndrome) is characterized by chronic pelvic pain, dyspareunia, abnormal uterine bleeding along with pelvic venous congestion. Diagnosis can be made by transuterine venography, transvaginal color Doppler sonography (TV-CDS) or by laparoscopy. Congested pelvic veins are seen. **Therapeutic options are**: Medroxyprogesterone acetate 50 mg daily is found to be effective. GnRH agonist with estrogen add back therapy is also recommended. Hysterectomy and bilateral salpingo-oophorectomy or embolization (UAE) is considered as the treatment of last resort for those who fail to respond with medical therapy.
- **Ancillary aids in diagnosis**

Blood: Complete hemogram helpful in the diagnosis of infection. Thyroid dysfunction (bowel or bladder pain), diabetes (neuropathy) to be ruled out.

Cervical and vaginal discharge is subjected to hanging drop preparation, Gram stain and culture, both aerobic and anaerobic. This can give a clue in the diagnosis of PID.

Endometrial biopsy to be done in suspected cases of genital tuberculosis (p. 113).

Sonography: It is of value in diagnosis of tumor, either fibroid or ovarian. TVS can detect adenomyosis and ovarian enlargement due to cysts. Color Doppler sonography (CDS) is helpful to detect ovarian torsion. Calculi in the urinary system can also be detected with sonography. It is also helpful in assessing the progress of the therapy in PID especially when laparoscopy is contraindicated or as an alternative to it.

Laparoscopy: It is an invaluable diagnostic tool in the investigation of chronic pelvic pain. It has been found that about 50% of cases with normal clinical pelvic findings have got detectable abnormality on laparoscopy. Conversely, one-third of women with detectable clinical pathology are ultimately proven to have normal pelvis on laparoscopy.

Its chief value is to detect minimal endometriosis and pelvic adhesions. The negative finding also have got value—assures the clinician that no abnormality exists. This can relieve the patient's psychosomatic factor related with CPP.

X-rays of lumbosacral region and hip joints helps to detect orthopedic lesions. CT scan or MRI are less commonly used in the diagnosis of CPP except in malignant conditions. Cystoscopy, sigmoidoscopy, colonoscopy may be helpful in some cases.

TABLE 34.8: Common nongynecologic causes of chronic pelvic pain.

Gastrointestinal	▪ Irritable bowel syndrome ▪ Appendicitis ▪ Constipation ▪ Diverticulitis ▪ Adhesions
Urological	▪ Interstitial cystitis (p. 342) ▪ Urethral syndrome (p. 346) ▪ Calculi, chronic urinary tract infection (UTI) ▪ Urinary tract stones
Orthopedic	Diseases of the lumbar bones, ligaments, muscles of the lumbosacral region, coccydynia
Neurological	Nerve entrapment or compression **Neuralgia:** Pudendal, ilioinguinal or genitofemoral nerve, pyriformis syndrome: It is due to the compression of the sciatic nerve by the pyriformis
Hernias	Inguinal, femoral, obturator
Musculoskeletal	Muscular strain, myofascial pain, levator ani syndrome, fibromyositis
Miscellaneous	Physical, sexual, psychiatric

Treatment Principles

- To have a definite diagnosis of the underlying disorders.
- To establish the relationship between the pathology and the symptoms.
- To evaluate psychosomatic factors—cause or effect.
- **Multidisciplinary approach** involving a psychologist is ideal especially when no pathology could be detected.

In detectable pathology: Conservative or radical surgery is to be done to remove the offending pathology. Hysterectomy is ideal for women with pelvic endometriosis or adenomyosis, when she has completed child bearing.

Medical management of pain

- **Assurance** and sympathetic handling too often cure or ameliorate the pain.
- **Nonsteroidal anti-inflammatory drugs (NSAIDs):** Ibuprofen, Naproxen: COX-2 inhibitors—Celecoxib, Ketorolac.
- **Neurolytic agents:** Tricyclic antidepressants—Amitriptyline, Imipramine, **Serotonin uptake inhibitors:** Sertraline, Fluoxetine, Paroxetine, **Ion channel blockers**: Gabapentin, Carbamazepine.
- **Narcotics (under supervision)**: Codeine, Methadone.
- **Others**: Oral contraceptive (OC) pills, progestogens, danazol or even GnRH analogs (p. 441) is indicated in young patients with minimal endometriosis, spasmodic dysmenorrhea or midmenstrual pain.
- **Minimal invasive surgery** includes laser therapy in pelvic endometriosis or laparoscopic adhesiolysis. Presacral neurectomy (PSN) and **laparoscopic** uterine nerve ablation (LUNA) are considered for midline dysmenorrhea when conservative management has failed.
- **Surgery** like ventrosuspension, plication of round ligaments (p. 506) in deep dyspareunia or even presacral neurectomy may be employed.
- **Hysterectomy** should be contemplated judiciously in selected cases.
- **Intractable pain of malignant origin:** Apart from narcotic analgesics, PSN or LUNA may relieve pain for few months.
- **Anticonvulsants:** May be used for CPP. **Gabapentin, pregabalin** and **lamotrigine** are commonly used for neuropathic pain.
- **Polypharmacy:** Sometimes combining drugs acting on different sites may improve pain.

RESIDUAL (TRAPPED) OVARIAN SYNDROME

The syndrome is characterized by chronic pelvic pain, deep dyspareunia and a fixed tender ovary felt at the vault of the vagina.

The syndrome is due to the ovary(ies) left intentionally at the time of hysterectomy. However, both the syndromes (trapped and remnant) have the identical symptoms though is differentiated by amount of ovarian tissue presented. Diagnosis and management are the same.

It may appear in 1–3% of all cases of hysterectomy with preservation of one or both the ovaries. **The pain is due to tension within the developing follicle of the ovary with periovarian adhesions. Pain may also be due to perioophoritis with a thickened ovarian capsule**. Ultrasonography (TVS) can detect characteristic ovarian enlargement.

The relief of pain may be achieved by ovarian suppression with hormones (high dose progestins, OC pills, danazol or GnRH agonists). Cure is by removal of the ovaries.

OVARIAN REMNANT SYNDROME

The syndrome is defined as the persistence of the ovarian function even after an apparently bilateral oophorectomy. Oophorectomy becomes technically difficult during hysterectomy in cases with extensive endometriosis or pelvic inflammatory disease. **Pain is due to the remnant of ovarian cortical tissue, left behind (retroperitoneally) unintendedly following a difficult oophorectomy.**

The presenting complaints are chronic pelvic pain (cyclic), deep dyspareunia and persistence of symptoms of endometriosis. **Confirmation is done** by serum FSH levels in premenopausal range. Laparoscopic visualization of the remnant ovarian tissue is difficult because of adhesions. Vaginal ultrasound and MRI are helpful to the diagnosis.

Ovarian suppression as mentioned above may be used for diagnosis. Cure is effective by surgical removal. Careful dissection is needed as it is adjacent to the ureter in the retroperitoneal space.

POSTMENOPAUSAL BLEEDING

INTRODUCTION

Bleeding per vagina following established menopause is called postmenopausal bleeding.

The significance of postmenopausal bleeding, whatever slight it may be, should not be underestimated. **As many as one-third of the cases are due to malignancy.** The same importance is also given to those cases where normal menstruation continues even beyond the age of 55 years.

CAUSES

The causes of postmenopausal bleeding are shown in Table 34.9:

- Senile endometritis (p. 138)
- Atrophic endometrium
- Endometrial hyperplasia (p. 275)
- Dysfunctional uterine bleeding
- Genital malignancy:
  - Carcinoma of the cervix, endometrium, vagina, vulva and fallopian tube.
  - Sarcoma uterus.
  - Granulosa cell tumor of the ovary

TABLE 34.9: Common causes of postmenopausal bleeding.

Senile endometritis	Decubitus ulcer
Genital malignancy	Retained pessary or IUCD
Endometrial hyperplasia	Urethral caruncle

(DUB: dysfunctional uterine bleeding; IUCD: intrauterine contraceptive device)

- Uterine polyp
- Tubercular endometritis
- Cervical erosion and polyp
- Senile vaginitis
- Decubitus ulcer
- Retained and forgotten foreign body such as pessary or intrauterine contraceptive device (IUCD)
- Withdrawal bleeding following estrogen intake
- Urethral caruncle, polyp, prolapse mucosa or carcinoma
- Unknown is about 25%. **The incidence however decreases with wider use of hysteroscopy**.

INVESTIGATIONS

Initial step is to establish the fact that it is vaginal bleeding and not bleeding per rectum or hematuria.

Detailed History

- Age of menopause.
- Menstrual pattern prior to menopause.
- Amount of bleeding, number of episodes.
- Sensation of something coming out of the introitus.
- Urinary problems like dysuria or frequency of urination.
- Intake of estrogen—even if the history of intake is present, full investigations should be carried out to exclude malignancy.
- Family history of endometrial and/or ovarian carcinoma (first degree relative).

General Examination

Obesity, diabetes and hypertension are often related to endometrial carcinoma.

Enlarged groin or supraclavicular lymph nodes may be palpated. Metastatic nodules in the anterior vaginal wall may be present. Breasts should be palpated because gynecological symptoms may be related to breast cancer.

Per abdomen: A lump in the lower abdomen may be due to pyometra or uterine sarcoma or adnexal mass.

Inspection of the perineum:

- If the uterus is outside the introitus, a decubitus ulcer may be detected (p. 172).
- Careful inspection of vulva may reveal a growth. If it is present, biopsy is to be taken.

Palpation: To separate the labia for better inspection of the urethral meatus to find out any caruncle, polyp or mucosal prolapse.

Speculum examination: To note the condition of the cervix and the vault of the vagina.

- Any visible cervical growth → biopsy is to be taken for histology.
- Cervix apparently looking normal → cervical and endocervical smear to exclude dysplasia or CIN (p. 268).
- Aspiration cytology—for endometrial carcinoma.

Pipelle endometrial sampling can be done with a long and narrow plastic cannula (Fig. 9.21). This is done as an outpatient department (OPD) procedure during speculum examination. Adequate sample is obtained with this procedure and the tissue is subjected for histological examination.

Bimanual Examination

- Uterus may be normal, atrophic or enlarged due to pyometra or sarcoma.
- Adnexal mass (infective or ovarian) may be palpable.

Special Investigations

Ultrasonography transvaginal probe (TVS) is more accurate because of its proximity to the target tissue (endometrium). Endometrial thickness less than 5 mm indicates atrophy. On the other hand, thick polypoid endometrium (9–10 mm), irregular texture, fluid within the uterus require further evaluation (to exclude malignancy). 3D sonography with Doppler studies are more informative.

- **Saline infusion sonography** (SIS) is more accurate compared to sonography alone and biopsy is taken (p. 99).
- **Hysteroscopic** evaluation and directed biopsy (p. 520).
- **Endometrial biopsy** may be done using pipelle cannula or the Sharman curette as an outpatient basis. Endometrial biopsy for diagnosis of endometrial carcinoma under guidance of sonohysterography or hysteroscopy has got the similar diagnostic accuracy. Thickness of endometrium ≤4 mm using TVS is suggestive of atrophic endometrium. Biopsy is indicated when the endometrium is thick.
- **Fractional curettage**, if the cervical cytology becomes negative (p. 299).
- **Laparoscopy** in suspected cases of ovarian or adnexal mass.
- **CT and MRI** are useful in selected cases of post-menopausal bleeding where malignancy is suspected (carcinoma cervix and endometrium).

Detection of a benign lesion should not prevent further detailed investigations to rule out malignancy.

Treatment

- **Once the cause is diagnosed**, the treatment is directed to it.
- **If no cause is detected** and there is only minimal bleeding once or twice, careful observation is mandatory, if conservatism is desired.
- **In cases of recurrences or continued bleeding** whatever may be the amount, it is better to proceed for laparotomy and to perform hysterectomy with bilateral salpingo-oophorectomy. Unexpectedly, one may find a pathology either in the ovary or fallopian tube or else, an uterine polyp—benign or malignant may be evident in the removed uterus.

LOW BACKACHE

Low backache is a frequent complaint of parous women. It may be the part of the gynecological complaints or the case may be referred by an orthopedic surgeon after excluding the pelvic pathology to account for the low backache. **The reasons to refer are:**

- The low backache often dates back to childbirth process or gynecological operation.
- The symptoms often aggravate in relation to period.
 To establish a correlation between the low backache and gynecologic pathology, **the following facts are to be remembered**.
- As the posterior peritoneum is poorly innervated, the pain is dull and diffuse.
- Backache of pelvic origin never reaches beyond the 4th lumbar vertebra.
- The pain pointed by fingertip is not of gynecologic origin.
- **Cornett sign:** Localized pain over the anterior abdominal wall (due to nerve entrapment or myofascial pain) is differentiated from the intra-abdominal pain by Cornett sign. Patient is asked to raise her head and shoulder from lying down posture. Anterior abdominal wall pain is relieved with this.

CAUSES

Common causes of backache of pelvic origin are as follows.

Uterine displacement:

- **Prolapse:** Uterine prolapse produces backache due to stretching of the ligaments supporting the uterus in position. If the ligaments are atrophic, there will be no pain. **Vaginal prolapse does not cause backache**.
 The pain in prolapse subsides when the patient is at rest and aggravates on standing.
- **Retroversion:** Retroverted uterus may produce backache only when it is fixed by inflammatory or endometriotic adhesions. **Mobile retroverted uterus does not produce backache**.

Chronic pelvic infection: Chronic PID producing adhesions and tubo-ovarian mass formation may be responsible for backache. There are associated menstrual abnormalities and dyspareunia.

Endometriosis: It involving the pelvic peritoneum, uterosacral ligament or rectovaginal septum produces backache and deep dyspareunia (p. 255).

Neoplasm: Benign neoplasm like ovarian tumor or fibroid will not ordinarily produce backache. However, cervical or broad ligament fibroid can cause backache by producing pressure on the nerve routes over the sacrum.

Pelvic malignancy produces backache by involving the nerve roots, metastasis in the vertebrae or involving the lateral pelvic wall.

BREAST IN GYNECOLOGY

Gynecologists are the primary health care personnel for women. The role of a gynecologist in women's breast care are:

- Creating breast self-awareness
- Performing clinical breast examination
- Giving instructions for breast self-evaluation
- Evaluation of all breast masses
- Organizing routine screening mammography
- Organizing diagnostic procedures, referral for specialized care.
- To evaluate individual women's risk factors based on family history medical examination.

Breast is one of the target organs for the various hormones, of particular estrogens, progesterone, and prolactin. As such, many a breast related complaint or disease is associated with endocrine dysfunctions.

Development: The breast develops at 6–8 weeks from the "milk ridge" which is an **ectodermal thickening** that extends longitudinally from the axilla to groin. Pectoral part of the ridge persists and the rest regresses.

At birth: There is only nipple with system of ducts without alveoli. Due to maternal estrogen, the growth becomes exaggerated with occasional mucoid discharge (witch milk). The involution usually is completed by 1–2 weeks after birth.

Puberty changes (p. 39): The breast duct growth is primarily stimulated by estrogen. The alveolar cells and sebaceous glands are stimulated by progesterone. The maturation of the breast components is accelerated by growth hormone, adrenal hormones, thyroid hormone, prolactin, and insulin.

ANATOMY OF THE ADULT BREAST

The breasts are bilateral glandular structures. In female, breasts constitute accessory reproductive organs as the glands are concerned with lactation following childbirth.

The shape of the breast varies in women. Adult breast weighs about 250 g. It usually extends from the second to sixth rib in the midclavicular line. It lies in the subcutaneous tissue over the fascia covering the pectoralis major or even beyond that to lie over the serratus anterior and external oblique. An axillary prolongation (axillary tail), if present, lies in the axillary fossa, sometimes deep to the deep fascia. Breasts are large modified apocrine or sweat glands.

Structures (Nonlactating Breasts)

The areola is placed about the center of the breast and is pigmented. It is about 2.5 cm in diameter. There are numerous sebaceous glands over it. It contains few involuntary muscles. The nipple is a muscular projection covered by pigmented skin. It is vascular and surrounded by unstriped muscles which make it erectile. It accommodates about 15–20 lactiferous ducts and their openings. Areolar glands (montogomery) produces an oily secretion to keep the nipple supple and protected. This is important in breastfeeding. The whole breast is embedded in the subcutaneous fat. The fat is, however, absent beneath the nipple and areola. **The breast tissue is composed of lobes (15–20), glandular tissues (20%), duct system and also fibrofatty tissues (Figs. 34.1A and B).** *For details see Dutta's Textbook of Obstetrics, 9th Edition.*

Blood supply: Arterial supply

- Lateral thoracic branches of the axillary artery
- Internal mammary arteries
- Intercostal arteries
- Thoracoacromial arteries

Veins: The veins follow the courses of the arteries.

Lymphatics: Axillary nodes 85%

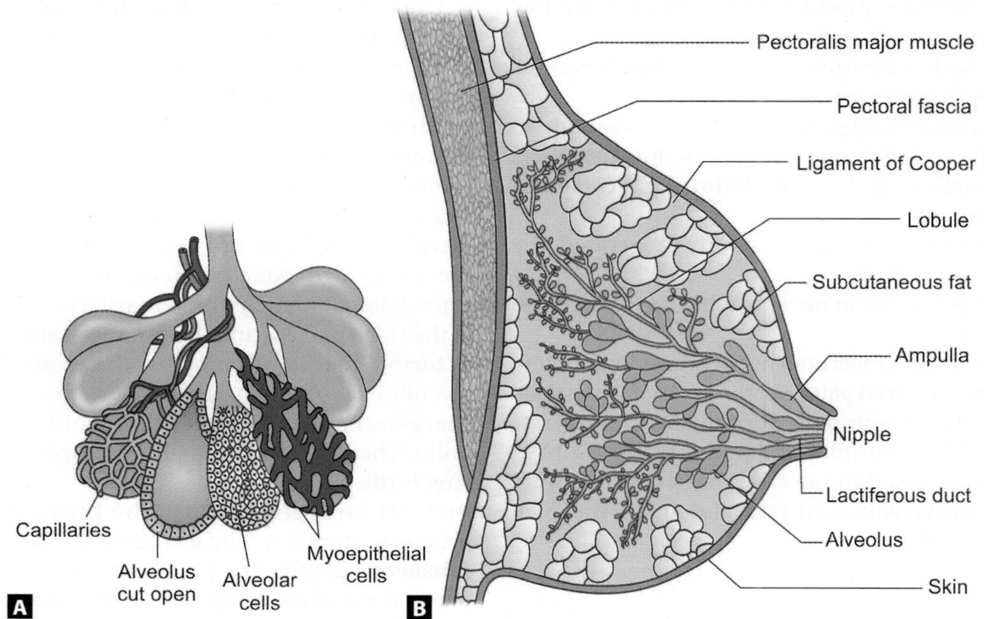

Figs. 34.1A and B: (A) Structure of the basic unit of the mammary gland; (B) Structure of adult female breast.

Lymphatic drainage: Initially drains into subareolar plexus of Sappy.

Outer quadrants: 75% lymphatics drain to ipsilateral axillary nodes. These lymphatics are the route for metastasis to the liver, ovary and peritoneum.

- Ipsilateral (75%)
- *Upper convexity*: Supraclavicular group.
- *Medial convexity*: Mediastinal glands (cross connection between the two breasts), internal mammary, supraclavicular notes. There is no contralateral drainage of lymph, until and unless there is ipsilateral obstruction.
- *Inferior convexity:* Mediastinal glands, abdominal nodes.

Sentinel node is the first lymph node draining the tumor bearing area.

Nerves: The nerve supply is from fourth, fifth, and sixth intercostal nerves.

ANATOMICAL DEFECTS

- **Small breasts (hypoplasia).** This may be due to:
  - Non or under production of ovarian estrogens.
  - Developmental defect in the breasts.

  In the former group, reassurance and cyclic estrogen or combined estrogen-progestogen preparations may be of help, if continued for a prolonged period. **In the latter group**, if the menstrual function is normal, it is no good to give hormone. Improvement of general health and breast augmention of the affected side may be done.
- **Huge enlargement (Fig. 34.2):** Some enlargement occurs during pregnancy and lactation. Breasts become pendulous in parous women due to stretching of the fibrous septa. Rarely, the breasts become hugely enlarged. The glandular tissues are affected but not the nipple. This may cause neck, back and shoulder pain.

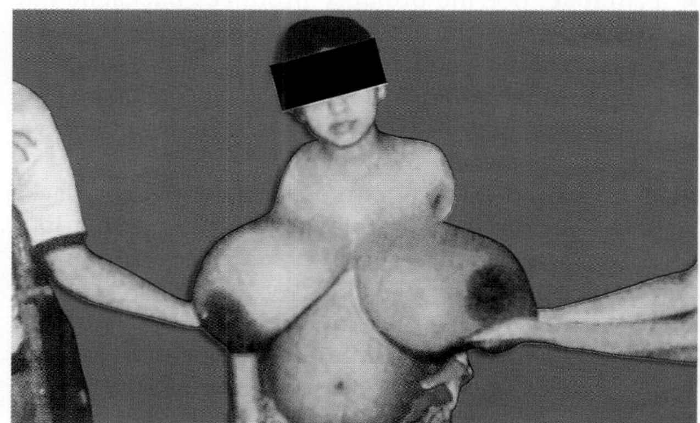

Fig. 34.2: Marked hypertrophy of the breast.
(*Courtesy:* Dr N Chowdhury)

  Young women are embarrassed also. Treatment by reduction mammoplasty is justified after the age of 17.
- **Asymmetry (Fig. 34.3):** During initial period of development, asymmetry is common. However, it soon rectifies within couple of years of menarche. Left is slightly larger than the right. Sometimes, the asymmetry persists and causes concern to the patient. Plastic surgery to increase the size of the smaller breast can be done if she is affected psychologically.
- **Accessory breasts (Fig. 34.3):** A breast (polymastia) or a part or a nipple (polythelia) may develop and tends to grow anywhere along a line extending from the axilla to the groin (milkline). **The most common site of extension is as a 'tail' into the axilla**. They can be the site of all diseases as found in a normal breast tissue. Excision may be needed because of discomfort, cosmesis or disease.

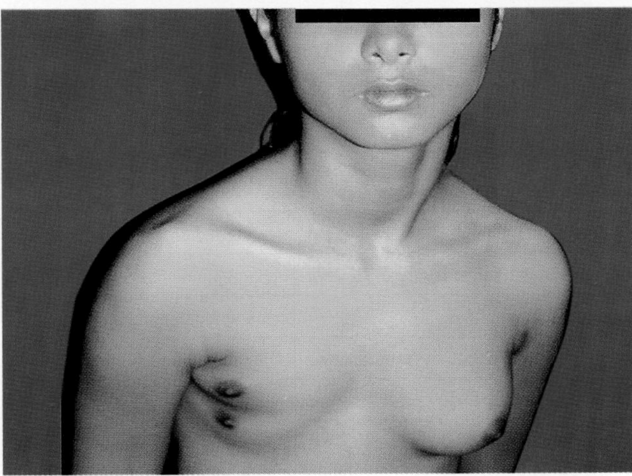

Fig. 34.3: Asymmetry of the breasts with polythelia (accessory nipple—right).

- **Athelia:** Complete absence (unilateral or bilateral) of nipple and areola may be familial (autosomal dominant). It may be associated with amastia. Reconstruction of nipple and areola is done.
- **Amastia:** Complete absence of both breast tissue and the nipple areola complex may occur. It may be associated with other ectodermal defect (cleft palate).

BENIGN BREAST DISORDERS

The majority (90%) of breast complaints and abnormalities are associated with benign breast disorders (BBDs).

Clinical Classification of BBDs

- Physiologic swelling and tenderness
- Nodularity
- Mastalgia (breast pain)
- Palpable breast lump
- Fibrocystic changes
- Fibroadenoma
- Nipple discharge including galactorrhea
- Breast infection and inflammation (associated with lactation)

Mastalgia

Mastalgia (breast pain) is a common problem for majority of women. It may be cyclic or noncyclic. Noncyclic mastalgia may be focal. This complain needs thorough evaluation to exclude breast malignancy. Mammography and other imagings could be valuable. Cyclic mastalgia is usually bilateral, diffuse, and severe during the luteal phase. It is relieved with menstruation. Cyclic mastalgia generally requires no specific evaluation.

Diagnosis is made from careful history-taking, examination and mammography (women ≥35 years of age). About 5% of women with breast cancer present with breast pain. Any complex cyst need a tissue diagnosis with core needle biopsy.

Drugs associated with mastalgia are: Hormones (estrogen, progestins), antihypertensives, spironolactone, fluoxetine.

The differential diagnosis includes a cyst, chest wall pain, costochondritis, mastitis, prolactinomas or drugs.

Management is primarily aimed to exclude cancer. The woman should be reassured. Drugs and measures commonly used with proven benefits are:

- **Acetaminophen or NSAIDs**
- **Bromocriptine**
- **Vitamin E**
- **Danazol 100–200 mg daily**
- **GnRH analogs (p. 441).**

Fibrocystic Changes

It is the most common benign lesion. It is generally observed between 20–50 years of age.

The etiology is not known. It may be due to altered estrogen progesterone ratio or relative decrease in progesterone or else, the breast tissues are more sensitive to prolactin. Stress factor may at times be related.

Histologically, a fibrocystic mass is characterized by adenosis, cyst formation, fibrosis, ductal epithelial proliferation and fluid retention. Fibrocystic breast disease may be of **proliferative** and **nonproliferative types**. The proliferative changes may be in the terminal ducts and the acini of the lobules. These conditions are referred to as ductal or lobular hyperplasia. Presence of nuclear atypia may lead to atypical ductal hyperplasia (ADH) or atypical lobular hyperplasia (ALH) respectively. Atypical hyperplasia have the relative risk of malignancy of about 4.5. Complex cyst need core needle biopsy to exclude malignancy.

The patients are usually premenopausal. The patient complains of breast pain present throughout the cycle but aggravated premenstrually. The pain is either dull continuous or intermittent and severe.

Examination reveals affection of both the breasts; one is more than the other. On palpation, coarsely nodular areas resembling ill-defined lumps either localized or diffused, are felt. These are prominent in premenstrual phase.

The patients become anxious of malignancy and the physicians too are confused to negate it. **Careful palpation, mammography, ultrasound and core needle biopsy is helpful to exclude malignancy.**

Treatment

- Assurance and re-examination at intervals.
- To wear a well-fitting brassiere day and night.
- Acetaminophen or NSAIDs may be helpful.
- To reduce the intake of methylxanthines (coffee, tea, chocolates, caffeinated soda) and tobacco.
- Vitamin E 400 mg daily may be helpful.
- In refractory cases, any of the following may be tried:
  - Cyclic combined estrogen-progestogen preparations.
  - Danazol 200 mg daily in divided doses.
  - Bromocriptine—2.5–5 mg daily at bed time.
  - GnRH agonist (p. 441)
  - Surgery—as indicated.

Fibroadenoma

This is the most common benign tumor of the breast occurring among the adolescents and younger (15–30 years) women. It is symptomless being accidentally discovered by self-palpation.

On palpation, an uniform, firm, mobile, painless, and well-defined mass is felt. Commonly they are bilateral and hormone dependent. Fibroadenoma with size >5 cm is known as giant fibroadenoma. Histologically, they have an epithelial and a fibrous component. A young patient however, may be reviewed **6 monthly** as the risk of malignancy is less than 0.2%.

Surgical excision and biopsy is indicated only when the mass enlarges and or report of core needle biopsy is inconclusive. Nonoperative management is done for small asymptomatic fibroadenoma in a young woman (<35 years). This is done only when clinical examination, imaging evaluation and biopsy are 100%, concordant. About 35% of fibroadenomas disappear and 10% become smaller. Symptomatic fibroadenomas are surgically excised. Ultrasound-guided cryoablation or HIFU is a treatment option.

EVALUATION OF A BREAST LUMP

Breast cancer is the most common (30%) of all cancers and is the second (next to lung cancer) common cause of cancer deaths in women. A breast cancer grows for 6–8 years before reaching a diameter of 1 cm. After that if doubles within a year. A breast mass detected by a woman who performs BSE at monthly examination is 2 cm.

It is difficult to distinguish a benign breast lump from a malignant one by clinical examination. However, findings on clinical examination should be supported with investigations like imaging studies and pathology report. Then it is helpful for management.

TABLE 34.10: Factors for breast carcinoma.

High risk factors for breast carcinoma
■ Early menarche
■ Obesity
■ Late menopause
■ Nulliparity
■ Late age of first birth (>35 years)
■ Never breastfed
■ Atypical lobular hyperplasia
■ Nipple discharge other than milk
■ High dose breast or chest irradiation
■ Combined oral contraceptives
■ Estrogen replacement therapy
■ Dense breasts
■ Low vitamin
■ Increased age
■ Breast carcinoma in first degree relative (mother, sister or daughter)
■ Carcinoma in the other breast
■ Previous cancer of endometrium, ovary, colon
■ Inherited mutations of *BRCA 1* and *BRCA 2* genes

Low risk factors for breast carcinoma
■ Born outside western countries
■ Oophorectomy
■ Lactation
■ Early age <20 years first birth
■ Vitamin D
■ Aspirin
■ Low fat diet

Genetic predisposition—is high when there is mutation of the *BRCA 1* (on chromosome 17 q) and/or *BRCA 2* (on chromosome 13 q) genes. *BRCA 1* and *BRCA 2* are the tumor suppressor genes. Hereditary breast cancer is seen in younger women and is often bilateral. Around 5% of breast cancers are familial.

TABLE 34.11: Clinical features of early malignancy.

- Nontender lump in the breast (mostly located in the upper and outer quadrant)
- Nonmilky nipple discharge especially bloody
- Retraction of the nipple (previously everted)
- Indrawing of the overlying skin
- Localized edema of the skin
- Persistent erosion or crusting of the nipple (refractory to medication)

Screening and Diagnostic Methods for Breast Carcinoma

Breast carcinomas are generally without any symptoms to start with. Screening can detect breast cancer at an earlier stage (Tables 34.10 and 34.11). Ideally, screening should be performed for all women from 40 years of age. Earlier detection improves the survival rate. Five-year survival is about 85% when axillary lymph nodes are not involved.

Different screening modalities are:

- **Breast self-examination (BSE):** The American College of Obstetricians and Gynecologists (ACOG) and American Cancer Society (ACS) recommends breast self-awareness which for some patients include BSE.
- **Clinical breast examination (CBE) by a physician**
  - Inspection
  - Palpation
  - ACOG recommends CBE for every 3 years from age 20–30 and annually thereafter (Table 34.12).
- **Breast imaging**
  - Screening mammography
  - Diagnostic mammography
  - Ultrasonography
  - Magnetic resonance imaging (MRI)
  - Digital mammography, positron emission tomography

TABLE 34.12: Breast cancer screening guidelines (ACOG–2000).

Age 20–39	*Age 40–49*	*Age ≥50*
BSE monthly	BSE monthly	BSE monthly
CBE at every 3 years	CBE annually	CBE annually
	MGY—annually	MGY annually

(BSE: breast self-examination; CBE: clinical breast examination; MGY: mammography)

- **Breast biopsy**
  - Fine needle aspiration biopsy
  - Stereotactic and ultrasound guided core biopsy
  - Open biopsy:
    - Excisional biopsy
    - Incisional biopsy.

Breast Self-examination

Breast self-examination should be made into a habit, **certainly by the age of 20**. The examination should be made on a monthly basis following the menses as the breasts become less tender and less engorged.

The procedures (as described above) are demon-strated to the patient. Circular method of palpation is easy to do. Inspection should be done standing in front of a mirror in a well lit-room. The patient should palpate her breasts with the opposite hand both in sitting position and lying supine with a pillow beneath her back. Axillary and supraclavicular areas are to be palpated. The nipples should be compressed for any discharge. She is instructed to contact physician whenever there is any abnormal finding.

Clinical Breast Examinations

Inspection (Figs. 9.1A to C, Ch. 9)

Inspection is performed while the patient is sitting with arms relaxed by her sides. Both the breasts are observed for contour, symmetry, nipple positions, and any skin changes. Patient is asked to press her hands on her hips so as to contract the pectoralis major muscles. Skin dimpling and nipple retraction if any, may be obvious with this method.

Palpation (Figs. 9.1D to F, p. 82)

Entire breast is palpated methodically by quadrant with the pads of the fingers (most sensitive) both in upright and in supine positions (p. 82).

Generally, a malignant mass is felt firm, nontender, fixed with ill-defined borders. Entire axilla and the supraclavicular areas are palpated for any lymph nodes. Nipple is compressed for any discharge. CBE is best done during the first half of the menstrual cycle.

Breast Imaging

- **Mammography** (MGY) is the most effective screening method for detection of nonpalpable and minimally invasive breast cancer. It uses X-ray photons. However, it has a false negative rate of 10–15%. It should be combined with CBE and BSE. Two views, one mediolateral oblique (MLO) side view and the other craniocaudal view (CC) are to be taken for each breast.

  Characteristic features suggestive of malignancy are—presence of a mass, asymmetric soft tissue densities and architectural distortion. Spiculated microcalcifications especially clustering or branching pattern are more suspicious but this is not a specific sign of malignancy. Radiation risks of mammography are negligible.
- Mammographic findings are summarized following the American College of Radiology Breast Imaging Reporting and Data System (BI-RADS). Category 4 and 5 are suspicion and warrant biopsy and category 6 is malignant.
- **Digital mammography (DM)** is more accurate in younger women (<50 years). DM can combine several images into **3D image (tomosynthesis)** to reduce the false negative rate.

  In the presence of any suspicious mass, one should always perform biopsy, irrespective of the mammographic findings.
- **Ultrasonography** is useful to differentiate a cystic lesion from a solid one. Solid masses with ill-defined borders and complex cystic lesions are considered suspicious. Ultrasound cannot detect microcalcifications. It also helps to take biopsy from a deep seated nonpalpable lesion.
- **MRI:** Interventional MRI can be used for MRI-guided surgery. However, MRI has low specificity (37–97%) besides that it is time consuming and expensive. Limitations of MRI are: It cannot detect microcalcifications and there is loss of image quality on respiratory movements. Therefore, MRI should be used combined with mammography USG and CBE to improve the detection rate (Fig. 34.4).
- **PET** (p. 101) has improved tumor detection rate. PET can differentiate malignant tissues from benign tissues and metastatic diseases. But it has reduced sensitivity for detection of masses <1 cm.

Breast Biopsy

- **Triple test:** It includes—CBE, imaging and needle biopsy, when all components are benign the risk of breast cancer is low (<1%) whereas if all are suggestive of cancer, the risk is high (99%). FNAC has a false negative rate of 20% and overall specificity is 98%.

  However, the lump should be excised regardless of the results of other two if any of the three assessments suggests malignancy.

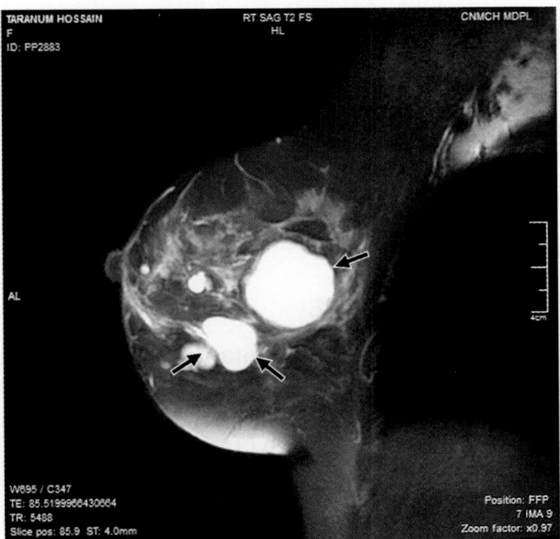

Fig. 34.4: Magnetic resonance imaging of the breast of a 36-year-old woman showing solid growths (within the breast tissues) (*see* arrows). MRI can detect 77% of breast cancers while used as a screening method as compared to mammography (40%).

- **Breast biopsy** is essential for the confirmation of diagnosis. Biopsy is generally done as an outpatient procedure.
- **Fine-needle aspiration cytology (FNAC)** is done for **cytologic evaluation** inserting a narrow gauge (22G) needle into a breast lesion. This is a simple and cheap procedure with no morbidity. Unfortunately false-negative diagnosis may be high (up to 20%) and it cannot differentiate a noninvasive carcinoma from an invasive one.
- **Core needle biopsy (CNB)** is done for histologic diagnosis. It is highly accurate (98%) and specific (100%) in confirming malignancy. CNB is performed under tactile, stereotactic or ultrasound guidance using local anesthesia or MRI. CNB helps definitive histologic diagnosis, tumor grade, lymphatic invasion and hormone receptor status. It is done using a larger needle (9 to 14 gauze) that FNA.
- **Open biopsy** is performed either as a primary procedure or when the results of FNAC/CNB are inconclusive. With excisional biopsy, the lesion is completely removed under local anesthesia. Incisional biopsy is done where only a portion of the mass is excised for confirmation of diagnosis.
- **Breast tissue sampling: It includes:** (a) Bloody nipple discharge; (b) Persistent breast mass; (c) Suspicious mammography; (d) Nipple retraction or elevation.

  Least invasive technique that can provide a diagnostic specimen should be used.

Staging of Breast Cancer

Breast cancer is staged clinically according to tumor size, regional lymph node involvement and distant metastasis **(TNM classification)**. American Joint Committee on Cancer Staging (2014) reclassified the nodal status by number of involved lymph nodes, use of sentinel lymph node biopsy. Complete staging includes a thorough history, physical examination, bilateral mammography, pretreatment chest radiography, routine blood values, pathology slides with estrogen receptor, progesterone receptor and HER 2 status along with breast MRI.

Staging helps to compare the results of trials through-out the world. This is also helpful to develop uniform treatment regimens.

For staging of breast cancer readers should consult any textbook of surgery.

NIPPLE DISCHARGE

A nipple discharge when spontaneous, persistent, and unrelated to lactation is considered abnormal. Any significant nipple discharge must be thoroughly evaluated with the following information (Table 34.13):

- Nature of discharge (milky, serous or bloody)
- Unilateral or bilateral
- From a single duct or multiple ducts
- Association of any mass in the breast
- History of any drug intake (phenothiazines or oral contraceptives)
- Premenopausal or postmenopausal.

TABLE 34.13: Common causes of nipple discharge.

Color	Probable diagnosis
Milky	▪ Physiologic (lactation) ▪ Pregnancy ▪ Oral contraceptives ▪ Inappropriate (galactorrhea p. 486)
Bloody sanguineous	▪ Intraductal papilloma ▪ Intraductal cancer ▪ Malignancy ▪ Duct ectasia ▪ Fibrocystic disease
Clear watery	Ductal cancer
Green, yellow	Ductal ectasia
Purulent	Infective
Serous or sticky	Fibrocystic disease

Nipple discharge may be due to benign conditions or due to breast cancer (20%).

Diagnosis

Careful history-taking, clinical examination and, mammography, sonography or MRI should be done. **Occult blood testing** and microscopic examination of the discharge should be done. **A glass slide smear** prepared with the discharge and fixed immediately is used for cytologic assessment. However, acellular smear cannot exclude malignancy. **Ductography or Ductoscopy** to visualize the individual discharging duct: for cytology and biopsy (microendoscopic) can be taken under local anesthesia.

Laboratory tests with prolactin; TSH and β hCG are done to exclude hyperprolactinemia, hypothyroidism and pregnancy-related discharge.

Pathologic nipple discharge once definitely diagnosed is treated with subareolar duct excision (microductectomy).

Surgical excision of the duct and its associated lobular unit may need to be done. It is both diagnostic and therapeutic.

Breast carcinoma is within the domain of general surgeon. As such, the interested readers are requested to consult 'Textbook of Surgery' for therapeutic protocol of breast carcinoma.

EMOTIONAL, PSYCHOSEXUAL ISSUES AND FEMALE SEXUALITY

SEXUAL FUNCTION DISORDERS

- Hypoactive sexual desire disorder
- Sexual aversion disorder
- Female sexual arousal disorder
- Female orgasmic disorder
- Sexual pain disorder
- Dyspareunia
- Vaginismus.

All the above disorders are associated with marked distress or interpersonal difficulty.

Hypoactive Sexual Disorder

It (loss of libido) may be due to depression or it may develop from a traumatic event (e.g. rape, sexual abuse or bereavement) in the past. Several drugs can cause disorders of desire (antipsychotics, lithium, antihypertensives, beta blockers, oral contraceptives, phenytoin sodium, etc.).

Treatment

Psychosexual therapy is essential to deal with the underlying psychologic problems. Psychiatric consultation is needed when there is depressive symptoms. Sometimes replacement with a different contraceptive pill may improve the problem. Postmenopausal loss of libido may be improved by using androgen containing hormone replacement therapy (HRT).

Vaginismus

Definition

Vaginismus is defined as the psychogenically mediated involuntary spasm of the vaginal muscles including the levator ani muscles and/or the thigh adductor muscles. This results in inability of penetrative sexual intercourse.

Etiology

- **Primary**
- **Secondary**

- **Primary:** Nothing has entered into the woman's vagina ever. However, the vagina is normal anatomically and physiologically. The cause is mostly psychosexual in origin. There is often presence of a subconscious fear of sexual intercourse (sexual phobias).
- **Secondary:** Vaginismus usually appear after childbirth or any other event in life. There is usually some local painful lesions. Such lesions include vulvitis, lacerations of the hymen, **tender scar on the perineum or narrow** vaginal introitus. The entity is usually transient and is relieved, when the cause is removed.

Clinical Presentation

The woman with vaginismus avoids vaginal examination and smear. She might present with painful sexual intercourse or with infertility.

Diagnosis

While diagnosis of the secondary one is not so difficult but to find out the cause of the primary one, examination under anesthesia may be required. If the two fingers can be easily introduced through the vaginal introitus, the caliber of the vagina is proved normal.

Treatment

- **Primary**
- **Secondary**

Primary: The following guidelines are prescribed:

- **Psychodynamic therapy:** Main causes of fear are removed. To educate and to gain confidence of the husband and wife. This may take time.
- **Behavioral therapy:** Dilatation of the vaginal introitus digitally followed by introduction of gradually increasing size of the dilators is to be done. Plastic vaginal trainers (pseudopenises) with graduated sizes can help her to remove her fear. This will gain her confidence that her vagina is anatomically of normal caliber.
- **Vaginal dilators:** Daily introduction of the dilators (pseudopenises) for 1–2 weeks and to keep it inside for 10–15 minutes is enough before she is allowed to attempt coital act.

Surgery: A classic case of vaginismus needs no surgery. However, surgery may be required, if the hymen is found tight—hymenectomy or Fenton's operation (operation to enlarge the introitus), if the introitus is narrow (Ch. 35, p. 497).

Secondary: The local lesion is to be treated medically or surgically.

Dyspareunia

Definition

Dyspareunia means that the coital act is difficult and or painful. Apareunia is inability to practice coitus. The two are most often interchangeable. Dyspareunia is the most common sexual dysfunction.

Etiology

- **Male**
- **Female**

Male causes

The following male factors are responsible:

- Impotence
- Premature ejaculation
- Congenital anatomic defect of the penis
- Lack of technique of coital act.

Female causes

Depending upon the site of pain, the dyspareunia may be either:

- Superficial or entrance
- Vaginal
- Deep.

Superficial: Any lesion of the lower part of the labia minora or around the fourchette may be responsible.

Causes of Superficial Dyspareunia

- Narrow introitus
- Tough hymen
- Bartholin's gland cysts
- Tender perineal scar
- Vulvar infection
- Urethral pathology
- Vulvar vestibulitis syndrome (p. 219)

Vaginal: Burning pain along the barrel of vagina either during or following intercourse is the presenting complaint. Common causes are:

- Vaginitis
- Vaginal septum
- Tender scar—following gynecologic operation or delivery
- Secondary vaginal atresia
- Tumor
- Vaginal atrophy (menopause).

Deep: The patient experiences pain while the penis penetrates deep into the vagina. As the vagina is insensitive

to pain, deep dyspareunia usually results from pathology of paravaginal tissues or other pelvic organs. Such lesions are:
- Endometriosis, especially on rectovaginal septum
- Chronic cervicitis
- Interstitial cystitis
- Chronic PID
- Retroverted uterus—mostly acquired and fixed
- Prolapsed ovary in the pouch of Douglas.

Treatment

Treatment depends upon the cause. Too often, sex education of both the partners relieves the symptom.

The infective lesions of the vulva and or vagina are to be treated. Tender scar on the perineum or the vagina is to be excised. The treatment of vaginismus has been mentioned earlier.

INTIMATE PARTNER VIOLENCE

Intimate partner violence (IPV) refers to injury inflicted by one intimate partner to the other. The main objective of their behavior is to cause pain or to control the other partner's behavior. IPV is one of the several (domestic violence, gender based violence or violence against women) abuses directed against women and girls.

Compared to older women younger women are at greater risk for IPV.

Violence against women may be battering, sexual assault, incest, physical trauma or elder abuse.

IPV during pregnancy: Screening for IPV is a component of antenatal care as many pregnant women (7–20%) may be the victims of IPV.

Domestic abuse may include physical, emotional, financial, and sexual abuse. Neglect is the prevalent form, perpetrated by the family members.

Patient's disclosure of IPV, need to be validated by the physician.

Patients should be consulted. Clinician should be careful with women's safety and health. The clinician should know the respective state law. Patients should be informed accordingly for the support and also for the community resources. Documentation of physical findings of violence is essential. Such records are important when clinical charges are pursued.

ABDOMINOPELVIC LUMP

Pelvic and lower abdominal masses need differentiation as regard their origin (ovary, cervix, uterus) or from other organs (bowel, retroperitoneal tissues). **This may occur at any age (Table 34.14) and are of different consistency (solid, cystic)**. However, some tumors are common in a particular age group. These masses need to be diagnosed by clinical evaluation. Different investigations should be done as too often they have confusing presentation.

TABLE 34.14: Common causes of lower abdominal lump.

Age group	Causes
Toddlers (<5 years)	▪ Ovarian tumor ▪ Mucocolpos ▪ Full bladder
5 years of age to puberty	▪ Ovarian tumor ▪ Full bladder ▪ Hematocolpos
Childbearing period	▪ Pregnancy ▪ Full bladder ▪ Ovarian tumor ▪ Fibroid ▪ Adenomyosis ▪ Chocolate cyst ▪ TO mass ▪ Pelvic hematocele ▪ Pelvic abscess ▪ Encysted peritonitis ▪ Pseudocyesis
Postmenopausal	▪ Ovarian tumor ▪ Pyometra ▪ Sarcoma uterus

Full Bladder

It is an axiom that prior to gynecologic examination, bladder must be kept empty. Not only full bladder may be confused with some abdominopelvic pathology but empty bladder ensures better evaluation of pelvic findings on bimanual examination.

Features of a full bladder
- Strictly suprapubic, may even reach up to the umbilicus
- Cystic or tense cystic
- Margins—ill-defined
- Tendency of urge for micturition on pressure
- Disappears after catheterization.

Pregnancy

Pregnancy with an uterine size of 16–18 weeks is most confusing. The confusion is accentuated with a history of oligomenorrhea, conception occurring during lactational amenorrhea or illegal pregnancy.

In fact, amenorrhea during childbearing period with a lump in the lower abdomen should be provisionally diagnosed as pregnancy unless proved otherwise.

Differentiating features are discussed in page 246 (Ovarian Tumor, Fibroid, Adenomyosis).

Encysted Peritonitis (p. 246 for details)

- History of Koch's infection
- Amenorrhea of longer duration may be present
- Swelling—ill-defined margins
- Feel—cystic/doughy
- Internal examination reveals: Uterus is separated from the cystic mass
- X-ray chest—a lesion may be found
- Mantoux test—may be positive
- Sonography Blood tests: PCR, NAAT.

Pseudocyesis

- Usually present in women having problem of infertility or approaching menopause with an intense desire to have a baby.

- History of amenorrhea.
- Abdominal examination reveals absence of positive signs of pregnancy.
- Examination under anesthesia (EUA)—uterus of normal size.
- Sonography—empty uterus, absence of fetal echo.

ADNEXAL MASS

An adnexal mass refers to any mass occupying the region of the uterine appendages (adnexa). Major concern is the ovarian neoplasm (malignancy).

Common Adnexal Masses

- **Ovarian**
  - Ovarian neoplasm
  - Ovarian cyst
  - Endometriomas
  - Tubo-ovarian mass
- **Tubal pathology**
  - Ectopic pregnancy
  - Hydrosalpinx
  - Tubal neoplasms
- **Uterine**
  - Myoma (broad ligament)
- **Gastrointestinal**
  - Diverticulitis
  - Appendicular mass (right)
- **Genitourinary**
  - Pelvic kidney

Evaluation of an Adnexal Mass

- **Clinical (bimanual pelvic) examination** for its size, shape, consistency, mobility, and tenderness.
- **Transvaginal ultrasonography**—whether the cyst is simple or complex, internal echoes, nodularity. **Doppler ultrasound** to study blood flow and to measure R1 and P1.
- **Computed tomography (CT):** It can differentiate loop of bowel, dermoid cyst, myomas.
- **Magnetic resonance imaging (MRI)** is also helpful and it has no risk of ionizing radiation.
- **Positron emission tomography (PET)** is more sensitive in detecting metastatic disease.
- **Tumor markers:** Numerous tumor markers have been studied for the detection and follow-up of ovarian malignancy namely CA-125, CA-15-3, TAG-72, CA-19-9 (p. 438).

Management of an Adnexal Mass

Whenever any adnexal mass is diagnosed the management will depend mainly on—(a) Nature of the mass; (b) Age of the woman.

Ovarian cysts in postmenopausal women—should be assessed for the risk of malignancy clinically and also using CA-125 and transvaginal sonography (TVS).

Important points on TVS for scoring are: Multilocular cyst, presence of a solid areas, metastases, ascites, and bilateral lesions.

According to RMI **(Risk of Malignancy Index)** the women are triaged into—**Low risk**: RMI <25, **Moderate risk**: RMI 25-250 and **High risk**: RMI >250 (p. 317).

Actual Management

Conservative management is ideal for a simple, unilateral unilocular ovarian cyst, <8 cm with low RMI (<25) and normal serum CA-125. Such women are followed up with TVS at an interval of 4 months. 50% of such cysts resolve spontaneously.

Surgical management: Besides those as described above, all need some form of surgical treatment (cyst aspiration, laparoscopy, and laparotomy).

Cyst aspiration for cytologic examination to differentiate benign from malignant tumors is done. It has the risks of intraperitoneal spread of malignant cells. In a postmenopausal women it is not recommended.

Laparoscopic approach should only be made with moderate risk women (RMI: 25-250). **Cystectomy** for young women and oophorectomy for postmenopausal women is recommended. Such women should be counseled preoperatively that a full staging laparotomy may be needed if evidence of malignancy is seen.

Laparotomy: All ovarian cysts that are suspicious of malignancy especially in a postmenopausal women (RMI >250), or with positive findings of laparoscopy, need a full staging laparotomy in a specialized center. **Procedure includes**: Laparotomy (midline incision) → peritoneal washings (for cytology) → staging → biopsies → total abdominal hysterectomy (TAH) + bilateral salpingo-oophorectomy (BSO) + total omentectomy (± selective pelvic and paraortic lymphadenectomy) (RCOG - 2006).

KEY POINTS

- **Leukorrhea** is defined strictly as an excessive normal vaginal discharge which stains the undergarment. It is nonpurulent, nonoffensive and never causes pruritus.
  The excess normal secretion occurs during puberty, menstrual cycle (around ovulation and premenstrual), pregnancy and sexual excitement. Abnormal vaginal discharge is mainly infective in origin (Table 34.2).
  Improvement of general health, sympathetic attitude towards ailments, local hygiene and appropriate therapy for the local ailments are enough to cure the state.
- **Pruritus** means sense of itching. It does not produce pain; nor there is any local tenderness.
  Local skin lesions, vaginal discharge, allergy, intestinal worms or diabetes are some of the important causes. Appropriate therapy is to be instituted depending upon the factors involved. Vulvectomy is not the treatment to cure pruritus.
- **The significance of postmenopausal bleeding** should not be underestimated. About one-third of the cases are due to pelvic malignancy, the most common being uterine (Table 34.9).

Contd...

Contd...

Apart from routine use of gynecological examination, the special investigations include cytology, transvaginal sonography, fractional curettage, hysteroscopic evaluation and/or laparoscopy. Even if no cause is detected, recurrence or persistent uterine bleeding dictates hysterectomy with BSO.

- **Pain** arising from the pelvic organs is often localized not to the organ but referred to the skin area supplied by the same spinal nerve (Table 34.3).
  The basic mechanism of **acute pain** is due to irritation of the peritoneum by either blood or infection.
  Apart from history and clinical examination, the investigations to pinpoint the diagnosis of acute pelvic pain include—examination of blood for hematocrit, midstream urine examination for UTI and urine for immunological test for pregnancy (Table 34.4). The diagnosis is established in most cases.
  Management in cases of definite diagnosis includes either immediate laparotomy or institution of medical therapy. In doubtful cases, diagnostic laparoscopy and observation are of help (Table 34.6).
  Chronic pelvic pain (CPP) is defined as six months or more of constant or intermittent pain (nonmenstrual pain) localized in the pelvis or lower back severe enough to cause functional disability or requiring medical or surgical treatment. CPP is often without any visible pathology (Table 34.7). Incidental detection of pathology may not be the cause of pain. Laparoscopy is done both for diagnostic and therapeutic purposes as "one-stop" procedure. In the absence of definite pathology, medical management of pain should be tried first.
  Medical treatment includes—analgesics, prostaglandin synthetase inhibitors, OC pills, progestogens, danazol or even GnRH analogs. Minimal surgery includes laser therapy in pelvic endometriosis and adhesiolysis endoscopically. Hysterectomy should be contemplated judiciously.
- **Trapped or residual ovarian syndrome** is manifested with chronic pelvic pain. The pain arises from the ovaries (preserved during hysterectomy) due to tension within the growing follicle or due to periovarian adhesions. The chronic pelvic pain in ovarian remnant syndrome is due to the remnant of ovarian cortical tissue, left behind unintendedly following a difficult oophorectomy.
- **The backache** pointed by fingertip is not of gynecologic origin. The pain in prolapse subsides when the patient is at rest and aggravates on standing. Mobile retroverted uterus does not produce backache.
- **Breast carcinoma** is one of the leading cause of death among female malignancies.
  The screening for breast carcinoma includes (p. 474)—breast self-examination, clinical breast examination, imaging studies, and breast biopsy. Baseline mammogram is to be done at 40 years. Mammography along with physical examination is to be done annually from the age of 40 and earlier in high risk group.
  Irrespective of mammographic findings, presence of any suspicious mass suggests biopsy.
- **FNAC** is a rapid diagnostic method with high degree of accuracy. Ultrasound-guided procedure allows the needle tip to reach the exact site.
- **High risk factors** for breast carcinoma are many (Table 34.10). Mutations in *BRCA-1* and *BRCA-2* genes (tumor suppressor genes) account for familial breast cancer (5%), which has an early age onset.
- **Causes of bloody nipple discharge** are (Table 34.13) malignancy, intraductal papilloma, fibrocystic disease and duct ectasia. Purulent discharge is due to infection and serous or sticky discharge is due to fibrocystic disease.
- **Female sexual dysfunction** includes different disorders. Dyspareunia means that the coital act is difficult and or painful. Apareunia is inability to practice coitus. Causes of deep dyspareunia are pelvic endometriosis, chronic cervicitis, chronic PID, fixed retroverted uterus or prolapsed ovary in the pouch of Douglas.
- **Prior to gynecological examination**, bladder must be kept empty. Full bladder should be excluded first in the differential diagnosis of abdominopelvic lump; similarly, pregnancy has to be excluded in childbearing period irrespective of the status of the women (Table 34.14)—married, unmarried, widow, divorced or separated.
- **Causes of abdominopelvic lump** varies with age. Tissue of origin may be ovary, cervix, uterus, bowel or the retroperitoneum.
- **Common causes** varies with age (Table 34.14). **Ovarian tumor** should be excluded in younger girls. **Pregnancy** is the most common cause for a woman in reproductive age and for a postmenopausal woman **genital malignancy** should be excluded.
- **Adnexal mass** may be due to the pathology of (a) **Ovary** (neoplasm, cyst, endometrioma, or tubo-ovarian mass); (b) **Uterine** (myoma); (c) **Tubal** (hydrosalpinx, ectopic pregnancy); (d) **Gastrointestinal** (appendicular mass) or genitourinary, (pelvic kidney) (p. 478).
- **Evaluation and management** need to consider the nature of the mass and age of the woman (p. 479).
- **An adnexal mass** needs to be critically evaluated to formulate the management. Clinical examination, imaging studies, tumor markers and the genetic markers (p. 479) are helpful to distinguish a **benign from a malignant tumor**. An adnexal mass may be followed up or may need medical or surgical intervention depending upon its nature (benign or malignant), size and the patient's age.

HIRSUTISM

NOMENCLATURE

Hirsutism: It is the excessive growth of androgen dependent sexual hair (terminal hair) in facial and central part of the body (male pattern) that worries a female (Figs. 34.5 and 34.6).

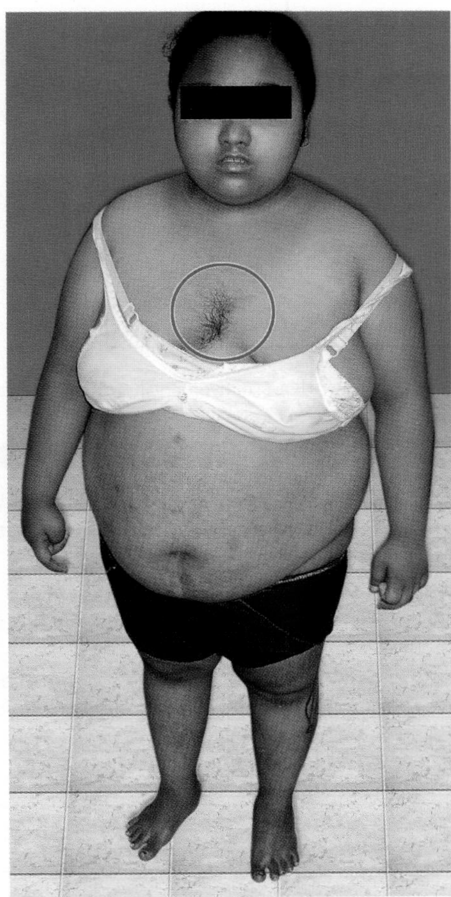

Fig. 34.5: Hirsutism: 15 years, young obese (BMI: 34) girl with excessive growth of hair in a male distribution (face, chest, and intermammary region, arms and legs).

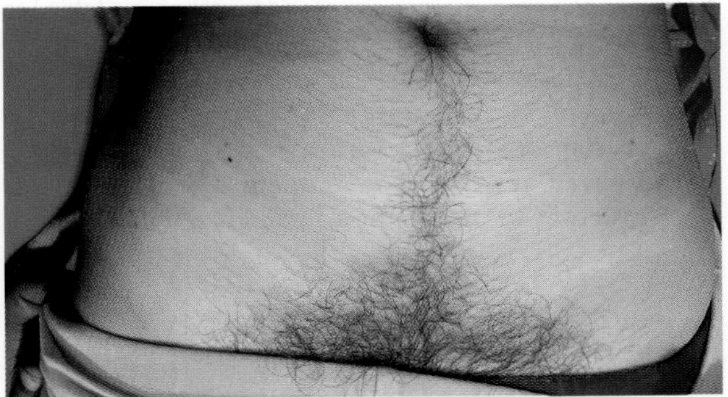

Fig. 34.6: Hirsutism: 24-year-old girl with secondary amenorrhea and male pattern of escutcheon.

Hypertrichosis: It connotes excessive growth of nonsexual (fetal lanugo type) hair in normal location.

Hyperandrogenism: It is a state of increased serum androgen level with or without any biological effect of hyperandrogenemia.

Virilism: It is defined as the presence of any one or more of the following features—deepening of the voice, temporal balding, amenorrhea, increased muscle mass, enlargement of clitoris (clitoromegaly) and breast atrophy. It is a more severe form of androgen excess. Virilism may be due to adrenal hyperplasia or tumors of adrenal or ovary.

In female major androgens are dehydroepiandrosterone sulfate (DHEA-S), dehydroepiandrosterone (DHEA), androstenedione, testosterone (T) and dihydrotestosterone (DHT). All androgenic activities are due to T and DHT.

The severity of hirsutism is roughly quantified by a modified scoring system of Ferriman and Gallwey (Table 34.16).

A score >8 is in the category of hirsutism. However, for an Asian woman the abnormal score is taken as >3.

Eleven sites in the body are included. Hair gradings are done from 1 to 4 at each site. Depending upon the extent of hair growth. The **body sites are:** (I) Upper lip, (II) Chin, (III) Chest, (IV) Upper back, (V) Lower Back, (VI) Upper abdomen, (VII) Lower abdomen, (VIII) Arm, (IX) Forearm, (X) Thigh, (XI) Leg. However, it is difficult to use clinically.

ANDROGEN SOURCES IN FEMALE

Testosterone is the second most potent androgen in circulation, the first one being DHT. The daily production rate of testosterone in normal female is 0.2–0.3 mg.

Approximately, 50% of testosterone arises from peripheral conversion of prohormones, predominantly androstenedione. The principal sites of peripheral conversion are skin, muscle, fat, liver, and lungs. The adrenal glands (zona reticularis and zona fasciculata) and ovaries (theca, stroma, and granulosa) contribute approximately equal amounts (25%) to the circulatory levels of testosterone.

Dehydroepiandrosterone sulfate (DHEA-S) arises exclusively from the adrenal glands while about 50% of DHEA is secreted from the adrenals.

Androstenedione arises from the adrenals and ovaries in equal amount.

The sources of androgens in normal female are schematically depicted in Flowchart 34.2.

Most of testosterone (80%) in the circulation is bound to sex hormone-binding globulin (SHBG) and is biologically inactive. About 19% is bound loosely with albumin and **only 1% of the testosterone remains free which is biologically active.** Normally total circulating testosterone level is 20–80 ng/dL.

To exert a biological effect, testosterone (T) is metabolically converted in target tissues to dihy-drotestosterone (DHT) by the enzyme 5α-reductase. DHT is the most potent androgen to stimulate the hair follicles and sebaceous glands (pilosebaceous unit). 3α-androstanediol glucuronide

Flowchart 34.2: Principal sources of androgen in a normal female.

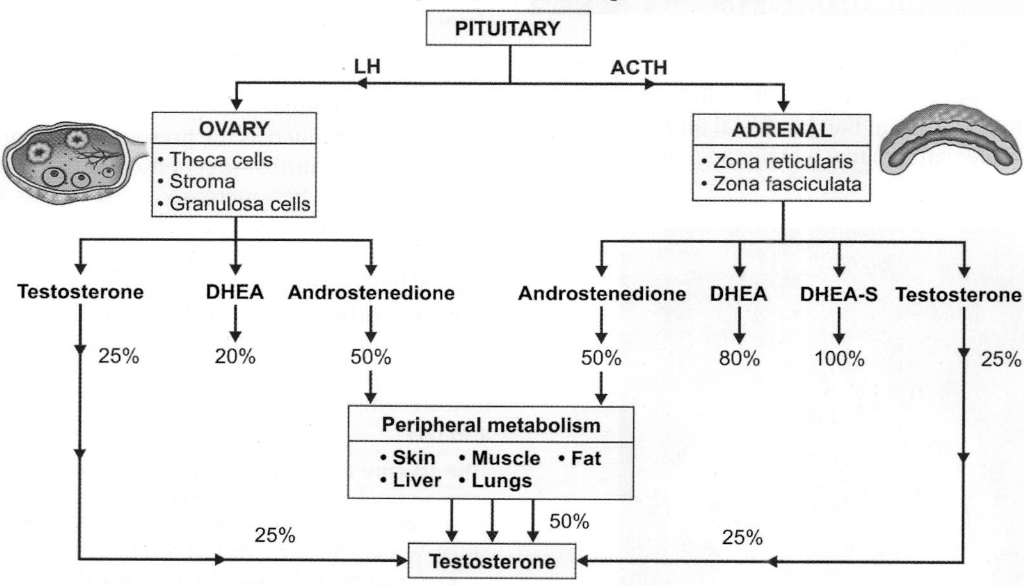

(LH: luteinizing hormone; ACTH: adrenocorticotropic hormone; DHEA: dehydroepiandrosterone; DHEA-S: dehydroepiandrosterone sulfate)

(3α-AG) is an important tissue metabolite of DHT. *3α-AG is thought to reflect the activity of the enzyme 5α-reductase at tissue level.*

T → (5α-reductase) → DHT → 3α-androstanediol (3α-A) → 3α-androstanediol glucuronide (3α-AG).

Therefore, the biochemical marker for each androgen compartment is different. ***For the ovary it is testosterone; for the adrenal gland it is DHEA–S and for the periphery it is 3α-AG.***

ANDROGENS AND PILOSEBACEOUS UNIT

The pilosebaceous unit (PSU) consists of sebaceous glands and hair follicles. Both are sensitive to androgens. The sebaceous glands are more sensitive to androgens than the hair follicles. Hyperstimulation of the sebaceous glands leads first to oily skin and subsequent infection results in acne.

The skin and hair follicle play an active role in serving as target organs for the androgens and also in producing androgens from circulatory prohormones.

MECHANISM OF EXCESSIVE HAIR GROWTH

The stimulus for the excessive hair growth is testosterone. Testosterone binds to the androgen receptors in the hair follicle. This is followed by activation of the enzyme 5α-reductase. This will convert testosterone to most potent androgen—dihydrotestosterone (DHT) and androstenediol which stimulate proliferation and growth of terminal hair (anagen phase). **Androgens convert vellus hair to terminal hair and hirsutism.** Once the black terminal hair is produced, the changes persist even in the absence of a continuing androgen excess. Increased hair follicle stimulation and increased 5α-reductase activity enable prohormones DHEA and androstenedione to be metabolized directly to DHT. **This latter phenomenon explains continued growth even if the initiating testosterone source has been removed (Table 34.15).**

TABLE 34.15: Adult body hair.

Hair type	*Phases of hair growth*
▪ **Vellus hair:** Fine unpigmented hair present over most body parts	▪ **Telogen:** Resting phase
▪ **Terminal hair:** Thick, coarse, pigmented hair present in certain parts of the body	▪ **Anagen:** Active phase of hair growth
▪ **Sexual hair:** Terminal hair sensitive to androgen, present in the midline of the body, upper lip, chin, chest, side burns, pubic area, the arms and thighs	▪ **Catagen:** Phase of rapid involution

PATHOPHYSIOLOGY OF HIRSUTISM

It involves combination of the following:

- **Increased concentration** of serum androgens, especially of testosterone.
- **Decreased level of SHBG** resulting in increased free testosterone (testosterone itself reduces SHBG level).
- **Increased responsiveness** of the target organ (skin) to the normal circulating androgens. This may be related to ethnic background. Oriental women have less number of hair follicles per unit area of skin compared to a Caucasian woman.
- **Increased activity** of 5α-reductase which converts testosterone to DHT in the skin and hair follicles.

T → Plasma T ↑ → SHBG ↓ → Free T ↑
↓
↑↑ 5α-reductase activity in hair follicle
↓
DHT
↓
Hirsutism

TABLE 34.16: Ferriman-Gallwey scoring system. Definition of hair grading at 11 sites.

Site	Grade	Definition
Upper lip	1	Few hairs at outer margin
	2	Small mustache at outer margin
	3	Mustache extending halfway from outer margin
	4	Mustache extending to midline
Chin	1	Few scattered hairs
	2	Scattered hairs with small concentrations
	3, 4	Complete cover, light and heavy
Chest	1	Circumareolar hairs
	2	With midline hair in addition
	3	Fusion of these areas, with 75% cover
	4	Complete cover
Upper back	1	Few scattered hairs
	2	Rather more, still scattered
	3, 4	Complete cover, light and heavy
Lower back	1	Sacral tuft of hair
	2	With some lateral extension
	3	75% cover
	4	Complete cover
Upper abdomen	1	Few midline hairs
	2	Rather more, still midline
	3, 4	Half- and full cover
Lower abdomen	1	Few midline hairs
	2	Midline streak of hair
	3	Midline band of hair
	4	Inverted V-shaped growth
Arm	1	Sparse growth affecting not more than 25% of limb surface
	2	More than this; cover still incomplete
	3, 4	Complete cover, light and heavy
Forearm	1–4	Complete cover of dorsal surface; two grades of light and two of heavy growth
Thigh	1–4	As for arm
Leg	1–4	As for arm

(*Source*: Ferriman D, Gallwey JD. Clinical assessment of body hair growth in women. J Clin Endocrinol Metab. 1961;21:1440-47)

Thus, the hair follicle becomes a secondary site of androgen metabolism at the expense of hair follicle stimulation and hirsutism.

Ferriman-Gallwey (1981) scoring system was developed to quantify the degree of hirsutism (Table 34.16). Abnormal hair distribution is assessed in eleven body areas and is scored from 1 to 4. Score of 8 or more has been accepted as hirsutism. As the procedure is cumbersome, it is not commonly clinically used. Usually, it is expressed as mild, moderate or severe depending upon location and diversity of hair growth.

CAUSES OF HIRSUTISM (TABLE 34.17)

Hirsutism may be associated with excess androgen production either from the ovaries or adrenals or excess stimulation of the endorgans, i.e. hair follicles. It represents one of the early manifestations in the spectrum of virilism. Whereas, virilism is almost always associated with hirsutism (except at birth) but hirsutism may not be associated with virilism. There may be racial or familial link. Increased hair growth is observed during puberty, pregnancy, and following menopause (Fig. 34.7).

TABLE 34.17: Causes of hyperandrogenism.

- **Ovarian**
  - Polycystic ovarian syndrome (PCOS) (p. 385)
  - Sertoli-Leydig cell tumor (p. 324)
  - Hilus cell tumor
  - Lipoid cell tumor
  - Stromal, hyperthecosis, luteoma of pregnancy
- **Adrenal**
  - Adrenal hyperplasia (congenital or late onset) (p. 392)
  - Cushing's syndrome (p. 392)
  - Adrenal tumor
- **Obesity (android)**
  - Insulin resistance and androgen excess (p. 386)
  - HAIR-AN syndrome (p. 385)
- **Exogenous (drug therapy):** Androgens, anabolics, oral contraceptives, synthetic progestogens, danazol, phenytoin, diazoxide, cortisone, etc.
- **Postmenopause**
- **Pituitary tumor**—secreting
  - Excess ACTH (Cushing's diseases)
  - Excess growth hormone (acromegaly)
- **Idiopathic:** Increased sensitivity of PSU to androgens

(ACTH: adrenocorticotropic hormone; PSU: pilosebaceous unit)

Obesity (android): Insulin resistance and androgen excess. Obesity (BMI >25) associated with distribution of fat primarily in the gluteal and femoral region is called **gynoid obesity**. Whereas in **android obesity,** fat distribution is in the trunk, and abdominal region. Android obese women are often associated with hyperinsulinemia (insulin resistance), impaired glucose tolerance and excess androgen production.

Obesity (android) → (↑) insulin → abnormal glucose tolerance/diabetes mellitus → (↑) androgen production → (↓) SHBG → (↑) free T and E_2.

INVESTIGATIONS (TABLE 34.18)

The following guidelines are prescribed in an attempt to pinpoint the diagnosis.

- **History of intake** of an offending drugs producing androgenicity is to be excluded first.
- **Family history** of excess hair growth is too often correlated.

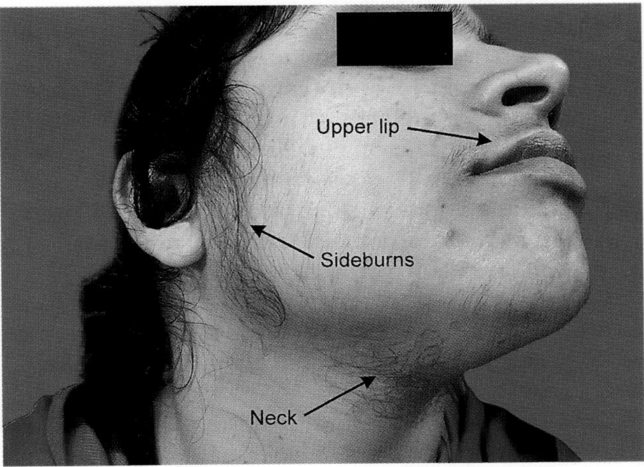

Fig. 34.7 Facial hirsutism.

TABLE 34.18: Diagnostic features for adrenal or ovarian causes of hyperandrogenism.

Adrenal		Ovarian	
Hyperplasia	***Tumor***	***Tumor***	***PCOS***
Perimenarcheal (early onset)	Any age	Any age	Early reproductive age
Insidious	Rapid onset	Rapid onset	Insidious
Hirsutes +	Hirsutes ++	Hirsutes ++	Hirsutes ±
Virilism ±	Virilism +	Virilism +	Virilism—nil
MH: Amenorrhea	MH: Amenorrhea	MH: Amenorrhea	MH: Oligomenorrhea or amenorrhea
Hormone status	**Hormone status**	**Hormone status**	**Hormone status**
▪ 17 hydroxyprogesterone ↑↑ (>800 ng/dL) ▪ DHEA-S ↑ ▪ Testosterone (T) ↑ Normal (<0.8 ng/mL) ▪ Dexamethasone suppression test: Positive	▪ DHEA-S ↑↑ (>700 µg/100 mL) ▪ T-normal or ↑ ▪ Dexamethasone suppression test—negative ▪ Intravenous pyelogram ▪ Sonography ▪ CT scan ▪ MRI (pituitary/adrenal)	▪ T ↑↑ (>200 ng/100 mL) ▪ DHEA-S Normal or ↑ ▪ Sonography ▪ Laparoscopy ▪ Biopsy	▪ LH: FSH—3 : 1 ▪ T ↑ (≤150 ng/dL) ▪ DHEA-S—may be ↑ ▪ Insulin resistance (IR): Raised fasting serum insulin ↑ (>25 µIU/mL). Fasting glucose/insulin ratio: <4.5 indicates insulin resistance. ▪ Sonography (p. 385) ▪ Laparoscopy (p. 386)

(MH: Menstrual history)

- **Mild hirsutes** are not infrequently found during puberty, pregnancy, and postmenopause. **During postmenopausal period**, there is decreased SHBG, more amongst obese patients, resulting in elevated testosterone (*see* above).
- **Physical examination:**
  - **BMI calculation:** (a) Modified Ferriman-Gallway score for grading hirsutism (p. 483); (b) Others for: Acne, acanthosis nigricans (p. 385), galactorrhea and clitoral size.
  - **Laboratory investigations includes:** Serum testosterone (free), free androgen index, DHEAS and 17OH progesterone.
  - **Hirsutism of rapid onset** and progressive in nature or symptoms of virilization, needs exclusion of a tumor (adrenal or ovarian). Serum DHEA-S >700 µg/dL may be seen with adrenal tumors. CT/MRI can confirm the diagnosis.
  - **Patients with primary amenorrhea** with or without virilism, require karyotyping to exclude 'Y' bearing dysgenetic gonads.
  - **Hirsutism of irrespective of age**, requires evalua-tion for adrenal or ovarian tumor.
  - **High serum level of testosterone** (>150 ng/dL) is mostly associated with an androgen producing tumor. Serum level of DHEA-S correlate well with daily urinary 17–KS secretion. Further evaluation should be done with ultrasonography, CT or MRI (Table 34.18) for ovarian or adrenal tumors.
  - **Mild hirsutism, young age:**
    - Raised levels of serum testosterone (>200 ng/dL) with normal DHEAS indicate ovarian tumor. **Diagnosis is confirmed** by ultrasonography, CT or MRI.
    - Gradually increasing hirsutism, even if associated with virilization, is unlikely to be a case of adrenal or ovarian tumor.
    - Serum testosterone levels >150 ng/dL is consistent with the diagnosis of ovarian stromal hyperthecosis.

    Mild hirsutism with irregular menses may be due to PCOS. Oral glucose tolerance test (OGTT) may be done to detect insulin resistance.
  - **Women with mild hirsutism of long duration**, regular menses, no virilization, require no investigation. **Moderate to severe hirsutism** needs serum total testosterone estimation (T). Raised serum T (>150 ng/dL) needs thorough evaluation with TVS, adrenal CT/MRI for exclusion of tumors (adrenal, ovary). Serum T level <150 ng/dL may be due to PCOS.
- **In Cushing's disease**, because of increased ACTH secretion from the anterior pituitary, there is increased glucocorticoid and androgen secretion from the adrenals. The findings include hirsutism, menstrual abnormalities, centripetal obesity, abdominal striae, dorsal neck fat pads, muscle wasting. If the plasma cortisol level is <1.8 µg/mL after overnight 1 mg dexamethasone suppression, Cushing's syndrome can be ruled out.
- **Late onset congenital adrenal hyperplasia (LOCAH)** is rarely associated with hirsutism. This is due to partial deficiency of 21-hydroxylase enzyme. Serum level of 17 α-hydroxyprogesterone (17-OHP) is elevated both baseline and after stimulation of ACTH.
- The diagnostic features of adrenal or ovarian causes are outlined in the Table 34.18.

MANAGEMENT PRINCIPLES OF HIRSUTISM

- To remove the source of excess androgen
- To suppress or neutralize the action of androgen
- To remove the excess hair.

Weight reduction: It is an important step of management (PCOS). Weight loss is associated with reduction of hyperinsulinemia and androgen excess. Ideal body mass index (BMI) should not be more than 25.

Removal of the source:

- Adrenal or ovarian tumor should be surgically treated.
- Cushing's disease can be treated by adrenalectomy, radiation to the pituitary or removal of ACTH-producing tumor by transsphenoidal surgery.
- In iatrogenic cases, the offending drug (Table 34.17) should be stopped.

To suppress or neutralize the excess androgen action

The drugs used are:

- Combined oral contraceptive pill
- Dexamethasone
- Antiandrogens.

Contraceptive Pill

Mode of Action

- Suppression of LH secretion from the pituitary (progestin effect).
- Antiandrogen at the level of hair follicle.
- Elevation of SHBG (estrogen effect).
- Progestins in OC pills inhibits 5 α-reductase activity in the skin.
- Inhibits adrenal androgen secretion (30%).

OC pills with **new progestins** (norgestimate, desogestrel, gestodine, drospirenone— Ch. 30) have very little androgenic effects. They increase the level of SHBG. They reduce free testosterone level significantly.

Case selection: Pill is suitable in cases of PCOS or idiopathic group especially in young and unmarried where only 'T' is elevated (Table 34.19).

Dexamethasone

It acts by suppressing pituitary-adrenal axis. It is used in adrenal or mixed adrenal and ovarian hyperandrogenism.

The dose varies from 0.25–1 mg daily at bed time. Aim of treatment is to suppress androstenedione and bring 17 hydroxyprogesterone to normal range. Ovulation usually returns soon.

GnRH agonists are used to suppress selectively ovarian steroid production by inhibiting LH secretion from the pituitary. This is used only when other antiandrogens have failed to give a response.

Antiandrogens

Cyproterone acetate is a derivative of 17-OHP. **It inhibits gonadotropin secretion and interferes with androgen action on the target organs by competing for the androgen receptors.** It blocks the action of DHT and T at both the nucleus and cytosol receptor level.

It should be administered along with ethinyl estradiol to prevent menstrual irregularities and ovulation. It is available as combined estrogen—progestin oral contraceptive (2 mg cyproterone acetate and 35 μg ethinyl estradiol).

TABLE 34.19: Hormone profile and drug therapy.

Hormone profile	*Drugs*
Elevated T (ovary)	Combined oral contraceptives (containing drospirenone or desogestrel)
Normal T and DHEA-S 3α-AG↑ (idiopathic)	Antiandrogens
DHEA-S↑, normal T	Dexamethasone

Improvement of hirsutism is observed after 3 months of therapy. This regimen gives contraceptive benefit also. **Important side effects are:** Nausea, fatigue, weight gain, loss of libido, and mastalgia.

Spironolactone: It is an aldosterone antagonist and acts as a potassium sparing diuretic.

Antiandrogen effects of spironolactone are:

- It inhibits ovarian and adrenal androgen biosynthesis.
- It competes with DHT for the androgen receptors in the hair follicle.
- It inhibits 5 α-reductase activity directly.

50–200 mg is given daily and the maintenance dose is 25–50 mg daily.

Important side effects are: Menstrual irregularity, fatigue, hyperkalemia, hypotension. (Add matter not found)

Flutamide: It is a nonsteroidal antiandrogen. It blocks the androgen receptors as well as it inhibits testosterone biosynthesis. Results are observed after 3 months of therapy. It is given in a dose of 250–750 mg/day. **Side effects are:** Nausea, dry skin, headache and hepatotoxicity. It is less commonly used.

Finasteride: It inhibits 5 α-reductase activity. It improves hirsutism significantly without any side effects. Daily dose is 5 mg.

Ketoconazole: page 452.

Insulin sensitizing drugs: Women with insulin resistance PCOS are treated with metformin and thiazolidinediones (rosiglitazone). These drugs decrease circulating insulin and androgen levels.

Glucocorticoids are used to suppress endogenous ACTH secretion to suppress adrenal androgen levels in cases with congenital adrenal hyperplasia (CAH). But they are less effective. Spironolactone containing COC pills may be the next choice.

Duration of therapy: Response of all the drugs are slow. Drugs should be continued for at least 6 months. Antiandrogens inhibit the growth of new hair follicle but fails to remove the hair that is already present.

Removal of hair: The excess hair is to be removed by **bleaching, twitching, depilation, epilation, waxing, lasers, shaving or electrolysis.** Laser and pulsed light therapy destroy hair follicles. Photo one epilation uses lasers to apply heat to the pigmented hair follicles. Skin pigmentation may occur. In electrolysis, individual hair follicle is destroyed. **Side effects are:** Pain, scarring, and pigmentation.

Eflornithine hydrochloride (13.9% cream) when used topically prevents hair growth by inhibiting the enzyme ornithine decarboxylase. This enzyme acts on the dermal papilla to stimulate hair growth. Treatment needs to be continued for a long time.

Acne is due to stimulation of the PSU with alteration in the bacteriologic flora. Androgens stimulate sebum production. High doses estrogen can inhibit it.

Treatment includes lowering the androgen levels (discussed above). The other therapies may be given with topical antibiotics, topical benzoyl peroxide, retinoid, and sometimes oral isotretinoin (analog of vitamin A). COCs are effective. Estrogen component of COC pills inhibits sebum production with usual dose of 30 μg. Acne vulgaris is due to the stimulation of androgens to the PSU. It is commonly treated with COC pills. Sometimes anti androgens are given. The overall response rate is about 90%. Oral isotretinoin is highly effective against severe recalcitrant acne. **It is teratogeneic**. Women must avoid pregnancy during therapy with isotretinoin. Consultation with a dermatologist may be sought.

Alopecia—is a cause for stress. The female pattern hairloss (androgenic alopecia) is seen on the frontal scalp and on the vertex.

Dermatologic diseases are to be excluded. Androgen excess or estrogen abnormalities and genetics may be the etiology. Exaggerated 5α-reductase activity is an important cause. **Antiandrogens:** Spironolactone and flutamide are effective. Minoxidil is used to stimulate hair growth. Overall response is about 30% only. Stem cell therapy may be helpful.

GALACTORRHEA

Definition: Galactorrhea is the secretion of a milky fluid which is inappropriate (unrelated to childbirth). The secretion contains fat globules when examined under microscope and is confirmatory for milk. A high prolactin level is encountered in one-third of cases with idiopathic amenorrhea.

Prolactin (PRL) is the most important hormone involved in the **pathophysiology of amenorrhea and/or galactorrhea**. Prolactin is under tonic hypothalamic inhibitory control of prolactin inhibitory factor (PIF).

Prolactin inhibits GnRH pulse secretion. Gonadotropin levels are suppressed. Hyperprolactinemia inhibits ovarian steroidogenesis. Hyperprolactinemia ultimately results in hypogonadotropic hypogonadism, oligomenorrhea, amenorrhea, anovulation, and many other clinical effects of hypoestrogenism.

PRL levels should be estimated in all women with galactorrhea, oligomenorrhea or amenorrhea (Table 34.20). Thyroid-stimulating hormone (TSH) level should be measured to rule out primary hypothyroidism.

Prolactinoma is present in about 50% of women with hyperprolactinemia. Serum prolactin level when raised on repeat assay beyond 20 ng/mL, suggests evaluation of sella turcica (p. 391). Level beyond 100 ng/mL is associated with high incidence of prolactinoma. Most of the prolactinomas are microadenomas. **About 33% of women with high prolactin levels, have galactorrhea**. However, galactorrhea can be seen in women with normal serum prolactin. About 30% of women with galactorrhea have normal menses. Women with 'big' prolactin (p. 391) may have normal menses with minimal or no galactorrhea.

TABLE 34.20: Indications of prolactin assay.

- Amenorrhea with or without galactorrhea
- Galactorrhea with or without amenorrhea
- Oligomenorrhea
- Raised serum thyroid-stimulating hormone (TSH) levels
- Women with PCOS/anovulation
- Unruptured luteinized follicle
- Delayed puberty
- Hirsutism.

It is known that prolactinomas may also secrete growth hormone (GH).

TREATMENT

Women with microadenoma or functional hyperprolactinoma who do not wish pregnancy may be followed up without treatment. Assessment of serum PRL and imaging should be repeated once a year. She should be given exogenous estrogen (COCs) if she has low estrogen levels.

MRI is recommended as it provides 1 mm resolution and can detect all microadenomas. Macroadenomas are uncommon. Macroadenomas are suspected if prolactin level is >100 ng/mL, or the woman complaints of headache or visual changes. Microadenomas are the common cause of hyperprolactinemia. Therapy is unnecessary as microadenomas remain stable in most cases. Breastfeeding may be initiated without any adverse effect on the tumors. During medical treatment of macroadenomas, MRI and visual field examination should be done to assess the effect of medication. Decision can be made as regard the continuation of medical treatment or to remove the tumor surgically.

Prolactin inhibitors: Dopamine, L Dopa, Bromocriptine, cabergoline.

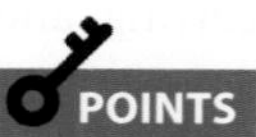

POINTS

- **The principal sources of androgen** in female are peripheral (50%), ovaries and adrenals (Flowchart 34.2).
  Most of the testosterone (80%) in the circulation is bound to SHBG; 19% is bound with albumin and 1% remains free which is biologically active.
  In the pilosebaceous unit, the testosterone is converted into potent dihydrotestosterone by the enzyme 5 α-reductase. Hirsutism may be associated with excess androgen production either form the ovaries or adrenals or excess stimulation of the hair follicles. Virilism is almost always associated with hirsutism except at birth but hirsutism may not be associated with virilism.
- **Causes of hirsutism** may be in the adrenals, ovaries, exogenous drug therapy or idiopathic (Table 34.17).
- **In adrenal hyperplasia**, 17-hydroxyprogesterone is elevated; in adrenal tumor, DHEA-S is elevated; in ovarian tumor, testosterone is elevated and in PCOS, LH: FSH ratio is increased. Dexamethasone suppression test is positive in adrenal hyperplasia but not in tumor. Sonography, CT scan, MRI, IVP, and laparoscopy may be extended to exclude organic lesion (Table 34.18).

Contd...

Contd...

- For each major compartment of androgen source, one biochemical marker is used. Testosterone reflects ovarian, DHEA-S reflects adrenal gland and 3 α–AG reflects peripheral tissue source.
- **Increased 5α-reductase activity** is seen in idiopathic hirsutism.
- **Women with PCOS** often suffer from android obesity (BMI >25). Biochemical abnormalities observed in women with PCOS are elevated levels of biologically active LH, hyperinsulinemia in 40% (insulin resistance), impaired glucose tolerance and excess circulating androgen (Ch. 29).
- **The most common cause of hirsutism** is PCOS. Women with a serum testosterone level > 200 ng/dL needs investigations (DHEA-S, 17-OHP, USG, CT, and MRI) to exclude tumors (ovary, adrenal) or CAH.
- **Treatment of hirsutism** depends on the source of excess androgen. Oral contraceptive therapy is instituted when serum testosterone is elevated (ovarian androgen). Dexamethasone is the drug of choice when DHEA-S is elevated (adrenal androgen). Antiandrogens (p. 451) are used when neither is elevated (peripheral androgen). Most women (80%) with idiopathic hirsutism have elevated levels of 3α-AG. The best treatment for such a woman is antiandrogen, spironolactone.
- **Antiandrogens** should be continued for a minimum of 3 months before any response is observed. This is due to the length of hair growth cycle. While the antiandrogen inhibits the growth of new hair follicle, it fails to remove the hair that is already present.
- **Source of excess androgen** may have to be removed surgically. Removal of hair is done by bleaching, twitching, epilation or electrolysis.
- **Medical management of hirsutism** needs at least 6 months to get the benefits of therapy. This is because the life cycle of a hair follicle is 6 months.
- **Women having mild hirsutism** of long duration, regular menses, no virilization, require no investigations. They may be treated with COCs or COCs containing drospirenone or desogestrel.
- **Prolactin** is the most important hormone, involved in the pathophysiology of galactorrhea.
- **About 5% of women** with hyperprolactinemia have hyperthyroidism.
- **Women with microadenomas** with hypoestrogenic state and not desiring fertility may be treated with COCs.
- **Most common cause** of mildly elevated PRL levels is stress and the next is the drugs.
- **In about 70% of women with hyperprolactinoma, galactorrhea and amenorrhea with low estrogen levels have prolactinoma.**
- With time macroadenomas enlarge but not the all the microadenomas.
- **Other common causes** are pituitary microadenoma (smaller than 10 mm), hypothalamic pathology, drug therapy: Phenothiazine antidepressants (sertraline, tricyclic antidepressants), antihypertensives (atenolol, methyldopa), H_2 receptor (cimetidine) blocker, hormones (DMPA, COCs) and primary hypothyroidism, chest wall irritation—10% (ill-fitting brassieres, burns, herpes zoster, breast surgery), neoplastic process—18% (bronchogenic carcinoma, renal carcinoma, lymphoma) (Ch. 29). Serum prolactin level of >100 ng/mL is too often associated with tumor (prolactinoma).
- **Bromocriptine** is the drug of choice for galactorrhea. Cabergoline is more effective and well-tolerated compared to bromocriptine. Pregnancy following bromocriptine has got no teratogenic effect on the offspring. There is no increased incidence of multiple pregnancy.
- **Most macroadenomas** enlarge with time whereas most microadenomas do not. Bromocriptine shrinks 80% of macroadenomas. Surgical treatment of prolactinomas (transnasal-transsphenoidal excision) is done for women who fail to respond with medical treatment.
- **Cabergoline** is more effective and well-tolerated compared to bromocriptine.

CHAPTER

35 Operative Gynecology

CHAPTER OUTLINE

INTRODUCTION

Perioperative management encompasses the care in the pre, intra and postoperative periods. The decision to operate and whether it should be emergently or electively is also important.

The prime objective of this Chapter is to make the readers familiar with the basic information about different aspects of practical gynecology. While the technical details may only concern the specialists, **the beginners should be familiar with the basic principles of operative gynecology.** The interested readers may go through the available textbooks of operative gynecology for further details.

PREOPERATIVE PREPARATIONS

The ultimate objective of surgery is to cure the ailments and/or to arrive at a diagnosis, if it is done for diagnostic purpose.

Preoperative evaluation should include a detailed history (general, medical, and surgical), a complete physical examination and laboratory investigations. Body mass index (BMI) is recorded for assessment of nutritional status. Past records of illness or surgery should be evaluated. An anesthesiologist should see the patient preoperatively. A physician or other specialists may be involved depending upon the patient's need. For any elective (planned) operation, the general condition of the patient must be improved, prior to operation any systemic disorder including anemia must be corrected.

INVESTIGATIONS

The objectives of preoperative investigations are:

- To evaluate the health status of an individual who may be otherwise healthy.
- To provide a baseline information in the event of any postoperative complication.
- To assess the severity of a pre-existing medical disorder that needs further attention.
- The investigations should preferably be done prior to admission.

Rationale for Preoperative Investigations

Any major gynecological surgery involves anesthesia, blood loss and disturbances in major organ function like cardiovascular and respiratory. The purpose of preoperative investigations is to assess the individual's physiological reserve and the ability to withstand the surgical stress.

Routine Investigations for Major Surgery

- **Blood:** Estimation of hemoglobin, hematocrit, total and differential leukocyte count, platelet count, blood group and cross matching are done. ***Other blood tests***: Liver function, renal function, serum electrolytes, blood sugar in aged women or in complicated cases.
- **Urine:** Routine and microscopic analysis includes examination for protein, sugar, casts and pus cells. If the pus cells are more than 5 per high power field, culture sensitivity is required.
- **Chest X-ray (CXR) and ECG:** For an healthy individual below the age of 40, these may not be essential. But women above 40 years of age should have CXR, ECG and serum electrolytes analysis.

If there is any history of systemic disease, relevant investigations should be carried out accordingly. Relevant investigations (e.g. echocardiography, coagulation profile) should be done as indicated. Special investigations appropriate to some lesions such as vesicovaginal fistula (VVF), malignancy have been mentioned in the concerned Chapters.

To protect the surgical staff, serological screening should be done for hepatitis B virus, C virus, and HIV. The screening for HIV should be done following patient counseling and permission (p. 128).

Admission

The patient is to be admitted on the day or 1–2 days prior to operation based on hospital protocol. Special cases need earlier admission. During this period, re-evaluation of the case and examination by anesthetist should be done.

Preoperative Work-up

Enquiry should be made about the details of medical or surgical history: Anemia, diabetes, hypertension, tuberculosis, urinary problems, kidney, liver disease, jaundice, asthma, obesity malignant disease, drug allergy, corticosteroid therapy, any infection (HIV), hepatitis B, C or medication used are to be noted. Cessation of smoking is important. Investigations in a patient are organized accordingly.

Benefits of preoperative evaluation are: (a) Decrease surgical morbidity; (b) Reduce preoperative delay or cancelation of surgery; (c) Optimize baseline health status; (d) Organize plan of anesthesia.

PREOPERATIVE COUNSELING AND INFORMED CONSENT

Preoperative discussion between a doctor and a patient (guardian in case of minor), should be in general terms. It should remove patient's anxiety and fear for operation. Pamphlets are useful as only a few (30%) patients can recollect verbal discussions. Informed consent is a legal document. It is an ethical principle to obtain a valid consent before any surgical intervention. **The following should be explained to her:**

- Diagnosis of the abnormality.
- Nature of the operation and its modifications depending on the findings during operation.
- The likelihood of success of surgery.
- The risks and complications of surgery.
- Alternative forms of treatment available.
- The option of no treatment.
- Informed consent must be in writing and signed in a prescribed proforma.
- Prognosis if the treatment is refused.
- Consent must be voluntary and without coercion.
- Consent form must be signed by the patient and the physician.

Diet: Light diet is given in the previous evening and nothing in the morning of the day of operation. No solid food by mouth for at least 6 hours before the operation is ideal, so that the stomach is empty at the time of anesthesia.

Preparation of the bowel: A cleansing enema is commonly given in the evening before the operation day. Rigorous bowel preparation is not routinely required unless bowel surgery is expected. However, in cases where satisfactory bowel preparation is needed, osmotic oral purgation using polyethylene glycol solution is used. Patient is asked to drink 1–2 liters of such mixtures. To avoid dehydration, intravenous fluids may be needed.

Night sedation: To ensure good sleep at night prior to the day of operation, either diazepam 5–10 mg or alprazolam 0.25–0.5 mg tablet is given at bed time.

Local antiseptic care: Abdominal preparation—routine shaving of the operative area before surgery is not recommended. Hair clipping reduces the rate of wound infection. Cleaning of the operative area with soap and water is generally done by the patient. The surgically prepared area should extend from the inferior rib cage to the midthigh. The abdomen is cleaned with a five minute scrub using povidone iodine solution before surgery.

Vaginal operation—the vaginal preparations include clipping of the pubic hair and up to middle of both the thighs. Presence of active vaginal or cervical infection requires eradication prior to surgery.

The perineum and the vulva are cleaned with savlon using a sponge held in a sponge forceps (Fig. 38.15). The vagina is cleaned with povidone iodine solution. This solution is then flushed away with sterile water poured into the vagina. Then a sterile sponge on a sponge forceps is used to clean the vagina.

Morning medication: In consultation with anesthetist, sedative like diazepam 5–10 mg orally, is given about 2 hours prior to sending the patient to the operation theater. Injection atropine sulfate 0.6 mg is usually (not as a routine) administered in the operation theater intravenously by the anesthetist.

Other medications: The patient is generally advised to take all regular medications on the morning of surgery with sips of water, unless contraindicated.

Surgical Site Infection and Prophylactic Antibiotics

Surgical infections may occur within 30 days of operation. Source of infection may be the contaminated instruments, surgeon's hand, theater air or from patient's endogenous flora at the operation site. Other risk factors are patient's age, diabetes mellitus, immunosuppression, prolonged hospital stay or prolonged operation. **Prophylactic antibiotic** is aimed to maintain adequate tissue levels of antibiotics for the duration of operation.

A broad spectrum antibiotic is selected to cover the common gram-positive, gram-negative and the anaerobic organisms. Generally, a third generation cephalosporin (ceftriaxone 1 g) is given by slow intravenous route just before induction of anesthesia. Second dose is repeated after 12 hours. Injection clindamycin 600 mg IV or metronidazole 500 mg IV is given to combat anaerobic infection.

Thromboprophylaxis is to be given to reduce the risk of venous thromboembolism (VTE). In major gynecological surgery, the risks of deep vein thrombosis and the pulmonary embolism (PE) are high. The risk of VTE is high particularly in patients with age >60 years, obesity (BMI >30 kg/m^2), positive family/personal history, antiphospholipid (APL) syndrome, severe infection, advanced cancer, prolonged immobility or thrombophilia. A patient should be adequately hydrated. Mechanical measures like compression stockings, intermittent pneumatic compression, leg exercises, early mobilization are recommended. **Low molecular weight heparin or unfractionated heparin** is used to reduce the risk of deep vein thrombosis (DVT) and PE. However, there may be increased bleeding due to use of heparin.

Preoperative Work-up in the Operation Table

- **IV infusion:** An infusion of Ringer's solution drip is started.
- **Anesthesia:** Local, regional or general anesthesia is administered with sole discretion of the anesthetist.

- **Patient position in gynecological surgery:** In abdominal operation, the position is dorsal. Dorsal lithotomy position is used for vaginal, laparoscopic and hysteroscopic surgeries. Dorsal lithotomy may cause injury to femoral, sciatic and peroneal nerves due to compression, stretching and ischemia. These complications are especially following a prolonged surgery. Hyperflexion of the hip causes compression of the femoral nerve against the inguinal ligament. Limited hipflexion, abduction and external rotation should be done (Fig. 9.3D).
- **Antiseptic dressings:** Bladder preparations—for minor operations the patient voids before being taken to the operating room. For major operations, soft rubber catheter or Foley's catheter is inserted in operating table. In **vaginal operation**, metal catheter is used after draping and Foley's catheter is introduced at the end of the operation (Fig. 38.7).
- **Draping:** Proper draping is done prior to surgery using sterile linen, towel and leggings (in vaginal operation). Towel clips are used (Fig. 38.40).

Formalities in Minor Vaginal Operations

- Examination of the cardiovascular system.
- Blood examination for hemoglobin estimation and total and differential count.
- Urine examination for protein, sugar and pus cells.
- The patient is to be admitted in the morning of the day of operation.
- Oral feeding is to be withheld for at least 6 hours prior to surgery.
- Vulvar cleaning is only done.
- The patient is asked to pass urine before entering the operation theater.
- Anesthesia.
- Lithotomy position (Figs. 9.3A to C).
- Antiseptic painting of the vulva and vagina.
- Draping.
- Examination under anesthesia.

Day Surgery

It includes selected surgical procedures where patients are admitted, operated and discharged **on the same day**. The operation should not be unduly complex or time consuming. Patients are screened before hand (*see* above).

Benefits of day surgery are: (a) Increased patient turn over; (b) Reduced hospital stay; (c) reduced inpatient work load; (d) Reduced concomitant cost; (e) Least disturbances of patient's daily work.

Assessment of suitability for day care surgery is important. After operation the patient should be seen both by the surgeon and the anesthetist. Before the discharge, follow-up procedures, analgesia and availability of emergency services are explained to the patient.

Common Gynecological Day Surgery Cases

- Dilatation and curettage.
- Termination of pregnancy (D and E).
- Biopsy procedures.
- Examination under anesthesia.
- Endoscopic procedures like (Ch. 36):
  - Diagnostic hysteroscopy, laparoscopy (p. 102)
  - Laparoscopic sterilization operation (p. 417)
  - Ovarian drilling diathermy (p. 504)
  - Transcervical resection/ablation of endometrium. (p. 162)

INTRAOPERATIVE CARE

INCISIONS

Most of the gynecological operations are done through transverse incisions.

- **Pfannenstiel incision (muscle separating):** It is commonly used.
  - **The main advantages of transverse incision are:** (a) Rapid wound healing; (b) Better postoperative convalescence; (c) Superior cosmetic result; (d) Good access to pelvic organs; (e) Less incidence of postoperative complications like: (i) Wound dehiscence and (ii) Incisional hernia.
  - **Disadvantages:** Incision is difficult to extend when exploration of the upper abdomen is needed.

Other transverse incisions are:

- **Cherney incision:** The rectus muscle is dissected from its insertion at the symphysis. During closure the rectus tendons are united to inferior portion of the rectus sheath with interrupted sutures.
- **Maylard incision** is a true transverse muscle cutting incision. The inferior epigastric vessels are ligated before incising the rectus. The muscles are approximated during closure.
- **Vertical (median or paramedian) incisions** give good access to whole of abdomen with excellent exposure. It spares all major nerves, vessels and muscles, as opposed to the transverse incision. It gives rapid entry to the abdominal cavity.
  - **Disadvantages:** It lacks all the advantages of transverse incision.

DRAINS

Drains are used to prevent any accumulation of blood, pus, lymph, bile or intestinal secretion. They are less commonly used in gynecological surgery when hemostasis is satisfactorily achieved. Early removal of drains is done to avoid infection and to improve mobilization. It is usually done by 2–3 days after surgery when drainage is <100 mL in 24 hours.

CLOSURE OF PERITONEUM

Traditionally closure of the pelvic and parietal peritoneum is done at the end of the operation to decrease adhesions. However, the current studies have suggested (RCOG-1998), that peritoneum rapidly spreads across any raw areas left after surgery and there is no need of peritoneal closure. However, it is surgeon dependent. Closure of the subcutaneous adipose layer is useful to close the dead space when it is ≥2 cm thick. A 2-0 plain catgut suture is optimum.

POSTOPERATIVE CARE

AIMS OF POSTOPERATIVE CARE

Aims are—(a) Support to restore patient's physiological functions; (b) Promote tissue healing; (c) Prevention/management of complications. Good postoperative care team involves surgical team, nursing staff, physiotherapists and dieticians.

RETURN FROM OPERATION THEATER

Immediate postoperative care: On return from the theater, the patient is taken to the recovery room or ward which is usually placed adjacent to the operation suite. Patient is accompanied by a responsible person—doctor or nursing staff. **The prerequisites prior to shifting are**:

- Vital signs such as pulse, respiration and blood pressure become steady.
- Patient recovers from anesthesia and is fully conscious.
- Anesthetist's consent should be available.
- Fluid balance and any bleeding from the surgical site are checked.

IN THE WARD

First 24 Hours (D–O)

Placement in the bed: The patient is gently placed on her side in the bed. This reduces the risk of inhalation of vomitus or mucous. If spinal anesthesia is given, the foot end is raised for about 12 hours.

Observation: The observation of the vital signs such as pulse, respiration and blood pressure is made half hourly in the initial period. The interval is gradually increased if these are found steady. Attention should be paid for any bleeding from the operated site.

Fluid replacement: Following any major operation, fluid is replaced intravenously. The amount of fluid to be replaced is decided upon the following factors: Intraoperative blood loss, operating time, urine output, insensible losses and the volume of fluid already replaced.

Blood transfusion, if needed is given during operation and soon after. **Blood transfusion should not be given unnecessarily**. Urine output of at least 30 mL/hour indicates adequate fluid replacement. On an average, after replacement of the fluid loss at operation, additional 2–2.5 liters of fluid are infused. As there is sodium retention following major surgery, the replacement is by 5% dextrose in water along with 0.5 to 1 liter of Ringer's solution.

Pain control: Adequate pain control ensures deep breathing, adequate oxygenation, early mobilization, prompt wound healing, reduced pulmonary complication and less hospital stay. Liberal analgesics should be given to relieve pain and to ensure sleep. A sedative is prescribed at night. For this purpose, intramuscular injection of pethidine hydrochloride 100 mg or morphine sulfate 10 mg is administered at an interval of 6–8 hours. Nonsteroidal anti-inflammatory agents (Ketorolac) are also effective analgesics. In some centers, **patient controlled analgesia (PCA)** infusion pumps are used. Patient is instructed to use a preset dose (1 mg) of morphine without any overdosage. Nausea or vomiting may be prevented by simultaneous administration of metoclopramide 10 mg or ondansetron 4 mg IM/IV.

Antibiotics: Perioperative prophylactic antibiotics as mentioned in preoperative care are to be considered. Alternatively, routine postoperative antibiotics are prescribed. This should be administered parenterally for 48 hours followed by oral route for another 3 days.

Bladder care: Women having major gynecological surgery, usually a Foley's catheter is inserted before the operation. It keeps the bladder empty throughout and reduces the risk of any bladder injury. It helps to monitor urine output, reduces the risk of urinary retention and pain. Generally, it is removed on third postoperative day. Prolonged catheterization is associated with urinary tract infection. Catheter is kept for 7–10 days in patients having any injury to the bladder. Following removal of catheter, postoperative urinary retention is a common problem. This is due to pain, spasm of the pelvic floor muscles, tissues edema or following regional anesthesia. Residual urine is measured after micturition with ultrasound scan or by a catheter. Recatheterization should be done if the residual urine is >100 mL. Catheter may have to be kept for 24–48 hours.

Mobilization: The patient should be encouraged to move freely in bed and to lie in any posture comfortable to her. Deep breathing and movements of the legs and arms are encouraged to minimize leg vein thrombosis and pulmonary embolism. It is advantageous to allow the patient to sit or to stand by the side of the bed by the evening. The patient can have sips of water to relieve the thirst.

First Postoperative Day

General care: The patient is expected to look better and fresh. Vital signs are noted at least twice daily. Abdominal auscultation is done for appearance of peristaltic sounds. Enquiry is to be made about the passage of flatus. Vaginal plug (if any) is to be removed early in the morning. The patient is encouraged to stand or to walk few steps by the side of the bed and to sit on the bedside or on a chair. Deep breathing exercises and leg and arm movements while on bed are encouraged.

Diet: Oral feeding in the form of plain or electrolyte water is given in small but frequent intervals. With the appearance of bowel sounds or passage of flatus, full liquid diet is prescribed.

However, early postoperative feeding is safe. Early feeding (<24 hours) does not cause any increase in paralytic ileus, vomiting or abdominal distension. Each case needs to be individualized.

Sedative and analgesics: Parenteral analgesics are gradually replaced with oral drugs (paracetamol, aspirin and NSAIDs) in combination.

Second Postoperative Day

- The patient feels comfortable and looks fresh
- She moves around in the room and goes to toilet

- Light solid diet of patient's choice is given
- Self-retaining catheter is removed.

Third and Fourth Postoperative Days

- Daily observation of vital signs twice daily is to be done as a routine.
- The diet is gradually brought to her normal.
- The bowels usually move normally, otherwise low enema or suppository may be given.

Fifth and Sixth Postoperative Days

The abdominal stitches are usually removed on the 5th day in transverse incision and on 6th day in vertical incision. **The stitches are to be removed in early morning with the patient in empty stomach**. The precaution is taken, so that emergency repair of the wound can be done, if burst abdomen occurs.

Care of the perineum: Following vaginal plastic operation, the perineal wound is dressed at least twice daily or following each act of micturition and defecation. The dressing is done with spirit and antibiotic powder or ointment. Local pain and edema may be relieved by hot compress with magnesium sulfate or infrared rays.

DISCHARGE

There is a trend towards shorter hospital stay these days. But complete recovery of all organ functions is needed before discharge. It may take 5–7 days when she is fit for discharge. **Written information** is given to the patient as regard the operative procedures.

While an uniform guideline is difficult to formulate, in an otherwise uneventful postoperative recovery, the patient may be discharged by 5–7 days following hysterectomy.

Examination Prior to Discharge

Abdominal operation

- Abdominal wound is to be thoroughly checked for evidences of sepsis, hematoma or dehiscence.
- Vaginal discharge if any, is to be noted. If the discharge is offensive, gentle vaginal exploration by a finger should be done to exclude a foreign body (gauze piece).

Vaginal operation

- Perineal wound is checked to assess the state of healing.
- Vaginal exploration with a finger is useful to detect accidentally a retained and forgotten gauze piece.

Advices Given on Discharge

Rest: Light household work can be resumed after 3 weeks and outside or office works to be resumed after 4–6 weeks. While some resume their work earlier comfortably, others may find it difficult. However, minimally invasive surgery (MIS) has got the advantage (p. 512).

Coitus: There is no fixed time bar. As soon as she is physically and psychologically fit, intercourse is permissible. However, it should not be resumed prior to the postoperative check up (i.e. 6 weeks) especially following vaginal plastic operation and hysterectomy.

Special instructions are mentioned in appropriate Chapters.

Follow-up is usually after 6 weeks or earlier if some complications occur.

GYNECOLOGICAL OPERATIONS

As mentioned in the introduction, **the technical details of the operation while concern to the specialists but the students should be acquainted with the principles involved.** Some considerations are however given in cases of minor operations. Such operations are common and some may have to do it following graduation during house officer job.

DILATATION OF CERVIX

This is an operation to dilate the cervix. While in some cases, dilatation of the external is enough but in majority, the entire canal including the internal is to be dilated.

The dilatation is done by graduated cervical dilators. When the internal os is to be dilated, prior introduction of uterine sound is mandatory to confirm the position of the uterus.

Indications of only dilatation are

- Prior to amputation of cervix (p. 179).
- Prior to hysteroscopy.
- Pyometra or hematometra (p. 138).
- Prior to introduction of uterine curette and insertion of intrauterine device (IUD), radium or laminaria tent.
- Spasmodic dysmenorrhea (p. 147).
- Dilatation may be difficult at times due to cervical stenosis. Difficulties may be overcome by:
  - Using a metal probe (lacrimal duct probe), cervical canal can be dilated.
  - Simultaneous use of sonography to guide the probe/uterine sound as it is being passed into the uterine cavity.
  - Use of tablet misoprostol (200/400 μg) vaginally 12–24 hours prior to the surgery is helpful as it softens the cervix.

DILATATION AND CURETTAGE

This is an operative procedure whereby dilatation of the cervical canal followed by uterine curettage is done. This is the most common gynecological operation done.

Indications

Indications of D&C

- **Diagnostic**
  - Infertility
  - Abnormal uterine bleeding (AUB)
  - Pathologic amenorrhea
  - Endometrial tuberculosis
  - Endometrial carcinoma
  - Postmenopausal bleeding
  - Chorionepithelioma
- **Therapeutic**
  - Dysfunctional uterine bleeding (DUB)
  - Endometrial polyp
  - Removal of IUD
  - Incomplete abortion
- **Combined**
  - DUB
  - Endometrial polyp

Principal Steps of Operation

- The patient is to empty the bladder prior to operation.
- The operation is done under general anesthesia or under diazepam sedation with or without paracervical block.
- She is placed in lithotomy position.
- Local antiseptic cleaning and draping done.
- Bimanual examination is performed.
- Posterior vaginal speculum is introduced.
- The anterior lip of the cervix is grasped with an Allis tissue forceps.
- An uterine sound is introduced to confirm the position and to note the length of the uterocervical canal.
- Cervical canal is dilated with graduated dilators.
  Hawkin-Ambler dilator should be held in such a way that the knob is inside the palm and the index finger rests on the body of the instrument. The tip of the finger should be placed at a distance of about 3 cm (slightly more than the length of the cervical canal) from the tip of the instrument. The finger tip acts as a guard. The tip of the instrument should pass beyond the internal os evidenced by the fact that it is grasped by it and does not fall even when the support of the instrument is withdrawn. The tip of the dilator should be directed anteriorly or posteriorly according to the position of the uterus.
- When the dilator is introduced, the cervix is made steady by traction of the vulsellum (Allis's tissue forceps).
- After the desired dilatation, the uterine cavity is curetted by an uterine curette either in clockwise or anticlockwise direction starting from the fundus down to internal os.
  In benign lesion, sharp curette and in suspected malignancy, blunt curette is used.
  The curette should be gentle but thorough. Vigorous curettage may damage the basal layer of the endometrium and uterine muscle.
- Vulsellum and the speculum are removed.
- The curetted material is **preserved in 10% formol-saline (normal saline in suspected tubercular endometritis), labeled properly and sent for histological examination.** Short history of the case and **first day of last menstrual period** especially in infertility cases and DUB should be positively mentioned.

Discharge

After a short period of observation (say 3–4 hours) with passing off of the anesthetic effect, the patient may go home.

Complications

- **Immediate**
- **Remote**

Immediate Complication

Although, it is a minor operation, but complications do occur. Such complications are:

- Injury to the cervix
- Uterine perforation
- Hemorrhage
- Injury to the gut
- Infection.

Injury to the cervix

The injury to the lip of cervix is caused by vulsellum bite or lateral tear by dilator. The bleeding from the vulsellum site is usually slight and stopped by gauze pressure or at best by a hemostatic suture.

Management of lateral tear

If slight, hemostasis is effective by intracervical or vaginal gauze plugging. The brisk hemorrhage is likely due to injury of the descending cervical artery and requires hemostatic sutures taking deep bite of the cervical tissue on the same side. If however, the tear extends upwards to involve the uterine artery, laparotomy has to be done along with resuscitative measures. Hemostasis is achieved by opening the anterior leaf of the broad ligament failing which ligation of the anterior division of the internal iliac artery may have to be done, if the uterus is to be preserved.

Uterine perforation

Uterus is perforated by uterine sound, or dilator or uterine curette. The perforation is more common in pregnant rather than nonpregnant uterus.

Diagnosis is made by:

- Sudden loss of resistance.
- Passage of the instrument more than the length of the uterine cavity.
- Undue mobility of the instrument.
- Vaginal bleeding.

Management: Attempt to confirm the perforation by reintroducing the instrument is to be condemned. Once perforation is suspected, following guidelines are to be followed:

- To stop the operative procedure.
- To watch the pulse and blood pressure and vaginal bleeding.
- To formulate the definitive treatment.

Noninfective/nonmalignant uterus

- Small perforation by sound or small dilator
  - To watch the vital signs.
  - To administer antibiotics.
  - To discharge the patient after 24–48 hours, if abdomen is soft, vital signs (pulse, BP) are stable and no untoward effects are noticed.
- Perforation by large dilator or curette.

Usually, the perforation is large and associated with varying degrees of internal hemorrhage. The gut may also be injured. As such laparotomy is justified. Repair of the rent or hysterectomy as the case may be is to be done. Associated gut injury is to be looked for and if found, to be tackled accordingly—repair or resection.

Laparoscopy can be performed in all cases at the earliest. This will help to complete the operative process under its guidance if the perforation is small, to minimize the period of observation and to guide the urgency of laparotomy.

Infective/malignant uterus

In suspected malignancy or in pyometra, prompt laparotomy is justified. This is to be followed by definitive surgery. However, if perforation occurs in potentially infected uterus of young woman, conservative treatment with antibiotics is justified and to watch for evidences of peritonitis.

Remote Complications

- Cervical incompetence due to injury to internal os. This may cause recurrent midtrimester abortion.
- Uterine synechiae due to injury to uterine muscle. This may cause secondary amenorrhea (p. 383).

DILATATION AND INSUFFLATION (D AND I)

This is an operation of dilatation of the cervix and introduction of air or CO_2 into the uterine cavity to know the patency of the fallopian tubes. It is also known as **Rubin test**. It is less commonly done these days.

Indications

To note the tubal patency in:

- Investigation for infertility
- Following tuboplasty operation.

It should be done in the first half of the cycle (between 8 and 12th day) and **should not be done** in the presence of pelvic infection (p. 106).

A positive test is evidenced by:

- A hissing sound is audible on the flank due to exit of air through the abdominal ostium.
- Drop in the manometer reading from 80–120 mm Hg.
- Patient complains of shoulder pain on sitting (due to irritation of the diaphragm by air and the pain sensation is carried by phrenic nerve).

Complications

- **Immediate**
- **Remote**

Immediate: The complications due to the use of uterine sound and cervical dilators are those of D&C operation. Special complications related to the operation include:

- **Air embolism:** About 7–10 mL of air is enough to produce embolism. Chance of air embolism is abolished with the use of CO_2.
- **Rupture of the tube:** If the tube is blocked and the pressure is raised beyond 200 mm Hg.
- **Flaring up of the pre-existing pelvic infection**.

Remote: Pelvic endometriosis, granuloma formation.

HYSTEROSALPINGOGRAPHY

Hysterosalpingography (HSG) is an operative procedure used to assess the **interior anatomy of the uterus and tube including tubal patency**. It is a radiographic study and a contrast media is used.

Indications

- **Assessment of tubal patency** in the investigation of infertility or following tuboplasty operation (p. 203).
- **Detection of uterine malformations** (unicornuate, bicornuate, septate uterus) (p. 35).
- **Diagnosis** of cervical incompetence (p. 37).
- Detection of translocated IUD whether lying inside or outside the uterine cavity (p. 403).
- Diagnosis of uterine synechiae (p. 384).
- Incidental diagnosis of submucous fibroid or an uterine polyp or hydrosalpinx or nodular tube is an additional gain.
- To confirm the diagnosis of secondary abdominal pregnancy.
- Following insertion of Essure to confirm tubal occlusion.

Principal Steps

The operation is done in the radiology department and without anesthesia.

- Patient is to empty her bladder.
- She is placed in dorsal position with the buttocks on the edge.
- Internal examination is done.
- Posterior vaginal speculum is introduced; the anterior lip of the cervix is held by Allis forceps and an uterine sound is passed.
- Hysterosalpingographic cannula is fitted with a syringe containing radio-opaque dye—either water soluble contrast medium, meglumine diatrizoate (Renografin-60) or a low viscosity oil-based dye, ethiodized oil (Ethidol). The dye is introduced slowly. About 5–10 mL of the solution is introduced. The passage of the dye into the interior may be observed by using a X-ray image intensifier and a video display unit.
- The speculum and the Allis forceps are removed but not the cannula.
- Two radiographic views are generally taken. The first one to show the filling of uterine cavity and the other at the completion of the procedure (after 10–15 minutes) showing tubal findings. The tubal patency is evidenced by peritoneal spillage (Fig. 17.3).

Advantages of Watery Medium over Oil-based Solution

- Permits rapid absorption
- Eliminates granuloma formation
- Negligible peritoneal irritation
- No risk of embolism when extravasated
- Better visualization of tubal mucosa.

Advantages of Oil-based Medium over the Watery Contrast Medium

- Better resolution of tubal architecture.
- Less uterine cramping pain.
- Higher subsequent pregnancy rate (better flushing of tubes).

Advantages of HSG over D&I

- Lesser false-negative report (cornual spasm can be overcome by prior IM injection of atropine sulfate 0.6 mg).
- Precise identification of the side and site of obstruction.
- Identification of uterine cavity abnormality.
- Flimsy intraluminal adhesions may be broken, as such chance of conception within 3–4 months is more.

Timings

HSG is done between D6 and D10 of the cycle. Antibiotic prophylaxis should be given. Doxycycline 100 mg PO twice daily is given, beginning the day before HSG and continuing for 5 days.

Complications

Apart from the inherent complications of the uterine sound (uterine perforation) hemorrhage, HSG has got the following complications even with the use of watery solution.

- Peritoneal irritation and pelvic pain.
- Vasovagal attack.
- Intravasation of dye within the venous or lymphatic channels (common in tubercular endometritis) (Fig. 11.7)
- Flaring up of pelvic infection (1–3%).

Contraindications to HSG

(a) Pelvic infection; (b) Women known to have hydrosalpinges (Fig. 38.58); (c) Presence of adnexal mass (PID); (d) Pelvic tenderness on bimanual examination; (e) Pregnancy; (f) Suspected pelvic tuberculosis; (g) Abnormal uterine bleeding.

CERVICAL BIOPSY

This is the common diagnostic procedure carried out both in the hospital and in the office.

Types

- **Surface (Ch. 9)**
- **Ring**
- **Punch**
- **Cone**
- **Wedge**

Punch Biopsy

Punch biopsy is done in the outpatient or as an office procedure, without anesthesia.

Using Cusco's bivalve speculum, biopsy is taken from the suspected area or a four quadrant using punch biopsy forceps. Alternatively, the biopsy may be taken from the unstained area (white) when the cervix is painted with Schiller's iodine or colposcopic directed. Hemostasis is usually achieved by pressure with a gauze piece.

Wedge Biopsy

This is done when a definite growth is visible. Necrotic area is to be avoided. **An area nearer the edge is the ideal site**.

- Posterior vaginal speculum is introduced.
- Anterior or posterior lip of the cervix is to be held by Allis forceps.
- With a scalpel, a wedge of tissue is cut from the edge of the lesion **including adjacent healthy tissue for comparative histologic study**.
- Hemostasis may be achieved by gauze packing or by sutures.

Ring Biopsy

Whole of the squamocolumnar area of the cervix is excised with a special knife. The tissue is subjected to serial section to detect cervical intraepithelial neoplasia (CIN) or early invasive carcinoma. This is almost replaced by directed biopsy either Schiller or colposcopy.

Cone Biopsy (Cold knife Conization)

The operation involves removal of cone of the cervix which includes entire squamocolumnar junction, stroma with glands and endocervical mucous membrane.

Indications

Conization is done both for **diagnostic and therapeutic purposes in CIN** (Table 23.5):

- Diagnosis/confirmation of CIN, microinvasive or invasive carcinoma
- Treatment of CIN
- Carcinoma in situ (CIS)
- Unsatisfactory colposcopic findings. The entire margins of the lesion are not visualized.
- Inconsistent findings—colposcopic, cytology and directed biopsy.
- Positive endocervical curettage.
- When biopsy cannot rule out invasive cancer from carcinoma in situ (CIS) or microinvasion.

Procedures (Fig. 35.1)

The procedure is usually done with conventional knife (cold knife cone). It is done under general or regional anesthesia. It is also done with the help of CO_2 laser used as scalpel under colposcopic guidance with advantages.

Principal Steps (Cold Knife Conization)

- The operation is done under general anesthesia/regional anesthesia
- Blood loss is minimized with prior hemostatic sutures at 3 and 9 o'clock positions on the cervix by ligating the descending cervical branches.
- No. 11 blade or a Beaver blade (triangular in shape with a 45° bend) is used.
- Incision is first made on the lower lip of the cervix to avoid the bleeding to obscure the vision.
- The cone is cut so as to keep the apex below the internal os (Fig. 35.1).
- After the cone is removed, a margin suture is placed at 12 o'clock position for identification of the cone.
- Routine endocervical curette above the apex of the cone is performed and uterine curettage is done, if indicated (Table 35.1).
- Cone margins are repaired by hemostatic sutures. Sturmdorf hemostatic suture should not be used as it interferes with future colposcopic examination.

The excised cervical tissue is sent for histological examination (serial section–minimum 6). **If the margins of the cone are involved in neoplasia**, hysterectomy should be seriously considered either within 48 hours or at a later date (6 weeks) to avoid infection.

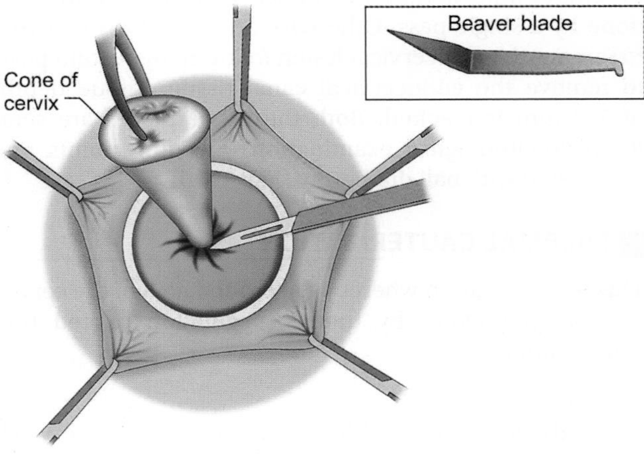

Fig. 35.1: Cone biopsy (knife).

TABLE 35.1: Advantages of laser over cold knife conization.

- Done in the outpatient under local anesthesia
- Less tissue damage and less blood loss
- Postoperative pain and discharge (morbidity)—less
- Regeneration of epithelium occurs earlier (3–4 weeks)
- All types of CIN can be treated
- Fertility and pregnancy outcome are not affected adversely

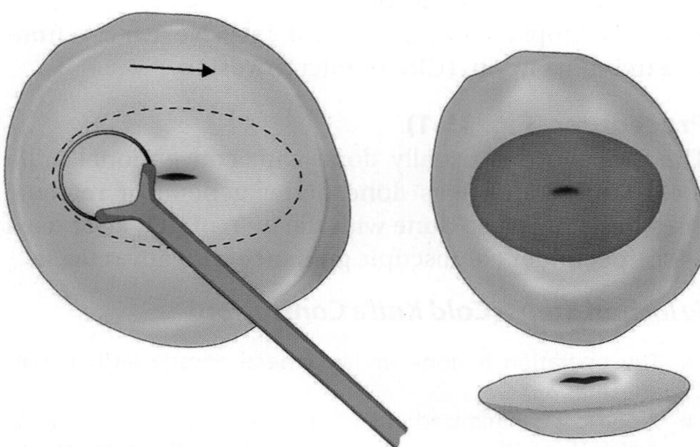

Fig. 35.2: The procedure of LLETZ and the excised tissue.

Complications

- Secondary hemorrhage.
- Cervical stenosis leading to hematometra.
- Infertility.
- Diminished cervical mucus.
- Cervical incompetence leading to recurrent miscarriage.
- Midtrimester abortion or preterm labor.

Large Loop Excision of the Transformation Zone (LLETZ) or Loop Electrosurgical Excision Procedure (LEEP)

Procedure: It is done under colposcopic guidance and with local anesthesia. Loop size is taken according to the size of the lesion. Cutting mode current (30–50 w) is passed. A deeper pass is made through the cervical stroma to remove a portion of the endocervical canal. It may be done by a single pass. Otherwise an initial pass is made to remove the ectocervical lesion followed by second pass to remove the endocervical canal tissue. Tissue depth of 5–8 mm is reached. Both the tissue pieces are sent for histopathological examination. Bleeding points are coagulated with ball diathermy (Fig. 35.2).

THERMAL CAUTERIZATION

This is an operation whereby the eroded area of the cervix is destroyed either by thermocoagulation or red hot cauterization.

Indication

Cervical ectopy with troublesome discharge. Prior cervical smear or biopsy if necessary, should be undertaken.

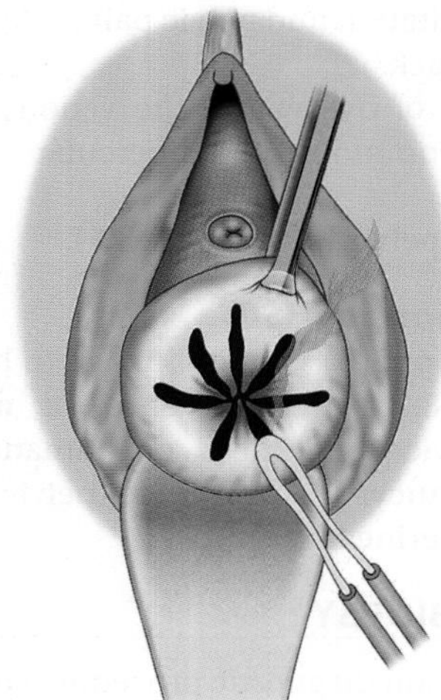

Fig. 35.3: Procedure of thermal cauterization.

Procedures (Fig. 35.3)

While the superficial cauterization can be done without anesthesia as an outdoor procedure but where extensive cauterization is required, it should be done under general anesthesia.

- Lower part of the cervical canal is dilated by one or two small dilators.
- The whole eroded area is cauterized by cautery point (Fig. 38.42) giving **linear radial strokes starting from inside the cervical canal to over the eroded area. The strokes should be made about 2 mm deep and at a distance of 1 cm.**
- The area is smeared with antibiotic ointment.

Healing

It takes about 2–3 weeks for sloughing of the burn area. Complete epithelialization by squamous epithelium occurs by 6–8 weeks.

Patient Information

There may be serosanguineous or even blood stained discharge for about 2–3 weeks.

Local (cream) and systemic antibiotic need to be given, when infection is there.

CRYOSURGERY

This is a procedure whereby destruction of the tissue is effective by freezing.

Indications

- Cervical ectopy (p. 220).
- Benign cervical lesions—such as cervical intraepithelial neoplasia (CIN), condyloma accuminata, leukoplakia, etc.
- Condyloma accuminata of vulva and VIN diagnosed colposcopically and not more than 2 cm in size.
- Vaginal intraepithelial neoplasia (VaIN), condyloma accuminata or vault granulation tissue following hysterectomy.
- As a palliative measure to arrest bleeding in carcinoma cervix or large fungating recurrent vulvar carcinoma.

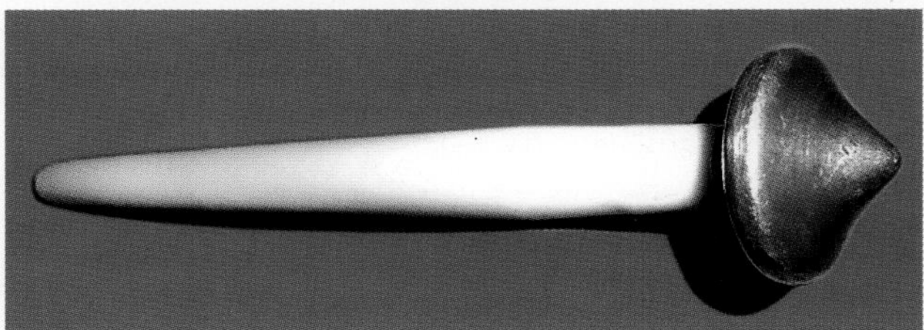

Fig. 35.4: Cryoprobe for cryodestruction of cervical lesions.

Principle

It consists of a 'probe' (Fig. 35.4), the tip of which is cooled to a temperature below freezing point (–60°C). **Freezing produces cellular dehydration by crystallization of intracellular water and ultimately death of cells.** This is effective by rapid expansion of gas which is passed through it. Carbon dioxide is widely used while nitrous oxide and liquid nitrogen are also used.

Procedures

This is an outpatient procedure and is done without anesthesia. Commonly used technique is freeze-thaw-freeze.

A probe that adequately covers the lesion is selected. The probe tip is lightly covered with water-soluble jelly to provide good thermal contact with the cervix.

The appropriate cryosurgery probe is applied to the cervix and the freezing activated. When a good iceball extending 4–5 mm beyond the edge of the probe is obtained, the freezing is stopped; the probe thawed (to raise the temperature above freezing point) and removed. The probe which adhered to the tissue should not be pulled out until the temperature rises again. Usually 90–180 seconds are required to obtain a satisfactory freeze. If necessary, a second time freezing technique may be employed to get a good result.

The application to the cervix freezes the tissue to a depth of about 3 mm.

Advantages over Thermal Cautery

- Anesthesia is not required
- Precise destruction of tissue
- There is no secondary hemorrhage
- Cervical stenosis is rare.

Drawbacks

There is excessive discharge for about 2–3 weeks.

Healing is complete in 6–10 weeks.

PERINEOPLASTY

Perineoplasty is the reconstruction of the narrow vaginal introitus to make it adequate for sexual function (Figs. 35.5A to C).

Indications are:

- Congenitally small introitus
- Rigid perineal body
- Rigid hymenal ring
- Narrowed introitus following overzealous perineorrhaphy or episiotomy repair.

Principal Steps

- A longitudinal incision is made in the midline from above (2 cm) the fourchette to the skin of the perineum below (2 cm) (Fig. 35.5A).
- The incision is deepened through the vaginal mucosa, skin, and the perineal body.
- Mobilization of the vaginal mucosa and perineal skin is done.
- Two gloves are worn on the left hand. Left index finger is passed into the rectum and it is hooked upwards and outwards, while the superficial perineal muscles are divided.
- Finally, the wound is sutured in layers transversely by using interrupted sutures (Figs. 35.5B and C).

In **Fenton's method,** a transverse incision is made along the fourchette.

Repair of complete perineal tear (p. 362).

AMPUTATION OF CERVIX

Amputation is an operative procedure whereby a part of the lower cervix is excised.

Indications

- Congenital elongation.
- Chronic cervicitis with hypertrophied cervix not relieved by conventional therapy.
- As a component part of Fothergill's operation to rectify the supravaginal elongation.

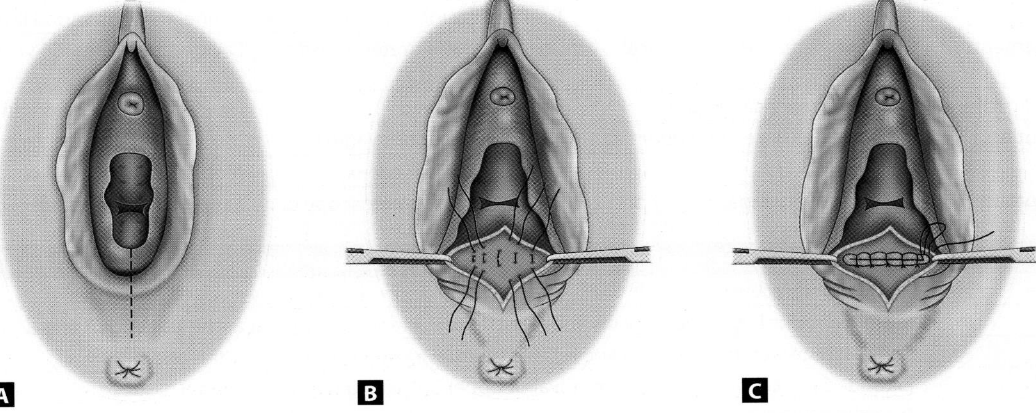

Figs. 35.5A to C: Perineoplasty. (A) Longitudinal incision on the perineum; (B and C) Divided perineal muscles are sutured transversely.

Guidelines

The following practical guidelines are formulated:

- Except in congenital elongation, prior exclusion of malignancy should be done (Pap smear, p. 89).
- High amputation is to be avoided in cases where future childbirth prospect is retained. High amputation may produce cervical incompetency.

Principal Steps

Initial steps are same as that of cold knife cone biopsy (p. 495).

- A circumferential incision is made around the cervix and vaginal mucosa is separated from the stroma of the cervix.
- A cone-shaped amputation is done and the cut margins are repaired with hemostatic mattress sutures.
- Raw surfaces of the cervix are covered by the Bonney-Sturmdorf suture using a cutting needle (Figs. 16.19A to D).

Complications

Immediate complications include:

- Hemorrhage—both primary and secondary.
- Sepsis.

Remote complications include:

- Cervical stenosis leading to hematometra.
- Cervical incompetency leading to midtrimester abortion.
- Secondary cervical dystocia during labor.

MAJOR SURGICAL OPERATIONS

Major surgical operations—vaginal or abdominal are in the domain of specialists conversant with gynecologic surgery. It is indeed difficult to make the students understand the techniques of the operations with language. As such, utmost attempt has been made to make them familiar with the **principal steps** of some such common operations with diagrams.

ABDOMINAL HYSTERECTOMY

Hysterectomy is the operation of removal of uterus. When the uterus is removed abdominally, it is called **abdominal hysterectomy.**

Types

Depending upon the extent of removal of the uterus and adjacent structures, the following types are described:

- **Total hysterectomy:** Removal of the entire uterus.
- **Subtotal:** Removal of the body or corpus leaving behind the cervix.
- **Panhysterectomy:** Removal of the uterus along with removal of tubes and ovaries of both sides. **The term 'hysterectomy with bilateral salpingo-oophorectomy' is preferred.**
- **Extended hysterectomy:** Panhysterectomy with removal of cuff of vagina.
- **Radical hysterectomy:** Removal of the uterus, tubes and ovaries of both the sides, upper one-third of vagina, adjacent parametrium, and the draining lymph nodes of the cervix.

Indications

The indications are grouped as shown in the Tables 35.3 and 35.4.

TABLE 35.2: Types of radical hysterectomy.

	Simple extrafascial hysterectomy	*Modified radical hysterectomy*	*Radical hysterectomy*
Piver and Rutledge classification	Type I	Type II	Type III
Querleu and Morrow classification	Type A	Type B	Type C
Indication	Stage IA1	Type IA1 with LVSI, IA2	Stage IB1 and IB2, selected Stage IIA
Uterus and cervix	Removed	Removed	Removed
Ovaries	Optional removal	Optional removal	Optional removal
Vaginal margin	None	1–2 cm	Upper one-quarter to one-third
Ureters	Not mobilized	Tunnel through broad ligament	Tunnel through broad ligament
Cardinal ligaments	Divided at uterine and cervical border	Divided where ureter transits broad ligaments	Divided at pelvic side wall
Uterosacral ligaments	Divided at cervical border	Partially removed	Divided near sacral origin
Urinary bladder	Mobilized to base of bladder	Mobilized to upper vagina	Mobilized to middle vagina
Rectum	Not mobilized	Mobilized below cervix	Mobilized below cervix
Surgical approach	Laparotomy or laparoscopy or robotic surgery	Laparotomy or laparoscopy or robotic surgery	Laparotomy or laparoscopy or robotic surgery
European Organization for Research and Treatment for Cancer			
Type I	Simple hysterectomy		
Type II	Modified radical hysterectomy (as above)+ Uterine arteries are ligated at the site of crossing ureters		
Type III	Radical hysterectomy (same as above) and uterine arteries are ligated at the origin		
Type IV	Extended radical hysterectomy, removal of upper 3/4 of vagina + paravaginal tissues		
Type V	Partial exenteration		
Type II–V	Completed with bilateral pelvic lymphadenectomy		

TABLE 35.3: Indications of abdominal hysterectomy.

Benign lesions	■ Done in the outpatient under local anesthesia ■ Dysfunctional uterine bleeding ■ Fibroid uterus ■ Tubo-ovarian mass ■ Endometriosis ■ Adenomyosis ■ CIN ■ Endometrial hyperplasia ■ Benign ovarian tumor in perimenopausal age
Malignancy	■ Carcinoma cervix ■ Carcinoma ovary ■ Carcinoma endometrium ■ Uterine sarcoma ■ Choriocarcinoma
Traumatic	■ Uterine perforation ■ Cervical tear ■ Rupture uterus
Obstetrical	■ Atonic postpartum hemorrhage (PPH) ■ Morbid adherent placenta ■ Hydatidiform mole >35 years ■ Septic abortion

TABLE 35.4: Common indications of abdominal hysterectomy.

Total	■ DUB ■ TO mass	■ Uterine fibroid ■ Endometriosis
Subtotal	■ Difficult TO mass ■ Endometriosis (rectovaginal septum) ■ Obstetric causes	
Panhysterectomy	■ Indications for total hysterectomy in perimenopausal age	
Extended Radical	■ Carcinoma endometrium ■ Carcinoma cervix-stage I and II	

Some Considerations of Hysterectomy (Benign Lesions)

Age and parity: An ideal condition is that the patient preferably be in the perimenopausal age group with family completed. However, the operation may have to be done under forced circumstances even in comparatively young age group or unmarried or nulliparous women (e.g. contemplating myomectomy).

Total or subtotal: The preferred surgery is always a total hysterectomy unless there is sufficient reason to leave behind the cervix. **The indications of subtotal (supracervical) hysterectomy are**:

- Difficult tubo-ovarian mass with obliteration of the anterior and posterior pouches.
- Pelvic endometriosis particularly involving the recto-vaginal septum.
- Emergency hysterectomy (cesarean hysterectomy).

Advantages of Subtotal (Supracervical) Hysterectomy

Controversy exists as regard the usefulness of subtotal hysterectomy. **The benefits mentioned are:** Reduced operative and postoperative morbidity, reduced vaginal shortening and vault prolapse, and increased sexual satisfaction. Hospital stay is shorter. Papanicolaou cervical smear must be normal before contemplating supracervical hysterectomy. It should be maintained as a routine follow-up (Table 9.1).

The risks of the cervical stump left behind are:

- Cervicitis with abnormal vaginal discharge
- Stump carcinoma may develop (1%).

Preservation of ovaries: Amidst controversy, it seems rational to preserve the ovaries in premenopausal women if they are found healthy (Table 35.5). Some however, remove the ovaries beyond 45 years and preserve the same before that age, if found healthy.

Special Considerations for Removal of Ovaries

- If the ovaries are diseased in inflammatory process, advanced endometriosis or involved in neoplastic conditions with the patient's age is 45 years or older.
- Hysterectomy done in a woman of any age who has a history of ovarian or breast cancer in first degree relative.
- Postmenopausal women as a routine.

Hormone replacement therapy is to be considered when ovaries are removed (p. 50).

Removal of Fallopian Tubes

The uterine tubes are removed:

- When the ovaries are removed (salpingo-oophorectomy).
- When the tubes are diseased but ovaries are conserved (salpingectomy) due to young age or salpingectomy for consideration of IVF (p. 206).
- **Risk reducing surgery:** Prophylactic salpingectomy to prevent ovarian cancer (p. 322).

Steps of Operation (Benign Lesion)

Preoperative Work-up

For detail p. 488.

Principal Steps (Figs. 35.6A to L)

- Abdomen is opened either by a low transverse or intraumbilical paramedian or midline incision.
- The uterus is drawn out of the wound.
- Doyen's retractor is placed in position.
- The patient is placed in Trendelenburg position.
- The bowels and omentum are packed off from the operative area.
- The pelvic organs are examined. The decision of preserving or removing the adnexae is made.
- The traction of the uterus is given by either using vulsellum or placing long artery forceps on either side of the uterine cornu (myoma screw is used in fibroid). The uterus is pulled to one side while clamps are placed on the contralateral side.
- **If the ovaries are to be removed** (Fig. 35.6A), paired clamps (two long straight artery forceps) are placed in the infundibulopelvic (IP) ligament. A window is created in the broad ligament medial to the IP ligament before the clamps are placed.

  The tissues in between are cut and replaced by transfixation sutures (Vicryl no. '0' or chromic catgut no. '1').

Contd...

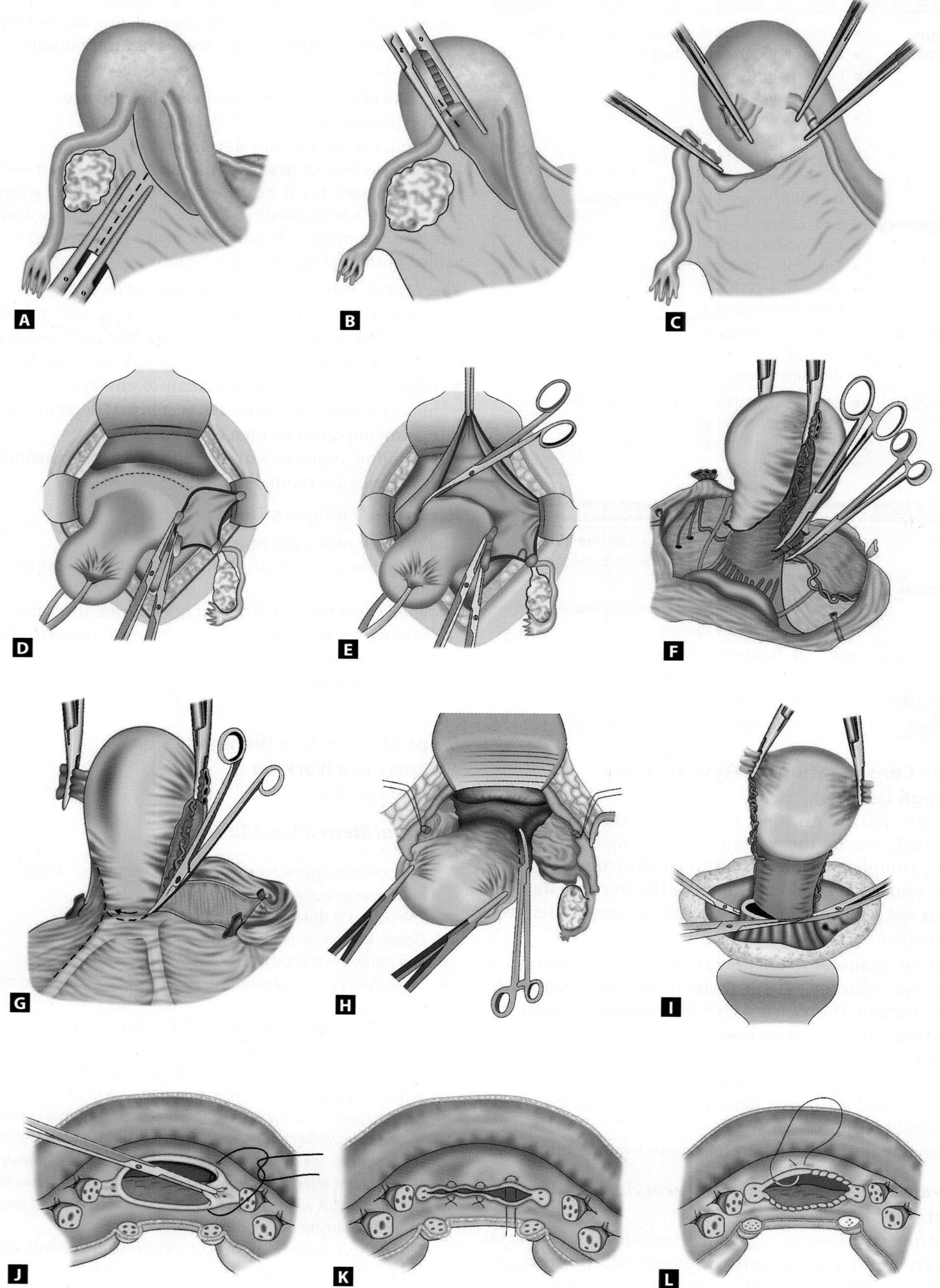

Figs. 35.6A to L: Principal steps of abdominal hysterectomy.

Contd...

- **If the ovaries are to be preserved** (Fig. 35.6B), the paired clamps are placed near the cornu of the uterus to include fallopian tube, mesosalpinx containing uterine vessels and ovarian ligament. The structures are cut in between the clamps and replaced by transfixation sutures (Vicryl no. '0' or chromic catgut no. '1').
- Paired clamps are placed on the round ligament, cut and replaced by sutures (Vicryl no. '0' or chromic catgut no. '1') (Fig. 35.6C).
- Similar procedures up to this stage are followed on the other side.
- **Loose peritoneum** of the uterovesical fold (Figs. 35.6D, E and 35.7 is cut and extended from one divided round ligament to the other. The bladder is pushed down and out with gauze added with scissors stripping till the anterior vaginal wall is reached. **This will minimize injury to the bladder and ureters in subsequent steps of operation.**
- Paired clamps are placed on the parametrium containing ascending branch of the uterine artery, close to the uterus at the level of internal os. The tissues in between are cut with the scalpel and replaced by ligature (Vicryl no. '0' or catgut no. '1'). Similar step is followed on the other side (Fig. 35.6F).
- The uterus is now pulled forwards to make the uterosacral ligaments prominent. Clamps are placed over the uterosacral ligaments as close to the cervix. The ligaments are cut. The peritoneum in between the ligaments is dissected down with scissors and finger. The clamps are replaced by sutures (same suture material) (Fig. 35.6G).
- Clamps are placed close to the cervix on the paracervical tissue (Mackenrodt's) containing descending cervical artery, cut and replaced by ligature (same suture material). Similar step is followed to the other side (Fig. 35.6H).
- Vault of the vagina is opened by a stab incision with a scalpel at the cervicovaginal junction. The remaining vault of the vagina is cut while traction is given with a single toothed vulsellum on the cervix (Fig. 35.6I).
- The edges of the cut vaginal vault are grasped by Allis forceps (Fig. 35.6J).
- Lateral vaginal angles are closed by transfixation suture (Fig. 35.6J).
- Vault is closed by interrupted sutures (Fig. 35.6K) or the free vaginal margin is reefed with a continuous locking suture (Fig. 35.6L).
- Pelvic peritonization may be done (optional) by running sutures using catgut no. '0'.
- Abdominal packs are removed; peritoneal toileting is done.
- Abdomen is closed in layers.

TABLE 35.5: Benefits and risks of ovarian conservation during hysterectomy.

Benefits	*Risks*
▪ Ovarian function continues till the expected time of spontaneous menopause ▪ Menopausal symptoms (p. 46) appear late and the severity is less ▪ Decreased incidence of vasomotor symptoms, osteoporosis and atherosclerotic changes	▪ Risks of developing ovarian neoplasms (benign or malignant). Relative risk (RR) of ovarian cancer is 0.6 even 10 years after hysterectomy ▪ Residual ovarian syndrome occurs in 1–3% of cases due to multiple cystic follicles and/or periovarian adhesions ▪ Chronic pelvic pain and dyspareunia ▪ Risk of relaparotomy in 3–5%

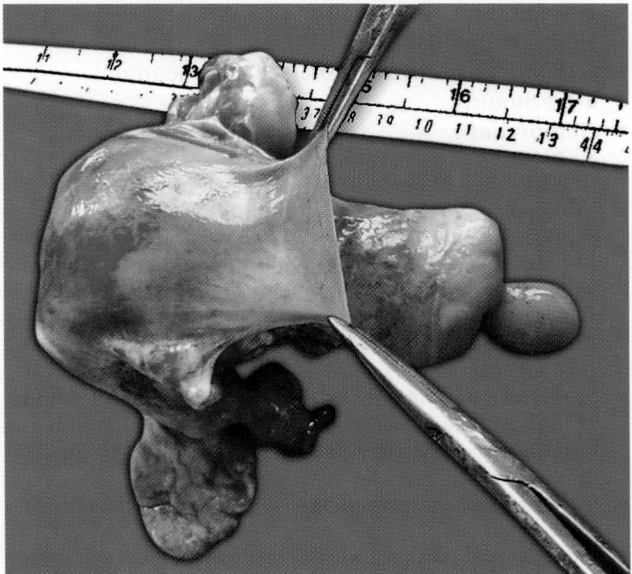

Fig. 35.7: Uterovesical fold of peritoneum dissected out during hysterectomy.

POSTOPERATIVE COMPLICATIONS AND CARE

COMPLICATIONS OF HYSTERECTOMY

- **Intraoperative** (during operation)
- **Postoperative:** (a) Immediate; (b) Late; (c) Remote

Intraoperative

- Hemorrhage
- Visceral injury: Intestine, bladder or ureter
- Anesthetic hazard: Atelectasis, pulmonary edema, embolism.

Postoperative

Immediate

- Hypovolemia (hemorrhagic) → shock.
- *Urinary*:
  - Retention due to pain and spasm
  - Cystitis
  - Anuria may be due to inadequate fluid replacement (prerenal) or ureteric obstruction (postrenal).

Late

- **Incontinence**
  - **Overflow** due to prolonged overdistension of the bladder.
  - **Stress** due to prolonged catheterization.
  - **True**—if occurs immediately after operation, it is caused by injury to the bladder or ureter (p. 349). If occurs 7–14 days after operation, it is due to sloughing and necrosis either of the bladder or ureters (VVF or UVF p. 351).
- **Pyrexia**—fever may be due to:
  - Cystitis (due to catheterization)
  - Abdominal wound infection

- Vault cellulitis, hematoma
- Thrombophlebitis
- Pulmonary infection, atelectasis, pneumonia
- Peritonitis.

- **Hemorrhage**
  - ***Primary***: It is due to slipping of the ligature usually that of the vaginal angle. Hemostasis can be achieved by the vaginal route under general anesthesia. Care is to be taken to prevent bite of the ureter in the suture. If the procedure fails, laparotomy has to be done for hemostasis.
  - ***Secondary***: This type of hemorrhage occurs between 7–14 days after operation and is due to sepsis. Bleeding source may be from the vault or internally (rare) from the sloughing uterine or ovarian artery.
- **From the vault**, hemostasis can be achieved by interrupted or mattress suture using 'Vicryl' under general anesthesia. In cases of recurrences, one may have to tackle the situation through abdominal route as mentioned below.
- **Intraperitoneal hemorrhage** which is fortunately rare, laparotomy has to be done along with resuscitative procedures. If the uterine artery is involved, anterior division of the internal iliac artery has to be tied to secure hemostasis.
- ***Hematomas:*** In the pelvis or rectus sheath may cause low grade temperature. Large hematomas should be drained.
- ***Wound dehiscence*** is seen commonly with vertical incision. Patients with infection, immune suppression, and malignancy are at high risk.
- ***Paralytic ileus and intestinal obstruction:*** Postoperative bowel dysfunction may be due to ileus or obstruction (Table 35.6).
- ***Necrotizing fascitis*** is a rare but life-threatening complication. Infection is in the superficial and subcutaneous tissues. There is extensive tissue necrosis. Supportive therapy, wide tissue debridement and antibiotics are the management.
- ***Phlebitis:*** Intravenous cannula related phlebitis causes pain, redness, and fever. Venous cannula should be removed and antibiotic should be continued.
- ***Deep vein thrombosis (DVT):*** It is not an uncommon problem. Calf veins are commonly affected. It is associated with low grade fever, pain, and swelling of the affected cuff. B-mode ultrasound can detect an intramural clot. Heparin is administered intravenously (30,000–40,000 units/24 hours) once the diagnosis is confirmed. Activated partial thromboplastin time (APTT) is maintained at 1.5–2.5 times the control. Heparin is replaced by warfarin orally after 5 days and it is continued for 4–6 weeks. Low molecular weight heparin (Fragmin) 2500 U SC every 24 hours or low dose heparin 5000 U SC every 12 hours, starting 1–2 hours before surgery, for 5–7 days is recommended as a preventive measure against venous thromboembolism.
- ***Pulmonary embolism*** is a rare but fatal complication. Patient commonly presents with sudden onset of chest pain, dyspnea, tachycardia, tachypnea, and hemoptysis. Arterial blood gas analysis, D-dimer level (negative) ventilation/perfusion scan and contrast pulmonary angiography, spiral CT are the diagnostic aids. Ventilation-perfusion scan reveals areas with decreased perfusion but adequate ventilation. Heparin is the drug of choice. Thrombolytic therapy (recombinant human plasminogen activator) clear the emboli more rapidly when infused IV. Pulmonary artery embolectomy or inferior vena cava filter placement may have to be considered for massive pulmonary embolus. Warfarin should be started orally after 2–3 days of heparinization. Heparin is withdrawn once the therapeutic level of warfarin is obtained. Dose of warfarin is aimed to prolong the prothrombin time. International normalized ratio (INR) is maintained at 2.0 to 3.0.

TABLE 35.6: Postoperative bowel dysfunction: Ileus versus obstruction.

Ileus	*Obstruction*
Distension: Present	Present
Pain: Mild due to distension	Progressively severe due to cramps
Bowel sounds: Absent	Peristaltic rushes
Vomiting: Present	Present
Onset: Within 48–72 hours of surgery	Delayed 5–7 days postoperative
X-ray: Loops of small and large bowel distended with gas	Distended bowel loops with air-fluid level
Treatment: Conservative: nasogastric suction, intravenous fluids, enemas, correction of electrolyte imbalance, and control of infection	Initial conservative; may need surgical intervention

Remote Complications of Hysterectomy

- **Vault granulation:** It is more with catgut and less with Vicryl.
- **Vault prolapse:** Less compared to vaginal.
- **Incisional hernia:** More with midline vertical incision than with low transverse one.
- Prolapse of the fallopian tube through the vault (rare).
- Depression, psychiatric symptoms.
- Sexual dysfunction.

Comments: Vaginal hysterectomy is the ideal method if not contraindicated. In the hands of an expert conversant with vaginal hysterectomy even in undescended uterus, vaginal hysterectomy is the method of choice. This route still offers benefits (Tables 35.7 and 35.8).

COMPLICATIONS OF VAGINAL HYSTERECTOMY AND OTHER OPERATIONS

- **Vaginal hysterectomy:** p. 185, 186.
- **Laparoscopic-assisted vaginal hysterectomy (LAVH)** (p. 518), does have some superiority over traditional vaginal hysterectomy even in an undescended uterus. Pelvic adhesions (endometriosis) can be dealt under vision with operative laparoscopy. The cost of the former is very high whereas perioperative morbidity is the same.
- **Pelvic floor repair (PFR)**—p. 180.
- **Fothergill's or Manchester operation**—p. 180.
- **Operations for vault prolapse**—p. 183.
- **Cervicopexy** (sling or Purandare's Operation)—p. 183.
- **Complications of vaginal operations**—p. 183.

TABLE 35.7: Abdominal hysterectomy.

Advantages	*Disadvantages*
▪ Scope of wide exploration of the abdominal and pelvic organs (ovaries, appendix, gallbladder, etc.)	▪ Difficult to perform in too obese patients
▪ Tubo-ovarian pathology can be tackled effectively and simultaneously	▪ Postoperative complications are slightly high. There is increased incidence of peritonitis, fever, pulmonary, and vascular complications
▪ Concurrent surgical procedures (appendicectomy) may be performed when needed	▪ More postoperative pain and more need of analgesia
▪ Operation can be done by a relatively less experienced surgeon with average skill	▪ More hospital stay
	▪ Delayed resumption in day-to-day activities
	▪ Morbidity and mortality are more compared to a vaginal hysterectomy
	▪ Presence of abdominal scar

TABLE 35.8: Vaginal hysterectomy (p. 182).

Advantages	*Disadvantages*
▪ Can be effectively done in obese patients	▪ More skill and experience are needed on the part of the surgeon
▪ Postoperative complications are less	▪ Exploration of abdominal and pelvic organs cannot be done
▪ Less morbidity and mortality	▪ Difficult in cases with restricted uterine mobility, limited vaginal space, and associated adnexal pathology
▪ Less postoperative pain and less need of analgesia	▪ Limitation in cases with: Uterus >12 weeks of size, presence of pelvic adhesions or, previous history of laparotomy with adhesions
▪ Less hospital stay	
▪ Early resumption of day-to-day activities	
No abdominal incision and scar	

OPERATIONS ON THE OVARY

OVARIAN CYSTECTOMY (FIGS. 35.8A TO C)

Removal of the ovarian cyst leaving behind the healthy ovarian tissue is called ovarian cystectomy.

It is the operation of choice especially when both the ovaries are involved with benign neoplasm in young women.

Principal Steps

- Incision (elliptical) is made with a scalpel through the ovarian cortex at the base of the ovarian cyst on the antimesenteric surface (Fig. 35.8A).
- The cyst wall is separated gently, using the handle of the scalpel or by scissors and the cyst is shelled out without rupture (Fig. 35.8B).
- The dead space is obliterated using (4–0) absorbable sutures. Ovarian surface is approximated using very fine interrupted sutures (Fig. 35.8C).

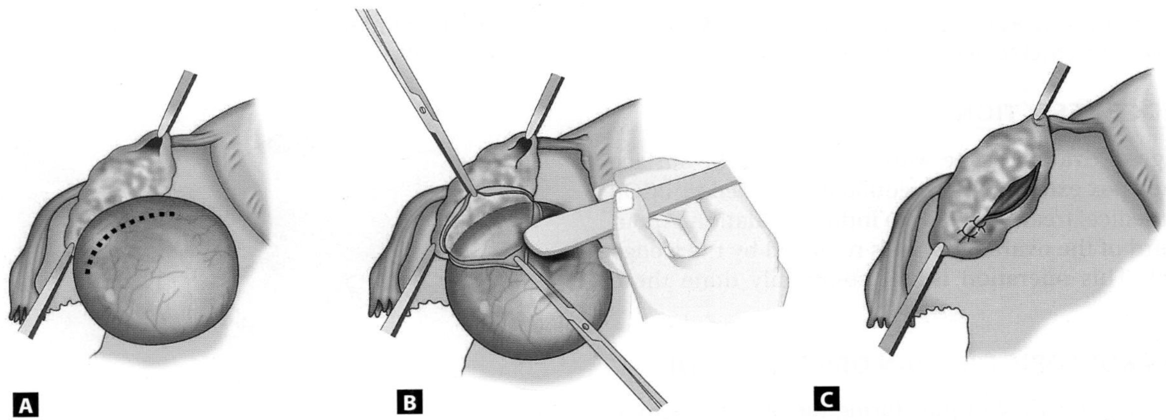

Figs. 35.8A to C: Steps of ovarian cystectomy: (A) Line of incision; (B) Enucleation of the cyst; (C) Closure of the ovarian incision.

OVARIOTOMY (FIGS. 35.9A TO D)

Removal of the tumor along with healthy ovarian tissue is called ovariotomy. The term is better replaced by oophorectomy. This is indicated when the tumor is big or complicated by torsion or hemorrhage and the other ovary is healthy.

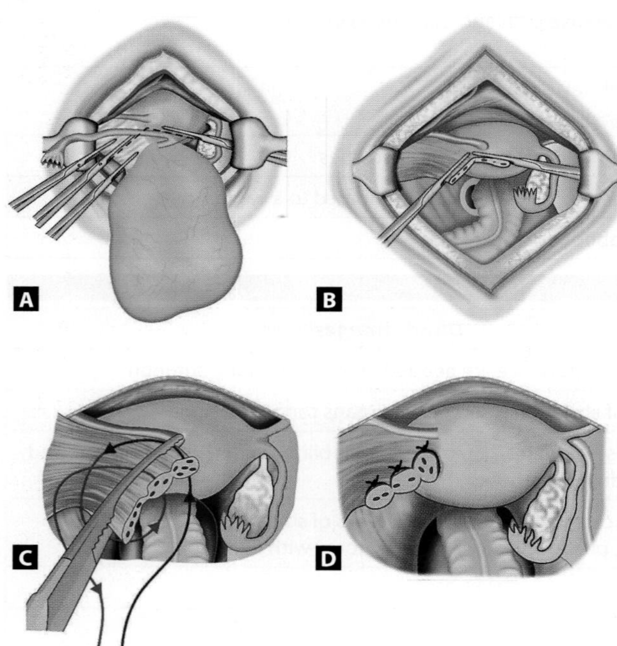

Figs. 35.9A to D: Steps of ovariotomy. (A) Clamps are placed on either side of the ovarian pedicle; (B) Removal of tumor with the clamps placed over the pedicle; (C) The clamps are replaced by sutures, the lateral one by transfixing. To note the placement of transfixation suture; (D) Look of the pedicle after the operation site.

Principal Steps

- Paired clamps are placed laterally over the infundibulopelvic fold of peritoneum with its contents. Medial pair of clamps are applied on the side of uterus to include the ovarian ligament and the fallopian tube (Fig. 35.9A).
- Pedicles are cut in between and the tumor is removed (Fig. 35.9B).
- Clamps are replaced by transfixing ligatures (Fig. 35.9C).
- Pedicles are checked carefully for hemostasis (Fig. 35.9D).

WEDGE RESECTION

A wedge of ovarian tissue with the base on the surface and the apex extending to medulla is removed in PCOS when medical treatment fails to induce ovulation. About one-third of the ovarian tissue is removed by the wedge method. This operation is not commonly done these days.

LAPAROSCOPIC OVARIAN DRILLING (LOD)

LOD is the procedure of puncturing the ovarian capsule by electrodiathermy needle or with laser beam (Fig. 38.49)

Procedure: It is done under general or regional anesthesia following patient positioning. Three ports are made in addition to the camera port at the umbilicus. The ovary is lifted up with a blunt grasper. The electrosurgical current used is around 40 Watts, cutting mode. Monopolar electrosurgery needle, with sharp tip is used to puncture the ovarian capsule, perpendicular to the surface.

OVARIAN BIOPSY

This is indicated for histological confirmation of any diagnosis (malignancy) or for the problem of intersexuality.

SALPINGECTOMY (FIG. 35.10)

One pair of long hemostatic forceps is placed on the medial end of the fallopian tube including the mesosalpinx as close to the uterus. A second pair of clamp is placed from the lateral aspect on the mesosalpinx. The clamp tips are to be approximated. The tube is excised and the clamps are replaced by ligatures. **The excised tube is to be sent for histology**.

SALPINGO-OOPHORECTOMY

Removal of the ovary and the fallopian tube:

Indications: (a) Pathologically enlarged ovary (>8–10 cm); (b) Adhesion pain (tubo-ovarian mass); (c) Pathological ovary where malignant potential is high.

Procedure: Identification of the ipsilateral infundibulo-pelvic (IP) ligament, ureter and the ovarian ligament is to be done. The peritoneum within the area bounded by the round ligament, IP ligament and external iliac vessels is tented with a tissue forceps and incised. It is extended both laterally and medially toward the uterus. A peritoneal window is created and enlarged with blunt dissection. The IP ligament is clamped (double). The IP ligament is cut in between the closed clamps and transfixed (1–0 Vicryl) Fig. 35.9A to D. On the medial side clamp (double) is placed on the ovarian ligament and the fallopian tube incorporating the mesosalpinx and mesovarium. The tip of the clamps meet/overlap each other (Fig. 35.9). The pedicle is cut in between the clamps. The freed adnexa is removed. The pedicle is transfixed (Fig. 35.9). The broad ligament leaves are closed. Specimen is sent for histopathology examination. Salpingo-oophorectomy can also be done laparoscopically.

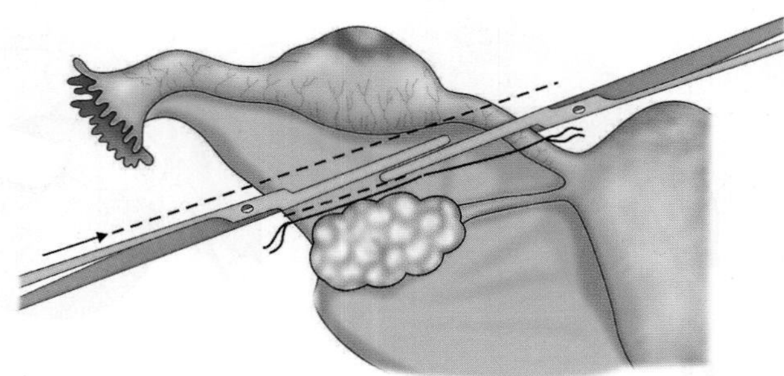

Fig. 35.10: Salpingectomy.

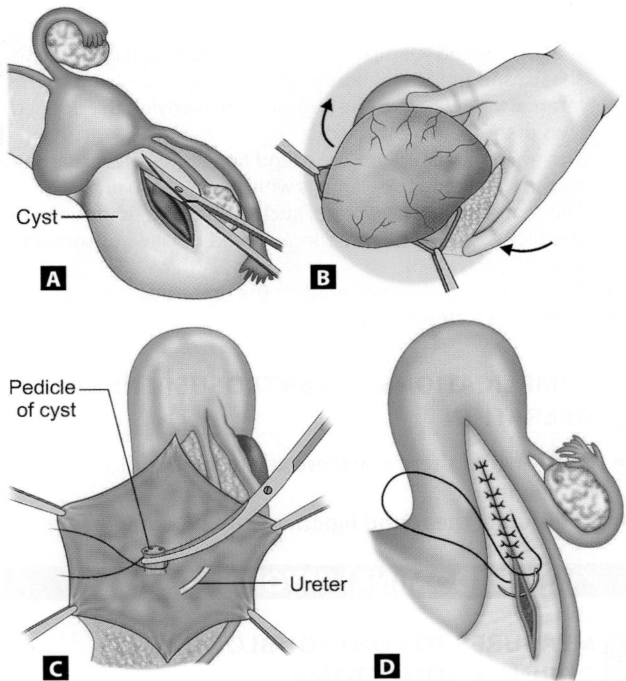

Figs. 35.11A to D: Broad ligament cyst: (A) Post-box incision on the anterior leaf of broad ligament parallel to the round ligament; (B) Enucleation of the cyst; (C) Hemostatic suture placed on the pedicle on the cyst. Note the position of the ureter; (D) Closure of the peritoneum.

BROAD LIGAMENT CYST OR LEIOMYOMA (FIGS. 35.11A TO D)

- Post box incision is made with a knife on the anterior leaf of the broad ligament making parallel to the round ligament (Fig. 35.11A).
- Fingers are used to separate the tumor from the leaves of broad ligament up to the base (Fig. 35.11B). In a case of fibroid, the capsule is incised and the myoma is enucleated from its bed by sharp and blunt dissection.

Contd...

Contd...

- Position of the ureter is checked and a clamp is placed on the tumor pedicle.
- The pedicle is cut and the clamp is replaced by a ligature (Fig. 35.11C).
- The leaves of broad ligament are closed with a continuous suture (Fig. 35.11D).

OPERATIONS FOR INVERSION OF THE UTERUS

HAULTAIN'S OPERATION (FIG. 35.12A)

Principle of the Operation

This is done abdominally. Correction of inversion is done after cutting the posterior rim of the cup-like depression (Fig. 35.12A).

Principal Steps

- Antiseptic cleaning of the vagina is done preoperatively.
- Abdomen is opened with the patient in Trendelenburg position.
- The ring of tissue is grasped by Allis forceps. A vertical incision is made on the midline at the posterior rim.
- A finger is passed through the incision and the inverted fundus is pushed up. An assistant may also push up inverted fundus through the vagina.
- Uterine incision is repaired with chromic catgut sutures in two layers.

KUSTNER'S OPERATION (FIGS. 35.12B AND C)

This is a vaginal procedure.

Principal Steps

- Uterus is drawn upwards and forwards by a single tooth vulsellum holding at the fundus.
- Pouch of Douglas is opened by a transverse incision made on the posterior vaginal wall.
- Left index finger is introduced along the hollow of the inverted uterus. Posterior uterine wall is cut through by a scalpel from fundus to the external os (Fig. 35.12B).

Contd...

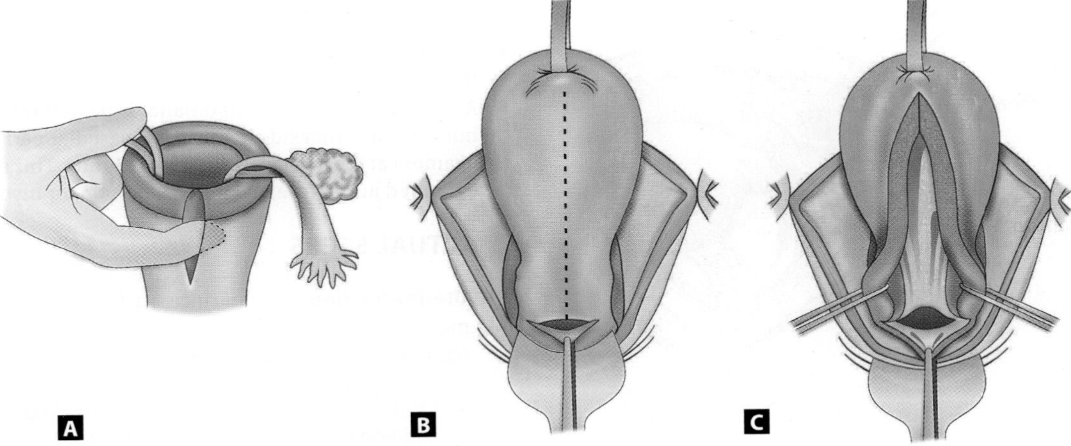

Figs. 35.12A to C: Operations for inversion of the uterus: (A) Haultain's operation; (B and C) Kustner's operation.

Contd...

- The inverted uterus is then turned inside out and inversion is corrected.
- Repair of the incised uterine wall is done with Vicryl (1–0) or chromic catgut sutures in two layers.
- Repair of the pouch of Douglas and posterior vaginal wall is done.

Spinelli's operation is a vaginal procedure and principle is the same as that of Kustner. Here uterovesical pouch is opened and uterine incision is made on the anterior wall.

VENTROSUSPENSION OPERATION

This operation is less commonly performed these days. It is done to prevent adhesions over the posterior uterine surface following: (a) Myomectomy operation; (b) Operation for endometriosis, where the uterus is bulky.

It may be done by: (a) Plication of the round ligaments; (b) modified Gilliam procedure; or (c) By laparoscopic suspension operation.

Actual steps: Abdomen is opened by suprapubic transverse incision.

Plication of the round ligaments

Reefing suture is passed through the substance of the round ligaments extending from the internal abdominal ring up to the myometrium at the cornu of the uterus. Suture material used is either chromic catgut or Vicryl. The suture is tied firmly at the end. Similar procedure is done on the other side. The round ligaments are shortened and the uterus is thus anteverted.

MODIFIED GILLIAM PROCEDURE

Principal Steps (Fig. 35.13)

- Each round ligament is sutured with no. 1 chromic catgut about 3–4 cm from the cornu of the uterus. This is left untied and used for traction.

Contd...

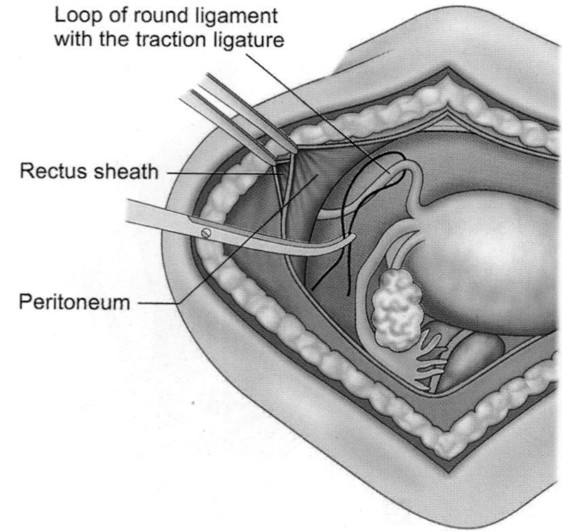

Fig. 35.13: Modified Gilliam procedure.

Contd...

- A long curved clamp is introduced between the rectus sheath and the lateral border of the rectus muscle up to the internal inguinal ring. The peritoneum overlying the opened jaws of the clamp is incised.
- The traction ligature on the round ligament is now grasped by the clamp and the clamp is withdrawn gradually.
- The loop of round ligament, such withdrawn, is sutured to the rectus sheath by three interrupted delayed absorbable sutures (Vicryl 1–0).
- Similar procedure is repeated on the other side.
- Abdomen is closed in layers.

COMPLICATIONS OF VENTROSUSPENSION OPERATION

- Pain—when there is excessive stretching of the round ligaments.
- Avulsion of the round ligament and bleeding—rare.

ABDOMINAL MYOMECTOMY

MEASURES TO CONTROL BLOOD LOSS DURING MYOMECTOMY

- Preoperative treatment with GnRH analog reduces the vascularity of the tumor and thereby reduces operative blood loss (p. 233).
- Use of vasoconstrictive agents—commonly used is vasopressin (synthetic). 20 units/mL of vasopressin diluted in 20–50 mL of normal saline is injected into the myometrium overlying the myoma.
- **Vasopressin** decreases blood loss significantly. Needle aspiration prior to injection is imperative to avoid intravascular injection. Anaesthetist is informed beforehand as sudden increase in blood pressure may occur. Blanching of myometrium is common. Plasma half-life is 10–20 minutes and injection should be stopped 20 minutes prior to uterine repair.

  Complications are due to inadvertent intravascular injection. This results in rise in BP, bradycardia, atrioventricular shock and pulmonary edema.
- Use of Victor Bonney's especially designed clamp (Fig. 38.22) to reduce uterine artery blood flow. This clamp is placed around the uterine vessels and the round ligament.
- Use of tourniquets—to occlude the uterine vessels and also the ovarian vessels at the infundibulopelvic ligament.
- A soft plastic tube (less traumatic) is passed through a small hole one on either side made in an avascular part of the broad ligament at the level of the uterine isthmus. This tourniquet is tightened just before making the incision for myomectomy.

ACTUAL STEPS

- **Uterine incision**—a single incision (linear or elliptical) in the midline on the anterior wall of the uterus is preferred. This has the following **advantages**:
  - Avoids any injury to the tube and ovary.
  - Lateral fibroids are removed by tunneling without any additional scar on the uterine surface.

Contd...

Contd...

- **Uterine incision**—a single incision (linear or elliptical) in the midline on the anterior wall of the uterus is preferred. This has the following **advantages:**
  - Avoids any injury to the tube and ovary.
  - Lateral fibroids are removed by tunneling without any additional scar on the uterine surface.
  - Fibroids from the cavity or posterior wall can be removed by transcavity approach. This avoids scar on the posterior wall and adhesion formation.
- **Incision is deepened** through the myometrium and the (pseudo) capsule, till the myoma is reached.
- **Myoma enucleation:** The myoma is grasped with a single toothed vulsellum and dissection is continued in the plane between the myoma and the capsule (to minimize blood loss). Myoma is enucleated (intracapsular) from its bed by sharp (scissors) and blunt (knife handle) dissection.
- **The myoma bed** (deep space) is obliterated by interrupted mattress or figure-of-eight suture using (1-0) Vicryl. Sometimes layers of sutures (tire stitch) may be required to approximate the myometrium (Fig. 35.14).
- When endometrial cavity is opened up it is repaired with a running suture of 4–0 or 5–0 delayed absorbable suture material.
- **Bonney's hood operation** is done to remove a large fundal myoma. A low transverse incision is made on the myoma over the anterior uterine surface. After enucleation of the myoma, the capsule is trimmed and is sewn over the anterior uterine wall. This minimizes adhesion formation (Fig. 35.15).
- The serous coat of the uterus is approximated with a thin absorbable suture (4–0 delayed absorbable suture). To prevent adhesion over the incision site, interceed (oxidized cellulose) or Gore-Tex (surgical membrane) can be used.

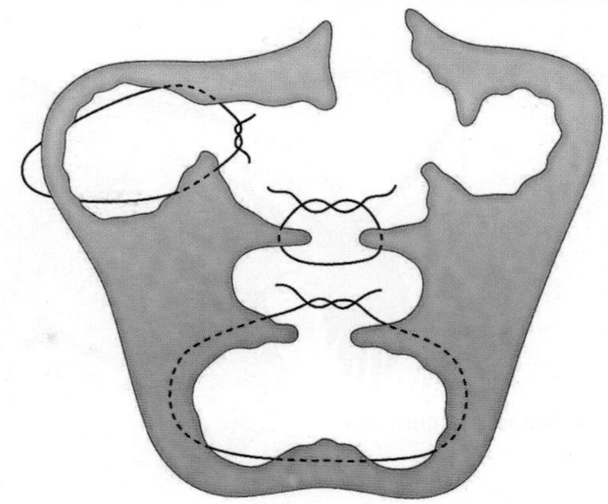

Fig. 35.14: Tire stitch to obliterate the myoma bed.

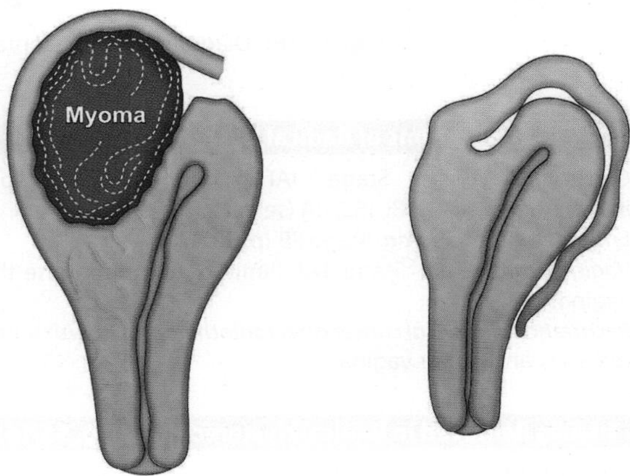

Fig. 35.15: Bonney's hood operation.

CERVICAL FIBROID

- *Anterior cervical myoma*—can be approached by making a transverse incision over the uterovesical peritoneum. Bladder is dissected down before the incision over the capsule of the fibroid is made. Fibroid is then enucleated (intracapsular).
- *Posterior cervical myoma*—approach is made by low posterior incision on the uterine surface through the pouch of Douglas.
- *Central cervical myoma*—the peritoneum of the uterovesical pouch is incised transversely and the bladder is dissected down. Hemisection of the uterus is done from above downwards to reach the myoma which is then enucleated (intracapsular). The dead space is obliterated without closure of the cervical canal. The bisected uterus is then repaired.

BROAD LIGAMENT MYOMA

For details p. 505.

COMPLICATIONS OF MYOMECTOMY

General complications of any abdominal procedure has been discussed (p. 501). The specific complications are:

Immediate

- Hemorrhage—intraperitoneal from the uterine wound. This may occur when hemostasis during operation is imperfect.
- Need of hysterectomy may be due to uncontrolled hemorrhage, and/or extensive myometrial injury.
- Postoperative fever is common due to hematoma formation at the myomectomy bed or due to tissue injury. The risk overall risk is less (0–2%).
- Risk of adhesion formation
- Recurrence of myoma
- Injury to bladder and ureter—especially with cervical and broad ligament myomas.
- Injury to the fallopian tubes—interstitial portion is commonly damaged during incision and suturing.
- Injury to bowel.
- Febrile morbidity—due to tissue reaction or infection.

Remote (Ch. 20, Table 20.9).

RADICAL HYSTERECTOMY
(SYN: CLASS IV RADICAL HYSTERECTOMY)

Wertheim's original operation was less extensive. With this procedure only a selective group of lymph nodes (e.g. enlarged and palpable) and only the medial half of the cardinal and uterosacral ligaments were removed.

The radical hysterectomy (type IV) is performed in most centers these days (p. 498).

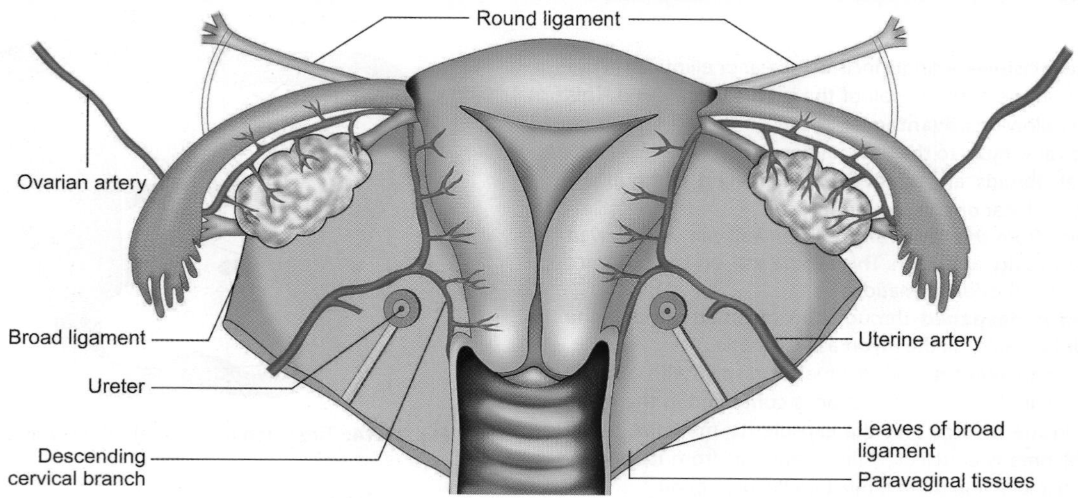

Fig. 35.16: Diagrammatic presentation of tissues removed in radical hysterectomy.

Indications of Radical Hysterectomy

- *Carcinoma cervix:* Stage IAI (lymphovascular space involvement)—IA2, IBI, IB2, IIA (selected)
- *Endometrial carcinoma:* Stage IIB (p. 301)
- *Vaginal carcinoma:* Stage I–II (limited to upper one-third vagina)
- *Recurrence of cervical cancer after radiotherapy:* Growth limited to cervix and upper vagina

Tissues Removed in Radical Hysterectomy (Fig. 35.16)

- Uterus, tubes +/- the ovaries
- Upper two-thirds of vagina
- Wide parametrial tissues
- Periureteral tissues
- Superior vesical arteries
- Cardinal ligaments up to lateral pelvic wall
- Uterosacral ligaments up to sacrum
- Paravesical and para rectal tissues
- Through pelvic lymphadenectomy

PRINCIPAL STEPS OF THE OPERATION

Preoperative work-up

- Continuous bladder drainage by Foley catheter.
- Vaginal packing under anesthesia.

Principal Steps

- Abdomen is opened by low midline vertical or transverse incision.
- Exploration of the abdomen and pelvis is done. Extent of spread of the disease (metastasis) helps to make the decision to proceed or to abort the operation.
- Liver, under surface of the diaphragm, kidneys, para-aortic lymph nodes, stomach, omentum, bladder, and ovaries are examined thoroughly.
- Traction of the uterus is given by long artery forceps, placed one on either side of the uterine cornu.

Contd...

Contd...

- The round ligament is clamped, cut, and ligated near the pelvic side wall. The infundibulopelvic ligament is also clamped, cut, and transfixed at this juncture (when ovaries are to be removed).

  In some doubtful cases, opening up of the peritoneum of the **uterovesical pouch is done first**. The cervix is then palpated for evidence of tumor extension. The operation is abandoned in favor of concurrent chemo and radiotherapy, if bladder is found involved with the tumor.
- The broad ligament leaves are opened up and the **paravesical and pararectal spaces** are created. **Bladder** is reflected off the cervix and the upper vagina and the **vesicocervical** and **vesicovaginal spaces** are created.

  Paravesical space is bounded anteriorly by the symphysis pubis, medially by the bladder superior vesical artery, laterally by the obturator muscle, external iliac vessels and the pelvic side wall and posteriorly by the cardinal ligament.

  Pararectal space is bounded anteriorly by the cardinal ligament, posteriorly by the sacrum, medially by the rectum and the uterosacral ligament, ureter and laterally by the hypogastric vessels.
- **The uterine artery** is identified and dissected out. A tunnel is created using a right-angled clamp. Tips of a right angle clamp are placed between the ureter and the paracervical tissues. The tips of the clamp sweeps through the paracervical tissue in a mode of opening and closing. The ureter is placed on gentle lateral traction by an umbilical tape (or a penrose drain). This is done carefully until a "tunnel" in the paracervical tissue is created ventromedially. The ureter passes through the tunnel to the bladder. Parametrial dissection is continued and unroofing of the ureteric tunnel is done. Pararvesical and pararectal spaces are now united. Rest of parametrial tissues are resected out. During dissection hemostasis is maintained using different methods including: (a) Clamping, cutting, suturing; (b) Stapler using; (c) Using electrodiathermy (bipolar). Ovarian transposition is done in cases where ovarian preservation is desired. Transposition is done out of the pelvis and above the anticipated field of radiation. It is transposed high up in the lateral peritoneum at the level of the kidney.

Contd...

Contd...

- The uterine artery is then clamped cut and ligated at its origin from the anterior division of internal iliac artery. Some prefer to ligate the anterior division of internal iliac artery just distal to its posterior division. Black silk ties are preferred. Hemoclip can also be used.
- **Mobilization of the ureter:** On the medial flap of peritoneum, the ureter is identified and is dissected free from rest of the parametrial tissue. Ureter can be retracted, when required, with an umbilical tape.
- The peritoneum of the pouch of Douglas is incised to expose the uterosacral ligaments. The rectum is rolled free and the **rectovaginal space** is created by sharp and blunt dissection.
- **The uterosacral ligament** is clamped close to the sacrum, cut, and ligated (with no.1 delayed absorbable suture).
- **The cardinal ligament** and paravaginal tissues are clamped close to the lateral pelvic wall, cut, and ligated.
- **The vaginal pack** is pulled out. Long right angled clamps are applied one on either side of vagina, low down to remove upper 3 cm of the vagina. The specimen is removed by cutting below the clamps (to avoid tumor spillage). The edges of the vagina are grasped with long Allis forceps.
- **The vaginal margins** are sutured if it is left open for drainage. Some prefer to close the vagina by interrupted sutures, so that postoperative suction (vacuum) drainage can be used.
- **Thorough pelvic lymphadenectomy** is done (external iliac, internal iliac, common iliac, obturator). **Para-aortic lymph nodes** are evaluated and sampling is done in women with positive pelvic lymph nodes (frozen section).
  The sensitivity of sentinel lymph node for prediction of lymph node metastasis is 100%.
- Hemostasis is checked. Pelvic peritonization may be done. Abdominal packs are removed.
- Abdomen is closed in layers. Continuous bladder drainage is maintained for 7–10 days.

Surgical steps are described for one side and similar steps are repeated on the other side.

- **Laparoscopic radical hysterectomy** is also being done for the management of early stage cervical carcinoma. MIS has similar rates of survival and complications as with laparotomy. Less intraoperative blood loss and shorter hospital stay are the advantages of MIS. Operative time depends upon the surgeon's skill. The surgical procedures of both the method's are the same.

The laparoscopic procedures used are:

- **Laparoscopic surgical staging only:** (a) Transperitoneally; or (b) Retroperitoneally.
- **Laparoscopically assisted radical vaginal hysterectomy (LARVH) with pelvic and para-aortic lymphadenectomy.** The abdominal part of the procedure includes division of: (a) Ovarian vessels; (b) Round ligaments; (c) Uterine artery by opening up of the pararectal and paravesical spaces; and (d) pelvic and aortic lymphadenectomy.
- **Laparoscopic radical hysterectomy with pelvic and para-aortic lymphadenectomy.**
- **Laparoscopically assisted radical vaginal trachelectomy (LARVT) with pelvic and para-aortic lymphadenectomy**—done in: (i) Selected young women; (b) Early stage disease (stage IA2 or IB1 ≤ 2 cm); (c) To preserve the reproductive function. This procedure includes: (i) Laparoscopic pelvic and aortic lymph node dissection; (ii) Vaginal radical trachelectomy if only there is no lymph node metastasis.
- **Robotic radical hysterectomy** has some more added advantages of MIS.

Involvement of para-aortic nodes without involvement of the pelvic nodes is extremely rare. If para-aortic nodes are found to be involved with metastatic tumor on frozen section biopsy in the beginning, the procedure of radical hysterectomy is abandoned. Concurrent chemotherapy and radiotherapy are then considered.

Complications of radical hysterectomy (p. 292).

OPERATIONS ON THE VULVA

SIMPLE (CONSERVATIVE) VULVECTOMY

Preoperative work up (p. 488).

Indications

- VIN (wide spread)
- Paget's disease of the vulva
- Vulvar granulomatous lesions (where malignancy is difficult to rule out).

Principal Steps (Fig. 35.17)

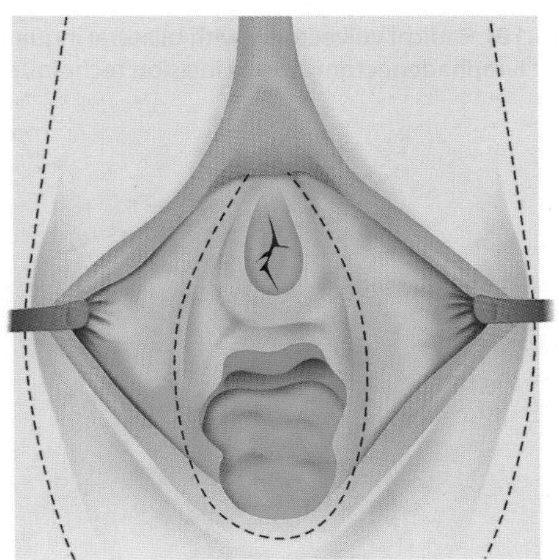

Fig. 35.17: Simple (Conservative) vulvectomy

- Lithotomy position.
- Outer incision—an elliptical incision is made commencing anteriorly on the mons pubis → encircling laterally along the medial side of labiocrural fold → posteriorly across the midline of perineum (Fig. 35.18).
- Inner incision—passes around the introitus and anterior to urethra (Fig. 35.18).
- Vulvar skin (not deeper tissues) is removed. Bleeding vessels (branches of internal pudendal artery) are ligated separately.
- Apposition of the skin edges is done (interrupted sutures) without tension.
- Continuous bladder drainage is maintained with a Foley's catheter for 3–4 days.

Tissues removed are—mons pubis, clitoris, labia majora and minora.

RADICAL VULVECTOMY WITH BILATERAL INGUINOFEMORAL LYMPHADENECTOMY

Survival outcome of patients with vulval cancer is improved following radical vulvectomy and bilateral inguinofemoral and pelvic lymphadenectomy (Figs. 35.18 and 35.19). En block excision was done by Taussig and Way (1940). Presently, there are several modifications for vulvar cancer surgery to minimize the morbidity the complications of radical vulveclomy are listed in Table 35.9. **Three separate incisions have been currently used to reduce the considerable morbidity of en bloc procedure (p. 282).**

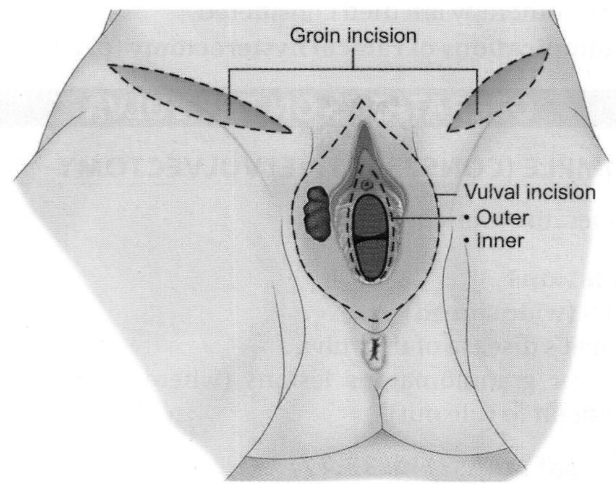

Fig. 35.18: Radical vulvectomy with bilateral inguinofemoral lymphadenectomy (three incision technique).

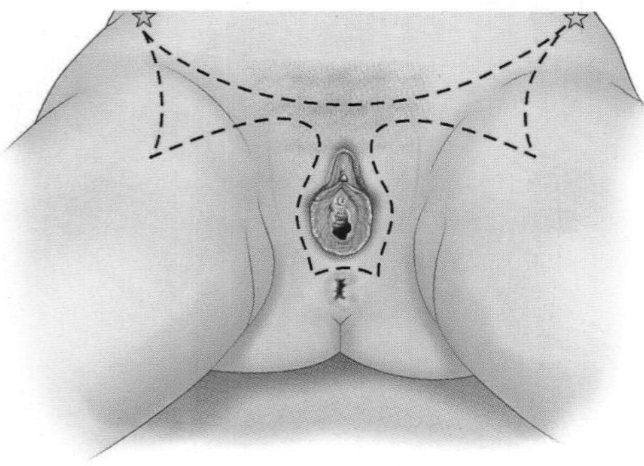

Fig. 35.19: Radical vulvectomy with bilateral inguinofemoral lymphadenectomy (en bloc incision).

TABLE 35.9: Complications of radical vulvectomy.

Early	*Late*
▪ Hemorrhage ▪ Seroma collection ▪ Fluid and electrolyte imbalance ▪ Groin wound infection, necrosis, and dehiscence ▪ Urinary tract infection ▪ Rectovaginal fistula ▪ Deep vein thrombosis ▪ Pulmonary embolism ▪ Psychological—depression ▪ Anesthetic: Atelectasis	▪ Leg edema, leg cellulitis ▪ Dyspareunia due to introital stenosis ▪ Femoral or inguinal hernia ▪ Osteitis pubis, osteomyelitis ▪ Loss of body image; depression ▪ Recurrence (10%)

PRINCIPAL STEPS

Three incision technique is preferred in most centers. These are—(a) Vulvar incision; (b) Groin incision one on either side (Fig. 35.17).

- **Groin incision** is a crescent-shaped one, starting about 2–4 cm medial and about 2 cm below the anterior-superior iliac spine. The incision curves gradually downwards above the inguinal ligament medially to the superficial inguinal ring or about 2 cm below and 2 cm medial to the pubic tubercle. Mons pubis is spared. A strip of skin (2–4 cm) width is excised. This incision helps more complete dissection and reduces skin necrosis.

Three incision technique is preferred in most centers. These are—(a) Vulvar incision; (b) Groin incision one on either side (Fig. 35.17).

- **Groin incision** is a crescent-shaped one, starting about 2–4 cm medial and about 2 cm below the anterior-superior iliac spine. The incision curves gradually downwards above the inguinal ligament medially to the superficial inguinal ring or about 2 cm below and 2 cm medial to the pubic tubercle. Mons pubis is spared. A strip of skin (2–4 cm) width is excised. This incision helps more complete dissection and reduces skin necrosis.

- Vulvar incisions are same as described in simple vulvectomy. Special points to note are:
  - Wide tumor free margin (at least 2 cm) is essential. If the tumor is close to urethra or vagina, lower 2 cm of urethra and lower vagina may be sacrificed.
- Dissection must be done down to the deep fascia.
- **Inguinofemoral lymphadenectomy**
  - Dissection is carried out down to external oblique fascia and fascia overlying the sartorius muscle.
  - The lymph nodes and the fatty tissues around the superficial circumflex iliac and the superficial epigastric vessels are resected off. The vessels are ligated.
  - At the caudal end of femoral triangle—the long saphenous vein is dissected and doubly ligated with 2–0 silk.
  - The surrounding lymph nodes (saphenofemoral junction) are dissected off the sartorius and the adductor fascia.
  - The lymph nodes, lateral and medial to femoral artery and vein are dissected out by sharp dissection.
  - Inguinal and femoral lymph nodes are removed and sent for frozen section biopsy. The **Cloquet node or node of Rosenmüller** at the femoral canal (medial to femoral vein) may be absent in more than 50% cases. If these nodes are positive, ipsilateral retroperitoneal pelvic lymphadenectomy is performed.
  - **Lymphatic drainage** occurs in a stepwise fashion. The **sentinel lymph node** when negative for tumor metastasis, it is rare for the other nodes in the basin to be involved. Identification of the **sentinel lymph node** (Cloquet node) can therefore guide the extent of surgery and also the surgical lymph node dissection. This can reduce the risk of surgical morbidity and mortality.
  - **Sentinel lymph node mapping and biopsy (SLNMB)** can reduce the radicality of the nodal dissection for metastasis. Physiologically first lymph node to receive tumor lymphatic drainage is the sentinel lymph node. When the SLNB is negative, the risk of metastasis within the entire lymph node basin is unlikely.

Contd...

SLNB is done by lymphoscintigraphy and isosulphan blue dye technique for vulval cancer. Lymphatic mapping is done by injecting radionuclide intradermally at the tumor border. A hand held gamma counter identifies the sentinel node subcutaneously and the skin is marked with a pen over the strongest signal. Thereafter isosulphan blue dye is injected at the same tumor border. The groin skin over the prior mark is incised about 5 minutes later. The sentinel node identified by the gamma control signal is also detected by the blue color. It is excised out

Contd...

Contd...

for histological examination. SLNB has the sensitivity of >90% and the false negative rate of 2%.

- However, radiation therapy is preferred to surgery for pelvic node dissection (p. 282).
- Closed system suction drains are placed in the groin area. Groin incision is closed by interrupted sutures.

Operations for urinary incontinence (p. 338).
Repair of vesicovaginal fistula (p. 352).
Repair of ureteric injuries (p. 355).
Vaginal reconstruction operation (vaginoplasty).

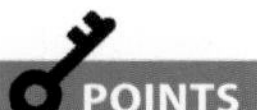

POINTS

- **Preoperative investigations** should preferably be done prior to admission in hospital.
- **For any operation**, preoperative counseling and informed consent are essential (p. 489).
- **In elective operations**, the patient should be made fit for surgery prior-hand.
- **Even in minor surgery**, examination of the cardiovascular system, complete hemogram and complete urine examination should at least be done.
- **Preoperative risk assessment** is essential to minimize surgical morbidity and other complications (p. 489).
- **Day care surgery** has many benefits. Here the patients are admitted, operated, and discharged on the same day (p. 490). Patients are screened before hand.
- **Postoperative care** should include record of vital signs, fluid replacement, output record, adequate pain control, antibiotic therapy, and vigilance to the close system suction drains at the catheter.
- **Only dilatation** of the cervix is indicated in—prior to amputation of the cervix, spasmodic dysmenorrhea, pyometra or hematometra.
- **Common indications of D and C** are infertility, DUB, incomplete abortion, and endometrial pathology.
- **Common complications** of D and C are injury to the cervix, uterine perforation, injury to the gut, and infection. Remote complications include cervical incompetence and uterine synechiae.
- **D and I** is indicated to note the patency of the tubes in cases of infertility or following tuboplasty operation.
- **HSG** is done in the radiology department without anesthesia (p. 494). Besides tubal patency test, it has many other benefits (p. 486). It is superior to D and I.
- **Types of cervical biopsy include**: surface, punch, wedge, ring, and cone type (p. 495).
- **CIN and cervical ectopy** are locally ablated. Destruction of the benign pathological cervical lesions (ectopy, CIN) can be done by thermal cauterization, cryosurgery or laser (p. 496).
- **Perineoplasty** is a simple reconstructive surgery for widening the narrow vaginal introitus for sexual function.
- **Complications of cervical conization** or amputation include postoperative hemorrhage and cervical stenosis or cervical incompetence.
- **Common indications of total hysterectomy** for benign lesions are DUB, fibroid, TO mass, and endometriosis (p. 498, Table 35.4).
- **Common indications of subtotal hysterectomy** are difficult TO mass, endometriosis of rectovaginal septum, and sudden deterioration of the general health while contemplating total hysterectomy.
- **Opportunistic bilateral salpingectomy** may be done as a primary preventive measure to ovarian cancer.
- **Bilateral salpingo-oophorectomy** in women following completed child bearing with *BRCA* mutation reduces the risk of ovarian cancer significantly and breast cancer also.
- **Premenopausal ovaries** are better to be preserved, if not pathological.
- **Conization of the cervix** is done either as a diagnostic or therapeutic procedure in CIN or in microinvasive carcinoma. Laser cone has got distinct advantages over the cold knife cone (Table 35.1).
- **Complications of abdominal hysterectomy** are intraoperative, postoperative (immediate, late, and remote) (p. 292). Postoperative bowel dysfunction (ileus and obstruction) need to be differentiated (Table 35.4).
- **Hysterectomy** can be abdominal, vaginal, laparoscopic or laparoscopic assisted vaginal. Each method has got advantages and disadvantages (p. 498). Each case needs to be individualized for any particular method. Hysterectomy may be classified into different types.
- **Laparoscopic ovarian drilling** is more commonly done compared to wedge resection in the management of PCOS cases (p. 504).
- **Operations for chronic inversion of the uterus** may be abdominal (Haultain) or vaginal (Kustner or Spinelli) (p. 504).
- **Ventrosuspension** operations are less commonly done these days. Plication of the round ligaments, modified Gilliam procedure or laparoscopic suspension operation are the different methods (p. 506).
- **Abdominal myomectomy** could be done either by open surgery or laparoscopically. Control of operative blood loss is an important step (p. 506). A single incision on the anterior wall is preferred. Hemorrhage is the single most important complication.
- **Radical hysterectomy** (Type IV) is the operation of choice for invasive carcinoma of the cervix. Extensive pelvic tissues are removed (p. 507). Complications of radical hysterectomy are other organ injury (bladder, ureter) besides the complications of simple hysterectomy.
- **Laparoscopic radical hysterectomy** is currently being done (p. 509). Laparoscopically assisted radical vaginal trachelectomy (LARVT) is a fertility sparing surgery, done for early stage (IA2 or IB1 ≤2 cm) diseases.
- **Radical vulvectomy** with bilateral inguinofemoral lymphadenectomy could be done either by three incision technique (preferred) or by en bloc procedure (butterfly incision).
- **Node of Cloquet** or Rosenmüller (deep femoral node) may be absent in more than 50% cases.
- **Pelvic node metastases** are rare unless inguinofemoral nodes are involved. However, radiation therapy is preferred to surgery for pelvic node dissection.
- **Complications of radical vulvectomy** may be early or late (p.292) and increase the morbidity.

CHAPTER

36 Endoscopic Surgery in Gynecology

CHAPTER OUTLINE

- History
- Basic Instruments
- Hemostasis during Laparoscopic Surgery
- Surgical Techniques
- Operative Laparoscopy
- Robotic Surgery in Gynecology
- Hysteroscopy

INTRODUCTION

The range of surgical procedures in gynecology, performed with the use of either a laparoscope or a hysteroscope is designated as **endoscopic surgery**. Endoscopic surgery is done through a small incision (hole) or no incision. Visualization is done by ensdoscopes (laparoscope/hysteroscope) and the surgery is done under vision. **This is also known as minimally invasive surgery (MIS) or minimally access surgery (MAS).** With very fast technological advancement, almost all of gynecological operations can be performed endoscopically.

HISTORY

First description of endoscopy is recorded by **Phillipp Bozzini** in 1805. He used a simple tube and candle light to visualize the interior of the urethra. **Pantaleoni** of Ireland first used a cystoscope in 1869 as an hysteroscope to diagnose a case of irregular vaginal bleeding. **Jacobaeus** of Sweden in 1910 first introduced a cystoscope in the peritoneal cavity and coined the term laparoscopy. In 1938, **Veress** first reported the spring loaded needle for creating pneumothorax in patients with tuberculosis. In 1947, **Raoul Palmer** of France introduced the use of gaseous distension of the peritoneal cavity using gas and the lithotomy (Trendelenburg) position. Landmark progress of the use of 'Coldlight' and fiberoptics were made by **Fourestier** and **others.** In 1967, **Steptoe** of England first published the monograph 'Laparoscopy in Gynecology' in english language. **Kurt Semm** of Germany is credited for his advanced operative laparoscopic procedures (myomectomy) in the 1970s. First laparoscopic hysterectomy was reported by **Reich,** et al in 1989.

ADVANTAGES OF LAPAROSCOPIC SURGERY

- Rapid postoperative recovery
- Less postoperative pain and reduced need of postoperative analgesia
- Excellent visualization of organs and tissues (Fig. 36.1)
- Shorter hospital stay and reduced concomitant cost
- Quicker resumption of day-to-day activity
- Less adhesion formation
- Minimal abdominal scars (cosmetic value)
- Reduced blood loss
- No large incisions
- Less risk of incisional hernia
- Increased patient's satisfaction.
- Less morbidity than laparotomy

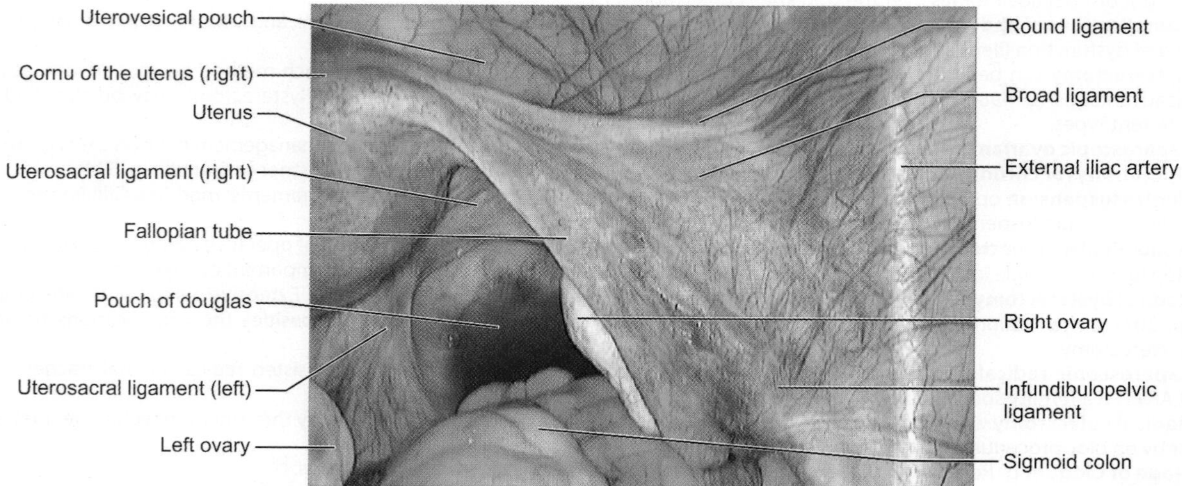

Fig. 36.1: Laparoscopic view of the lateral , anterior and the posterior pelvis. Peritoneal fold of the broad ligament is seen. .

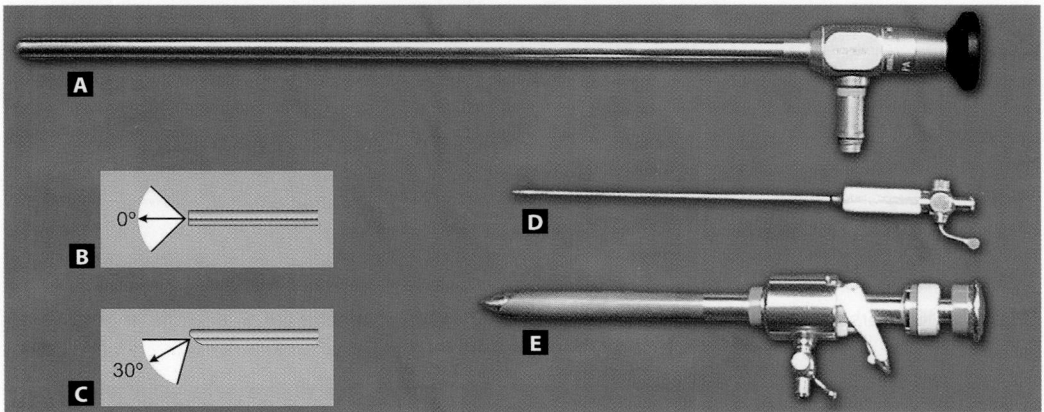

Figs. 36.2A to E: Laparoscopic instruments: (A) Telescope; (B) Telescope: 0-degree viewing angle; (C) Telescope: 30-degree viewing angle; (D) Veress needle; (E) Trocar and cannula (conical tip) with multifunctional valve.

- Excellent visualization with magnified image using videocam and camera.

Difficulties with MIS

- Counter intuitive movements.
- Indirect palpation of tissues.
- Limited number of ports for access of abdominal organs.
- Restricted movement of tools.
- Need of three-dimensional vision.

BASIC INSTRUMENTS AND ELECTROSURGICAL UNITS FOR LAPAROSCOPIC SURGERY (FIGS. 36.2A TO E)

- **Telescope:** Caliber varies from 4–12 mm with rod lens system. Angle of view may be either straight forward (0°) or fore oblique (30°) (Figs. 36.2A to C).
- **Veress needle:** It is used for creating pneumoperitoneum by carbon dioxide. It is spring loaded to prevent visceral injury. The blunt tip point springs out when it enters the peritoneal cavity (Fig. 36.2D).
- **Trocar and cannula:** It is inserted through the abdominal wall following pneumoperitoneum. The trocar is removed and the telescope is introduced through the cannula (sleeve). Disposable trocar and veress needles are available (Fig. 36.2E).
- **Light source:** High intensity light (xenon or halogen source) beam (cold light) is transmitted to the telescope for excellent visualization. Fiberoptic cables are used to transmit the cold light from source to the telescope.
- **Imaging system includes:** Laparoscope, light source, fiberoptic cord, camera unit and monitors.
- **Camera unit:** It includes camera head, cable, and camera control. **The camera** head is attached to the eye piece of the laparoscope. The image resolution depends on the number of pixels (2,50,000–3,80,000) on the chip. High definition digital camera uses resolution up to 1,100 lines to produce more vivid picture.
- **Monitor:** High resolution video color monitors with 700 lines provide optimal picture visualization. For best surgeon ergonomics placement of the monitor should be 10–20° below the surgeons eye level to prevent neck strain.
- **Insufflator:** The rate of gas flow rate (L/min) and intra-abdominal pressure (mm Hg) are displayed on the insufflator. It is used to create controlled pneumoperitoneum as there is some amount of gas (CO_2) leak through the different ports. Either low flow rate (0.5–1 L/min) or high flow rate is used depending on the need.

ACCESSORY INSTRUMENTS (FIGS. 36.3A TO J)

- **Scissors** of different sizes and designs are used for dissection and to cut tissue (Fig. 36.4).
- **Grasping forceps** of different designs with are used to hold tissues (Fig. 36.5).
- **Probes:** Blunt probe is used for manipulation of visceras (e.g. intestines and ovaries) to visualize other structures.
- **Aspirator and irrigator:** Blunt and sharp aspirators are used for aspiration of fluid from the peritoneal cavity or ovarian cysts. **Irrigation** is done for washing the peritoneal cavity with normal saline at the end of a surgical procedure.
- **Needle driver (Fig 36.6):** It is used to drive needle through tissues and knots are tied within the abdomen.

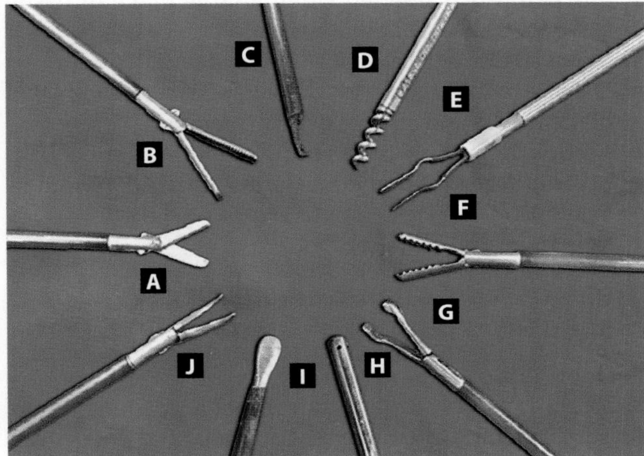

Figs. 36.3A to J: Ancillary instruments: (A) Scissors; (B) Bowel grasper; (C) Monopolar L-hook; (D) Myoma screw; (E) Bipolar coagulating forceps; (F) Grasping forceps (alligator jaws); (G) Grasper (Babcock); (H) Suction and irrigation cannula; (I) Spatula; (J) Dissecting grasping forceps (Maryland).

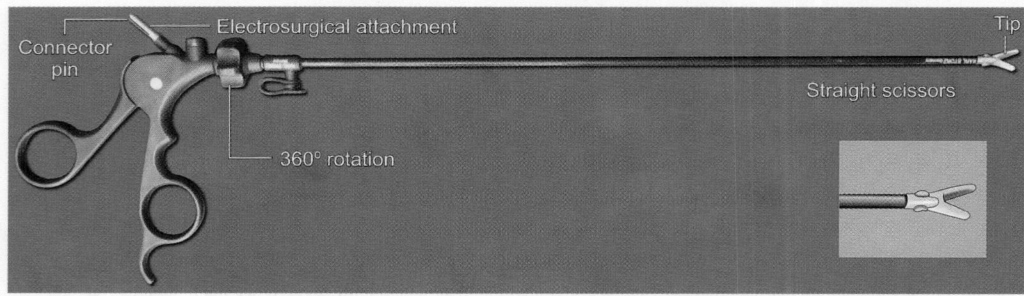

Fig. 36.4: Scissors straight with handle with unipolar coagulation connector pin. Size 5 mm, length 36 cm. It is rotating and dismantable.

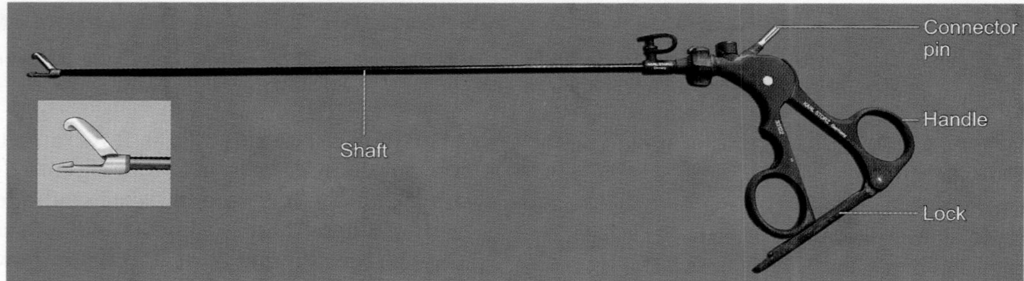

Fig. 36.5: Toothed grasping forceps with handle and lock; size: 5 mm; length: 36 cm. It is rotating and dismantable. It has a connector pin for unipolar coagulation.

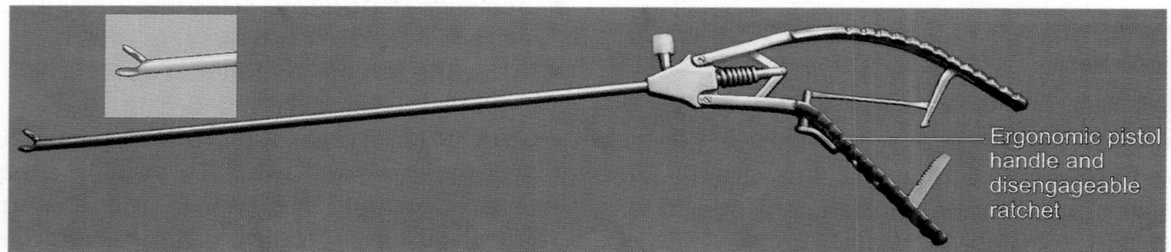

Fig. 36.6: Needle driver with ratchet (hemostat type) straight jaws, metal outer sheath; length 36 cm.

Laparoscopic suturing needs much practice to load the needle into the needle driver and to place the sutures accurately.

- **Morcellator** is needed when a large piece of tissue (myoma) is morcellated into small pieces so as to be removed through the laparoscopic sleeve.
- **Uterine manipulator** is used for adequate visualiza-tion of the uterus and adnexa during operation.
- **L-hook** for cutting tissues using monopolar energy.
- **Myoma screw**—for myomectomy (laparoscopic modi-fication).
- **Specimen retrieval bag.**

HEMOSTASIS DURING LAPAROSCOPIC SURGERY

Perfect hemostasis is mandatory at the end of any endoscopic surgery. Hemostatic measures depend on the vessel diameter. For small vessels monopolar energy can be used and for larger vessels, the bipolar.

Electrocoagulation: Electrosurgical units are used for cutting and coagulation of biological tissues. **Cutting mode** provides uninterrupted low voltage to vaporize tissues (100°C). Lateral thermal spread is minimal. **Coagulation mode** creates peak voltage three times higher than of cutting made. It causes rapid tissue desiccation and carbonization. In **blended mode** cutting and coagulation currents are combined creating alternate high and low voltage current.

Monopolar electrosurgery: The current (electrons) is pushed from the generator through the active electrode to the contact tissue. The current returns back to generator through the neutral electrode after it has passed through the patient.

It is used for tissues cutting, dissection, vaporization, desiccation and coagulation. It is delivered through a needle point tip or scissors. Monopolar instruments may cause electrosurgical burns through insulation failure, direct coupling or capacitive coupling. The return electrode should be broad enough to reduce the current density far below the level of tissue burning. It should be in good contact with the patient.

Bipolar electrosurgery: Here the current flows from the generator between the two jaws of the forceps or scissors, holding the target tissue (Fig. 36.10). There is no need for ground plate. Bipolar energy is very effective for hemostasis. It works by conducting electrical current with high power density that is confined between the jaws of the forceps. It has low contact temperature and high compressive effects. Damage to tissue is more precise compared to unipolar mode.

It is used for hemostasis and tissue desiccation. Fine tip "micro bipolar" forceps aid hemostasis near vulnerable organs like ureter, bowels. Burns are less as the current is confined between the two blades.

Advanced bipolar devices are LigaSure and EnSeal. Both are used for tissue dissection and desiccation. There is reduced thermal spread, improved tissue seal, less plume formation and reduced tissue sticking.

LigaSure is a bipolar electrosurgical device used to cut, vaporize, coagulate and seal blood vessels. It delivers electrical energy as high current and low voltage output. The problem of sticking and charring to tissues are less. Lateral thermal spread is also less. It seals blood vessels, up to 7 mm in size.

EnSeal vessel fusion is a bipolar system that deliver a locally regulated current. Tissue temperature remains within 120°C as there is generation of resistance in the plastic jaws of the instrument. The device has a mechanical blade that can be advanced gradually to desiccate and cut tissue bundles.

Laser coagulation (p. 103): Lasers used in gynecological surgery are CO_2, KTP-532 and Nd:YAG lasers. For effective cutting, vaporization and coagulation of tissue, power density is an important factor. The depth of tissue penetration depends on the type of laser used, e.g. for CO_2 (most commonly used) 0.1 mm, KTP-532—0.4–0.8 mm and Nd:YAG is 0.6-4.2 mm (p. 103).

Harmonic scalpel: It is an ultrasound energy source to break hydrogen bonds in tissues. It uses vibration at the rate of 55,000 cycles per second. Harmonic Ace (Ethicon) has minimal lateral thermal injury. It converts ultrasonic energy to mechanical energy at the active blade (Fig. 36.7). The active blade vibrates to deliver the high-frequency ultrasonic frictional force. The inactive upper arm holds tissues against the active blade. This is effective in cutting or coaptation (sealing) of vessels up to 5 mm diameter. There is no risk of electrical injury.

Harmonic energies are preferred. Advanced bipolar method achieve vessel sealing by desiccation up to 7 mm in diameter. However, thermal spread of any device is a concern. Micro bipolar probes and needle-tip monopolar probes are useful for delicate tissues as the thermal spread is minimal.

Liquid topical hemostatic agents (vessel sealants) are also being used. Moreover, an **oxidized regenerated cellulose fabric** sheet can also be used.

Mechanical clips and staples: Titanium clips and staples are used for hemostasis by securing blood vessels. Disposable stapling cartridge with a self-contained knife blade (Endo GIA 30) is used for laparoscopic hysterectomy producing quick cut and hemostasis. Newer angled staplers made of polyglactin are used.

Sutures and ligature: Like an open surgery sutures can be used to ligate blood vessels and to secure vascular pedicles. Different methods of suturing and knot tying are used—(a) intracorporeal knot tying; (b) extracorporeal knot tying; or (c) endoloops pretied ligature (Roeder loops).

Laparoscopic knot tying creates increased friction and suture fraying. Synthetic delayed absorbable suture has high tensile strength, less tissue reaction, greater knot reliability and ease of handling.

Barbed suture has advantage of maintaining the tensile pressure on continuous suture line. The outer surface of this synthetic suture has multiple barbs that are placed evenly. These barbs pass smoothly through the tissues while apposing, but flare up once come out to the other side. These barbs prevent suture from slipping back once the tissue margins are apposed. Barbs suture does not need any knot tying; It is commonly used during myomectomy or for closure of vaginal cuff following TLH.

Knots: The length of suture depends on the extent of suturing and knot tying. Generally, 8–10 cm is needed for intracorporeal knot tying. Intracorporeal knot tying has a steeper learning curve. Alternative to manual knot tying disposable clips can be placed at the end of a suture line for security.

INDICATIONS OF LAPAROSCOPIC SURGERY

Almost all gynecologic surgical procedure can be performed with MIS. The laparoscopic surgical procedures are graded according to the extent of surgery and also to the competence of the surgeon. They are labeled as follows:

- Diagnostic laparoscopy (p. 102)
- Therapeutic (operative) laparoscopy.

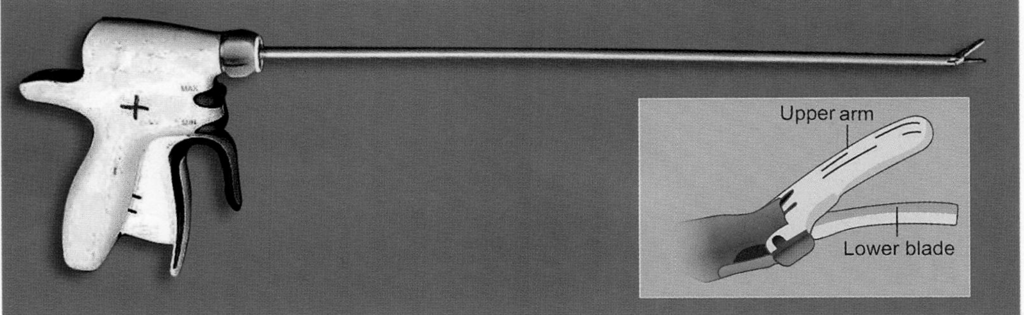

Fig. 36.7: Laparoscopic Harmonic scalpel.

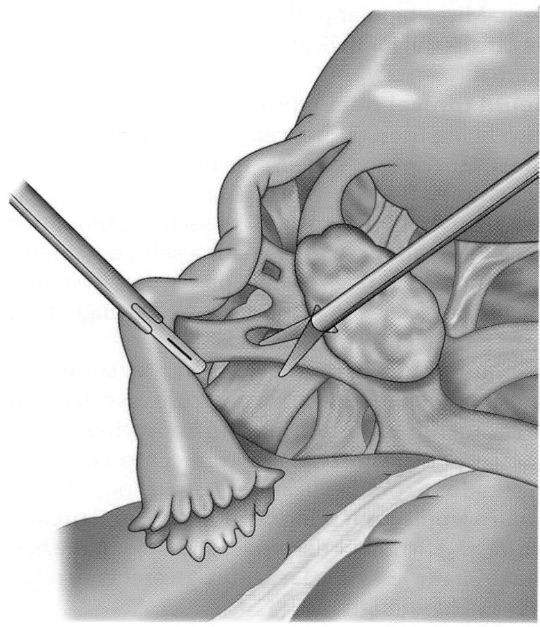

Fig. 36.8: Laparoscopic adhesiolysis (salpingolysis and ovariolysis).

- **Minor procedures**
  - Tubal sterilization (p. 415, Fig. 36.12).
  - Adhesiolysis (without bowel involvement) (Fig. 36.8)
  - Aspiration of simple ovarian cysts.
  - Ovarian biopsy.
- **Moderate procedures (Figs. 36.9A to C)**

Ovary	*Uterus*
▪ Diathermy for polycystic ovarian syndrome (PCOS) (Fig. 36.10) ▪ Drainage of endometriomas ▪ Ovarian cystectomy ▪ Salpingo-ovariolysis (Fig. 36.8). **Ectopic Pregnancy** ▪ Salpingostomy (Figs. 36.9A to C) ▪ Segmental resection ▪ Salpingectomy ▪ Salpingo-oophorectomy **Endometriosis:** Ablation or excision by diathermy or laser.	▪ Myomectomy ▪ Laparoscopic assisted vaginal hysterectomy (LAVH) ▪ Adhesiolysis—including bowel involvement (Fig. 36.8) **Extensive procedures** ▪ Major endometriosis ▪ Myomectomy ▪ Retroperitoneal lymphadenectomy ▪ Hysterectomy ▪ Urinary incontinence ▪ Sacrocolpopexy.

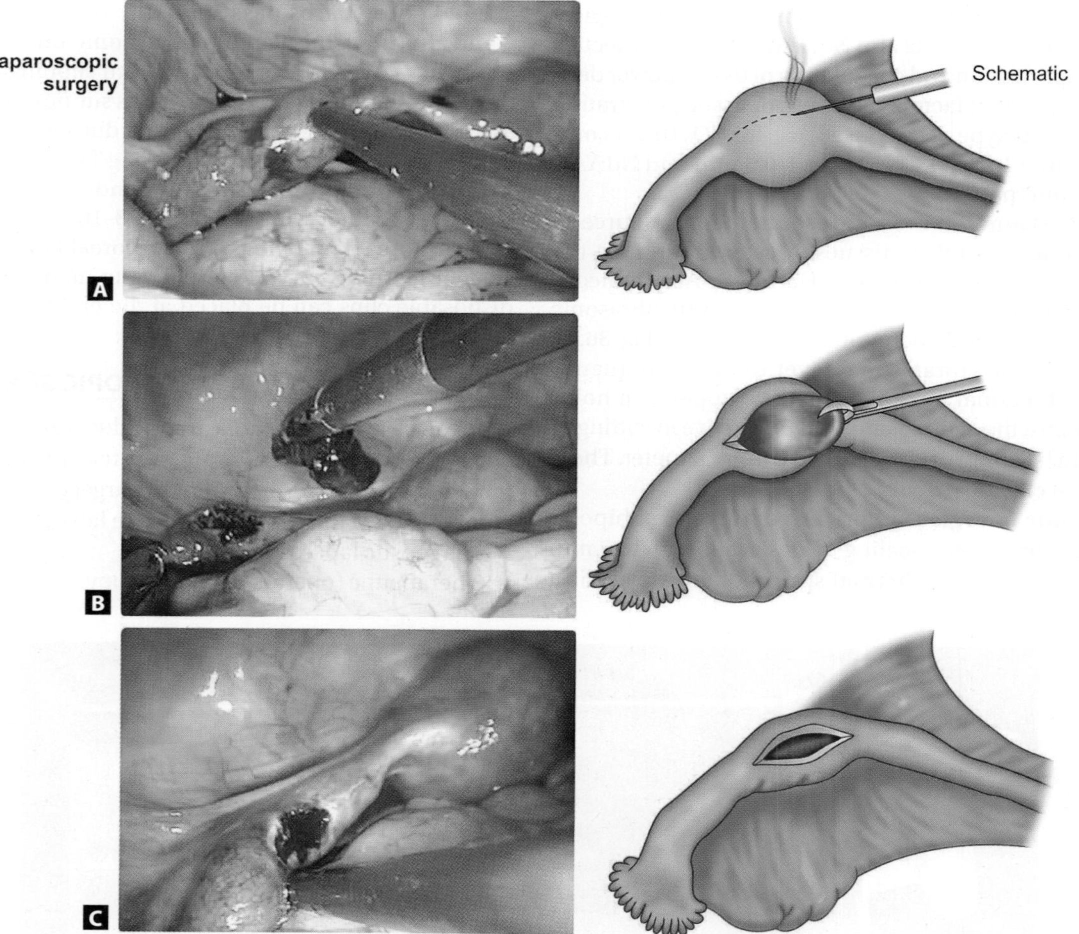

Figs. 36.9A to C: Laparoscopic linear salpingostomy for unruptured tubal ectopic pregnancy. (A) Linear incision on the antimesenteric border; (B) Gestation sac is removed; (C) Incision margins left unsutured. *Left*: Operation and *Right*: Schematic.

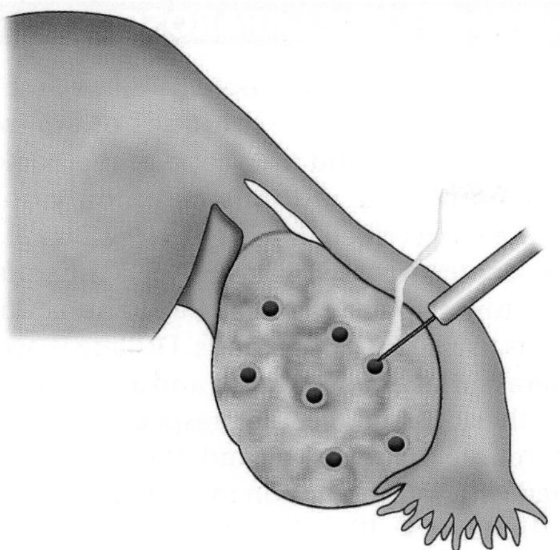

Fig. 36.10: Surgical treatment of PCOS by drilling.

CONTRAINDICATIONS (TABLE 36.1)

One should be familiar with the contraindications to maximize the patient safety and minimize the procedure related morbidity.

OPERATIVE PROCEDURES FOR LAPAROSCOPY

Preoperative screening is essential and contraindications are excluded (Table 36.1). Informed consent is taken and it should include the permission for open surgery if necessity arises. **General anesthesia** is generally preferred. Depending on the surgery local or regional may be used. There is significant hemodynamic changes during laparoscopy due to—(a) Raised intra-abdominal pressure (CO_2 insufflation); (b) Head-down position; (c) Lung compression due to pneumoperitoneum and bradycardia due to vagal stimulation (visceral manipulation). Cardiac output may fall by 10–30%. Procedures like sterilization could be performed under local anesthesia. The operating table should have the facilities for rotating at different angles. Low lithotomy position of the patient with buttocks protruding slightly from the edge of the table is used.

TABLE 36.1: Contraindications of laparoscopy.

Absolute	*Relative*
■ Severe cardiopulmonary disease ■ Patient hemodynamically unstable ■ Significant hemoperitoneum ■ Intestinal obstruction ■ Tubercular peritonitis ■ Anticoagulation therapy	■ Extensive peritoneal adhesion ■ Large pelvic tumor ■ Morbid obesity ■ Large hiatal hernia ■ Advanced malignancy ■ Generalized peritonitis ■ Inflammatory bowel disease ■ Pregnancy
■ **Laparoscopy in pregnancy** can be done in all the trimesters but optimally in the second trimester. Intra-abdominal pressure is maintained between 8 to 12 mm Hg to avoid maternal reduction of cardiac output, acidosis and decrease in placental perfusion.	

SURGICAL TECHNIQUES

- Patient positioning
- Production of pneumoperitoneum
- Introduction of trocar and cannula
- Introduction of laparoscope
- Creation of accessory ports
- Surgical procedures to carry out
- Deflation of the peritoneal gas
- Closure of the parietal wound (ports).

Position of patient

The patient is placed in lithotomy position. The buttocks are at the edge or slightly over the table's edge. Stirrups should have ample padding to support the lower leg. Head end of the patient is lowered (Trendelenburg 15–30°) after insertion of the primary trocar. This is done to displace the bowel out of the pelvis. For good view and hand-eye coordination, both for the surgeon and the assistants, the video monitor is placed at the foot-end of the table. The electrosurgical unit and the suction irrigator should be placed behind the surgeon or assistant. The bladder is emptied by a Foley's catheter. Pelvic examination is done methodically. An uterine manipulator is introduced through the cervical canal for manipulation to visualize the tubes and uterus at a later step.

Pneumoperitoneum

A small skin incision (1.25 cm) is made just below the umbilicus. The Veress needle is introduced through the incision with 45° angulation into the peritoneal cavity. The abdomen is inflated with about 1–4 L of gas (carbon dioxide). Symmetrical distension of abdomen with loss of liver dullness is suggestive of proper pneumoperitoneum. Volume of gas varies from 1–4 L depending upon the patient. But in any case intra-abdominal pressure should not exceed 20 mm Hg. The flow rate of the gas is about one liter per minute with a pressure not exceeding 20 mm Hg. Otherwise this interferes with diaphragmatic excursion and venous return due to caval obstruction.

Correct placement of Veress needle is verified by:

- **Hanging drop method:** A small amount of sterile saline is placed on the top of the Veress needle. The saline drops in the peritoneal cavity while there is negative intraperitoneal pressure.
- **Syringe barrel test:** A 10 mL syringe with normal saline is attached to the Veress needle. Aspiration is done to rule out blood or bowel contents. The saline is then pushed down and aspiration is again done. If the needle placement is correct, the fluid cannot be withdrawn as it goes in the peritoneal cavity.
- **Intra-abdominal** pressure is low (<10 mm Hg) on correct placement and there is free flow of gas.
- **Obliteration of liver dullness** (on percussion).

Other possible sites of Veress needle insertion: (a) Left subcostal margin (3 cm below in midclavicular line—**Palmer's point**). Stomach must be decompressed and splenomegaly to be ruled out; (b) Transvaginal—through the pouch of Douglas.

Laparoscopic insufflator: Operative laparoscopic procedures needs high flow. Automatic sensors of the insufflator shut off gas flow when the intra-abdominal pressure reaches 15–20 mm Hg.

Port entry (Fig. 36.11): Peritoneal cavity is entered through three main sites: (a) At the umbilicus (most common); (b) Suprapubic (2–4 cm above); (c) Palmer's point (midclavicular line) on the left. In obese patients the needle is inserted more vertically.

Introduction of trocar and cannula

The abdominal wall is elevated (inflated to 15 mm of Hg) and the trocar with cannula is inserted through the same incision. The

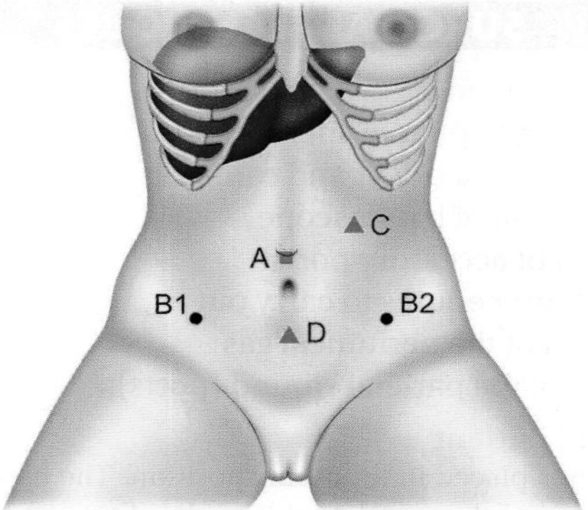

Fig. 36.11: Port entry: (A) Primary port—umbilical port. (B1 and B2) Accessory ports—lateral ports one on each side 3–4 cm medial to anterior superior iliac spine but lateral to inferior epigastric artery; (C) Palmer's point; (D) Suprapubic port.

angle of insertion is similar to that of the Veress needle, directing towards the hollow of the sacrum. There is escape of gas when the trocar is within the peritoneal cavity. The trocar is removed and the laparoscope is then introduced. **Open laparoscopy** was introduced (Hasson, 1971) to reduce the risk of blind insertion of the Veress needles and trocars. Peritoneal cavity is opened through a small incision (1 cm) at the umbilicus pneumoperitoneum is done through a special cannula inserted in the incision. The laparoscope is then introduced. Direct trocar entry (trocar and cannula with safety valve) has been done.

Secondary trocar insertion is needed for both the diagnostic and operative procedures (Fig. 36.11). Sites selected are either on the flank (3-4 cm lateral to the medial umbilical ligament) or lateral to the lateral margin of rectus abdominis muscle or on the suprapubic region. This is done under direct vision with illumination to avoid trauma to abdominal organs and the inferior epigastric vessels.

Laparoscopic procedures of tissue dissection: (a) Blunt dissection; (b) Sharp dissection (using scissors). For control of bleeding, bipolar diathermy is used for hemostasis; (c) Aquadissection with hydraulic pressure is used to create tissue planes; (d) Electrodissection using unipolar or bipolar diathermy for dissection and coagulation; (e) Laser dissection (p. 103); (f) Harmonic scalpel. Operative laparoscopy needs uterine manipulations, tissue traction, irrigation and suction procedures.

Methods of hemostasis (p. 514).

Removal of specimens: Large volume of tissues after laparoscope could be removed by any of these methods: (a) Morcellation; (b) By enlarging any of the suprapubic trocar incision site; (c) Through the colpotomy incision. The specimen is put in a EndoCatch bag and is taken out without spilling.

Examination of the pelvis: After introduction of the laparoscope, a systematic inspection of the pelvic and abdominal organs is done. The patient is put to Trendelenburg position for proper visualization of the pelvic organs.

Visualization: Diagnostic procedures may be performed with direct optical visualization. Operative procedures are carried out with video camera (Fig. 36.16).

OPERATIVE LAPAROSCOPY

- **Tubal sterilization with single puncture technique:** The various operative techniques of laparoscopic procedures are beyond the scope of the book. As the laparoscopic sterilization is commonly done, this procedure is described in page 415 (Fig. 36.12).
- **Laparoscopic ovarian drilling (LOD):** The surface cysts are punctured up to a depth of 4 to 10 mm. Monopolar current is used for 3 to 4 seconds. Drilling is avoided on the lateral surface of the ovaries and also at the hilum to avoid adhesions and bleeding respectively. Usually 5-7 punctures are made. At the end, the ovarian surface is irrigated with saline solution to cool it.
  Complications: Bleeding and later on adhesion formation and rarely ovarian failure may be there.
- **Total laparoscopic hysterectomy (TLH):** Uterus is freed of all its attachment laparoscopically. The uterus is removed either vaginally (commonly) or abdominally following morcellation. Vagina is closed with sutures laparoscopically (details *see* below).
- **Laparoscopic assisted vaginal hysterectomy (LAVH):** *See* below.

Benefits of laparoscopy prior to vaginal hysterectomy are: (a) Diagnosis of any other pelvic pathology; (b) Adhesiolysis or excision of endometriosis; (c) Adnexa is freed laparoscopically; (d) Dissection of bladder from uterus; (e) Desiccation and transection of uterine artery; (f) Entire uterus may be freed from its attachments.

PROCEDURE OF LAPAROSCOPIC HYSTERECTOMY

Three or four puncture sites are made. One 10 mm umbilical port is used for the laparoscope, connected to the video camera. Three other secondary ports are made, each of 5 mm size. Two of them are placed on the ipsilateral side and the third on the opposite side. These are placed lateral to the inferior epigastric artery or in the midline above the bladder. The left lower puncture is the major portal for

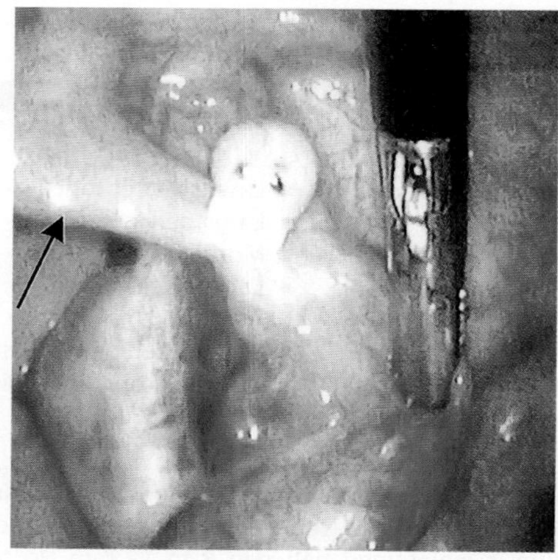

Fig. 36.12: Laparoscopic view showing tubal sterilization with silastic (Fallope) rings.

operative manipulation. The right is used for retraction with atraumatic grasping forceps.

Bipolar coagulation or harmonic scalpel are used to transect pelvic ligaments and to achieve hemostasis. Bipolar coagulation desiccates the blood vessels. Scissors are used to transect the pedicles following coagulation. The round ligament, infundibulopelvic ligament are similarly coagulated and transected. Sutures, staples or clips can also be used. The leaves of the broad ligament are opened up with the scissors. The peritoneum of the vesicouterine pouch is dissected with the scissors. Hydrodissection may be used to develop the space.

- **LAVH**, the laparoscopic procedure is stopped at this point. The rest of the operation is completed vaginally. Uterine vessel ligation is done from below. This is exactly the same as that of vaginal hysterectomy (p. 223). Uterus is removed through the vagina.
- **Total laparoscopic hysterectomy (TLH):** Dissection is continued as in LAVH to expose the uterine vessels. After careful identification of the uterine vessels and the ureter, the uterine vessels are desiccated using bipolar diathermy and then cut. Harmonic scalpel use causes coagulation and cutting simultaneously.

Uterus is then freed from the rest of attachment. The cardinal ligaments on each side are divided. Colpotomy device and vaginal occluding device (colpotomizer system) help to detect the site of colpotomy and maintain pneumoperitoneum simultaneously. Wet laparotomy sponge may be placed in the vagina for this purpose. Vagina is transected using monopolar energy or by harmonic. Bipolar cautery is used for hemostasis. The specimen is removed (*see* above). Vaginal vault is closed. Extracorporeal sutures may be used.

After completion of the procedure, laparoscope is used to check the pelvis for hemostasis. Peritoneal cavity is irrigated with Ringer's lactate solution and suctioned until clear fluid is obtained. Bleeding vessels are coagulated. 500 mL of Ringer's solution are left in the peritoneal cavity. The laparoscopic instruments are then removed and the pneumoperitoneum is deflated. The trocar incisions (ports) are closed.

Postoperative Care

General postoperative care is similar to any other major gynecological surgery. Care specific to laparoscopic hysterectomy are:

- **Prophylactic antibiotics** are used in a case of hysterectomy (p. 491)
- **Laparoscopic ports** should be kept clean and dry for next 7–10 days.
- **Diet** may be started by next 12 hours.
- **Discharge:** Patient may be discharged by next 48–72 hours.
- **Day-to-day physical activity** may be started by 10–12 days time.
- **Intercourse should be** avoided for next 6 weeks.

COMPLICATIONS OF LAPAROSCOPY

Complications are grouped into: (a) Specific to laparoscopy itself; (b) Due to anesthesia; (c) Common to any surgical procedures.

- **Complications due to laparoscopy itself:**
  - **Extraperitoneal insufflation**
    - Surgical emphysema
    - Omental emphysema
    - Cardiac arrhythmia.
  - **Injury to blood vessels**—mesenteric, omental, injury to major pelvic or abdominal artery or vein (iliac, aorta and the vena cava). Inferior epigastric vessels may be injured during insertion of accessory trocars.
  - **Injury to bowel**—with Veress needle or trocar especially when there is adhesions.
  - **Injury to organs** like bowel, bladder or ureter. Damage may be mechanical during dissection or thermal by electrical or laser energy.
  - **Electrosurgical complications**—causing thermal injury (electrode burns, insulation defects) to bowel, ureter.
  - **Gas (carbon dioxide) embolism**—resulting in hypotension, cardiac arrhythmia.
- **Anesthetic complications peculiar to laparoscopy are:**
  - **Hypoventilation** (pneumoperitoneum and Trendelenburg position lead to basal lung compression and reduced diaphragmatic excursion).
  - **Hypercarbia** and metabolic acidosis (when CO_2 is used for pneumoperitoneum), tachycardia and arrhythmia.
  - **Basal lung atelectasis**.
  - **Others**—esophageal intubation, aspiration, and cardiac arrest.
- **Complications common to any surgical procedure**
  - Hemorrhage
  - Wound dehiscence
  - Infection
  - Port site hernia.

Death rate in diagnostic laparoscopy is about 5/100,000 procedures. With experience, the fatality is markedly reduced to even zero. **Causes of death are** cardiac arrest, gas embolism, and consequences of intestinal injury.

ROBOTIC SURGERY IN GYNECOLOGY

Robotic technology facilitates the laparoscopic surgery with the use of a computer interface. Robotic technology enhances surgeon's accuracy; dexterity, shorter working times, and reduces the number of complications compared to conventional laparoscopic surgery.

The technology and instruments in robotic surgery: The surgeon controls the robotic arms with his two hands. Foot switches (five) to control are: clutch, camera, focus, energy sources (monopolar and bipolar-cutting and coagulation).

Robotic equipments: The surgeon sits at the console which is away from the patient. The assistant sits by the side of the

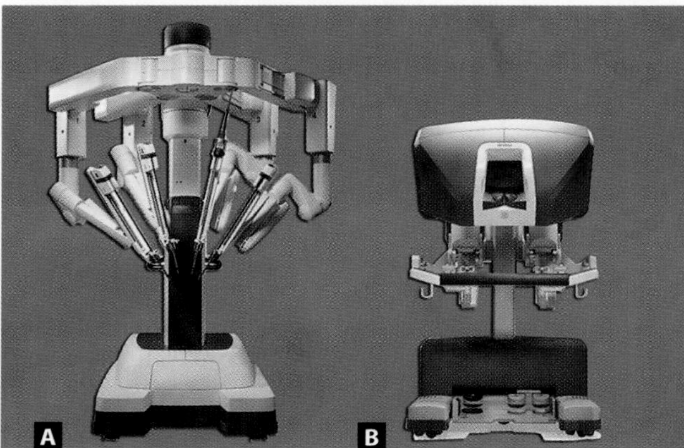

Figs. 36.13A and B: (A) da Vinci system robot (Robotic column with four arms). All the arms always works in a direction towards the robotic column and not away from it; (B) Robotic console: Surgeon controls the robotic arms using both the hands (above) and within the five foot switches (below). Surgeon sits at the console. Console is away from the patient. One assistant sits with the patient.

patient. The stereoscopic view of robotic laparoscopy is different from laparoscopic image. Robotic system consists of a robotic column with robotic arms (Figs. 36.13A and B) and a surgeons' console.

Currently, the only commercially available robot is the da Vinci system (Figs. 36.13A and B).

Initial abdominal entry and port placement are similar to laparoscopy. Of the four arms, one controls the laparoscope and the others hold the robotic instruments. The second surgeon in the console is generally for training.

Advanced video technology within an 8 mm laparoscope gives a high definition and magnified view.

The instrument tips mimic those used in open surgery and in laparoscopy. These are: Graspers, cutting instruments and needle drivers.

TECHNOLOGY OF ROBOTIC SURGERY

Advantages

- Robotic image is stereoscopic (3D) which is different from laparoscopic view.
- Robotic movements are intuitive. The instrument tips are articulated such, as to have seven degrees of movements. It mimics the movements of human wrist and fingers. So, any complex maneuver can be done within a limited space.
- It helps suturing and intracorporeal knot tying with ease unlike that of laparoscopy.
- High precision and absence of tremor are of particular benefits in cases of ureteric anastomosis, fistula repair or retroperitoneal lymphadenectomy.
- Increased accuracy and enhanced dexterity are the distinct benefits compared to laparoscopic surgery.
- Significant reduction in surgeon's morbidity and stress compared to laparoscopic surgery.
- More rapid patient's recovery.
- Decreased postoperative morbidity.
- Patient selection criteria are similar to laparoscopy.

Disadvantages

- Absence of tactile feedback.
- Long initial set up time needed during each case.
- Cost (both initial or maintenance) is prohibitive for robotic programs.

HYSTEROSCOPY

Hysteroscopy is a procedure that allows direct visua-lization inside the uterus (Fig. 36.14). It can be used for diagnostic as well as therapeutic purposes.

Basic instruments and electrosurgical units for hysteroscopic surgery (Figs. 36.15A to C)

Telescope: Rigid telescopes are commonly used. Rigid telescopes vary in diameters: 3–5 mm for diagnostic purpose and 5–7 diameters are usually needed for operative procedures. Cervical dilatation is needed. The telescope may be either straight on (forward view) (0°) or fore oblique view 30°, 70° or 90°.

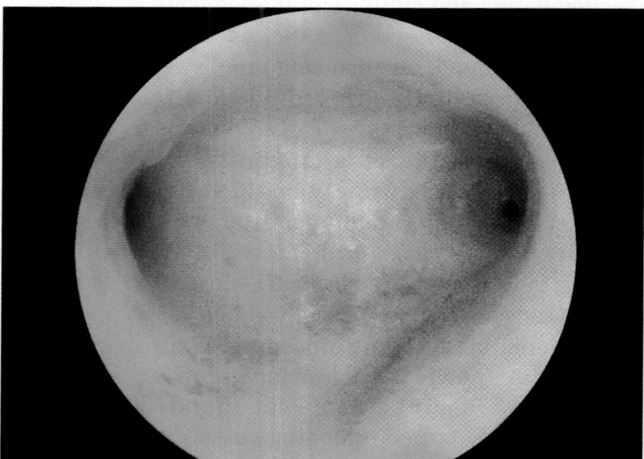

Fig. 36.14: Panoramic view of the uterine cavity with a hysteroscope. Tubal ostium is seen one on either side.

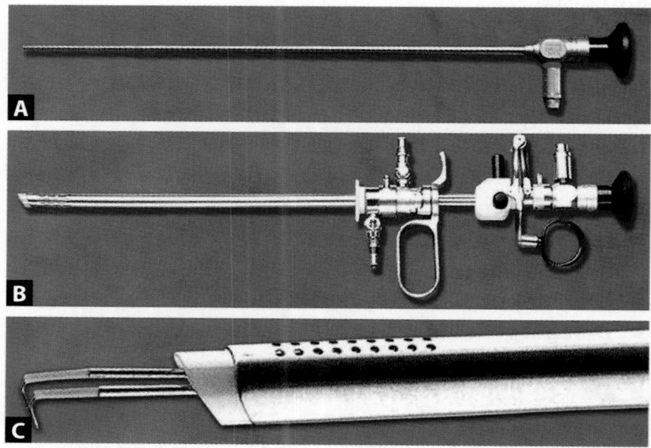

Figs. 36.15A to C: (A) Hysteroscope; (B) Hysteroscope with working element for operative interventions (outer diameter: 8 mm); (C) Resectoscope (with an angled cutting loop).

Flexible telescopes: The tip of the hysteroscope can bend up to 110°. It has the advantage of easy uterine entry through the angle between cervix and uterus. It helps easy aligning the catheter for tubal cannulation (Fig. 36.14).

Microhysteroscope acts as a high powered microscope by switching the lens to 150X. Light contact with the mucous membrane is needed.

Telescope sheath: A sheath is required to introduce the telescope. Sheath used for diagnostic purposes are smaller (5 mm) than that for operative sheath (7–10 mm). Operative instruments are introduced through the sheath. Operative hysteroscopy needs separate inflow and outflow sheaths. The inflow sheath carries the distension medium to the tip of the telescope, from where it is withdrawn via the outer sheath. This helps to maintain the clear view.

Distending media: The uterine cavity is distended with a media to separate the uterine walls and to have a panoramic view. The media used could be either a gas or a liquid.

Carbon dioxide (CO_2): It is commonly used for diagnostic purposes. It is soluble in blood and is safe. Visibility is poor in presence of bleeding.

Liquid media is used for operative procedures. Liquid media should distend the cavity optimally, allow good endoscopic view, should be nonconductive and nontoxic.

Normal saline can be used both for diagnostic and operative procedures. It allows good image quality, bipolar electrosurgery and acts as both distension and conduction media. It is not suitable for monopolar electrosurgery. Constant flow is to be maintained to flush the operative area. Risk of fluid overload is there.

Glycine 1.5% is used for excellent visualization. It is hypoosmolar. Resectoscope (monopolar electrosurgery) can be used as it does not conduct electricity. Fluid can be pressurized via a roller pump or by a pressure infusion bag cuff system with a maximum flow rate of 100 mL/min and maximum pressure of 100 mm Hg. Risk of fluid overload is there.

Mannitol (5%) and glycine (2.2%) are iso-osmolar, so can be used safely. They can be used with electrosurgical devices also.

Hyscon (32% dextran) is nonconductive. Risk of anaphylactic reaction and hypertonic fluid over load is there.

While using liquid distension media, volume of fluid instilled, volume of return fluid and the fluid deficit must be calculated. Significant fluid deficit (saline 1.5–2L) warns the surgeon to discontinue the procedure. Glycine—a fluid deficit of >500 mL, may cause hyponatremia and hypoosmolar state.

A fluid deficit of (≥500 mL is alarming) to prevent hyponatremia and hypoosmolality. Fluid deficit ≥IL, require measurement of serum electrolytes and diuretic (frusemide) therapy.

A pressure of about 50–70 mm Hg is required for adequate distention of the uterine cavity. This pressure should not exceed the mean arterial pressure to avoid extravasation.

Accessory instruments are: Scissors, forceps, grasping forceps (Fig. 36.3). Monopolar and bipolar electrodes (a ball, needle or cutting loop) are used for operative hysteroscopy.

Image-recorder: The recorded images are useful as teaching aids to the trainees. They can also be used as an evidence (in defense) for medicolegal purpose.

Camera: The hysteroscopic image is visualized on the monitor with the help of a camera. The camera used for laparoscopy is used. The monitor is checked before hand for visualization of appropriate image. A high resolution camera and color monitor is required for both the surgeon and the assistants.

Light source: Xenon or mercury halide can provide high intensity light sources for excellent illumination.

ANESTHESIA AND THE PROCEDURES (FIG. 36.16)

Diagnostic Procedures (BSGE – 2018)

These are carried out as an outpatient under paracervical block with 1% xylocaine (10–15 mL). Initial steps are same as in dilatation and curettage (p. 492). Telescope inserted within the diagnostic sheath, is gradually inserted through the cervical canal while the light is on. The distension media (normal saline) is flushed through the sheath. Uterine cavity is evaluated thoroughly with a closer view at fundus, lateral, anterior, posterior walls and the tubal ostia. Endocervical canal is seen while withdrawing the hysteroscope from the uterus.

Operative Procedures

These are carried out under general anesthesia or regional anesthesia (spinal or epidural).

INDICATIONS OF DIAGNOSTIC HYSTEROSCOPY

- **Abnormal uterine bleeding (AUB):**
  - Menorrhagia (Fig. 36.17).
  - Postmenopausal bleeding (p. 469).

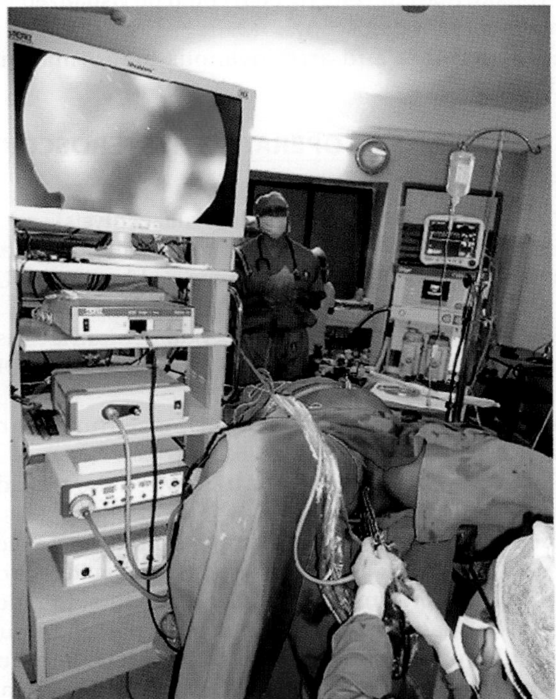

Fig. 36.16: Hysteroscopic procedures in progress.

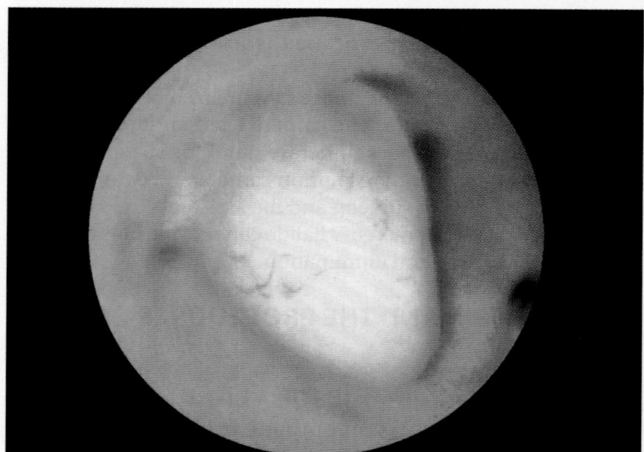

Fig. 36.17: Hysteroscopic view of a submucous fibroid.

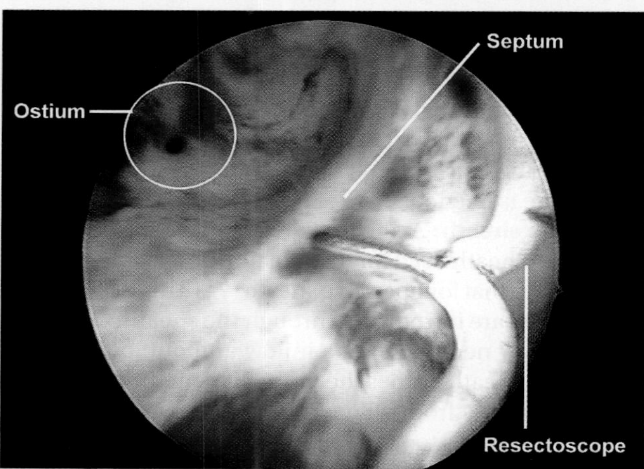

Fig. 36.18: Patient with complete septum. Resection of the septum is being done using the resectoscope.

- **Infertility:** When associated with abnormal hysterosalpingogram (filling defect, synechiae).
- **Müllerian anomalies** like arcuate, subseptate, septate, bicornate uterus or uterus didelphys can be diagnosed with hysteroscopy. The procedure is combined with laparoscopy for confirmation.
- **Recurrent miscarriage:** Intrauterine pathology such as fibroids, polyps, Asherman's syndrome (Fig. 38.76) can be diagnosed and treated.
- **Misplaced intrauterine device (IUD)** (Fig. 30.8).
- **Chronic pelvic pain** due to obstructive uterine anomaly, submucous fibroids, bicornuate uterus may be diagnosed. Laparoscopy is done to exclude other pelvic pathologies.
- **Transformation zone** (p. 268) could be visualized with microcolpohysteroscopy.
- **Hemangioma** and arteriovenous malformation—diagnosis.

INDICATIONS OF OPERATIVE HYSTEROSCOPY

- **Polypectomy** and myomectomy.
- **Lysis** of intrauterine adhesions (synaecholysis).
- **Endometrial ablation** (laser or roller ball) for patients suffering from dysfunctional uterine bleeding (DUB) (p. 161).
- **Endometrial resection**—where endometrium is excised using a resectoscope (Fig. 15.4) for patients with DUB (p. 162).
- **Metroplasty** (resection of uterine septum) under laparoscopic guidance (Fig. 36.18).
- **Removal** of foreign body or IUD, when the thread is missing.
- **Biopsy** of suspected endometrium under direct vision.
- **Tubal cannulation**—under hysteroscopic guidance can release any proximal tubal obstruction (due to mucus plugs or spasm). A special catheter is passed through the tubal ostium up to the interstitial part of the tube.
- **Sterilization**—by destroying the interstitial portion of the tubes using Nd:YAG laser or electrocoagulation.
- Tubal occlusions with 'Essure" by inserting the coil in the proximal part of the tube are done hysteroscopically (p. 424).
- Hysteroscopy: Superior to HSG in the diagnosis of intrauterine disease.
- **Laser coagulation** of endometrial hemangioma and arteriovenous malformation in cases with unresponsive bleeding.

Pretreatment Evaluation and Protocol

- It should preferably be done in the postmenstrual phase with normal sized uterus.
- It should be preceded by diagnostic hysteroscopy.
- Pretreatment with danazol, GnRH analog or progestogen for 4–6 weeks to make the endometrium thin prior to endometrial ablation/resection.

LEVELS OF HYSTEROSCOPIC PROCEDURES (RCOG – 1994)

- **Level 1 (diagnostic procedures)**
  - Diagnostic hysteroscopy plus target biopsy
  - Removal of simple polyp
  - Removal of IUCD.
- **Level 2 (minor operative procedures)**
  - Fallopian tube cannulation (proximal)
  - Minor Asherman's syndrome—adhesiolysis
  - Removal of pedunculated fibroid or large polyp.
- **Level 3 (complex operative procedures)**
  - Resection of uterine septum
  - Major Asherman's syndrome—synaecholysis
  - Transcervical resection of endometrium (TCRE)
  - Resection of submucous leiomyoma.

CONTRAINDICATIONS OF HYSTEROSCOPY

- **Pelvic infection:** Hysteroscopy can cause spread of infection. The distension media flowing through the tube spreads the infection in the peritoneal cavity.
- **Pregnancy:** However, hysteroscopy can be done to remove an IUCD when the threads are missing.

- **Cervical cancer:** Trauma to the friable cervix can cause excessive bleeding.
- **Cardiopulmonary disorders** are at higher risk of anesthesia as hysteroscopy carries its own risk of gas embolism, fluid overload and pulmonary edema.
- **Cervical stenosis** can cause cervical trauma. PGE_2 gel inserted 2 hours before surgery, softens the cervix and help easy dilatation.

OPERATIVE HYSTEROSCOPY

Transcervical resection of endometrium (TCRE) or laser ablation of endometrium (LAE) is done as an alternative to hysterectomy for dysfunctional uterine bleeding.

Principle

This operation is to destroy the endometrium up to a depth of 3–5 mm. There would be no further regeneration of endometrium as the basal layer of endometrium as well as the basal and spiral arterioles are destroyed.

Procedure

Hysteroscopic resection procedure is done on monopolar current. It needs nonelectrolyte solutions like glycine or mannitol. Bipolar electrosurgery systems (versapoint) allow use of tools in a saline solution. Resectoscope has a cutting loop, ball tip and pointed coagulation electrode attachments.

Endometrial resection is done from cornu to cornu (fundus) and all the walls. Ablation is not needed below the level of the internal os. TCRE or LAE is completed by about 30 minutes time and patient can go home on the same day.

Total resection or ablation of endometrium should result in amenorrhea. **Selection of the patient** is very important. Presence of pelvic pain is a contraindication. Before TCRE or LAE endometrium is suppressed using danazol or GnRH analog for 4–6 weeks. Therapeutic response following TCRE or LAE has been observed in 80–85% of cases.

HYSTEROSCOPIC MYOMECTOMY (FIG. 36.19)

It is done for submucous myomas as an alternative to hysterectomy or laparotomic myomectomy for a patient with intractable symptoms.

Indications

- **Infertility**
- **Menorrhagia**

Surgical Technique

Preoperative GnRH agonist therapy is used (p. 443). Resectoscope is normally used for myoma resection. Electrosurgical working element with 90° cutting loop (Figs. 36.14A to C) is usually used to shave off any submucous leiomyoma (Fig. 20.9). Myometrium is desiccated through contact coagulation for 30–40 seconds to control bleeding. Bleeding can also be controlled using roller ball coagulation. Uterine tamponade with the inflated bulb of a Foley catheter is also effective.

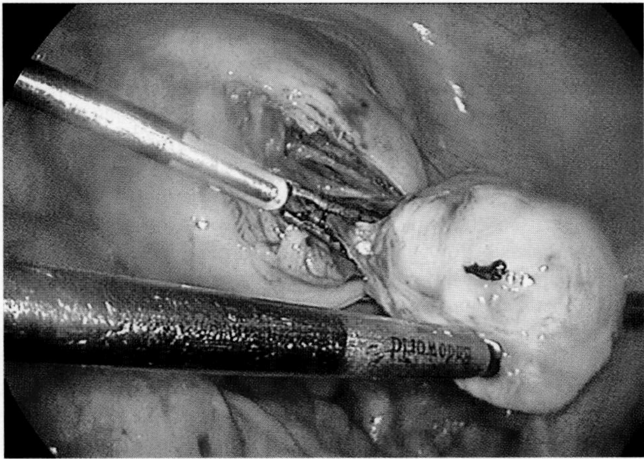

Fig. 36.19: Laparoscopic myomectomy. Myoma screw (Fig. 36.3D) is used for traction of the myoma.

(*Courtesy:* Dr Parul Kodtawala, Ahmedabad)

Common Complications

Uterine perforation and hemorrhage.

COMPLICATIONS OF HYSTEROSCOPY

Complications may arise from any of these following:

- **Perioperative**
- **Late**

Perioperative Complications

- **Distension media:**
  - Fluid overload
  - Pulmonary edema, cerebral edema
  - Hyponatremia
  - Neurological symptoms
  - Ammonia toxicity due to excess glycine absorption
  - Gas embolism (CO_2)
  - Coagulopathies
  - Seizures
- **Operative procedures**
  - Uterine perforation.
  - Hemorrhage—intraoperative or postoperative.
  - Injury to intra-abdominal organs.
- **Electrosurgical:** Thermal injury to intra-abdominal organs due to laser or electricity.
- **Others:** Infection, anesthetic complications, and treatment failure.

Late Complications

- **Abnormal uterine bleeding** due to failure of TCRE especially in the young age group.
- **Hematometra and pyometra**—may occur due to infection after hysteroscopic surgery with cervical stenosis. Ablation near internal os level should not be done.
- **Pregnancy**—may occur following TCRE (rare).
- **Post ablation tubal sterilization syndrome** (PATSS).

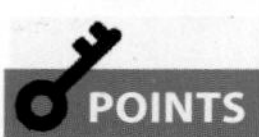

POINTS

- **Endoscopy** is the procedure to visualize the interior of a viscous or space with the use of a telescope. In gynecology as much as 80% of operations can be performed endoscopically with the use of either a laparoscope or a hysteroscope.
- **During laparoscopy**, the magnification of the object depends upon the distance of the laparoscope from the object. With 'Storz' it is nearly 10 times when working distance is 3 mm and is 1 when the distance is 30 mm.
- **Laparoscopic surgery** could be diagnostic (p. 102) or therapeutic (p. 516). Before any procedure is undertaken, contraindications must be carefully excluded (Table 36.1). Informed consent should include the permission for open surgery if necessity arises.
- **Hemostasis** during laparoscopic surgery can be achieved using electrocoagulation (monopolar/bipolar), laser coagulation, ligatures, sutures (extracorporeal/intracorporeal), EnSeal, harmonic scalpel or by stapler and clips (p. 514).
- **Thermal damage** caused by electrosurgery or laser depends on the degree of heat applied to the tissues. Tissue damage with heat is as follows: 45°C = Tissue death; 70°C = Coagulation; ≥ 90°C = Desiccation; ≥100°C = Vaporization; ≥200°C = Carbonization (charring).
- **Laparoscopic tubal sterilization** is the most common surgical procedure. In LAVH the uterine arteries are clamped and secured through vaginal route. In TLH entire procedure is done laparoscopically.
- **Complications of laparoscopy** may be due to the procedure itself or due to anesthesia (p. 519).
- **Hysteroscopy** is superior to HSG. The distending media commonly used in hysteroscopy is normal saline or glycine (1.5%).
- **The contraindications** (p. 522) of hysteroscopy are pelvic infection, pregnancy, and abnormal uterine bleeding. Complications include fluid overload, pulmonary edema, and injury to genital or abdominal organs or electrosurgical injuries.
- **Hysteroscopic surgery** should be done in the postmenstrual phase. Pretreatment with danazol or GnRH analog for 4–6 weeks facilitate endometrial ablation or resection.
- **Hysteroscopy** may be diagnostic (target biopsy, detection of IUCD) or therapeutic (tubal cannulation, removal of polyp, resection of uterine septum and for release of intrauterine adhesions).
- **Major indications of hysteroscopy are:** AUB, removal of endometrial polyps, submucous myomas, retained IUCDs and the others (*see* above)
- **Complications of hysteroscopy include:** Uterine perforation, bleeding, fluid over load and pulmonary edema (p. 523)
- **Absolute contraindications of laparoscopy are:** Hemoperitoneum, hemodynamic instability, bowel obstruction, severe cardiovascular disease (p. 522).
- **Complications of operative laparoscopy** are many (p. 519). Thermal bowel injuries often go unrecognized intraoperatively. Delay in diagnosis is life-threatening.

CHAPTER

37 Current Topics in Gynecology

CHAPTER OUTLINE

- Stem Cells and Therapies
- Properties of Stem Cells
- Use of Embryonic Stem Cells in Regenerative Medicine

STEM CELLS AND THERAPIES IN GYNECOLOGY

Reproductive tissues are the important source of stem cells (progenitor cells). Stem cells have the potential to be used in the field of regenerative medicine.

Potentials for the use of Stem Cells in Regenerative Medicine

- Treatment of inherited genetic disorders
- Treatment of hematological diseases.

A stem cell has the ability to renew (reproduce) itself for long periods.

Properties of Stem Cells

- Ability to self-renew (undergoing numerous cell divisions) maintaining the undifferentiated state.
- Multipotency: Capacity to differentiate into a mature cell type.

Totipotent stem cells are produced by first few divisions of the fertilized egg cell. Totipotent stem cells (from the morula) can differentiate into embryonic and extraembryonic cell types. Totipotent cells can produce a complete and viable organism.

Pluripotent stem cells are descendent of totipotent cells. These cells can differentiate on tissues derived from any of the three germ layers including fetal tissues (placenta, umbilical cord, amnion, amniotic fluid cells).

Embryonic stem (ES) cells are pluripotent. These cells are derived from the inner cell mass of a blastocyst.

Multipotent stem cells can differentiate into various tissues originating from a single germ layer (mesenchymal cells or hematopoietic stem cells that produce red blood cells, white blood cells, platelets).

Unipotent cells produce only their own cell type. They have greater self-renewal property than fully mature cells.

Theoretically, the more primitive or potent stem cells are the potential for uncontrolled cell division is more strong. Unfortunately, the potential for oncogenesis is also high. It is the major concern about the oncogenic potential of pluripotent stem cells (embryonic stem cells). Nonpluripotent cells source are not inherently oncogenic.

Embryonic stem cells have the potentials to be used in regenerative medicine.

Multipotent stem cells can be obtained from several fetal tissues (following medical termination of pregnancy or at birth).

USE OF EMBRYONIC STEM CELLS IN REGENERATIVE MEDICINE

Gynecology

- **Regeneration of urogenital tract tissues**
  - **Treatment of stress urinary incontinence (SUI):** Currently SUI is treated by mechanical support to the bladder (TOT) (*see* p. 339) Biomaterials (autologous stem or urethral tract progenitor cells) are injected into the urethral sphincter. This is aimed to restore and regenerate rhabdomyosphincter muscle content and function. These autologous cells commonly integrate into the sphincter complex. These cells then differentiate and ultimately lead to sphincter regeneration. This ongoing research might be of immense benefits in regenerative medicine.
  - **Bladder reconstruction:**
    - Acellular natural or synthetic biomaterials are used as an implant which becomes incorporated through ingrowth of cells from the adjacent native host cells of the bladder. The biomaterials used are—small intestinal submucosa and bladder-derived acellular matrix.
    - Implantation of scaffolds (cell-seeded collagen-coated PGA scaffolds) preincubated with autologous cells (wrapped in omentum within a vascular bed). Reports are available, indicating possibility of creating full thickness bladder wall.
- **Biomaterials** can be used for the use of pelvic organ prolapse (POP) and urinary incontinence. The purpose is to generate new muscles/tissues which can perform in an integrated manner with the existing tissues to provide mechanical support to the pelvic organs. Currently synthetic meshes are used for POP and SUI. Mesh erosion, infection are the known complications.

Hybrid biomaterials (synthetic and naturally-derived polymers) may be fabricated to restore pelvic floor function and cure of SUI. Biomaterials should have good biocompatibility and appropriate biomechanical and biochemical properties.

- **Müllerian ducts reconstruction:**
  - Progenitor cells with ability of self-repair (bone marrow stem cells) can be used for uterine malformations.
  - Autologous cells (from vaginal biopsy) can be expanded and functional vagina can be reconstructed for a woman with vaginal agenesis.

However, till date it is essential to understand its known limitations, putative benefits and the unknown risks. Until there is sufficient evidence on the efficacy of therapy, each case should be considered on an individual basis.

CHAPTER

38 Practical Gynecology

CHAPTER OUTLINE

INSTRUMENTS

SPATULA, BROOM (PLASTIC) AND CYTOBRUSH (FIGS. 38.1A TO C)

Ayre's spatula, the broom (plastic) and the endocervical brush are used for collection of cells for cytology screening.

Sampling the transformation zone at the SCJ is done. Three types of plastic devices are used: (a) Spatula; (b) Endocervical brush (cytobrush); and (c) Broom.

Procedure

- **For cervical cells:** Spatula—projected end of the spatula goes within the external os. The spatula is rotated 360° to collect cells from the entire ectocervix (Fig. 9.15).
- **For endocervical cells:** The cytobrush goes within the cervical canal and is rotated to collect cells (Fig. 9.18).
- (a) **Spatula** to sample the ectocervix; (b) **Cytobrush** is for the endocervical canal. Cytobrush when used the outermost bristles to remain just visible within the external OS. This avoids inadvertent sampling of the lower uterine segment. The brush is rotated only one quarter to one-half turn. Spatula and the cytobrush are used in combination; (c) **Plastic broom** samples both endo and ectocervical epithelium. Broom device has longer bristles in the center. These longer bristles are flanked by the shorter bristles. When the central longer bristles are inserted into the endocervical canal, the shorter bristles splay out over the ectocervix during rotation. Five rotations in the same direction are made. Reverse rotation may cause loss of the collected cells. Broom is used for liquid based cytology (LBC) Pap and HPV testing.
- **For cytohormonal study (p. 90)**, the rounded end of the spatula is used (Fig. 9.15).

Self-assessment

Q. ***How do you prepare the slide?***

Ans. Slide preparation: The cells collected by the spatula is quickly spread evenly over a major (two-thirds) part of a glass slide. The endocervical brush is rolled over the remaining area of the slide. **Cytofixation** is quickly done by spraying aerosol (95% ethyl alcohol or ethyl alcohol with polyethylene glycol) over it or immersing the slide in a fixative. Once dried up, the slide is then stained (in the laboratory) either with Papanicolaou or Sorr's method. It is examined under the microscope by a cytopathologist.

Q. Who are the women (at risk), that they need cervical cytology screening?

Ans.
- Any sexually active women 25 years (30 years, Government of India) and up to 65 years of age.
- Others: P. 90.

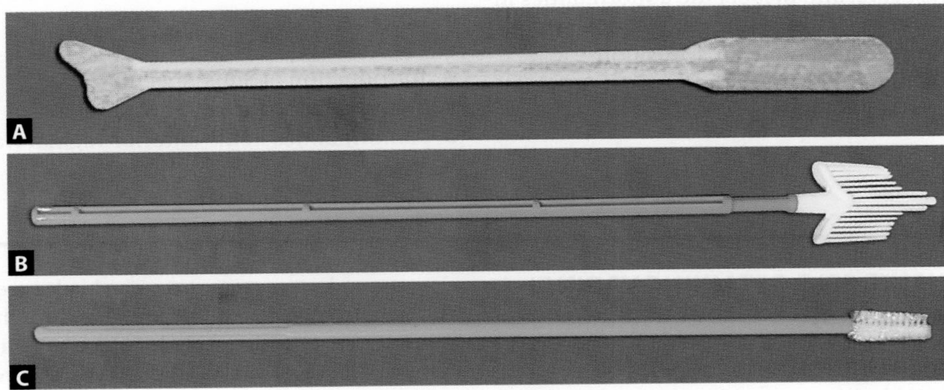

Figs. 38.1A to C: (A) Plastic spatula; (B) Broom; (C) Cytobrush.

Q. How cervical cytology is reported (the Bethesda system)?

Ans. (1) Squamous cell abnormalities: (A) Atypical squamous cells (ASC)—(a) ASC-US, (b) ASC-H; (B) LSIL; (C) HSIL; (D) SCC. (2) Glandular cell abnormalities (*see* details Ch. 9).

Q. What is a dyskaryotic smear? What are the different types of dyskaryotic smear?

Ans. Dyskaryosis is the morphological abnormalities of the nucleus. Abnormalities may be nuclear enlargement in size and shape, irregularity in outline, multinucleation, and hyperchromasia. Dyskaryotic smear may be: (a) Mild; (b) Moderate; and (c) Severe (p. 91).

Q. What is koilocytosis?

Ans. It is the nuclear abnormalities observed in human papilloma virus (HPV) infection. The typical changes are: Perinuclear halo, nuclear irregularity, hyperchromasia and multinucleation (Fig. 23.3).

Q. What is CIN? How do you diagnose CIN?

Ans. It is the histological observation where part or whole of thickness of cervical squamous epithelium is replaced by cells with varying degree of atypia. Basement membrane remains intact. Diagnosis of CIN is made by: (a) Cytology; (b) VIA; (c) Colposcopy; (d) Cervicography; (e) Biopsy; and (f) Conization of cervix.

Q. How do you manage a case of CIN?

Ans. (a) Local ablative methods; (b) Excisional methods (LLETZ); (c) Conization; or by (d) Hysterectomy.

Q. What is the Bethesda system classification for cervical cytology?

Ans. P. 92 (Table 9.2).

Q. How to take cervical smear?

Ans. Cervix is exposed with a Cusco's bivalve speculum without any lubricant. Prior bimanual examination should not be done. Rest p. 89.

Q. How to send samples for LBC and HPV?

Ans. Smear is taken using a broom (covering both the ecto and the endocervix). The broom end is dipped into the LBC for cytology and the HPV testing also.

Q. How HPV infection and CIN are related and how it could be prevented?

Ans. P. 271.

SIMS' DOUBLE BLADED POSTERIOR VAGINAL SPECULUM (FIG. 38.2)

Description and Identification

This is a metallic instrument.

The instrument was designed by Marion Sims'. The blades are of unequal breadth to facilitate introduction into the vagina depending upon the space available (narrow blade in nulliparous and the wider blade in parous women). This double bladed speculum has a groove in the handle (located in between the blades). This groove is in continuity at either end, with the concave inner surface of each blade. The purpose of the groove is to allow drainage of blood, urine [in a case with vesicovaginal fistula (VVF)], or secretions to collect samples and for tests.

Uses

- It is commonly used in vaginal operations such as D&C, D&E, anterior colporrhaphy, vaginal hysterectomy, etc. to retract the posterior vaginal wall.
- To visualize the cervix and inspect the abnormalities in the anterior vaginal wall like cystocele, VVF or Gartner's cyst after placing the patient in Sims' position.
- To collect the materials from the vaginal pool for cytology, Gram stain or culture.

Sterilization

Boiling or autoclaving.

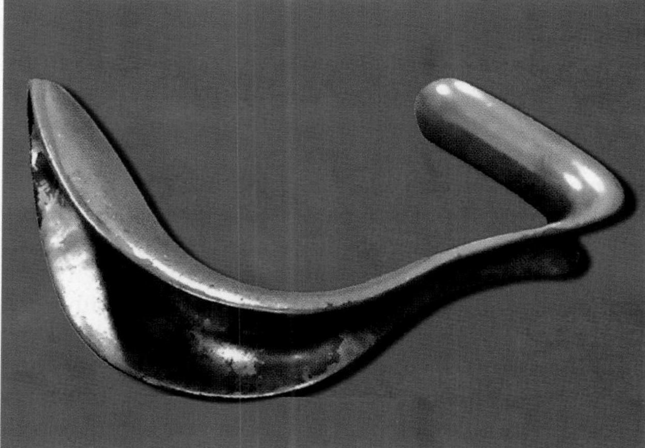

Fig. 38.2: Sims' speculum.

Self-assessment

- Who was Marion Sims'? (See author's Bedside Clinic)
- Sims' position.
- Sims' triad (p. 353).
- Introduction of Sims' speculum.
- Why the blades are of unequal sizes?
- Abnormalities in the anterior vaginal wall.
- Indications of D&C (p. 492).
- Steps of D&C (p. 492).

CUSCO'S BIVALVE SELF-RETAINING VAGINAL SPECULUM (FIG. 38.3)

Description and Identification

It is a **metallic** (could be plastic also) instrument. It has two blades joined by screws that allow the blades to open and close around a transverse axis. The blades are concave inside. The handle is designed to open and close the blades and to adjust the space with the blades with a separate rod and screw system. This also makes the blades **self-retaining** during examination. This speculum does not need any assistant to hold it.

The blades are opened to retract the anterior and posterior vaginal wall so as to have a good look to the cervix. A light source from behind is essential. **It is commonly used in the OPD.**

Uses

- To visualize the cervix and vaginal fornices.
- To collect cervical smear for cytologic screening and vaginal pool materials.
- To have cervicovaginal swabs for Gram stain and culture.
- To insert or to remove intrauterine contraceptive device (IUCD) or to check the threads.
- To perform minor operations like punch biopsy, surface cauterization or snipping a small polyp.

Sterilization

Boiling or autoclaving.

Self-assessment

- Use of two blades (*see* above).
- Lesions in the cervix.
- Ectopy (erosion) cervix (Ch. 19)
- Bethesda system cytology reporting (p. 92).
- Polyps.

Q. What is cervical ectopy?

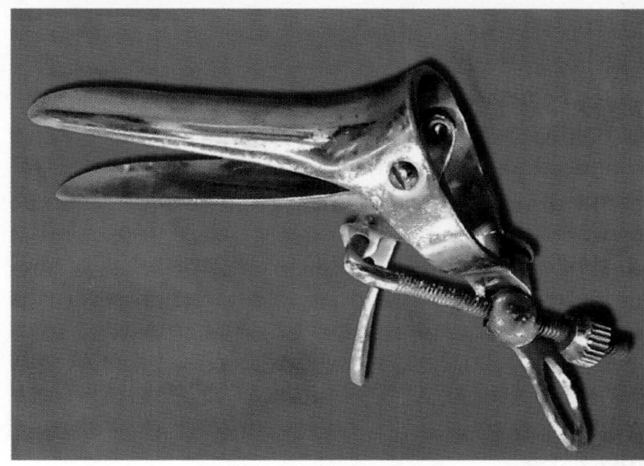

Fig. 38.3: Cusco's speculum.

Ans. It is the replacement of squamous epithelium of the ectocervix by columnar epithelium of endocervix by the process of metaplasia (Ch. 19).

Q. What are the different types of polyps?

Ans. Polyps may be benign (mucous, fibroid or placental) or malignant. It may be sessile or pedunculated (Ch. 20).

AUVARD'S SELF-RETAINING POSTERIOR VAGINAL SPECULUM (FIG. 38.4)

Description and Identification

It is a metallic instrument. It is made heavy as a ball with lead is attached with it. The handle is longer. The upper surface of the blade is concave. In continuity to this concavity there is a groove that runs all along the handle. This is to drain out any blood that is collected on the upper surface of the blade. The blade has two small holes, two on each side. Labial stitches can be placed through the holes to prevent it slipping down.

Uses

- It is used as posterior vaginal wall retractor in operations like anterior colporrhaphy, vaginal hysterectomy, etc.
- It should be used when the operation is done under general or regional anesthesia as the instrument is heavy. It requires no assistant. **Disadvantage:** It is heavy. Prolonged use may cause perineal pain in the postoperative period.

Sterilization

Autoclaving or boiling.

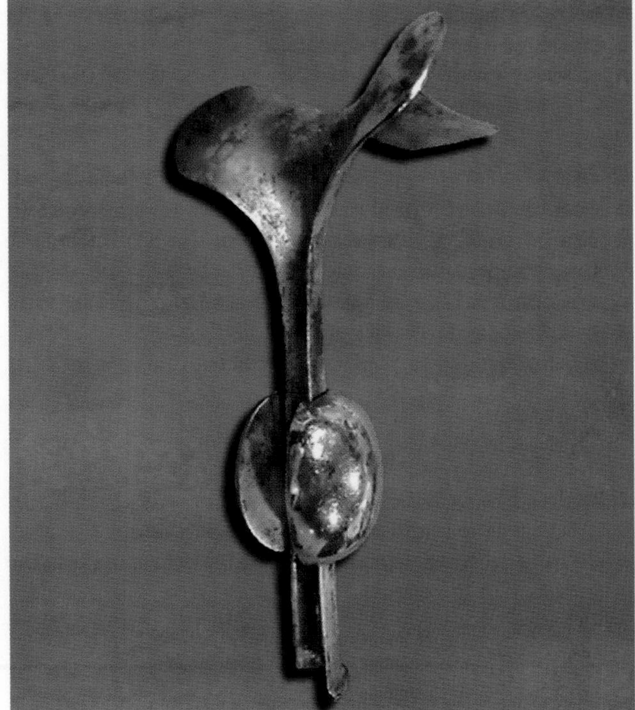

Fig. 38.4: Auvard's speculum.

FEMALE RUBBER CATHETER (FIG. 38.5)

Description and Identification

It is made of red rubber. There is an opening close to its tip to drain urine from the bladder. It is made of different sizes.

Uses

- To empty the bladder in retention of urine.
- To administer oxygen (where nasal probes not available).
- To use as a tourniquet in myomectomy operation as an alternative to myomectomy clamp.

Sterilization

Boiling.

Self-assessment

- Causes of retention of urine (Table 25.8).
- Procedure of catheterization (Fig. 9.13).

Q. What are the causes of acute and chronic retention of urine?

Ans. (a) Postoperative (common); (b) Obstructive (urethral kinking—big cystocele, compression over the bladder neck, urethra: vaginal packing, impacted ovarian tumor in the POD); (c) Failure of detrusor contraction; (d) External sphincter spasm; and (e) Others (Table 25.8).

Q. What are the different types of urinary incontinence?

Ans. P. 335.

Q. What are the different menstrual abnormalities that can manifest with retention of urine? (p. 343, Table 25.8).

Ans.

a. **Primary amenorrhea** (cryptomenorrhea) → hematocolpos (p. 377) → retention.
b. **Secondary amenorrhea** → retroverted gravid uterus → urinary retention.

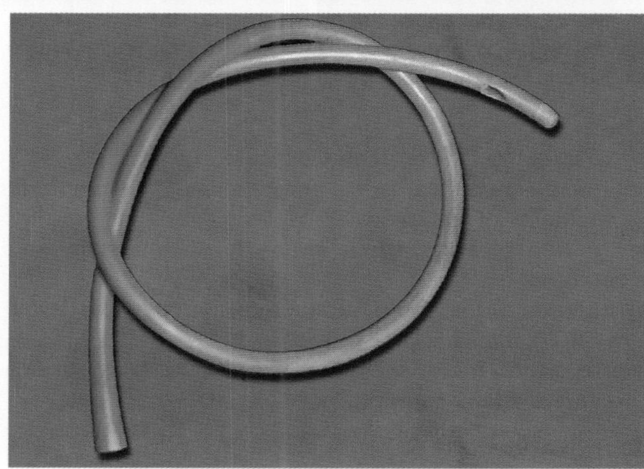

Fig. 38.5: Simple rubber catheter.

c. **Menorrhagia** → impacted uterine fibroid in the pouch of Douglas (POD) → urinary retention.
d. **Irregular bleeding and pain** → pelvic hematocele, pelvic abscess → retention.
e. **No menstrual abnormality** → impacted ovarian tumor, cervical fibroid or ovarian mass.

FEMALE METAL CATHETER (FIG. 38.6)

Description and Identification

It is a metallic catheter with a flat handle at its on end. The other end has several openings on its either side. This perforated end is introduced through the urethra into the bladder to drain urine.

Uses

- To empty the bladder prior to major vaginal operations. Not only it facilitates the operation but minimizes the injury to the bladder.
- To confirm the diagnosis of Gartner's cyst from cystocele (p. 175).
- It is not used in obstetrics to avoid trauma.

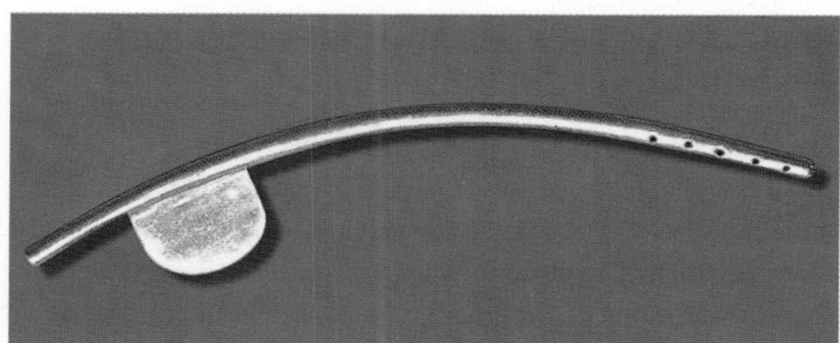

Fig. 38.6: Female metal catheter.

- At the end of the operation to make sure about absence of any bladder injury.

Sterilization

By autoclaving or boiling.

Uses in PFR (p. 180)

- To empty the bladder prior to the operation.
- To note the lower limit of the bladder before making the incision on the vagina.
- Prior to cutting the vesicocervical ligament.

Self-assessment

- What is the length of female urethra? (p. 10).
- Differentiation of Gartner's cyst from cystocele (p. 172).
- Management of injury to bladder during operation: Bladder mucosa is apposed with 3-0 delayed absorbable suture (Vicryl) as a continuous layer. A second layer of (musculofascial) suture with the same material is used to reinforce the first layer. Continuous bladder drainage is maintained for 10 days.

FOLEY'S CATHETER (FIG. 38.7)

Description and Identification

It is made of silicon rubber. The catheter tip has two slit openings one on either side for drainage of urine. The other end goes to the urinary bag for collection of urine. The catheter has two channels within. One channel for drainage of urine and the other channel is used to push some water through it. Water inflates the catheter bulb that makes the catheter self-retaining. The bulb capacity is written on the catheter. The catheters are of different sizes. The commonly used sizes in female are 14F, 16F or 18F.

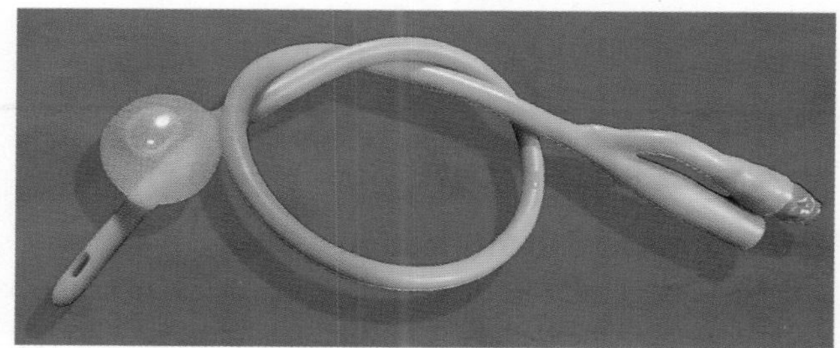

Fig. 38.7: Foley's catheter with balloon inflated.

Uses

It is used in gynecology for:

- **Continuous drainage of bladder.** Common indications of use are:
  - Vaginal/abdominal hysterectomy.
  - Pelvic floor repair.
  - Repair of VVF.
  - Urinary retention due to pelvic tumor/retroverted gravid uterus.
  - Radical hysterectomy.
  - To monitor urine output in a critically ill-patient.
- During hysterosalpingography and sonohysterosalpingography (SIS). The catheter is introduced into the uterocervical canal. The balloon is inflated to occlude the internal os. The media (dye/saline) is pushed and sonography is then done.
- To assess the patency of the fallopian tube during laparotomy. The catheter is introduced in the uterocervical canal. The balloon is inflated to occlude the internal os. The dye is then pushed through the catheter. Spillage of dye from the fimbrial end is then verified.

Sterilization

It is available in a sterile package following sterilization with Ethylene Tetra Oxide (ETO). It is disposable.

Self-assessment

Q. Why the term Foley's is attached?

Ans. This catheter goes with the name of Federic E B Foley, who originally designed it. It was designed initially as a hemostatic bag catheter (*see* Dutta's Bedside clinic p. 556).

- What are the urinary complications following abdominal hysterectomy?
- Common urinary complications of vaginal hysterectomy.
- Mention the postoperative management following repair of VVF.
- Common causes of retention of urine due to pelvic tumor or retroverted gravid uterus (Ch. 25).
- What is sonohysterosalpingography (SIS)?

CERVICAL DILATORS (FIGS. 38.8A AND B)

Description and Identification

It is a single ended (Hawkin-Ambler) or double ended (Hegar's) metallic cervical dilator. The disk shaped end is the handle and the other pointed side, is the dilating end. It has a smooth curvature with the tip directing upwards to follow the curvature (anteversion and anteflexion) of the uterus.

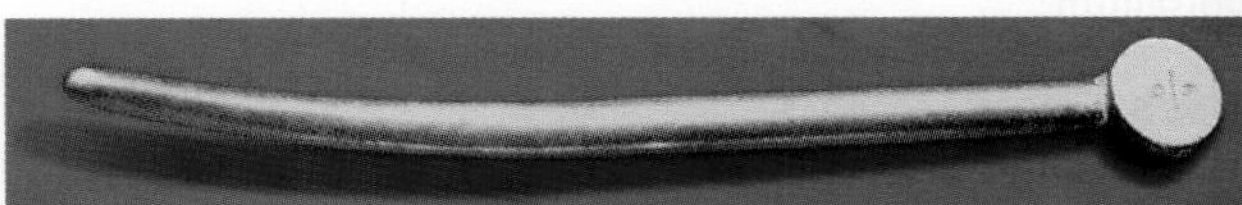

Fig. 38.8A: Hawkin-Ambler dilator.

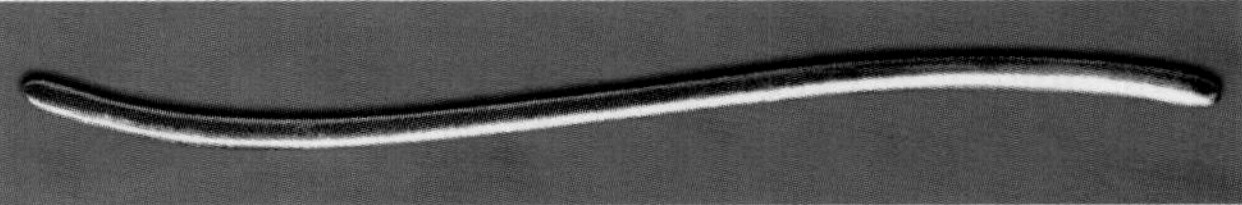

Fig. 38.8B: Das's dilator.

Varieties

- Hawkin-Ambler: There are 16 sets starting from 3/6 and ends with 18/21 (Fig. 38.8A).
- Hegar's: There are 12 sets, the smallest one is of 1–2 mm. This is used mainly in gynecological operations.
- Das's dilator (named after Sir Kedarnath Das) (Fig. 38.8B). Both the sides of the instrument are used. The side with smaller diameter is used first.

Uses

- To dilate the cervix to facilitate intrauterine introduction of instruments (curette), devices (IUCD), hysteroscope or radium.
- To dilate the cervix to facilitate drainage of intrauterine collection—pyometra, hematometra or lochiometra.
- To confirm patency of cervical canal after amputation of the cervix.
- To dilate the urethra in urethral stricture.

Sterilization: Boiling or autoclaving.

Self-assessment

- Indications of dilatation of the cervix only (Ch. 35).
- Indications of amputation of cervix (Ch. 35).
- Causes of pyometra (Ch. 13).
- Complications of dilatation operation (Ch. 35).

MULTIPLE TOOTHED VULSELLUM (FIG. 38.9)

Description and Identification

It is a long metallic instrument. It is designed to have small teeth (3–4) arising from each blade. The teeth fit in spaces between them. It is used to grasp tissues firmly with less trauma. The handle has a catch that also makes the grip firm.

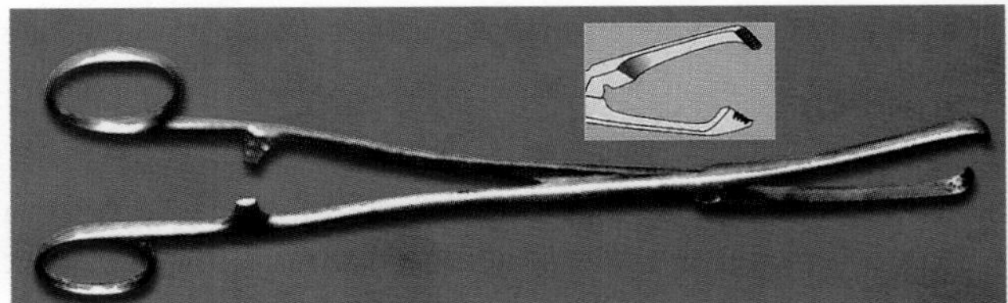

Fig. 38.9: Multiple toothed vulsellum.

Uses

- To hold the parous cervical lip in operations like D&C, anterior colporrhaphy or vaginal hysterectomy. Its function is to make the cervix steady by traction.
- To remove a polyp by twisting as an alternative to Lane's tissue forceps.
- To hold the fundus of the uterus and to give traction while the clamps are placed in operation of total abdominal hysterectomy for benign lesion.

Sterilization

Autoclaving and boiling.

Self-assessment

When the posterior cervical lip is to be held?

Usually, the anterior lip is held but in some conditions, the posterior lip is to be held. Such conditions are:

- In amputation cervix or vaginal hysterectomy when the posterior cervicovaginal mucous membrane is cut.
- Posterior colpotomy for drainage of pus (pelvic abscess).
- During vaginal ligation of tubes.
- When there is growth in the anterior lip (cancer cervix).
- Culdocentesis.

SINGLE TOOTHED VULSELLUM (FIG. 38.10)

Description and Identification

It is a long metallic instrument. It is similar to multiple toothed vulsellum. This instrument is designed to have two long teeth, one arising from each blade. Compared to a multiple tooth vulsellum, depth of tissue penetration is more in single toothed vulsellum.

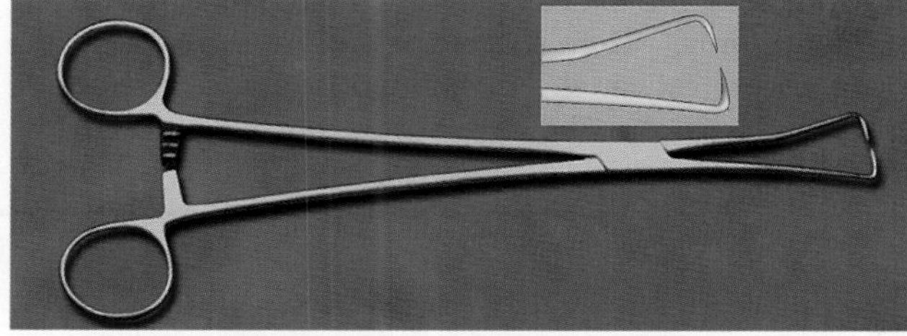

Fig. 38.10: Single toothed vulsellum.

Uses

- To hold the cervix after opening the vault of vagina and to give traction while the remaining vault is being cut in total abdominal hysterectomy.
- To hold the new cervical stump after amputation of the cervix and in Fothergill's operation (Ch. 16).
- To hold the cervical stump left after (abdominal) subtotal hysterectomy (Ch. 35).
- Sometimes to hold the anterior lip of nulliparous cervix in operation of D&C (Allis' tissue forceps preferred).

Sterilization

Autoclaving and boiling.

Self-assessment

- What are the indications of amputation cervix? (Ch. 35).
- Indications of subtotal hysterectomy (Ch. 35).
- Mention common indications of abdominal hysterectomy.
- Common indications of vaginal hysterectomy (p. 179).
- Indications of Fothergill's operation (Ch. 16).
- Principal steps of Fothergill's operation.
- Complications of Fothergill's operation.

ANTERIOR VAGINAL WALL RETRACTOR (FIG. 38.11)

Description and Identification

It is a long metallic instrument. Its both the ends are flattened, fenestrated, and transversely serrated. The flattened ends are of different sizes. The long shaft of the instrument is used as the handle.

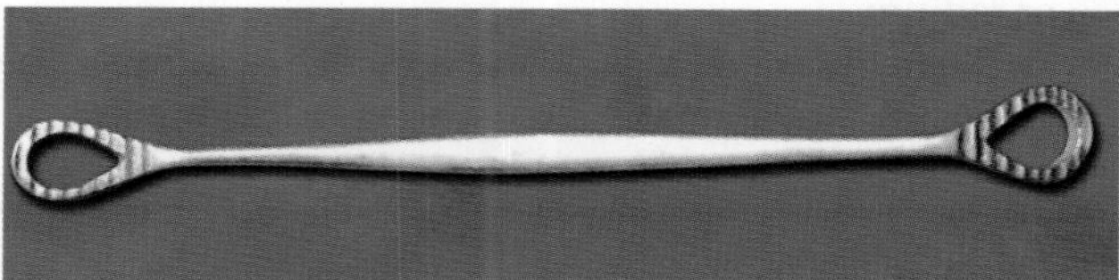

Fig. 38.11: Anterior vaginal wall retractor.

Uses

- To retract the sagging anterior vaginal wall to have a good look on the cervix while retracting the posterior vaginal wall by the Sims' speculum.
- It is used for examination of the cervix in a case with cystocele.

Sterilization

Autoclaving and boiling.

OLIVE POINTED MALLEABLE GRADUATED METALLIC UTERINE SOUND (FIG. 38.12)

Description and Identification

It is a long metallic instrument. It has one flattened end that works as the handle. The other end is olive pointed (as described above). The instrument is graduated both in inches and centimeter and it is malleable. Its curvature could be changed (anteverted or retroverted) to adapt the position of the uterus and for ease of introduction.

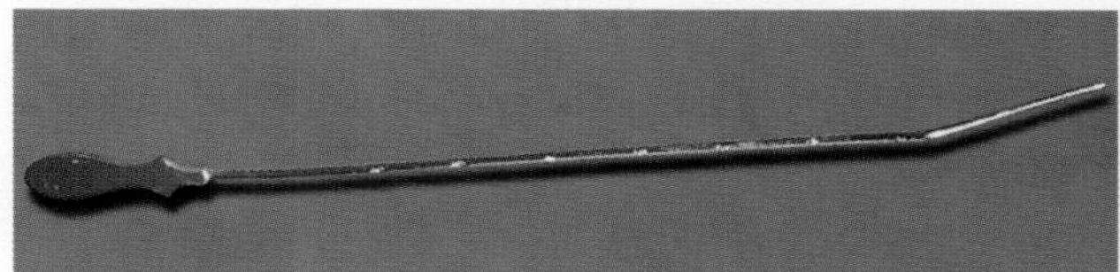

Fig. 38.12: Olive pointed malleable graduated metallic uterine sound.

Uses

- To confirm the position of the uterus.
- To note the length of the uterocervical canal.
- It acts as a first dilator.
- To sound the uterine cavity in a case of IUCD with missing threads.
- To differentiate a polyp from inversion.

Originally, it was used to detect stone in urinary bladder by way of touching (sounding).

Sterilization

Autoclaving and boiling.

Self-assessment

- Describe the normal position of the uterus and length of the uterocervical canal (7.5 cm).
- **Conditions** where the length of the uterocervical canal is increased.

Ans. Fibroid uterus, elongation of cervix, endometrial carcinoma, adenomyosis.

- ***What are the causes of reduced length of uterocervical canal?***

Ans. (a) Postmenopausal uterus; (b) Hypoplastic uterus; (c) Uterine inversion; (d) Submucous fibroid (sessile).

- Causes of elongation of the cervix.

Q. Common complications of using uterine sound.

Ans. Uterine perforation and hemorrhage.

Q. How do you recognize uterine perforation?

Ans. (a) Sudden loss of resistance (sense of giving a way); (b) Passage of the instrument more than the length of the uterine cavity; (c) Vaginal bleeding.

- Management of uterine perforation.

UTERINE CURETTE (FIGS. 38.13A TO C)

Description and Identification

It is a long metallic instrument with a small fenestrated end at each side and a shaft in between. The shaft is used as the handle. The edge of the fenestration is sharp at one end and on the other end it is blunt. The blunt and the sharp edges are directed in opposite direction.

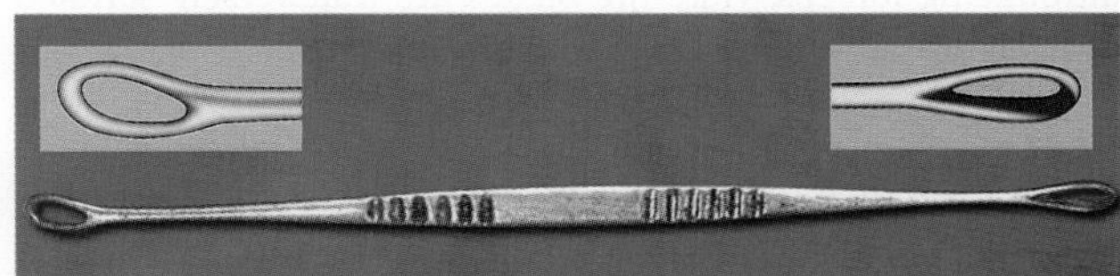

Fig. 38.13A: Sharp at one end, blunt at the other end.

Types

- Sharp at one end, blunt at the other (Fig. 38.13A)
- Sharp or blunt at both ends
- Handle with only sharp at one end
- Flushing curette (blunt) (Fig. 38.13B)
- Sharman's curette (Fig. 38.13C).

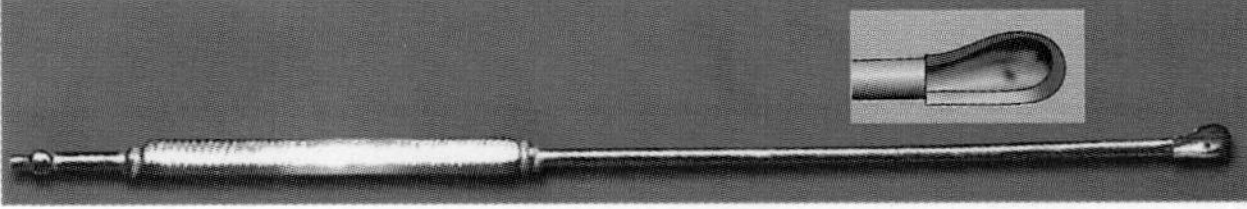

Fig. 38.13B: Flushing curette.

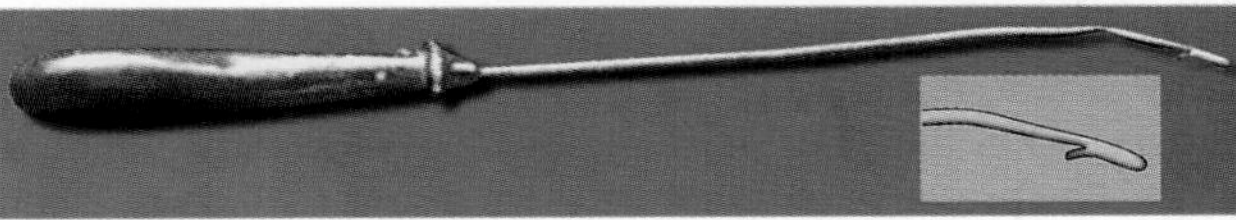

Fig. 38.13C: Sharman's curette.

Uses

Sharp Curette (Fig. 38.13A)

- Infertility (Ch. 17)
- Dysfunctional uterine bleeding (DUB) (Ch. 15)
- TB endometritis
- Endometrial hyperplasia.

Blunt Curette

- Suspected choriocarcinoma.
- Suspected endometrial carcinoma.

Flushing Curette (Fig. 38.13B)

- Following D&E (*see* Dutta's Bedside Clinic p. 258).

Sharman's Curette (Fig. 38.13C)

Infertility work up, where only a strip of endometrium is enough to study the hormonal reflection. It is done as an outpatient procedure and without anesthesia.

Sterilization

By autoclaving or boiling.

Self-assessment

Q. What is the purpose of doing endometrial biopsy in a woman with infertility?

Ans. To detect evidence of ovulation—by seeing the secretory changes in the endometrium (Ch. 8).

Q. Which day of the menstrual cycle endometrial biopsy is usually done?

Ans. Biopsy should be done on D21–D23 when the cycle is regular. When the cycles are irregular, it is done within 24 hours of the mens.

Q. What are the methods to assess the endometrium?

Ans. (A) Endometrial thickness is assessed by: (a) Transvaginal sonography (TVS); (b) Saline infusion sonography (SIS); and (c) Hysteroscopy. **(B) Histologic evaluation** of endometrium is done by: (a) Pipette; (b) Uterine curettage and (c) Hysteroscopic targeted biopsy.

Q. In the endometrial biopsy, what is the earliest evidence of ovulation?

Ans. Subnuclear vacuolation is the earliest evidence appearing within 36–48 hours of ovulation (Ch. 8).

Q. What are the other methods of diagnosis of ovulation?

Ans. BBT, cervical mucus study, vaginal cytology, serum progesterone, serum LH and estradiol, sonography and laparoscopy (Ch. 17).

Q. What are the ovarian causes of infertility?

Ans. Anovulation, LPD and LUF (Ch. 17).

Q. What are the risks of overzealous curettage of the endometrium?

Ans. (a) Excess curettage destroys the basal layer of the endometrium. This will cause uterine synechiae formation (Asherman's syndrome); (b) Women may suffer amenorrhea or hypomenorrhea; (c) Risk of developing morbid adherent placenta, in subsequent pregnancy is more.

UTERINE DRESSING FORCEPS (FIG. 38.14)

Description and Identification

This instrument has a smooth curvature which is directed upwards close to its anterior half.

The instrument is often confused with laminaria tent introducing forceps. Here the blades are transversely serrated while in the latter, there is a groove on either blade.

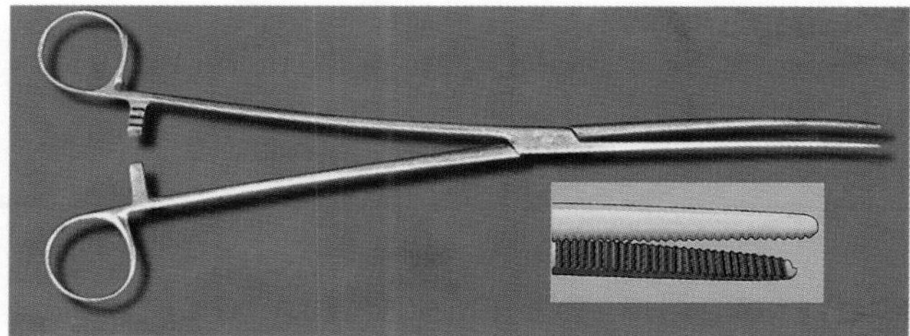

Fig. 38.14: Uterine dressing forceps.

Uses

- To swab the uterine cavity following D&E operation with a small gauze piece.
- To dilate the cervix in lochiometra or pyometra.
- To plug the uterine cavity with gauze twigs in continued bleeding after removal of polyp.

Sterilization

Autoclaving or boiling.

Self-assessment

- Causes of pyometra (Ch. 12).
- Management of polyps (Ch. 20).

SPONGE HOLDING FORCEPS (FIG. 38.15)

Description and Identification

It is a long metallic instrument. The uterine ends are oval shaped, fenestrated with transverse serrations on their inner surfaces. The other end is the handle with two finger rings and the catch. The presence of transverse serrations at the uterine end and the catch at the handles ensures firm grip of the instrument.

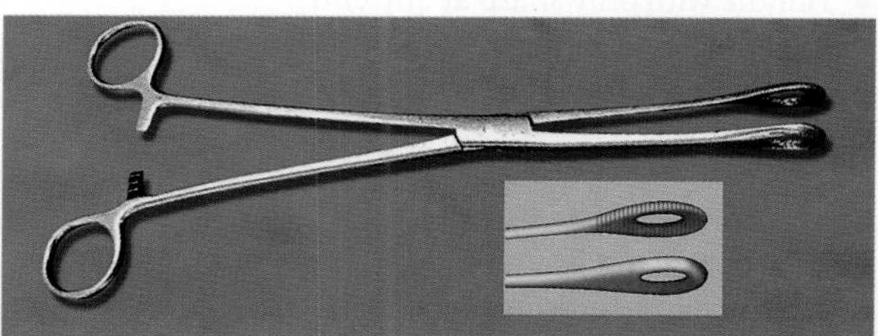

Fig. 38.15: Sponge holding forceps.

Uses

- Antiseptic dressing before any abdominal or vaginal operation.
- To clean the vagina with gauze pieces before and after vaginal operations.
- To hold the cervix in circlage operation during pregnancy.
- To remove cervical polyp by holding and twisting.
- Rubber guarded sponge forceps may be used to occlude ovarian vessels at the infundibulopelvic ligament temporarily, during myomectomy.

Sterilization

Autoclaving or boiling.

Self-assessment

Q. Name a few common abdominal operations.

Ans. Abdominal hysterectomy, myomectomy, ovariotomy.

Q. Name a few common vaginal operations.

Ans.
- D&C
- PFR
- Vaginal hysterectomy
- Fothergill's operation.

OVUM FORCEPS (FIG. 38.16)

Description and Identification

It is a long metallic (steel) instrument with two ends and a shaft. The handle has no catch. For this reason, risk of crushing any tissue, if it is grasped inadvertently, is less. The fenestrated end has no serrations inside. This way (absence of catch and serrations) ovum forceps differs from a sponge holding forceps.

It is often confused with sponge holding forceps but it has no catch. As such, it minimizes trauma to the uterine wall if accidentally caught and also it has got no crushing effect on the conceptus.

Uses

- To remove the products of conception in D&E after its separation partially or completely.
- To remove molar tissue in hydatidiform mole.
- To remove uterine polyp (small).

Sterilization

Autoclaving or boiling.

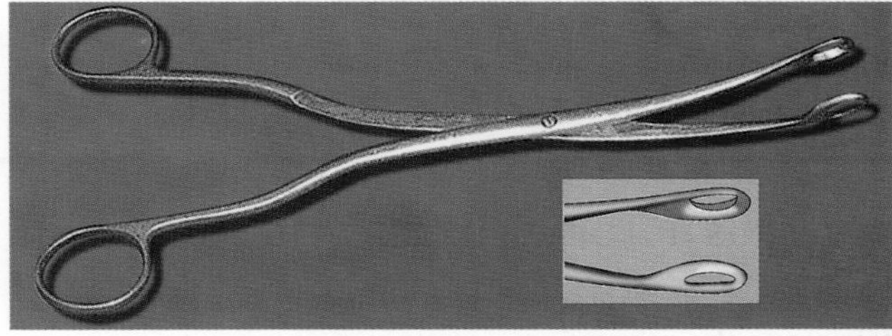

Fig. 38.16: Ovum forceps.

Methods of Use

The cervical canal is dilated first. The instrument is introduced with the blades closed and opened inside the cavity. The products are caught and then with twisting movements and simultaneous traction, the products are removed.

Complications

It may produce injury to the uterine wall to the extent of even perforation. Not infrequently, a segment of intestine or omentum may even be pulled out through the rent.

ALLIS TISSUE FORCEPS (FIG. 38.17)

Description and Identification

It is a metallic instrument having two ends. One end is the handle with the provision of catch. The other end has the arrangement of multiple teeth (4–6). The blades allow some space within in locked position so that the tissue hold is not crushed. This forceps may be of different sizes.

Uses

- To hold the margins of the vaginal flaps in colporrhaphy operation.
- To hold the peritoneum or rectus sheath during repair of the abdominal wall.
- To hold the margins of the vagina in abdominal hysterectomy.
- To hold the anterior lip of the cervix in D&C operation.
- To catch the torn ends of the sphincter ani externus in complete perineal tear (CPT) repair.
- To remove a small polyp.
- To take out the tissue following wedge biopsy.

Sterilization

Autoclaving or boiling.

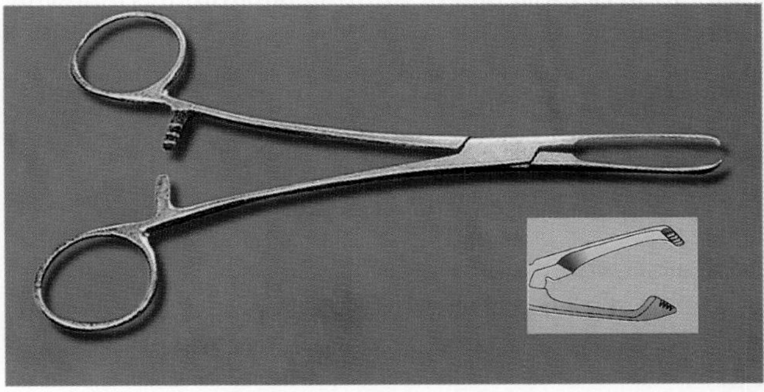

Fig. 38.17: Allis tissue forceps.

Self-assessment

Q. What are the common symptoms associated with genital prolapse?

Ans. Woman may remain asymptomatic if the prolapse is mild. The common symptoms are genital organs protruding out of the vaginal opening, difficulties in walking, sitting, urination or defecation. Prolapse may interfere with sexual intercourse or may cause vaginal bleeding due to ulceration of mucosa. It may cause incontinence of urine, pelvic pressure or backache.

LANES TISSUE FORCEPS (FIG. 38.18)

Uses

- To hold parietal wall (bulk of tough tissues) for retraction during abdominal operations with transverse incision (hysterectomy).
- To hold the polyp or fibroid in polypectomy or myomectomy operation.
- To hold the towels during draping.

Sterilization

Autoclaving or boiling.

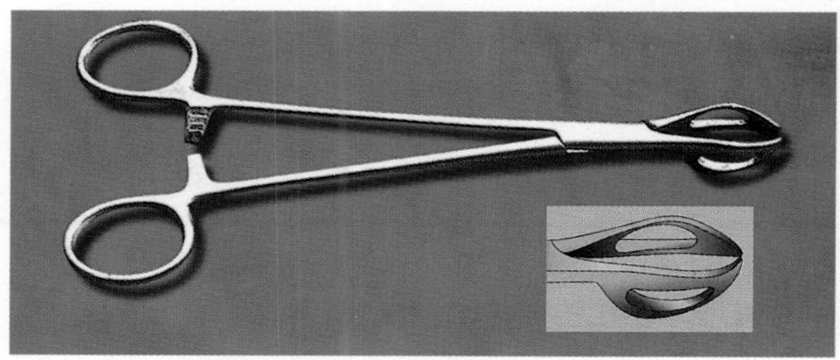

Fig. 38.18: Lanes tissue forceps.

UTERUS HOLDING FORCEPS (FIG. 38.19)

The blades are protected with rubber tubes to minimize trauma to the uterus.

Uses

To fix and steady the uterus when conservative surgery is done on the adnexa (tuboplasty).

Self-assessment

What are the different surgical procedures for proximal and distal tubal disease?

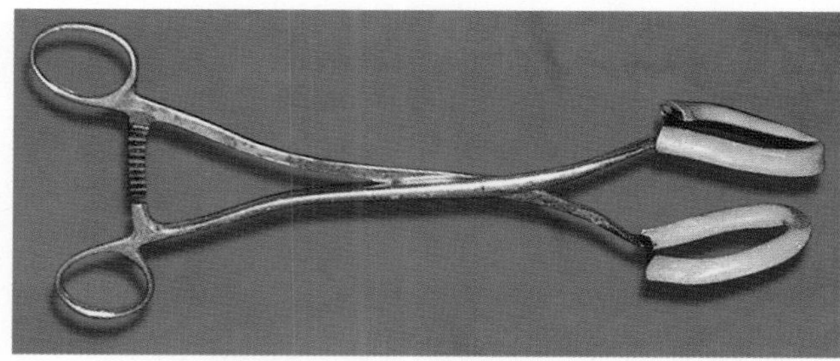

Fig. 38.19: Uterus holding forceps.

CERVICAL OCCLUSION CLAMP (FIG. 38.20)

The blades are guarded with rubber tubes to avoid trauma to tissues.

Uses

Evaluation of tubal patency during laparotomy (following tuboplasty).

Procedure

Cervix is occluded with the instrument and methylene blue dye is injected into the uterine cavity through the fundus using a syringe and a needle.

Self-assessment

- Different methods to assess tubal patency (Ch. 17).
- Different types of tubal reconstructive surgery.

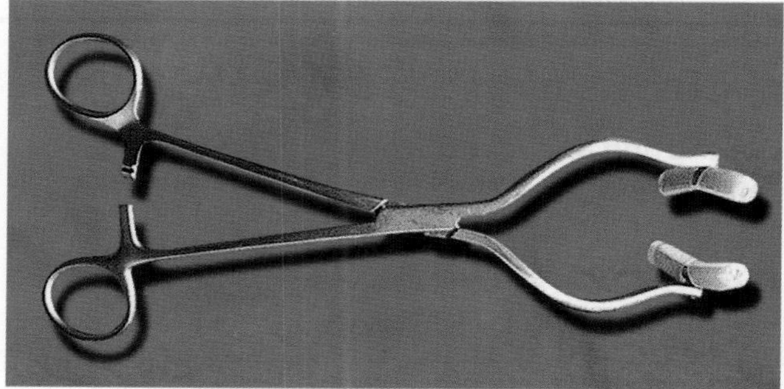

Fig. 38.20: Cervical occlusion clamp.

MYOMA SCREW (FIG. 38.21)

Description and Identification

It has one spirally designed side that ends at a sharp point. Others end is the handle. The sharp spirally designed end goes inside the myoma during operation.

Uses

- To fix the myoma after the capsule is cut open and to give traction while the myoma is enucleated out of its bed (myomectomy).
- To give traction in a big uterus (multiple fibroid) requiring hysterectomy while the clamps are placed.
- To liftout a big uterus for ease of operation through the abdominal incision.

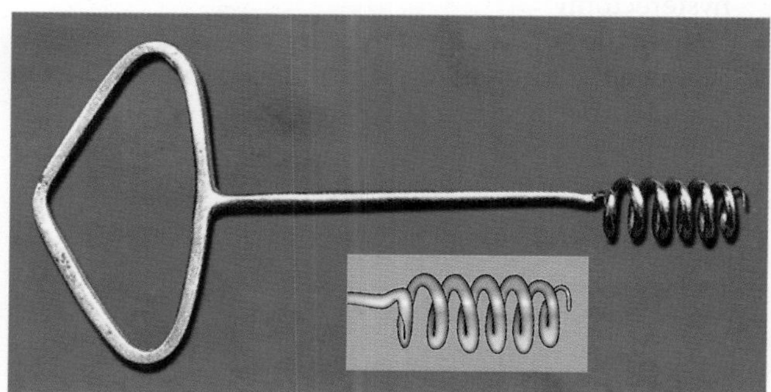

Fig. 38.21: Myoma screw.

Self-assessment (Ch. 20 and 35)

- Indications of myomectomy
- Steps of myomectomy
- Complications of myomectomy
- Important considerations before myomectomy.

Sterilization

Autoclaving or boiling.

BONNEY'S MYOMECTOMY CLAMP (FIG. 38.22)

Uses

- The clamp is used in myomectomy operation. It curtails the blood supply to the uterus temporarily, thereby minimizing the blood loss during operation. Simultaneous, bilateral clamping of the infundibulopelvic ligaments by rubber guarded sponge holding forceps may be employed.
- The instrument is placed at the level of internal os with the concavity fitting with the convexity of the symphysis pubis. The round ligaments of both sides are included inside the clamp to prevent slipping of the instrument and preventing the uterus from falling back. The clamp is removed after suturing the myoma bed but before closing the peritoneal layers.

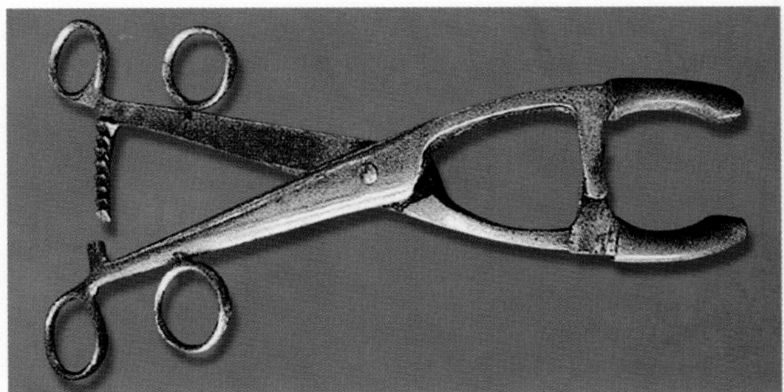

Fig. 38.22: Bonney's myomectomy clamp.

- It is seldom used nowadays. Alternative methods are: Preoperative use of GnRH analog (p. 434), and/or intraoperative use of tourniquets, vasocon-strictive agents (vasopressin) and others.

HYSTEROSALPINGOGRAPHY CANNULA (LEECH WILKINSON VARIETY) (FIG. 38.23)

Description and Identification

It is a long metallic instrument having two ends and a channel inside.

The uterine end is shaped like a cone and is spirally designed. The other end has a valve device through which a radiopaque dye could be pushed in.

During HSG, a syringe is required to push the dye. Iodine containing radio-opaque dye (urograffin) is used. It is done in the radiology department without anesthesia.

Uses

- Hysterosalpingography (HSG) (p. 494)
- For hydrotubation
- Laparoscopic chromopertubation.

Hydrotubation: Medicated solution is pushed transcervically in conditions such as following tuboplasty operation or suspected flimsy fimbrial adhesions. The drugs instilled are dexamethasone 4 mg with gentamicin 80 mg in 10 mL normal saline. It is instilled in the proliferative phase for at least 3 cycles.

Sterilization

Autoclaving or boiling.

Self-assessment

- What is HSG? (p. 494 and 499)

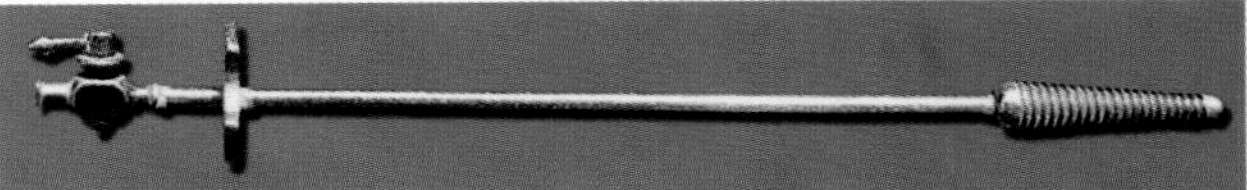

Fig. 38.23: Hysterosalpingography cannula.

- Timing of HSG.
- Advantages of HSG over laparoscopic chromopertubation.

Q. How do you compare the oil-based versus water-based media used in HSG?

Ans. Water-based media is commonly used. It causes less cramping pain and discomfort. Oil-based media gives better image and has higher pregnancy rates. Granuloma is more with oil-based media. Embolization is minimal with either media.

Q. What are the indications of HSG?

Q. Advantages of laparoscopy over HSG.

Q. What are the complications of HSG?

Q. What are the other alternatives to HSG?

Ans. Diagnostic laparoscopy and dye test; sono-hysterosalpingography test.

Q. What is saline infusion sonography?

KOCHER'S ARTERY FORCEPS (FIG. 38.24)

Description and Identification

This is a hemostatic forceps and may be of straight or curved variety. This instrument has a tooth at the end of one blade and a groove on the other, so as to have a firm grip on the tissue pedicle. It has transverse serrations along the shaft. The handles have the provision of catch.

This instrument is named after Professor Emil Theodor Kocher. He was the professor of Surgery, Berne, Switzerland.

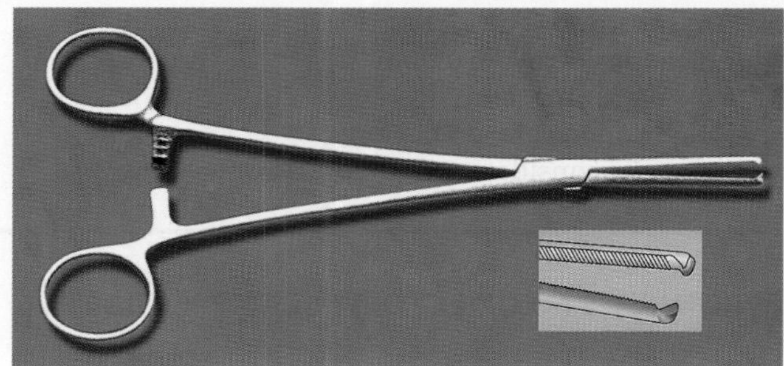

Fig. 38.24: Kocher's artery forceps.

Uses

- To use as a clamp in hysterectomy operation
- To hold vascular pedicles before cutting.

Sterilization

Autoclaving or boiling.

Self-assessment

- What added advantage it has got?
  Due to the presence of tooth, it gives a firm grip to the pedicle hold.
- Indications of abdominal hysterectomy.
- Mention the different sites where the clamps are placed in total abdominal hysterectomy.
- The important steps of Fothergill's operation (Ch. 16).
- Complications of Fothergill's operation (Ch. 16).

LANDON'S BLADDER RETRACTOR (FIG. 38.25)

Description and Identification

It is a metallic instrument. One end is flattened with a rectangular shape. The other end is the handle. The handle is fenestrated and has a circular gap in the middle for good grip with the fingers.

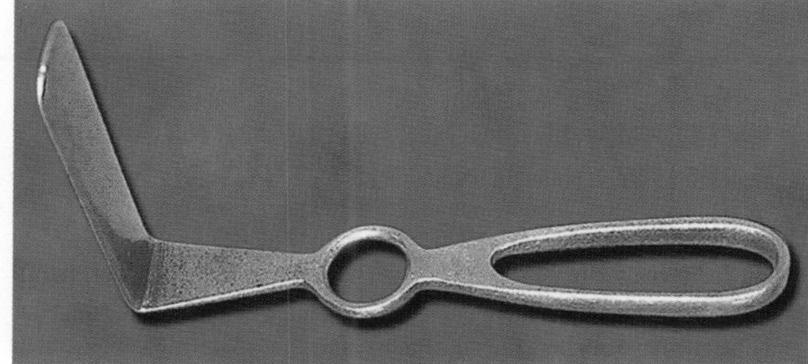

Fig. 38.25: Landon's bladder retractor.

Uses

- In vaginal hysterectomy.
- To keep the bladder up, to facilitate opening of the uterovesical peritoneum.
- To introduce it through the opening of the uterovesical pouch and to retract the bladder while the clamps are placed. This prevents injury to the bladder.
- To inspect the suture lines after completion of vaginal plastic operations by retracting the anterior or posterior vaginal wall.
- Intravaginal plugging can be done under its guidance.
- To use as lateral vaginal wall retractor while the clamps are placed.

Sterilization

Autoclaving or boiling.

Self-assessment

Q. What are the nonsurgical treatments of prolapse?

Ans. Conservative treatments include: (a) To avoid aggravating factors (obesity, chronic cough, constipation); (b) Pelvic floor exercise; (c) Estrogen replacement therapy (postmenopausal women); (d) Pessary in some cases.

Q. Mention the different sites where the clamps are placed during vaginal hysterectomy (p. 182).

Q. Mention the important postoperative complications following vaginal hysterectomy with PFR (p. 180).

INSUFFLATION CANNULA (FIG. 38.26)

Description and Identification

The instrument is not complete. It requires a 'Y' rubber tube. One end is attached to a bulb and the other end to a manometer.

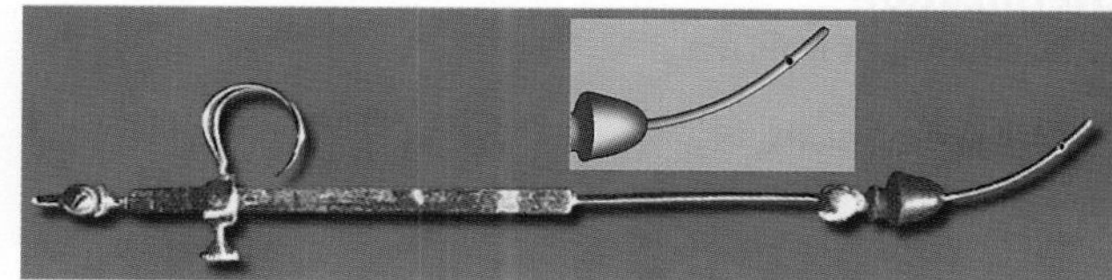

Fig. 38.26: Insufflation cannula.

Use

- To know the patency of the tube (Rubin's test) in infertility investigation or following tuboplasty.

Self-assessment

- Ideal time of operation in relation to menstrual cycle .
- Complications of D&I (Ch. 35).
- Advantages of HSG over D&I (Ch. 35).

ABDOMINAL RETRACTORS (FIGS. 38.27A TO C)

Description and Identification

Retractors are used to retract tissues out of the operative field. This is needed for better exposure of the operative field during surgery. Retractors are held in place and retracted either by an assistant (manual retractor) or by counter pressure with some device (self-retaining retractor). Manual retractor can be used alone or in combination with a self-retaining retractor. Manual retractors can be placed according to need.

DOYEN'S RETRACTOR (FIG. 38.27A)

Description and Identification

This is a long and heavy metallic instrument. One end is the handle and the other end is flattened and curved with concavity inwards.

Uses

- To retract the abdominal wall in abdominal pelvic surgery to expose the field of operation.
- As an alternative, self-retaining retractor may be used.

BALFOUR SELF-RETAINING RETRACTOR (FIG. 38.27B)

Two lateral blades and an additional (third) blade. All the blades are detachable and may be of different sizes.

Uses

- To retract the abdominal wall all around.
- To expose the field of operation widely (no assistant is needed for manual retraction).

DEAVER'S RETRACTOR (FIG. 38.27C)

Description and Identification

It is a metallic instrument. It is designed flattened, and curved.

It is a manual retractor either used alone or in combination with a self-retaining one. It has got different sizes.

Sterilization

Autoclaving or sterilization.

Uses

- It is used in abdominal operation to retract the viscera as and when required in order to facilitate the operative procedures like abdominal hysterectomy. For that purpose, it may also be used as a lateral retractor.
- To retract the parietal wall during abdominopelvic surgery (hysterectomy).
- To retract the bladder or intestines during the surgery.

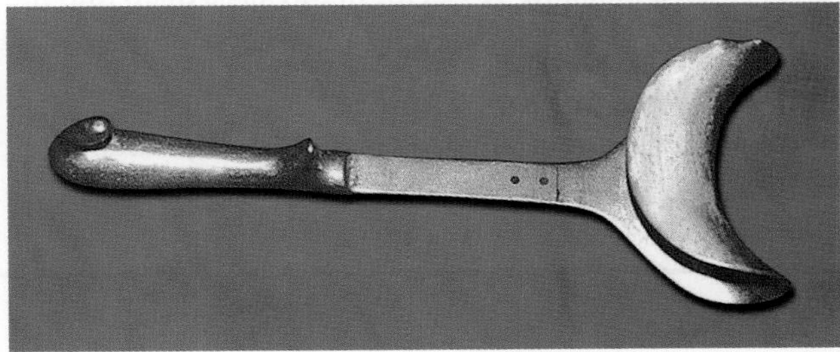

Fig. 38.27A: Doyen's retractor.

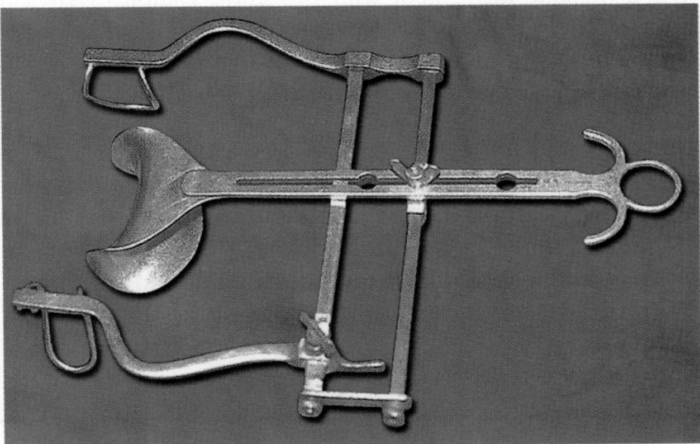

Fig. 38.27B: Balfour self-retaining retractor.

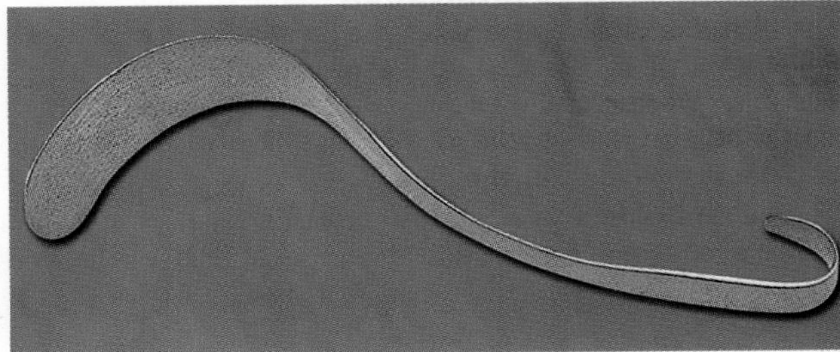

Fig. 38.27C: Deaver's retractor.

LONG STRAIGHT HEMOSTATIC FORCEPS (SPENCER WELL'S) (FIG. 38.28)

Description and Identification

It is a long hemostatic forceps. It is designed to have the blades with longitudinal ridges on the inner surfaces. This ensures firm pedicle grip. The handles have the provision of catch. Both the straight and curved varieties are available.

Uses

- It is used to hold the vascular pedicles as a clamp in (a) hysterectomy; (b) salpingectomy; or (c) salpingo-oophorectomy operation.
- To catch a bleeding vessel for hemostasis deep into the pelvis.

Self-assessment (Ch. 16 and 35)

- Mention the important pedicles hold in total abdominal hysterectomy.
- Indications of salpingectomy.
- Pedicles hold in vaginal hysterectomy.
- Pedicles hold during salpingo-oophorectomy.
- Complications of abdominal hysterectomy during the operation.

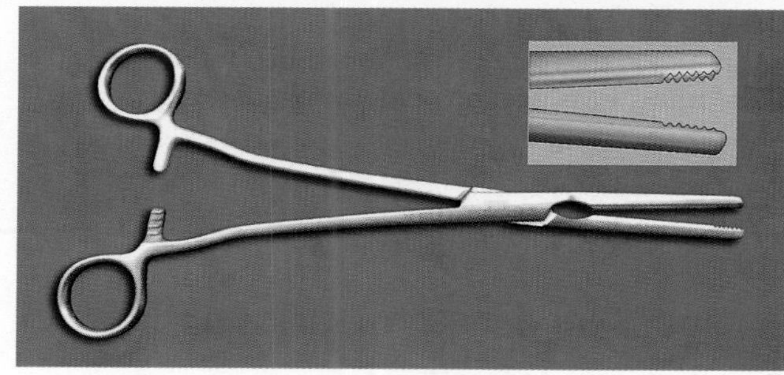

Fig. 38.28: Long straight hemostatic forceps.

BABCOCK'S FORCEPS (FIG. 38.29)

Description and Identification

It is a metallic instrument with two ends. Handles have got catches. The other end has fenestrated blades. The blades are curved and allow some space within, in locked position, so that structure hold in between is not crushed.

Uses

- To hold the fallopian tube in tuboplasty operation.
- To hold lymph nodes during dissection in radical hysterectomy (lymphadenectomy).
- To hold the appendix, bowel during appendicectomy.
- To hold the ureter during dissection (Wertheim's operation).

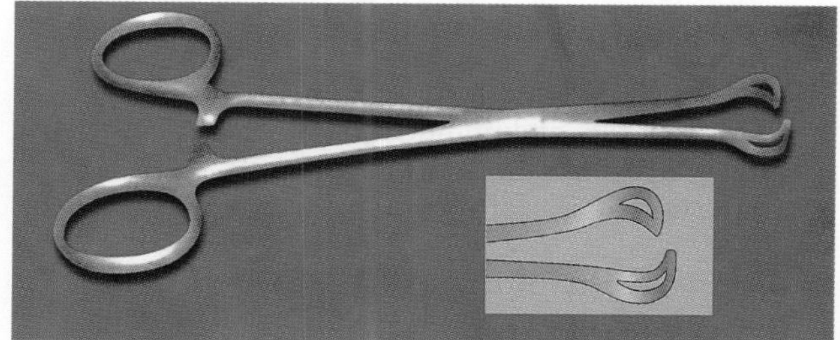

Fig. 38.29: Babcock's forceps.

Sterilization

Autoclaving or boiling.

NEEDLE HOLDER (FIG. 38.30)

Description and Identification

The instrument blades are short, the handles are long. Needle holders with long handles are useful for suturing at a depth. The inner surface of the blades have crisscross serrations and a longitudinal groove in the middle. This ensures firm grip and prevents the needle from rotating.

Needle holders may be long and heavy or small and delicate. It may be straight (Wangensteen) or curved (Heaney) variety.

Uses

- The curved variety may be helpful to see tissues at a depth (vaginal surgery).
- To catch-hold the needle, the needle should be caught at the junction of its anterior 2/3rd and posterior 1/3rd.
- The needle holder grasps the needle at its junction of anterior 1/3rd and posterior 2/3rd.

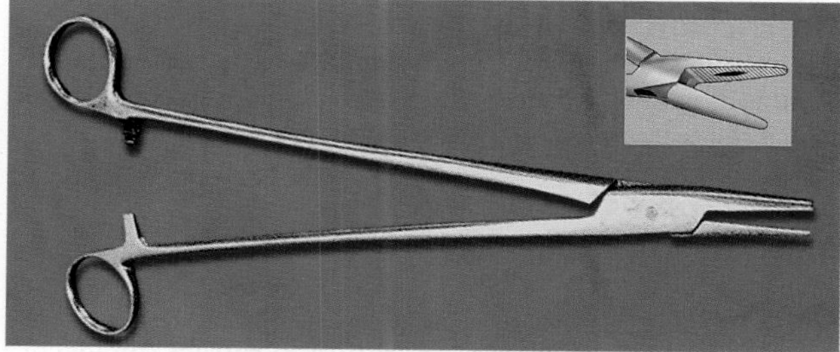

Fig. 38.30: Needle holder.

Sterilization

Autoclaving or boiling.

BARKELAY BONNEY VAGINAL CLAMP (FIG. 38.31)

Uses

To occlude the vaginal canal prior to cutting the vagina in Wertheim's hysterectomy.

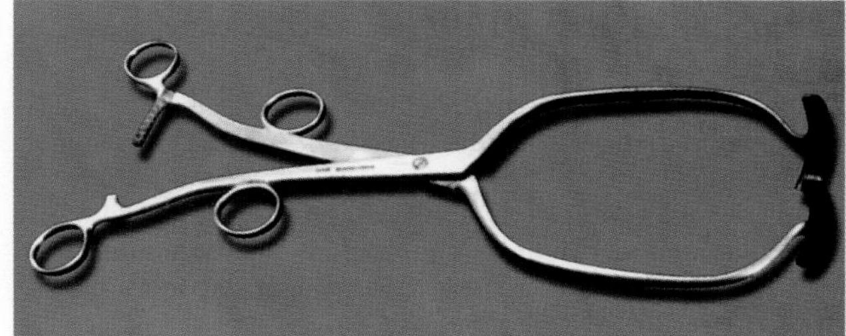

Fig. 38.31: Barkelay Bonney vaginal clamp.

PUNCH BIOPSY FORCEPS (FIG. 38.32)

Description and Identification

It is long metallic instrument with two ends. At one end the oval blades with sharp cutting edges are there. The incised bit of tissue remains within these two blades. The other end is the long handles. There is no catch in the handle.

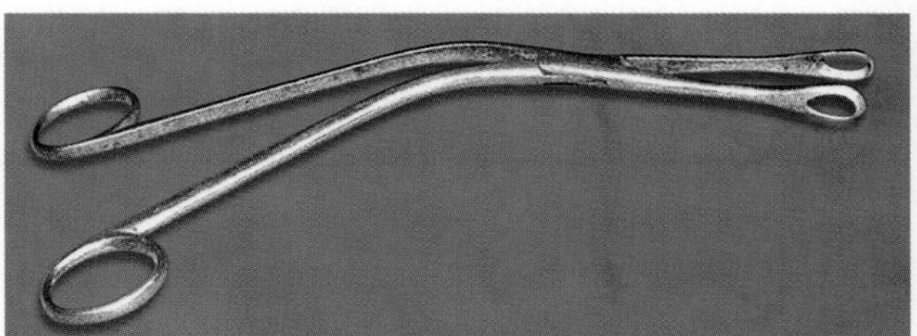

Fig. 38.32: Punch biopsy forceps.

Uses

- To take biopsy from the cervix.
- The biopsy is taken as an outdoor procedure without anesthesia. The site of biopsy is either from the suspected area or Schiller's iodine or colposcopically directed.

Sterilization

Autoclaving or boiling.

Self-assessment

- Mention the different types of cervical biopsy (p. 487). Biopsy can also be made under colposcopy directed or following Schiller's test.
- Procedure of sending the material for histology (Ch. 9).
- Schiller's test (Ch. 23).
- VIA
- Histology of carcinoma cervix (Ch. 24).
- Early diagnosis of carcinoma cervix (Ch. 24).
- Complications of cervical biopsy (p. 495).
- Complications of cone biopsy.

DISSECTING FORCEPS (FIGS. 38.33A AND B)

Toothed Variety

Uses

- To hold tough structures like rectus sheath, cut margins of vaginal vault following hysterectomy or margins of vaginal flaps in PFR or the skin margins during suturing.
- To hold the needle during tissue suturing to make it steady and to be pulled out by the needle holder.
- To hold the suture ends during stitch removal.

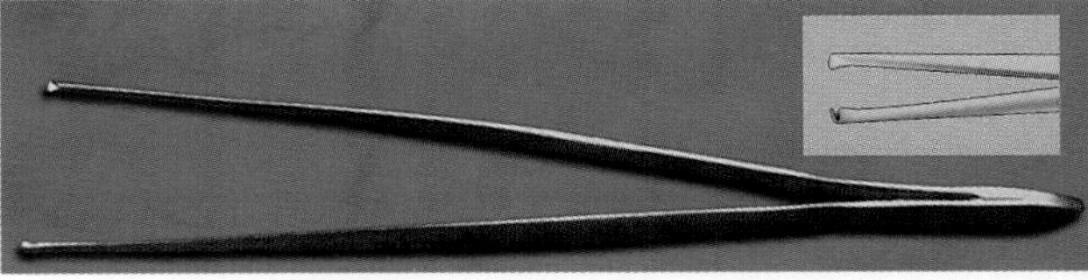

Fig. 38.33A: Toothed dissecting forceps.

Plain or non-toothed Variety

Uses

- To hold soft tissues like muscles, peritoneal margins during suturing.
- To hold bleeding vessels for cauterization.

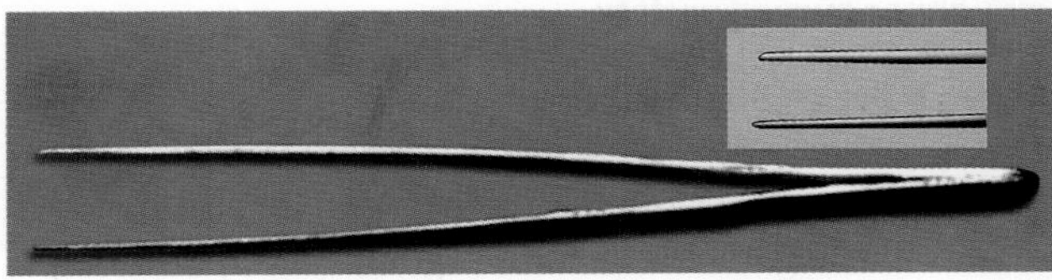

Fig. 38.33B: Non-toothed dissecting forceps.

SCALPEL (FIGS. 38.34A TO C)

Description and Identification

The instrument has a—handle (Bard Parker's) and a detachable blade.

Blades with sizes (10, 11, 12, 15, 20, 22) are specific to a particular number of handle. The size 10 is most commonly used size. The size 11 (bayonet-shaped) in used for stab incisions.

Uses

- To cut the abdominal wall—skin, subcutaneous tissue, rectus sheath, and opening the peritoneum.
- To cut the mucous coat in vaginal plastic operation and to cut tissues during surgery.
- To cut pedicles during hysterectomy.
- To make incision for drainage of abscess (Bartholin's abscess).

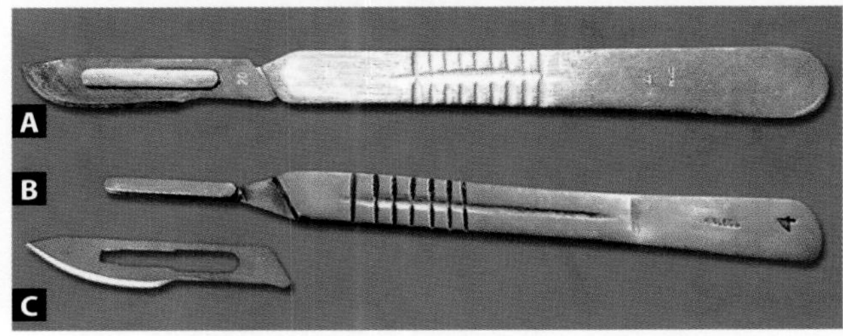
A
B
C

Figs. 38.34A to C: (A) Scalpel; (B) Handle (BP); (C) Blade (detachable).

- To make stab incision (size 11) to create laparoscopic ports.

Sterilization

Blades are disposable (sharp). The handles are autoclavable.

NEEDLES (FIG. 38.35)

Curved needles need less space for suturing. These are suitable for most surgical procedures. Curved needles are available in various curvatures like 1/2 circle, 3/8 circle, etc. Less the arc the needle has, more shallow a bite the needle takes.

Round Bodied (Curved)

It is used while suturing soft structures like:

- Peritoneum, muscles.
- Suturing the pedicles in hysterectomy.
- Suturing the pubocervical fascia.
- Tubectomy or salpingectomy operation.

Cutting (Curved)

It is used while suturing tough structures like:

- Suturing the vaginal wall margins in PFR.
- Closure of the vaginal vault following hysterectomy.
- Repair of the rectus sheath.
- Suturing the skin.

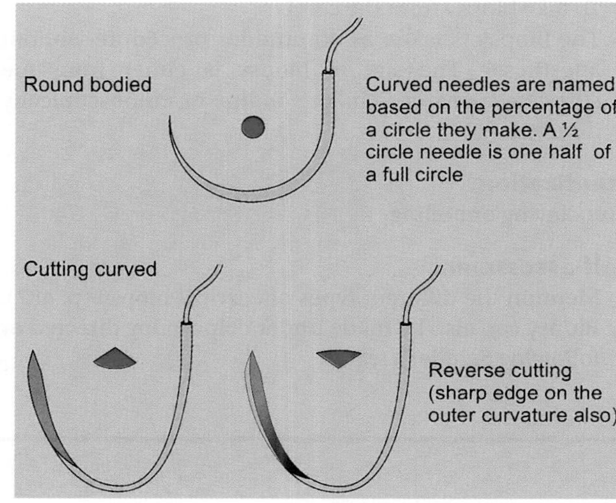
Round bodied
Curved needles are named based on the percentage of a circle they make. A ½ circle needle is one half of a full circle
Cutting curved
Reverse cutting (sharp edge on the outer curvature also)

Fig. 38.35: Curved needles. All the needles are swaged or eyeless.

SCISSORS (FIGS. 38.36 TO 38.39)

Scissors are used to dissect and cut tissues. It may be straight or curved variety.

Mayo's Type (Fig. 38.36)

This is used in almost every operation requiring tissue dissection and excision. It is mainly used for cutting tough tissues like, e.g. rectus sheath, vaginal vault, peritoneum, cutting sutures, ligaments.

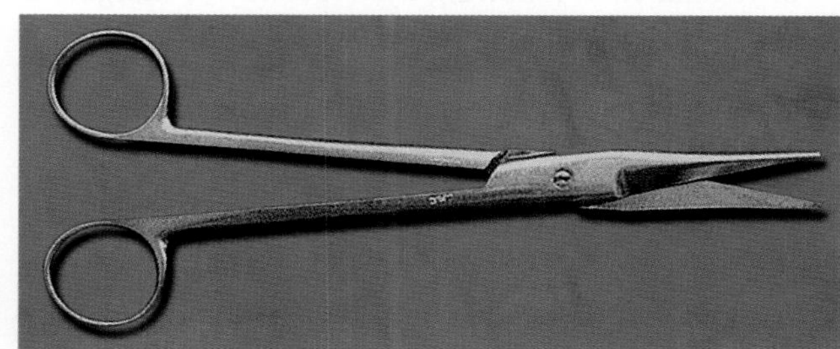

Fig. 38.36: Scissors (Mayo's type).

Bent on Flat (Bonney) Type (Fig. 38.37)

This is used conveniently in anterior colporrhaphy to dissect the vesicovaginal space and also for tissue dissection.

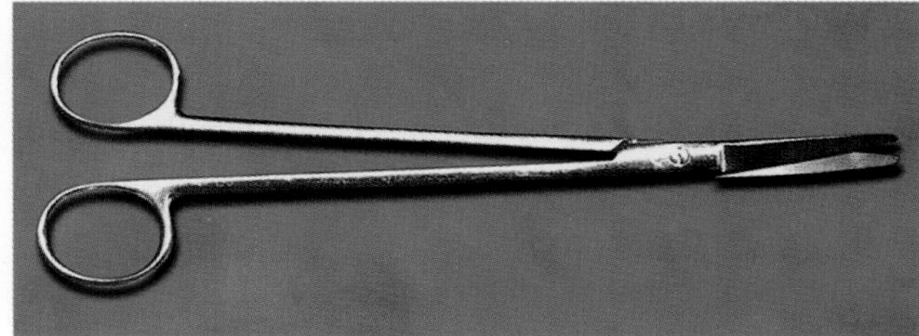

Fig. 38.37: Scissors (Bonney)—bent on flat type.

Metzenbaum (Fig. 38.38)

This is used to dissect and cut tissue such as peritoneum and adhesions.

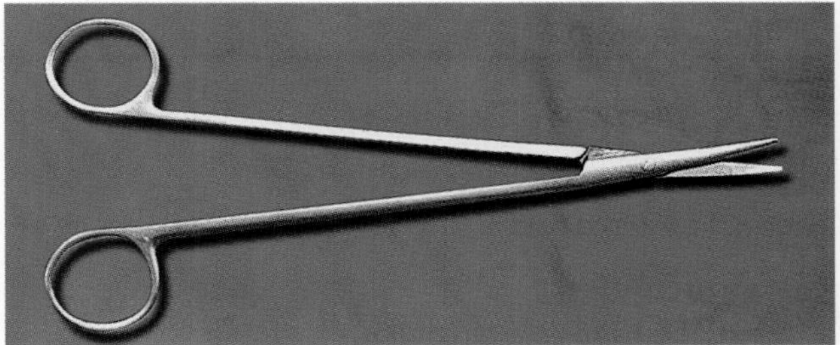

Fig. 38.38: Scissors (Metzenbaum).

Perineorrhaphy (Fig. 38.39)

It is comfortably used in perineorrhaphy operation; also used in episiotomy.

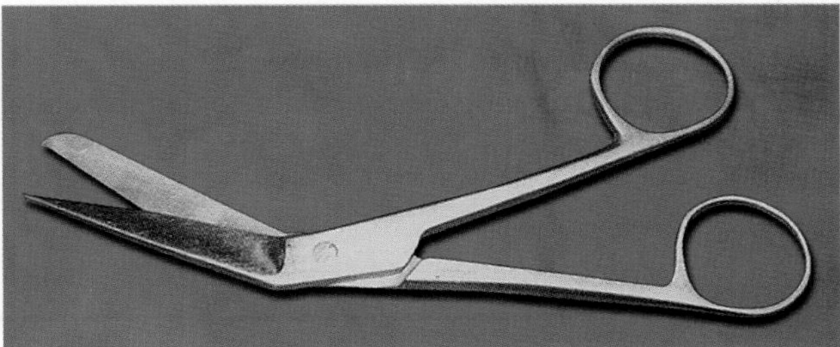

Fig. 38.39: Scissors (perineorrhaphy).

Sterilization

Immersing in Cidex (glutaraldehyde) solution for 24 hours.

Self-assessment (Ch. 16)

- Indications of PFR.
- Complications of PFR.
- Principal steps of perineorrhaphy, PFR, CPT repair.
- Complications in abdominal wound.

Q. What is wound dehiscence?

Ans. When the separation of the layers of abdominal wound is up to the peritoneum—it is called a complete dehiscence. If the intestines come out of the wound, it is called **evisceration or burst abdomen.**

Burst abdomen usually occurs between seven and ten days of the operation. Predisposing factors are malnutrition, infection, cough due to chronic lung disease or abdominal distension.

Management: In the operation theater, under general anesthesia, necrotic tissues and clots are removed. The bowel is cleansed thoroughly with warm normal saline and placed back in the abdominal cavity.

Through and through nylon (No. 2) sutures are passed 2 cm apart and about 3 cm from the skin margins to close the wound. Sutures are left in place for three weeks. Antibiotic (broad spectrum) is started and modified according to the culture and sensitivity report. Predisposing factors are to be taken care of.

TOWEL CLIPS (FIG. 38.40)

Uses

- These are used in draping the operative area—abdominal or vaginal. The towels or sheets are fixed to the skin and to each other with these clips.
- To fix the electrodiathermy cables, suction irrigation tubings, endoscopic surgery cables.

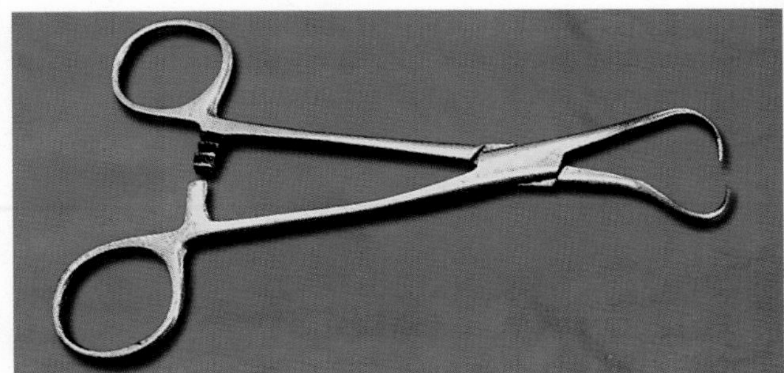

Fig. 38.40: Towel clip.

Sterilization

Autoclaving.

Self-assessment

- How the antiseptic cleaning in abdominal or vaginal operation is done in the operation table prior to draping?

LOOP HOOK (FIG. 38.41)

Uses

To remove IUCD from the uterine cavity when the threads are missing.

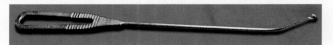

Method of Use

The cervical canal is dilated if needed. The hook is introduced within the uterine cavity. The IUCD is felt and is grasped within the hook. It is then pulled out.

Fig. 38.41: Loop hook.

Precautions

Location of the IUCD within the uterine cavity must be confirmed by sonography. Trauma (perforation) to the uterus is to be avoided. Hysteroscopic removal can also be done.

ELECTROCAUTERY (FIG. 38.42)

Uses

Thermal cauterization of the cervix for cervical ectopy.

Self-assessment

- Steps of thermal cauterization.
- How tissue healing occurs?
- How the patient is counseled for the postoperative care?
- What are the complications of the procedure?

Ans. Excessive vaginal discharge, slight vaginal bleeding and pelvic pain.

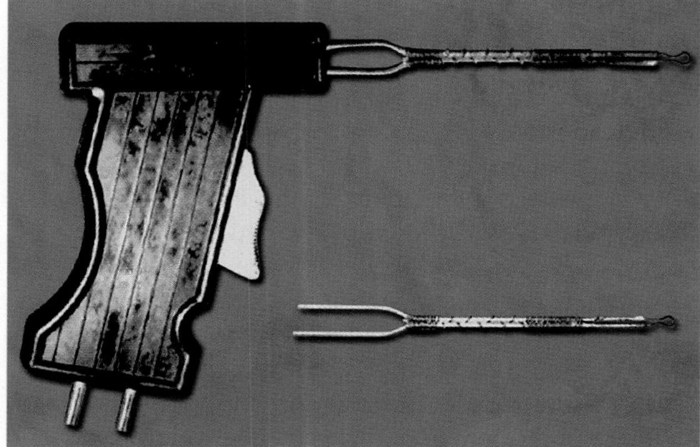

Fig. 38.42: Electrocautery.

CRYOPROBE (FIG. 38.43)

Uses

Tissue destruction is done by freezing (p. 496) at '– 90°C'.

Self-assessment

- ***What are the indications of cryotherapy?***

Ans. (a) **Cervical lesions:** Ectopy, cervical intro epithelial (CIN), vulvar intraepithelial neoplasia (VIN) (Ch. 23), vaginal intraepithelial neoplasia (VaIN) (Ch. 23).

- ***What is the principle of using cryotherapy?***

Ans. The cryoprobe is held in contact with the tissue and the tip is cooled to '–90 °C' (CO_2 is commonly used). Freezing produces cellular dehydration by crystallization of intracellular water and ultimately death of cells occur. Tissue damage occurs up to 5 mm depth.

- ***What are its advantages over thermal cautery?***

Ans. (a) No anesthesia is needed; (b) Precise tissue destruction; (c) No secondary hemorrhage.

- ***What are the disadvantages?***

Ans. Excessive vaginal discharge for about 10–14 days.

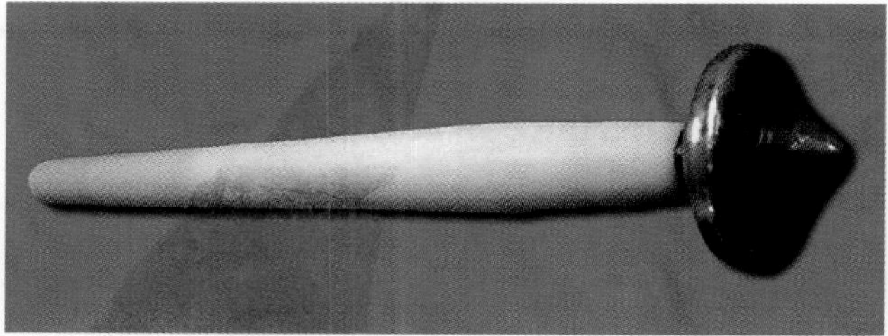

Fig. 38.43: Cryoprobe.

LAPAROSCOPIC INSTRUMENTS (FIGS. 38.44A TO C AND CH. 34)

A. **Telescope:** Commonly used are 5 mm or 10 mm diameter and viewing angle may be 0 or 30 degrees.

B. **Trocar and cannula.**

C. **Veress needle.**

The Veress needle consists of a spring loaded blunt perforated trocar within a sharp cannula. Resistance allows the sharp cannula to protrude but when the resistance disappears, the blunt trocar protrudes out. This prevents injury to the viscera.

Uses

It is used in laparoscopy operation to produce pneumoperitoneum. The common site of puncture is through a small incision made in the lower rim of the umbilicus.

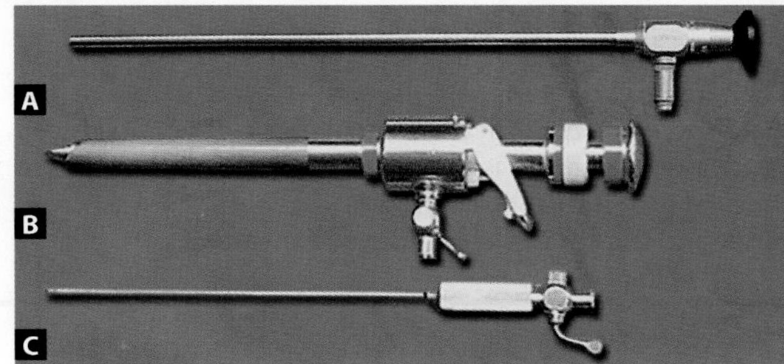

Figs. 38.44A to C: Telescope 10 mm 0-degree, trocar and cannula, Veress needle.

TROCAR AND CANNULA (FIG. 38.45)

The instrument is introduced through the same infraumbilical incision (through which Veress needle is passed), at an angulation of 45° towards the pelvis.

After its introduction, trocar is withdrawn and the telescope is introduced. It is then attached to the cold light source.

Self-assessment

- Indications of laparoscopy.
- Complications.
- Distension media used.
- Advantages and disadvantages of laparoscopic sterilization operation over conventional methods (p. 406).

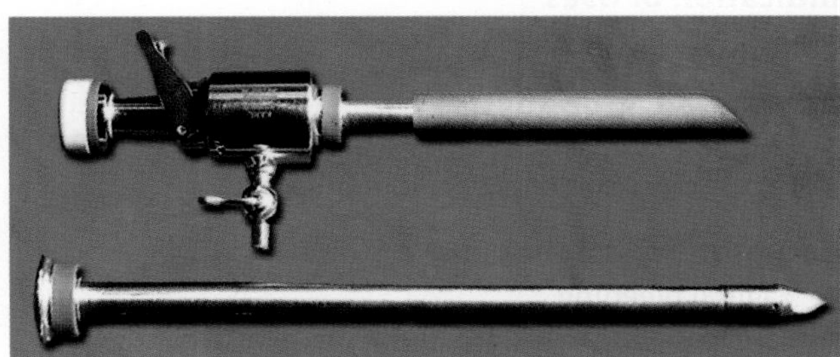

Fig. 38.45: Cannula and trocar (pyramidal tip)—separated.

HYSTEROSCOPIC INSTRUMENTS (FIGS. 38.46A TO C AND CH. 34)

A. **Telescope:** 4 mm 0 degree
B. **Telescope with working element**
C. **Electrode (coagulating roller ball electrode).**

Self-assessment

- Indications of hysteroscopy
- Distension media used
- Complications
- Contraindication of hysteroscopy.

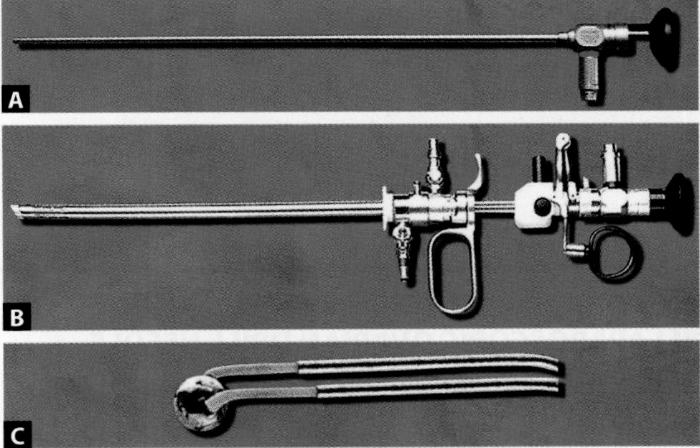

Figs. 38.46A to C: Hysteroscopic instruments.

HODGE-SMITH PESSARY (FIG. 38.47)

It is made up of rubber silicone or ebonite. It is sterilized by immersing it in Cidex for 12 hours.

Indications of Use

P. 167.

Contraindications of Use

- **Fixed RV uterus**
- **Presence of infection**

Self-assessment

How pessary works?

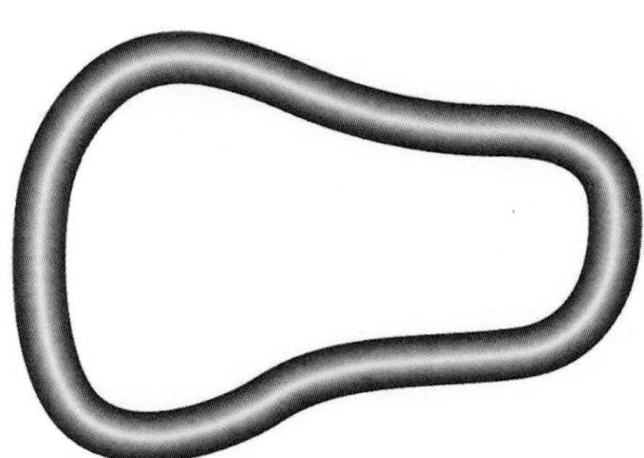

Fig. 38.47: Hodge-Smith pessary.

Method of Insertion

The patient lies in dorsal position with an empty bladder. The pessary is held collapsed or folded to make the insertion easy. A lubricant may be used. It is introduced inside the vagina and is pushed high. The broad end lies in the posterior fornix, the narrow end behind the symphysis pubis and the concavity is directed upwards.

Instructions to the Patient

- To have vaginal douche at least twice a week
- To check after 1 month
- To be removed or reintroduced after 3 months.

RING PESSARY (FIG. 38.48)

It is made up of silicon and rubber. It is sterilized by keeping in Cidex for 12 hours.

Indication of Uses

Ch. 16

Contraindications of Use

- Presence of sepsis.
- Gross relaxation of pelvic floor muscles.

Complications of Pessary

- Vaginal bleeding
- Pessary ulcers needs treatment with local estrogen
- Pelvic pain (with large size pessary)
- Vaginal discharge

Measurements

As in Hodge-Smith pessary.

Instructions

As in Hodge-Smith pessary.

Self-assessment

- Mechanism of action (p. 167).
- How the patient is followed up and what symptoms are usually enquired?

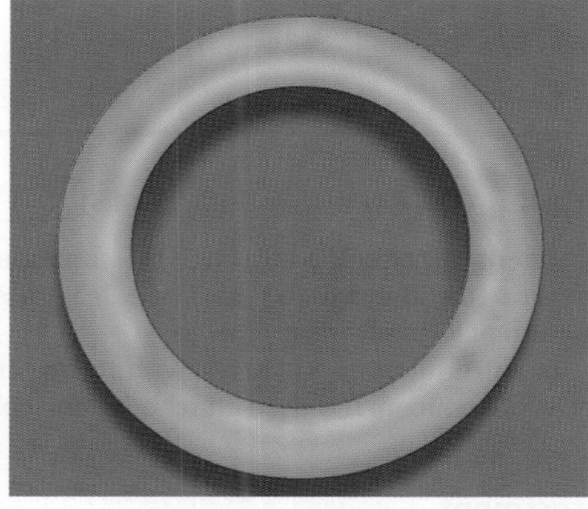

Fig. 38.48: Ring pessary.

Ans. Pessary removal, examination, cleaning and reinsertion is done usually at an interval of 8–10 months. It is done initially by the doctor/nurse and later on by the patient herself once she is taught about the procedure. In every follow up visit, patient is asked about any symptoms like: Vaginal bleeding, pain, offensive discharge and voiding difficulty.

- ***What are the complications of pessary use?***

Ans. Vaginal discharge, bad odor, vaginal erosion, ulceration, pessary incarceration, forgotten pessary rarely vaginal cancer (rare).

LAPAROSCOPIC OVARIAN DRILL NEEDLE (FIG. 38.49

Needle used for laparoscopic ovarian drilling. Monopolar diathermy current is passed.

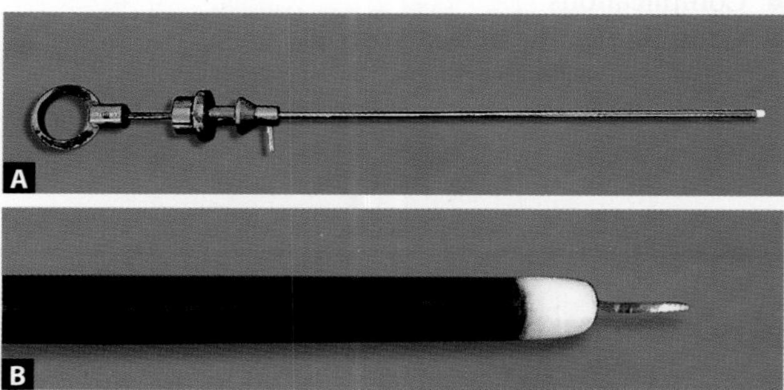

Fig. 38.49: Laparoscopic ovarian drill needle.

PROCESSING OF INSTRUMENTS

- **Disinfection:** It is done by any one of the methods: Immersing instruments in (a) boiling water for 20 minutes; (b) 2% glutaraldehyde (Cidex) solution for 20 minutes; or (c) 0.5% chlorine solution for 20 minutes [0.5% of chlorine solution is made by adding 3 teaspoons (15 g) of bleaching powder in one liter of water].
- **Cleaning:** Instruments are disassembled and washed on all surfaces in running (preferably warm) water. The cannulas should be flushed repeatedly.
- **Sterilization:** Either by—(a) Autoclaving at 121°C (250°F), under pressure of 15 lbs/in^2 (106 kPa) for 30 minutes; or (b) Immersing in 2% glutaraldehyde (Cidex) solution for 10 hours.

STERILIZATION OF INSTRUMENTS

Blunt instruments: All blunt instruments are sterilized either by boiling for half an hour or in an autoclave for 20 minutes with 20 lbs pressure at 120°C.

Sharp instruments: Sharp instruments like knife, needle, etc. are sterilized by keeping in Lysol for 24 hours.

SUTURE MATERIALS

The suture materials used in a particular surgical step depend on the strength of the tissues to be sutured and the time required for the wound to regain its strength. Depending on diameter, sutures are categorized into no. 0, 1, 2, etc. Sutures when smaller than no. 0, are indicated as 1-0, 2-0, and so forth. Due considerations also to be given on tensile strength of the suture, the rate at which the suture material loses its strength in vivo and the interaction expected between suture and tissues (Table 38.1).

CLASSIFICATION

The suture materials may be classified either as absorbable or nonabsorbable. Their biological origin or synthetic preparations are mentioned briefly.

- **Absorbable**
- **Nonabsorbable**

Absorbable

- **Biological (Natural)**
- **Synthetic**

Biological

- **Catgut and collagen**

Sutures: Sutures may be monofilament (Dexon, PDS, nylon) or polyfilament (Vicryl, silk). It is based on the number of fiber strands. Monofilament (single-stranded fiber) sutures need 5 to 6 throws to make knots secured. Polyfilament sutures are braided and their knots are secured with usual (2 to 3) throws. Risks of infection are high with polyfilament sutures. However, the tensile strength of polyfilament sutures is high.

The catgut (derived from the word kitgut—strings of a musical instrument known as kit) is obtained from the submucosa of sheep or ox intestines. Collagen is derived from ox Achilles tendon. Both are available in plain and chromic form. **Treatment with chromic sulfate produces chromic catgut and the untreated material produces plain catgut.** Chromic catgut is degraded and phagocytosed by proteolytic enzymes of white blood cells (inflammatory cells) slowly. Chromic catgut loses half of its tensile strength by 10 days and maintains some strength up to 21 days. Plain catgut loses 70% of its tensile strength by 7 days.

Synthetic

Dexon

Dexon (polyglycolic acid) is a copolymer of glycolic acid and is degraded by hydrolysis with minimal inflammation. It loses half of its tensile strength in 15 days and is absorbed in 4 months.

Vicryl (coated)

Vicryl (polyglactin): It is a copolymer of lactide and glycolide (90 : 10). It loses its tensile strength in 30 days. It is absorbed by 70 days. It produces less tissue reaction than catgut.

Vicryl rapide (coated) (Fig. 38.50): It is also a polyglactin suture. It is similar to plain catgut. Absorption is rapid with minimal tissue inflammation. 70% of its tensile strength is lost by 7 days. It is used for soft tissues, episiotomy repair and skin.

TABLE 38.1 Sutures.

Nature	Type	*Wound support (weeks)*	*Complete absorption (weeks)*	Mode of absorption	*Tissue where used*
Absorbable	Plain catgut	1–2	4–8	Phagocytosis, enzymatic degradation	Subcutaneous tissue and its blood vessels
	Chromic catgut	3	8–12	Phagocytosis, enzymatic degradation	Vascular pedicle, vaginal wall, rectus sheath
Delayed abs	Dexon	3	8–12		Subcuticular, fascial structure, skin
	Vicryl	3–4	8–10	Hydrolysis	Microsurgery, vaginal vault
	PDS	6–7	16–24	Hydrolysis	Rectus sheath, uterine muscles
	Vicryl rapide	1–2	5–6	Hydrolysis	Episiotomy, subcuticular tissues
Nonabsorbable	Nylon			Less tissue reaction, less prone to infection	Skin herniorrhaphy
	Prolene			Least tissue reaction	Herniorrhaphy, Rectus sheath
	Silk		50–100	Fibrous encapsulation (2–3 weeks)	Skin of the abdomen Ligation of internal iliac artery
	Dacron				

All the synthetic absorbable materials are sterilized by ethylene oxide.

The tensile strength of the above sutures is much greater than that of catgut. But these sutures need more throws to secure knots compared to catgut.

Polydioxanone suture (PDS)

It is a pliable monofilament made of polydioxanone. It loses half of its tensile strength in 28 days. Tissue inflammation is minimal. Monofilament sutures have no interstices to lodge any bacteria. So infections are rare. **Polyglyconate sutures** have got similar properties. These are used for fascial closure.

Nonabsorbable

- **Biological**
- **Synthetic**

Biological

- **Silk** suture can be handled and tied easily. It has excellent knot security. It is sterilized by gamma radiation. It is a foreign protein and initiates strong inflammatory response and loses half of its tensile strength by 1 year. It should not be used in contaminated or infected tissue.
- **Cotton** is the weakest nonabsorbable suture. It loses 50% of the tensile strength by 6 months. Wet cotton is stronger (10%) than dry cotton. It is rarely used now.

Synthetic

- **Terelene or dacron:** These are extruded from a homopolymer.

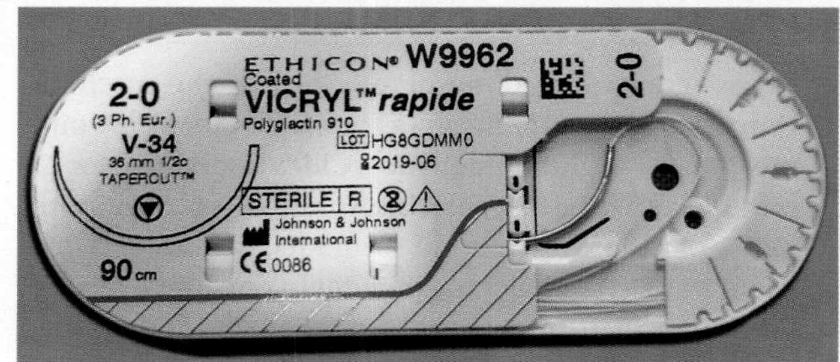

Fig. 38.50: Vicryl rapide 2–0 suture, length 90 cm with round bodied needle, 36 mm, half circle.

- **Polyamide (nylon):** This is a man-made monofilament or multifilament. It is very much nonreactive in tissues. Monofilament nylon has greater tensile strength, incites less tissue reaction and is less prone to infection than braided nylon.
- **Polypropylene (prolene):** It is a hydrocarbon polymer and is monofilament. It has least tissue reaction. Knot security is greater. It is sterilized by ethylene oxide.
- **Steel** suture is nonreactive and has highest tensile strength. It is not commonly used now in obstetrics and gynecology. This is used in orthopedic and dental surgery.

Nonabsorbable sutures maintain their tensile strength for a long time. However, there may be suture related pain or rarely sinus formation.

SPECIMENS

DESCRIPTION

The description of a specimen includes:

- Identification of the organ/organs.
- To describe the pathology as seen on naked eye examination.

Identification of the Organ

Uterus

The uterus is identified by:

- Pear-shaped structure
- Adnexal attachment
- Cervical opening
  - Circular in nulliparous
  - Transverse slit in parous.

Anterior surface is identified by

- Attachment of round ligament
- Loose attachment of uterovesical peritoneum.

Posterior surface is identified by

- Attachment of ovarian ligament with or without ovary.
- Cut margin of the posterior peritoneum which is densely attached and placed at a lower level than the cut edge of the anterior peritoneum.

Uterine Tubes

Tubular structures with abdominal ostium surrounded by fimbriae and mesosalpinx.

Ovary

Fallopian tube is usually attached to the ovarian specimen. If the uterine tube is not mounted, even then the specimen is likely to be ovarian as there is no other pelvic organs resembling it, exception being a parovarian cyst (Fig. 38.65).

SPECIMEN—1 AND 2

Description (Figs. 38.51 and 38.52)

This is a specimen of uterus with tubes and ovaries of both the sides (Fig. 38.51).

There is alteration in the size (enlarged) and shape (irregular) of the uterus due to multiple fibroids. The fibroids are of different sizes. Some are cut open to show whorled appearance (Fig. 38.52B). A capsule is seen (Fig. 38.51) surrounding the fibroid. Part of the tumor is covered by endometrium [submucous fibroid (Fig. 38.52A)] or a part is covered by serous coat [subserous fibroid (Fig. 38.52B)]. One subserous fibroid has got a pedicle (Fig. 38.52B)— pedunculated.

The tubes and the ovaries are looking normal in all the specimens.

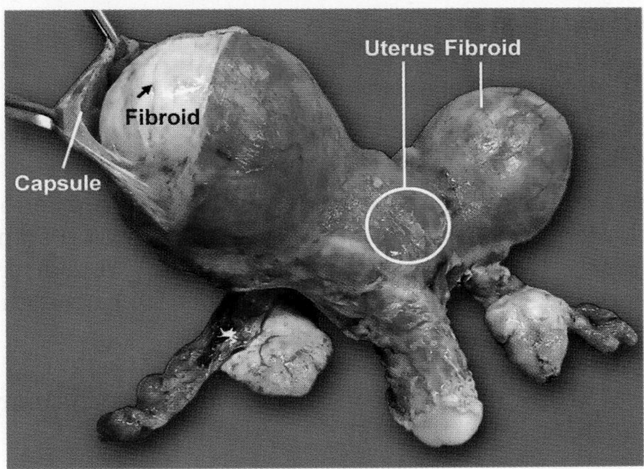

Fig. 38.51: Multiple fibroid uterus, hysterectomy and bilateral salpingo-oophorectomy had been done. Tissue dissection had been done to show the capsule of the fibroid.

Operation done: Total hysterectomy with bilateral salpingo-oophorectomy.
Diagnosis: Multiple fibroids of the body of the uterus.

Self-assessment

- What are the different types of uterine fibroid? (Ch. 20).
- Causes of menorrhagia.
- Causes of infertility (Ch. 17).
- Causes of pelvic pain (Ch. 34).
- How to differentiate a fibroid from an ovarian tumor on clinical examination?
- Place of medical management (p. 227).
- Different types of surgical management available (p. 229).

Q. What could be the presentation of the woman in the clinic?

Ans. As with these specimens with total hysterectomy, the women are unlikely to suffer from infertility and as bilateral oophorectomy had been done, their probable age would be ≥45 years.

Q. What are the indications, conditions to be fulfilled before myomectomy? What are the contraindications?

Ans. Ch. 20.

Q. What are the different treatment options available for fibroids?.

Ans. (1) **Surgery**: (A) Hysterectomy; (B) Myomectomy—**Surgical procedures** may be: (a) Laparotomy, (b) Laparoscopy, (c) Hysteroscopy (p. 227); (C) Myolysis. (2) Medical therapy. (3) Interventional radiology—uterine artery embolization.

Q. How do you differentiate fibroid uterus from adenomyosis?

Ans. Ch. 20.

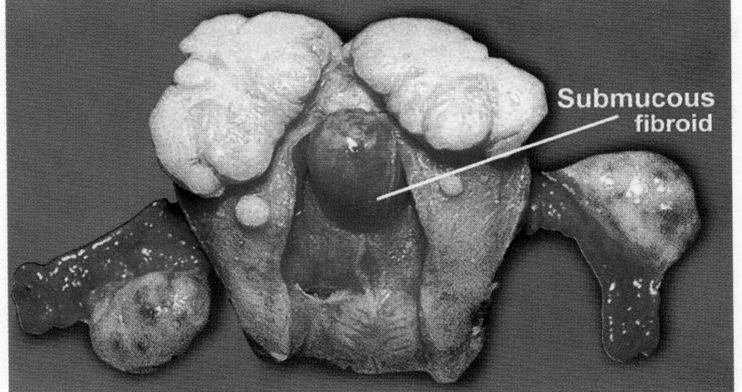

Fig. 38.52A: Fibroid uterus—subserous, interstitial and, submucous variety. Specimen 38.49B has got a huge subserous (arrow) and also a pedunculated subserous variety of fibroid (arrow). Both the specimens are cut-opened to show the endometrial cavity. Both the cavities are increased and distorted.

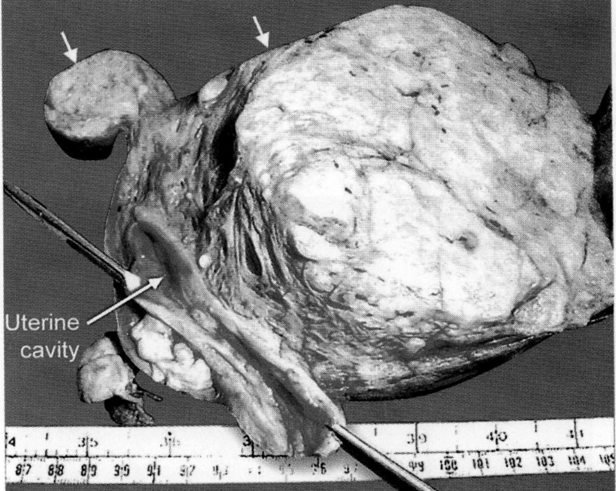

Fig. 38.52B: Uterine cavity is shown with Allis tissue forceps.

SPECIMEN—3

Description (Fig. 38.53)

This is a specimen of uterus, with tubes and ovaries of both the sides.

Anterior surface of the uterus is cut open to show a mass arising from the fundus protruding into the uterine cavity. Another mass is seen to come out of the uterus through the cervical canal with a long pedicle.

Operation done: Total hysterectomy with bilateral salpingo-oophorectomy.
Diagnosis: Submucous fibroid polyps—sessile and pedunculated.

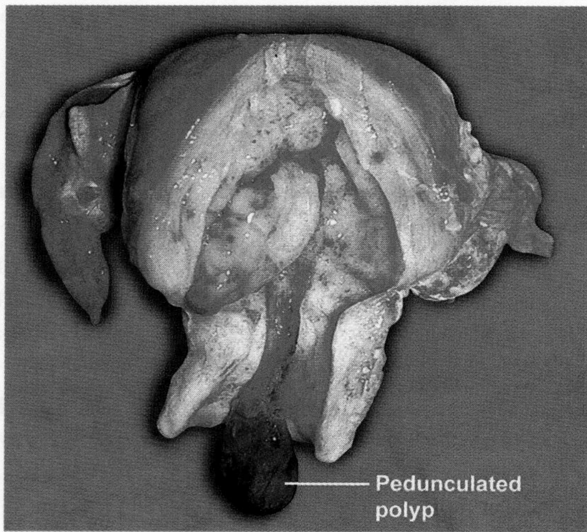

Fig. 38.53: Submucous fibroid polyps (sessile and pedunculated). Patient suffered menorrhagia, metrorrhagia and dysmenorrhea.

Self-assessment

- Clinical presentation of such a case (p. 228)
- Confirmation of diagnosis.

Q. When do myomas require to be removed (indications of myomectomy)?

Ans. (a) Any myoma growing during the follow-up period; (b) Menorrhagia not responding to medical therapy; (c) Excessive pain or pressure symptoms; (d) Woman with infertility or recurrent miscarriage when no cause other than fibroid is present.

- What are secondary changes in a fibroid? (p. 227).
- What are management alternative to hysterectomy? (p. 231).

SPECIMEN—4

Description (Figs. 38.54A and B)

This is a specimen of uterus (Fig. 38.52A) with tubes and ovaries of both the sides. There is a huge mass arising from the posterior cervical wall. The small uterus sits on the top of the huge mass (*lantern on dome of St. Paul's cathedral*).

The anterior surface of the uterus (Fig. 38.52B) is cut open to show the anterior cervical wall and the uterine cavity.

Operation done: Total hysterectomy with bilateral salpingo-oophorectomy with removal of the mass.

Diagnosis: Cervical fibroid (posterior).

Self-assessment

- Types of cervical fibroid (p. 234).
- Modes of presentation in a case with cervical fibroid (p. 234).
- What are the surgical risks in such a case?
- Approach for surgical removal of cervical myoma (p. 507).
- Displacements of the ureter and risks of ureteric injury (p. 355).
- Common gynecological pathologies where ureteric injury is more likely (p. 355).

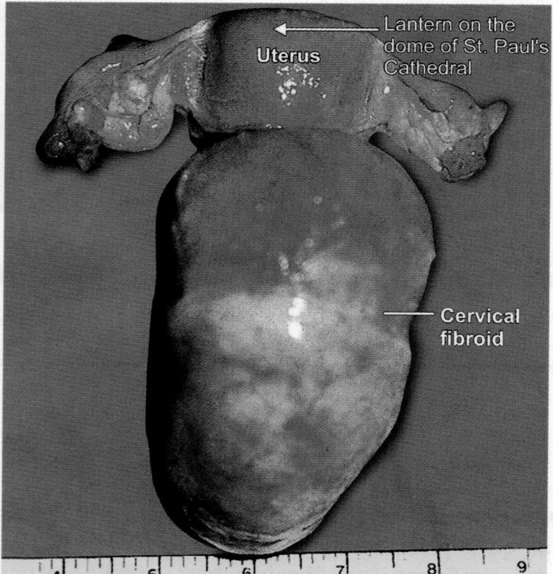

Fig. 38.54A: A huge posterior cervical fibroid.

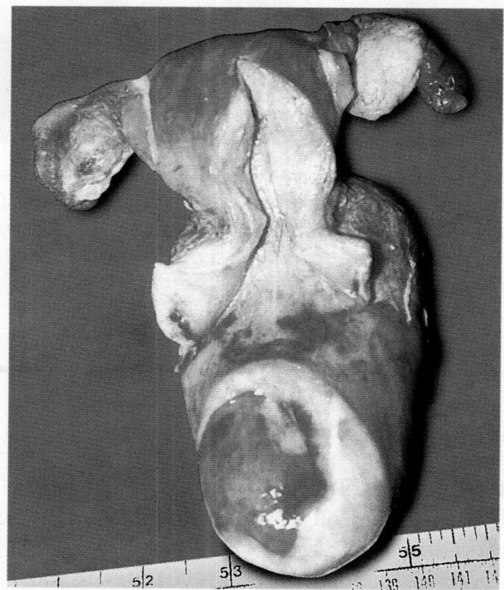

Fig. 38.54B: Same specimen as in Fig. 38.52A, is seen from the anterior surface.

SPECIMEN—5

Description (Fig. 38.55)

This is a specimen of the uterus and the tubes and ovaries of both the sides. The uterus is enlarged and is cut open to show a diffuse growth located at one wall. The growth presents a striated appearance with scattered dark hemorrhagic spots. It has got no capsule. (c.f. — fibroid — whorled appearance and a capsule).

Operation done: Total hysterectomy with bilateral salpingo-oophorectomy.

Diagnosis: Adenomyosis.

Self-assessment

- Describe the clinical presentation of pelvic endometriosis (p. 255).
- Causes of infertility in endometriosis (p. 257; Table 22.4).
- Clinical features of adenomyosis (p. 263)
- Histological picture of adenomyosis.
- Mention treatment options for pelvic endometriosis (p. 258).
- Treatment for adenomyosis (p. 264).

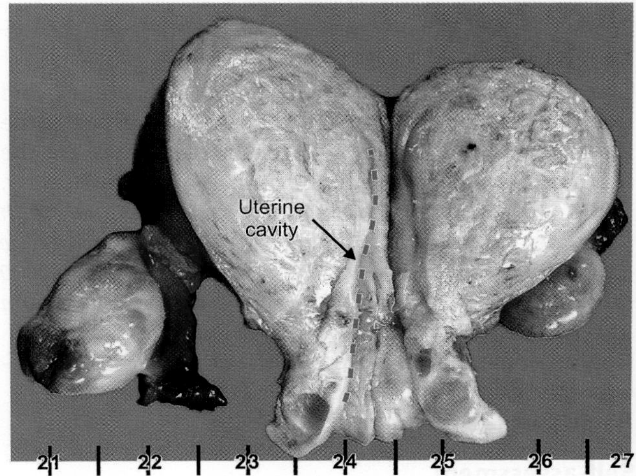

Fig. 38.55: Specimen of adenomyosis.

SPECIMEN—6

Description (Fig. 38.56)

This is a specimen of the uterus with tubes and ovaries of both the sides. The ovaries are hugely enlarged, lobulated with a yellowish tinge. The uterus is also enlarged. Vesicular mass is seen protruding out through the incised uterus.

Operation done: Total hysterectomy with bilateral salpingo-oophorectomy.

Diagnosis: Hydatidiform mole with large theca lutein cysts of both the ovaries.

Self-assessment

- High-risk factors for gestational trophoblastic neoplasia (GTN).
- Clinical features of GTN.
- Management of GTN.
- Place of uterine curettage in GTN.
- **Management of theca lutein cysts**: Once hydatidiform mole or GTN is treated, there is spontaneous regression (within a few months) of the cysts. Rarely, they are removed when complications like torsion or intracystic hemorrhage occur.

Q. ***What are the common sites of metastasis?***

Ans. P. 303–309.

Q. ***What is the place of prophylactic chemotherapy and what are its limitations?***

Ans. P. 303–309.

Q. ***WHO FIGO scoring system for risk assessment.***

Ans. P. 303–309.

Q. ***Reproductive behavior of women following treatment of GTN.***

Ans. P. 303–309.

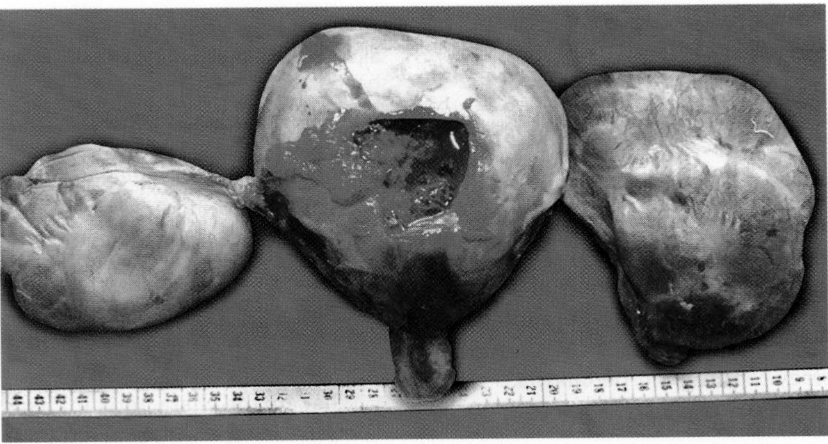

Fig. 38.56: Hydatidiform mole with bilateral large theca lutein cysts.

SPECIMEN—7

Description (Fig. 38.57)

This is the specimen of a uterus with the tubes and ovaries. The uterus is enlarged. The anterior surface of the uterus is cut open to show a purplish growth invading the myometrium. The tube and the ovary are looking healthy.

This 37-year-old parous lady was admitted with irregular bleeding P/V following a miscarriage. She underwent D/C thrice. Her serum βhCG level was 96,000 mIU/mL. Following courses of chemotherapy the serum hCG level remained persistently elevated.

Operation done: Total hysterectomy with bilateral salpingo-oophorectomy. Histology confirmed chorio-carcinoma.

Diagnosis: Choriocarcinoma.

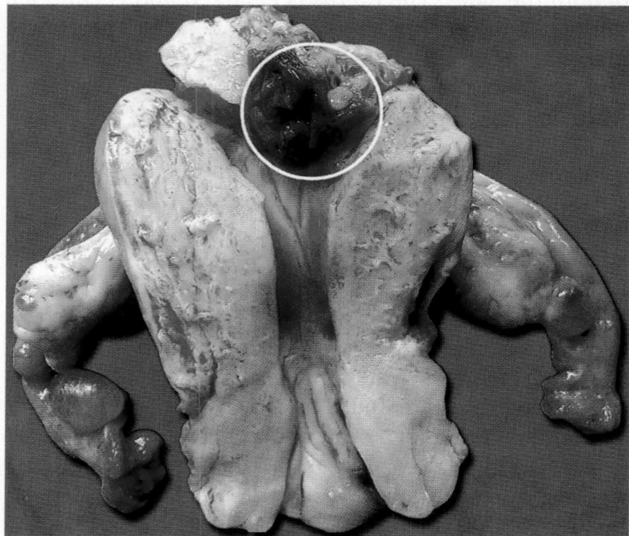

Fig. 38.57: Choriocarcinoma resistant to chemotherapy. Lesion is seen to invade the myometrium.

Self-assessment

Q. How the selection of chemotherapy regimen is done?

Ans. P. 303.

- Place of hysterectomy in GTN (p. 303–309).
- Prognosis of GTN following treatment and the risk of recurrence.
- Response to chemotherapy and subsequent reproductive behavior.
- Patient follow-up following treatment.

SPECIMEN—8

Description (Fig. 38.58)

This is a specimen of uterus, tubes and ovaries of both the sides. The left tube is markedly enlarged especially towards the outer half. The shape looks like a 'retort.' The inside fluid appears to be clear.

Diagnosis: Hydrosalpinx of the left tube.

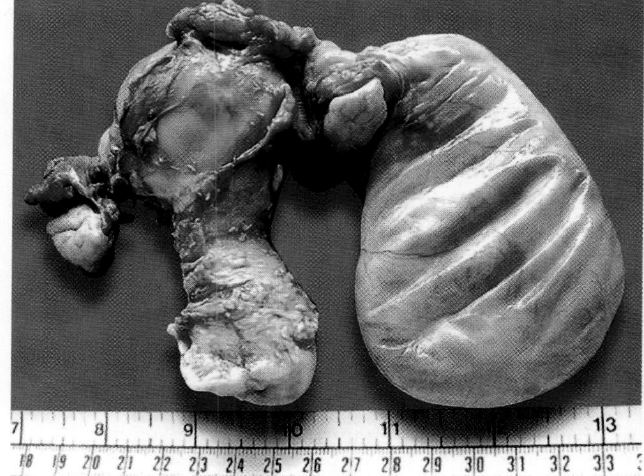

Fig. 38.58: Specimen of total hysterectomy with bilateral salpingo-oophorectomy showing a large hydrosalpinx (retort-shaped) of the left tube.

Self-assessment (Ch. 12 and 35)

- Pathogenesis of hydrosalpinx
- Organisms involved in pathology
- Mode of affection in gonococcal infection
- Mechanism of the 'retort' shape
- Steps of salpingectomy.

SPECIMEN—9

Description (Fig. 38.59)

This is a specimen of the uterus, tubes, and ovaries of both the sides. The tubes of both sides are coiled, wall is thickened and matted with the ovaries. There are adhesions over the surfaces of the tubes and uterus. TAH and BSO had been done. Histology confirmed tuberculosis.

Diagnosis: Bilateral tubo-ovarian (TO) mass.

Self-assessment (Ch. 11 and 13)

- Mention the pathogenesis of TO mass (p. 110).
- Mention the clinical diagnostic criteria of PID.
- What is the mode of spread of infection in tubercular, pyogenic and other infections?
- How infertility could be explained with genital tuberculosis?
- Mention the complications of acute PID and its late sequelae.
- What are the characteristic changes on HSG of the tube when infected with tuberculosis?
- What are the contraindications and indications of surgery in a woman with pelvic tuberculosis?

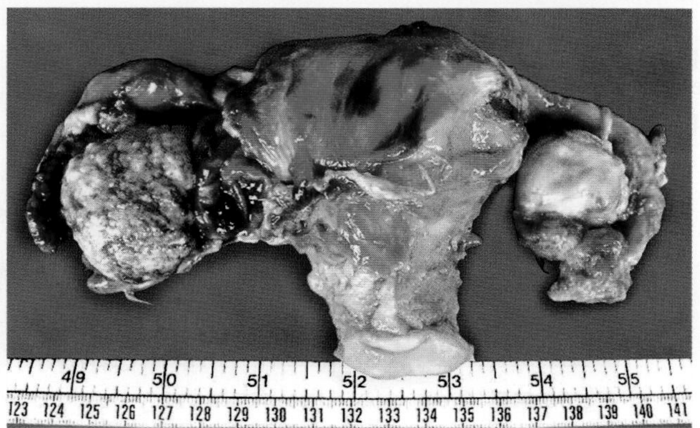

Fig. 38.59: Specimen of uterus, tubes, and ovaries showing bilateral tubo-ovarian mass due to genital tuberculosis. Areas of caseation calcification are seen.

41-year-old woman presented with chronic pelvic pain, abnormal uterine bleeding and occasional vaginal discharge. She had the history of genital tuberculosis for which she received complete treatment. She underwent laparotomy. Total abdominal hysterectomy and bilateral salpingo-oophorectomy was done. Histology confirmed genital tuberculosis.

SPECIMEN—10

Description (Fig. 38.60)

This is a specimen of a noncommunicating horn of a bicornuate uterus (cut-opened) with the tube. The tube is elongated, sausage shaped and purplish in color. The cut-open uterus shows the cavity which was filled with blood. The tube is filled with blood.

Operation done: Excision of the noncommunicating horn and salpingectomy.

Diagnosis: **Rudimentary (noncommunicating) horn of a bicornuate uterus with hematosalpinx**.

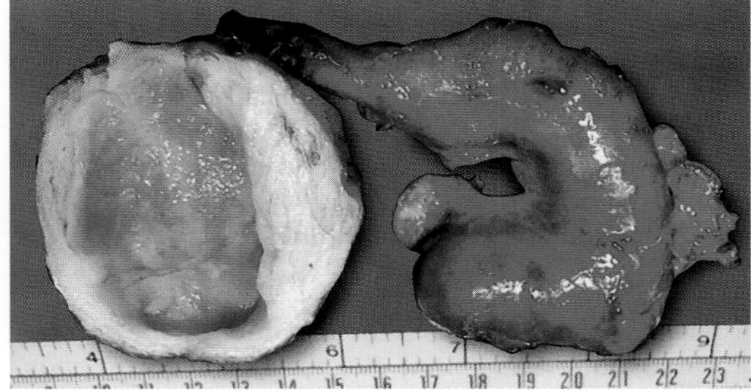

Fig. 38.60: Hematosalpinx of the right tube.

Self-assessment

- **Causes of hematosalpinx**: Tubal ectopic pregnancy, endometriosis, cryptomenorrhea and rarely primary tubal carcinoma (0.3% of all genital malignancies).
- **Causes** of cryptomenorrhea.
- **Clinical presentation** of a care with tubal carcinoma: Triad of lower abdominal pain (colicky), profuse watery discharge (hydrops tubae profluens), and vaginal bleeding. Preoperative diagnosis is rare and often mistaken as an ovarian tumor.

SPECIMEN—11

Description (Figs. 38.61A and B)

These are the specimens of the uterus with tube and ovary of the right side. The ovarian cysts (right) are cut open to show inspissated sebaceous material, hair and other mature (mesenchymal) tissues. Teeth is present in about a third (Figs. 38.61A and B).

Operation done: Total hysterectomy with bilateral salpingo-oophorectomy.

Diagnosis: **Dermoid cyst of the right ovary**.

Self-assessment (Ch. 21)

- Name the tissues arising from the three germ cell layers. Ans: **Ectodermal**: Skin, hair, teeth, **Mesodermal:** Bone, cartilage; **Endodermal**: Thyroid, intestine.
- Frequency of bilaterality (15–20%) and association with pregnancy (20-40%).
- Common complications.
- Management in a young patient.
- Risk of malignant change.
- What are strumal carcinoids?

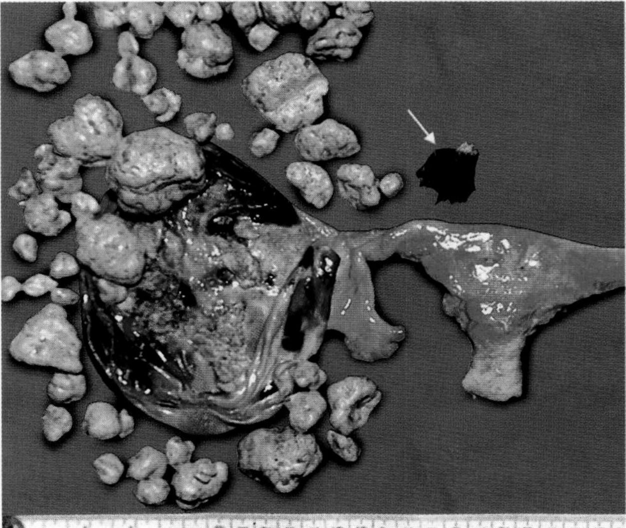

Fig. 38.61A: Gross appearance of a dermoid cyst of the ovary showing hair, teeth (arrow) and butter balls (sebum aggregated to form spherules).

Q. How carcinoid tumors of the ovary are treated?

Ans. Excision of the tumor (ovariotomy) causes rapid fall in the serum level of serotonin and disappearance of 5-hydroxyindole acetic acid in the urine. There is rapid remission of symptoms.

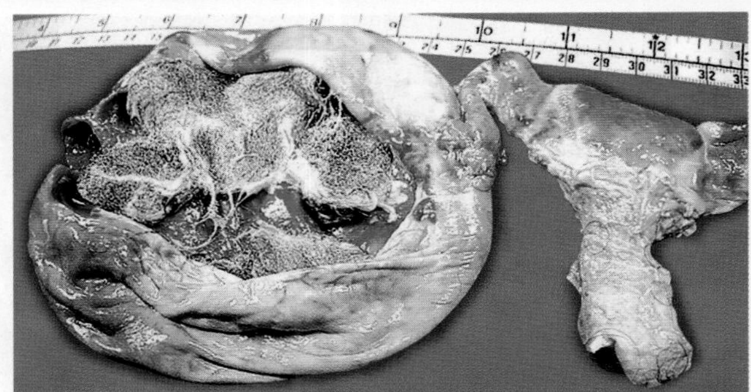

Fig. 38.61B: Gross appearance of dermoid cyst of the ovary with hair and sebaceous material (cut section).

SPECIMEN—12

Description (Fig. 38.62)

This is a specimen of the uterus with tubes and ovaries of both the sides. The left sided ovarian cyst is cut open to show many septa. There are few smaller cysts projecting inside.

Operation done: Total hysterectomy with bilateral salpingo-oophorectomy.

Diagnosis: Mucinous cyst adenoma.

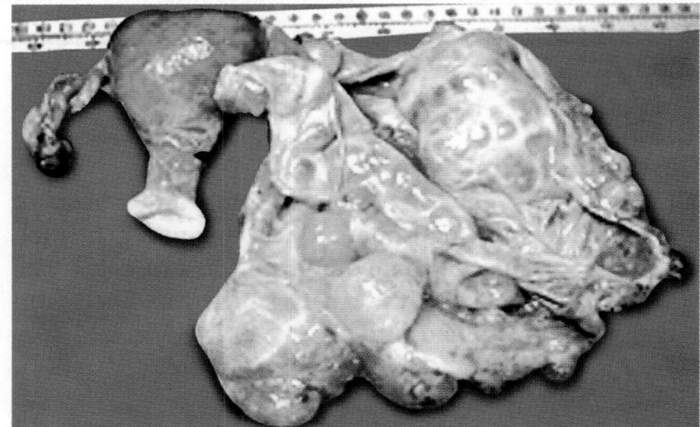

Fig. 38.62: Left sided mucinous cyst adenoma (*gross appearance on cut specimen*).

Self-assessment (Ch. 21)

- Mention the common epithelial tumors of the ovary.
- Discuss the differential diagnosis of a pelvic abdominal lump.
- Clinical presentation of a benign ovarian tumor.
- Features of a functional cyst.
- How a benign ovarian tumor could be differentiated from a malignant one clinically?
- How laparotomy findings could be helpful to differentiate a benign tumor from a malignant one?
- What are Psammoma bodies?
- What are the complications of a benign ovarian tumor?
- Management of a benign ovarian tumor.
- Structures forming the ovarian pedicle.

SPECIMEN—13 (CH. 21 AND 24)

Description (Fig. 38.63)

This is a specimen of uterus with tubes and ovaries of both the sides. The right ovary is hugely enlarged and cut opened to show its solid texture islands of yellow tissue separated by fibrous septa.

Operation done: Total hysterectomy with bilateral salpingo-oophorectomy.

Diagnosis: Solid ovarian tumor. Theca cell tumor of the ovary was confirmed on histology.

Self-assessment

- *Mention the common solid tumors of the ovary.*

  Benign: Fibroma, Thecoma, Brenner tumor. Sex cord-stromal tumors.

  Malignant: Primary ovarian carcinoma, dysgerminoma, carcinoid, immature teratoma, mesonephroma. Krukenberg tumor and primary lymphoma.
- ***What is Meig's syndrome?***

Ans. It is a triad of findings including ascites, pleural effusion and benign ovarian fibroma. The cause is unknown. The ascites and pleural effusion resolve spontaneously when the ovarian tumor is removed.

- ***What are the hormone producing tumors of the ovary?***
  - **Feminizing tumors:** Granulosa cell and theca cell.
  - **Masculinizing tumors:** Sertoli-Leydig cell and Hilus cell.
  - **Others:** Struma ovarii (thyroid hormones) carcinoids are rare specialized germ cell ovarian tumors that secrete 5-HT.
- ***What are the germ cell tumors of the ovary?***

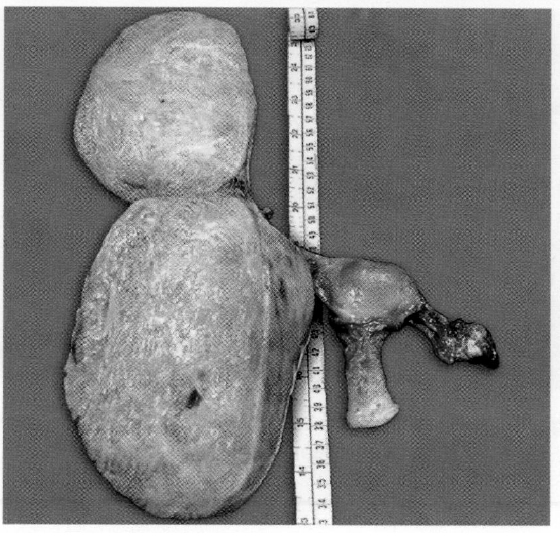

Fig. 38.63A: Gross appearance (cut section) of a solid ovarian tumor (right).

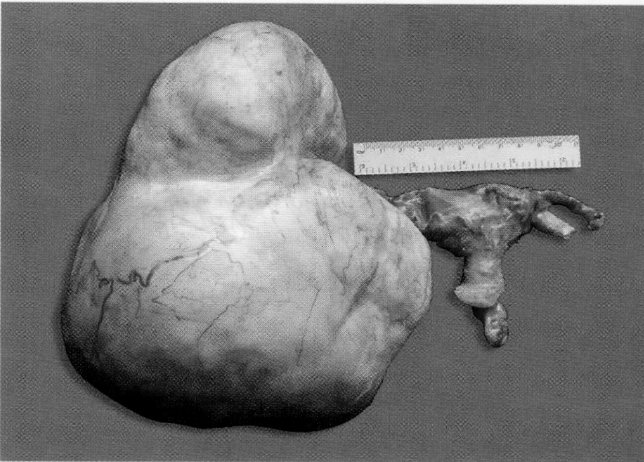

Fig. 38.63B: Gross appearance of a solid ovarian tumor. Total hysterectomy with bilateral salpingo-oophorectomy was done. Histology confirmed fibroma of the ovary.

SPECIMEN—14

Description (Figs. 38.64A to C)

A. This is a pathological specimen of the uterus and both the ovaries. The one ovary is enlarged lobulated with the walls irregular and shaggy. Cut section shows solid areas with hemorrhage and necrosis at places.
B. Omentectomy done.
C. Ascitic fluid (hemorrhagic) is collected.

Diagnosis: Most likely malignant ovarian tumor.

Self-assessment (Ch. 24)

- Clinical features of a malignant ovarian tumor.
- What are the common malignant ovarian tumors?
- How omentectomy is helpful in the management of ovarian malignancies?
- Is epithelial ovarian cancer hereditary?

Ans. About 10–15% of all epithelial ovarian cancers are familial. There are three different syndromes of hereditary ovarian cancer: (a) Breast/ovarian familial cancer (75–90%); (b) Site specific ovarian cancer (5%); and (c) Lynch II syndrome (2%)—

- Mention the high-risk factors as well as the protective factors for ovarian malignancy.
- Principles of surgical approach (guidelines) in a malignant ovarian tumor.
- What are the tissues removed in cytoreductive surgery? Histology confirmed malignant Brenner tumor.
- ***How serum CA-125 measurement is helpful?***

Ans. It is helpful with a known case of ovarian cancer: (a) To know the response of treatment; (b) To know if the tumor is resistance to chemotherapy; (c) Early detection of tumor recurrence (p. 311).

SPECIMEN—15

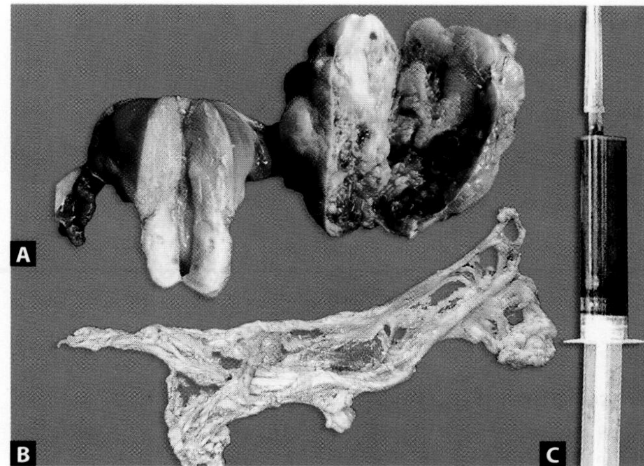

Figs. 38.64A to C: Photograph of a surgical specimens showing: (A) Uterus, ovaries (one is hugely enlarged), cut opened to show the areas of hemorrhage and necrosis; (B) Infracolic omentectomy; (C) Ascitic fluid (hemorrhagic) was collected for malignant cell cytology. Histology confirmed malignant Brenner tumor. Omentum was free of metastasis.

Description (Fig. 38.65)

This is a specimen of the uterus with tubes and ovaries of both the sides. The ovaries are enlarged with capsules ruptured. There is exophytic growth on the surface that infiltrates the surrounding organs. The cut surfaces show solid texture, extensive areas of hemorrhage and necrosis.

Operation done: Total hysterectomy with bilateral salpingo-oophorectomy and omentectomy.

Diagnosis: Bilateral ovarian carcinoma (mucinous cyst adenocarcinoma).

Self-assessment (Ch. 24)

- ***What are the common sites of metastases?***
- ***Methods of spread in a case of ovarian malignancy.***
- ***Place of neoadjuvant chemotherapy for ovarian malignancy.***
- ***What are the findings during laparotomy to differentiate a benign ovarian tumor from a malignant one?***
- ***What are the treatment modalities in a case with ovarian malignancy?***
- ***What is the place of prophylactic oophorectomy during hysterectomy?***

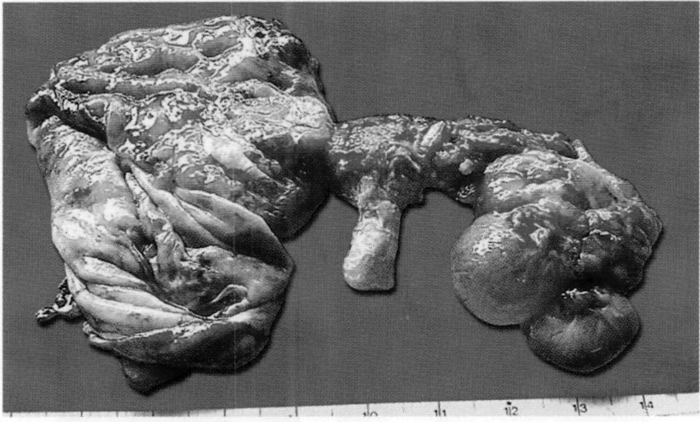

Fig. 38.65: Bilateral mucinous adenocarcinoma of the ovaries (gross appearance on cut specimen).

SPECIMEN—16

Description (Fig. 38.66)

This is a per-operative photograph of the uterus with tubes and ovaries of both the sides. The ovaries are found enlarged with lobulated appearance and are free of adhesions. The shape of the ovary is maintained. The color is pinkish with smooth surfaces. Uterus and tubes are found normal.

Operation done: Total hysterectomy with bilateral salpingo-oophorectomy.

Diagnosis: Probably **Krukenberg's tumor**.

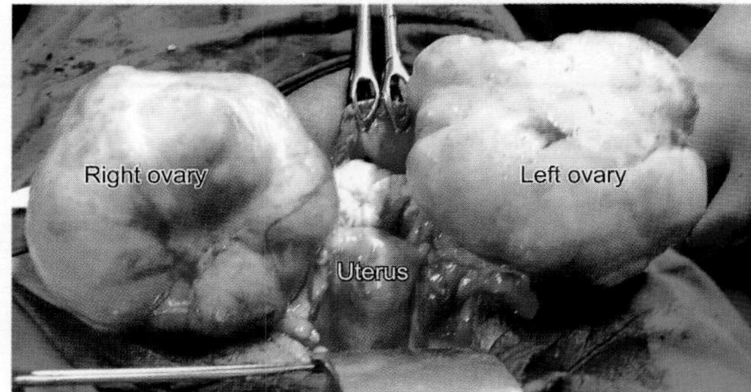

Fig. 38.66: Per-operative photograph of a case with bilateral ovarian tumors. Histology confirmed metastatic ovarian tumor (Krukenberg tumor).

Self-assessment

- ***What is a Krukenberg tumor?***

Ans. This is a metastatic adenocarcinoma of the ovary. Almost all metastasize from the stomach. Few arise from the breast, colon or biliary tract.

- ***Suggestive appearance for diagnosis.***
- ***Primary sites?***
- ***Mode of spread to the ovaries?***
- ***Histological picture?***
- ***Prognosis?***
- ***What is the survival rate?***

SPECIMEN—17

Description (Fig. 38.67)

This is a per-operative photograph of the uterus with the tubes and ovaries. A hugely enlarged cyst is attached to the fimbrial end of the left tube which is stretched out. Left ovary is seen clearly (*see arrow*) behind the tube.

Operation done: Total hysterectomy with bilateral salpingo-oophorectomy with removal of the cyst is done.

Diagnosis: **Parovarian cyst (left)**.

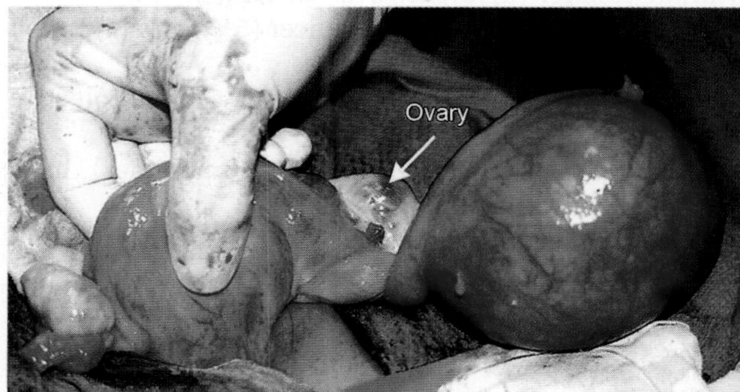

Fig. 38.67: At a glance, it seems to be ovarian but careful inspection reveals the ovary is separated from the cyst (*see* arrow). The pedicle is seen to undergo torsion.

Self-assessment (Ch. 21)

- Diagnosis of a parovarian cyst.
- Embryological origin of the cyst: From the remnant of the Wolffian body situated in the mesosalpinx.
- Usually, the cyst is unilocular, has a thin wall and is filled with a clear fluid.
- Clinical features and management: Same as ovarian tumor.
- Management: Excision of the cyst.
- Risk of malignancy—rare.

SPECIMEN—18

Description (Fig. 38.68)

This is a pathological specimen of the uterus, tubes and ovaries of both the sides with upper vagina and the parametrium. The growth arising from the cervix is huge (>4 cm) and exophytic.

Operation done: Radical hysterectomy for carcinoma cervix. Uterine artery is dissected from the internal iliac artery. Dissected pelvic lymph nodes are seen.

Diagnosis: Carcinoma cervix (invasive) (FIGO Stage IIA).

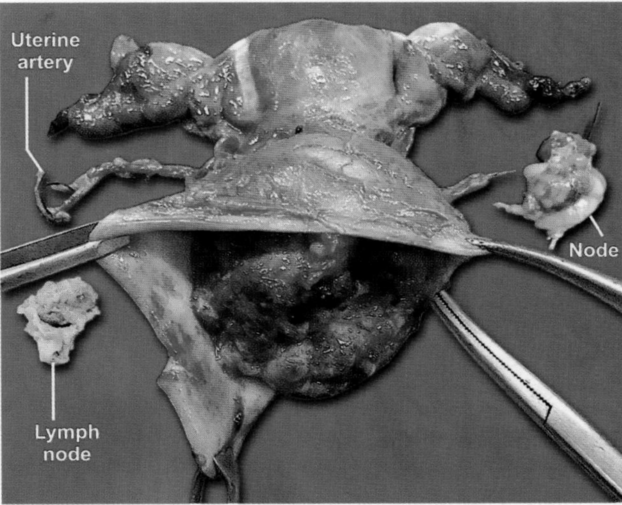

Fig. 38.68: A specimen of carcinoma (squamous cell) of the cervix showing marked exophytic growth. Radical hysterectomy had been done. Uterine arteries are ligated at their origin from the internal iliac artery. Both the ovaries and upper third of vagina had been removed (seen in the photograph). Pelvic lymph adenectomy done (one enlarged node on either side is seen).

Self-assessment (Ch. 24)

- Histological types.
- Diagnosis of early carcinoma.
- Lymphatic drainage of the cervix.
- Management of CIS, microinvasive and early stage carcinoma.
- Advantages and disadvantages of radiotherapy.
- Principal steps of radical hysterectomy.
- Tissues removed in radical hysterectomy.
- Significance of sentinel node biopsy.
- Staging procedures allowed by FIGO.
- Complications of radical hysterectomy.
  - **Complications during surgery:** (a) Injury to ureter, bladder, rectum, major pelvic vessels, fistula formation; (b) Hemorrhage; (c) Anesthetic complications; (d) Even mortality (<1%)
  - **Postoperative complication:** Similar to abdominal hysterectomy

  Others are: (a) Bladder dysfunction; (b) Neuropathies; (c) Lymphocyst formation; (d) Dyspareunia; (e) Recurrence.
- Preventive measures for carcinoma cervix—Primary and secondary prevention.
- Mention the different treatment modalities for carcinoma cervix.

  A. **Surgery:**
     a. Radical hysterectomy
     b. Fertility sparing surgery (LARVT)

  B. **Radiotherapy:** EBRT and brachytherapy

  C. **Radiotherapy followed by surgery** in cases with bulky tumor, endocervical cancer

  D. **Neoadjuvant chemotherapy (NACT)**

  E. **Neoadjuvant chemotherapy followed by surgery**

  F. **Concurrent chemoradiation**
- Causes of death in carcinoma cervix.
- Differential diagnosis of carcinoma cervix.
- Place of laparoscopic assisted vaginal trachelectomy.

SPECIMEN—19

Description (Fig. 38.69)

This is a specimen of the uterus with tubes and ovaries of both the sides. The uterus is uniformly enlarged. The anterior surface is cut open to show a fungating growth confined to the body. The tubes and ovaries are healthy.

Operation done: Total hysterectomy with bilateral salpingo-oophorectomy.

Diagnosis: Endometrial carcinoma.

Self-assessment (Ch. 24)

- Clinical presentation.
- Discuss the methods of diagnosis.
- Histological types of endometrial carcinoma.
- Lymphatic drainage of body of the uterus.
- High-risk women for endometrial cancer: Nulliparity, corpus cancer syndrome (obesity, diabetes and hypertension), late menopause.
- Surgical procedures in the management.
- Place of chemotherapy and radiotherapy.

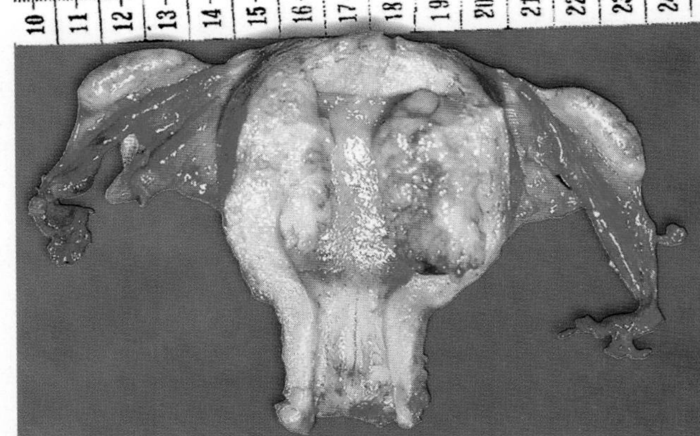

Fig. 38.69: The uterus is cut open to show a diffuse and partly necrotic growth of adenocarcinoma filling the uterine cavity.

SPECIMEN—20

Description (Fig. 38.70)

This is a specimen of the vulva. The vulva shows a large exophytic growth and biopsy revealed squamous cell carcinoma.

Operation done: Radical vulvectomy. Vulvectomy specimen is obtained by the skin sparing 'long horn' incisions. Tips of the horns rest on the anterior superior iliac spines. The upper margin of incision is interspinous, the lower margin is along the inguinal skin creases and the labiocrural folds. Three incision techniques are currently used in most of the centers.

Diagnosis: Carcinoma of the vulva.

Self-assessment (Ch. 24)

- Common sites of vulvar malignancy.
- Different histological types.
- Lymphatic drainage of the vulva and its clinical significance.
- Clinical presentation.
- Types of vulvectomy.

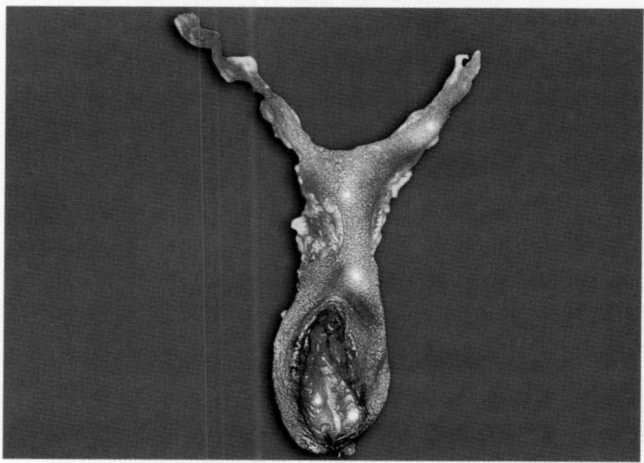

Fig. 38.70: Carcinoma of the vulva—radical vulvectomy done using 'long horn' incisions.

- Advantages of three separate incisions.
- Complications of radical vulvectomy.
- Significance of a sentinel node.
- Prognostic factors for vulvar carcinoma.

IMAGING STUDIES IN GYNECOLOGY

PLATES: SKIAGRAPHS, ULTRASONOGRAPHS, COMPUTED TOMOGRAPHS, AND MAGNETIC RESONANCE IMAGINGS

HYSTEROSALPINGOGRAM

Figure 38.71

Hysterosalpingogram (HSG) showing radio-opaque shadow demarcating the uterine cavity. The radio-opaque dye is visible in the lumen of both the tubes. There is peritoneal spillage on both sides.

Diagnosis: Normal hysterosalpingogram (normal cavity) with bilateral patent tubes (free peritoneal spill).

Self-assessment (Ch. 35)

- Indications and contraindications of HSG.
- Timing of HSG in relation to the menstrual cycle.
- Steps of the procedure.
- Complications of HSG.
- Prospect of fertility in this case:

Ans. As the tubes are patent, the couple should be investigated to assess the ovulatory status and male factors for infertility.

- Other methods for assessment of tubal patency.
  a. Laparoscopy and chromopertubation
  b. Sonohysterosalpingography
  c. Falloposcopy
  d. Salpingoscopy are done in a special situation
  e. Insufflation test is not done these days.

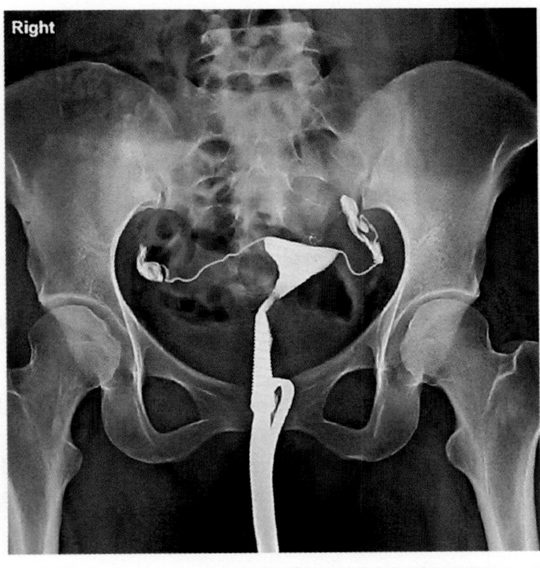

Fig. 38.71: Hysterosalpingogram with bilateral peritoneal spillage.

Figure 38.72

Hysterosalpingogram showing radio-opaque shadow demarcating the uterine cavity. No radio-opaque shadow is visible on either tube.

Diagnosis: Hysterosalpingogram showing bilateral cornual block.

Self-assessment

- Alternative investigations
- Management if tubes are damaged
- Results of tuboplasty
- Different methods of assisted reproductive technology (ART).

Management if tubes are normal:

- To assess the male factors and ovarian factors for infertility.
- What other information can be obtained from HSG?
- What are the causes of tubal block?

Ans: Salpingitis, salpingitis isthmica nodosa, benign polyps within the tubal lumen, tubal endometriosis, tubal spasm, and intratubal mucous debris.

- How to treat a patient with proximal tubal obstruction (block for infertility)?

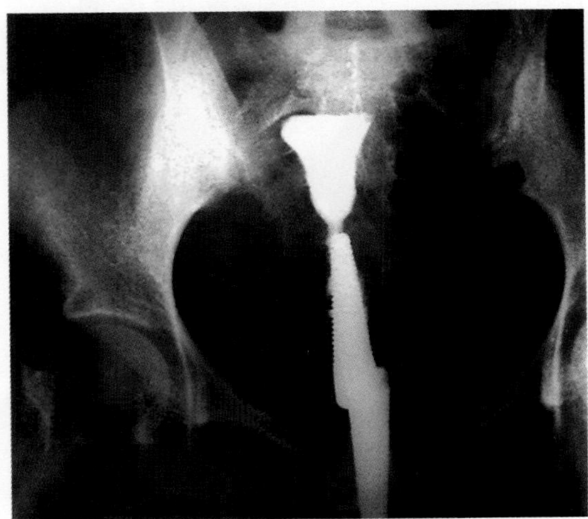

Fig. 38.72: Hysterosalpingogram showing bilateral cornual block. She had a history of MTP.

Ans: Hysteroscopic cannulation of the proximal tube can be done. It is done under laparoscopic guidance. If it is not possible, IVF may be the option.

Figure 38.73

Hysterosalpingogram showing radio-opaque shadow filling the uterine cavity. The tubes of both sides are distended with the radio-opaque dye. There is no evidence of peritoneal spillage.

Diagnosis: Bilateral hydrosalpinx (fimbrial block).

Self-assessment

- Causes of bilateral fimbrial block.
- Is this woman a suitable case for HSG?

Ans. Ideally this woman suffering from hydrosalpinx (chronic PID) should not have undergone HSG, had this been diagnosed before hand? Infection may flare up following HSG.

- Management for distal and proximal tubal block.
- ***What is the appearance of the tube on HSG when infected with tuberculosis?***
- ***What is the reproductive outcome in a woman with pelvic tuberculosis?***
- Indications of IVF–ET.
- Does the presence of hydrosalpinx impair the result of IVF?

Ans. Hydrosalpinx reduces the pregnancy rates of IVF by about 50%. Endometrial receptivity is reduced resulting in implantation failure. Pretreatment (IVF), salpingectomy improves the outcome.

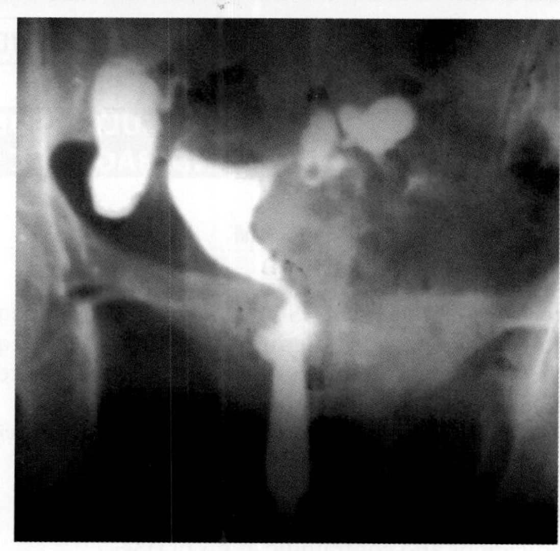

Fig. 38.73: Hysterosalpingogram showing bilateral hydrosalpinx (fimbrial block). Bilateral salpingostomy was done. Thereafter, she had an ectopic pregnancy.

Figures 38.74A and B

Hysterosalpingogram showing a radio-opaque shadow filling both the horns of the uterus. The radio-opaque dye is visible within the tubes. There is peritoneal spillage on both the sides (Fig. 38.74).

Diagnosis: It seems to be a case of bicornuate uterus with bilateral patent tubes.

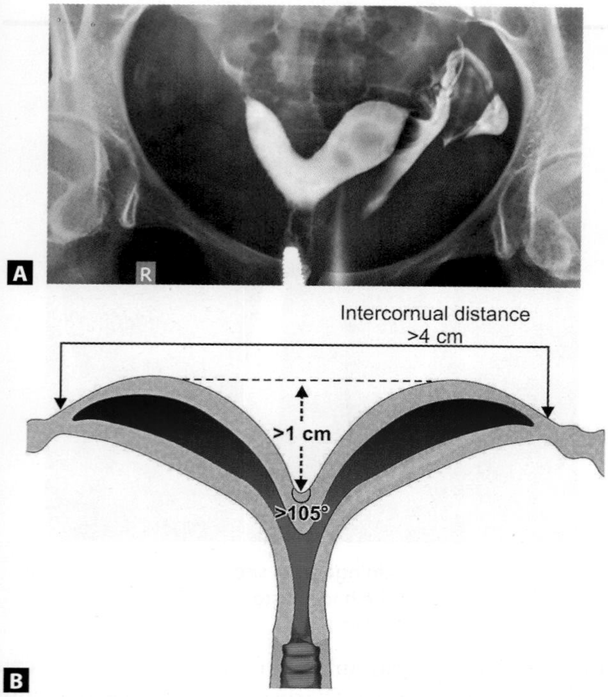

Figs. 38.74A and B: (A) Hysterosalpingogram showing bicornuate uterus. Metroplasty was done for recurrent midtrimester miscarriage. Subsequently, she had a live birth at term, delivered by lower segment cesarean section; (B) Diagrammatic.

Self-assessment

- How one can differentiate bicornuate from septate uterus? (Table 38.2).

Ans. Use of HSG, 3D sonography and/or MRI provide internal and external uterine architecture assessment. MRI is superior. When hysteroscopy is combined with laparoscopy, both the internal and external architecture of the uterus is clearly revealed. This is one of the way to confirm the diagnosis. Surgical intervention should be made on definitive diagnosis

- Management options of a patient with septate uterus.
- **Gynecological symptoms** in bicornuate uterus (Ch. 4).

TABLE 38:2: Differentiation of bicornuate from septate uterus.

Study and parameter	*Bicornuate*	*Septate*
HSG: Cornu position	Widely diverging horns	No such
Intercornual angle: coronal plane MRI/3D USG	≥105°	≤75°
Intercornual distance	>4 cm	<4 cm
Fundal contour	Fundal cleft ≥1 cm form the intercornual line	Convex, flat or minimally indented
Intervening myometrium	Thick	Thin (fibrous), low signal intensity on MRI T_1 and T_2 images

- **Management** of a bicornuate uterus is difficult. **Metroplasty** or unification (Strassman or Tompkins) operation has been recommended.
- Reproductive behavior of a woman with uterine anomalies (bicornuate uterus) is often adversely affected.

Figure 38.75

Hysterosalpingogram showing a radio-opaque shadow filling a single horn of the uterus. There is peritoneal spillage from the tube.

Diagnosis: It seems to be a case of unicornuate uterus with patent tube.

Self-assessment

- Confirmation of diagnosis.
- Discuss the types of Müllerian anomalies.
- What is the reproductive outcome in a case with unicornuate uterus?

Ans. Poor—due to reduced uterine capacity, less muscle mass and inability to expand. Rupture may occur during pregnancy.

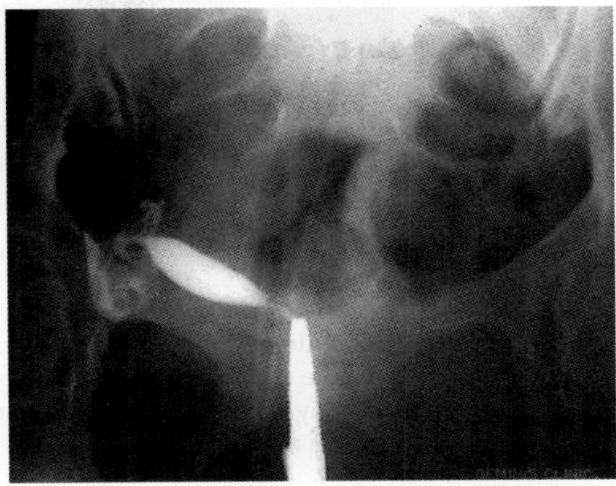

Fig. 38.75: Hysterosalpingogram showing a unicornuate uterus.

Figure 38.76

Hysterosalpingogram showing irregular filling of radio-opaque dye.

Diagnosis: Uterine synechiae (Asherman's syndrome).

Self-assessment (Ch. 29)

- Common causes of uterine synechiae
- Other methods of diagnosis
- Management of uterine synechiae
- Uterine causes of amenorrhea
- How a woman with uterine synechiae could be treated for her problem of infertility?

Ans: Adhesiolysis could be done surgically to restore the normal uterine cavity size and configuration. It could be done by dilation and curettage. Hysteroscopic adhesiolysis could be done using scissors or electrosurgical cutting. In severe cases where adhesiolysis is not possible gestational surrogacy is the option.

- ***In what conditions of amenorrhea karyotyping is needed?***

Ans. (a) Patients with uterus but no breasts and high FSH level—gonadal failure; (b) Patients with no uterus but breasts present—androgen insensitivity syndrome; (c) Premature ovarian failure if <30 years of age; (d) Short stature (<60") with Turner stigmata—Turner's syndrome.

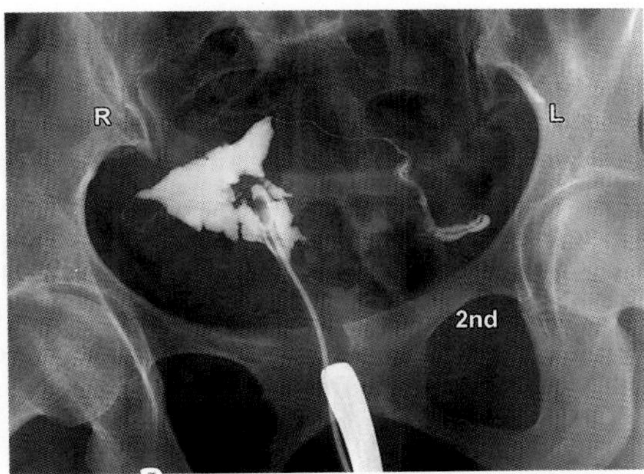

Fig. 38.76: Hysterosalpingogram showing intrauterine adhesion. A case of tuberculous endometritis.

(Courtesy: Dr H Roy, Patna)

Figure 38.77

Ultrasonographic view of a septate uterus.

Self-assessment

- What are the different types of uterine abnormalities? (p. 35).
- What may be the clinical presentation of such a case? (p. 35).
- What are the different obstetric complications? (p. 35).
- What are the different modes of diagnosis?

Ans. Uterine malformation could diagnosed with the help of HSG, 3D ultrasonography, and MRI imaging parameters. All are discussed in p. 560, Table 38.2.

- What are the treatment options available? (p. 36).

Ans. Treatment option is hysteroscopic resection of the septum under laparoscopic guidance. It is safe and effective. It has the advantages over the abdominal metroplasty. Successful pregnancy and live birth rate is about 87%.

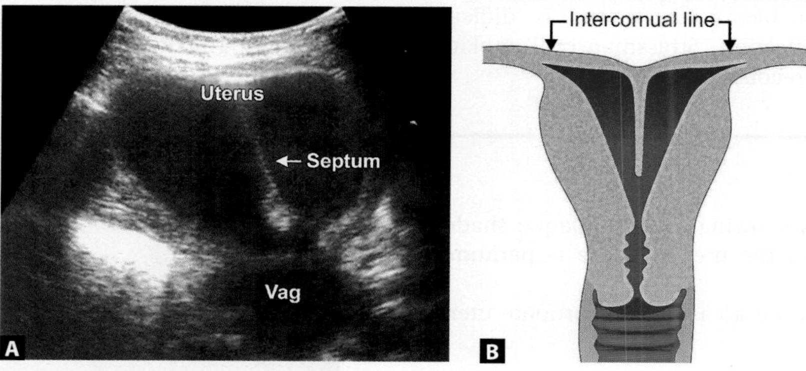

Figs. 38.77A and B: (A) Ultrasonographic and (B) diagrammatic view of a septate uterus.

- How arcuate uterus is diagnosed and managed?

Ans. Arcuate uterus: Mild indentation of the myometrium over the fundus towards the endometrium is observed. Fundal cleft on MRI there may be small <1.0 cm. It is a normal variant of the uterus with no clinical significance.

Treatment approach: Bicornuate uterus: Metroplasty, unification of the uterine horns are done. Successful pregnancy with viable birth is reported in 85% of pregnancies.

Figure 38.78

Ultrasonographic view of a fibroid uterus.

Self-assessment (Ch. 20)

- What are the causes of symmetrical enlargement of the uterus?
- How a couple should be counseled before proceeding to myomectomy?
- What are the principal steps of myomectomy?
- What are the measures that can be adopted to minimize blood loss in myomectomy operation?

Ans. A. Before the operation: Drugs used are: (a) Danazol; (b) GnRH agnosits; (c) LNG-IUS; (d) NSAID; (e) COCs.

B. During the operation: (a) Use of clamp; (b) Tourniquet; (c) Vasoconstrictive agents: Vaso-pression is available in synthetic form. One vial contains 20 units/mL. 20 U is diluted in 20–100 mL of normal saline. It is injected over the planned incision site, between the myoma capsule and the myometrium. It reduces operative blood loss significantly.

Side effects: Rise in blood pressure, bradycardia, atrioventricular block and pulmonary edema.

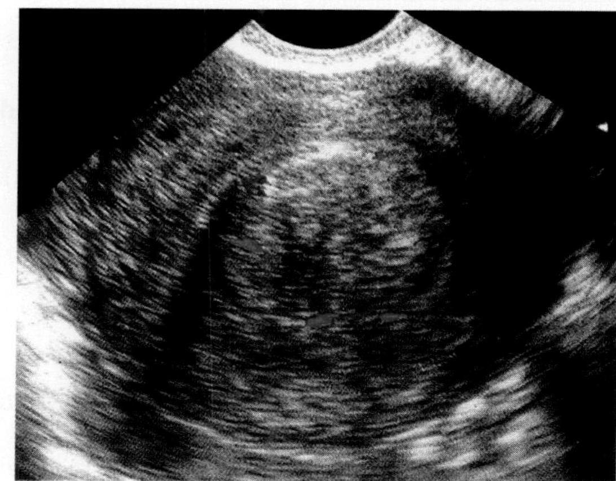

Fig. 38.78: Ultrasonographic (TV) view of a leiomyoma.

- What are the different types of surgery for myomectomy?
- What are the common complications of myomectomy?
- What are the long-term results of myomectomy in respect of recurrence and others?

Figure 38.79

Ultrasonographic view of an adenomyosis of the uterus.

Self-assessment (Ch. 22)

- Mention the different modalities of treatment options for pelvic endometriosis.

Ans: (a) Expectant; (b) Medical (hormones and others); (c) Surgery (conservative, definitive); (d) Combined (medical and surgical).

- **What are the common sites of pelvic endometriosis?**

- Mention the indications and the different types of surgery that can be done for endometriosis.
- How do you manage a case of chocolate cyst (ovarian endometrioma) of the ovary?
- What are the different hormones used in the management of endometriosis?
- Treatment of scar endometriosis.
- How leiomyoma uterus could be differentiated from adenomyosis? (Table 38.3).

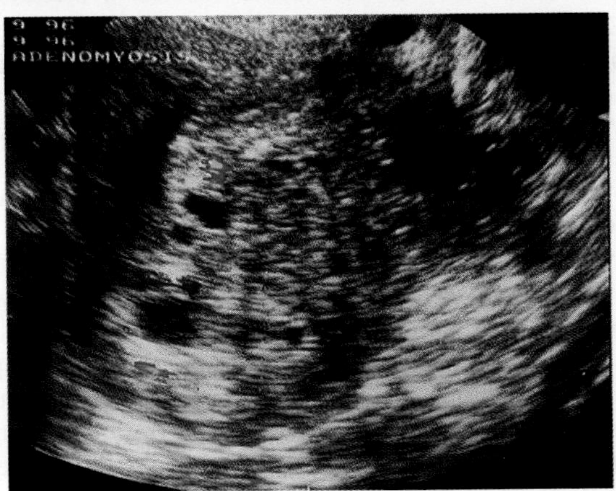

Fig. 38.79: Sonographic view of adenomyosis showing diffusedly enlarged uterus with cystic spaces.

TABLE 38.3: Differentiating features of fibroid uterus and adenomyosis.

	Leiomyoma uterus (Fig. 38.78)	*Adenomyosis (Fig. 38.79)*
Age	▪ Usually observed in the **reproductive age**	▪ Commonly seen in women **older than 40 years**
Pathology	▪ It is the benign neoplasia of the smooth muscle and fibrous tissue of the uterus	▪ It is due to the presence of functioning endometrium within the muscle layers of the uterus
Uterus	▪ Irregularly enlarged depending upon the site, size and number of myomas. It is firm and nontender (unless degeneration)	▪ Diffusely enlarged due to myohyperplasia. Uterus is soft and tender
Symptoms	▪ Menorrhagia and dysmenorrhea—often present	▪ Menorrhagia—present. Dysmenorrhea often begins a week before and it continues even after the period is over
Diagnosis	▪ **Sonography (TVS)**—homogeneous echogenic area over the fibroid ▪ **Cut section:** Capsule present, smooth and whitish surface with whorled appearance ▪ **Histology:** Proliferation of smooth muscle and fibrous tissue	▪ **USG:** Cystic spaces within the myometrium ▪ **MRI:** Endometrial-myometrial junctional zone >12 mm is diagnostic ▪ *Capsule absent*. Diffuse trabeculated appearance, cystic spaces with hemorrhagic spots ▪ Proliferation of endometrial glands and stroma. Phagocytic cells laden with hemosiderin pigment are present

Figure 38.80

Ultrasonographic view of Cu T inside the uterine cavity. Thread was missing in this case.

Self-assessment

- What are the possible causes of missing thread?
- How do you investigate such a case with missing thread?
- What are the indications of removal of IUDs?
- What are the complications of IUD use?
- What are the specific of the third generation of IUDs over the others?

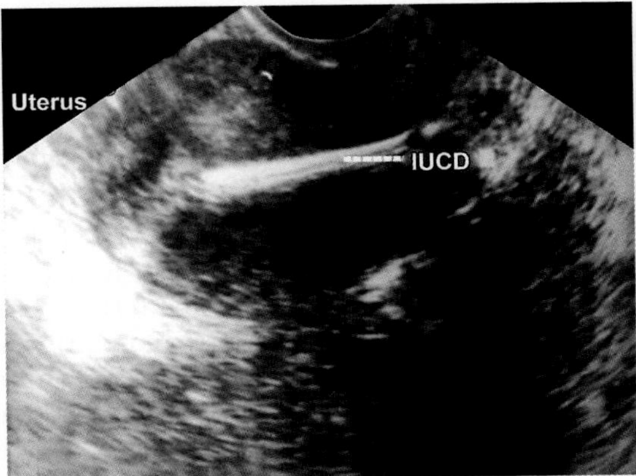

Fig. 38.80: Ultrasonographic view of a Cu T inside the uterine cavity, in a case of missing thread.

Figure 38.81

Hysterosalpingogram showing markedly dilated tube with retention of dye.

Diagnosis: **Bilateral hydrosalpinges.**

Self-assessment

- ***What are the other methods of diagnosis?***

Ans. USG, laparoscopy.

- Dangers of HSG in such a case.

Ans: (a) Pelvic pain; (b) Flaring up of pelvic infection. Otherwise it is a contraindication for HSG.

- What are the common types of tubal reconstructive surgery? (Ch. 17).
- What factors are related to the success of tuboplasty? (Ch. 17).
- What are the guidelines for tubal surgery? (Ch. 17).
- What are the cases with good and poor result following tuboplasty?

Ans. Factors associated with good outcomes: (a) Salpingolysis; (b) Fimbrioplasty; (c) Salpingostomy; (d) Tubotubal anastomosis following laparoscopic sterilization operation. **Factors associated with poor outcomes:** (a) Dense pelvic adhesions; (b) Loss of fimbria; (c) Bilateral hydrosalpinx >3 cm; (d) Length of reconstructed tube <4 cm.

Result of tuboplasty is best in cases with reversal of tubal sterilization. It is done by tubo-tubal anastomosis following microsurgical techniques.

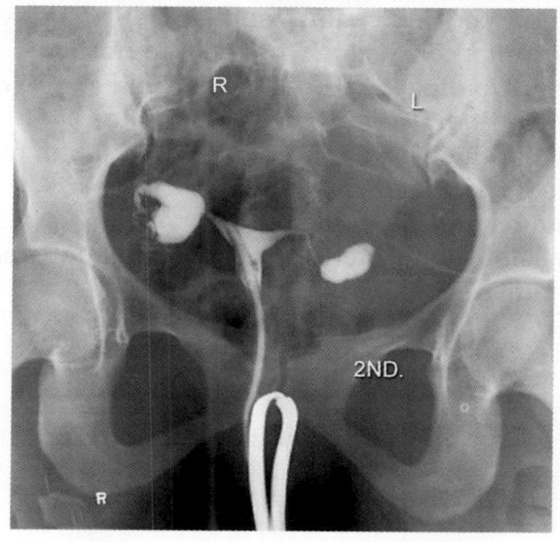

Fig. 38.81: Hysterosalpingogram showing markedly dilated tube with retention of dye. Bilateral hydrosalpinges.
(*Courtesy:* Dr H Roy, Patna)

Figure 38.82

Ultrasonographic view of the ovary following hyperstimulation syndrome (OHSS). Multiple follicles are seen.

Self-assessment (Ch. 32)

- What are the different grades and the clinical features of OHSS?
- How could this problem be prevented?
- Indications of use of gonadotrophins in infertility.
- What is ovarian reserve?
- Who are the high responders?
- What is coasting?
- How do you manage a case of OHSS?

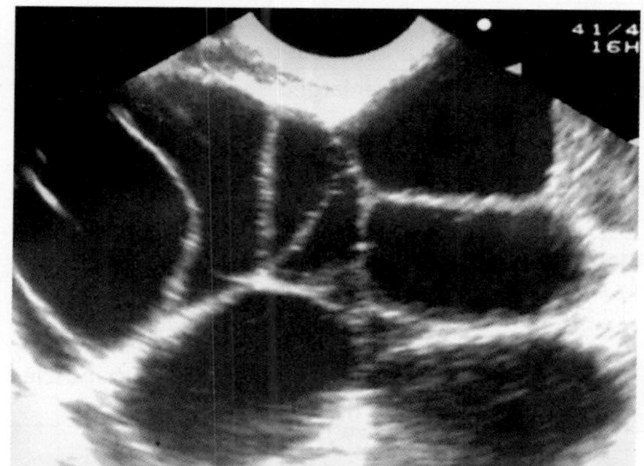

Fig. 38.82: Sonographic view of OHSS.

Figures 38.83A and B

Calcific degeneration of a fibroid uterus.

Self-assessment

- What are the secondary changes in a fibroid? (Ch. 20).
- What are the degenerations in fibroid? (Ch. 20).

Ans: Secondary changes in a fibroid are (a) Degeneration of different types like: Hyaline (most common), calcific (Figs. 38.83A to C). Others infection and necrosis (Fig. 38.83C); (b) Atrophy; (c) Vascular; and (d) Sarcomatous (<1%).

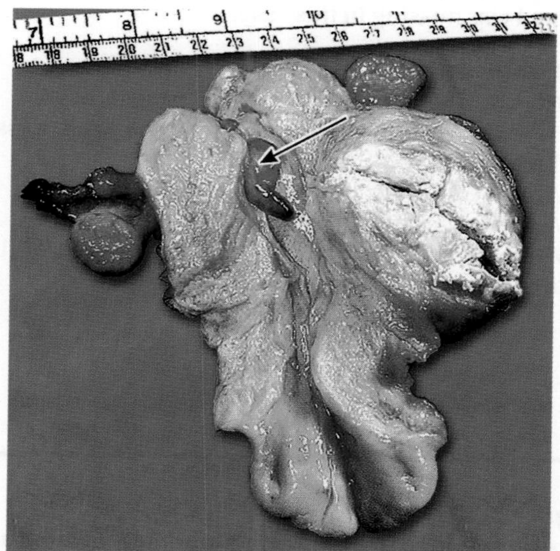

Fig. 38.83A: Specimen of a uterus, tubes, and ovaries cut opened to show multiple fibroids of the uterus. The uterine cavity is enlarged. The fibroid is cut to show the calcific degeneration (womb stone) within it.

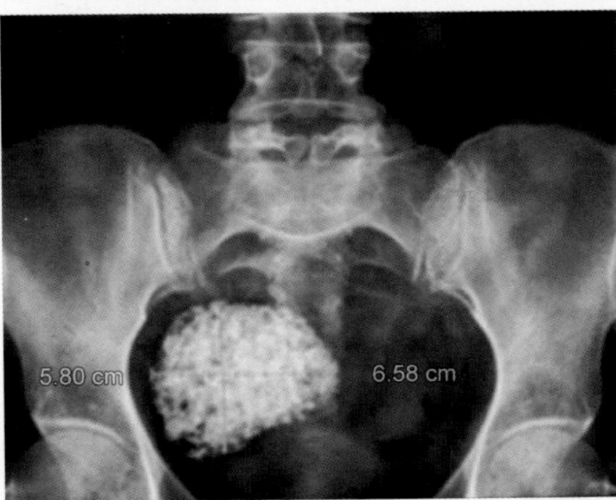

Fig. 38.83B: Plain X-ray of the pelvis and lower abdomen showing the calcific degeneration of a fibroid (popcorn appearance).

- How this patient presents in the clinic?

Ans: Persistant vaginal discharge is the common presentation. Often it is foul smelling and purulent. Patient may present with irregular bleeding or blood mixed discharge. Patient suffers chronic ill health and lower abdominal pain.

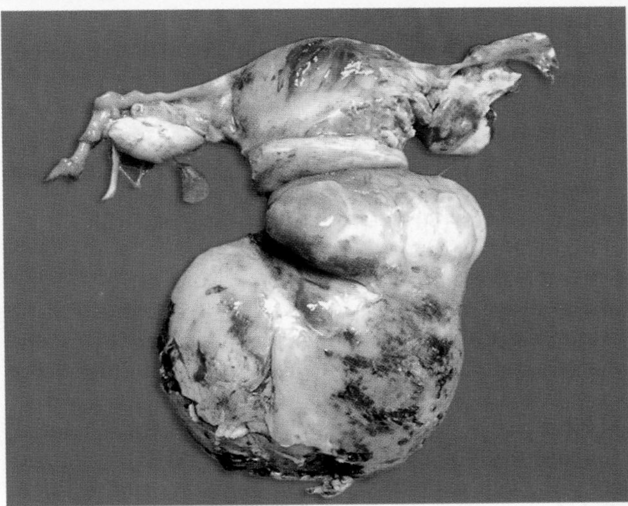

Fig. 38.83C: A large cervical polyp with infective and degenerative changes.

(*Courtesy*: AGMC and GB Pant Hospital, Department of Obstetrics and Gynecology, Agartala, Tripura)

- What operation has been done to this patient?

Ans: Total abdominal hysterectomy with bilateral saalpingo oophorectomy.

Figures 38.84A and B

Dermoid cyst of the ovary: X ray and the CT view.

Self-assessment

- Describe the cut section of an ovarian dermoid cyst.
- Typical findings of an ovarian dermoid cyst in CT.

Ans. Characteristics of a dermoid cyst in CT include the mixture of low density areas due to fat, high density areas from dental elements or calcification (arrow) and a fat-fluid level.

- ***What is the limitation of USG?***

Ans. Compared to CT or MRI, USG is not sufficient for accurate staging of any pelvic malignancy.

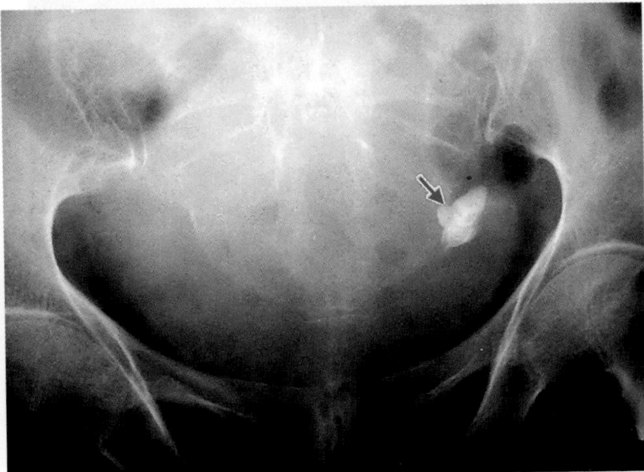

Fig. 38.84A: Straight X-ray of the abdomen and pelvis with an ovarian tumor showing (arrow) the shadow of a tooth (dermoid cyst).

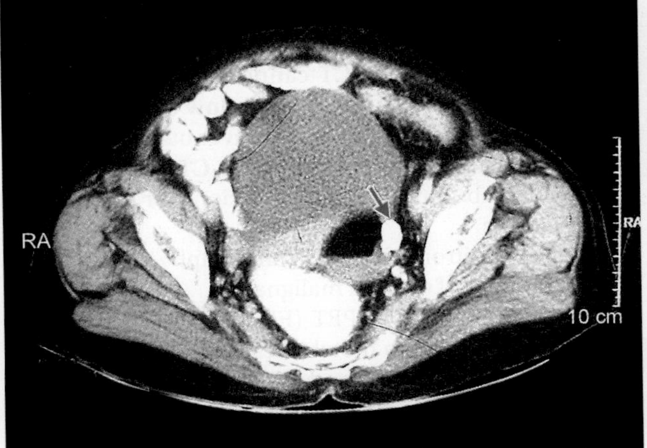

Fig. 38.84B: Computed tomographic view of the abdomen and pelvis of the same women as in Figure 38.86 showing the tooth (dermoid cyst of the ovary).

Figure 38.85

CT of the brain in a patient with choriocarcinoma, showing metastasis.

Self-assessment

- ***What are the common sites of metastasis in choriocarcinoma?***

Ans. (a) Lungs (80%); (b) Anterior vaginal wall (30%); (c) Brain (10%); (d) Liver (10%) and others.

- ***What is the significance of metastasis?***

Ans. (a) Site of metastasis is related to the prognosis of the disease, e.g. metastasis in lungs and pelvis is of low score, whereas brain metastasis puts the patient into high score disease.

(b) Number of metastasis is also prognostically related. More the number, higher the score. (WHO prognostic scoring). Such patients need combination drug regimen, whole brain radiation therapy.

- ***How do the patients usually present?***

Ans. Common symptoms are: Ill health, irregular vaginal bleeding. Symptoms due to metastases are: Cough, breathlessness, hemoptysis (lung); headache, convulsion, paralysis or coma for cerebral metastases and epigastric pain, jaundice for liver metastases.

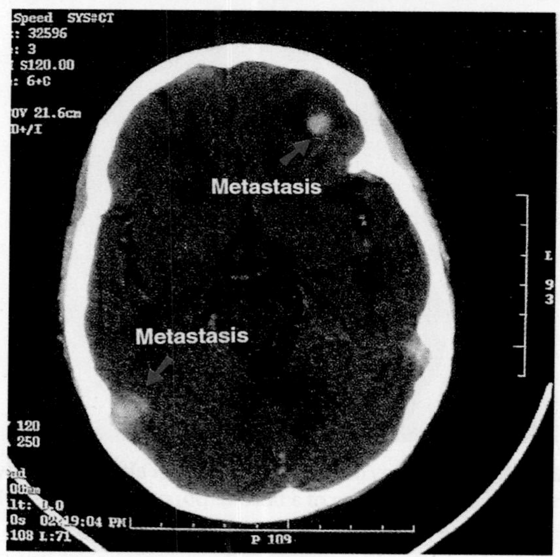

Fig. 38.85: CT view of the brain, in a patient with choriocarcinoma, showing metastasis (arrow).

Figure 38.86

Computed tomographic view of an ovarian tumor.

Self-assessment

- What special advantages CT has got in gynecology? (p. 100).

Ans: CT scanning is done for preoperative evaluation of cases with **gynecologic malignancy** including advanced ovarian cancers. It is done to detect the spread of the disease (cervical cancer). **Metastatic spread** in the liver, omentum, retroperitoneal lymph nodes and also in other sites. This helps to plan the surgery and the extent of cytoreduction. However, CT cannot detect any implant <2 cm in diameter. CT is used for **follow up of cases** following therapy (surveillance). Intravenous contrast use enables superior evaluation of organs. **CT-guided biopsy** for any intra-abdominal mass suspicions for malignancy could be done.

- Place of positron emission tomography (PET) in the management of ovarian malignancy.

Ans: Fluorodeoxyglucse-PET (FDG-PET) is injected IV. This is taken up by the metabolically active tumor cells. The combination of PET and CT allows superior imaging compared to CT alone and MRI for lymph node metastasis. However, PET is unable to detect lymph node metastasis <5 mm. PET is useful for planning radiation field in patients with distant metastasis.

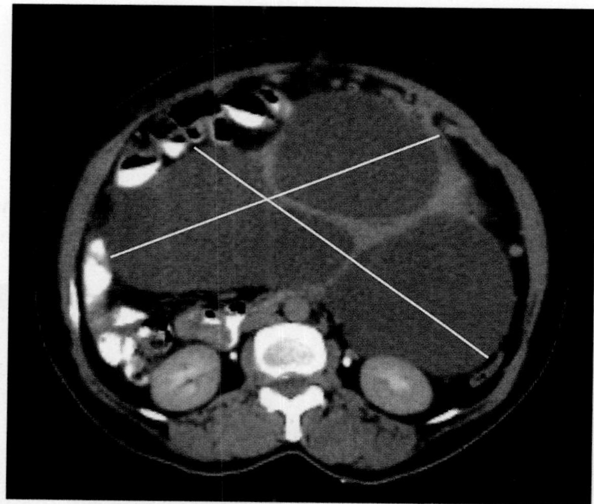

Fig. 38.86: Computed tomographic (CT) view of an ovarian tumor.

- ***What is the value of CT in the evaluation of pelvic or periaortic lymph node metastasis?***

Ans. For most pelvic malignancies lymph nodes more than 8 mm in maximum short-axis dimension (MSAD) are regarded as abnormal. CT is helpful to detect retroperitoneal metastatic nodes. However, results may be false-negative due to micrometastasis or false-positive due to lymphadenitis or reactive hyperplasia.

Figure 38.87

MRI view of a fibroid uterus.

Self-assessment

- ***What are the advantages of MRI in the diagnosis of fibroid uterus?***

Ans. MRI is more accurate compared to USG. It can differentiate adenomyosis from fibroids. MRI can detect: Submucous myoma, adnexal pathology, various types of degenerations and the sarcomatous change also. However, MRI is not used as a routine for the diagnosis. It is expensive.

MR-guided high intensity focused ultrasound (MRgHIFU), therapy is done for treatment of leiomyomas. MRgHIFU is found to be safe, effective, feasible and minimally invasive.

- ***What is the place of MRI in the management of Müllerian anomalies?***

Ans. MRI can differentiate varieties of Müllerian anomalies more accurately compared to 3D sonography. Bicornuate uterus could be differentiated from a septate uterus. T_2 weighted images and coronal planes are more informative.

MRI can detect the presence of endometrial tissue within the rudimentary horn. Moreover, MRI can detect whether the rudimentary horn is communicating with the other functioning horn. Noncommunicating rudimentary horn may manifest with cyclic pain due to formation of hematometra.

MRI can identify uterine agenesis, cervicovaginal agenesis and uterus didelphys.

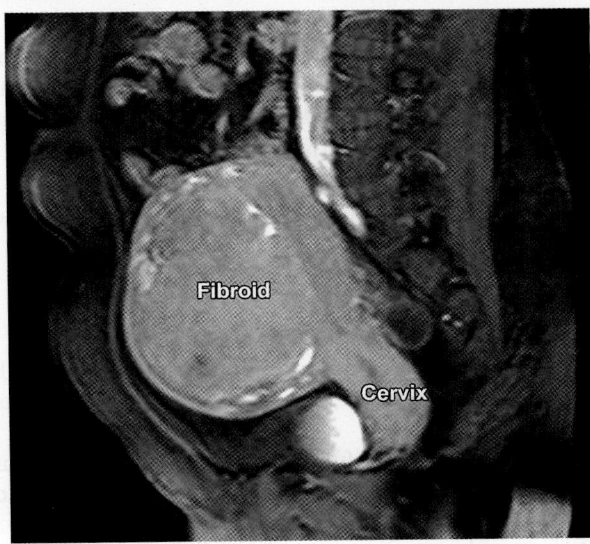

Fig. 38.87: Magnetic resonance image of a fairly large size fibroid arising from the body of the uterus.

Figure 38.88

MRI view of a normal uterus.

Self-assessment

- ***How normal endometrium and myometrium could be studied with MRI?***

Ans. With MRI endometrium is shown as the inner zone of high-signal-intensity stripe. The deeper myometrium is recognized as a very-low-signal intensity zone. The junctional zone demarcates the two. The myometrium appears as the intermediate signal-intensity zone. In postmenopausal women, the contrast between the junctional zone and the myometrium decreases.

- ***What special advantages MRI has got in gynecology?***

Ans.

1. MRI offers multiplaner images.
2. Gadolinium enhanced T_1-weighted images can determine.

   (a) Depth of myometrial invasion in a case with endometrial carcinoma; (b) Pelvic and periaortic (retroperitoneal) nodal metastasis in cervical, ovarian and endometrial carcinoma; (c) Invasion of malignant process in the parametrium in cases with cervical cancer can be done accurately; (d) It can detect recurrence of pelvic tumor; (e) MRI is superior to CT for evaluating cervical cancer as regard the tumor size, extension to the bladder, rectum, parametrium and lymph node involvement. MRI is performed before doing radical trachelectomy (fertility sparing surgery).
3. MRI is safe in pregnancy.

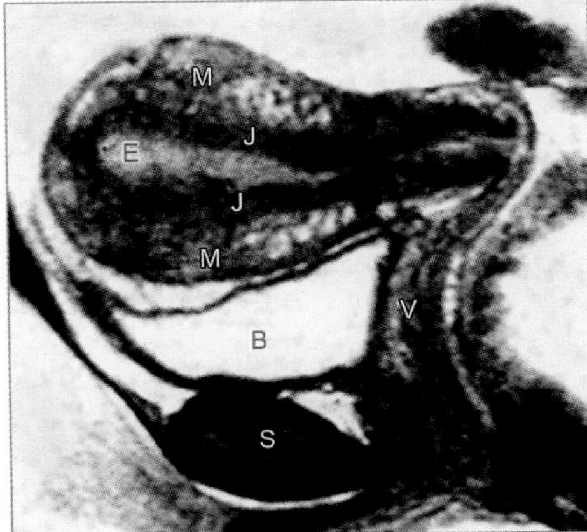

Fig. 38.88: MRI plate of a normal uterus on a sagittal T_2-weighted spin-echo image showing endometrium (E), the junctional zone (J), the myometrium (M) urinary bladder (B) and the vagina (V).

Figure 38.89

MRI is useful in selected cases with endometrial carcinoma to get some additional information. It has got more value compared to computed tomography (CT) scans. Accuracy of MRI is up to 90%.

The additional benefits of MRI are:

- Assessment of endometrial carcinoma with its spread and invasion to:
  - Myometrium
  - Cervix
  - Pelvic and para-aortic lymph nodes.
- MRI can distinguish an endometrial cancer with its cervical extension from a primary endocervical adenocarcinoma.
- MRI is especially useful in cases like serous and clear cell tumors, where the frequency of extrauterine spread of disease is high.
- It can guide whether a case is required to be referred to a gynecological-oncologist or could be operated by a gynecologist for staging laparotomy and surgery.
- As a diagnostic aid is there any limitation for MRI? (p. 101)

MRI is useful (discussed above) but it has got limitations also. The only accurate method to assess the depth of myometrial invasion is by histological examination of the hysterectomy specimen.

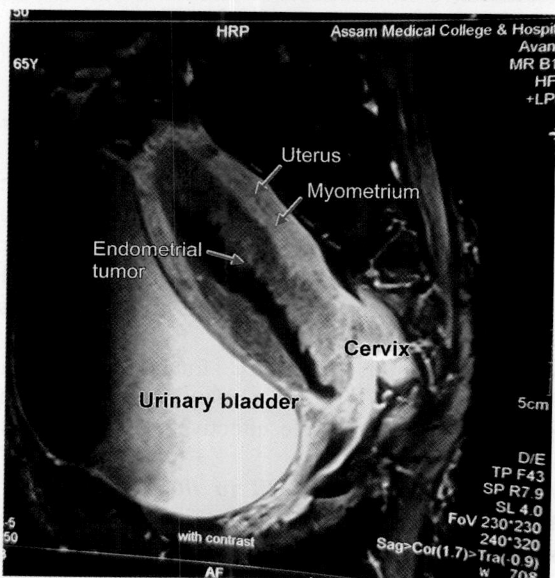

Fig. 38.89: Magnetic resonance image (MRI) in the sagittal plane of a 65-year-old woman with endometrial adenocarcinoma Gadolinium-enhanced sagittal T_2-weighted image shows endometrial tumor with invasion to the myometrium, more on the anterior wall and the fundus (more than 50%). There is extension of the cancer to the cervix (*see* arrow).

(*Courtesy:* Department of Obstetrics and Gynecology, Department of Radiology, Assam Medical College, Dibrugarh, Assam, India).

NOMOGRAM FOR CALCULATING BODY SURFACE AREA OF ADULTS

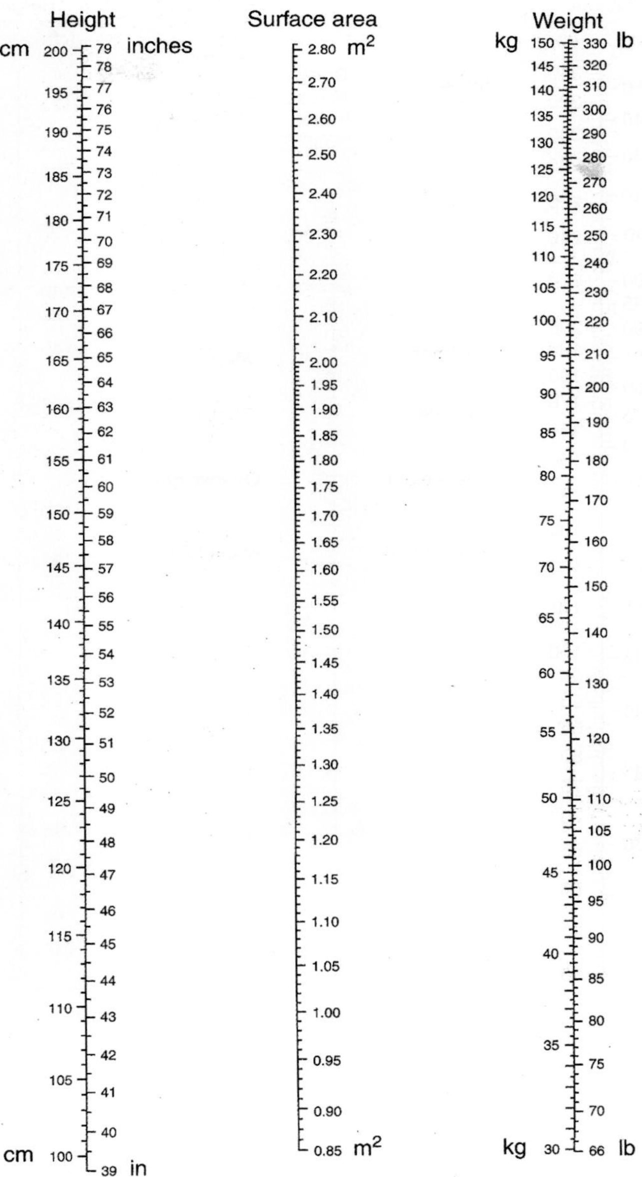

NOMOGRAM FOR CALCULATING BODY MASS INDEX

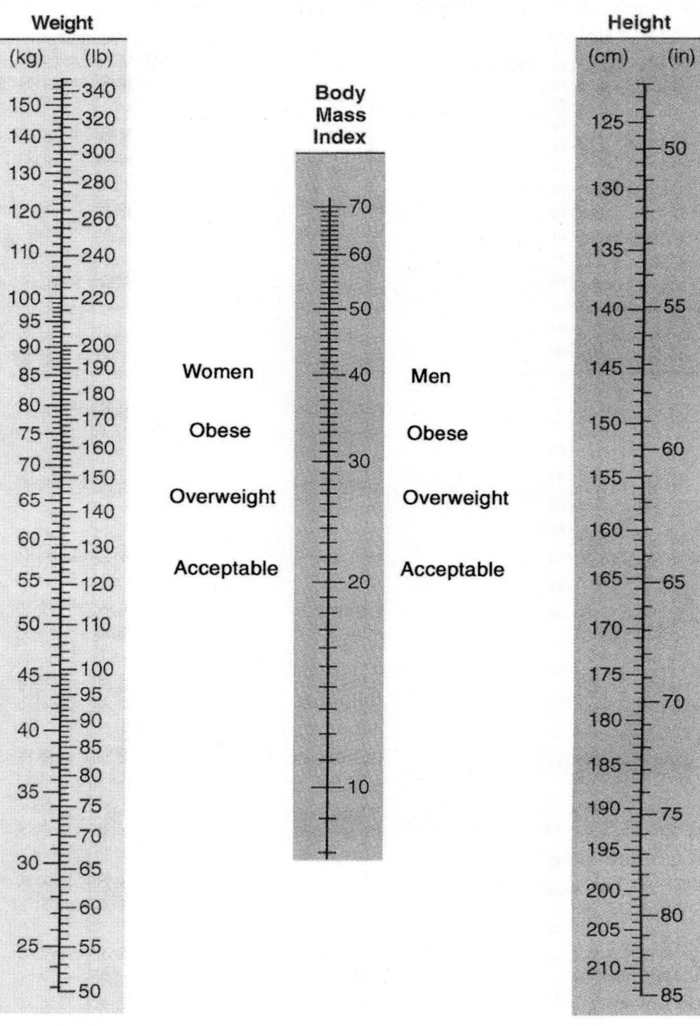

Index

Page numbers followed by *f* refer to figure, *t* refer to table, and *fc* refer to flowchart.

B

D

E

F

G

K

L

M

N

O

P

Q

R

T

U

V